Comprehensive

Clinical Hepatology

ELSEVIER CD-ROM LICENCE AGREEMENT

PLEASE READ THE FOLLOWING AGREEMENT CAREFULLY BEFORE USING THIS PRODUCT. THIS PRODUCT IS LICENSED UNDER THE TERMS CONTAINED IN THIS LICENCE AGREEMENT ('Agreement'). BY USING THIS PRODUCT, YOU, AN INDIVIDUAL OR ENTITY INCLUDING EMPLOYEES, AGENTS AND REPRESENTATIVES ('You' or 'Your'), ACKNOWLEDGE THAT YOU HAVE READ THIS AGREEMENT, THAT YOU UNDERSTAND IT, AND THAT YOU AGREE TO BE BOUND BY THE TERMS AND CONDITIONS OF THIS AGREEMENT. ELSEVIER LIMITED ('Elsevier') EXPRESSLY DOES NOT AGREE TO LICENSE THIS PRODUCT TO YOU UNLESS YOU ASSENT TO THIS AGREEMENT. IF YOU DO NOT AGREE WITH ANY OF THE FOLLOWING TERMS, YOU MAY, WITHIN THIRTY (30) DAYS AFTER YOUR RECEIPT OF THIS PRODUCT RETURN THE UNUSED PRODUCT AND ALL ACCOMPANYING DOCUMENTATION TO ELSEVIER FOR A FULL REFUND.

DEFINITIONS As used in this Agreement, these terms shall have the following meanings:

'Proprietary Material' means the valuable and proprietary information content of this Product including without limitation all indexes and graphic materials and software used to access, index, search and retrieve the information content from this Product developed or licensed by Elsevier and/or its affiliates, suppliers and licensors.

'Product' means the copy of the Proprietary Material and any other material delivered on CD-ROM and any other human-readable or machine-readable materials enclosed with this Agreement, including without limitation documentation relating to the same.

OWNERSHIP This Product has been supplied by and is proprietary to Elsevier and/or its affiliates, suppliers and licensors. The copyright in the Product belongs to Elsevier and/or its affiliates, suppliers and licensors and is protected by the copyright, trademark, trade secret and other intellectual property laws of the United Kingdom and international treaty provisions, including without limitation the Universal Copyright Convention and the Berne Copyright Convention. You have no ownership rights in this Product. Except as expressly set forth herein, no part of this Product, including without limitation the Proprietary Material, may be modified, copied or distributed in hardcopy or machine-readable form without prior written consent from Elsevier. All rights not expressly granted to You herein are expressly reserved. Any other use of this Product by any person or entity is strictly prohibited and a violation of this Agreement.

SCOPE OF RIGHTS LICENSED (PERMITTED USES) Elsevier is granting to You a limited, non-exclusive, non-transferable licence to use this Product in accordance with the terms of this Agreement. You may use or provide access to this Product on a single computer or terminal physically located at Your premises and in a secure network or move this Product to and use it on another single computer or terminal at the same location for personal use only, but under no circumstances may You use or provide access to any part or parts of this Product on more than one computer or terminal simultaneously.

You shall not (a) copy, download, or otherwise reproduce the Product or any part(s) thereof in any medium, including, without limitation, online transmissions, local area networks, wide area networks, intranets, extranets and the Internet, or in any way, in whole or in part, except for printing out or downloading nonsubstantial portions of the text and images in the Product for Your own personal use; (b) alter, modify, or adapt the Product or any part(s) thereof, including but not limited to decompiling, disassembling, reverse engineering, or creating derivative works, without the prior written approval of Elsevier; (c) sell, license or otherwise distribute to third parties the Product or any part(s) thereof; or (d) alter, remove, obscure or obstruct the display of any copyright, trademark or other proprietary notice on or in the Product or on any printout or download of portions of the Proprietary Materials.

RESTRICTIONS ON TRANSFER This Licence is personal to You, and neither Your rights hereunder nor the tangible embodiments of this Product, including without limitation the Proprietary Material, may be sold, assigned, transferred or sublicensed to any other person, including without limitation by operation of law, without the prior written consent of Elsevier. Any purported sale, assignment, transfer or sublicense without the prior written consent of Elsevier will be void and will automatically terminate the Licence granted hereunder.

TERM This Agreement will remain in effect until terminated pursuant to the terms of this Agreement. You may terminate this Agreement at any time by removing from Your system and destroying the Product and any copies of the Proprietary Material. Unauthorized copying of the Product, including without limitation, the Proprietary Material and documentation, or otherwise failing to comply with the terms and conditions of this Agreement shall result in automatic termination of this licence and will make available to Elsevier legal remedies. Upon termination of this Agreement, the licence granted herein will terminate and You must immediately destroy the Product and all copies of the Product and of the Proprietary Material, together with any and all accompanying documentation. All provisions relating to proprietary rights shall survive termination of this Agreement.

LIMITED WARRANTY AND LIMITATION OF LIABILITY Elsevier warrants that the software embodied in this Product will perform in substantial compliance with the documentation supplied in this Product, unless the performance problems are the result of hardware failure or improper use. If You report a significant defect in performance in writing to Elsevier within ninety (90) calendar days of your having purchased the Product, and Elsevier is not able to correct same within sixty (60) days after its receipt of Your notification, You may return this Product, including all copies and documentation, to Elsevier and Elsevier will refund Your money. In order to apply for a refund on your purchased Product, please contact the return address on the invoice to obtain the refund request form ('Refund Request Form'), and either fax or mail your signed request and your proof of purchase to the address indicated on the Refund Request Form. Incomplete forms will not be processed. Defined terms in the Refund Request Form shall have the same meaning as in this Agreement.

YOU UNDERSTAND THAT, EXCEPT FOR THE LIMITED WARRANTY RECITED ABOVE, ELSEVIER, ITS AFFILIATES, LICENSORS, THIRD PARTY SUPPLIERS AND AGENTS (TOGETHER 'THE SUPPLIERS') MAKE NO REPRESENTATIONS OR WARRANTIES, WITH RESPECT TO THE PRODUCT, INCLUDING, WITHOUT LIMITATION THE PROPRIETARY MATERIAL. ALL OTHER REPRESENTATIONS, WARRANTIES, CONDITIONS OR OTHER TERMS, WHETHER EXPRESS OR IMPLIED BY STATUTE OR COMMON LAW, ARE HEREBY EXCLUDED TO THE FULLEST EXTENT PERMITTED BY LAW.

IN PARTICULAR BUT WITHOUT LIMITATION TO THE FOREGOING NONE OF THE SUPPLIERS MAKE ANY REPRESENTATIONS OR WARRANTIES (WHETHER EXPRESS OR IMPLIED) REGARDING THE PERFORMANCE OF YOUR PAD, NETWORK OR COMPUTER SYSTEM WHEN USED IN CONJUNCTION WITH THE PRODUCT, NOR THAT THE PRODUCT WILL MEET YOUR REQUIREMENTS OR THAT ITS OPERATION WILL BE UNINTERRUPTED OR ERROR-FREE.

EXCEPT IN RESPECT OF DEATH OR PERSONAL INJURY CAUSED BY THE SUPPLIERS' NEGLIGENCE AND TO THE FULLEST EXTENT PERMITTED BY LAW, IN NO EVENT (AND REGARDLESS OF WHETHER SUCH DAMAGES ARE FORESEEABLE AND OF WHETHER SUCH LIABILITY IS BASED IN TORT, CONTRACT OR OTHERWISE) WILL ANY OF THE SUPPLIERS BE LIABLE TO YOU FOR ANY DAMAGES (INCLUDING, WITHOUT LIMITATION, ANY LOST PROFITS, LOST SAVINGS OR OTHER SPECIAL, INDIRECT, INCIDENTAL OR CONSEQUENTIAL DAMAGES ARISING OUT OF OR RESULTING FROM: (I) YOUR USE OF, OR INABILITY TO USE, THE PRODUCT; (II) DATA LOSS OR CORRUPTION; AND/OR (III) ERRORS OR OMISSIONS IN THE PROPRIETARY MATERIAL.

IF THE FOREGOING LIMITATION IS HELD TO BE UNENFORCEABLE, OUR MAXIMUM LIABILITY TO YOU IN RESPECT THEREOF SHALL NOT EXCEED THE AMOUNT OF THE LICENCE FEE PAID BY YOU FOR THE PRODUCT. THE REMEDIES AVAILABLE TO YOU AGAINST ELSEVIER AND THE LICENSORS OF MATERIALS INCLUDED IN THE PRODUCT ARE EXCLUSIVE.

If the information provided in the Product contains medical or health sciences information, it is intended for professional use within the medical field. Information about medical treatment or drug dosages is intended strictly for professional use, and because of rapid advances in the medical sciences, independent verification of diagnosis and drug dosages should be made.

The provisions of this Agreement shall be severable, and in the event that any provision of this Agreement is found to be legally unenforceable, such unenforceability shall not prevent the enforcement or any other provision of this Agreement.

GOVERNING LAW This Agreement shall be governed by the laws of England and Wales. In any dispute arising out of this Agreement, you and Elsevier each consent to the exclusive personal jurisdiction and venue in the courts of England and Wales.

Comprehensive
Clinical Hepatology

Second Edition

Edited by

Bruce R Bacon MD

James F King MD Endowed Chair in Gastroenterology;
Professor of Internal Medicine;
Director, Division of Gastroenterology and Hepatology
Saint Louis University Liver Center
Saint Louis University School of Medicine
St Louis, MO, USA

John G O'Grady MD, FRCPI

Consultant Hepatologist
Institute of Liver Studies
King's College School of Medicine
London, UK

Adrian M Di Bisceglie MD

Professor of Internal Medicine;
Chief of Hepatology
Division of Gastroenterology and Hepatology
Saint Louis University Liver Center
Saint Louis University School of Medicine
St Louis, MO, USA

John R Lake MD

Professor of Medicine and Surgery;
Director, Gastroenterology Division;
Director, Liver Transplantation Program
University of Minnesota Medical School
Minneapolis, MN, USA

Emeritus Editor

Peter D Howdle MD FRCP
Professor of Clinical Education;
Consultant Gastroenterologist;
Head of Academic Unit of General Surgery, Medicine and
Anaesthesia
St James's University Hospital
Leeds, UK

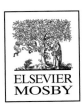

ELSEVIER
MOSBY

ELSEVIER
MOSBY

An imprint of Elsevier Limited

© 2006, Elsevier Limited.

First published 2006

First edition 2000
Second edition 2006

ISBN 0 3230 3675 9

British Library Cataloguing in Publication Data
A catalogue record for this book is available from the British Library

Library of Congress Cataloging in Publication Data
A catalog record for this book is available from the Library of Congress

Printed in China
Last digit is the print number: 9 8 7 6 5 4 3 2 1

Working together to grow
libraries in developing countries

www.elsevier.com | www.bookaid.org | www.sabre.org

ELSEVIER   **BOOK AID**   Sabre Foundation
International

Commissioning Editor: **Rolla Couchman, Karen Bowler**
Project Development Manager: **Martin Mellor Publishing Services Ltd, Louise Cook**
Project Manager: **Kathryn Mason**
Production Assistant: **Gemma Lawson**
Design Manager: **Andy Chapman**
Illustration Manager: **Mick Ruddy**
Illustrator: **Richard Tibbitts**
Marketing Managers (UK & Rest of world/USA): **Amy Hey, Laura Meiskey**

Contents

List of Contributors vii

Foreword xi

Acknowledgements xiii

Section I: Normal Structure and Function

1 Anatomy 1
   Bernard C. Portmann

2 Cellular Biology of the Normal Liver 17
   Gary Guangsheng Fan, Clifford J. Steer

3 Functions of the Liver 43
   Bruce A. Luxon

Section II: Evaluation of Patients with Liver Disease

4 History and Physical Examination 61
   Peter D. Howdle

5 Laboratory Tests 73
   Joanne C. Imperial, Emmet B. Keeffe

6 Jaundice 83
   Steven D. Lidofsky

7 Liver Biopsy 101
   Kyle E. Brown, M. Kay Washington, Elizabeth M. Brunt

8 Imaging of the Liver 123
   B. Kirke Bieneman, Adrian M. Di Bisceglie

Section III: Clinical Manifestations of Liver Disease

9 Portal Hypertension and Gastrointestinal Hemorrhage 137
   Anastasios A. Mihas, Arun J. Sanyal

10 Ascites, Hyponatremia, Hepatorenal Syndrome and Spontaneous
   Bacterial Peritonitis 153
   Andrés Cárdenas, Pere Ginès and Vicente Arroyo

11 Hepatic Encephalopathy 169
   Andres T. Blei

12 Malnutrition in Cirrhosis 177
   Arthur J. McCullough

13 Associated Systemic Conditions 191
   Michael A. Heneghan, James P. O'Beirne

Section IV: Specific Diseases of Liver and Biliary Tree

14 Hepatitis A and E 205
   Martin Tagle, Maria de Medina, Eugene R. Schiff

15 Hepatitis B and D 213
   Patrick Marcellin

16 Hepatitis C 235
   Adrian M. Di Bisceglie

17 Miscellaneous Infections of the Liver 249
   Rachel Baden Herman, Margaret J. Koziel

18 Autoimmune Hepatitis 263
   Christian P. Strassburg, Arndt Vogel, Michael P. Manns

19 Primary Biliary Cirrhosis 277
   Raoul Poupon, Renée Eugénie Poupon

20 Primary Sclerosing Cholangitis 289
   K.V. Narayanan Menon, Russell H. Wiesner

21 Alcoholic Liver Disease 311
   Timothy R. Morgan, Samuel W. French

22 Fatty Liver, Non-alcoholic Steatohepatitis 327
   Brent A. Neuschwander-Tetri

23 Hemochromatosis 341
   Bruce R. Bacon

24 Wilson Disease 351
   Peter Ferenci

25 The Porphyrias, α_1-Antitrypsin Deficiency, Cystic Fibrosis, and
   Other Metabolic Diseases of the Liver 369
   Herbert L. Bonkovsky, James H. Reichheld

26 Pediatric Liver Disease 397
   Deirdre A. Kelly

27 Benign Tumors of the Liver 423
   John Karani

28 Biliary Diseases, Gallstones and Cystic Disease 435
   Gregory T. Everson, Fernando E. Membreno

29 Malignant Tumors 451
   Philip J. Johnson

30 Vascular Diseases of the Liver 471
   Dominique-Charles Valla

31 Liver Diseases in Pregnancy 485
   Rebecca W. Van Dyke

32 Drug and Toxin-Induced Liver Disease 495
   Suzanne Norris

33 Acute Liver Failure 515
   John G. O'Grady

34 The Liver in Systemic Disease 535
   Andrew Ross, Lawrence S. Friedman

35 Non-Cirrhotic Portal Hypertension 547
   Shiv Kumar Sarin

36 Hepatobiliary Surgery 565
   Andrew M. Smith, J. Michael Henderson

Section V: Liver Transplantation

37 Indications and Patient Selection 583
   John R. Lake

38 The Transplant Operation: what the hepatologist should
   know 603
   Michael L. Schilsky, Milan Kinkhabwala, Jean Crawford Emond

39 Immunology and Immunosuppression 619
   Geoffrey W. McCaughan

40 Early Management 641
   Federico G. Villamil, Andres E. Ruf

41 Long Term Management 653
   James Neuberger

42 Recurrent Viral Hepatitis in Liver Transplant Recipients 667
   Scott Biggins, Norah A. Terrault

Index 689

Contributors

Vicente Arroyo MD
Professor of Medicine
Director, Institute for Digestive Diseases
Hospital Clinic I Provincial de Barcelona
Universitat de Barcelona, Spain

Bruce R. Bacon MD
James F. King MD Endowed Chair in Gastroenterology;
Professor of Internal Medicine;
Director, Division of Gastroenterology and Hepatology
Saint Louis University Liver Center
Saint Louis University School of Medicine
St. Louis, MO, USA

Rachel Baden Herman MD
Clinical Fellow
Division of Infectious Diseases
Beth Israel Deaconess Medical Center
Havard Medical School
Boston, MA, USA

B. Kirke Bieneman MD
Assistant Professor
Department of Radiology
Saint Louis University Liver Center
Saint Louis University School of Medicine
St. Louis, MO, USA

Scott W. Biggins MD
Gastroenterology Fellow
Medicine/Gastroenterology
University of California San Francisco
San Francisco, CA, USA

Andres T. Blei MD
Professor of Medicine
Northwestern University Medical School;
Attending Physician
Northwestern Memorial Hospital
Chicago, IL, USA

Herbert L. Bonkovsky MD
Professor of Medicine and Molecular, Microbial and
Structural Biology;
Director, General Clinical Research Center/Office of
Clinical Research;
Director, The Liver-Biliary-Pancreatic Center
University of Connecticut Health Center
Farmington, CT, USA

Kyle E. Brown MD, MSc
Assistant Professor
Division of Gastroenterology/Hepatology
University of Iowa Carver College of Medicine;
Staff Physician
GI Section
Iowa City Veterans Administration Medical Center
Iowa City, IA, USA

Elizabeth M. Brunt MD
Professor of Pathology
Saint Louis University Liver Center
Saint Louis University School of Medicine
St. Louis, MO, USA

Andrés Cárdenas MD MMSc
Assistant Professor of Medicine
Division of Gastroenterology and Hepatology
Hospital Pablo Tobon Uribe
University of Antioquia
Medellin, Colombia

Maria de Medina MSPH
Senior Research Associate
Center for Liver Diseases
Department of Medicine
Division of Hepatology
University of Miami School of Medicine
Miami, FL, USA

Adrian M. Di Bisceglie MD
Professor of Internal Medicine
Chief of Hepatology
Division of Gastroenterology and Hepatology
Saint Louis University Liver Center
Saint Louis University School of Medicine
St. Louis, MO, USA

Jean Crawford Emond MD
Professor of Surgery
Columbia College of Physicians and Surgeons
Director Center for Liver Disease
New York Presbyterian Hospital
New York, NY, USA

Gregory T. Everson MD
Professor of Medicine;
Director of Hepatology
University of Colorado School of Medicine and Health
Sciences Center
Denver, CO, USA

Gary Guangsheng Fan MD, PhD
Anesthesiologist
White Memorial Medical Center
Los Angeles, CA, USA

Peter Ferenci MD
Professor of Internal Medicine
Department of Gastroenterology and Hepatology
Clinic of Internal Medicine IV
Vienna, Austria

Samuel W. French MD
Professor of Pathology and Chief, Anatomic Pathology
Harbor-UCLA Medical Center
Torrance, CA, USA

Lawrence S. Friedman MD
Professor of Medicine
Harvard Medical School;
Assistant Chief of Medicine
Massachusetts General Hospital
Boston, MA, USA
and
Chair
Department of Medicine
Newton-Wellesley Hospital
Newton, MA, USA

Pere Ginès MD
Associate Professor of Medicine
Liver Unit, Institute for Digestive Diseases
Hospital Clinic I Provincial de Barcelona
Universitat de Barcelona
Barcelona, Spain

J. Michael Henderson MB, ChB, FRCS(Ed), FACS
Professor
The Cleveland Clinic Lerner College of Medicine
Case Western Reserve University
Cleveland, OH, USA

Michael A. Heneghan MD, MMedSC, MRCPI
Consultant Hepatologist
Institute of Liver Studies
Kings College Hospital
London, UK

Peter D. Howdle BSc, MD, FRCP
Professor of Clinical Education;
Consultant Gastroenterologist;
Head of Academic Unit of General Surgery, Medicine
and Anaesthesia
St James's University Hospital
Leeds, UK

Joanne C. Imperial MD
Associate Clinical Professor of Medicine
Division of Gastrenterology and Hepatology
Department of Medicine
Stanford University School of Medicine
Stanford, CA, USA

Philip J. Johnson MD, FRCP
Clinical Head;
Professor of Oncology and Translational Research;
Director, Clinical Trials Unit
Institute for Cancer Studies
University of Birmingham
Birmingham, UK

John Karani MD
Consultant Radiologist
King's College Hospital
London, UK

Emmet B. Keeffe MD
Professor of Medicine
Chief of Hepatology;
Co-Director, Liver Transplant Program
Stanford University Medical Center
Stanford, CA, USA

Deirdre A. Kelly MD, FRCP, FRCPI, FRCPCH
Consultant Pediatric Hepatologist;
Professor of Paediatric Hepatology
University of Birmingham
Birmingham, UK

Milan Kinkhabwala MD
Associate Professor of Surgery
Weill Medical College of Cornell University
New York, NY, USA

Margaret J. Koziel MD
Associate Professor of Medicine
Harvard Medical School and Staff Physician
Division of Infectious Disease
Beth Israel Deaconess Medical Center
Boston, MA, USA

John R. Lake MD
Professor of Medicine and Surgery
Director, Gastroenterology Division
Director, Liver Transplantation Program
University of Minnesota Medical School
Minneapolis, MN, USA

Steven D. Lidofsky MD, PhD
Associate Professor of Medicine and Pharmacology
University of Vermont
Burlington, VT, USA

Bruce A. Luxon MD, PhD
Professor of Internal Medicine
Division of Gastroenterology and Hepatology
Saint Louis University Liver Center
Saint Louis University School of Medicine
St. Louis, MO, USA

Michael P. Manns MD
Professor and Chairman
Department of Gastroenterology, Hepatology and
Endocrinology
Hanover Medical School
Hanover, Germany

Patrick Marcellin MD, PhD
Head of the Claude Bernard Viral Hepatitis Research
Centre
Hôpital Beaujon
Clichy, France
and
Professor of Hepatology
University of Paris
Paris, France

Geoffrey W. McCaughan MD, PhD
Professor
Royal Prince Alfred Hospital and University of Sydney
Sydney, Australia

Arthur J. McCullough MD
Director of Gastroenterology
MetroHealth Medical Center;
Professor of Medicine
Case Western Reserve University
Cleveland, OH, USA

Fernando E. Membreno MD, MS
Instructor of Medicine
Gastroenterology and Hepatology Section
Eastern Colorado Health Care System
Denver, CO, USA

K.V. Narayanan Menon MD, FRCP(Edin),
FRCP(Glas)
Assistant Professor of Medicine
Mayo Medical School;
Consultant
Division of Gastroenterology and Hepatology
Mayo Clinic
Rochester, MN, USA

Anastasios A. Mihas MD, DMSc, FACP, FACG
Chief, Clinical Research;
Associate Director of Hepatology
McGuire Veterans Affairs Medical Center;
Professor of Medicine
Virginia Commonwealth University School of Medicine
Richmond, VA, USA

Timothy R. Morgan MD
Chief, Hepatology and Gastroenterology Section
Department of Gastroenterology
VA Medical Center
Long Beach, CA, USA

James Neuberger DM, FRCP
Consultant Physician
Liver Unit
Queen Elizabeth Hospital;
Professor of Medicine
University of Birmingham
Birmingham, UK

Brent A. Neuschwander-Tetri MD
Professor of Internal Medicine
Division of Gastroenterology and Hepatology
Saint Louis University Liver Center
Saint Louis University School of Medicine
St. Louis, MO, USA

Suzanne Norris MD, PhD, FRCPI
Consultant Hepatologist
St James's Hospital;
Honorary Lecturer
Trinity College Dublin
Dublin, Ireland

James P. O'Beirne MB, BS, MRCP
Clinical Fellow in Hepatology
Institute of Liver Studies
Kings College Hospital
London, UK

John G. O'Grady MD, FRCPI
Consultant Hepatologist
Institute of Liver Studies
King's College School of Medicine
London, UK

Bernard C. Portmann MD, FRCPath
Consultant Histopathologist and Professor of
Hepatopathology
King's College Hospital NHS Trust, and Guy's, King's
and St Thomas' School of Medicine
University of London
London, UK

Raoul Poupon MD
Professor of Medicine
Assistance Publique
Hôpitaux de Paris
University Paris VI
Hôpital Saint-Antoine
Paris, France

Renée Eugénie Poupon PhD
Director of Research
Faculté de Médecine Necker
Paris, France

James H. Reichheld MD
Consultant Gastroenterologist and Hepatologist
Lowell General Hospital and Saints' Memorial Medical
Center;
Director of Endoscopy
Lowell General Hospital
Lowell, MA, USA
and
Clinical Instructor
Tufts New England Medical Center
Boston, MA, USA

Andrew S. Ross MD
Clinical Fellow
Section of Gastroenterology, Hepatology, and
Nutrition
The University of Chicago Hospitals
Chicago, IL, USA

Andres E. Ruf MD
Assistant Director of Hepatology;
Assitant Director of Liver Transplantation
Fundacion Favaloro
Buenos Aires, Argentina

Arun J. Sanyal MBBS, MD
Charles Caravati Professor of Medicine;
Chairman
Division of Gastroenterology, Hepatology and Internal
Medicine
VCU Health System
Richmond, VA, USA

Shiv Kumar Sarin MD, DM
Professor and Head
Department of Gastroenterology
G B Pant Hospital;
President
Asian Pacific Association Study of the Liver (APASL);
Adjunct Professor of Molecular Medicine
Jawaharlal Nehru University
New Delhi, India

Eugene R. Schiff MD, MACP, FRCP, MACG
Professor of Medicine;
Chief, Division of Hepatology;
Director, Center for Liver Diseases
University of Miami School of Medicine
Miami, FL, USA

Michael L. Schilsky MD
Associate Professor of Medicine;
Medical Director
Center for Liver Disease and Transplantation
New York Weill Cornell Medical Center
New York, NY, USA

Andrew M. Smith BSc, MD, FRCS
Hepatobiliary Fellow
The Cleveland Clinic Lerner College of Medicine
Case Western Reserve University
Cleveland, OH, USA

Clifford J. Steer MD
Professor of Medicine and Genetics, Cell Biology and
Development;
Director, Molecular Gastroenterology Program
University of Minnesota Medical School
Minneapolis, MN, USA

Christian P. Strassburg MD
Assistant Professor of Experimental Gastroenterology
Hanover Medical School
Hanover, Germany

Martin Tagle MD
Associate Professor of Medicine
Universidad Peruana Cayetano Heredia;
Staff Gastroenterologist and Hepatologist
British American Hospital
Lima, Peru

Norah A. Terrault MD, MPH
Assistant Professor
Medicine/Gastroenterology
University of California San Francisco
San Francisco, CA, USA

Dominique-Charles Valla MD
Professor of Hepatology
University of Paris VII;
Head, Department of Hepatology
Hôpital Beaujon
Clichy, France

Rebecca W. Van Dyke MD
Professor of Medicine
University of Michigan Medical School;
Attending Physician
University of Michigan Hospitals;
Staff Physician
Veterans Administration Health Care System
Ann Arbor, MI, USA

Federico G. Villamil MD
Director of Hepatology and Medical Director of Liver
Transplantation
Liver Unit
Fundacion Favaloro;
Professor of Medicine
Favaloro University
Buenos Aires, Argentina

Arndt Vogel MD
Fellow in Hepatology
Department of Hepatology, Gastroenterology and
Endocrinology
Hanover Medical School
Hanover, Germany

M. Kay Washington MD, PhD
Professor
Department of Pathology
Vanderbilt University Medical Center
Nashville, TN, USA

Russell H. Wiesner MD
Medical Director of Liver Transplantation
Mayo Clinic
Rochester, MN, USA

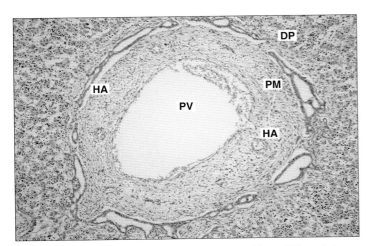

Figure 1.2 The embryonal ductal plate highlighted in a stillborn fetus with autosomal recessive polycystic kidney disease. Note the persistent ductal plate (DP) encircling the portal mesenchyme (PM) with a centrally placed portal vein branch (PV). HA, hepatic arteriole.

GROSS ANATOMY OF THE LIVER

The liver is the largest solid organ in the body with a median weight of approximately 1600 g in men and 1400 g in women. It lies in the right upper quadrant of the abdomen essentially under the protection of the rib cage. Its high location and intimate relationship with neighboring organs are of major importance to clinicians examining patients with liver disease and taking percutaneous needle biopsies (**Fig. 1.3**):

- The right kidney and the right colonic flexure lie in close contact with the inferolateral-lateral surface of the right lobe; the stomach imprints the inferior aspect and margin of the left lobe which extends to variable degrees into the left hypochondrium as far as the left mid-clavicular line.
- The lung and pleural sac overlie the dome of the right lobe for some distance laterally, a disposition which is responsible for dullness to percussion.
- The anterior edge of the liver comes into contact with the anterior abdominal wall below the costal margin and the xiphisternum, where it can be palpated during inspiration.
- The entire liver is covered by the fibrous capsule of Glisson, except posteriorly where it lies in direct contact with the diaphragm, the so-called 'bare area' which is surrounded by reflections of the peritoneum – the coronary and left and right triangular ligaments (**Fig. 1.4b, c**).

Anatomic landmarks seen on external examination are illustrated in Figure. 1.4. On the upper surface, the falciform ligament running anteroposteriorly attaches the liver to the diaphragm and to the anterior abdominal wall. Visually it divides the organ into two uneven lobes, the right lobe being about six times the size of the left; these have no functional significance (Fig. 1.4a). The anterior portion of the falciform ligament – the round ligament (ligamentum teres) – runs within the fissure of the umbilical vein and connects the left branch of the portal vein to the umbilicus (Fig. 1.4b); it contains small vestigial veins that re-open and even become varicose when intrahepatic portal venous block develops secondary to liver cirrhosis. Posteriorly the falciform ligament merges with the coronary ligaments surrounding the bare area (Fig. 1.4c).

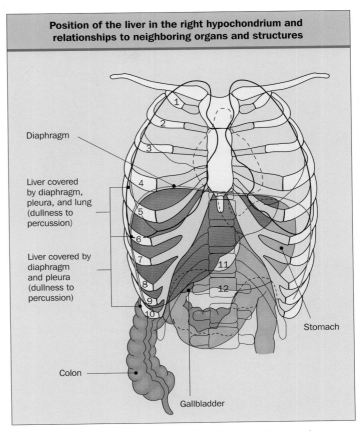

Position of the liver in the right hypochondrium and relationships to neighboring organs and structures

Diaphragm

Liver covered by diaphragm, pleura, and lung (dullness to percussion)

Liver covered by diaphragm and pleura (dullness to percussion)

Colon

Stomach

Gallbladder

Figure 1.3 Position of the liver in the right hypochondrium and relationships to neighboring organs and structures.

On the inferior surface, the caudate lobe bulges posteriorly between the fossa for the ductus venosus and the vena cava. The quadrate lobe lies anteriorly, lined by the gallbladder to its right and the fissure of the umbilical vein to its left (Fig. 1.4b)

Between caudate and quadrate lobes is the porta hepatis. In this deep fissure the portal vein and hepatic artery enter, and bile ducts leave, the liver contained in the peritoneal fold of the hepatoduodenal ligament. At that level the Glisson capsule is reflected inwardly to form the fibrous sheaths that invest the portal vessels and ducts throughout the liver, down to their smallest ramifications, the so-called portal tracts.

Vessels and functional anatomy of the liver

The liver receives 75% of its blood through the portal vein that carries blood from the entire capillary system of the digestive tract, spleen, pancreas and gallbladder, and 25% through the hepatic artery, the second major branch of the celiac axis. Functionally, the liver is divided into two roughly equal parts ('true' lobes) on the basis of its blood supply and bile drainage. The line of demarcation between right and left hepatic arterial and portal venous inflow is located along a plane that passes some 4 cm to the right of the falciform ligament, joining the tip of the gallbladder to the groove of the vena cava (Fig. 1.4a). The recognition of this plane of demarcation between true left and right lobes is of major importance in staging primary hepatic tumors. The liver can be further divided into eight functional segments based on vascular distribution as illustrated in

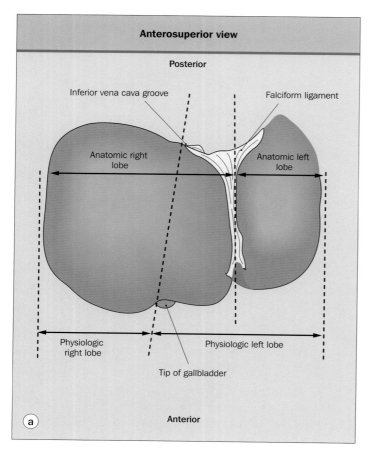

Anterosuperior view

Posterior

Inferior vena cava groove

Falciform ligament

Anatomic right lobe

Anatomic left lobe

Physiologic right lobe

Physiologic left lobe

Tip of gallbladder

Anterior

a

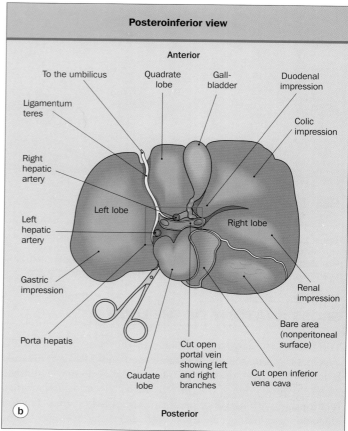

Posteroinferior view

Anterior

To the umbilicus

Quadrate lobe

Gall-bladder

Duodenal impression

Ligamentum teres

Colic impression

Right hepatic artery

Left lobe

Left hepatic artery

Right lobe

Gastric impression

Renal impression

Porta hepatis

Bare area (nonperitoneal surface)

Caudate lobe

Cut open portal vein showing left and right branches

Cut open inferior vena cava

b

Posterior

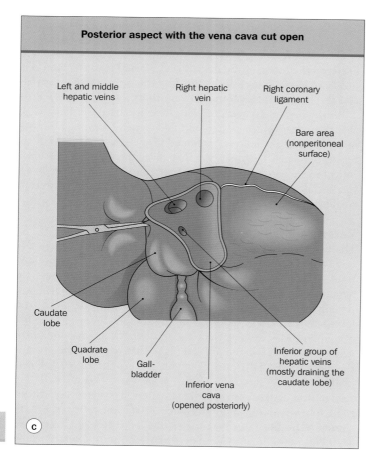

Posterior aspect with the vena cava cut open

Left and middle hepatic veins

Right hepatic vein

Right coronary ligament

Bare area (nonperitoneal surface)

Caudate lobe

Quadrate lobe

Gall-bladder

Inferior vena cava (opened posteriorly)

Inferior group of hepatic veins (mostly draining the caudate lobe)

c

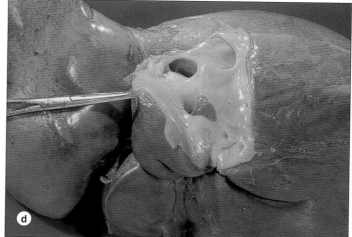

d

Figure 1.4 External appearances and surface markings of the liver.
(a) Anterosuperior view. (b) Posteroinferior view. (c and d) Posterior aspect with the inferior vena cava cut open to show the outlets of the hepatic veins.

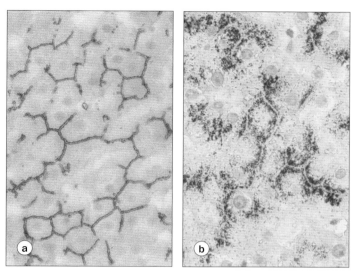

Figure 1.12 Bile canaliculi in light microscopy. (a) Histochemical demonstration of ATPase in pericanalicular cytoplasm. (b) Canalicular network outlined in iron overload due to pericanalicular accumulation of hemosiderin (Perls' stain).

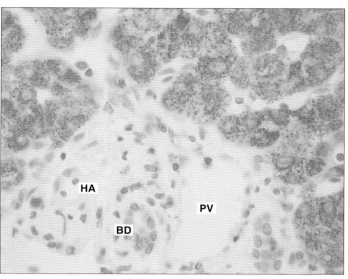

Figure 1.14 Normal hepatocyte cytoplasm shows distinctive brown granules after immunostaining for hepatocyte specific antigen, which appears to detect antigenic material unique to hepatocellular mitochondria. PV, portal venule; HA = hepatic arteriole; BD, bile duct (HepPar-1, immunoperoxidase).

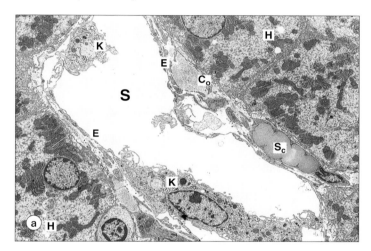

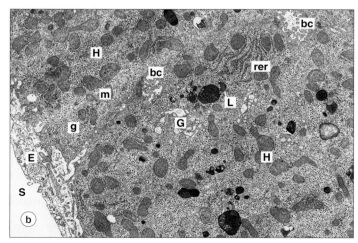

Figure 1.13 Electron micrograph of a sinusoid with its lining cells (a), and hepatocytes with organelles (b). H, hepatocyte; bc, bile canaliculus; m, mitochondrion; L, lysosome; G, golgi apparatus; g, glycogen; rer, rough endoplasmic reticulum; S, sinusoidal lumen; E, endothelial cell; K, Kupffer cell; Sc, hepatic stellate cell; Co, collagen in Disse space. (a) (× 2600). (b) (× 6400). Courtesy of Professor P Bioulac-Sage.

xenobiotics, the SER harboring the cytochrome P450 oxidation system whose induction is expressed by a proliferation of SER membranes (see Ch. 32). Other cell functions associated with SER include metabolism of fatty acids, phospholipids and triglycerides, and synthesis of cholesterol and possibly of bile acid.

The mitochondria are particularly numerous in the hepatocytes, their inner membranes and cristae being concerned with the oxidative phosphorylation and fatty acid oxidation whereas their matrix contains the enzymes involved in the citric acid and urea cycles.

Although not yet fully characterized, a monoclonal antibody referred to as hepatocyte specific antigen or hepatocyte paraffin-1 (HepPar-1) appears to identify an antigen unique to hepatocellular mitochondria. This commercialized antibody is widely used when there is a need to identify hepatocytes or hepatocellular neoplasms (**Fig. 1.14**).

The lysosomes, first recognized in the liver, are membrane-bound vesicles that are involved in the digestion and catabolism of various exogenous and endogenous substances, a function that is reflected in their heterogeneous content – autophagic vacuoles, storage products, lipofuscin, hemosiderin and copper complexes. They are rich in acid hydrolase, for example acid phosphatase, which can be used for their histochemical identification; they are involved in a number of storage disorders (see Ch. 25).

The peroxisomes (microbodies) are membrane-bound ovoid bodies that contain oxidases and use molecular oxygen for the production of H_2O_2. This is in turn hydrolyzed by peroxisomal catalase, an enzyme that can be used for the ultrastructural identification of these organelles. Peroxisomes are involved in the metabolism of fatty acid and alcohol; they proliferate following administration of hypolipidemic drugs, such as clofibrate.

The cytoskeleton comprises:

• The microfilaments (6 nm) are composed of filaments of actin and myosin which, associated in bundles, form a three-dimensional meshwork throughout the cytoplasm; they are attached to the plasma membrane, extend into the microvilli, and are particularly abundant in the pericanalicular ectoplasm, being attached to the junctional complex on either side of the canaliculus; they play a major role in bile secretion and flow regulation, as exemplified by intrahepatic cholestasis produced by drugs that cause depolymerization of the pericanalicular actin belt, in particular cytochalasin B and norethandrolone.

- The intermediate filaments (8–10 nm) are a family of self-assembling protein fibers that act as an intracellular scaffold with a role in integrating cytoplasmic space and organelle movement; like in other epithelial cells in the body they react as cytokeratins, more specifically hepatocyte cytokeratins 8 and 18, in contrast to cytokeratins 7 and 19 which characterize biliary epithelium; intermediate filaments contribute to the formation of Mallory bodies as a result of their depolymerization in alcoholic and other liver diseases.
- The microtubules (20 nm) are hollow, unbranched structures that play a role in cell division (formation of mitotic spindle), in the movement of transport vesicles, and in the transport and export of proteins and lipoproteins.

Glycogen is abundant, reflecting a principal role of the liver in the synthesis of glycogen from glucose, or lactic and pyruvic acid, and its breakdown and release as glucose into the circulation. When depletion occurs, glycogen starts disappearing from the perivenular region. In electron microscopy it appears as dense β-particles, 15–30 nm in diameter, and α-particles, aggregates of the smaller particles arranged in rosettes.

Cells of the hepatic sinusoid

Sinusoids with an average diameter of about 10 μm, which may distend to about 30 μm, are lined by endothelial cells which delineate the space of Disse running underneath their fenestrated cell process at the sinusoidal surface of the hepatocytes; hepatic stellate cells lie in the space of Disse, the Kupffer cells and liver-associated lymphocytes lie on the luminal aspect of the endothelium (see Figs 1.10 and 1.13).

The endothelial cells form an attenuated cytoplasmic sheet perforated by numerous holes (fenestrae), which constitute the sieve plate. They seem to form no intercellular junctions and do not lie on a basement membrane, a unique configuration that allows free passage of solutes from the sinusoidal lumen into the space of Disse. Unlike vascular endothelium elsewhere in the body, they do not bind ulex europaeus, do not express FVIII-related antigen or CD34 in the normal human liver, but their membrane is immunoreactive for intercellular adhesion molecule-1 (ICAM-1). The natural ligand for this adhesion molecule, leukocyte function-associated antigen-1 (LFA-1), is present on Kupffer cells. In pathologic situations such as capillarization of the sinusoids in the cirrhotic liver and in benign and malignant hepatocellular neoplasms, endothelial cells do acquire CD34 immunoreactivity.

The Kupffer cells are members of the mononuclear-phagocytic system forming the largest part of the fixed tissue macrophages in the body. They account for 2.1% of the non-parenchymal cells on a volume basis and have an increased density, a larger size and are more phagocytic in the periportal areas. Irregularly stellate in shape, they float freely in the lumen of the sinusoids, anchored by their process to the endothelial cells. Their major function is the clearance of particles, immune complexes,

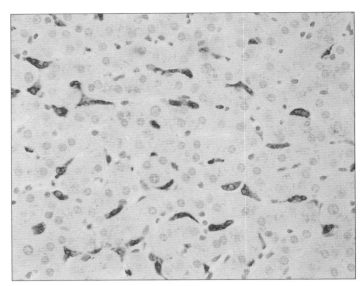

Figure 1.15 Kupffer cells are clearly identified due to dark brown appearance of their cytoplasm following immunostaining for CD68 antigen.

injured red cells and endotoxins. Their release of mediators, including interleukins 1 and 6, tumor necrosis factor-α (TNF-α), interferons and eicosanoids, constitutes part of the host response to infection and explains some of the clinical manifestations of endotoxemia. Kupffer cells are difficult to identify by light microscopy alone and proper identification rests on using their immunoreactivity to CD68 (**Fig. 1.15**) or their expression of class II histocompatibility antigens, in particular human leukocyte antigen-DR (HLA-DR).

The hepatic stellate cells (perisinusoidal, fat-storing or Ito cells) lie in the space of Disse, their long cytoplasmic processes surrounding the sinusoids. Their nucleus and perikaryon are often embedded within recesses between hepatocytes; their cytoplasm contains many small lipid droplets that are rich in vitamin A. Besides their role in storing vitamin A, they represent resting fibroblasts which are a major source of extracellular matrix in the normal and diseased liver. Their phenotypic transformation into transitional myofibroblasts in acute and chronic liver disease is associated with the acquisition of α-smooth muscle actin reactivity. Stellate cells are a potential source of hepatocyte growth factor and their contractility has led to a speculative role in controlling sinusoidal blood flow. They are not obvious in conventional light microscopy, but they become evident in semi-thin sections due to their microvesicular fatty cytoplasm (**Fig. 1.16**).

Liver-associated lymphocytes initially described as pit cells in the rat liver are now well recognized in human liver. They seem to be recruited from the peripheral blood to the liver sinusoids where they acquire natural and lymphokine-activated killer cell activity.

Other constituent tissues
Extracellular matrix

The connective tissue represents only 5–10% of the normal liver weight, a figure largely below that of the rest of the body, and 30% of the total protein mass is made of collagen. The other

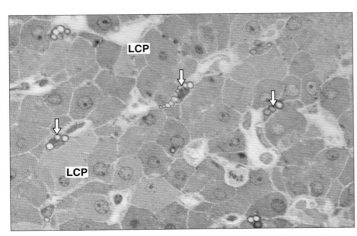

Figure 1.16 Hepatic stellate cells. Semi-thin section of a 2-year-old child's liver showing a two cell-thick plate arrangement with nuclei disposed toward the sinusoidal border of the hepatocytes and easily-identifiable stellate cells due to their microvesicular cytoplasm (arrowed). LCP: liver cell plate.

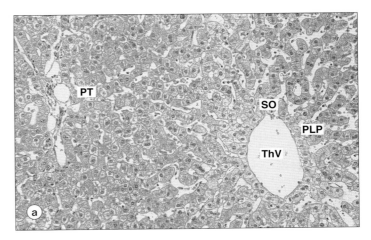

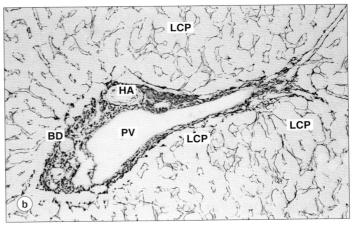

Figure 1.17 Liver histology at low magnification. (a) A terminal portal tract (PT) and a terminal hepatic venule (ThV) are shown, the latter in direct contact with the perivenular hepatocyte limiting plate (PLP). Note two sinusoidal outlets (SO). (b) Silver impregnation to show the reticulin network (black) and a small amount of type I collagen (gold brown) supporting portal vessels and bile duct. HA, hepatic arteriole; PV, portal venule; BD, bile duct; LCP, spaces occupied by liver cell plates.

structural components of the extracellular matrix are glycoproteins and proteoglycans.

Type I, III, IV, V and VI collagens are found in the normal liver. Type I and III, which represent more than 95% of the total collagen weight, are mainly located in Glisson capsule and its intrahepatic extension supporting the portal vein, hepatic artery and bile-duct branches – the portal tracts. Some extension of the capsular tissue accompanies the major hepatic vein branches, but there is no fibrous coat around the terminal hepatic venules which lie in direct contact with the perivenular hepatocyte plate (**Fig. 1.17**a).

Discrete strands of collagen are also present in the space of Disse. Type V collagen is closely associated with smooth muscle cells within vessel walls and may also form core fibrils upon which growth of large fibrils of type I collagen is initiated. Type VI forms microfilaments which serve as a flexible network that anchors blood vessels and nerves into the surrounding connective tissue. Type IV differs in that its terminal propeptides are not removed, but serve to cross-link the molecule into a three-dimensional lattice. It is an essential component of the vascular and bile duct basement membranes.

The matrix glycoproteins are highly cross-linked and insoluble. They have well-defined domains that interact with cell surface receptors and other components of the extracellular matrix. Laminin is a major component of basement membranes where it interacts with type IV collagen; both components are normally present in small amounts in the space of Disse, where increased deposition is associated with so-called capillarization of the sinusoids. Fibronectin mediates cell adhesion to collagen.

The proteoglycans are macromolecules that consist of a central protein core to which proteoglycans and oligosaccharides are attached. They are classified according to the type of glycos-aminoglycan. In the liver, heparan sulfate is the most abundant and is present in the portal tracts, in basement membrane and on the surface of hepatocytes.

The extracellular matrix in the normal liver is considered of major importance in regulating and modulating hepatocyte function; it serves to provide cohesiveness between cells, induces cell polarization, allows intercellular communication, and affects gene expression and cellular differentiation.

In the lobular parenchyma, the extracellular matrix is confined to the space of Disse. It is of unusually low density and thus invisible ultrastructurally, but visualized in light microscopy after impregnation with a silver method – the so-called reticulin network (Fig. 1.17b).

Lymphatics

The liver is the largest single source of lymph in the body, producing 15–20% of the total volume. Hepatic lymph has a high protein and cell content and is formed mainly by drainage from the perisinusoidal space of Disse into the first-order lymphatic plexus of the portal tracts. Traced towards the porta hepatis, the plexus, composed of flattened endothelial tubes with a primarily periarterial distribution, progressively enlarges, and in larger tracts becomes associated with portal vein and bile duct tributaries. Large collectors are thickened at the porta hepatis due to the acquisition of a muscle layer. They mainly drain into the hepatic nodes, located along the hepatic artery and celiac nodes. Other efferent routes include:

- via the falciform ligament and epigastric vessels to the para-sternal nodes,

- from the liver surface to the left gastric nodes, and
- from the bare area to the posterior mediastinal nodes.

In conditions such as portal hypertension there is a significant increase in production of hepatic lymph, with a protein content identical to that of the plasma, indicating unrestricted passage of protein into the space of Disse. There ensues a considerable enlargement of the capsular plexus due to important anastomoses between intrahepatic and capsular lymphatics, with lymph exudating from the capsular plexus to form protein-rich ascites.

Nerve supply

There are two main separate but intercommunicating nerve plexuses around the hepatic artery and portal vein that distribute with the branches of these vessels. These include preganglionic parasympathetic fibers derived from both vagal and sympathetic fibers with cell bodies in the celiac ganglia. Immunohistochemical studies of human liver using antibodies to common neural proteins such as protein gene product (PGP) 9.5 have demonstrated nerve fibers, not only around vessels and bile ducts in the portal tracts, but in the acini, running along the sinusoids. There is evidence that sympathetic nerves play a role in carbohydrate metabolism and possibly in regulating sinusoidal blood flow.

Light microscopy as seen in biopsy specimens

With reference to the three-dimensional model of Elias (see Fig. 1.6) it is easy to extrapolate that the liver cell plates appear as single cell thick anastomosing 'cords' in conventional light microscopy (see Fig. 1.9). These are two-cell thick up to the age of 5 years (see Fig. 1.16), a pattern that in adults reappears as an indication of liver regeneration, sometimes associated with an acinar or rosette arrangement. Hepatocytes appear as polygonal cells with clearly outlined cell margins and centrally placed nuclei which contain one or two nucleoli. There are occasional binucleated cells. Variation in nuclear size increases with increasing age, a pleomorphism that is more marked in acinar zone 2 (mid-zonal areas). The cytoplasm is granular and eosinophilic, but slightly basophilic aggregates of RER can be identified in a perinuclear and pericanalicular distribution (see Fig. 1.9). At low magnification relatively regularly spaced portal tracts and hepatic venules are expected (see Fig. 1.17a), but the boundaries between acini or acinar zones are not evident. Thus the sleeve of parenchyma surrounding the portal tracts is referred to as periportal parenchyma or acinar zone 1, the one surrounding the hepatic venules as perivenular parenchyma or acinar zone 3, intermediate areas between these zones being considered as acinar zone 2 or mid-zonal. Appearances of the portal areas depend on their size and the plane along which they are cut (**Fig. 1.18a–c**).

However, at any level the size of the arteriole roughly matches that of the bile duct. The portal venules are of variable shape and size and they are thin-walled, their lumen being generally much larger than that of the corresponding arterial branch. Large tracts (Fig. 1.18c) may show a considerable amount of collagen (Fig. 1.18d), especially around the bile duct, and, when

sampled by the biopsy needle, this can easily be misinterpreted as fibrotic liver.

Intrahepatic and extrahepatic biliary passages

The bile canaliculi, as already described, form a complicated anastomosing network running half way within the thickness of the liver cell plates. They drain into minute periportal channels, also known as canals of Hering, which have a basement membrane and are lined by both hepatocytes and bile duct cells. The canal of Hering is supposed to harbor progenitor cells which, in various pathologic situations, are able to differentiate into bile ducts or liver cells and from which so-called ductular reaction is likely to arise. Bile ductules, lined by flattened cholangiocytes, in which inconstant intralobular and short intraportal segments are recognized, join the canal of Hering to the interlobular bile ducts (**Fig. 1.19**). Canals of Hering and bile ductules are hardly visible on hematoxylin-eosin stained sections, but clearly revealed by cytokeratin immunostaining (Fig. 1.19b). The interlobular bile ducts, lined by a single layer of low cubic cells (see Fig. 1.18a, b) will by subsequent anastomoses increase in size from 15–20 μm to 100 μm to form septal bile ducts that are lined by tall columnar cells with basally located nuclei (Fig. 1.18c). The portal tract fibrous tissue shows some condensation around these ducts, which through further anastomoses form successively the area and segmental bile ducts. The latter, similar to the extrahepatic bile ducts and neck of gallbladder are invested with intramural mucinous and extramural seromucinous glands, the peribiliary glands (**Fig. 1.20**). They anastomose further to give rise to the left and right hepatic ducts, which in turn join to form the common hepatic duct, itself joined by the cystic duct of the gallbladder to become the common bile duct or choledochus (**Fig. 1.21**).

The common bile duct runs between the layers of the lesser omentum, lying anterior to the portal vein and to the right of the hepatic artery. It passes behind the first part of the duodenum in a groove on the back of the head of the pancreas, before entering the second part of the duodenum. The duct runs obliquely through the posteromedial duodenal wall, usually joining the main pancreatic duct to form a variable length common channel, the ampulla of Vater. In about 30% of individuals, the bile and pancreatic ducts open separately into the duodenum. The ampulla of Vater makes the duodenal mucous membrane bulge inwards to form an eminence, the duodenal papilla (Fig. 1.21).

During its passage through this collecting system, canalicular bile is modified by a process of absorption and secretion of water and electrolytes, and addition of seromucinous fluid by the peribiliary glands. There is evidence of immunoglobulin A secretion by the bile duct epithelium which normally expresses HLA class I, γ-glutamyltranspeptidase, carcinoembryonic antigen and epithelial membrane antigen. These represent phenotypic differences between bile duct epithelium and liver cells additional to their different cytokeratin profiles already mentioned.

CHAPTER
2

Cellular Biology of the Normal Liver

Gary Guangsheng Fan and Clifford J Steer

INTRODUCTION

More than 50 years ago, EB Wilson believed that 'the key to every biological problem must finally be sought in the cell'. With the recent dramatic advances in technology and our understanding of cell function, cellular biology of the liver is beginning to take its rightful place as an application to clinical hepatology. In this chapter, we present an overview of how hepatic cells are formed and how they function and cooperate to form the amazing liver. In higher organisms, organ systems are like cellular cities in which groups of cells perform specialized functions and are linked by intricate systems of communication. Cells occupy a halfway point in the scale of biologic complexity (**Fig. 2.1**). A fetal liver has three main cellular compartments, which are:
- parenchymal cells (hepatocytes, bile duct cells);
- sinusoidal cells (endothelial and Kupffer cells); and
- perisinusoidal cells (stellate and hematopoietic cells).

In a human embryo, the hepatic diverticulum consists of a cranial and caudal portion. Hepatocytes develop from the cranial portions, while the caudal bud is the origin of extrahepatic bile duct cells and epithelial cells that form the gallbladder. Generally, the proliferation of hepatic cells occurs by diffusion away from the thickening endoderm, but the formation of the extrahepatic ducts always proceeds from the caudal portion of the diverticulum. Studies in rat embryos suggest that the emerging hepatic tissue is composed of bipotential progenitor epithelial cells that are capable of differentiating either along the hepatocytic or biliary epithelial cell lineage.

The formation of intrahepatic bile ducts is initiated by hepatocytes. It has been suggested that the sinusoidal lining cells in early fetuses may be undifferentiated vascular stem cells. During development, these stem cells diverge, with one group committed to becoming an endothelial cell line and a second to becoming a Kupffer cell line. For mammals, the main function of the fetal liver is hematopoiesis, which begins soon after the appearance of the hepatic diverticulum. The hematopoietic cells are initially scattered throughout the liver, but are ultimately replaced by the developing and differentiating adult hepatic cells. An adult liver is occupied by hepatocytes and non-hepatocytes, in which hepatocytes constitute 78% of the tissue volume, non-hepatocytes account for 6.3% of the tissue volume, and the extracellular space for approximately 16% (**Table 2.1**).

The architecture and ultrastructure of the normal liver are unique to this organ (Fig. 2.1). The structure of the muralium simplex consists of polygonal-shaped parenchymal cells or hepatocytes. These cells enclose a chicken wire-like network of bile canaliculi in the central plane and are flanked by sinusoids on both sides of the muralium. The equivalent of an apical pole for the exocrine secretion of bile by the hepatocyte corresponds to the canalicular membrane, which surrounds the parenchymal cell periphery in a belt-like fashion. This structural organization implies that the biliary secretory polarity of the hepatocyte is oriented towards a peripheral ring around the middle of the parenchymal cell. In contrast, metabolic uptake and secretion occur at, or towards, the surfaces facing the sinusoids, implying bidirectional metabolic secretory activity. This complex secretory polarity requires a well-organized intracellular system for adequate and correct addressing of secretory products to their respective destinations. Hepatocytes are large polyhedral cells of approximately 20–30 μm diameter, which are arrayed in plates one or two cells thick along the hepatic sinusoids. As a metabolically highly active cell, the hepatocyte contains a vast array of organelles (**Table 2.2**). In human hepatocytes, approximately 30% of the cells are binucleate. While adult parenchymal cells display considerable heterogeneity in size, they all share at least one common constituent. The hepatocyte plasma membrane guarantees separation from but, at the same time, links the cell with its environment and matrix.

HEPATOCELLULAR PLASMA MEMBRANE

The plasma membrane encloses the cell, defines its boundaries and maintains the essential differences between the cytosol and the extracellular environment. All biological membranes have a common general structure which comprises a very thin film of lipid and protein molecules, held together mainly by non-covalent interactions (**Fig. 2.2**). Cell membranes are dynamic, fluid structures, and most of their molecules are able to move about in the plane of the membrane. The lipid molecules are arranged as a continuous double layer which is about 5 nm thick. This lipid bilayer provides the basic structure of the membrane and serves as a relatively impermeable barrier to the passage of most water-soluble molecules. Protein molecules within the lipid bilayer mediate most of the other functions of the membrane, transporting specific molecules across it, or catalyzing membrane-associated reactions such as adenosine triphosphate (ATP) synthesis. In the plasma membrane some proteins serve as structural links that connect the membrane to the cytoskeleton and/or to either the extracellular matrix or an adjacent cell, while others serve as receptors to detect and transduce chemical signals in the cell's environment.

Cell membranes are asymmetric structures. The lipid and protein compositions of the inner and outer faces differ from one another in ways that reflect the different functions performed at the two surfaces. The protein–lipid ratio varies enormously in different type cells. In hepatocytes, plasma membrane contains 54% protein, 36% lipid and 10% carbohydrate (by dry weight) (**Table 2.3**). Hepatocytes express the greatest abundance of

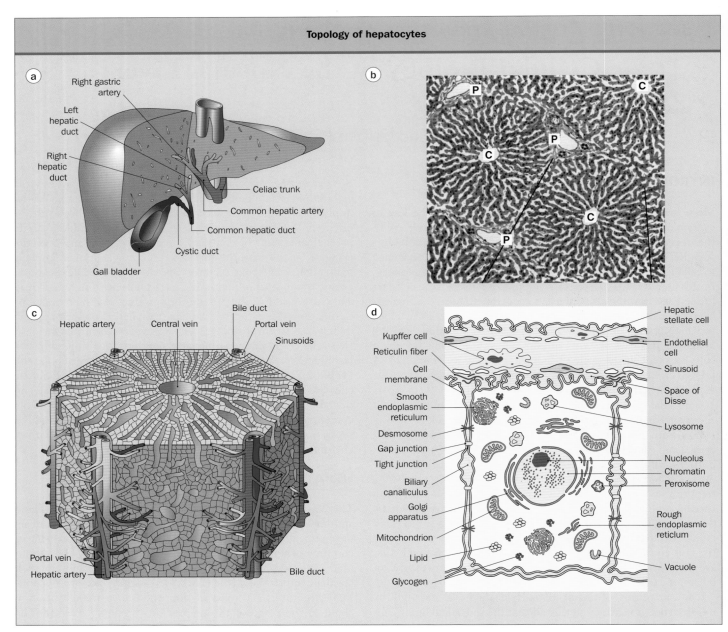

Topology of hepatocytes

(a)
Right gastric artery
Left hepatic duct
Right hepatic duct
Celiac trunk
Common hepatic artery
Common hepatic duct
Cystic duct
Gall bladder

(c)
Bile duct
Hepatic artery
Central vein
Portal vein
Sinusoids
Portal vein
Hepatic artery
Bile duct

(d)
Kupffer cell
Reticulin fiber
Cell membrane
Smooth endoplasmic reticulum
Desmosome
Gap junction
Tight junction
Biliary canaliculus
Golgi apparatus
Mitochondrion
Lipid
Glycogen
Hepatic stellate cell
Endothelial cell
Sinusoid
Space of Disse
Lysosome
Nucleolus
Chromatin
Peroxisome
Rough endoplasmic reticlum
Vacuole

Figure 2.1 The topology of hepatocytes and liver lobules in a normal liver. (a) A cross-section of an adult liver. (b) A magnified normal lobular section. The central veins (C) are surrounded by anastomosing cords of block-like hepatocytes. At the periphery of the lobule, typical portal areas (P) consist of branches of the portal vein, the hepatic artery and the bile duct. (c) A schematic view of the relationship of the different liver cells to each other and to the sinusoids. The principal organelles and inclusions in the cytoplasm are shown. (d) Schematic view of a liver lobule.

Relative number and volume of different cell types in the adult liver		
Cell type	Number (%)	Volume (%)
Hepatocytes	60	78
Non-hepatocytes	40	6.3
Endothelial cells	20	2.8
Kupffer cells	14	2.1
Stellate cells	6	1.4
Extracellular space		15.7

Table 2.1 Relative number and volume of different cell types in liver

membrane carbohydrates, where they occur almost exclusively on the outer surface.

Membrane lipids

Lipid contribution to membranes is highly varied depending on the species and cell type. However, in most eukaryotic cells there are three major classes of membrane lipid molecules: glycerophospholipids, cholesterol and sphingolipids (**Fig. 2.3**). The polar head groups of the phospholipids face the surrounding water and the fatty acyl chains form a continuous hydrophobic interior. In such a lamellar structure, each layer of phospholipid is called a *leaflet*. In addition, the lipid compositions of the inner and outer leaflets are different. Most of the sphingolipids are present in the outer leaflet, while some of the glycerophospholipids are restricted to the inner leaflet. Cholesterol and

Relative volumes occupied by the major intracellular compartments in a hepatocyte

Intracellular compartment	Cell volume (%)	Approximate number per cell
Cytosol	54	1
Mitochondria	22	1700
Rough ER cisternae	9	1
Smooth ER cisternae plus Golgi cisternae	6	
Nucleus	6	1
Peroxisomes	1	400
Lysosomes	1	300
Endosomes	1	200

Table 2.2 Relative volumes occupied by the major intracellular compartments in a hepatocyte. All the cisternae of the rough and smooth endoplasmic reticulum are thought to be joined to form a single large compartment. The Golgi apparatus, in contrast, is organized into a number of discrete sets of stacked cisternae in each cell, and the extent of interconnection between these sets has not been clearly established. ER, endoplasmic reticulum.

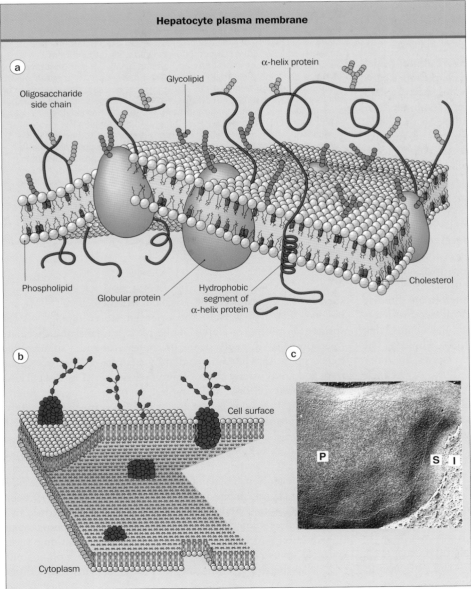

Hepatocyte plasma membrane

(a) α-helix protein
Glycolipid
Oligosaccharide side chain
Phospholipid
Globular protein
Hydrophobic segment of α-helix protein
Cholesterol

(b) Cell surface
Cytoplasm

(c) P S I

Figure 2.2 The hepatocyte plasma membrane.
(a) Schematic diagram of the membrane. The phospholipid molecules in the top layer, which faces the external medium, are shown as yellow spheres. The bottom layer, which faces the cytoplasm inside the cell, has a different phospholipid composition and is also shown in yellow. In some transmembrane proteins the polypeptide chain crosses the bilayer as a single α helix (blue); in others the polypeptide chain crosses the bilayer multiple times, either as a series of α helices or as a β sheet in the form of multipass proteins. Other membrane-associated proteins do not span the bilayer but instead are attached to either side of the membrane. Rigid cholesterol molecules (red) tend to keep the tails of the phospholipids relatively fixed and orderly in the regions closest to the hydrophilic heads; the parts of the tails closer to the core of the membrane move about freely. Side chains of sugar molecules attached to proteins and lipids are shown in green.
(b) The path followed by a fracture that splits a membrane into bilayers. (c) The membrane structure visible in a freeze-fracture preparation. P, membrane particles in bilayer; S, external membrane surface; I, ice crystals. Part (a) reproduced from Bretscher (85) by permission of Sci Am. Parts (b) and (c) reproduced from Wolfe (93) by permission of Brooks/Cole.

Lipid, protein, and carbohydrate content in cellular membranes			
		Dry mass (%)	
Membrane	Protein	Lipid	Carbohydrate
Plasma membrane	54	36	10
Nuclear envelope	66	32	2
Endoplasmic reticulum	62	27	10
Golgi complex	64	26	10
Mitochondrion			
outer membrane	55	45	Trace
inner membrane	78	22	

Table 2.3 Lipid, protein, and carbohydrate content in cellular membranes.

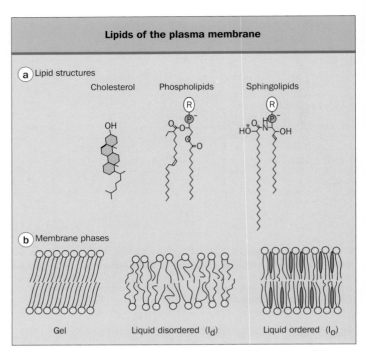

Figure 2.3 The lipids of the plasma membrane. (a) Structures of the major lipid classes of eukaryotic cells. Sterols like cholesterol are based on a four-ring structure. Glycerophospholipids are derived from diacylglycerol and typically carry acyl chains of 16–18 carbon atoms, one of which contains a cis double bond. The head group (R) is either neutral (serine or inositol) to give a net acidic charge, or basic (ethanolamine or choline) to give a neutral or zwitterionic lipid. Sphingolipids are based on a ceramide, and in mammals the head group is either choline (sphingomyelin), or in the case of the glycosphingolipids the phosphate is replaced with glucose, which is further elaborated to make a wide range of glycolipids. The acyl chain attached to the sphingoid base is typically saturated, varying in length from 16 to 26 carbons depending on the lipid and tissue (C26 is shown here). (b) Structures of lipid bilayers. Simple phospholipid bilayers below their T_m form a solidified gel phase, which melts above the T_m to a fluid phase (liquid-disordered (l_d), sometimes referred to as 'liquid-crystalline'). The presence of cholesterol (hatched ovals) orders the acyl chains of the latter phase, and indeed can fluidize the former phase, arriving at an intermediate state for which the term liquid-ordered (l_o) was coined. Reproduced from Munro (03) by permission of Elsevier.

sphingolipids are present at low levels in internal membranes and at high levels in the plasma membrane and endosomes. The high cholesterol bilayer is thus termed 'liquid-ordered' (l_o), in contrast to the 'liquid-disordered' state without cholesterol (l_d).

The most complex of the glycolipids, gangliosides, contain oligosaccharides with one or more sialic acid residues, which give gangliosides a net negative charge. The glycolipids may serve as receptors for normal extracellular molecules that mediate cell-recognition processes and protection of the membrane from the harsh conditions, and assist cells in binding to the extracellular matrix. Charged glycolipids may be important for their electrical effects. Their presence alters the electrical field across the membrane and the concentrations of ions, especially calcium, at its external surface.

The fluidity of a cell membrane is biologically important. For example, certain membrane transport processes and enzyme activities can be shown to cease when the bilayer viscosity is experimentally increased beyond a threshold level. All cell membranes contain a mixture of different fatty acyl chains and are fluid at the temperature at which the cell is grown and functions. Membrane cholesterol is a major determinant of bilayer fluidity. The net effect of cholesterol on membrane fluidity varies, depending on the lipid composition. Cholesterol restricts the random movement of portions of the fatty acyl chains lying closest to the outer surfaces of the leaflets. However, it separates and disperses the fatty acyl tails and causes the inner regions of the bilayer to become slightly more fluid. At the high concentrations found in eukaryotic plasma membranes, cholesterol tends to restrict fluidity at growth temperatures near 37°C. At temperatures below the *phase transition*, cholesterol maintains the membrane in a fluid state by preventing the hydrocarbon fatty acyl chains of the membrane lipids from binding to each other. This offsets the drastic reduction in fluidity that would otherwise occur at low temperatures.

The raft model of plasma membrane lipids

The plasma membrane contains more lipid species than are needed to form a simple bilayer. In plasma membranes, glycosphingolipids lie outside and most phosphatidylserine (PS) is located within the cell. PS asymmetry gives the cytoplasmic

surface of the plasma membrane a net negative charge above and beyond that arising from the oriented water dipoles on the surface. In the outer leaflet of the plasma membrane there are microdomains or small islands of cholesterol and a sphingolipid rich l_o phase that are surrounded by a l_d phase. They are called *rafts* and are typically about 50 nm in diameter (**Fig. 2.4**). These small islands of lipid are coupled to cholesterol-rich microdomains in the inner leaflet by an unknown mechanism. Rafts include transmembrane proteins, external glycosylphosphatidylinositol (GPI)-anchored proteins, and fatty acid-anchored proteins (such as Src tyrosine kinase) on the inner face. Raft lipids and associated proteins diffuse together laterally on the membrane surface. Some signaling receptors can move into the rafts upon ligand engagement, or 'cluster' smaller rafts into larger ones.

It is becoming evident that rafts play an important role in a wide range of biological processes, including numerous signal transduction pathways, apoptosis, cell adhesion and migration, synaptic transmission, organization of the cytoskeleton, and protein sorting during both exocytosis and endocytosis. In addition

number of cellular functions are dependent on actin filaments, including receptor-mediated endocytosis and various transport processes.

Endoplasmic reticulum

Much of the cellular sorting and distribution system of proteins is through the ER and Golgi complexes. After synthesis and initial processing in the ER, proteins are transported to the Golgi complex where the majority is chemically modified before being sorted into vesicles and targeted to their final destinations. The ER is a collection of membranous tubules, vesicles and flattened sacs that extend throughout the cytoplasm of eukaryotic cells. It is the source of all membranes within the cell and the largest intracellular membrane compartment. ER membranes are continuous and unbroken, and enclose a *lumen* or channel that is separate from the surrounding cytoplasm. The surface membrane of the *RER* is distinguished by the presence of ribosomes facing the surrounding cytoplasm. It is the site of synthesis, folding, assembly and co-translational membrane translocation of proteins. In contrast, the *smooth ER* has no ribosomes and functions in lipid biosynthesis, detoxification and calcium regulation. RER commonly extends into large, flattened sacs called *cisternae*. Smooth ER membranes form primarily tubular sacs that are generally smaller in dimension than RER cisternae. At some points the smooth ER and RER membranes may connect, forming a continuous inner channel enclosed by both systems. In addition to the RER and smooth ER, there are at least four other morphologically distinct domains of the ER, including the nuclear envelope, transitional elements, crystalloid ER and luminal ER bodies containing protein aggregates. Each of these domains is associated with distinct functions **(Table 2.4)**.

Golgi complex

All newly synthesized proteins that are exported out of the ER system are funneled through the Golgi complex before being sorted to different final destinations within the cell. A Golgi complex consists of a localized stack of flattened, sac-like membranes. Ribosomes are characteristically absent from Golgi membranes as well as the spaces between and immediately surrounding the Golgi sacs. An entire Golgi complex often appears to be cup-shaped in cross-section, giving the structure convex and concave faces. The individual sacs of a Golgi complex, called cisternae, as in the ER, are typically dilated or swollen at their margins. Dispersed around the Golgi cisternae are numerous vesicles of varying sizes. Some of these bud from, or fuse with the edges of the cisternae. Golgi complexes are usually closely associated with the RER, separated only by a layer of small, protein-filled vesicles. Some of these vesicles arise as buds from the RER and others join with the face of the nearest Golgi sac. At least some of these structures are considered to be *transition vesicles* transporting proteins from the ER to the Golgi complex. The side of the Golgi complex facing the ER is known as the *cis* or *forming* face. The opposite *trans* or *maturing* face of the Golgi complex typically contains larger vesicle structures. Sacs in the region between the cis and trans faces form the medial segment of the Golgi complex. *Shuttle vesicles* are believed to move proteins and glycoproteins between the Golgi sacs.

ER and Golgi compartments	
Compartment	*Function*
ER	
RER	Protein synthesis and translocation Protein folding and assembly Lipid synthesis
SER	Lipid synthesis Detoxification Ca^{2+} storage and release
Nuclear envelope	Compartmentalization of nuclei Nucleocytoplasmic transport Attachment to lamins
Transitional elements	Membrane export out of the ER
Crystalloid ER	Storage of specific membrane proteins
Luminal ER bodies	Storage of luminal protein aggregates
Golgi	
CGN	Receives material from ER
Golgi stacks	Processing of N-linked and O-linked glycoproteins Phosphorylation of glycoproteins Elongation of GAGs and glycolipids Addition of lipid to secretory lipoproteins
TGN	Terminal glycosylation Tyrosine sulfation Proteolytic cleavages Sorting to lysosomes and plasma membrane Concentration of content

Table 2.4 Endoplasmic reticulum and Golgi compartments. CGN, cis-Golgi network; TGN, trans-Golgi network; RER, rough endoplasmic reticulum; SER, smooth endoplasmic reticulum; GAGs, glycosaminoglycan side chains.

The Golgi complex has three major functions within cells:
- the receipt and sorting of membrane and soluble components arriving from the ER;
- N- and O-linked glycosylation and processing of glycoproteins and glycolipids; and
- sorting of membrane and soluble components that exit the Golgi to different destinations within the cell.

Each of these functions is predominantly associated with specific morphologic domains or subcompartments of the Golgi complex **(Table 2.4)**.

Lysosomes

All of the proteins that pass through the Golgi apparatus, except those that are retained as permanent residents, are sorted in the trans-Golgi network according to their final destination. The sorting establishes a link for some of the proteins to lysosomes, a ubiquitous cytoplasmic organelle interconnected with other subcellular compartments through selective membrane budding and fusion processes. Lysosomes are membrane-bound sacs containing a combination of hydrolytic enzymes (>50) capable of breaking down most biologic substances. In general, the hydrolytic reactions catalyzed by lysosomal enzymes occur at pH 4.5–5, which is a typical environment for primary lysosomes. The boundary membranes of lysosomes contain characteristic proteins, among them a H^+-ATPase active transport pump that continually moves H^+ from the surrounding cytoplasm into the lysosomal interior, thereby maintaining the acidic pH characteristic of these organelles. Newly synthesized lysosomal proteins are transferred into the lumen of the ER, transported through the Golgi apparatus, and then carried from the trans-Golgi network to the lysosomal compartment by vesicular trafficking.

Lysosomal hydrolases contain N-linked oligosaccharides that are covalently modified in the cis-Golgi network so that their mannose residues are phosphorylated. These mannose 6-phosphate (M6P) groups are recognized by the M6P receptor in the trans-Golgi network that segregates the hydrolases and helps to package them into budding transport vesicles, en route to late endosomes as they transform into lysosomes. These transport vesicles act as shuttles that move the M6P receptor to and from the trans-Golgi network and the endosomal compartment. The low pH in the late endosome dissociates lysosomal hydrolases from the M6P receptor, making the transport of the hydrolases unidirectional.

Exocytosis and endocytosis

Exocytosis provides the route by which proteins that are synthesized within the cell are exported to the cell's exterior. Some of the final steps of the pathway are similar to those exhibited by endocytosis, a route of entry for selected materials from outside the cell. However, endocytosis is more than a simple reversal of exocytosis and utilizes receptors and other elements that are not typically associated with exocytosis.

In the exocytotic pathway the secreting proteins take a route from ER to cis-Golgi, to *medial*-Golgi, from medial- to trans-Golgi, and finally from the trans-Golgi network to the cell surface. This transport is mediated by a novel class of coated vesicles. Unlike the coated vesicles that are involved in endocytosis, these transporting vesicles do not contain clathrin. Liver cells can secrete more than one type of protein in a secretory vesicle. For example, two commonly secreted but unrelated proteins, albumin and transferrin, have been found to be packaged in the same secretory vesicles at the Golgi complex and released together to the extracellular medium.

Endocytosis is defined as the process by which cells bind and internalize macromolecules from the environment (**Fig. 2.8**). Cells can take up materials from the surrounding medium through three distinct but closely related pathways: pinocytosis, phagocytosis and receptor-mediated endocytosis (RME). Pinocytosis is a constitutive type of process described as the nonselective uptake of extracellular fluid by small smooth-surfaced invaginations in the plasma membrane. Phagocytosis is the ingestion of particles and, not infrequently, internalization of expansive regions of the cell surface. In contrast, RME is the process by which cells specifically bind and internalize a variety of macromolecules or ligands.

Of the three endocytotic pathways, RME has been studied in greatest detail in liver cells. It proceeds in several steps. After binding to specific receptors that are randomly distributed on the hepatocyte sinusoidal plasma membrane, the ligand–receptor complexes are concentrated in distinctive regions of the membrane called *coated pits*. The major building block of the coat

material is the *triskelion*, a three-legged structure composed of three clathrin molecules. Invagination of the coated pits proceeds rapidly until they pinch free from the plasma membrane and sink into the underlying cytoplasm as a coated vesicle. As the vesicle forms, the membrane quickly loses its clathrin coat and becomes an endosome. At this stage, some ligand–receptor complexes may return to the surface membrane by diacytosis, and participate in additional rounds of endocytosis. The endosomal vesicles may be spheric or extend into elongated and variously branched tubules. As they travel along microtubules deeper into the cytoplasm, vesicles often fuse into larger structures.

During vesicle movement and fusion, the ligands within the interior space are released from their receptors and begin to be sorted into separate compartments. Hydrogen ions pumped into the intravesicular space typically result in ligand–receptor dissociation. A small fraction of internalized ligand is transported directly to the bile canalicular membrane. The majority of ligands remain within the acidified vesicle interior. Although the basis for sorting is presently unknown, it presumably involves an interaction between recognition sites on the endocytotic vesicles. The sorted molecules may proceed to the Golgi complex as smaller vesicles that pinch off from the endocytic vesicle.

Molecules that are sorted into vesicles that travel to the Golgi complex may remain there or may be distributed further to the ER or perinuclear space. They may also be resorted and secondarily routed in vesicles to the plasma membrane or to lysosomes. Fusion of vesicles with lysosomes exposes their contents to degradation by the lysosomal enzymes. Most hepatocyte receptors, devoid of bound ligand, return to the plasma membrane attached to small vesicles, and are reintroduced by membrane fusion. Not all receptors recycle, however; some undergo lysosomal degradation together with their associated ligands.

In most cells coated pits occupy approximately 2% of the surface membrane area. It has been estimated that about 2500 clathrin-coated vesicles invaginate from the plasma membrane of a cultured fibroblast every minute. In the liver, the coated pit regions are particularly abundant along the hepatocyte sinusoidal membrane base of the microvilli (**Fig. 2.9**). It is now well-established that the coat structure of both coated pits and coated vesicles consists of a highly ordered array of specific macromolecules organized into polygonal lattices consisting primarily of a single protein, clathrin. Clathrin subunits associate into triskelions. This remarkable structure consists of three molecules of clathrin heavy chain (180 kDa) and three molecules of clathrin light chain (33–36 kDa). Triskelions assemble in an overlapping network to form the lattice lining a coated pit. The structure and assembly of a coat structure is illustrated in and consists of a geometric array of 12 pentagons and a variable number of hexagons depending on the size of the coat.

Caveolae or plasmalemmal vesicles are a characteristic feature of the plasma membrane of many mammalian cell types and especially fibroblasts, endothelial cells and smooth muscle cells (**Fig. 2.10**). Morphologically, caveolae are 50–60 nm invaginations of the plasma membrane with a characteristic flask shape. Unlike clathrin-coated pits, caveolae exhibit a characteristic spiral coat on the cytoplasmic side of the caveolae, consisting in part of the integral membrane protein caveolin. A number of molecules have now been localized to caveolae including GPI-anchored

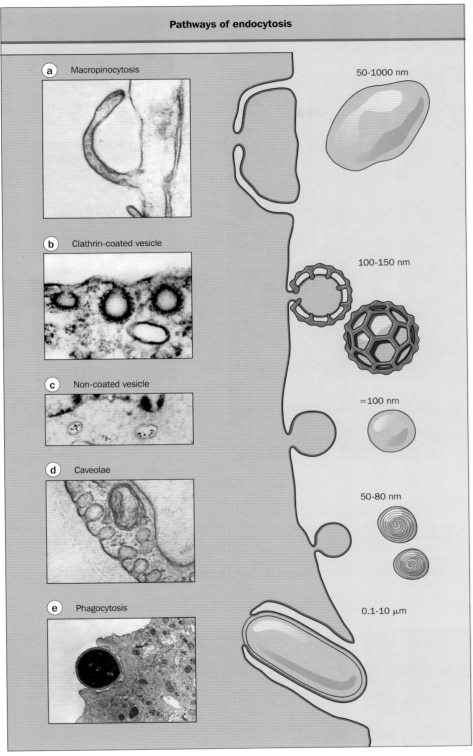

Pathways of endocytosis

a   Macropinocytosis

50-1000 nm

b   Clathrin-coated vesicle

100-150 nm

c   Non-coated vesicle

=100 nm

d   Caveolae

50-80 nm

e   Phagocytosis

0.1-10 μm

Figure 2.8 Pathways of endocytosis. Electron micrographs and diagrams illustrating five structurally and mechanistically distinct pathways for entry into the cell. Receptor-mediated endocytosis has been studied in greatest detail. After ligands bind to the specific receptors, the ligand/receptor complexes are concentrated in coated pits. The pits invaginate and sink into the underlying cytoplasm as endocytotic vesicles. During vesicle movement and fusion, the ligands within the vesicles are sorted and, in many cases, released from their receptors. The sorted molecules may proceed to the Golgi complex or to lysosomes. After release from their ligand, some receptors are recycled to the plasma membrane; others are degraded in the vesicles that fuse with lysosomes. Reproduced from Pollard & Earnshaw (02) by permission of Elsevier.

proteins, the β-adrenergic receptor, as well as tyrosine kinase and substrates. Caveolae exhibit a number of different functions including potocytosis, signal transduction, calcium regulation, and non-clathrin-dependent endocytosis and transcytosis.

Mitochondria

Mitochondria are respiratory organelles that constitute about 20% of the cytoplasmic volume of hepatocytes. Their primary function is to conserve the energy from the oxidation of substrates by oxygen as the high-energy phosphate anhydride bonds of ATP. They contain the enzymes of the tricarboxylic acid cycle, fatty acid oxidation and oxidative phosphorylation. Other functions include parts of the urea cycle, gluconeogenesis, fatty acid synthesis, and regulation of intracellular calcium concentrations. Normal human hepatocytes contain numerous mitochondria throughout the cytoplasm (**Fig. 2.11**). All mitochondria

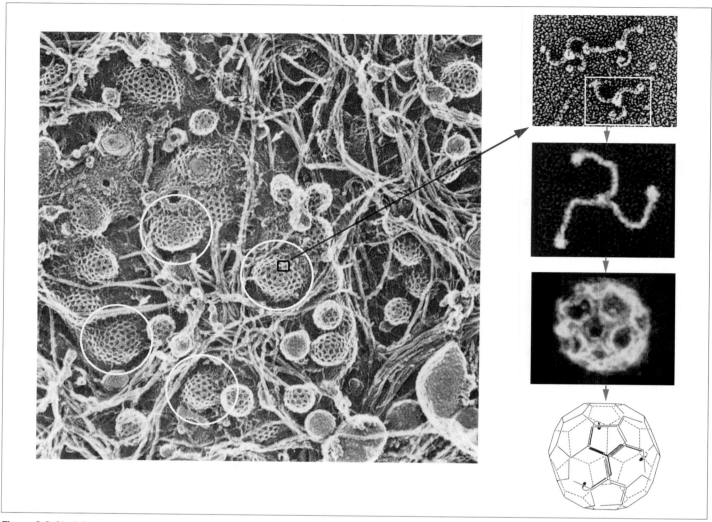

Figure 2.9 Clathrin-coated cell membrane. (Left) Schematic view of a coated membrane region from within the cell. Clathrin basketworks (encircled) form coated membranes, pits and vesicles. Smooth-surfaced membranes and intermediate filaments are particularly numerous. (Right) Electron micrographs of clathrin triskelions (× 230 000), a clathrin shell reformed from triskelions and a schematic representation of the clathrin coat lattice. Each structure is composed of 12 pentagons and a variable number of hexagoris forming an outer cage of clathrin, an inner layer of clathrin terminal domains and an innermost shell consisting of an array of proteins that interact directly with receptors in the coated regions. Reproduced from Steer in Zakim & Boyer (96) by permission of Elsevier.

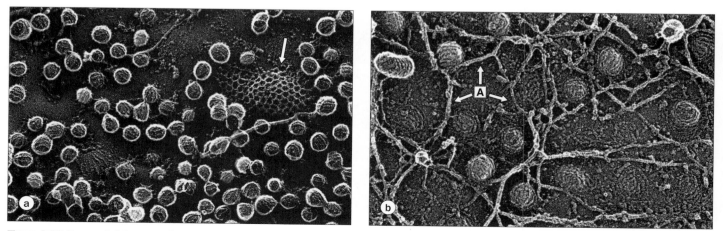

Figure 2.10 Freeze-etch images of caveolae. They are smaller and are usually more round than clathrin-coated pits [(a), arrow]. Caveolae are coated with ridges of material on their surface that resemble fingerprints. Typically, they occur in clusters and often in actin filament (A)-rich regions of the cell (b). × 130 000 for (a); × 177 000 for (b). Reproduced from Steer in Zakim & Boyer (96) by permission of Elsevier.

Extracellular matrix proteins in normal liver					
Collagen type	Associated anchorage protein	Associated proteoglycans	Cell-surface receptor	Source	Localization
I	Fibronectin	Chondroitin sulfate	Integrin	Fibroblasts	Vascular space, Glisson capsule, space of Disse
III	Fibronectin	Heparan sulfate Heparin	Integrin	Hepatocytes, fibroblasts	Vascular space, Glisson capsule, space of Disse
IV	Laminin	Heparan sulfate	Laminin	Epithelial cells, hepatocytes	Vascular, lymphatic, canalicular structure, and sinusoids
V	Fibronectin	Heparan sulfate Heparin	Integrin	Fibroblasts	Periportal tissue, basal lamina of bile ducts
VI	Fibronectin	Heparan sulfate	Integrin	Fibroblasts	Periportal spaces, space of Disse

Table 2.5 Extracellular matrix proteins in normal liver.

modulin and perlecan. The extracellular matrices are highly structured. The distribution and organization of the extracellular matrix of the liver is unique and during development is produced along the migration path of the hepatocytes. The absence of a continuous basement membrane between the hepatocytes and liver endothelial cells is another unique feature of the liver.

SIGNAL TRANSDUCTION

Each cell of the human body is programmed during development to respond to a specific set of signals that act in various combinations to regulate its behavior as well as its life span and rate of replication. Most of these signals are paracrine, in which local mediators are rapidly taken up, destroyed or immobilized, so that they act only on neighboring cells. Centralized control is, in general, exerted by endocrine signaling, in which secreted hormones are carried in the blood to target cells throughout the body. In synaptic signaling, neurotransmitters are secreted by nerve cells which act locally on the postsynaptic cells in contact with their axons.

The liver plays a critical role in the adaptive response to systemic changes such as inflammation and alteration of energy requirements. Hepatocytes are particularly sensitive to signals generated in these environments. Some small hydrophobic signaling molecules, including the steroid and thyroid hormones and the retinoids, diffuse across the plasma membrane of hepatic cells and activate intracellular receptor proteins, which directly regulate the transcription of specific genes. Some dissolved gases such as nitric oxide act as local mediators by diffusing across the plasma membrane of the target cell and activating an intracellular enzyme, usually guanylyl cyclase, which produces cyclic guanosine monophosphate (GMP) in the target cell. But most extracellular signaling molecules are hydrophilic and are able to activate receptor proteins only on the surface of the target cell (**Table 2.6**). These receptors act as signal transducers, converting the extracellular binding event into intracellular signals that alter the behavior of the target cell. Plasma membrane receptors exhibit a variety of topologies and, of course, are res-

Cell surface receptors in normal liver		
Ligand	Binding sites/cell	Cell type
ASGP	150–250,000	Hepatocyte
LDL	20–50,000	Hepatocyte
Transferrin	31,000	Hepatocyte
Insulin	16,000	Hepatocyte
EGF	300,000	Hepatocyte
M6P (CI)	19,000	Hepatocyte
IgA Fucose	200,000	Hepatocyte Kupffer cell Endothelial cell
GlcNAc (Avian)	33,000	Hepatocyte
Mannose	50–150,000	Kupffer cell Endothelial cell

Table 2.6 Cell surface receptors in normal liver. CI, cation-independent; ASGP, asialoglycoprotein; LDL, low-density lipoprotein; EGF, epidermal growth factor; GlcNAc, N-acetylglucosamine; M6P, mannose 6-phosphate.

ponsive to many different ligands (**Fig. 2.15**). In general, there are three main families of cell-surface receptors, each of which transduces extracellular signals in a different way. Ion-channel-linked receptors open or close briefly in response to their respective stimuli. G-protein-linked receptors indirectly activate or inactivate plasma-membrane-bound enzymes or ion channels via trimeric GTP-binding proteins (G-proteins). Enzyme-linked receptors act either directly as or indirectly through enzymes that are usually protein kinases. In general, kinases regulate the phosphorylation state of specific proteins in the target cell. Through cascades of highly regulated protein phosphorylations, elaborate sets of interacting proteins relay most signals from the

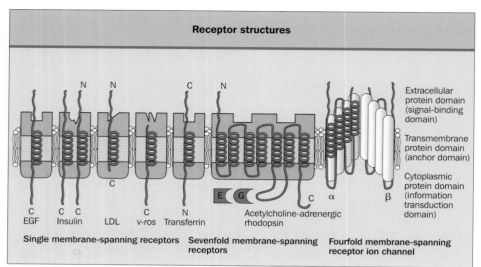

Figure 2.15 Topology of different receptor structures in the membrane. E, effector protein; G, G protein; C, C-terminus; N, N-terminus; EGF, epidermal growth factor; v-ros, viral ros receptor; LDL, low-density lipoproteins. Reproduced from Hesch (91) by permission of Springer and author.

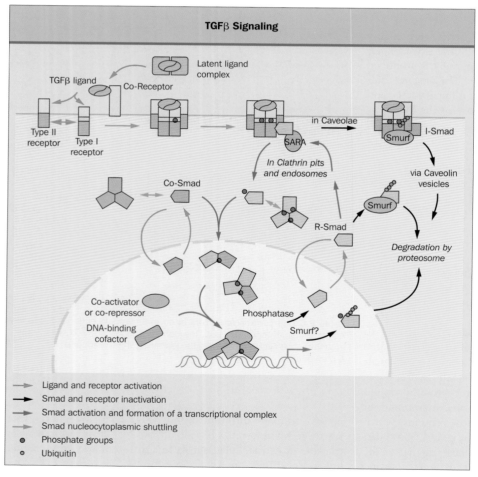

Figure 2.16 Schematic diagram of TGF-β signaling from cell membrane to the nucleus. The arrows indicate signal flow and are color coded: orange for ligand and receptor activation, gray for Smad and receptor inactivation, green for Smad activation and formation of a transcriptional complex, and blue for Smad nucleocytoplasmic shuttling. Phosphate groups and ubiquitin are represented by green and red circles, respectively. Accessory receptors, such as homo-oligomeric TGF-β receptor (TBR) III, may present TGF-β to homo-oligomeric TBR II, which is a constitutively active serine/threonine kinase. The TGF-β–TBR-II complex recruits TBR-I into the complex, after which TBR-I is phosphorylated by TBR-II and activated. In such a state, TBR-I propagates signals to downstream components. Reproduced from Shi (03).

cell surface to the nucleus, thereby altering the cell's pattern of gene expression and, as a consequence, its behavior.

Transforming growth factor (TGF)-β signaling is one of the better understood examples in this class of signal transduction pathways (**Fig. 2.16**). The isoforms of TGF-β exist as homodimers that are excreted from hepatocytes and liver nonparenchymal cells as latent molecules (pro-TGF-βs). The pro-TGF-β undergoes plasmin-mediated activation when bound to the mannose 6-phosphate receptor. There are three types of TGF-β receptor. Type I and II receptors form heterodimers that transmit the TGF-β signal into the hepatocyte. The type III receptor does not appear to transduce an intracellular signal, but serves as a

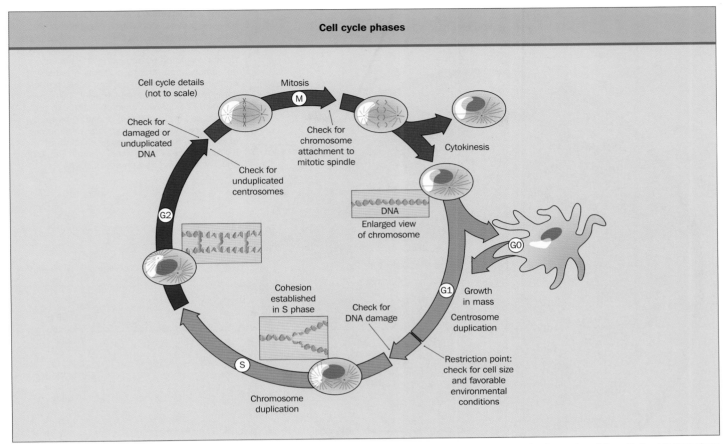

Cell cycle phases

Figure 2.17 Cell cycle phases. Diagram of cellular morphology and chromosome structure across the cell cycle. Reproduced from Pollard & Earnshaw (02) by permission of Elsevier.

repository for TGF-β on the plasma membrane. The type II receptor binds ligand with high affinity, resulting in the recruitment of a type I receptor to form a receptor-ligand complex. Upon dimerization, the type II receptor phosphorylates the type I receptor in a cluster of glycine and serine residues near the membrane, known as the GS domain. Phosphorylation of the GS domain stimulates intracellular responses to the bound ligand. Thus, the GS region serves as an important regulatory domain in receptor activation for TGF-β signaling.

Regulation of the cell cycle

Cells reproduce by duplicating their contents and then dividing. This *cell division cycle* is the fundamental means by which all living things are propagated. Within the liver, the normal state of hepatocytes is a quiescent or non-proliferative one, but they exhibit a tremendous capacity to replicate. For example, after loss of hepatic tissue, hepatocytes, which may have been quiescent for years, dramatically enter into the cell cycle and proliferate until the liver mass is completely restored. Then, just as acutely, they become quiescent again. A typical cell division cycle in somatic cells consists of four major phases (**Fig. 2.17**). The *G1 phase* is the interval between the completion of mitosis and the beginning of DNA synthesis; *S phase* (synthesis phase) is the period of replication of the nuclear DNA; the *G2 phase* is the interval between the end of DNA synthesis and the beginning

of mitosis; and finally, the *M phase* is the period of mitosis in which nuclear division takes place.

In mitosis, the nuclear envelope breaks down, the contents of the nucleus condense into visible chromosomes, and the cell's microtubules reorganize to form the *mitotic spindle* that will eventually separate the chromosomes. As mitosis proceeds, the cell seems to pause briefly in a state called *metaphase*, in which the chromosomes, already duplicated, are aligned on the mitotic spindle, poised for segregation. The separation of the duplicated chromosomes marks the beginning of *anaphase*, during which the chromosomes move to the poles of the spindle, where they decondense and reform intact nuclei. The cell is then pinched in two by a process called *cytokinesis*, which marks the end of M phase. In most cells the M phase takes only about an hour, which represents only a small fraction of the total cell cycle division time. The much longer period that elapses between one M phase and the next is known as *interphase*, and represents the time required to grow before the next division. Cells which have not yet committed themselves to DNA replication can pause in their progress. They enter a specialized resting state, called *G0*, where they can remain for days, weeks, or years before resuming proliferation.

There are four checkpoints that control transitions between cell cycle stages. They modulate progression of cells through the cycle in response to external or internal signals. The restriction

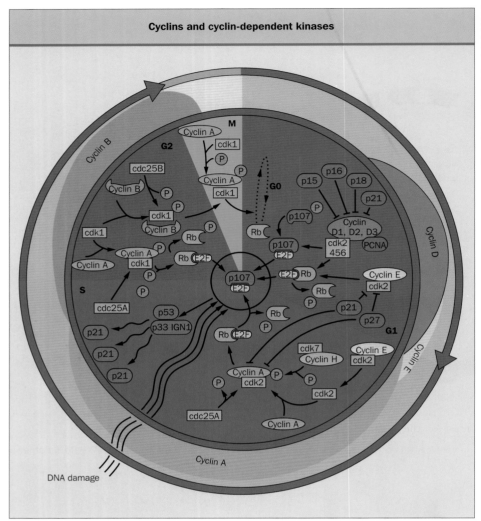

Cyclins and cyclin-dependent kinases

Figure 2.18 Cyclins and cyclin-dependent kinases (cdks). Modulation of cyclins A, B1, D and E provides a mechanism to regulate cdk activity throughout the cell cycle. Cdk activity is further regulated by activating or inhibitory phosphorylation, and by a variety of small proteins, which bind to cyclins, cdks, or their complexes and inhibit cdk activity. The active cyclin-cdk complexes drive cells through the various cell cycle phases, or checkpoints, by phosphorylation of the retinoblastoma family of proteins. Reproduced by permission of BD-Biosciences-PharMingen. Applied Reagents and Technologies (brochure, p.2).]

point is at late G1 and sensitive to the size and physiologic state of the cell and to its interactions with the surrounding extracellular matrix. Cells that do not receive appropriate growth stimuli from their environment arrest at this point and may commit suicide by apoptosis. The restriction point is also called a molecular 'gate' to cell cycle progression that regulates the expression of genes required for cell cycle progression. The gate is based upon the retinoblastoma protein (pRb) and E2F, a family of essential transcription factors, regulated by phosphorylation or dephosphorylation. Two DNA damage checkpoints monitor the integrity of DNA in late G1 or G2 phase. The cells with damaged or partially replicated DNA arrest their progression through the cycle. The damage can either be repaired or undergo programmed cell death (apoptosis). The metaphase checkpoint exists in mitosis and delays the onset of chromosome segregation until all chromosomes have attached properly to the mitotic spindle.

The sequence of the cell cycle events is governed by a control system that delicately balances the expression and activity of a set of interacting proteins. These include the cyclins, cyclin-dependent kinases, the tumor-suppressor protein retinoblastoma and p53, transcription factor E2F and p21. These proteins can induce and coordinate the essential downstream processes that duplicate and divide the cell's contents. The cell cycle control system is primarily based on the regulation of certain protein kinases. Cyclins and cyclin-dependent kinases (cdks) are essential for cell-cycle regulation in eukaryotes (**Fig. 2.18**). The cyclins (regulatory subunits) bind to cdks (catalytic subunits) to form active cyclin–cdk complexes in different cell cycle phase. Cdk subunits by themselves are inactive and binding to a cyclin is required for their activity. A number have been identified in eukaryotic cells and participate in diverse processes ranging from transcriptional regulation, cell differentiation and cell cycle regulation. Up to date, more than 16 different cyclins have been identified in humans. Cdk activity is further regulated by a number of modulating pathways, and at least four different mechanisms regulate Cdk activity.

When hepatocytes are stimulated to replicate, an early response is the transcription and translation of G1 cyclins. These G1 cyclins bind to appropriate kinases to form the activated cyclin–cdk complexes that subsequently phosphorylate a set of specific downstream targets. The potential downstream targets of the G1 specific cyclin–cdk complexes include p53, retinoblastoma and p107 (a retinoblastoma-family protein). Retinoblastoma is a nuclear tumor-suppressor phosphoprotein that is hypophosphorylated throughout most of G1 and becomes prog-

pit cells are short-lived and continuously replaced by cells originating from extrahepatic sources. They were originally called large granular lymphocytes. In human liver they are present at very low numbers in contrast to rat liver. The human pit cells have pronounced polarity, abundant cytoplasm containing dense granules, a conspicuous cytocenter, and locomotory shape with hyaloplasmic pseudopods and a uropod. The number of typical granules is significantly smaller than in the rat hepatocyte,

however, and rod-cored vesicles are extremely rare. Another characteristic for human pit cells is the 'parallel tubular arrays', in which the tubular structures frequently associate with dense granules. They are thought to function in the liver:

- against cancer because of their strong cytotoxic activity against various tumor cell lines in vitro;
- in antiviral activity similar to that of natural killer cells; and
- in control of growth and differentiation of liver cells.

FURTHER READING

Intracellular organelles

Altan-Bonnet N, Sougrat R, Lippincott-Schwartz J. Molecular basis for Golgi maintenance and biogenesis. Curr Opin Cell Biol 2004; 16:364–372.

Conner SD, Schmid SL. Regulated portals of entry into the cell. Nature 2003; 422:37–44.

Hinshaw JE, Carragher BO, Milligan RA. Architecture and design of the nuclear pore complex. Cell 1992; 69:1133–1141.

Kim JS, He L, Qian T, et al. Role of the mitochondrial permeability transition in apoptotic and necrotic death after ischemia/reperfusion injury to hepatocytes. Curr Mol Med 2003; 3:527–535.

Morré DJ. Cell-free analysis of Golgi apparatus membrane traffic in rat liver. Histochem Cell Biol 1998; 109:487–504.

Newmeyer DD, Ferguson-Miller S. Mitochondria: releasing power for life and unleashing the machineries of death. Cell 2003; 112:481–490. *An interesting view on the potential role of the mitochondrion in cell death and survival. The functions of these remarkable organelles reveal a versatility and complexity that were previously unsuspected. They are many, and they are powerful.*

Reddy JK. Peroxisome proliferators and peroxisome proliferator-activated receptor α. Biotic and xenobiotic sensing. Am J Pathol 2004; 164:2305–2321.

Sherlock S, Dooley J. Diseases of the liver and biliary system. 10th edn. London: Blackwell; 1997:10–11.

Steer CJ. Receptor-mediated endocytosis: mechanisms, biologic function, and molecular properties. In: Zakim D, Boyer TD, eds. Hepatology: a textbook of liver disease. 3rd edn. Philadelphia: Saunders; 1996: 149–214.

Svitkina TM, Verhovsky AB, Borisy GG. Plectin sidearms mediate interaction of intermediate filaments with microtubules and other components of the microskeleton. J Cell Biol 1996; 135:991–1007.

Treem WR, Sokol RJ. Disorders of the mitochondria. Semin Liver Dis 1998; 18:237–253.

Wolfe SL. Molecular and cell biology. Belmont: Brooks/Cole; 1993.

Transport and cholestasis

Graf J, Haussinger D. Ion transport in hepatocytes: mechanisms and correlations to cell volume, hormone actions and metabolism. J Hepatol 1996; 24(suppl 1):53–77.

Li MK, Crawford JM. The pathology of cholestasis. Semin Liver Dis 2004; 24:21–42. *A scholarly review of what can go wrong in the hepatic formation of bile.*

Nakielny S, Dreyfuss G. Transport of proteins and RNAs in and out of the nucleus. Cell 1999; 99:677–690.

Ohno M, Fornerod M, Mattaj IW. Nucleocytoplasmic transport: the last 200 nanometers. Cell 1998; 92:327–336.

Pauli-Magnus C, Meier PJ. Pharmacogenetics of hepatocellular transporters. Pharmacogenetics 2003; 13:189–198.

Zegers MMP, Hoekstra D. Mechanisms and functional features of polarized membrane traffic in epithelial and hepatic cells. Biochem J 1998; 336:257–269.

Liver injury and regeneration

Fausto N. Liver regeneration and repair: hepatocytes, progenitor cells, and stem cells. Hepatology 2004; 39:1477–1487. *An excellent review of the many factors and cell types that may be responsible for repair and regeneration of the liver. It is not quite as simple as we once thought.*

Friedman SL. Molecular regulation of hepatic fibrosis; an integrated cellular response to tissue injury. J Biol Chem 2000; 275:2247–2250.

Mitaka T, Mizuguchi T, Sato F, et al. Growth and maturation of small hepatocytes. J Gastroentol Hepatol 1998; 13:S70–77.

Murray AW. Recycling the cell cycle: cyclins revisited. Cell 2004; 116:221–234.

Taub R, Greenbaum LE, Peng Y. Transcriptional regulatory signals define cytokine-dependent and -independent pathways in liver regeneration. Semin Liver Dis 1999; 19:117–127.

Wisse E, Luo D, Vermijlen D, et al. On the function of pit cells, the liver-specific natural killer cells. Semin Liver Dis 1997; 17:265–286. *They probably originate in bone marrow as lymphoid cells, and migrate to the liver where they act as natural killer cells against a growing list of intruders.*

Yin XM, Ding WX. Death receptor activation-induced hepatocyte apoptosis and liver injury. Curr Mol Med 2003; 3:491–508. *This article comprehensively reviews the mechanisms of induction and regulation of death receptor-initiated apoptosis in hepatocytes and how these molecular events affect our understanding of the pathogenesis of diseases.*

Zaret KS. Regulatory phases of early liver development: paradigms of organogenesis. Nat Rev Genet 2002; 3:499–512.

Liver fibrogenesis

Hui AY, Friedman SL. Molecular basis of hepatic fibrosis. Expert Rev Mol Med 2003; 1–23.

Sato M, Suzuki S, Senoo H. Hepatic stellate cells: unique characteristics in cell biology and phenotype. Cell Struct Funct 2003; 28:105–112.

Shi Y, Massagué J. Mechanisms of TGF-β signaling from cell membrane to the nucleus. Cell 2003; 113:685–700.

Membrane organization and function

Braet F, Wisse E. Structural and functional aspects of liver sinusoidal endothelial cell fenestrae: a review. Comp Hepatol 2002; 1:1.

Bretschner MS The molecules of the cell membrane. Sci Am 1985; 253:100–108.

Hesch RD. Classification of cell receptors. Curr Topics Pathol 1991; 83:13–51.

Holthuis JC, Pomorski T, Raggers RJ, et al. The organizing potential of sphingolipids in intracellular membrane transport. Physiol Rev 2001; 81:1689–1723.

Hynes RO. Integrins: bidirectional, allosteric signaling machines. Cell 2002; 110:673–687.

Munro S. Lipid rafts: elusive or illusive? Cell 2003; 115:377–388.

Pollard TD, Earnshaw WC. Cell biology. Philadelphia: Saunders. 2002.

Simons K, Toomre D. Lipid rafts and signal transduction. Nat Rev Mol Cell Biol 2000; 1:31–39.

Staehelin LA, Hull BE. Junctions between living cells. Sci Am 1978; 238:140–153.

Trembley JH, Kren BT, Steer CJ. Cyclins and gap junctions. In: Strain A, Diehl AM, eds. Liver growth and repair. London: Chapman & Hall; 1998:311–365.

CHAPTER

3

Functions of the Liver

Bruce A. Luxon

OVERVIEW

The liver is a unique organ anatomically located to serve its dual role as a metabolic and biochemical transformation factory. The liver receives blood containing substances absorbed or secreted by the gastrointestinal organs including the pancreas, intestine, stomach and spleen. The liver uses these substances as raw materials and modifies them or synthesizes completely new chemicals. These are then returned to the bloodstream or to bile for excretion.

On a cellular level, the liver allows maximal interaction between the blood and liver cells. In its unique design, liver cells are organized into cell plates, each plate being formed by one-cell-thick cords, which are surrounded by blood vessels (sinusoids). The perfusion of these sinusoids is unidirectional, proceeding from the portal tract to the hepatic venule. The specialized capillaries found in the sinusoids have large fenestrations, which allow free exchange between plasma and the extracellular space. Because blood flow proceeds sequentially down the length of the sinusoid, hepatocytes located in different positions along these cell plates contain differing amounts of enzymes and thus have distinct functional capabilities. As blood traverses the liver from its entry point at the portal inlet to its

exit at the hepatic vein, the composition of sinusoidal blood is modified by removal and addition of compounds.

In this chapter, we describe the basic elements of the organization of the liver and emphasize how these elements determine its unique physiology. The structure of the liver lobule is then first described and emphasis is placed on the concept of the liver cell plate. The remaining sections deal with the functional organization of the cell plate, with emphasis on the uptake of compounds from plasma into hepatocytes, their metabolism, excretion into bile and biotransformation.

MORPHOLOGIC CONSIDERATIONS

Hepatocytes are arranged in single-cell thick plates extending from the portal tract to the terminal hepatic venule (**Fig. 3.1**). Adjacent plates of hepatocytes are separated by the hepatic sinusoids, lined by endothelial cells with several characteristic ultrastructural features. Slender processes extending from the cell body contain pores (fenestrae), which are arranged in sieve plates. The fenestrae are dynamic structures under the regulation of an actin cytoskeleton. Unlike other endothelia, sinusoidal endothelial cells lack an underlying basement membrane, allowing direct exchange between plasma and the

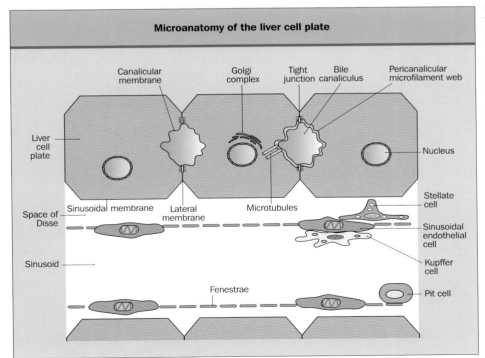

Microanatomy of the liver cell plate

Canalicular membrane · Golgi complex · Tight junction · Bile canaliculus · Pericanalicular microfilament web

Liver cell plate

Nucleus

Sinusoidal membrane · Lateral membrane · Microtubules

Stellate cell

Space of Disse

Sinusoidal endothelial cell

Sinusoid

Kupffer cell

Fenestrae

Pit cell

Figure 3.1 Microanatomy of the liver cell plate. The relationship of the four non-parenchymal cells to the hepatocytes is shown on the right. Kupffer cells and pit cells lie within the sinusoidal lumen. Endothelial cells separate the sinusoidal lumen from the space of Disse. Stellate cells (lipocytes) lie within the space of Disse. Intracellular organelles and features that play a role in bile secretion are shown within the hepatocytes.

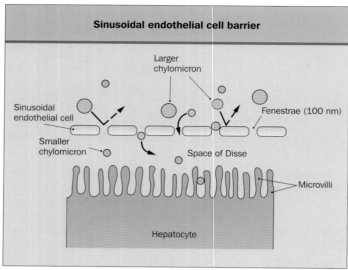

Figure 3.2 Sinusoidal endothelial cell barrier. Sinusoidal endothelial cells provide an important barrier to larger molecules such as chylomicrons. Fenestrae have a diameter of approximately 100 nm and exclude large chylomicrons. Smaller molecules permeate into the space of Disse and reach the microvilli of hepatocytes. Modified from Roll et al in Kaplowitz (96) by permission of Lippincott, Williams & Wilkins.

perisinusoidal space of Disse. This feature facilitates the transfer of protein-bound solutes, such as drugs, bilirubin and bile acids, from sinusoidal blood to the hepatocyte and promotes the excretion of, for example, lipoproteins and other proteins from the hepatocyte to the sinusoid (**Fig. 3.2**). In cirrhosis, a continuous basement membrane accumulates between hepatocytes and endothelial cells, obliterating the fenestrae and impairing solute transfer in both directions. Defenestration also occurs early in liver cancer and in chronic alcohol abuse, contributing to the hyperlipoproteinemia associated with alcoholism.

Hepatocyte membranes

Neighboring hepatocytes are joined by junctional complexes that serve to demarcate the canalicular space from the basolateral, or sinusoidal, domain. Differences in the structure and function of the sinusoidal and canalicular membrane define the hepatocyte as a polarized cell. A lipid composition of a higher cholesterol–phospholipid and a lower phospholipid–sphingomyelin molar ratio in the canalicular than in the sinusoidal domain confers a relative resistance to the detergent actions of bile acids on the canalicular membrane. Morphologically similar to other transporting epithelia, the surface area of the sinusoidal and canalicular membranes is increased by microvilli. Major alterations in canalicular microvilli occur in intrahepatic and extrahepatic forms of cholestasis, including a reduction in the number of microvilli and the development of giant microvilli secondary to edema and bleb formation, which occlude the canalicular lumen to some degree. These findings suggest that canalicular microvilli, like their morphologic counterparts in the enterocyte, play a role in solute transport.

The sinusoidal membrane is primarily involved in the bidirectional exchange of solutes and has uptake mechanisms for amino acids, glucose and organic anions such as bile acids, fatty

acids and bilirubin; receptor-mediated endocytotic processes; Na^+,K^+-ATPase and glucagon-stimulatable adenylate cyclase activity; and export processes for albumin, lipoproteins and clotting factors. The predominant function at the canalicular membrane surface is secretion, although limited reabsorptive capacity has been demonstrated. Certain membrane enzymes are selectively localized to the canalicular domain, including alkaline phosphatase, leucine aminopeptidase and glutamyltranspeptidase.

From adjacent canaliculi, bile enters small terminal bile ductules, the canals of Hering, which consist of fusiform cells in close association with neighboring hepatocytes. These short channels traverse the limiting plate to form successively larger ductules and intralobular bile ducts, composed of cuboidal epithelial cells. Interlobular bile ducts, ranging in size from 30 to 40 mm, convey bile to the extrahepatic bile duct, the gallbladder and the duodenum. Cholangiocytes along the intrahepatic biliary tree are morphologically and functionally heterogeneous; regulated transport of water and electrolytes primarily occurs in the medium and large interlobular bile ducts.

Hepatocyte membrane junctions

The junctional complexes that join adjacent hepatocytes consist of several discrete structures. The tight junctions (i.e. zonulae occludens) function as a barrier to unrestricted movement of solutes from the space of Disse to the canalicular lumen. The tight junction, seen with freeze-fracture electron microscopy, is a network of anastomosing intramembrane strands or fibrils in the outwardly facing cytoplasmic leaflet (**Fig. 3.3**a). This barrier for entry into bile acts as if it is associated with a net negative charge, since the paracellular movement of negatively charged solutes from blood to bile is impaired. Likewise, negatively charged species, such as conjugated bile acids, secreted across the canalicular membrane may be retained in the canalicular lumen by this selective permeability barrier. Tight junction permeability, altered in intrahepatic and extrahepatic cholestasis, is determined by at least three tight junction-specific proteins. Rows of the transmembrane protein, occludin, act as the intercellular seal. Occludin is linked on its cytoplasmic surface zonula occludens to ZO1 and ZO2 (Fig. 3.3b). Adjacent to the tight junction is the adherens junction or zonula adherens (Fig. 3.3b). The adhesion molecules, the cadherins, form zipper-like connections between hepatocytes. The cytoplasmic domains of cadherins interact with catenins, which are cytoplasmic proteins linked to the actin cytoskeleton.

Located distal to the tight junction is the nexus or gap junction. One of the proposed functions for gap junctions is mediation of intercellular communication under physiologic conditions. Individual gap junction proteins, termed connexins, form hexameric channels that allow the exchange of ions and small molecules, such as calcium, cyclic AMP and inositol trisphosphate, between adjacent hepatocytes.

Spot desmosomes, or macula adherens, are also found in the junctional complex, where they are also involved in cell–cell adhesion. Composed of desmogleins, these structures serve a bridging function, maintaining contact between hepatocytes during pathologic situations that interfere with the function of gap junctions. Actin-containing microfilaments are numerous in the pericanalicular cytoplasm, where they insert into the canalicular microvilli and into the junctional complex to form a pericanalicular web. Coordinated and periodic contractions of

bile pigments (**Table 3.1**). The volume of hepatic bile excreted is between 500 and 600 mL/day. The relative proportions of the major organic solutes of bile are illustrated in **Figure 3.8**. Bile acids are the major organic solutes in bile and are derived from two sources. Primary bile acids (i.e. cholic and chenodeoxycholic acid in humans) are synthesized from cholesterol in the liver. Microsomal 7-α-hydroxylase is the rate-limiting enzyme in bile acid synthesis. The secondary bile acids (i.e. deoxycholic, lithocholic and ursodeoxycholic acid in humans) are produced from primary bile acids by bacterial enzymes in the intestine (Fig. 3.9). Bile acids consist of two components that determine their physiologic and physicochemical properties: a steroid nucleus with its hydroxyl substituents and an aliphatic side chain.

The terminal carboxylic acid group of the side chain is modified after the synthesis of the primary bile acids and during the hepatic phase of the enterohepatic cycling of the secondary bile acids by enzymatic conjugation to taurine or glycine. Conjugation decreases the ability of bile acids to traverse cell membranes by passive diffusion. Glycine and taurine conjugates of bile acids also demonstrate selective resistance to hydrolysis by pancreatic enzymes during small intestinal transit. The net

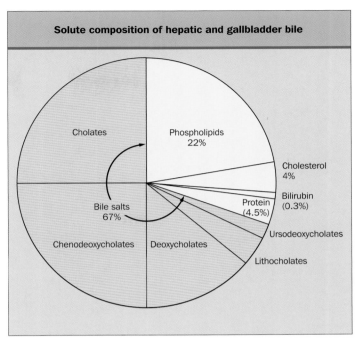

Figure 3.8 Typical solute composition in percentage by weight of hepatic and gallbladder bile in healthy humans.

Composition of hepatic bile	
Component	Concentration (mmol/L)
Electrolytes	
Na+	141–165
K+	2.7–6.7
Cl–	77–117
HCO3–	12–55
Ca2+	2.5–6.4
Mg2+	1.5–3.0
Organic anions	
Bile acids	3–45
Bilirubin	1–2
Lipids	
Lecithin	140–810 (mg/dL)
Cholesterol	97–320 (mg/dL)
Proteins	2–20 (mg/mL)
	0.02–0.2 (g/L)
Peptides and amino acids	
Glutathione	3–5
Glutamate	0.8–2.5
Aspartate	0.4–1.1
Glycine	0.6–2.6
Modified from Boyer in Andreoli et al (86) by permission of the author and Springer Science and Business Media.	

Table 3.1 Composition of hepatic bile.

effect of conjugation is to permit bile acids to accumulate at an intraluminal concentration in the small intestine high enough to facilitate fat digestion and absorption.

The presence of hydrophilic (i.e. hydroxyl substituents and the amide linkage on the aliphatic side chain) and lipid-soluble or hydrophobic (i.e. the steroid nucleus) regions allows conjugated bile salts to act as amphiphilic molecules that form micelles or polymolecular aggregates above a critical micellar concentration. Bile salt micelles can solubilize other biologically important amphiphilic solutes, such as cholesterol and phospholipids, to form mixed micelles. This detergent-like property of bile acids is important in stabilizing the physical state of bile and in promoting fat digestion and absorption.

The dihydroxy bile acid ursodeoxycholic acid (UDCA) is used in the treatment of chronic cholestatic disorders, such as primary biliary cirrhosis. Under normal conditions, UDCA represents less than 3% of the bile acid pool; it is more hydrophilic than the other major dihydroxy bile acids, chenodeoxycholic acid and deoxycholic acid. The mechanism of action of UDCA is not clear, but it stimulates the biliary secretion and inhibits the intestinal reabsorption of endogenous bile acids, becoming the predominant bile acid in serum and in bile after long-term administration. It may, therefore, protect against bile duct and hepatocyte injury from hydrophobic bile acids, such as chenodeoxycholic acid, deoxycholic acid and lithocholic acid, and other potential hepatotoxins.

As shown in Table 3.1, the predominant biliary cation is Na+ and the concentrations of inorganic electrolytes in bile are similar to their plasma concentrations. The inorganic electrolytes are largely responsible for the osmotic activity of bile. This is because the osmotic activity of most of the organic solutes, such as bile acids, is lost by aggregation into mixed micelles.

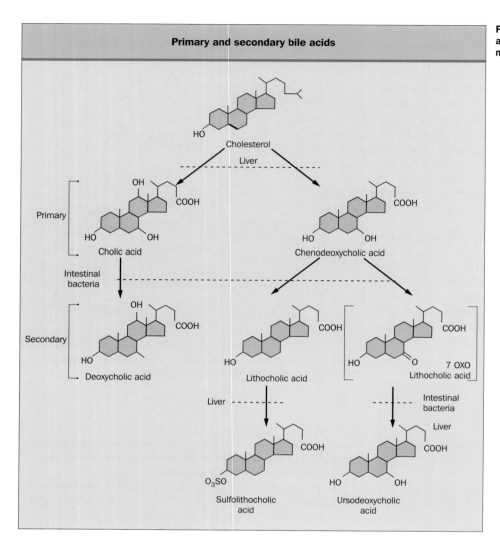

Figure 3.9 Major primary and secondary bile acids and their sites of synthesis and metabolism.

In contrast to the passive, hydrostatic forces that govern glomerular filtration by the kidney, bile formation by hepatocytes is an osmotic process that involves the active secretion of osmotically active inorganic and organic solutes into the canalicular lumen, followed by passive water movement. In this important respect, hepatic bile secretion can be characterized by the same processes found in more conventional secretory epithelia.

Canalicular bile formation is classically measured using metabolically inert solutes, such as erythritol and mannitol, which are assumed to enter bile passively only at the level of the canaliculus and not to undergo modification by biliary ductular cells. Using these markers, canalicular bile formation has been traditionally divided into two components (**Fig. 3.10**): bile acid-dependent bile flow (BADBF), which is defined as the slope of the line relating canalicular bile flow to bile salt excretion; and bile acid-independent bile flow (BAIBF), which is attributed to the active secretion of inorganic electrolytes and other solutes and defined as the extrapolated y-intercept of this line.

Bile acid transport

The sinusoidal uptake of conjugated bile acids, such as taurocholate, is primarily mediated by a secondary active transport process, which is driven by the inwardly directed Na^+

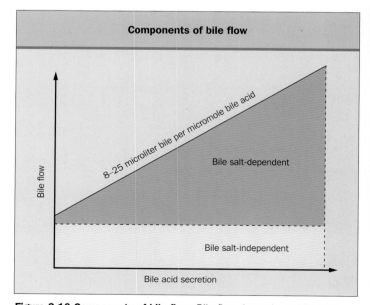

Figure 3.10 Components of bile flow. Bile flow depends on bile acid secretion as well as bile acid independent components. Slope of line indicates that 8–25 μL of bile are produced for each μmol of bile salt transported into bile. Adapted from Zakim (03) by permission of Elsevier.

gradient maintained by Na⁺,K⁺-ATPase activity. The negative electrical potential difference (PD) across the membrane maintained by Na⁺,K⁺-ATPase activity is also an important driving force, because Na⁺-taurocholate cotransport is electrogenic (i.e. associated with the net entry of positive charge). This bile salt transporter has been cloned from both rat and human liver and termed the Na⁺-taurocholate cotransporting polypeptide, ntcp and NTCP, respectively. Expression and function of ntcp is downregulated in several models of experimental cholestasis, including a model of sepsis-associated cholestasis. Findings in patients with extrahepatic biliary atresia suggest similar regulation of NTCP.

The uptake of unconjugated bile acids at the sinusoidal membrane, in contrast, is a Na⁺-independent process mediated, in part, by the organic anion transporting polypeptide, oatp1. The Na⁺-independent uptake of bile salts exhibits a broad substrate specificity that includes electroneutral steroids, such as ouabain and progesterone; cyclic oligopeptides, such as phalloidin, somatostatin analogs and cyclosporin; and a wide variety of xenobiotics. Hepatic uptake of amatoxins, the toxic product in toadstools of the genus *Amanita* and the cause of most accidental mushroom poisonings, is also mediated by this multispecific organic anion transport process.

The mechanism for intracellular transport of bile acids from the sinusoidal to the canalicular pole of hepatocytes is not as well understood. Intracellular binding of bile acids has been proposed as a mechanism for hepatic transport and a protective mechanism against potential toxic effects of free bile acids. Two unrelated families of cytosolic proteins with high affinities for bile acids have been identified: ligandins and Y9 proteins. The Y9 bile acid

binders belong to the monomeric reductase gene family that also binds derivatives of polycyclic aromatic hydrocarbon carcinogens. These cytosolic proteins may be involved in the intracellular transport of bile acids and carcinogens to the canalicular membrane or to intracellular organelles by diffusion.

Canalicular excretion represents the rate-limiting step in the hepatic transport of bile acids. Canalicular secretion of anionic bile acids was believed to occur by passive facilitated diffusion down an energetically favorable electrochemical gradient. However, the magnitude of the membrane potential is too small to account for the bile salt concentration gradient that exists across the canalicular membrane, and alternative mechanisms have been identified for carrier-mediated bile acid secretion at this membrane domain. A member of the P-glycoprotein family encoded by the *spgp* gene is an ATP-dependent canalicular bile acid transporter. A defect in this canalicular bile acid transporter is responsible for a form of progressive familial intrahepatic cholestasis, PFIC type 2. The vectorial movement of bile acids from sinusoidal blood to canalicular bile is schematically depicted in Figure. 3.11.

Electrolyte transport

In contrast to the information regarding BADBF, less is known about the hepatocellular mechanisms that underlie BAIBF. Inhibition of Na⁺,K⁺-ATPase activity does not appear to have a significant effect on BAIBF and indirect evidence points to a primary role for bicarbonate (HCO₃⁻) transport. In other epithelia, such as the pancreas, HCO₃⁻ transport has been attributed to Na⁺–H⁺ exchange (i.e. antiport) activity. With the identification and characterization of sinusoidal Na⁺–H⁺

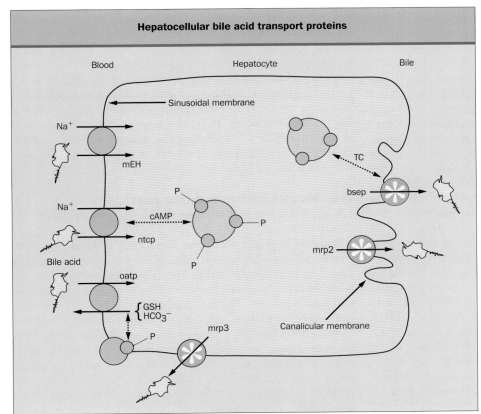

Figure 3.11 Major known hepatocellular bile acid transport proteins. Solid arrows indicate transport of the indicated substrate. Dashed arrows denote regulatory pathways of vesicular transport and phosphorylation. * indicates ATP-dependent transport. bsep, bile salt export pump; GSH, glutathione; mEH, microsomal epoxide hydrolase; mrp2/mrp3, multidrug resistance-associated protein 2/3; ntcp, Na⁺-taurocholate cotransporting polypeptide; oatp, organic anion transporting protein; TC, taurocholate; P, phosphorylated transporter. Adapted from Wolkoff et al (03) by permission of Elsevier.

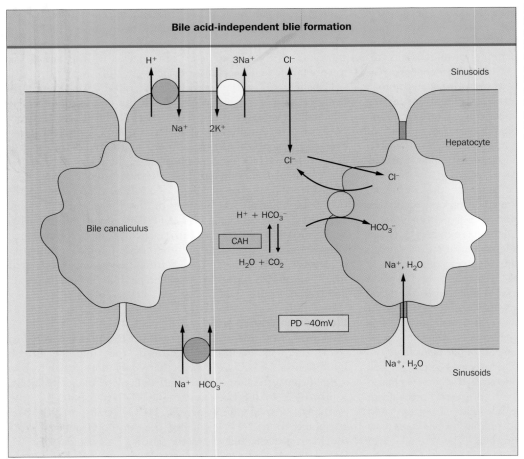

Bile acid-independent blie formation

PD −40mV

Figure 3.12 Bile acid-independent bile formation. Sinusoidal Na⁺–H⁺ exchange and canalicular Cl–HCO₃⁻ exchange are functionally coupled by means of cytosolic carbonic anhydrase (CAH) to generate net biliary bicarbonate secretion. A sinusoidal Na⁺–HCO₃⁻ symport in conjunction with canalicular Cl–HCO₃⁻ exchange may also play a role in biliary HCO₃⁻ secretion. Adapted from Moseley et al (86) by permission of The American Physiological Society.

exchange and canalicular Cl–HCO_3^- exchange, a model was proposed (Fig. 3.12) in which these two transport processes are functionally coupled by way of cytosolic carbonic anhydrase to generate net biliary bicarbonate secretion. A sinusoidal Na^+–HCO_3^- symport in conjunction with canalicular Cl–HCO_3^- exchange may also play a role in biliary bicarbonate secretion. Support for this model comes primarily from studies examining the effects of certain cholestatic and choleretic agents on membrane transport. Ethinyl estradiol, which causes a diminution in BAIBF, inhibits Na^+–H^+ exchange activity; UDCA, which results in a HCO_3^--rich choleresis, stimulates Na^+–H^+ exchange activity. Amiloride and acetazolamide, inhibitors of Na^+–H^+ exchange and carbonic anhydrase activity, respectively, produce a concentration-dependent inhibition of UDCA-stimulated bile flow and biliary HCO_3^- output.

Inorganic electrolytes may not provide a sufficient driving force for BAIBF, however, because their biliary secretion depends primarily on passive diffusion and solvent drag. This has led to the alternative suggestion that non-bile salt organic anions may provide a major driving force for canalicular BAIBF. The tripeptide glutathione (γ-L-glutamyl-L-cysteinylglycine; GSH) may fulfil this role. It is present in bile in high concentrations (see Table 3.1) and, as a result of intrabiliary catabolism of GSH by γ-glutamyltranspeptidase located on the luminal membranes of bile ductule cells and the bile canalicular membrane, the concentration of this solute in the canalicular lumen may be substantially higher than that measured in excreted bile. At concentrations that exceed free (i.e. non-micelle associated) bile acids and bile pigments, GSH may generate a potent osmotic driving force for canalicular bile formation. Because biliary secretion of GSH is a carrier-mediated process, the requirement that the solute providing the driving force for BAIBF is not governed by passive diffusion or solvent drag is met. Additional indirect evidence supports a role for GSH in BAIBF, including the strong correlation of GSH excretion with drug-induced changes in BAIBF and with ontogenic changes in bile formation. However, other unidentified solutes, in addition to GSH, may also contribute to BAIBF.

Bilirubin metabolism and transport

For a full discussion of bilirubin metabolism and transport, see Chapter 6.

Bilirubin is generated by the breakdown of heme. Approximately 80% of bilirubin is derived from heme released by senescent erythrocytes, while the remainder comes from the heme moieties of other hemoproteins, such as myoglobin and tissue cytochromes. The microsomal enzyme, heme oxygenase, converts heme to biliverdin, which is then converted to bilirubin by biliverdin reductase. The unconjugated bilirubin produced by these enzymatic reactions is transported in the plasma tightly bound to albumin. Competition for albumin binding by certain drugs displaces unconjugated bilirubin and, in the neonate, may result in the diffusion of bilirubin across the blood–brain barrier and bilirubin encephalopathy, or kernicterus.

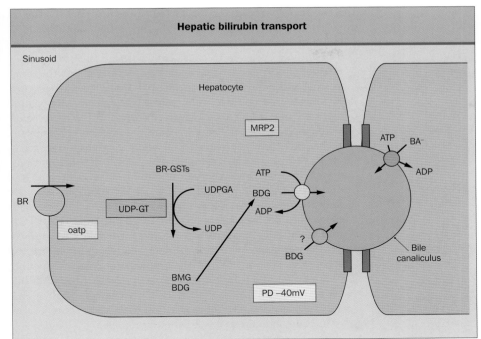

Hepatic bilirubin transport

Figure 3.13 Hepatic bilirubin transport.
Unconjugated bilirubin (BR), disassociated from albumin, is taken up at the sinusoidal membrane by a Na^+-independent process and mediated by organic anion transporting polypeptide (oatp). Within the hepatocyte, bilirubin and other organic anions bind to cytosolic glutathione S-transferases or ligandins. Conjugation of bilirubin to its monoglucuronides and diglucuronides (BMG and BDG), catalyzed by bilirubin-UDP-glucuronosyl-transferase (UDP-GT), is required for canalicular secretion. Canalicular secretion involves a homolog of the multidrug resistance protein, MRP2.

Bilirubin uptake and secretion is mediated by transport processes distinct from those identified for bile acid transport (**Fig. 3.13**). Sinusoidal uptake of bilirubin and other non-bile acid organic anions is a Na^+-independent process mediated, in large part, by oatp1. Glutathione efflux from the hepatocyte appears to provide the driving force for uptake via oatp1. Within the hepatocyte, bilirubin and other organic anions bind to cytosolic glutathione S-transferases or ligandins. Conjugation of bilirubin to its monoglucuronides and diglucuronides, catalyzed by bilirubin-UDP-glucuronosyl-transferase (UDP-GT), is required for canalicular secretion. Canalicular secretion, in turn, involves a homolog of the multidrug resistance protein, MRP2. A point mutation in MRP2 is the molecular basis for the Dubin-Johnson syndrome, an autosomal-recessive disorder characterized by a conjugated hyperbilirubinemia. Sepsis-associated cholestatic jaundice may be, in part, the result of down regulation of this rate-limiting step in overall hepatic bilirubin transport.

Impaired hepatic uptake at the sinusoidal membrane occurs in Gilbert syndrome and following the administration of certain drugs, such as rifampin (rifampicin). Reduced activity of UDP-GT leads to impaired bilirubin conjugation and is observed in the neonate and in patients with Gilbert and Crigler-Najjar type I and II syndromes. Activity of UDP-GT can be induced by phenobarbital, effectively reducing the jaundice in Crigler-Najjar type II syndrome.

Hepatic bilirubin uptake and conjugating activity are preserved in most forms of liver disease. Accordingly, conjugated hyperbilirubinemias can occur in a wide spectrum of hepatic diseases, including disorders associated with acute and chronic hepatocellular and cholestatic injury and with extrahepatic biliary obstruction.

Ductular events
Experimental approaches, such as the isolation of intact segments from small interlobular bile ducts, the site of injury in the vanishing bile duct syndromes, have led to a better understanding of the biology and pathology of the biliary epithelium; the biliary tract is no longer considered merely a conduit for bile. The mechanism for the HCO_3^- rich fluid secretion by bile duct epithelial cells has been examined at both a cellular and molecular level. As shown in **Figure 3.14**, the binding of the hormone secretin, and possibly of other agonists, to receptors localized to the basolateral domain of the bile duct epithelial cell leads to an increased intracellular level of the second messenger cAMP. Chloride exits from the apical membrane through cAMP-responsive cystic fibrosis transmembrane conductance regulator (CFTR)-associated Cl^- channels. The resulting cell depolarization facilitates the uptake of HCO_3^- at the basolateral membrane, mediated by a Na^+–HCO_3^- symport (or a Na^+–Cl^-–HCO_3^- cotransporter). Intracellular HCO_3^-, increased by either this mechanism or by enhanced carbonic anhydrase activity, then enters the bile duct lumen by means of apical Cl^-–HCO_3^- exchange. A clinical correlation of the secretory activity of the biliary epithelium can be found in the increased response to secretin and increased bile flow observed in patients with chronic liver diseases associated with ductular proliferation.

Gallbladder function
The physiologic functions of the gallbladder include concentration and storage of bile during interdigestive periods, evacuation by smooth muscle contraction in response to cholecystokinin, moderation of hydrostatic pressure within the biliary tract, bile acidification, and absorption of organic components of bile. Although not essential for bile secretion, the gallbladder concentrates bile as much as 10-fold. This process is largely the result of electroneutral Na^+-coupled Cl^- transport and passive water movement (**Fig. 3.15**). The exact mechanism is unclear; experimental evidence supports either coupled NaCl entry or a Na^+–H^+ and Cl^-–HCO_3^- exchange operating in parallel. The net result of this concentrative process

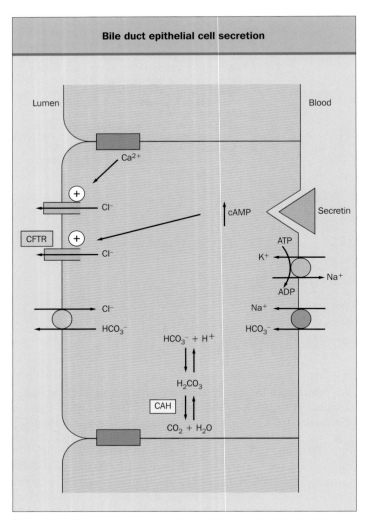

Bile duct epithelial cell secretion

Figure 3.14 Bile duct epithelial cell secretion. See text for details. CFTR, cystic fibrosis transmembrane conductance regulator; CAH, carbonic anhydrase; cAMP, adenosine 39,59-cyclic monophosphate.

enterohepatic circulation (**Fig. 3.16**). Intestinal conservation of bile acids is approximately 90% efficient, reflecting the additive effects of both passive and active reabsorptive processes. The bile acid pool cycles 5–15 times daily through this pathway.

Passive absorption of bile acids occurs throughout the small intestine and depends on intestinal pH and bile acid structure. The most hydrophobic bile acids (i.e. glycine-conjugated dihydroxy bile acids) are passively absorbed in the more acidic environment of the duodenum, where the fraction in protonated (uncharged) form is greatest. Bile acids are transported across the ileal brush border membrane by a Na^+-dependent transporter, referred to as the apical sodium-dependent bile acid transporter (ASBT). Trihydroxy (i.e. cholic acid) bile acids are favored over dihydroxy (i.e. chenodeoxycholic acid) bile acids and conjugated over unconjugated species. Similar to NTCP, ASBT is not fully operative at birth and the inability to conserve bile salts may contribute to the diminished bile salt pool size and 'physiologic steatorrhea' of the immediate postnatal period. Mutations in ABST have been associated with idiopathic bile acid diarrhea, a chronic diarrheal illness characterized by bile acid malabsorption, lack of association with other forms of ileal dysfunction, and a response to cholestyramine.

Intracellular transport of bile acids in enterocytes is mediated by several cytosolic and microsomal proteins. The best characterized of these proteins is the ileal lipid-binding protein, a member of the fatty acid-binding protein family. At the basolateral membrane of the ileum, bile acids leave the enterocyte by a Na^+-independent anion exchange process, recently attributed to a member of the organic anion transporting polypeptide family, oatp3.

The small fraction of bile acids that escapes active or passive absorption in the small intestine undergoes bacterial modification in the colon. The secondary bile acids formed are also reabsorbed to various degrees, depending on their physicochemical properties, their interaction with luminal constituents, and the permeability characteristics of the colon. Lithocholate and deoxycholate, formed from the 7-dehydroxylation of chenodeoxycholate and cholate, respectively, are the major fecal bile acids in humans.

Bile acid synthesis

Continuous bile acid synthesis from cholesterol is required to maintain the bile acid pool in the enterohepatic circulation. The maximal rate of synthesis is on the order of 4–6 g/day. The importance of bile acid synthesis in health is evident if the effects of a cessation in synthesis are considered. Fecal loss would not be repleted, cholesterol would not be excreted, bile acid-dependent bile formation would stop, and fat-soluble substances would not be absorbed.

CENTRAL METABOLIC MECHANISMS

Apart from its unique role in biliary metabolism, the liver is central to the metabolism of lipids, carbohydrates and proteins, as well as being closely involved in drug metabolism. Some of these metabolic pathways are summarized in **Figure 3.17**.

Cholesterol and lipoprotein metabolism

The liver plays a pivotal role in normal cholesterol and lipoprotein metabolism. Cholesterol homeostasis is maintained

is the formation of gallbladder bile, isotonic to plasma and composed of higher concentrations of Na^+, bile salts, K^+ and Ca^{2+} and lower concentrations of Cl^- and HCO_3^- than hepatic bile.

Despite the considerable concentration gradient for bile salts and bile pigments, the absorption of highly ionized organic solutes such as taurocholate, sulfobromophthalein and iodipamide is minimal. In acute cholecystitis, increased permeability to water and to highly ionized solutes has been demonstrated and enhanced absorption of iodipamide may account for the non-visualization of the gallbladder that occurs in this setting.

Mucus is released by the exocytosis of secretory granules in the apical portion of gallbladder epithelial cells. Gallbladder mucin synthesis and release are markedly accelerated in animal models of cholesterol cholelithiasis before crystal and stone formation. Formation of an insoluble mucin–bilirubin complex may provide a nidus for cholesterol monohydrate nucleation.

Enterohepatic circulation

It is best to consider bile acid secretion as a cyclic flow of molecules anatomically limited to the hepatocyte, biliary tree, small intestine, enterocyte and portal blood, known as the

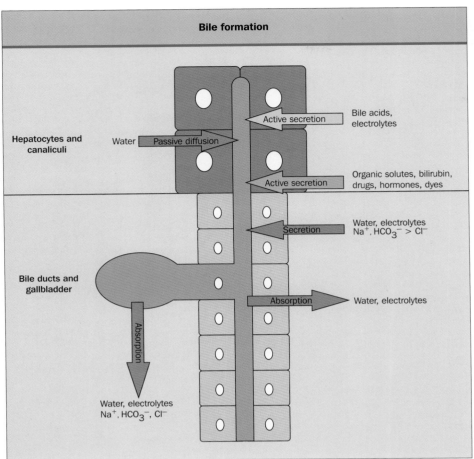

Bile formation

Hepatocytes and canaliculi

Water — Passive diffusion →

Active secretion ← Bile acids, electrolytes

Active secretion ← Organic solutes, bilirubin, drugs, hormones, dyes

Bile ducts and gallbladder

Secretion ← Water, electrolytes Na^+, HCO_3^- > Cl^-

Absorption → Water, electrolytes

Absorption

Water, electrolytes Na^+, HCO_3^-, Cl^-

Figure 3.15 Bile formation. Bile formation involves the active transport of electrolytes, bile acids and organic solutes such as bilirubin. Water follows passively into the canaliculi (top). Bile is modified in the bile ducts and gallbladder by secretion and subsequent absorption of electrolytes and water. Modified from Scharschmidt in Zamkin et al (90) by permission of Elsevier.

by pathways that either increase or decrease hepatic cholesterol. Pathways that increase hepatic cholesterol include uptake from lipoproteins [chylomicrons and low-density lipoprotein (LDL)] and de novo synthesis of cholesterol, regulated by the enzyme, 3-hydroxy-3-methylglutaryl (HMG)-coenzyme A (CoA) reductase. Cholesterol present in the liver exists either as cholesterol esters, a storage form, or free cholesterol. Concentrations of these two forms of cholesterol are governed by acyl-CoA:cholesterol acyltransferase which esterifies free cholesterol, and cholesterol ester hydrolase which hydrolyzes cholesterol esters. The two major pathways that decrease hepatic cholesterol are synthesis of bile acids from free cholesterol and biliary excretion of free cholesterol.

The pathways responsible for cholesterol homeostasis are tightly regulated. Cholesterol inhibits HMG-CoA reductase and bile acids decrease bile acid biosynthesis from cholesterol by inhibition of cholesterol 7α-hydroxylase.

The major lipoprotein secreted by the liver is very-low-density lipoprotein (VLDL). The amounts of free fatty acids taken up by the liver and diet are the principal regulatory factors in the rate of production, composition and rate of secretion of VLDL.

Biliary bile acids promote endogenous lipid secretion and stabilize the physicochemical state of bile. Biliary output of non-esterified cholesterol and phosphatidylcholine (PC) (i.e. lecithin), the two major lipids in bile, is curvilinearly related to bile acid output. Lecithin secretion exceeds cholesterol secretion.

Bile salts appear to promote biliary secretion of phospholipids following their secretion into bile by preferential partitioning into microdomains of the outer leaflet of the canalicular membrane that are also enriched with biliary-type PCs. These bile salts in the canalicular lumen induce vesiculation of the canalicular membrane. The inner or cytoplasmic leaflet of the canalicular membrane is resupplied with biliary-type PCs derived from smooth ER membranes by PC transfer protein and sterol carrier protein 2. Translocation of phospholipid from the inner to the outer leaflet of the canalicular membrane bilayer is mediated by the product of the *mdr2* gene, the mouse homolog of human *MDR3*.

The pathway for phospholipid secretion proposed in **Figure 3.18** appears to be specific for PCs; although the mechanism is unclear, a largely separate secretory pathway exists for cholesterol secretion. However, the initiating event in the pathogenesis of cholesterol cholelithiasis may involve disruption of the coupling of biliary cholesterol excretion to simultaneous secretion of phospholipid and bile acids.

Drug metabolism

The liver plays a major role in drug metabolism or biotransformation. Products of hepatic biotransformation destined for urinary elimination are transported back into sinusoidal blood. Organic lipophilic drugs undergo biliary excretion, because these substances are poorly filtered at the glomerulus and minimally secreted by the renal tubule. Hepatic uptake of

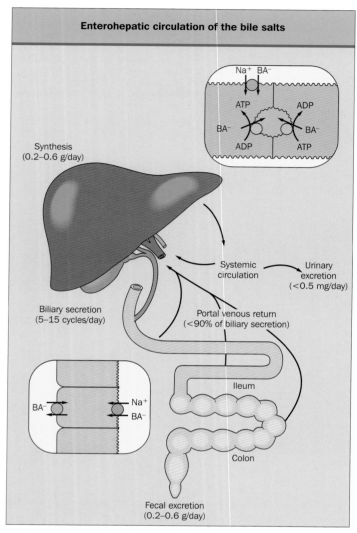

Enterohepatic circulation of the bile salts

Synthesis
(0.2–0.6 g/day)

Systemic
circulation

Urinary
excretion
(<0.5 mg/day)

Biliary secretion
(5–15 cycles/day)

Portal venous return
(<90% of biliary secretion)

Ileum

Colon

Fecal excretion
(0.2–0.6 g/day)

Figure 3.16 Enterohepatic circulation of bile salts and typical kinetic values for healthy humans. Insets depict bile acid transport at the level of the hepatocyte and the enterocyte. BA, bile acid.

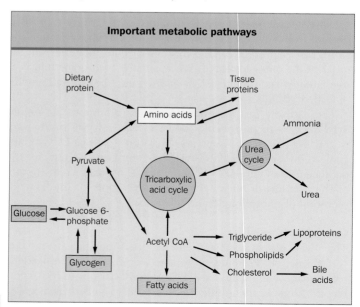

Important metabolic pathways

Dietary
protein

Tissue
proteins

Amino acids

Ammonia

Pyruvate

Urea
cycle

Tricarboxylic
acid cycle

Urea

Glucose

Glucose 6-
phosphate

Acetyl CoA

Triglyceride

Lipoproteins

Phospholipids

Glycogen

Cholesterol

Bile
acids

Fatty acids

Figure 3.17 Important metabolic pathways of proteins, carbohydrates and lipids in the liver.

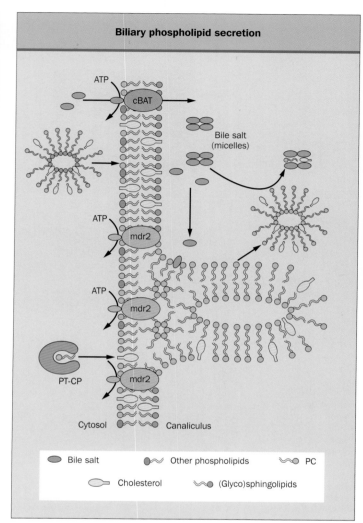

Biliary phospholipid secretion

ATP

cBAT

Bile salt
(micelles)

ATP

mdr2

ATP

mdr2

PT-CP

mdr2

Cytosol

Canaliculus

Bile salt   Other phospholipids   PC

Cholesterol   (Glyco)sphingolipids

Figure 3.18 Biliary phospholipid secretion. Phosphatidylcholine (PC) is delivered to the cytoplasmic leaflet of the canalicular membrane by phosphatidylcholine transfer protein (PC-TP). PC is then translocated to the outer leaflet by mdr2, resulting in relative phospholipid excess in microdomains of the canalicular membrane. In the presence of bile salts, secreted into the lumen by the canalicular bile acid transporter (cBAT), SPGP, these microdomains are destabilized and vesicular structures develop that pinch off to yield biliary lipid vesicles.

many drugs is mediated by the same transport processes that are involved in hepatic bile formation discussed above. In addition, the hepatic uptake of organic cations, a class of substances that accounts for about 70% of drugs used in clinical practice, is mediated by a membrane potential-dependent carrier on the sinusoidal membrane, termed OCT1 (**Fig. 3.19**). Once the liver takes up drugs, they are processed or metabolized by several families of enzymes located in the endoplasmic reticulum, the cytosol, and, to a lesser extent, other organelles. The P450 cytochromes are a family of hemoproteins situated predominantly in the endoplasmic reticulum of the hepatocyte in a membrane-bound form. Drug metabolism by the P450 system, although typically detoxifying, occasionally produces toxic intermediates such as electrophiles and free radicals that, if not further metabolized, can lead to covalent binding to cellular proteins and membrane lipid peroxidation, respectively. Conjugation

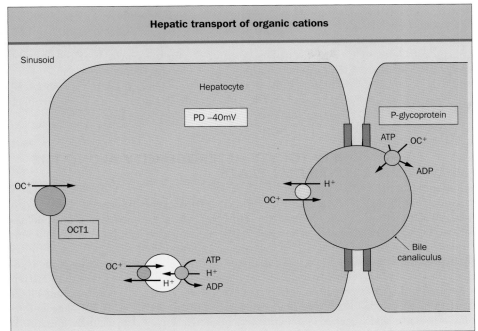

Hepatic transport of organic cations

Sinusoid

Hepatocyte

PD −40mV

P-glycoprotein

ATP OC⁺

ADP

H⁺

OC⁺

OC⁺

OCT1

Bile canaliculus

OC⁺ ATP H⁺ ADP

Figure 3.19 Hepatic transport of organic cations. The uptake of organic cations (OC⁺) is mediated by a membrane potential-dependent carrier on the sinusoidal membrane, termed OCT1. Organic cations may then be sequestered into acidified intracellular organelles by an H⁺-ATPase-dependent organic cation–H⁺ exchanger. In addition to P-glycoprotein-mediated organic cation efflux, biliary secretion of small-molecular-weight organic cationic drugs may be mediated by an organic cation–H⁺ exchanger.

with glutathione is mediated by cytosolic enzymes, the glutathione S-transferases, and plays an important role in the detoxification of electrophiles produced by the P450 system. However, glucuronidation and sulfation are more frequently employed in hepatic biotransformation and are mediated by microsomal UDP-glururonyl transferases and cytosolic sulfotransferases, respectively.

Hepatic biotransformation can thus be classified into two phases. Phase I reactions involve oxidation or reduction of the parent compound, often generating a carboxyl, hydroxyl, or epoxide group that can subsequently be conjugated in a phase II reaction with, for example, glucuronic acid, glutathione, sulfate, or acetate. However, many drugs do not undergo sequential phase I and II reactions. The effect of phase I reactions is increased polarity, or water solubility, and, therefore, enhanced excretory potential. Phase II reactions further increase the water solubility of a compound. Although the products of phase II reactions tend to be less toxic and less active than the parent compound, phase I reactions may produce toxic intermediates. Exposure to specific substrates of a hepatic drug-metabolizing enzyme may induce the activity of that enzyme. Such induction may be clinically relevant if the enzyme induced produces a toxic intermediate. One of the best examples of such a phenomenon is acetaminophen (paracetamol) hepatotoxicity. Although metabolized largely by sulfation and glucuronidation (phase II reactions), a small percentage of the drug is oxidized by cytochrome P450 to a reactive metabolite. Chronic alcohol exposure induces this form of cytochrome P450, providing an explanation for the enhanced susceptibility of chronic alcoholics to acetaminophen hepatotoxicity.

A specific example of a biliary excretory mechanism for drugs is the multidrug transport protein, known as P-glycoprotein or 9170, encoded by the *MDR1* gene. Originally described in tumor-derived tissue culture systems resistant to cytotoxic hydrophobic agents, such as vinblastine, vincristine and daunomycin, this ATP-dependent drug efflux system is located on the canalicular membrane and the apical surface of biliary epithelial cells lining small biliary ductules. This selective localization suggests that this membrane transport protein may serve as a pathway for the detoxification of physiologic metabolites and chemotherapeutic agents. In addition to P-glycoprotein-mediated drug efflux, biliary secretion of small-molecular-weight organic cationic drugs may be mediated by an organic cation–H⁺ exchanger, a process that shares similarities with renal drug transport (see Fig. 3.19).

Carbohydrate metabolism

Carbohydrate metabolism by the liver appears to be compartmentalized. In the fed state, the liver is involved in glycogen synthesis from glucose and glycolysis, metabolic processes that are preferentially located in perivenular hepatocytes. In the postabsorptive or fasted state, there is a shift from glucose uptake to glucose production mediated by glycogenolysis and gluconeogenesis predominantly in periportal hepatocytes.

Glucose is not the only ingested carbohydrate that is metabolized by the liver. Fructose is metabolized by the liver via a unique pathway and the metabolism of galactose depends on a conversion to glucose that occurs almost exclusively in the liver. Portosystemic shunting in cirrhosis results in impaired galactose elimination capacity, a finding that may have prognostic importance.

Fatty acid metabolism

Fatty acids continuously cycle between the liver and adipose tissue. During the fed state, hepatocytes synthesize fatty acids that are then incorporated into lipoproteins to be delivered to adipocytes. During fasting, fatty acids derived from triglycerides stored in adipocytes are delivered to the liver where they undergo oxidation to ketone bodies in mitochondria and, in the case of very long chain fatty acids, in peroxisomes. In cirrhosis, fatty acids are preferentially used as an energy source, even in the non-fasted state. Mitochondrial oxidation of fatty acids depends on the availability of the amino acid carnitine. Carnitine deficiency may play a role in valproate-induced hepatotoxicity and defects in mitochondrial fatty acid oxidation underlie disorders such as acute fatty liver of pregnancy, Reye syndrome and Jamaica vomiting sickness.

Ammonia metabolism

Urea synthesis in the liver, through the Krebs–Henseleit cycle, is required for the disposal of the toxic product of nitrogen metabolism, ammonia. Glutamine synthesis plays a minor role in overall ammonia metabolism. Removal of ammonia from the circulation is compartmentalized in the liver. Carbamoylphosphate synthetase, the key regulatory enzyme in urea synthesis from ammonia, is expressed in all but the last one or two hepatocytes surrounding the terminal hepatic venule. The last one or two perivenous hepatocytes, in contrast, express glutamine synthetase and avidly scavenge any remaining ammonia from the circulation to form glutamine, which is subsequently released into the terminal hepatic venule and the systemic circulation. Elevated serum ammonia levels are often observed in both acute and chronic forms of liver disease. The striking elevations seen in fulminant hepatic failure are the result of impaired conversion of ammonia to urea in the setting of severe hepatocellular necrosis, whereas the hyperammonemia present in patients with cirrhosis and portal hypertension reflects loss of glutamine synthetic capacity by the perivenous scavenger cells in the liver as well as portosystemic shunting of ammonia derived from colonic bacteria. Additional factors that influence the level of serum ammonia in patients with cirrhosis include intestinal production of ammonia by bacterial deamination of blood or dietary protein, renal production of ammonia by glutaminase in response to metabolic alkalosis or hypokalemia, intestinal production of ammonia from urea by urease-forming bacteria in the setting of diminished renal function, and hepatic production of ammonia from amino acids in response to increased glucagon secretion.

Protein synthesis

Albumin is the single most abundant serum protein and the liver synthesizes and exports up to 12 g of albumin/day. Besides serving as a vehicle for the transport of many drugs, serum albumin is a critical factor in the maintenance of plasma oncotic pressure. Albumin synthesis is regulated by changes in nutritional status, osmotic pressure, systemic inflammation and corticosteroids.

The liver also plays an important role in normal blood coagulation. Normal serum activities of the vitamin K-dependent coagulation-factor proenzymes (factors II, VII, IX and X), as assessed by the one-stage prothrombin time, depend on intact hepatic synthesis and adequate intestinal absorption of lipid-soluble vitamin K. Vitamin K is required for the post-translational formation of γ-carboxyglutamyl residues that are essential for physiologic activation of the factors. Prolonged prothrombin times can be observed in both hepatocellular disorders that impair hepatic synthetic function, such as hepatitis and cirrhosis, and in cholestatic syndromes that interfere with lipid absorption. Hepatocellular injury can be differentiated from cholestatic causes of prothrombin time prolongation by the

parenteral administration of vitamin K; intact hepatic function is established by an improvement in prothrombin time greater than 30% within 24 h of administration.

The liver is also a major site for the synthesis of antithrombin III, protein C and protein S. Despite reductions in these plasma inhibitors of hemostasis in chronic liver disease, thrombosis is a rare complication, presumably because of a disproportionate deficiency in procoagulants in most patients.

HEPATOCYTE HETEROGENEITY ALONG THE LIVER CELL PLATE

Along the liver cell plate, hepatocytes in general appear histologically uniform. However, when examined on a morphologic or histochemical basis, hepatocytes exhibit marked heterogeneity. This heterogeneity (also called zonation) is manifested by cells located in the periportal zone that differ from those downstream in the perivenous zone. Hepatocytes demonstrate zonation with respect to key enzymes, cell receptors, subcellular structures and cell matrix interaction (**Fig. 3.20**). The heterogeneity is expressed by activation of the cellular genome in response to various inputs, including concentration gradients in hormones, oxygen, metabolic substrates and neural input.

In the 1960s and 1970s, it became clear that there was a zonal organization for specific groups of enzymes and the concept of 'metabolic zonation' became popular. In the original model of metabolic zonation, only two zones of equal size were defined. Later, as the concept of zonation became more prevalent, the periportal and perivenous compartments were subdivided into a proximal and distal part creating four zones.

Zonation of specific metabolic pathways

Numerous experimental approaches using perfused livers, isolated hepatocytes and hepatocyte cultures have been used to study differences in the metabolic specialization of hepatocytes. There are clear zonal differences in the metabolism of carbohydrates, amino acids and ammonia, and fatty acids. Bile formation as well as the metabolism of xenobiotics demonstrate zonation. In the following sections, there is a brief overview of the current understanding of the zonation of each of these pathways (**Table 3.2**).

Carbohydrate metabolism

Zonation of carbohydrate metabolism is divided into two phases: absorptive and postabsorptive phase. During the absorptive phase, the perivenous cells primarily take up glucose. In these cells, it is used to synthesize glycogen. Following replacement of glycogen stores, glucose is converted to lactate and released into the hepatic veins. Lactic acid is then taken up by the periportal cells, where it is used as a substrate for gluconeogenesis. This concept is consistent with the observation that glycogen stores are refilled first in the perivenous hepatocytes whereas glycogen degradation starts periportally.

In the postabsorptive phase, glycogen is degraded to glucose in the periportal hepatocytes. As the glucose proceeds down the sinusoid, it is taken up by perivenous cells and degraded to lactate. Lactate is again released into the circulation, and, if unused by the peripheral circulation, it is used as a substrate for gluconeogenesis by periportal cells.

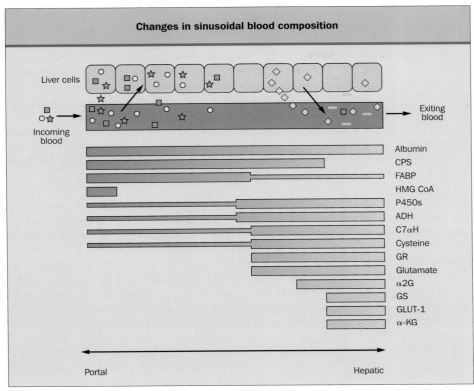

Changes in sinusoidal blood composition

Figure 3.20 Changes in sinusoidal blood composition. Sinusoidal blood composition changes as incoming solutes are removed by liver cells (top). As solutes are taken up by hepatocytes, their concentration decreases. 'Perivenular' plasma contains increased concentrations of material that have been secreted by zone 3 hepatocytes. Hepatic gene expression along the liver cell plate (bottom). The 20 to 30 hepatocytes lining the liver sinusoid contain varying amounts of key enzymes. (CPS, carbamoyl phosphate synthetase; FABP, zfatty acid-binding protein; HMG-CoA, 3-hydroxy-3-methylglutaryl-coenzyme A reductase; P-450s, cytochromes of the P-450 family; ADH, alcohol dehydrogenase; C7αH, cholesterol 7 α-hydroxylase; Cysteine, cysteine transporter; GR, glucagon receptor; Glutamate, glutamate transporter; α2G, α2-globulin; GS, glutamine synthetase; GLUT-1, glucose transporter; α-KG, α-ketoglutarate transporter.) Modified from Gumucio et al in Kaplowitz (96) by permission of Lippincott, Williams & Wilkins.

Heterogeneity of hepatocyte metabolism and biotransformation

Physiologic function	Periportal (zone 1) cells Metabolic function	Enzyme involved	Physiologic function	Pericentral (zone 3) cells Metabolic function	Enzyme involved
Oxidation		Succinate dehydrogenase			
Glucose formation	1. Gluconeogenesis 2. Glucose from glycogen 3. Glycogen from pyruvate	Glucose-6 phosphatase Phosphoenolpyruvate carboxykinase	Glucose uptake	1. Glycolysis 2. Glycogen from glucose 3. Glycogen to pyruvate	Glucokinase
Urea formation	Urea from amino acid nitrogen and from NH₃	Carbamoyl phosphate synthetase	Glutamine formation		
Protective metabolism	1. Glutathione peroxidation 2. Glutathione conjugation	Glutathione peroxidase Glutathione level	Xenobiotic metabolism	1. Mono-oxygenation 2. Glucuronidation	Cytochrome P450 UDP-glucuronosyl-transferase
Plasma protein synthesis		Albumin	Plasma protein synthesis		α-Fetoprotein
		α₂-Macroglobulin Fibrinogen			Angiotensinogen α₁-Antitrypsin
Cholesterol synthesis	Hydroxymethyl glutaryl-coenzyme A reductase				
Bile formation	Taurocholate uptake carrier Bile acid export carrier				

Table 3.2 Heterogeneity of hepatocyte metabolism and biotransformation.

Fatty acid metabolism

The zonation of fatty acid metabolism is less pronounced than that described for carbohydrate metabolism. Perivenous cells appear to synthesize preferentially VLDL, whereas periportal cells perform β-oxidation and ketogenesis. Fatty acid-binding protein, the chief intracellular transport protein for long chain fatty acids, is located predominantly in periportal cells. It is unclear whether the presence of this intracellular carrier promotes the preferential β-oxidation and ketogenesis seen in periportal cells. HMG-CoA reductase is located almost exclusively in periportal cells.

Amino acid and ammonia metabolism

Nutrient proteins in the form of amino acids are supplied to hepatocytes via the portal vein. Periportal cells preferentially convert the ammonia to urea. If the quantity of ammonia presented to the periportal region is sufficient to escape ureagenesis, perivenous hepatocytes take up the ammonia and convert it to glutamine. Glutamine is then released into the systemic circulation and returned to periportal cells, where again the ammonia is preferentially formed into urea. The periportal and perivenous systems have different kinetics with the periportal system being a high-capacity, low-affinity pathway and the perivenous pathway having a high affinity but a low capacity. Work using perfused livers has demonstrated that the removal of ammonia in periportal cells (urea synthesis) is restricted to incoming ammonia concentrations higher than 50 μM and that glutamine synthesis in the perivenous cells occurs at concentrations of ammonia below 50 μM.

Zonation of xenobiotic metabolism

The cytochrome P-450 system is responsible for the metabolism of many xenobiotics. This process often involves mono-oxygenation followed by conjugation with either glucuronic or sulfuric acid. Sulfate formation predominates in periportal cells, whereas glucuronide formation is the major conjugation reaction in perivenous cells. The mono-oxygenation also occurs preferentially in the perivenous zone, leading to the formation of potentially toxic electrophiles. The perivenous zone, therefore, is predisposed to the toxicity of reactive oxygen intermediates. The combination of this predilection as well as the decreased ability of the cell to detoxify oxygen intermediates by glutathione leads to the perivenous necrosis caused by some hepatotoxins.

Regulation of hepatocyte heterogeneity

It is generally assumed that hepatocyte zonation develops as a consequence of the heterogeneity in the microenvironment of individual cells. This is controlled by various signals such as substrate concentration (including oxygen), hormones, neuro-mediators, nerves and cell-to-biomatrix interactions. The differential expression patterns seen in the zonation may be attributed to different rates of mRNA transcription, mRNA degradation, mRNA translation, or end-protein degradation.

The expression of the genes for the enzymes of gluconeogenesis is regulated at the pretranslational level. Similarly, the amino acid metabolizing enzymes are regulated at the pretranslational level. Each of these alterations in gene expression occurs during a normal feeding rhythm. In contrast, glycolytic enzymes appear to be regulated mainly at the post-translational level during a normal feeding pattern. Each of these generalities regarding the regulation of zonal gene expression may change depending on the nutritional conditions.

Ammonia detoxification also appears to be regulated at the pretranslational level. Both the mRNA and the proteins of the key ureagenic enzymes are located exclusively in the periportal cells. In contrast, the mRNA and the protein for glutamine synthesis are located exclusively in parenchymal cells in the distal perivenous area. Neither these mRNA nor the enzyme levels themselves seem to vary with the nutritional state, suggesting that the organism needs to maintain tight control over ammonia despite external influences.

Physiologic significance of hepatocyte heterogeneity

The pattern of organization described earlier indicates the complexity of the liver's ability to respond to a large variety of input and output solute concentrations and the overall metabolic demands of the organism. Two control elements seem to dictate the degree of zonal responses: the sequential delivery of substrates and the zonal patterns of gene expression. Because of the unidirectional perfusion of the liver acinus, periportal cells are exposed to a high concentration of incoming solutes. Solutes using transport systems that have a great capacity for uptake (ammonia and bile acids) are preferentially taken up by the first hepatocytes that they encounter. Refluxed material or substances escaping uptake by periportal cells are subsequently presented to 'downstream' cells. The removal of ammonia, either as urea or by glutamine synthesis, is an example of this complexly controlled system. Each of these systems allows minute adjustments in the outflow concentration of substances of a splanchnic origin as well as new products formed by the synthetic machinery of the liver.

In summary, the zonation of hepatocytes allows the liver acinus to accomplish the regulation of substrate production and the metabolism of proteins and hormones in a dynamic fashion. Zonation appears to depend on the unidirectional perfusion of substrates as well as on basic gene expression by hepatocytes. Each of these control mechanisms is dynamic, responding to the overall needs of the organism.

FURTHER READING

Hepatic endothelial cells

Arias IM. The biology of hepatic endothelial cell fenestrae. Progress in Liver Disease 1990; 9:11–26. *A superb review of the biology of the hepatic endothelial cell and its unique features that facilitate hepatic transport.*

Roberts SK, Ludwig J, LaRusso NF. The pathobiology of biliary epithelia. Gastroenterology 1997; 112:269–279. *A review of the advances made in understanding the mechanisms of bile formation by the bile duct epithelial cells or cholangiocytes and the role of these cells as targets in a variety of hepatobiliary diseases.*

Bile salt transport

Trauner M, Boyer JL. Bile salt transporters: molecular characterization, function, and regulation. Physiologic Reviews 2003; 83:633–671. *A comprehensive summary of the current knowledge of the molecular characterization, function and regulation of bile salt transporters in normal physiology and in cholestatic liver disease.*

Wolkoff AW, Cohen DE. Bile acid regulation of hepatic physiology I. Hepatocyte transport of bile acids. American Journal of Physiology Gastrointestinal Liver Physiology 2003; 284:G175–179. *A concise review of the regulation of bile acid transporters and their role in promoting bile flow.*

Lipid transport

Oude, Elferink RPJ, Tytgat GNJ, Groen AK. The role of MDR2 P-glycoprotein in hepatobiliary lipid transport. FASEB J 1997; 11:19–28. *Fascinating review of the physiologic role of this canalicular ATP-binding cassette transporter and its role in human liver disease.*

Tight junctions

Nusrat A, Turner JR, Madara JL. Molecular physiology and pathophysiology of tight junctions IV. Regulation of tight junctions by extracellular stimuli: nutrients, cytokines and immune cells. American Journal of Physiology Gastrointestinal Liver Physiology 2000; 279:G851–857. *Part of a four series review of the physiology and pathophysiology of tight junctions. This section emphasizes the role of cytokines and leukocytes in modulating tight junction function.*

patients with severe chronic liver disease, there is a high mortality from infections (38%). In acute liver failure, fungal infections are an important complicating problem (see Ch. 33). Blood, urine, sputum and ascites should be cultured routinely and a chest X-ray should be obtained.

Facial signs

There are no particular facial characteristics denoting liver disease, but there are rare instances of specific features (e.g. Alagille syndrome – widely set eyes, prominent forehead, flat nose and small chin associated with congenital hepatic duct hypoplasia). Other facial signs include:

- telangiectasia as one of the common cutaneous stigmata of chronic liver disease,
- pseudo-Cushingoid appearance and parotid swelling in alcoholic liver disease,
- subconjunctival hemorrhage (see Fig. 4.3) which is commonly seen in severe acute liver failure,
- xanthelasma around the eyes suggesting chronic cholestatic liver disease (e.g. PBC) and,
- conjunctival pallor, suggesting anemia which is common in liver disease.

A specific sign in the eye is the Kaysler-Fleischer (K-F) ring (**Fig. 4.7**). This is a ring due to the deposition of copper-containing pigment in the Descemet's membrane at the periphery of the posterior surface of the cornea. The K-F ring is usually greenish-brown in color; although visible to the naked eye, it is best seen by an ophthalmologist using a slit-lamp. It is present in more than 90% of all patients who have Wilson disease with neurologic signs, and in the majority of those with hepatic involvement (see Ch. 24). It may be absent (or very difficult to visualize) in approximately 50% of adolescents with acute presentations of Wilson disease. A similar ring may rarely be found in cases of chronic cholestasis or cirrhosis.

Fetor

Hepatic fetor or fetor hepaticus complicates severe hepatocellular disease with associated encephalopathy. It is described as a sweet, slightly fecal smell of the breath which is presumed to be of intestinal origin, being particularly prevalent in patients with an extensive portal collateral circulation.

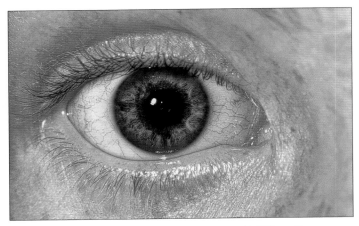

Figure 4.7 A Kayser-Fleischer ring in a patient with Wilson disease.

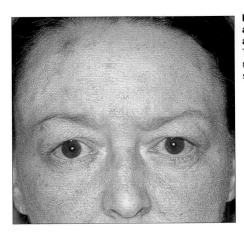

Figure 4.8 Jaundice in a patient with alcoholic liver disease. There is also a spider nevus and paper money skin.

Skin signs

Jaundice is the physical sign most often regarded as synonymous with hepatobiliary disease (Figs 4.2 and **4.8**). It is detectable by the physician when the serum bilirubin level exceeds approximately 45 μmol/L (2.6 mg/dL). Patients are referred to as being 'jaundiced' or 'icteric'. The earliest sign is a yellow discoloration of the sclerae but as the serum bilirubin rises the jaundice is obvious in the skin and, if prolonged, the skin can develop a greenish tinge. Bilirubin binds preferentially to elastic tissues, but body fluids such as ascites, sweat or urine can also become yellow. There are several mechanisms affecting the depth of jaundice, although in general hepatobiliary diseases cause deeper jaundice than does hemolysis. The severity of the jaundice does not necessarily correlate with the prognosis of the underlying pathology.

Very rarely a yellow pigmentation of the skin may be due to excessive consumption of foods containing carotene or lycopene (e.g. tomatoes and carrots). Some drugs may also cause discoloration (e.g. mepacrine). However, in these circumstances, the sclerae remain white.

There are other signs in the skin that are strongly associated with liver disease. Hyperpigmentation is common in chronic liver disease, and is due to the increased deposition of melanin. It is seen particularly in primary biliary cirrhosis and hemochromatosis (bronze diabetes). Local areas of hyperpigmentation occur at sites of irritation, trauma or in more exposed areas. In addition, patients with marked hyperbilirubinemia can have general hyperpigmentation. Vitiligo is much more obvious in pigmented patients, and it is associated with autoimmune disease (e.g. PBC and chronic hepatitis). Pruritus is a frequent symptom of cholestatic conditions and associated scratch marks on the skin are commonly observed. These are in accessible areas and so the center of the back is usually spared. The nails in such patients are highly polished; this may be a striking phenomenon on examination.

Lichen planus is associated with PBC and the increased plasma lipids in chronic cholestatic conditions lead to xanthelasma around the eyes and xanthomata over pressure areas such as buttocks, knees and elbows (**Fig. 4.9**). Porphyria cutanea tarda is associated with hepatitis C, with up to 80% of these patients being hepatitis C virus (HCV) positive.

Excessive bruising and purpura occur in patients where the coagulation factors and platelet count are disturbed. Often sites of venipuncture show excessive extravasation of blood. Needle

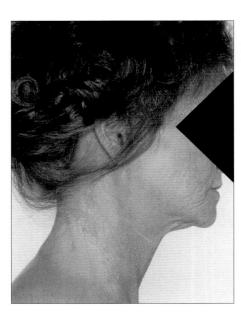

Figure 4.9 Extensive xanthoma in the neck of a pigmented patient with primary biliary cirrhosis.

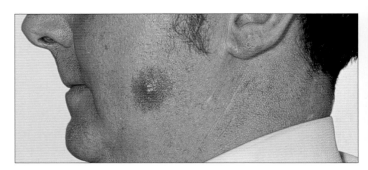

Figure 4.11 A large spider nevus on the cheek.

marks from intravenous drug abuse should be noted, since they may suggest the cause of viral hepatitis. Tattoos similarly should be noted. Leukocytoclastic vasculitis, a necrotic rash with transient erythema multiforme, may be an early manifestation of both hepatitis B and C infection.

Vascular 'spiders' are commonly seen in association with chronic liver disease. There are several synonyms: spider telangiectasia, spider nevi, arterial spiders, spider angiomas. The lesion consists of a central arteriole with numerous small radiating vessels resembling a spider's legs, hence the various names for this lesion (**Fig. 4.10**). Pressure on the central prominence causes blanching of the whole lesion. Occasionally such lesions can be seen or felt to pulsate. The spiders can vary in size from 1 mm to 1–2 cm in diameter (**Fig. 4.11**). They are found in the drainage area of the superior vena cava and are commonly found in the neck, face, arms and hands. Approximately 2–3% of normal individuals have two or three spiders, but any more than that, especially if they are developing or enlarging, suggests parenchymal liver disease. Spiders can occur briefly in acute hepatitis, but usually reflect cirrhosis. They can develop during pregnancy, but fade after delivery. There are two other lesions

associated with spiders: white spots on the arms and buttocks on exposure to cold; these indicate the position of a spider's central arteriole. Secondly, in the area of the spiders, there may be numerous, random small vessels. These resemble the pattern on the paper used for US dollar bills, hence the skin is called 'paper money skin' (see Fig. 4.8).

The skin may occasionally reveal several relatively specific signs. The CREST syndrome (*c*alcinosis, *R*aynaud's phenomenon, *e*sophageal dysfunction, *s*clerodactyly, *t*elangiectasia) suggests primary biliary cirrhosis; hereditary hemorrhagic telangiectasia may cause cirrhosis and hepatic vascular ectasia; striae and a facial rash occur with autoimmune hepatitis.

Examination of the limbs

Examination of the limbs in liver disease patients may reveal proximal myopathy associated with alcohol abuse or vitamin D deficiency, bone tenderness related to osteopenia of chronic liver disease or the arthritides associated with primary biliary cirrhosis or hemochromatosis.

Pitting edema, particularly in the legs, is common, especially in patients with chronic liver disease who have already developed ascites (**Fig. 4.12**).

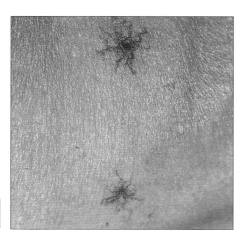

Figure 4.10 Spider nevi on the neck.

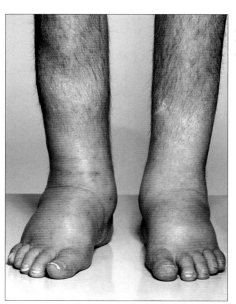

Figure 4.12 Peripheral edema in a patient with chronic liver disease.

Hand and nail signs

Examination of the hands can reveal several signs in patients with liver disease. None of these signs, however, are specific to liver disease. The hands may be warm and the palms bright red. This palmar erythema is a mottled red discoloration affecting the thenar and hypothenar eminences, the pulps and bases of the fingers (**Fig. 4.13**). The feet may be similarly affected. This appearance is associated with acute and chronic liver disease but can also occur in rheumatoid arthritis, thyrotoxicosis, fever and pregnancy.

Dupuytren's contracture has been traditionally associated with alcoholic cirrhosis. In this condition there is a thickening and shortening of the palmar fascia causing flexion deformities of the fingers. The abnormality is now known to have a multifactorial origin but to be strongly associated with cigarette smoking and alcohol consumption rather than primary liver disease. It affects approximately 10% of men over 65 years of age and consequently will be commonly seen in older males who drink regularly, whether or not liver disease is present.

Reference has already been made to the highly polished nails associated with pruritus. The nails can also appear white (leukonychia). This is due to opacity of the nail bed and occurs in up to 80% of patients with chronic liver disease. The distal border may retain a 1–2 mm pink edge, but the lunulae are often obscured by the white nail bed (**Fig. 4.14**). An alternative appearance is one of transverse white lines, parallel to the lunula, band leukonychia (Muehrcke lines) (**Fig. 4.15**). Both these forms of leukonychia are said to be related to a low serum albumin, such as occurs in chronic liver disease. Other conditions in which leukonychia is found include nephrotic syndrome, diabetes mellitus, pulmonary tuberculosis, rheumatoid arthritis and multiple sclerosis. Blue discoloration of the lunulae has been described in Wilson disease and argyria.

Finger clubbing occurs in chronic liver disease and even regresses after hepatic transplantation. It is associated, however, with many other conditions. It may be associated with hypoxia

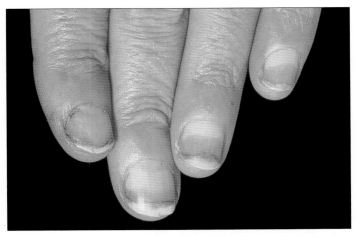

Figure 4.14 Leukonychia of the proximal nail bed in a patient who has alcoholic liver disease.

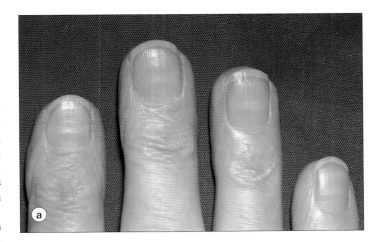

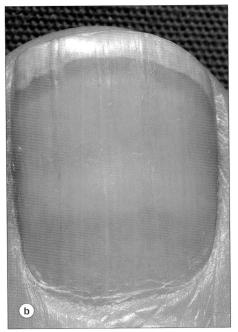

Figure 4.15 (a) Band leukonychia in a patient who has hemochromatosis.
(b) Close up.

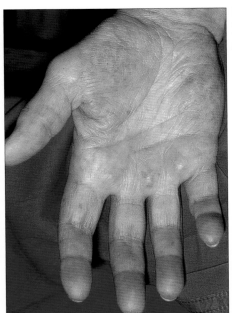

Figure 4.13 Palmar erythema in a patient who has chronic liver disease.

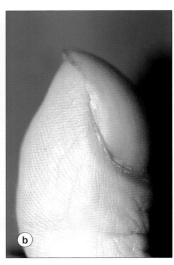

Figure 4.16 (a) Clubbing of the fingers in a patient who has chronic alcoholic liver disease. (b) Close up.

and pulmonary hypertension and, in these conditions, hypertrophic osteoarthropathy with periostitis occurs. This is seen radiologically in up to 40% of patients with chronic liver disease (**Fig. 4.16**).

Cardiovascular examination

Patients in the early stages of liver disease have a normal cardiovascular system on clinical examination. Alcohol has an effect on blood pressure and this may contribute towards hypertension in some cases. Patients who have advanced hemochromatosis and alcohol abuse can develop cardiomyopathies with the consequent heart failure.

Cardiovascular changes develop as patients with chronic liver disease slowly deteriorate. Similar hemodynamic effects occur rapidly if the patient has acute liver failure. In these conditions a hyperdynamic circulation develops and the patient manifests warm peripheries, a bounding pulse, tachycardia at rest and systemic hypotension. There is an evident precordial impulse and an ejection flow murmur. As the disease progresses the blood pressure falls further and this contributes to the progressive compromise of renal, hepatic and cerebral blood flow and ultimately to terminal multisystem failure. The deterioration in the hemodynamic parameters may be reversible in acute-on-chronic liver failure, i.e. when an acute deterioration is triggered by a potentially reversible or treatable complication like sepsis or gastrointestinal hemorrhage. These circulatory changes are the result of increased cardiac output and reduced peripheral vascular resistance. The cause is thought to be the release of a variety of vasodilators, often acting via the induction of nitric oxide synthase.

Pulmonary hypertension rarely produces symptoms. However, significant asymptomatic pulmonary hypertension is found in 2–10% of patients with portal hypertension. The incidence depends on the pressure threshold used to define pulmonary hypertension. It can contribute to the signs of right heart failure and low cardiac output which may be found in severely affected patients. When severe, it represents a contraindication to liver transplantation.

Respiratory examination

There is a variety of pulmonary pathologies that can affect patients who have liver disease and these produce abnormal physical signs. Cyanosis occurs in up to 30% of cases of chronic liver disease. Reduced chest expansion, evidence of pleural effusions, dyspnea, orthopnea and signs of intrapulmonary fluid, infection or pulmonary fibrosis can all be found in patients with acute or chronic liver disease. The hepatopulmonary syndrome is another important cause of dyspnea (see Ch. 13). In this condition there is evidence of intrapulmonary arteriovenous (A-V) shunts, vasodilatation leading to ventilation–perfusion mismatching, and capillary wall thickening leading to diffusion defects. The impairment of oxygenation is classically worsened by rising from the lying to the standing position (orthodeoxyia).

Pleural effusions occur in approximately 6% of cirrhotic patients but are more common in decompensated cirrhosis, usually occurring on the right and in association with ascites. However, they can occur bilaterally and in the absence of ascites, or can still be present when ascites has responded to diuretic treatment. A right-sided effusion is the norm in the post-operative phase following liver transplantation.

More specific associations between the lung and liver are seen in autoimmune conditions such as fibrosing alveolitis and Sjögren syndrome. In α_1-antitrypsin deficiency emphysema may be present and in cystic fibrosis chronic suppurative lung disease is usual.

Abdominal examination
Observation

Observation of the abdomen may reveal wasting due to severe malnutrition or cachexia due to malignancy. Alternatively, distention, especially in the flanks, may be present, suggestive of ascites. Normal abdominal wall movement may be restricted by intra-abdominal pathology causing tenderness and pain. The abdominal skin may show petechiae, scratch marks or striae, all of which are related to possible liver disease (Figs 4.1 and 4.4).

Dilated abdominal wall veins are a notable finding in liver disease (see Figs 4.1, 4.6 and **4.17**). Prominent superficial veins

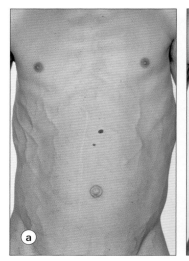
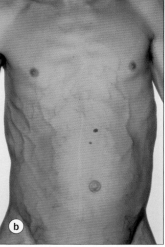

Figure 4.17 Abdominal wall veins in a patient with chronic liver disease. (a) Routine photograph. (b) Infrared photograph.

occur around the umbilicus if the portal venous blood flow is obstructed beyond the origin of the umbilical veins from the left branch of the portal vein, as occurs in intrahepatic pathology. Such portal hypertension allows the umbilical and paraumbilical veins to open up and produce dilated veins on the abdomen and the umbilicus. Blood in these veins flows away from the umbilicus. The appearance is classically called 'caput medusae' since the serpiginous veins are supposed to resemble snakes on the head of the mythological gorgon Medusa. However, this classical appearance is rarely observed in practice, and the term 'caput medusae' has come to be used to describe the more common finding of dilated veins that flow away from the umbilicus in patients with cirrhosis. Dilated veins due to an obstructed inferior vena cava are usually contrasted with paraumbilical veins. In inferior vena caval obstruction the distended veins are more commonly seen in the sides of the abdomen and the flow is upwards from legs to chest.

Palpation

Palpation of the abdomen may reveal general features such as abnormal masses or an area of tenderness. These may be associated with hepatobiliary problems, for example intra-abdominal malignancy or biliary infection. More specifically, the clinician needs to palpate the liver and spleen. The shape and size, the contour and the consistency of the liver are all important features. Normally the liver may just be palpable. A Riedel's lobe (anatomical variant of the right lobe) or downward displacement by pulmonary disease may inappropriately suggest the liver is enlarged. True hepatomegaly is usually indicative of liver disease, unless it is a manifestation of right ventricular failure or related conditions (**Table 4.1**).

The development of cirrhosis often leads to shrinkage of a previously enlarged liver, perhaps with compensatory hypertrophy of the left lobe. The cirrhotic liver becomes irregular and firm. An enlarged, hard, irregular liver suggests malignancy.

Splenomegaly is an important physical sign in liver disease (**Table 4.2**). The spleen is normally palpable although, in one study, it was felt in 3% of 2200 healthy college students. It enlarges due mainly to portal hypertension and hyperplasia of the reticuloendothelial component and can thus be felt in chronic or acute liver disease. In the presence of chronic liver disease,

Common causes of hepatomegaly	
Causes	Examples
Chronic liver disease	Multiple causes often leading to cirrhosis
Inflammation	Viral, bacterial (including abscess), parasitic
Venous congestion	Cardiac, venous occlusion (e.g. hepatic vein)
Tumors	Primary hepatobiliary, secondary carcinoma, hematologic malignancies
Biliary disease	Extrahepatic obstruction, congenital cystic disease
Metabolic	Fatty liver, amyloidosis, storage diseases

Table 4.1 Common causes of hepatomegaly. The differential diagnosis of hepatomegaly

Common causes of splenomegaly	
Causes	Examples
Venous congestion	Liver disease, hepatic/portal vein occlusion
Infection	Viral, bacterial, parasitic
Inflammation	Rheumatoid arthritis, sarcoidosis, systemic lupus erythmatosus
Hematologic disturbances	Chronic hemolysis, hemoglobinopathies, myeloproliferative disease, leukemia, lymphoma
Miscellaneous	Storage diseases, amyloidosis

Table 4.2 Common causes of splenomegaly. The various etiologies of splenomegaly

splenomegaly is the most important sign of portal hypertension. When splenomegaly is present, the peripheral blood may show features of hypersplenism. The splenic size is most easily assessed by ultrasound examination.

Palpation of the kidneys is usually unhelpful in liver disease, although 70% of cases with adult renal polycystic disease may develop liver cysts.

Percussion

Percussion of the abdomen is useful in assessing the size of the liver, especially when it is small, and in detecting the presence of ascites (see Figs 4.1 and 4.6). The cardinal sign of ascites is 'shifting dullness' present on both sides of the abdomen. At least 2 L of ascites must be present before it can be thus detected. A fluid thrill requires marked ascites before it is detected. An everted umbilicus is frequently associated with gross ascites (see Figs 4.1 and 4.6).

Auscultation

Auscultation of the abdomen in relation to liver disease may reveal three types of sounds:

- *Arterial bruits* heard over the liver suggest the presence of a vascular hepatocellular carcinoma or other malignancy, an A-V malformation, very rarely tortuous arteries in a cirrhotic liver, or severe alcoholic hepatitis.
- *Venous hums* are occasionally heard in portal hypertension and reflect turbulent flow in collateral veins. A venous hum at the umbilicus in association with dilated abdominal wall veins and occasionally a venous thrill is termed the Cruveilhier-Baumgarten syndrome. This rare and unusual association may be due to a congenitally patent umbilical vein or portal hypertension in well-compensated cirrhosis.
- *Friction rubs* over the liver suggest inflammation or infiltration. They may be caused by tumor or abscess invading the peritoneum or by hepatic infarction. A transient rub is often heard over the site of a liver biopsy. In the Fitz-Hugh-Curtis syndrome a rub is heard as a result of perihepatitis often caused by chlamydial infection.

Examination for endocrinologic abnormalities

Endocrine changes may occur in the presence of liver disease and are common when there is an alcoholic cause. In patients with cirrhosis, hypogonadism is common, which in men produces feminization leading to testicular atrophy, a female body habitus and distribution of body hair, and gynecomastia (see Fig. 4.4). The latter particularly occurs in alcoholics, but is also seen in patients taking spironolactone. This combination of factors may be frequently present in patients with liver disease. Gonadal atrophy in women produces very few clinically detectable physical signs, although the premenopausal patient loses female characteristics such as breast and pelvic fatty tissue.

It is important to recognize that alcohol abuse can produce features of pseudo-Cushing's syndrome and that some of the above features in men with hemochromatosis can occur before evidence of chronic liver disease.

Neurologic examination

Neurologic abnormalities due to underlying liver disease are rare, apart from hepatic encephalopathy. The neurologic examination is usually, therefore, unremarkable. Specific associations should be borne in mind, for example the neurologic features of Wilson disease, the effects of vitamin A and E deficiency, and the neurologic consequences of viral hepatitis or alcohol abuse.

The clinical features of encephalopathy vary from subtle signs with mild cognitive impairment (minimal hepatic encephalopathy) to coma. A clinical grading system from 1 to 4 is useful (**Table 4.3**), particularly when frequent observations need to be made to follow the development of the condition or the effect of treatment. Early changes may be monitored by serial use of a number connection test where the time taken by a patient to join together sequential but randomly spaced numbers is recorded. The time taken increases progressively as the severity of the encephalopathy increases.

One of the most characteristic signs of encephalopathy is that of a flapping tremor ('asterixis' or 'liver flap'). This is demonstrated best with the arms outstretched, the wrists dorsiflexed and the fingers separated. This position may have to be maintained for 3–5 min to elicit a flapping tremor. The flapping tremor consists of brief, rapid flexion and extension movements of the fingers or wrists. If it is severe, a similar tremor may be seen in the arms, head and feet. The tremor is seen best on sustained posture; it is absent at rest and disappears if coma develops. The 'liver flap' is not specific for liver disease and can occur in renal failure, respiratory failure, metabolic disturbances and drug intoxication.

When neurologic deterioration of this nature occurs, the clinician should evaluate the patient carefully because intracranial lesions such as infection, hemorrhage or tumor can produce a similar clinical picture, as can metabolic and drug-induced pathology. In patients who have chronic liver disease and consequent hemostatic disturbances, even minor head injury can lead to significant intracranial bleeding. Hepatic encephalopathy can progress rapidly to coma in acute liver failure and is a severe prognostic sign. In cases of chronic liver disease, it is often precipitated by a number of factors, particularly if there is significant portal-systemic shunting (**Table 4.4**).

More focal neurologic signs may rarely be present in chronic hepatic encephalopathy as a result of irreversible neurologic degeneration in the cerebral cortex, the basal ganglia, the cerebellum or the spinal cord, such as occurs in the acquired hepatocerebral degeneration syndrome or in hepatic myelopathy.

DIAGNOSIS AND PROGNOSIS

The evaluation of the patient with liver disease needs careful clinical assessment and the use of various investigations in order to arrive at a definitive diagnosis and management plan. Analysis of the information obtained also allows an assessment of the severity of the disease and the prognosis for the patient. Grading the overall severity of liver disease is now more important than it used to be because of the routine use of liver transplantation in the management of patients. An estimate of prognosis is essential if the timing of transplantation is to be optimal.

Hepatic encephalopathy: precipitating factors in chronic liver disease	
Causes	*Examples*
Gut factors	Constipation, high protein intake, upper gastrointestinal bleeding
Electrolyte/water imbalances	Vomiting, diarrhea, diuretic treatment, renal failure, paracentesis
Infection	Chest, urinary, spontaneous bacterial peritonitis
Drugs	Hypnotic/sedative drugs, alcohol
Severe factors affecting major metabolic functions	Hypoxia, hypotension, hypoglycemia

Table 4.4 Hepatic encephalopathy: precipitating factors in chronic liver disease. A number of clinical conditions not involving the liver can worsen hepatic encephalopathy

Clinical grading of hepatic encephalopathy		
Clinical grade	*Clinical signs*	*Flapping tremor*
Grade 1 (prodrome)	Alert, euphoric, occasionally depression. Poor concentration, slow mentation and affect, reversed sleep rhythm	Infrequent at this stage
Grade 2 (impending coma)	Drowsiness, lethargic, inappropriate behavior, disorientation	Easily elicited
Grade 3 (early coma)	Stuporous but easily rousable, marked confusion, incoherent speech	Usually present
Grade 4 (deep coma)	Coma, unresponsive but may respond to painful stimulus	Usually absent

Table 4.3 Clinical grading of hepatic encephalopathy. The spectrum of encephalopathy is divided into four clinical grades

Child's grading of disease severity in chronic liver disease with Pugh's 1973 modifications			
Criteria assessed	*Points scored for increasing abnormality*		
	1	2	3
Encephalopathy (grade)	None	1–2	3–4
Ascites	Absent	Slight	Moderate
Serum bilirubin [μmol/L (mg/dL)]	<35 (<2)	35–50 (2–3)	>50 (>3)
In primary biliary cirrhosis	<70 (<4)	70–170 (4–10)	>170 (>10)
Serum albumin [g/L (g/dL)]	>35 (3.5)	35–28 (3.5–2.8)	<28 (<2.8)
Prothrombin time [prolongation (s)]	1–4	4–10	>10
Total score	5–6	7–9	10–15
Child's grade equivalent	A	B	C
Overall mortality in Pugh's series (%)	29	38	88
Modified from Pugh et al (73).			

Table 4.5 Child's grading of disease severity in chronic liver disease with Pugh's 1973 modifications. The Child-Pugh score is universally used to quantify the severity of liver disease

Various classifications have been used to assess severity of disease. In patients with chronic liver disease Child's grading with Pugh's modification is frequently used. This system uses a combination of clinical and laboratory parameters. Each feature is scored from one to three points and the total score equated with a Child's grade (from A to C) (**Table 4.5**). The Child grade has been equated with survival (**Table 4.6**), C being the most severe with an overall mortality of 88% (Table 4.5). MELD is a score of disease severity that is based exclusively on laboratory parameters, and this is increasingly replacing the Child's classification in some clinical situations.

There are some important clinical points that have a bearing on survival in individual patients who have chronic liver disease when they are assessed. Serious factors include:

- persistent jaundice,
- intractable ascites,
- spontaneous bacterial peritonitis,
- progressive encephalopathy,
- persistent hypotension,
- low serum albumin,
- persistent hyponatremia, and
- prolonged prothrombin time.

Survival in chronic liver disease			
	Percentage survival in chronic liver disease		
Child's grade	*At 1 year*	*At 5 years*	*At 10 years*
A	84	44	27
B	62	20	10
C	42	21	0
Modified from Christensen et al (84).			

Table 4.6 Survival in chronic liver disease. The risk of death in patients with chronic liver disease correlates well with the Child's grade

In clinical practice, the experienced physician uses his or her skills to elicit many of the features described in this chapter. Clinical diagnoses are dependent upon a process of pattern recognition and the astute physician integrates all the information obtained in evaluating the patient. It is perhaps useful to remember that the liver is affected by a variety of etiologies but often reacts in a similar, diffuse pathologic fashion. As a result, a number of clinical effects can be reliably predicted (**Figs 4.18 and 4.19**).

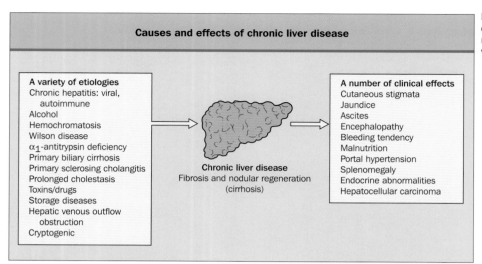

Figure 4.18 Causes and effects of chronic liver disease. This figure shows the common clinical manifestations of chronic liver disease together with the common etiologies of cirrhosis.

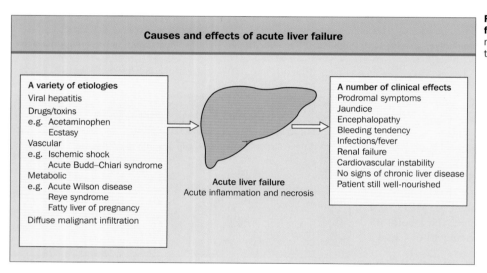

Figure 4.19 Causes and effects of acute liver failure. This figure shows the common clinical manifestations of acute liver failure together with the common etiologies of acute liver injury.

FURTHER READING

Historical interest

Bean WB. Vascular spiders and related lesions of the skin. Oxford: Blackwell; 1958. *An interesting historical record of skin lesions in a variety of conditions. Of special note are the extensive descriptions of vascular spiders and palmar erythema, particularly in liver disease. Professor Bean obviously made many careful observations.*

Christensen E, Schlichting P, Fauerholdt L, et al. Prognostic value of Child-Turcotte criteria in medically treated cirrhosis. Hepatology 1984; 4:430–435

Pugh RNH, Murray-Lyon IM, Dawson JL, et al. Transection of the oesophagus for bleeding oesophageal varices. Br J Surg 1973; 60:646–649. *A modification and refinement of Child's grading system which produced a good predictor of survival in patients with chronic liver disease undergoing esophageal transection and variceal ligation for bleeding varices.*

Sherlock S, Summerskill WHJ, White LP, et al. Portal-systemic encephalopathy. Neurological complications of liver disease. Lancet 1954; 2:453–457. *Eighteen patients are described with chronic liver disease and the now 'classical' features of encephalopathy. These changes were related to portal-systemic shunting of nitrogenous substances to the brain. A good description of this common clinical problem in hepatology.*

General review

Hislop WS, Bouchier IAD, Allan JG, et al. Alcoholic liver disease in Scotland and North Eastern England: presenting features in 510 patients. Q J Med 1983; 52:232–243.

Saunders JB, Walters JRF, Davies P, et al. A 20-year prospective study of cirrhosis. Br Med J 1981; 282:263–266. *A useful description of the causes and prognosis of cirrhosis in an English health district during the 1960s–1970s. Alcoholic cirrhosis was seen to increase rapidly in prevalence.*

Specific complications

Forton DM, Patel N, Prince M, et al. Fatigue and primary biliary cirrhosis: association of globus pallidus magnetisation transfer ratio measurements with fatigue severity and blood manganese levels. Gut 2004; 53:587–592.

Hoeper MM, Krowka MJ, Strassburg CP. Portopulmonary hypertension and hepatopulmonary syndrome. Lancet 2004; 363:1461–1468. *A comprehensive review with extensive bibliography. A good description of the pathogenesis and clinical features of these two conditions.*

Lewis M, Howdle PD. The neurology of liver failure. Q J Med 2003; 96:623–633.

CHAPTER
5

Laboratory Tests

Joanne C. Imperial and Emmet B. Keeffe

A broad array of biochemical tests is used to provide indirect evidence of hepatobiliary disease. The term *liver function tests* (LFTs) is firmly entrenched in routine medical language, although this terminology has been criticized because the tests most commonly employed in the evaluation of liver disease (i.e. serum aminotransferase and alkaline phosphatase) assess hepatocyte integrity rather than synthetic function. Biochemical tests on routine automated chemistry panels that may indicate liver disease can be divided into those that truly evaluate liver function, such as serum albumin or prothrombin time, and those that are simply markers of hepatobiliary disease, such as alanine aminotransferase (ALT), aspartate aminotransferase (AST), alkaline phosphatase (ALP) and γ-glutamyltransferase (GGT). The clinical approach to the diagnosis of conditions that are associated with mild elevation of liver enzymes that are markers of hepatocellular necrosis, i.e. AST and ALT and enzymes indicating cholestasis, i.e. ALP and GGT, is the focus of this review.

Screening biochemical testing of healthy, asymptomatic populations has revealed that up to 6% have abnormal serum aminotransferases. However, the prevalence of liver disease in the general population, excluding simple fatty liver, is lower (i.e. 2–4%). The relatively low prevalence of liver disease, as well as the fact that abnormal liver test results are often minor, and that the screened patient is often asymptomatic, may explain the frequent failure of physicians to perform confirmatory testing or additional evaluations. Despite this tendency to dismiss minor abnormalities of liver tests results, it is important that all such abnormalities be investigated and that, at least, a plausible explanation for the abnormality be determined. Elevated liver enzyme levels may be explained by significant liver disease, which may be treatable, as well as by insignificant liver disease, especially fatty liver, or occasionally diseases of other organs, such as muscle or bone. Additionally, even abnormal markers of hepatic synthetic function (albumin and prothrombin) can be attributable to non-hepatic causes (**Table 5.1**). On rare occasions, minor elevation of liver enzyme levels is explained by a laboratory error, artifact or macroenzyme formation. Taking into account these considerations, the clinical challenge is to determine the etiology of an abnormal liver test result in an asymptomatic individual using a stepwise and cost-effective approach.

Non-hepatic causes of abnormal liver tests		
Test	Non-hepatic causes	Discriminating tests
↓Albumin	Protein-losing enteropathy	Serum globulins, α_1-antitrypsin clearance
	Nephrotic syndrome	Urinalysis, 24 h urinary protein
	Malnutrition	Clinical setting
	Congestive heart failure	Clinical setting
↑Alkaline phosphatase	Bone disease	GGT, SLAP, 5′-NT
	Pregnancy	GGT, 5′-NT
	Malignancy	Alkaline phosphatase electrophoresis
	Myocardial infarction	MB-CPK
	Muscle disorders	Creatine kinase
↑Bilirubin	Hemolysis	Reticulocyte count, peripheral smear, urine bilirubin
	Sepsis	Clinical setting, cultures
	Ineffective erythropoiesis	Peripheral smear, urine bilirubin, hemoglobin electrophoresis, bone marrow examination
	Shunt hyperbilirubinemia	Clinical setting
↑Prothrombin time	Antibiotic and anticoagulant use, steatorrhea, dietary deficiency of vitamin K (rare)	Response to vitamin K, clinical setting

GGT, γ-glutamyltranspeptidase; SLAP, serum leucine aminopeptidase; 5′-NT, 5′-nucleotidase. Modified from Moseley (96).

Table 5.1 Non-hepatic causes of abnormal liver tests.

TESTS THAT REFLECT HEPATOBILIARY INJURY

Aminotransferases

The aminotransferases (previously called aminotransferases) are the most frequently utilized and specific indicators of hepatocellular integrity. These enzymes – AST (formerly serum glutamic oxaloacetic transaminase, or SGOT) and ALT (formerly serum glutamic pyruvic transaminase, or SGPT) – catalyze the transfer of the α-amino groups of aspartate and alanine, respectively, to the α-keto group of ketoglutaric acid. ALT is localized primarily in the liver, but AST is present in a wide variety of tissues, including the heart, skeletal muscle, kidney, brain and liver. Whereas AST is present in both the mitochondria and cytosol of hepatocytes, ALT is localized to the cytosol. The evaluation of an asymptomatic individual with an isolated elevation of ALT is outlined in **Figure 5.1**.

Although no uniform definition of 'mild', 'moderate' or 'severe' elevation of liver enzymes exists, a working definition has been suggested (**Table 5.2**). Diagnostic clues can often be obtained by assessing the degree of elevation. Mild elevations are typically found in non-alcoholic fatty liver disease (NAFLD), including simple fatty liver and non-alcoholic steatohepatitis (NASH), as well as in chronic viral hepatitis. Moderate elevations may be seen in chronic viral hepatitis, alcoholic hepatitis and a number of miscellaneous chronic liver diseases with or without cirrhosis, including extrahepatic biliary obstruction. Marked elevation of aminotransferases are typical of severe acute viral hepatitis, toxic or drug-induced hepatic injury, and shock or ischemia to the liver. The finding of extremely high aminotransferase levels, i.e. greater than 2000–3000 U/L, should always raise concern

for acetaminophen overdose, use of excessive therapeutic doses of acetaminophen by the alcoholic patient or shock and/or ischemia to the liver. In the great majority of liver diseases, however, AST and ALT elevations are mild or moderate.

The height of the elevation of aminotransferase levels does not appear to correlate with the extent of necrosis on liver biopsy specimens and therefore has no prognostic value. In fact, rapidly declining aminotransferase levels may be a reflection of decreased numbers of viable hepatocytes and indicate a poor prognosis in

Characteristics of elevated concentrations of liver enzymes				
Test	Normal*	Mild†	Moderate†	Marked†
AST	11–32	<2–3	2–3 to 20	>20
ALT	3–30	<2–3	2–3 to 20	>20
ALP	35–105	<1.5–2	1.5–2 to 5	>5
GGT	2–65	<2–3	2–3 to 10	>10

*Units for normal are U/L; normal ranges vary with the assay used and should be obtained from the laboratory performing the test.
†Numbers in the table refer to multiples of the upper limits of normal.
ALT, alanine aminotransferase; AST, aspartate aminotransferase; ALP, alkaline phosphatase; GGT, γ-glutamyltranspeptidase.
Reproduced from Keeffe (94).

Table 5.2 Characteristics of elevated concentrations of liver enzymes.

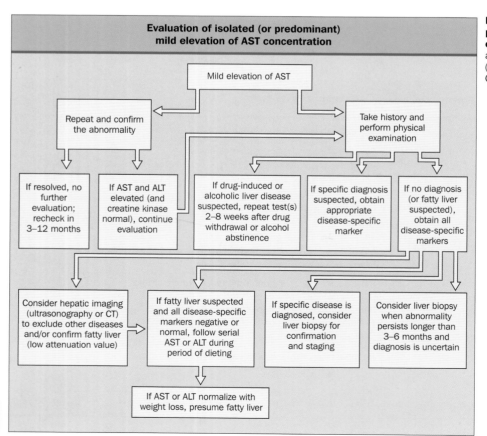

Evaluation of isolated (or predominant) mild elevation of AST concentration

Mild elevation of AST

Repeat and confirm the abnormality

Take history and perform physical examination

If resolved, no further evaluation; recheck in 3–12 months

If AST and ALT elevated (and creatine kinase normal), continue evaluation

If drug-induced or alcoholic liver disease suspected, repeat test(s) 2–8 weeks after drug withdrawal or alcohol abstinence

If specific diagnosis suspected, obtain appropriate disease-specific marker

If no diagnosis (or fatty liver suspected), obtain all disease-specific markers

Consider hepatic imaging (ultrasonography or CT) to exclude other diseases and/or confirm fatty liver (low attenuation value)

If fatty liver suspected and all disease-specific markers negative or normal, follow serial AST or ALT during period of dieting

If specific disease is diagnosed, consider liver biopsy for confirmation and staging

Consider liver biopsy when abnormality persists longer than 3–6 months and diagnosis is uncertain

If AST or ALT normalize with weight loss, presume fatty liver

Figure 5.1 Evaluation of isolated (or predominant) mild elevation of AST concentration. AST, aspartate aminotransferase. Reproduced from Keeffe (94) by permission of The American Gastroenterological Association.

fulminant hepatic failure. In patients with extrahepatic biliary tract obstruction, serum levels of AST and ALT may increase to greater than 300 U/L but usually decline rapidly after peaking within the first 24–48 h after obstruction. Although elevations in aminotransferase levels may be the first clue to liver disease and screening has proved useful for detecting subclinical liver disease in asymptomatic persons, patients with normal levels may also have significant liver damage. For instance, recent studies have demonstrated that asymptomatic carriers of hepatitis C virus (HCV) may have evidence of chronic hepatitis and even cirrhosis on liver biopsy despite having repeatedly normal aminotransferase levels. Another characteristic feature of chronic hepatitis C is the episodic, fluctuating pattern of serum ALT levels: periods of elevated enzyme activity alternating with periods of normal or near-normal ALT levels.

The ratio of AST to ALT may be helpful diagnostically, particularly in patients with alcoholic liver disease who characteristically have a ratio of greater than 2.0 (**Fig. 5.2**). The reason for the elevation of the AST level out of proportion to the ALT level appears to be a differential reduction in hepatic ALT caused by a deficiency of the cofactor, pyridoxine-5-phosphate. In fact, oral administration of this cofactor to patients with alcoholic liver disease has been shown to result in an increase in serum ALT levels. Although an AST:ALT ratio of greater than 2.0 strongly suggests the diagnosis of alcoholic liver disease, it does not preclude other diagnoses. Other biochemical clues to the presence of alcoholic liver disease include elevations of

GGT, erythrocyte mean corpuscular volume and desialyated transferrin. Conversely, NAFLD is typically associated with an ALT level greater than the AST level. In viral hepatitis, the ratio of AST to ALT is also usually less than 1.0 but may rise to values greater than 1.0 as cirrhosis develops.

It is important to note that certain clinical situations are associated with relatively low levels of aminotransferases. Yauda and associates have shown that values higher than 20 U/L are definitely abnormal and possibly indicative of liver disease in patients undergoing hemodialysis, which suggests that the upper normal limits of AST and ALT in these patients should be reduced considerably. There is considerable evidence that hepatitis C viremia without biochemical evidence of hepatic dysfunction is common in patients with renal failure. **Figure 5.3** outlines the evaluation of elevated liver enzymes in hemodialysis patients. The reduced sensitivity of antibody to HCV (anti-HCV) in this population warrants direct measurement of serum HCV RNA when clinical suspicion of HCV infection is high.

Clinical studies of patients with chronic, asymptomatic and mild-to-moderate elevation of AST or ALT is limited, particularly studies that include liver biopsy as part of the evaluation process. One of the earliest, most comprehensive studies of the significance of mild-to-moderate elevation of AST is a Scandinavian investigation by Hultcrantz et al (1986) of 149 asymptomatic patients, all of whom had elevation of liver enzymes for >6 months and underwent liver biopsy. These patients were not only asymptomatic, but also had normal physical examinations; the remainder of the standard liver profile was normal except for a minority of patients with less than twofold elevation of ALP. The histologic diagnoses on liver biopsy included:

- fatty liver in 63%;
- CAH (chronic active hepatitis) or CPH (chronic persistent hepatitis) presumably viral, in 20%; and
- miscellaneous liver disease in 17%.

Fatty liver was associated with high body weight, alcohol intake, hyperlipidemia and diabetes mellitus. These patients had all undergone evaluation with hepatic imaging and a number of immunoserologic tests. The authors found that hepatitis B serology, serum ferritin and α_1-antitrypsin levels were the only useful specific tests. It is important to note that this study was performed prior to the availability of serologic testing for HCV infection with anti-HCV.

In a study of the cause of an elevated ALT in 100 blood donors, which represents a different population from patients referred to a tertiary care center, as in the above investigation, presumptive fatty liver was once again the most common diagnosis based on exclusion of viral, autoimmune and genetic diseases and on the association with daily alcohol use and/or obesity. This study did not include liver biopsies as part of the evaluation, but relied on clinical diagnoses. A practical finding of this study was that ALT was elevated on only one occasion in one-third of the subjects, i.e. at the time of blood donation and elevated intermittently (36%) or persistently (28%) in the other two-thirds of the subjects. These same authors later applied testing for anti-HCV by the second generation enzyme-linked immunosorbent assay-2 (ELISA-2) to this group, and anti-HCV was detected in 17 of the 100 blood donors. The anti-HCV positive donors had a higher mean ALT, a persistent rather than transient or intermittent ALT elevation, more often admitted use of injection drugs, were lean rather than obese and were less likely to be regular alcohol

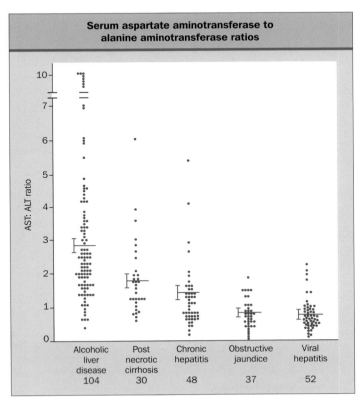

Figure 5.2 Serum aspartate aminotransferase (AST) to alanine aminotransferase (ALT) ratios in patients with biopsy proven liver disease. Of patients with alcoholic liver disease, 70% had ratios greater than 2.0 compared with 26% of patients with postnecrotic cirrhosis, 8% with chronic active hepatitis, 4% with viral hepatitis, and none with obstructive jaundice. Reproduced from Cohen et al (79) by permission of Springer Science and Business Media.

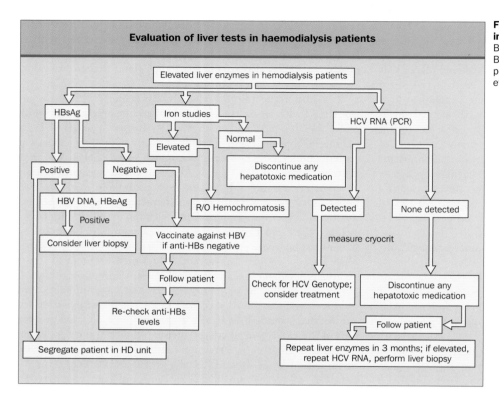

Figure 5.3 Algorithm for evaluation of liver tests in a hemodialysis (HD) patient. HBsAg, hepatitis B surface antigen; anti-HBs, antibody to hepatitis B surface antigen; HBV, hepatitis B virus; PCR, polymerase chain reaction. Modified from Rosen et al (96).

drinkers. Thus, chronic hepatitis C is more often the explanation of asymptomatic elevation of ALT in persons who are not obese or use alcohol, while anti-HCV is likely to be negative in those subjects who are obese or drink alcohol regularly. These latter patients are more likely to have fatty liver.

The two studies cited above document that fatty liver, now referred to as NAFLD is frequently the cause of mildly elevated levels of AST or ALT (as well as ALP and GGT). This observation appears to be especially true in the healthy blood donor population, where obesity has been proposed as the major cause of persistent elevation of ALT. NAFLD is often associated with obesity, hyperlipidemia, or diabetes mellitus and can be predicted by reduced attenuation values on computed tomography (CT) of the liver. A study by Palmer & Schaffner (1990) of overweight adults with abnormal aminotransferases and no primary liver disease by specific immunoserologic testing demonstrated that weight reduction of >10% corrected abnormal LFTs and decreased hepatosplenomegaly. These authors recommend that, after other causes of liver disease are eliminated by clinical and biochemical parameters, weight reduction should be tried before proceeding with more expensive and invasive tests, such as liver biopsy.

The prevalence and clinicopathologic features of NAFLD, with or without NASH, are now recognized as a major cause of liver disease in the USA. NASH has traditionally been thought to most commonly affect obese, diabetic, especially insulin-resistant, middle-aged women, but recent experience documents that men are also affected and obesity and diabetes may be absent. In some patients, it may progress to clinically significant liver disease, including decompensated cirrhosis requiring liver transplantation and even hepatocellular carcinoma. AST and ALT levels are mildly to moderately elevated, while bilirubin, albumin and prothrombin time are usually normal. The absence

of elevated AST and ALT levels does not rule out the possibility of histologically significant liver disease, however. This entity is pertinent to this review, since 48–100% of patients have no symptoms of liver disease. Thus, liver biopsy is essential to establish a diagnosis and/or stage the disease in this population of patients with a negative immunoserologic work-up. Pathologic features of NASH include acinar zone 3 (central vein) injury with hepatocellular fat accumulation, Mallory bodies and perivenular and pericellular fibrosis. This lesion may be histologically indistinguishable from that of alcoholic liver disease. Fibrosis or cirrhosis occurs in approximately 15–50% of patients.

In a large prospective study of French blood donors from 1987 to 1989, non-A, non-B hepatitis was assessed with third generation tests for anti-HCV and serum HCV RNA by polymerase chain reaction (PCR) and fatty liver was once again found to be common. In this study, 184 subjects (1.7%) had elevated ALT×2 over 6 months and 88 agreed to follow-up. Of these, 45 subjects had persistently elevated ALT over 6 months and underwent liver biopsy. Findings included:

- fatty liver in 29/45 (65%), with 23 cases explained by alcohol, obesity or hyperlipidemia; ALT normalized in 22 patients with dietary management; and
- chronic hepatitis in 16/45 (35%); 12 of 16 patients had documented chronic hepatitis C, but 4 patients remained unexplained, suggesting the possibility of another virus (non-A, non-B, non-C virus).

A unique condition that can present with persistently elevated aminotransferase levels and/or fatty liver is heterozygous familial hypobetalipoproteinemia. This entity is related to apolipoprotein B (ApoB) deficiency, which can be suspected when hypocholesterolemia is found on a routine chemistry panel. These patients are generally otherwise healthy.

Finally, elevated serum ALT levels may be unexplained or associated with muscle injury from rigorous exercise in individuals undergoing military basic training. In a study of US Air Force recruits, 99 of 19 877 individuals (0.5%) had an ALT elevation greater than 55 U/L. In the majority (88%) of subjects, the cause of the elevation was not apparent after clinical evaluation and screening serologic and immunologic laboratory tests. The elevated ALT was presumably related to individual variation from a non-Gaussian distribution, non-hepatic (muscular) disease, or undetected liver disease.

The development and current wide availability of testing for viral, autoimmune and genetic liver diseases now generally results in a specific etiologic diagnosis of liver disease prior to biopsy. For example, serologic markers for hepatitis A, B, C and D are commercially available and facilitate the specific diagnosis of acute and chronic viral hepatitis (**Table 5.3**). Seroprevalence studies show that 1.4% of the US population is reactive to anti-HCV, with 70–85% being viremic, and approximately 0.3% of the US population is HBsAg carriers. Hemochromatosis is a relatively common disease that occurs in 1 in 250 individuals in the general population and can be diagnosed by the finding of an elevated serum ferritin and a high percentage iron saturation, or the detection of the *HFE* gene. A subsequent liver biopsy with measurement of quantitative iron content and calculation of the hepatic iron index provides confirmation of disease. Wilson disease is rare, occurring in approximately 1 in 30 000 population, but can be specifically diagnosed by the finding of low serum ceruloplasmin and high urinary copper excretion. Liver biopsy with determination of quantitative copper content provides a confirmatory diagnosis. α_1-antitrypsin deficiency can be diagnosed by the finding of a reduced α_1-antitrypsin level, typically to 20% of normal, and confirmed by phenotyping or by liver biopsy showing the characteristic periodic acid-Schiff, diastase-resistant inclusions.

Most common liver diseases	
Common	*Uncommon*
Non-alcoholic fatty liver disease	Drug-induced liver disease
Chronic hepatitis C	Autoimmune hepatitis
Chronic hepatitis B	α_1-antitrypsin deficiency
Alcoholic liver disease	Wilson disease
Hemochromatosis	Miscellaneous conditions

Table 5.4 Most common liver diseases.

A reasonable diagnostic approach to the evaluation of a patient with a mild isolated (or predominant) elevation of AST (and/or ALT) is shown in Figure 5.1. In the application of the above algorithm, the most common hepatic conditions should be kept in mind, i.e. fatty liver, chronic hepatitis C, chronic hepatitis B, alcoholic liver disease, and hemochromatosis, as should those that are less common, i.e. drug-induced liver disease, autoimmune hepatitis, α_1-antitrypsin deficiency and Wilson disease (**Table 5.4**). Depending on logistic and cost issues, an asymptomatic patient with mildly elevated ALT might be evaluated sequentially for the above two groups of liver conditions rather than in a shotgun fashion.

TESTS THAT REFLECT CHOLESTATIC LIVER INJURY

Alkaline phosphatase and γ-glutamyltranspeptidase

The usual markers to identify cholestasis are ALP and GGT, with 5' nucleotidase and leucine aminopeptidase used less

Types of hepatitis viruses						
	Hepatitis A	*Hepatitis B*	*Hepatitis C*	*Hepatitis D*	*Hepatitis E*	*Hepatitis G*
Virus	HAV	HBV	HCV	HDV	HEV	HGV
Size	27 nm	42 nm	30–60 nm	35 nm	37 nm	30–60 nm
Genome	ssRNA	dsDNA	ssRNA	ssRNA	ssRNA	ssRNA
Antigens	HAAg*	HBsAg HBeAg HBcAg*	HCAg*	HDAg*	HEAg*	None available
Antibodies	IgM anti-HAV Anti-HAV	IgM anti-HBc Anti-HBc Anti-HBs Anti-HBe	Anti-HCV	IgM anti-HDV Anti-HDV	anti-HEV	None available
Viral markers	HAV RNA*	HBV DNA DNA polymerase	HCV RNA†	HDV RNA	none	HGV RNA

*Research test.
†See the text for a discussion of HCV genotyping.
ss, Single stranded.
Modified from Lindsay et al in Kaplowitz (96).

Table 5.3 Types of hepatitis viruses.

commonly. Serum ALP is the name applied to a group of enzymes that catalyze the hydrolysis of phosphate esters at an alkaline pH. The enzymes are widely distributed and may originate from bone, liver, intestine, or placenta. In children and adolescents, in whom bone growth is active, the serum ALP may increase up to threefold. In patients with hepatobiliary disorders, elevated ALP levels result from increased hepatic production with leakage into the serum, rather than failure to clear or excrete circulating ALP. Markedly elevated levels of ALP suggest the possibility of disorders such as extrahepatic biliary obstruction, infiltrative diseases of the liver, including primary and metastatic tumors, primary biliary cirrhosis (PBC), primary sclerosing cholangitis, or drug-induced cholestasis. The degree of elevation does not differentiate extra- and intrahepatic etiologies of cholestasis. In partial extrahepatic biliary obstruction, ALP may be elevated in the absence of hyperbilirubinemia or pruritus. ALP may also be mildly elevated in parenchymal liver disease, particularly alcoholic liver disease.

Mild to moderate ALP abnormalities are seen in infiltrative processes such as amyloidosis, granulomatous disease and some neoplasms. Patients with Hodgkin disease and renal cell carcinoma may have elevated ALP without any direct involvement of bone or the hepatobiliary system. Mild elevation of ALP is also common in physiologic situations, such as pregnancy and physiologic bone growth and is seen not uncommonly in subjects >50 years of age. In most cases, the ALP elevation is evident on the basis of history and physical examination and hepatic imaging tests.

Low serum levels of ALP have been associated with congenital hypophosphatasia, hypothyroidism, pernicious anemia and zinc deficiency. Moreover, patients with fulminant Wilson disease complicated by hemolysis can present with undetectable levels of serum ALP. Whether this is due to replacement of the cofactor, zinc, by copper and subsequent inactivation of ALP remains unknown.

The significance of isolated mild elevation of ALP (<1.5–2 × normal) is problematic and has undergone only limited investigation. Rubenstein et al (1986) found that most ambulatory patients with unexplained ALP elevation detected during multiphasic screening had no overt disease during a 2-year follow-up period. Lieberman & Phillips (1990) evaluated the clinical outcome of hospitalized patients with isolated ALP elevation. A total of 87 patients with isolated ALP were identified and 45 of these patients (52%) had normalization of ALP, usually within 1–3 months. For 12 patients (14%) there was no apparent explanation for the transient rise in ALP, while miscellaneous diagnoses explained the transient rise in the remainder of patients. In the 42 patients with persistent ALP elevation, 14 had terminal malignancies and all but 7 of the remaining patients had obvious diagnoses.

Finally, elevation of ALP >1.5–2-fold, particularly when associated with abnormalities of other liver tests, points to the presence of an underlying hepatobiliary disease. A reasonable diagnostic approach to the evaluation of a patient with a mild isolated or predominant elevation of ALP is shown in **Figure 5.4**.

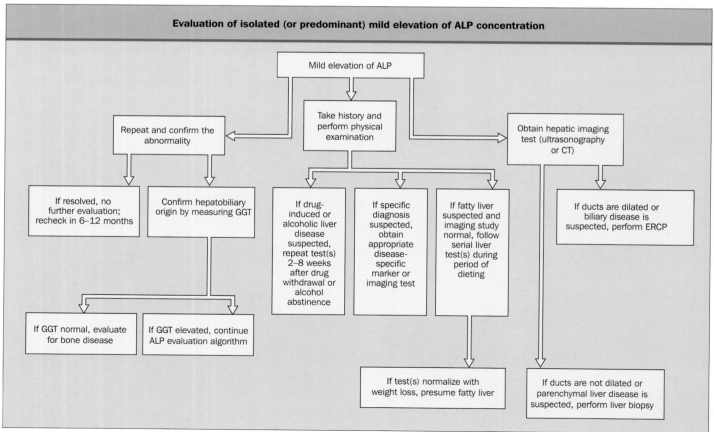

Figure 5.4 Evaluation of isolated (or predominant) mild elevation of ALP concentration. ERCP=endoscopic retrograde cholangiopancreatography. Reproduced from Keeffe (94) by permission of The American Gastroenterological Association.

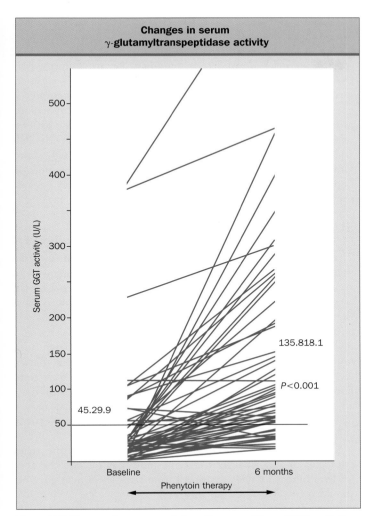

Figure 5.5 Changes in serum γ-glutamyltranspeptidase (GGT) activity. Changes monitored from baseline to 6 months of phenytoin therapy in 58 patients. Of the total group, 52 patients demonstrated a rise and six patients a fall in GGT activity. Reproduced from Keeffe et al (86) by permission of Springer Science and Business Media.

Serum GGT is useful to confirm whether an elevated ALP is secondary to hepatobiliary disease or is of extrahepatic origin. Some automated chemistry batteries include GGT, which may lead to the clinical problem of whether or not to evaluate an isolated elevation. Unfortunately, because the enzyme is ubiquitous, an elevated GGT has poor specificity and may be due to induction by alcohol, phenytoin (**Fig. 5.5**), or other drugs. Although the diagnostic yield of an isolated elevation of GGT has not been studied, the consensus is that extensive evaluation is usually not appropriate beyond a routine history, physical examination and general chemistry panel. 5'-Nucleotidase, on the other hand, is specific for liver disease and its measurement is particularly helpful in diagnosing liver disease in children and pregnancy, those clinical settings in which ALP is elevated physiologically.

TESTS THAT REFLECT HEPATIC SYNTHETIC FUNCTION

Bilirubin

Bilirubin is an endogenous organic anion derived primarily from the degradation of hemoglobin released from red blood cells.

Hyperbilirubinemia is classified as either unconjugated or conjugated. (Ch. 6). In patients with hyperbilirubinemia due to hepatocellular dysfunction or cholestasis, the serum bilirubin is predominantly conjugated and hence water soluble, allowing easy renal excretion. Extreme hyperbilirubinemia (i.e. >25 mg/dL) usually signifies severe liver disease in association with another cause of unconjugated hyperbilirubinemia (i.e. hemolysis) or renal dysfunction.

The level of serum bilirubin has been utilized to predict the natural history of specific liver diseases. Dickson and others have reported that serum bilirubin is the most important variable for predicting survival in patients with PBC. The level of hyperbilirubinemia also has prognostic significance in patients with fulminant hepatic failure and acute alcoholic hepatitis, comprising the majority of the discriminant function scores derived by Maddrey and associates. Moreover, recent studies of candidates for liver transplantation have shown that serum bilirubin is an important component of the Model for End-stage Liver Disease (MELD) scale and a reliable measure of disease severity and mortality risk in patients with end-stage liver disease awaiting liver transplantation. The MELD scale is a tool originating from the Mayo Clinic, originally used to determine prognosis after a TIPS (transjugular intrahepatic shunt), and now applied to liver transplantation for assessment of clinical status while waiting for transplantation. MELD has replaced CPT score as a predictor of pre and post transplant survival and disease severity for patients awaiting liver transplantation.

SERUM ALBUMIN

Albumin is quantitatively the most important circulating protein synthesized by the liver, accounting for three-quarters of the plasma colloid oncotic pressure. The liver is the only site of synthesis with approximately 12–15 g produced daily in the normal adult. Plasma albumin concentration is decreased in severe acute and chronic liver disease and is one of the criteria for the CTP (Child-Turcotte-Pugh) classification widely used to grade severity of cirrhosis. In addition to liver disease, hypo-albuminemia may also result from gastrointestinal and renal losses, hormonal changes, increased catabolism and hyper-gammaglobulinemia, which may lead to feedback inhibition of albumin synthesis. Prealbumin (or thyroid-binding prealbumin) appears to be a more sensitive index of hepatic protein synthesis than albumin, particularly in acute liver failure because its half-life is shorter (1.9 days).

PROTHROMBIN TIME AND SERUM COAGULATION FACTOR LEVELS

With the exception of factor VIII, all the clotting factors are synthesized within hepatocytes. The clotting factors that determine prothrombin time (PT) are short-lived (hours), making the test suited for evaluating acute liver injury; indeed, PT is one of the key elements in prognostic scores for fulminant hepatic failure and acute alcoholic hepatitis. In general, a prolongation of ≥ 2 s more than control is considered abnormal. Unfortunately, the PT is not a sensitive index of chronic liver disease, because it may be normal even in patients with cirrhosis; moreover, its specificity is low in the presence of malabsorption, because factors II, VII and X are dependent on vitamin K. It is now generally accepted that the international normalized ratio should replace the PT, because the latter is based on different types of thromboplastin that have considerable variation in different countries.

OTHER QUANTITATIVE TESTS OF LIVER FUNCTION

Patients with essentially normal conventional serum liver tests may have significantly diminished hepatic function; conversely, hepatic function may be well preserved in some patients with abnormal serum liver tests. Although quantitation of functional reserve is not performed routinely in clinical practice, quantitative serum liver tests may provide useful data regarding the prognosis and effects of therapeutic interventions. Some examples of these tests are described below.

Indocyanine green (ICG) is a dye removed from the circulation by the liver after intravenous injection. Because it is taken up exclusively by hepatocytes, the clearance of low doses of ICG is used to measure liver blood flow. With administration of higher doses of ICG, the uptake process becomes saturated; the maximal removal of ICG can be calculated and this reflects functional hepatic mass rather than blood flow in the liver.

The metabolism of aminopyrine is sensitive to alterations in the redox state, thyroid disease, infection, amino acid deficiency and glutathione deficiency as well as folate and vitamin B_{12} deficiency. The aminopyrine breath test has been used to predict short-term prognosis and mortality in patients with alcoholic hepatitis, and in one study was a better predictor of outcome than standard serum liver tests. The caffeine breath test is comparable to the aminopyrine test, except without the need for radioisotope usage. Caffeine clearance appears to be impaired in advanced liver disease and has limited utility for screening mild or early liver disease.

The ^{14}C-galactose breath test is a simple test that may provide good prognostic information in fulminant hepatic failure where the galactose elimination capacity (GEC) is reduced. In addition, serial measurements of the GEC were more accurate in predicting death in patients with PBC than the Mayo score. However, in multivariate analysis of survival in other patients with cirrhosis, determination of GEC appeared to provide little additional information compared with the Child-Pugh score. Unlike the ICG, the GEC is not suitable for assessment of hepatic reserve before hepatic resection for malignancy because some tumors may metabolize galactose.

SUMMARY

The differential diagnosis of abnormal serum liver tests includes hepatic and extrahepatic conditions and is greatly narrowed by a comprehensive history and physical examination and by the recognition of classic patterns of liver injury. The limitations of these liver tests, including problems with specificity and sensitivity, must always be taken into account. Patients with essentially normal conventional serum liver tests may have significantly impaired hepatic function; conversely, hepatic function may be well preserved in some patients with abnormal serum liver tests. Furthermore, other indices of hepatic function, such as bilirubin and PT, are important prognostic indicators of the natural history of specific conditions such as PBC, alcoholic hepatitis and end-stage liver disease.

Serologic tests are invaluable tools in diagnosing the many etiologies of abnormal liver enzymes and may obviate the need for liver biopsy in many cases. All abnormalities of liver enzymes should be investigated.

FURTHER READING

General
Moseley FH. Evaluation of abnormal liver function tests. Med Clin North Am 1996; 80:888.

Serum aminotransferases
Ahmed A, Keeffe EB. Asymptomatic elevation of aminotransferase levels and fatty liver secondary to heterozygous hypobetalipoproteinemia. Am J Gastroenterol 1998; 93:2598–2599.

Cohen JA, Kaplan MM. The SGOT/SGPT ratio – an indicator of alcoholic liver disease. Am J Dig Dis 1979; 24:835–838.

Daniel S, Ben-Menachem T, Vasudevan G, et al. Prospective evaluation of unexplained chronic liver transaminase abnormalities in asymptomatic and symptomatic patients. Am J Gastroenterol 1999; 94:3010–3014. *Fatty liver is the most frequent cause of elevated aminotransferases in asymptomatic patients.*

Flora KD, Keeffe EB. Evaluation of mildly abnormal liver tests in asymptomatic patients. J Insur Med 1990; 22:264–267.

Flora KD, Keeffe EB. Significance of mildly elevated liver tests on screening biochemistry profiles. J Insur Med 1990; 22:206–210.

Friedman LS, Dienstag JL, Watkins E, et al. Evaluation of blood donors with elevated serum alanine aminotransferase levels. Ann Intern Med 1987; 107:137–144.

Hultcrantz R, Glaumann H, Lindberg G, et al. Liver investigation in 149 asymptomatic patients with moderately elevated activities of serum aminotransferases. Scand J Gastroenterol 1986; 21:109–113.

Katkov WN, Friedman LS, Cody H, et al. Elevated serum alanine aminotransferase levels in blood donors: the contribution of hepatitis C virus. Ann Intern Med 1991; 115:882–884.

Keeffe EB. Diagnostic approach to mild elevation of liver enzyme levels. Gastrointest Dis Today 1994; 3:1–9.

Kundrotas LW, Clement DJ. Serum alanine aminotransferase (ALT) elevation in asymptomatic US Air Force basic trainee blood donors. Dig Dis Sci 1994; 38:2145–2150.

Lindsay KL, Hoofnagle JH. Serologic tests for viral hepatitis. In: Kaplowitz N, ed. Liver and biliary diseases, 2nd edn. Baltimore: Williams & Wilkins; 1996:221–234.

Mofrad P, Contos MJ, Haque M, et al. Clinical and histologic spectrum of non-alcoholic fatty liver disease associated with normal ALT values. Hepatology 2003; 37:1286–1292. *Points out that significant liver disease due to NAFLD may be present in the face of normal serum aminotransferases.*

Neuschwander-Tetri BA, Caldwell SH. Nonalcoholic steatohepatitis: Summary of an AASLD Single Topic Conference. Hepatology 2003; 39:1201–1219.

Palmer M, Shaffner F. Effect of weight reduction on hepatic abnormalities in overweight patients. Gastroenterology 1990; 99:1408–1413.

Pratt DS, Kaplan MM. Evaluation of abnormal liver-enzymes results in asymptomatic patients. N Engl J Med 2000; 342:1266–1271.

Rosen HR, Friedman LS, Martin P. Hepatitis C in renal dialysis and transplant patients. Viral Hepatitis Rev 1996; 2:97–110.

Williams ALB, Hoofnagle JH. Ratio of serum aspartate to alanine aminotransferase in chronic hepatitis: relationship to cirrhosis. Gastroenterology 1988; 95:734–739. *Documents that as liver disease due to viral hepatitis progresses to cirrhosis, AST becomes higher than ALT.*

Yasuda K, Okuda K, Endo N, et al. Hypoaminotransferasemia in patients undergoing long-term hemodialysis: clinical and biochemical appraisal. Gastroenterology 1995; 109:1295-1300.

Serum alkaline phosphates and γ-glutamyltranspeptidase

Keeffe EB, Sunderland MC, Gabourel JD. Serum γ-glutamyl transpeptidase activity in patients receiving chronic phenytoin therapy. Dig Dis Sci 1986; 31:1056–1061.

Lieberman D, Phillips D. 'Isolated' elevation of alkaline phosphatase: significance in hospitalized patients. J Clin Gastroenterol 1990; 12:415–419.

Rubenstein LV, Ward NC, Greenfield S. In pursuit of the abnormal serum alkaline phosphatase: a clinical dilemma. J Gen Intern Med 1986; 1:38–43.

Wolf PL. Clinical significance of an increased or decreased serum alkaline phosphatase level. Arch Pathol Lab Med 1978; 102:497–501.

Other diagnostic tests

Czaja AJ, Freese DK. Diagnosis and treatment of autoimmune hepatitis. Hepatology 2002; 36:479–497.

Dickson ER, Grambsch PM, Fleming TR, et al. Prognosis in primary biliary cirrhosis: model for decision making. Hepatology 1989; 10:1–7.

Kamath PS, Wiesner RH, Malinchoc M, et al. A model to predict survival in patients with end-stage liver disease. Hepatology 2001; 33:464–470. *Description of MELD score which is now widely used to allocate livers for transplantation.*

Kim WR, Wiesner RH, Poterucha JJ, et al. Adaptation of the Mayo primary biliary cirrhosis natural history model for application in liver transplant candidates. Liver Transpl 2000; 6:489–494.

Maddrey WC, Boitnott JK, Bedine MS, et al. Corticosteroid therapy of alcoholic hepatitis. Gastroenterology 1978; 75:193–199.

Marcellin P, Martinot-Peignoux M, Gabriel F, et al. Chronic non-B, non-C hepatitis among blood donors assessed with HCV third generation tests and polymerase chain reaction. J Hepatol 1993; 19:167–170.

Wiesner, RH, McDiarmid SV, Kamath PS, et al. MELD and PELD: Application of survival models to liver allocation. Liver Transpl 2001; 7:567–580.

CHAPTER
6

Jaundice

Steven D. Lidofsky

INTRODUCTION

Jaundice, which gives rise to a yellow appearance of the skin, occurs as a consequence of bilirubin deposition into subcutaneous tissues. In darker skinned individuals (or early in the course of jaundice), this yellow discoloration may be more readily apparent in the sclerae and mucous membranes. Yellow pigmentation of the skin can also result from excessive ingestion of vegetables that are abundant in the content of carotene or other carotenoids. Distinction of these conditions from true jaundice is generally straightforward, however, as scleral icterus and hyperbilirubinemia are not seen with ingestion of vegetable products. Jaundice is classically associated with liver and biliary tract disease, but it is important to emphasize that there are extrahepatobiliary causes of jaundice as well.

The cause of jaundice can be identified in the vast majority of cases. Indeed, with a simple history, physical examination and routine biochemical screening tests, the presence versus absence of biliary tract obstruction can be correctly distinguished 75% of the time. Additional tests are often necessary to make a precise diagnosis, however. The diversity of currently available laboratory and imaging techniques requires judicious selection in order to minimize cost and patient discomfort.

This chapter covers five principal areas. It begins with a discussion of bilirubin formation and metabolism, especially as it relates to the pathophysiology of jaundice. It then presents a rational clinical classification of the causes of jaundice. Some of the causes described are delineated with brevity, as they are discussed in greater detail in other chapters in this book. This section is followed by clinical clues to various types of jaundice. With this as a background, the chapter moves toward a presentation of the strengths and weaknesses of different modalities for the diagnosis of jaundice. The chapter concludes with a general approach, built upon the conceptual framework already established, to the management of the jaundiced patient.

PATHOPHYSIOLOGY

Overview

Jaundice is a manifestation of an elevated serum bilirubin concentration. Serum bilirubin levels are generally less than 1–1.5 mg/dL (17–25 μmol/L) and jaundice is not usually detectable until bilirubin concentration exceeds 3 mg/dL (50 μmol/L). The level of bilirubin elevation is a critical determinant of overall prognosis in several hepatobiliary disorders. These include acute liver failure, alcoholic hepatitis, primary biliary cirrhosis and sclerosing cholangitis. An understanding of the origins of an elevated bilirubin concentration is particularly germane to the management of these clinical entities, as is

elucidating the cause of jaundice in patients who do not have a defined illness.

Bilirubin formation

Bilirubin is a potentially toxic compound that is an end-product of heme degradation. It has the chemical structure of a tetra-pyrrole, which renders it highly water-insoluble due to internal hydrogen bonding. As such, the elimination of bilirubin from the circulation requires chemical conversion in the liver to water soluble conjugates that are normally excreted into bile. This multistep process is schematically illustrated in **Figure 6.1**. An abnormality at any of these steps can lead to hyperbilirubinemia and jaundice.

Daily bilirubin production is considerable. Most (70–80%) is derived from hemoglobin degradation from senescent erythrocytes and a small proportion comes from premature destruction of developing erythrocytes in the bone marrow (ineffective erythropoiesis). The liver represents the dominant source of the remaining 20–30% of bilirubin formed. The principal intracellular sources for this are heme-containing enzymes such as catalase and cytochrome oxidases. Other heme-containing proteins (e.g. myoglobin) are present in extrahepatic tissues. However, the overall contribution of such proteins to bilirubin production is minimal due to their low mass or slow degradation rate.

Heme is converted to bilirubin via a two-step process (**Fig. 6.2**). First, heme is converted to biliverdin by the microsomal enzyme heme oxygenase. Second, biliverdin is converted to bilirubin by the cytosolic enzyme biliverdin reductase. Degradation of heme derived from erythrocyte hemoglobin primarily takes place in macrophages in the spleen, liver and bone marrow. By contrast, hepatocytes produce bilirubin from heme derived from free hemoglobin, haptoglobin-bound hemoglobin and methemalbumin.

Bilirubin metabolism

Bilirubin metabolism is a complex process in which several inherited disorders and associated gene products have been identified. This is illustrated in Figure 6.1. Bilirubin circulates in plasma tightly bound to albumin. Extraction of bilirubin from plasma occurs in the liver, where bilirubin is metabolized and transported into bile through the actions of hepatocytes.

Bilirubin uptake occurs at the sinusoidal (basolateral) membrane of hepatocytes. The mechanism appears to be carrier-mediated. This process is competitively inhibited by certain organic anions such as bromsulfophthalein (BSP) and indocyanine green. In addition, the drug rifampin (rifampicin) may lead to hyperbilirubinemia by a similar process. A candidate gene product, the organic anion transporting polypeptide OATP2 (SLC21A6),

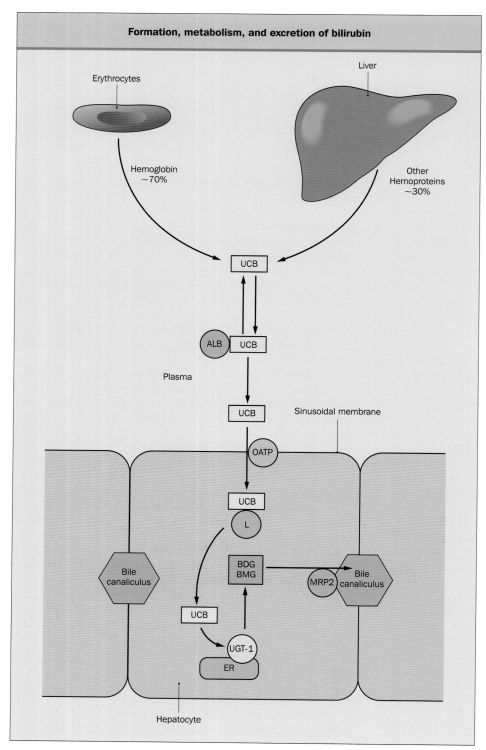

Formation, metabolism, and excretion of bilirubin

Erythrocytes

Liver

Hemoglobin
~70%

Other
Hemoproteins
~30%

UCB

ALB UCB

Plasma

UCB

Sinusoidal membrane

OATP

UCB

L

Bile
canaliculus

BDG
BMG

MRP2 Bile
canaliculus

UCB

UGT-1

ER

Hepatocyte

Figure 6.1 Formation, metabolism and excretion of bilirubin. Unconjugated bilirubin (UCB), formed from breakdown of hemoglobin from erythrocytes and heme-containing proteins from other tissues (principally liver), circulates in plasma bound to albumin (ALB). It is taken up by the hepatocyte (possibly via a member of the OATP family of transport proteins), diffuses through the cytosol bound to ligandins (L) and undergoes conjugation in the endoplasmic reticulum (ER) by bilirubin glucuronyltransferase (UGT-1). Mono- and diglucuronidated bilirubins (BMG, BDG) are exported into the bile canaliculus via the transport protein MRP2.

has been proposed to mediate sinusoidal bilirubin uptake, but its role remains controversial.

Once sinusoidal uptake has occurred, bilirubin is directed to the endoplasmic reticulum by several cytosolic binding proteins, which serve to facilitate intracellular diffusion of this hydrophobic molecule. These cytosolic proteins include the ligandins and fatty acid binding protein. Bilirubin conjugation occurs in the endoplasmic reticulum. There it is principally converted to water-soluble monoglucuronides and diglucuronides via covalent linkage with uridine diphosphate (UDP)-glucuronic acid. This is accomplished by the enzyme bilirubin UDP-glucuronosyl transferase (bilirubin UGT-1), the *HUG-Br1* gene product. Conjugation serves to convert hydrophobic bilirubin into a water-soluble form that can be readily excreted into bile.

Three inherited disorders of bilirubin metabolism are associated with defects in bilirubin UGT-1 activity (**Fig. 6.3**). In

Inherited disorders of hepatic bilirubin metabolism and transport					
	Gilbert syndrome	Type I Crigler-Najjar syndrome	Type II Crigler-Najjar syndrome	Dubin-Johnson syndrome	Rotor syndrome
Incidence	<10% of population	Extremely rare	Uncommon	Uncommon	Rare
Genetic defect	Mutations in promoter region of HUG-Br1	Absent HUG-Br1 expression	Mutations in coding region of HUG-Br1	Absent expression of MRP2	Unknown
Inheritance	Autosomal recessive	Autosomal recessive	Autosomal recessive	Autosomal recessive	Autosomal recessive
Mechanism	Decreased bilirubin conjugation	Absent bilirubin conjugation	Markedly decreased bilirubin conjugation	Impaired canalicular excretion of conjugated bilirubin via multispecific anion transporter	Unknown
Serum bilirubin concentration (mg/dL) (µmol/L)	<3–4 (51–68), virtually all unconjugated	Usually >20 (340), unconjugated	Usually <20 (340), virtually all unconjugated	Usually <7 (120), about 50% conjugated	Usually <7 (120), about 50% conjugated
Other laboratory abnormalities	Bilirubin decreases with phenobarbital	No change in bilirubin with phenobarbital	Bilirubin decreases with phenobarbital	Normal total urinary coproporphyrin (>80% type I)	Elevated total urinary coproporphyrin (<80% type I)
Liver histology	Normal	Normal	Normal	Dark pigment, predominantly centrilobular	Normal
Prognosis	Good	Poor, death in infancy from kernicterus unless specific therapy employed	Good	Good	Good
Treatment	None required	Phototherapy initially, liver transplantation necessary for long-term survival	Phenobarbital for marked hyperbilirubinemia	None available; avoid estrogens (worsens hyperbilirubinemia)	None

Table 6.2 Inherited disorders of hepatic bilirubin metabolism and transport.

icteric liver disease is briefly outlined here. Two broad categories of liver disease can be defined: that in which hepatocellular injury is the predominant mechanism; and that in which reduced bile formation (cholestasis) predominates. The latter types of diseases are the most problematic from a diagnostic standpoint, because they are often difficult to distinguish clinically from obstruction of the bile ducts. The following discussion is arbitrarily organized according to the above classification. Clearly, however, there are instances in which hepatocellular injury and cholestasis contribute similarly to the development of jaundice.

Acute hepatocellular injury

A variety of disorders can produce acute or subacute hepatocellular injury, including viral hepatitis, exposure to hepatotoxins, hepatic ischemia and certain metabolic derangements. In these situations there is usually evidence of severe hepatocyte injury with widespread necrosis and/or apoptosis and often associated inflammatory cell infiltration. This severe damage leads to metabolic dysfunction and destruction of excretory mechanisms, resulting in jaundice.

Five major hepatotropic viruses have been isolated. Hepatitis A and E viruses are transmitted enterally. Each typically pro-duces a self-limited illness that does not progress to chronic liver disease. By contrast, hepatitis B, C and D viruses are transmitted parenterally and illness produced by these agents may be prolonged and progress to chronic disease. The diagnosis of each these disorders is aided by serologic testing (see Chs 14, 15 and 16).

Toxins and drugs can produce hepatocellular injury, either in a dose-dependent fashion, or idiosyncratically. The most common agent to produce acute dose-dependent hepatocellular injury is acetaminophen (paracetamol). A wide variety of drugs produce idiosyncratic hepatocellular injury and jaundice. These include isoniazid, HMG-CoA reductase inhibitors and minocycline (see Ch. 32). In a patient with ethanol dependency, alcoholic hepatitis should always be a diagnostic consideration when there is jaundice and biochemical evidence of hepatocellular injury. Of note, alcoholic hepatitis can also have an atypical cholestatic presentation that can create diagnostic confusion (see Ch. 21).

Several forms of hepatic ischemia produce hepatocellular injury and jaundice. These include hepatic ischemia caused by systemic hypotension, and/or hypoxia, or occlusive vascular disorders. Thrombosis of the hepatic veins (Budd-Chiari syndrome) should be suspected in patients with hypercoaguable states and, in particular, myeloproliferative disorders. Hepatic veno-occlusive disease should be suspected in a patient receiving cytotoxic agents in the setting of bone marrow transplantation (see Ch. 30).

Jaundice is a recognized complication of Wilson disease, an inherited disorder of copper excretion into bile with copper overload and hepatocellular injury. Patients with Wilson disease can also develop a Coombs negative hemolytic anemia, which contributes to the disproportionate hyperbilirubinemia that is often present (see Ch. 24). Several mitochondriopathies are associated with impaired fatty acid metabolism and hepato-cellular injury from fatty acid overload. These include Reye syndrome, which classically follows a viral illness in children, valproic acid toxicity and fatty liver of pregnancy.

Chronic hepatocellular injury

Jaundice is a well-recognized indicator of significant hepatic dysfunction in the setting of liver diseases produced by chronic hepatocellular injury. In such situations, there are a variety of pathogenetic mechanisms that cause liver damage. In general, there is hepatocyte necrosis and/or apoptosis, as well as inflammation of varying severity, and progressive hepatic fibrosis that ultimately leads to cirrhosis. The hepatocytes are therefore severely affected at a functional level, and biliary excretion is also substantially affected at both the canalicular and more distal levels due to the grossly deranged architecture. As a rule, jaundice is unusual in chronic hepatocellular injury unless cirrhosis has developed. Although the broad categories of chronic hepato-cellular injury are similar to those of acute injury, there are differences in the specific details. For example, causes of chronic viral hepatitis are largely limited to hepatitis B, C and D viruses. The major hepatotoxin-associated chronic hepatocellular disease is alcoholic cirrhosis, whereas drug toxicity is a much less common cause of chronic as opposed to acute hepatocellular injury. Non-alcoholic fatty liver disease (which is histologically indistinguishable from alcoholic liver disease) has emerged as a leading cause of chronic hepatocellular injury in industrialized nations; it is most prevalent in overweight individuals, in parti-cular those with type 2 diabetes mellitus. The possibility of industrial exposure to toxic compounds such as vinyl chloride should be a diagnostic consideration in jaundiced patients with an appropriate background; carbon tetrachloride, a classic industrial hepatotoxin, is no longer used in the USA.

Two metal storage diseases merit consideration. Wilson disease clearly produces chronic hepatocellular injury (see Ch. 24). However, the most common metal storage disease worldwide is the iron overload disorder genetic hemochromatosis, with an estimated prevalence of 0.5% in Caucasian populations. Hepatocytes are a major target of iron-mediated injury in hemochromatosis, although cholangiocytes can be affected when iron overload is significant (see Ch. 23). Miscellaneous causes of chronic hepatocellular injury include autoimmune hepatitis and α_1-antitrypsin deficiency.

Cholestasis

Cholestasis is a term referring to a reduction in bile flow or bile formation. It can therefore occur anywhere from the sinusoidal membrane of the hepatocyte to the exit of the common bile duct into the duodenum. Thus, cholestasis can be classified as

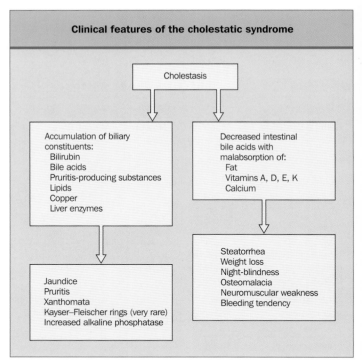

Figure 6.5 Clinical features of the cholestatic syndrome.

intra- or extrahepatic, and there are many causes of each. This classification is adhered to here with a discussion of hepatic disorders that cause intrahepatic cholestasis and of obstruction of the bile ducts that causes extrahepatic cholestasis.

Functionally, if bile flow is interrupted, at whatever level, there will be decreased hepatic secretion of water and organic anions (including bile acids and bilirubin). Normal bile flow is obviously necessary for bilirubin excretion, and thus, many of the pathologic processes affecting overall bile production also affect bilirubin clearance (see Figs 6.1 and 6.4). Morphologically, bile will accumulate in the liver and biliary system and evidence of this can be seen on liver biopsy.

Clinically, there will be features resulting from the decreased secretion and retention of bile, such as jaundice, pruritus and evidence of malabsorption (**Fig. 6.5**).

As indicated, in the diagnosis of jaundice, one of the most difficult differentials is between intra- and extrahepatic cholestasis.

Hepatic disorders with prominent cholestasis (intrahepatic cholestasis)
Overview
The following diseases are characterized by biochemical abnormalities that mimic obstruction of the bile ducts. These disorders have the greatest potential to generate diagnostic con-fusion. Such disorders can be categorized histologically accord-ing to those that infiltrate the liver, those that mainly involve injury to intrahepatic bile ductules or portal triads, and those in which major histologic changes are not evident.

Infiltrative diseases
Many forms of infiltrative liver diseases are often associated with striking cholestasis and jaundice. Infiltrative diseases of the

liver can be conveniently divided into granulomatous diseases, amyloidosis and neoplastic replacement of hepatic parenchyma. The latter should be suspected if there is a known underlying malignancy. These disorders are likely to produce cholestasis by compression or obliteration of small bile ductules. Granulomatous diseases of the liver include:

- infections, such as tuberculosis, *Mycobacterium avium* complex (particularly in the immunocompromised host), leprosy, brucellosis, Q fever, syphilis, fungal diseases, parasitic diseases and mononucleosis;
- toxins, such as beryllium, quinidine, allopurinol and sulfonamides; and
- systemic disorders, including sarcoidosis, lymphoma (in particular, Hodgkin disease) and Wegener granulomatosis.

Tuberculosis and sarcoidosis are the most common forms of granulomatous liver diseases to produce jaundice. Although amyloidosis is in the differential diagnosis of infiltrative liver diseases, jaundice is extremely uncommon in that setting.

Disorders involving bile ductules
Inflammation and loss of small intrahepatic bile ductules are characteristic of primary biliary cirrhosis. When jaundice occurs, the disease is generally advanced. In particular, the presence of a serum bilirubin concentration of greater than 10 mg/dL (170 μmol/L) carries an extremely poor prognosis without liver transplantation. A distinct form of bile ductular injury occurs with hepatic involvement in graft versus host disease, encountered primarily after bone marrow transplantation but occasionally in organ transplant recipients as well. Certain drugs can produce inflammation of the portal tracts with resultant cholestasis. These include chlorpromazine, erythromycin (particularly the estolate salt), chlorpropamide and methimazole. Cholestasis generally resolves within several months after drug discontinuation.

Cholestasis with minimal histologic abnormalities
Jaundice may accompany conditions characterized by minimal hepatocellular injury or histologic abnormalities. The mechanism of cholestasis in these conditions is not well understood at present and may be multifactorial. In benign recurrent cholestasis, an autosomal recessive disorder that has been mapped to the same gene (*PFIC1*) that is mutant in progressive familial intrahepatic cholestasis type I (Byler disease), there is a defect of canalicular secretion of several classes of organic anions, including bile acids, into bile.

Sex hormones can produce a histologically bland intrahepatic cholestasis. Estrogens reduce bile formation through several mechanisms. These include:

- inhibition of the hepatocellular plasma membrane sodium pump, an important modulator of solute transport from blood to bile;
- impaired acidification of intracellular organelles, which may disrupt the targeting of organic anion transporters to their proper membrane domain;
- inhibition of the activity of the bile salt export pump (BSEP) (ABCB11), and;
- decreased membrane fluidity, which may perturb the function of such transporters.

Each of these mechanisms may contribute to jaundice resulting from the use of oral contraceptives. However, jaundice is rare with the low doses of estrogen in modern contraceptives. Anabolic steroids can produce a syndrome that is clinically indistinguishable from that of estrogen-induced cholestasis. Of interest, the anabolic steroids methyltestosterone and norethandrolone may impair the integrity of hepatocellular microfilaments and thus increase back diffusion of biliary solutes through tight junctions into serum.

The features of cholestasis associated with total parenteral nutrition (TPN) can resemble those of cholestasis associated with estrogens and anabolic steroids. However steatohepatitis can also be seen with TPN. It has been proposed that TPN-induced cholestasis is also related to an altered enterohepatic circulation as well as diminished neuroendocrine stimulation of bile flow.

Cholestasis and jaundice may also develop during bacterial infections. Several mechanisms have been proposed, each related to cytokines, including tumor necrosis factor-α and interleukin-1β released during infection. Tumor necrosis factor-α reduces expression of MRP2, interleukin-1β reduces expression of BSEP, and each reduces expression of the basolateral bile acid uptake protein NTCP (SLC10A1), all of which result in decreased bile flow. Sepsis-related cholestasis in the critically ill patient may be extremely difficult to distinguish from obstruction of the bile ducts. Helpful diagnostic clues are discussed below.

Atypical presentations of cholestasis
Viral hepatitis may on occasion produce profound cholestasis with marked pruritus. Unless there are risk factors for viral hepatitis, no features reliably distinguish this disorder from those of other cholestatic syndromes or biliary tract obstruction. A high level of suspicion and appropriate serologies will aid in establishing the diagnosis. The course can be quite prolonged. Similarly, alcoholic hepatitis can uncommonly have a cholestatic presentation. This is one setting in which urgent liver biopsy may be required to make the diagnosis.

Jaundice in pregnancy
Several cholestatic disorders associated with pregnancy merit discussion. Each of these characteristically occurs in the third trimester. Intrahepatic cholestasis in pregnancy typically presents with pruritus. Infrequently, it is associated with jaundice. It generally resolves within 2 weeks of delivery and tends to recur with subsequent pregnancies. Two far more serious syndromes are acute fatty liver of pregnancy and pre-eclampsia with HELLP syndrome (*h*emolysis, *e*levated *l*iver function and *l*ow *p*latelets). The former histologically resembles Reye syndrome with microvesicular steatosis in hepatocytes. The latter is a microvascular disorder of the third trimester that is characterized by hemolysis, coagulopathy and low platelet counts. Each requires prompt delivery.

Jaundice in the postoperative patient
Postoperative jaundice is often multifactorial and includes both cholestatic disorders and those that produce hepatocellular injury. Potential contributors include inhalational anesthetic agents, other potentially hepatotoxic drugs, hepatic ischemia, blood transfusions, TPN and sepsis. These can be distinguished from benign postoperative cholestasis, a self-limited (less than 1–2 weeks) syndrome characterized by transient conjugated

hyperbilirubinemia without biochemical evidence of hepatocellular injury.

The liver transplant recipient represents a special case, in which the differential diagnosis of jaundice may not only include the disorders common to all postoperative patients, but those that relate to transplantation in particular. Specific diagnostic considerations include graft dysfunction due to ischemia-reperfusion injury or vascular occlusion, graft rejection, obstruction of the bile ducts, bile leak, viral hepatitis (e.g. cytomegalovirus, recurrent hepatitis B or C), immunosuppressive drug toxicity (e.g. azathioprine) and lymphoproliferative disorders.

Obstruction of the bile ducts

Obstructive disorders of the biliary tree include occlusion of the bile duct lumen by gallstones, intrinsic disorders of the bile ducts and extrinsic compression.

Choledocholithiasis

The most common cause of biliary obstruction is choledocholithiasis. Two types of gallstones are associated with this problem: cholesterol gallstones and pigment gallstones. Cholesterol gallstones typically originate in the gallbladder, migrate into the common bile duct and either impact at the ampulla of Vater or produce partial obstruction in a ball-valve fashion. Calcium bilirubinate (black pigment) gallstones characteristically develop in patients with unconjugated hyperbilirubinemia. Black pigment stones, like cholesterol stones, can form in the gallbladder, but they may also form in situ at any level of the biliary tree including the common bile duct. A distinct type of bilirubinate stone, so-called brown pigment gallstones, also forms in situ within the biliary tree. Obstruction of the bile ducts by these stones leads to repeated bouts of cholangitis (recurrent pyogenic cholangitis) in patients from certain regions in Asia, in association with biliary parasitic infestations, and in patients with prior biliary tract surgery.

Diseases of the bile ducts

Intrinsic disorders of the bile ducts may be inflammatory, infectious, or neoplastic. Primary sclerosing cholangitis, an inflammatory disorder of the bile ducts, characterized by focal and segmental strictures, is extensively discussed elsewhere in this book (see Ch. 20). A similar picture of focal narrowing and localized obstruction of the bile ducts is seen in patients infected with human immunodeficiency virus (so-called AIDS cholangiopathy), but jaundice is distinctly unusual in this setting. Biliary strictures may also follow hepatic arterial infusion of certain chemotherapeutic agents or result from surgical injury to the bile duct or hepatic artery. Neoplasms of the biliary tree, including cholangiocarcinoma, are discussed elsewhere in this book (see Chs. 28 and 29).

Extrinsic compression of the bile ducts

Extrinsic compression of the biliary tree may result from neoplastic involvement or inflammation of surrounding viscera. Rarely, marked enlargement of surrounding vessels (e.g. arterial aneurysms, cavernous transformation of the portal vein) can compress the bile ducts as well.

Painless jaundice is a classic sign of carcinoma of the head of the pancreas. Occasionally, hepatocellular carcinoma or peri-portal lymph nodes enlarged by any metastatic tumor or lymphoma obstruct the extrahepatic bile ducts. An unusual complication of cholecystitis, Mirizzi syndrome, occurs when a large gallstone becomes impacted in the cystic duct leading to compression of the common bile duct. Pancreatitis may also produce extrinsic biliary compression as a result of edema, pseudocyst formation, or fibrosis.

CLINICAL FEATURES

Overview

In a jaundiced individual, associated clinical features can be very helpful in distinguishing isolated disorders of hyperbilirubinemia from intrinsic liver disease or from biliary tract obstruction. Important clues can be obtained from the history and physical examination. These, in conjunction with standard biochemical tests, will substantially improve the efficiency of subsequent diagnostic studies.

It should be remembered that jaundice is only one of the features of cholestasis, but that other effects of cholestasis are encountered in such patients. Some of these features can be present without jaundice (see Fig. 6.5).

History

The absence of any symptoms other than jaundice is consistent with hemolysis or an isolated disorder of bilirubin metabolism. However, it does not exclude intrinsic liver disease or biliary tract obstruction. Clues to the presence of liver disease versus biliary tract obstruction are featured in **Table 6.3**.

Symptoms compatible with a viral prodrome, such as anorexia, malaise and myalgias, make viral hepatitis a strong possibility, as does a history of known infectious exposure, injection drug use, or receipt of blood products. The presence of arthralgias and rash, and other autoimmune disorders, heightens the suspicion for autoimmune hepatitis. Symptoms of pruritus are encountered with several disorders of intrahepatic cholestasis, such as primary biliary cirrhosis. Important clues to chronic liver disease include a history of fluid retention or confusion. A history of rapid fluid retention and jaundice raises the concern of Budd-Chiari syndrome or veno-occlusive disease. A careful history may suggest that environmental hepatotoxins, ethanol, or medications underlie hepatic dysfunction that is responsible for jaundice. Finally, a family history of liver disease suggests the possibility of a hereditary disorder, such as hemochromatosis, Wilson disease, or α_1-antitrypsin deficiency.

There are several historic clues to the presence of biliary tract obstruction. A history of fever, especially when accompanied by rigors, or abdominal pain, particularly in the right upper quadrant, is suggestive of cholangitis due to obstructive diseases (particularly choledocholithiasis). A history of prior biliary surgery also increases the likelihood that biliary tract obstruction is present. Although weight loss is often a non-specific symptom, it is suggestive of malignancy in an older individual with jaundice. Obstructive jaundice from gallstone disease is also more common in the elderly.

Physical examination

Like the history, physical examination can offer important clues that distinguish intrinsic liver disease from biliary tract obstruction. Several signs suggest that liver disease is the cause of jaundice. These include evidence of portal hypertension (i.e.

Features that differentiate biliary tract obstruction from cholestatic liver disease in the diagnosis of jaundice		
	Favors biliary obstruction	*Favors liver disease*
History	Abdominal pain Fever, rigors Poor biliary surgery Older age	Malaise, myalgias, arthralgias, suggestive of viral syndrome Known infectious exposure Receipt of blood products, intravenous or nasal use of illicit drugs Exposure to known hepatotoxin Family history of liver disease
Physical examination	Fever Abdominal tenderness Palpable abdominal mass Surgical scar	Ascites Signs of chronic liver disease (e.g. prominent abdominal veins, gynecomastia, spider angiomata, asterixis, encephalopathy) Ascites Signs of specific liver disease (e.g. Kayser-Fleischer rings, xanthelasmas)
Routine laboratory studies	Predominant elevation of alkaline phosphatase Prothrombin time that is normal or normalizes with vitamin K administration Elevated serum lipase	Predominant elevation of serum aminotransferases Prolonged prothrombin time that does not correct with vitamin K administration Decreased albumin concentration

Table 6.3 Features that differentiate biliary tract obstruction from cholestatic liver disease in the diagnosis of jaundice.

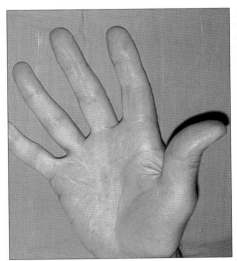

Figure 6.6 Xanthomata (fatty deposits) in the skin creases and palm of a patient with primary biliary cirrhosis.

A caveat

All clues in the history and physical must be interpreted with caution, because fever and abdominal pain accompany diseases other than biliary obstruction, and patients with prior biliary surgery may develop viral hepatitis. Conversely, anorexia and malaise are not exclusively symptoms of viral hepatitis, and patients with parenchymal liver disease can certainly develop gallstones. Nonetheless, when these clues are evaluated with physical findings and routine laboratory tests, jaundice is correctly characterized as obstructive or non-obstructive in most cases.

DIAGNOSIS AND EVALUATION

Overview

A general algorithm for evaluating the patient with jaundice is presented in **Figure 6.7**. The sequential approach involves: a careful patient history, physical examination and screening laboratory studies; formulation of a working differential diagnosis; selection of further specialized tests to narrow the diagnostic possibilities; and development of a strategy for treatment or further testing if unexpected diagnostic possibilities are suggested.

Screening laboratory studies

Essential laboratory studies include serum total bilirubin, alkaline phosphatase, aminotransferases [asparate aminotransferase (AST) and alanine aminotransferase (ALT)], albumin, and prothrombin time. Serum alkaline phosphatase activity reflects the presence of a number of related enzymes of different tissue origins. In liver, alkaline phosphatase is a membrane-associated protein that is present on the apical domain of the plasma membrane of hepatocytes and cholangiocytes. Under physiologic conditions, this protein is

ascites, splenomegaly, or prominent abdominal veins) or other characteristic features, such as spider angiomata, gynecomastia and asterixis. Certain physical findings may suggest particular liver diseases. Examples of such classic signs include hyperpigmentation in hemochromatosis, xanthomas in primary biliary cirrhosis (see **Fig. 6.6**), and Kayser-Fleischer rings in Wilson disease. By contrast, certain findings suggest biliary tract obstruction. For example, high fever or abdominal tenderness (particularly right upper quadrant) suggests cholangitis. A palpable abdominal mass or palpable gallbladder suggests a neoplastic cause of obstructive jaundice. Finally, an abdominal scar in the midline or right upper quadrant may be the only clinical clue to prior biliary surgery.

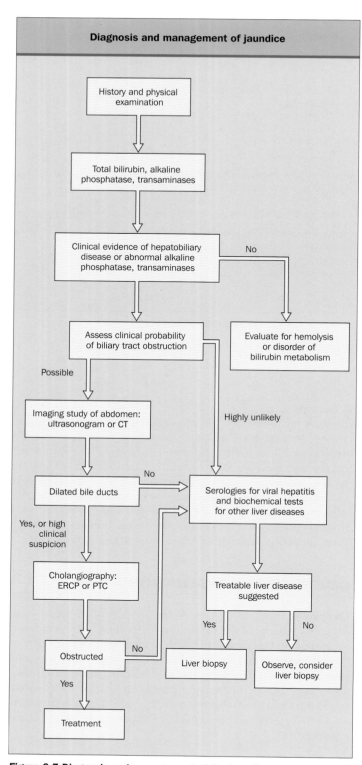

Diagnosis and management of jaundice

History and physical examination

Total bilirubin, alkaline phosphatase, transaminases

Clinical evidence of hepatobiliary disease or abnormal alkaline phosphatase, transaminases

No → Evaluate for hemolysis or disorder of bilirubin metabolism

Possible → Assess clinical probability of biliary tract obstruction

Imaging study of abdomen: ultrasonogram or CT

Highly unlikely

Dilated bile ducts

No → Serologies for viral hepatitis and biochemical tests for other liver diseases

Yes, or high clinical suspicion

Cholangiography: ERCP or PTC

Treatable liver disease suggested

Yes   No

Obstructed   No → Liver biopsy   Observe, consider liver biopsy

Yes

Treatment

Figure 6.7 Diagnosis and management of the jaundiced patient.

increased serum alkaline phosphatase activity may reflect release of alkaline phosphatase isoenzymes that are released from extrahepatobiliary tissues. Hence, other more specific markers, such as the serum activities of the canalicular enzymes γ-glutamyltranspeptidase, leucine aminopeptidase, or 5′-nucleotidase are useful to confirm the hepatobiliary origin of alkaline phosphatase. In a jaundiced patient, a predominant increase in (hepatic) alkaline phosphatase activity relative to those of serum aminotransferases suggests the possibility of biliary tract obstruction. It should be noted that intrahepatic cholestatic disorders can produce an identical biochemical picture. By contrast, in hemolysis or an isolated disorder of bilirubin metabolism, alkaline phosphatase and serum aminotransferases are normal.

Measurements of aminotransferases, in particular, AST and ALT, are useful in the evaluation of jaundice. Serum AST reflects a mixture of isozymes released from both the cytosol and mitochondria of hepatocytes as well as AST released from other tissues. ALT is a cytosolic enzyme found predominantly in hepatocytes. Both AST and ALT ordinarily circulate in low concentrations in serum. However, hepatocyte damage, due to ischemia, viral infection, or toxins, significantly increases serum aminotransferase activity. Thus, predominant elevation of serum aminotransferase activity in comparison with alkaline phosphatase activity suggests that jaundice is due to intrinsic hepatocellular disease. By contrast, in hemolysis or an isolated disorder of bilirubin metabolism, serum aminotransferases are normal.

Of note, a serum activity of AST that exceeds that of ALT by at least a factor of two, but is less than 10 times the upper limit of normal, represents a clue to the diagnosis of alcoholic liver disease. However, acute Wilson disease may present with similar biochemical abnormalities. There are exceptions to the above generalizations. For example, transient biliary obstruction from choledocholithiasis is occasionally associated with a brief but dramatic elevation (exceeding 10 to 20 times normal) of serum aminotransferase activity.

Serum albumin is a useful marker of hepatic synthetic function, as it is decreased in the presence of significant liver disease. However, other conditions such as malabsorption, nephrotic syndrome and systemic inflammation can depress serum albumin levels. Thus test results are best interpreted in conjunction with the prothrombin time. The prothrombin time is a measure of the plasma activities of the coagulation factors I, II, V, VII and X, each of which is synthesized in the liver. Prolongation of the prothrombin time can result from impaired hepatic synthesis of these proteins but may also reflect deficiency of vitamin K, which is essential for post-translational γ-carboxylation of lysine residues of factors II, VII, IX and X. Vitamin K absorption requires an intact enterohepatic circulation (hence an unobstructed biliary tree) of bile acids. Thus, parenteral administration of vitamin K will generally normalize a prolonged prothrombin time in patients with obstructive jaundice but not in patients with liver disease. In hemolysis or an isolated disorder of bilirubin metabolism, serum albumin and prothrombin time are (generally) normal.

In most cases, the measurement of the total bilirubin concentration is sufficient to aid in the diagnosis of jaundice, especially when it is interpreted in conjunction with the alkaline phosphatase and aminotransferases. In patients with liver disease

enzymatically cleaved and released into bile, but small amounts are released into serum as well. Biliary obstruction or intrahepatic cholestasis increases serum alkaline phosphatase activity by increasing its synthesis, targeting to the basolateral domain of the plasma membrane and release into serum. However,

or biliary tract obstruction, there are either signs or symptoms of hepatobiliary disease, or more than one of the above laboratory tests is abnormal. By contrast, patients with hemolysis or isolated disorders of bilirubin metabolism have no signs or symptoms of hepatobiliary disease, and the only abnormality in screening laboratory studies is hyperbilirubinemia.

Although some laboratories provide colorimetric estimates of conjugated and unconjugated bilirubin, these are not usually necessary in practice (with the exception of neonatal jaundice, in which unconjugated hyperbilirubinemia has therapeutic implications). In general, such tests may have greatest utility in distinguishing unconjugated hyperbilirubinemias (e.g. hemolysis, Gilbert and Crigler-Najjar syndromes), from isolated conjugated hyperbilirubinemias (e.g. Rotor and Dubin-Johnson syndromes). These are uncommon issues. Moreover, accurate distinction between these conditions usually requires more sophisticated chromatographic tools that are available only in specialized centers. Thus, reliance on the relative concentrations of unconjugated versus conjugated bilirubin is not helpful in most cases.

Decision analysis

In aggregate, history, physical examination and screening laboratory studies provide a good estimate of the likelihood that obstructive jaundice is present or absent. For example, an asymptomatic hyperbilirubinemic patient who has an unremarkable physical examination and normal serum alkaline phosphatase, ALT, AST, albumin and prothrombin is unlikely to have liver disease or biliary obstruction. Further testing for specific disorders, such as hemolysis or isolated defects in bilirubin metabolism, is warranted (see Fig. 6.9).

If classic features of liver disease are present on the basis of history, physical examination and screening laboratory studies, and biliary tract obstruction is not suspected, then a further evaluation for causes of liver disease should ensue. On the other hand, if the history, physical examination and laboratory studies suggest that biliary tract obstruction is possible, an imaging study is appropriate to confirm either the presence or absence of biliary tract obstruction. Selection of an imaging study depends on the likelihood of obstruction, diagnostic accuracy, cost, complication rate and availability, especially if simultaneous therapeutic intervention is anticipated.

Imaging studies (see Ch. 8 also)
Abdominal ultrasonography

Abdominal ultrasonography is often the initial imaging study in the evaluation of hepatobiliary disease, because it determines the caliber of the extrahepatic biliary tree, evaluates the liver panenchyma and it reveals intra- or extrahepatic mass lesions. The sensitivity of abdominal ultrasonography for the detection of biliary obstruction in jaundiced patients ranges from 55 to 91%, and the specificity from 82 to 95% (**Table 6.4**). Ultrasonography can also demonstrate cholelithiasis (although common duct stones may not be well seen) and space occupying lesions in the liver greater than 1 cm in diameter. Ultrasonography has three major advantages. First, it is non-invasive. Second, it is portable (this may be invaluable in the evaluation of the critically ill patient). Third, it is relatively inexpensive. However, there are several potential disadvantages with ultrasound. For example, studies may be difficult to interpret in obese patients or patients in whom overlying bowel gas obscures the biliary tree. Also, dilatation of the common bile duct, which usually indicates biliary tract obstruction, is common in patients who have undergone previous cholecystectomy. A final caveat is that in patients with cirrhosis and other conditions associated with poorly compliant hepatic parenchyma such as primary sclerosing cholangitis, intrahepatic ducts may not dilate with obstruction.

Computed tomography of the abdomen

Computed tomography (CT) of the abdomen with intravenous contrast is an excellent alternative to ultrasound in evaluating the possibility of biliary tract obstruction in jaundiced patients. Abdominal CT has a diagnostic accuracy comparable to that of ultrasound in the diagnosis of biliary obstruction, with a sensitivity and specificity of 63–96% and 93–100%, respectively (see Table 6.4). Abdominal CT has several advantages over ultrasound. First, it detects space occupying lesions as small as 5 mm. Second, it is not operator-dependent as in ultrasonography. Third, it provides technically superior images in obese individuals and in patients in whom the biliary tree is obscured by bowel gas. Additional caveats that apply to the accuracy of ultrasonography for the diagnosis of biliary obstruction also apply to abdominal CT. Other considerations in the utilization of abdominal CT in patients with jaundice are its lack of portability, requirement for use of intravenous contrast and expense.

Endoscopic retrograde cholangiopancreatography

Endoscopic retrograde cholangiopancreatography (ERCP) permits direct visualization of the biliary tree as well as the pancreatic ducts. In contrast to abdominal ultrasonography and CT, ERCP is more invasive. The procedure involves passage of an endoscope into the duodenum, introduction of a catheter into the ampulla of Vater and injection of contrast medium into the common bile duct and/or pancreatic duct. Importantly, conscious sedation and even in some cases general anesthesia is necessary.

The technique of ERCP is highly accurate in the diagnosis of biliary obstruction, with a sensitivity of 89–98% and specificity of 89–100% (see Table 6.4). It offers the possible implementation of other diagnostic maneuvers in addition to simple visualization and radiography. For example, it permits biopsies and brushings for cytology of periampullary lesions. Moreover, if a focal cause for biliary obstruction is identified (e.g. choledocholithiasis, biliary stricture), maneuvers to relieve obstruction (e.g. sphincterotomy, stone extraction, dilatation, stent placement) can be performed during the same session. It should be noted that acquisition of biopsy material and therapeutic intervention via ERCP are largely limited to lesions that are distal to the bifurcation of the right and left hepatic bile ducts.

The technical success rate of ERCP is higher than 90%; the rate limiting step is cannulation of the ampulla of Vater. This may be a particularly important consideration in patients with prior abdominal surgery and altered anatomy (e.g. choledochojejunostomy, gastrojejunostomy). As an invasive procedure, ERCP should be employed thoughtfully. The morbidity and mortality associated with ERCP from untoward events such as respiratory depression, aspiration, bleeding, perforation, cholangitis and pancreatitis, are 3 and 0.2%, respectively. These

Imaging studies for the evaluation of jaundice					
Test	Sensitivity (%)	Specificity (%)	Morbidity (%)	Mortality (%)	Comments
Abdominal ultrasonogram	55–91	82–95	–	–	Advantages: Non-invasive, portable, less expensive Disadvantages: Bowel gas may obscure common bile duct; interpretation difficult in obese individuals and in those with ileus
Abdominal CT	63–96	93–100	–	–	Advantages: Non-invasive, not operator-dependent, interpretation less affected by obesity or ileus Disadvantages: Not portable, intravenous contrast required (potential for nephrotoxicity)
ERCP	89–98	89–100	3	0.2	Advantages: Provides direct imaging of bile ducts, permits direct visualization of periampullary mucosa, potential for simultaneous tissue acquisition or therapeutic intervention, especially useful for lesions distal to bifurcation or hepatic ducts Disadvantages: Cannot be performed if altered anatomy precludes endoscopic access to ampulla (e.g. gastro- or choledochojejunostomy)
PTC	98–100	89–100	3	0.2	Advantages: Provides direct imaging of bile ducts, potential for simultaneous tissue acquisition or therapeutic intervention, especially useful for lesions proximal to common hepatic duct Disadvantages: More difficult with non-dilated intrahepatic bile ducts

CT, computed tomography; ERCP, endocrine retrograde cholangiopancreatography; PTC, percutaneous transhepatic cholangiography

Table 6.4 Imaging studies for the evaluation of jaundice.

rates are increased when interventional procedures are concomitantly employed. A final consideration is cost, as ERCP is more expensive than non-invasive imaging procedures.

Percutaneous transhepatic cholangiography

Percutaneous transhepatic cholangiography (PTC) is a procedure that complements ERCP. It requires the passage of a needle through the skin and subcutaneous tissues into the hepatic parenchyma and advancement into a peripheral bile duct. When bile is aspirated, a catheter is introduced through the needle and radio-opaque contrast medium is injected. It has accuracy comparable to that of ERCP in the diagnosis of biliary tract obstruction in the setting of jaundice, with a sensitivity and specificity of approximately 98–100% and 89–100%, respectively (see Table 6.4). As in ERCP, interventional procedures, such as balloon dilatation and stent placement to relieve amenable focal obstructions of the biliary tree, can be performed at the time of PTC.

Percutaneous transhepatic cholangiography is potentially technically advantageous under conditions in which the level of biliary obstruction is proximal to the common hepatic duct or in which altered anatomy precludes ERCP (see above). However, when the intrahepatic ducts are not dilated, multiple passes are frequently required and PTC may be technically unsuccessful in up to 25% of attempts. The morbidity and mortality of PTC from bleeding, perforation and cholangitis are 3 and 0.2%, respectively. Like ERCP, it is more expensive than abdominal ultrasonography or CT.

Other imaging studies

Magnetic resonance cholangiography (MRC) is a technical refinement of standard magnetic resonance imaging that permits rapid clear-cut delineation of the biliary tree without the requirement for intravenous contrast. Emerging evidence suggests that its accuracy for detecting biliary tract obstruction approaches that of ERCP. Endoscopic ultrasonography (EUS) appears to

CHAPTER
7

Liver Biopsy: Indications, Technique, Complications and Interpretation

Kyle E. Brown, Kay Washington and Elizabeth M. Brunt

INDICATIONS

Liver biopsy evaluation remains the gold standard for diagnosing and staging a variety of liver disorders (**Table 7.1**). The most common indications for biopsy are to assess fibrosis in chronic hepatitis C and to evaluate elevated liver tests. Liver biopsy evaluation is also indicated to assess response to treatment and/or progression of disease. Finally, biopsy can be useful in evaluation of systemic conditions, including sarcoidosis, amyloidosis and fever of unknown origin.

TECHNIQUE OF PERCUTANEOUS LIVER BIOPSY

The importance of obtaining adequate tissue cannot be over-emphasized. While 'skinny needles' may be adequate in sampling mass lesions, larger bore needles are preferred for sampling diffuse parenchymal disease. Two types of needles are used for percutaneous liver biopsy (PLB): cutting needles (e.g. Tru-Cut) and aspiration-type needles such as the Menghini, Jamshidi and Klatskin. The use of cutting needles causes less fragmentation of fibrotic tissue and may provide superior specimens in cases of cirrhosis, but has been associated with higher complication rates than aspiration needles in some studies.

The aspiration biopsy is performed while the patient is recumbent with his or her right arm extended. Liver span is identified by percussion. A site several centimeters caudad to the top of the liver in the right mid-axillary line is selected, usually in the 8th or 9th intercostal space. The site is prepped, draped and infiltrated with local anesthetic extending to the liver capsule; a 2–3 mm skin incision is made so that the needle can pass easily. The needle is attached to a syringe containing 2–3 mL of sterile saline. It is inserted over the superior margin of the rib (in order to avoid the intercostal artery) with its tip directed toward the xiphoid process. Once through the intercostal tissues, 1–2 mL of the saline is expelled to flush the needle. The patient holds his or her breath in expiration. With the syringe plunger retracted to create negative pressure, the needle is passed quickly into the liver and withdrawn. The specimen is transferred to a specimen container. If additional tissue is required, one or two additional passes can be made through the same entry site without significantly increasing the risk of complications. The patient is placed in the right lateral decubitus position for 1 h and kept at bed rest for an additional 2–3 h while vital signs are monitored frequently. Outpatients may be observed for 6–8 h afterward, as virtually all complications become evident within this period.

CONTRAINDICATIONS AND COMPLICATIONS

Liver biopsy-related mortality occurs in 0.1–0.01% of cases. Hemorrhage is the most common cause of fatalities. Although serious bleeding complicates 0.06–0.35% of cases, clinically insignificant intrahepatic or subcapsular hematomas are found in about a quarter of patients undergoing ultrasound examination a day after biopsy. Less common complications of liver biopsy include perforation of the gallbladder, bile peritonitis, puncture of the intestine or kidney, pneumothorax, hemobilia, hemothorax, arteriovenous fistula and sepsis.

To diminish the risk of bleeding, patients are usually instructed to discontinue medications that interfere with platelet function at least 7 days before the biopsy. These include non-steroidal anti-inflammatory agents, clopidogrel and ticlopidine. Prior to performing the procedure, the adequacy of hemostatic mechanisms is estimated using the platelet count and prothrombin time (PT). Although acceptable levels are somewhat arbitrary, platelets $<50\,000/\text{mm}^3$ or PT >3 s above control would be regarded as contraindications to PLB in most cases. While blood product transfusion may correct these abnormalities, use of transjugular biopsy (TJB) is probably more prudent. Bleeding times are not checked in our center unless platelet dysfunction is suspected, such as in uremic patients. In these cases, options include DDAVP just prior to biopsy, performing the biopsy immediately after dialysis or TJB; however, data regarding the efficacy of these approaches are lacking. Other situations in which TJB is preferable include massive ascites, morbid obesity, hemophilia and inability to cooperate.

Ultrasound guidance has been advocated as a means of reducing complications from PLB. While ultrasound may be

Indications for liver biopsy
Grading and staging of chronic liver disease
Hepatitis C and B
Non-alcoholic fatty liver disease (NAFLD)
Alcoholic liver disease
Autoimmune hepatitis
Evaluation of elevated liver tests of unclear etiology
Aid in diagnosis and evaluation of cholestatic disease
Primary biliary cirrhosis
Primary sclerosing cholangitis
Evaluation of hepatomegaly
Evaluation of liver diseases related to iron overload
Aid in diagnosis of Wilson disease
Evaluation of a liver mass (CT or ultrasound guided biopsy)
Assessing suitability of potential donor livers
Evaluation of engrafted liver post-liver transplantation
Evaluation of fever of unknown origin

Table 7.1 Indications for liver biopsy.

helpful in avoiding inadvertent puncture of adjacent organs or unsuspected liver lesions (e.g. hemangioma), it is less clear that ultrasound alters the risk of hemorrhage. Data suggest that use of ultrasound results in less pain and fewer hospitalizations; however, no differences in transfusion requirement, surgery or mortality have been observed. Indeed, given the relatively low rate of serious complications associated with 'blind' PLB, none of the randomized studies to date have adequate statistical power to assess these outcomes. Despite the lack of clear evidence for its cost-effectiveness, ultrasound is commonly used and will likely increase as hand-held devices become more readily available.

PROCESSING, STAINS AND GENERAL MORPHOLOGIC APPROACH

Processing and stains

'Routine' handling for histopathologic interpretation of most liver diseases begins with immediate fixation in 10% neutral buffered formalin; it is recommended that the specimen should not be placed on a biopsy sponge due to well-described artifacts. In some clinical settings, special handling of the tissue is necessary for evaluation (**Table 7.2**). A 1 mm² portion of the biopsy may be postfixed in 2.5% glutaraldehyde for further processing if ultrastructural evaluation is necessary. Pathologists' practice for utilization of histochemical stains may differ; however, in general, 'routine' stains are utilized to highlight features in addition to those easily noted on the standard hematoxylin and eosin stain. In our practice, routine stains include: trichrome and reticulin stains for demonstrating fibrosis and cord architecture respectively; iron stain for hemosiderin; and diastase-pretreated periodic acid-Schiff (PAS-d) stain. Each of these stains can serve multiple purposes in evaluation and the findings for these stains will be discussed in the following sections. **Table 7.3** lists additional histochemical and immunohistochemical stains, the disease processes for which they are useful, and the expected reactivity. Sophisticated techniques, such as in situ hybridization and polymerase chain reaction are available in limited numbers of research facilities and are variably available for diagnostic testing.

General interpretation

Interpretation of liver biopsy is a multistep process that incorporates architectural and cellular assessment. A standard liver biopsy is estimated to represent only 1/50 000–1/65 000 of the organ; thus, assessment of sample adequacy is the initial step in interpretation. To a large extent, adequacy depends on the nature of the process under consideration, whether a focal, space-occupying lesion, or diffuse parenchymal disease. The former may be able to be diagnosed with a small fragment of representative tissue, while the latter requires larger cores. An adequate sample is also one that is not entirely subcapsular.

Even with adequate sample size, there are recognized difficulties in interpretation due to inherent inhomogeneity of parenchymal involvement in liver disease, including the full spectrum of acute and chronic hepatitic and vascular processes, and the chronic cholestatic diseases. For these reasons, pathologists commonly recommend more than five portal tracts, or a core length of 1.5–2.0 cm for adequacy of evaluation of parenchymal disease. **Figure 7.1** illustrates this difficulty.

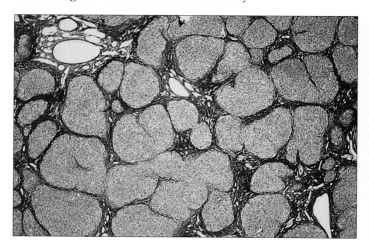

Figure 7.1 Explant liver, cirrhosis. The distorted, remodeled hepatic architecture of cirrhosis, characterized by nodules of hepatocytes surrounded by scar tissue, is easily recognized. However, a liver biopsy could sample various areas within this section and 'miss' the diagnostic lesions of cirrhosis (Masson trichrome).

Tissue processing for specialized analysis		
Disease process	*Diagnostic evaluation*	*Tissue preparation*
Hereditary hemochromatosis	Iron concentration; µg/g dry weight	Fresh tissue or paraffin block*
Wilson disease	Copper concentration; µg/g dry weight	Fresh tissue or paraffin block*
Microvesicular steatosis Fatty liver of pregnancy Reye syndrome	Microvesicular steatosis best seen with Oil Red O or Sudan Black stains	Frozen sections of fresh or formalin-fixed tissue; cannot be done on paraffin-embedded tissue
Porphyria cutanea tarda	Intracytoplasmic needle-shaped crystals	Unstained tissue sections examined under polarized light; ferric ferricyanide reduction test
Inborn errors of metabolism Bacterial, viral, fungal, mycobacterial infections	Enzymatic assays Culture and identification	Fresh tissue obtained at biopsy* Fresh tissue supplied to the microbiology laboratory or PCR analysis on fresh or fixed tissue
*Submission of tissue to a reference laboratory is necessary. PCR, polymerase chain reaction.		

Table 7.2 Tissue processing for specialized analysis.

Histochemical and immunohistochemical stains			
Histochemical stains	*Use in diagnostic liver pathology*	*Pathologic processes*	*Comments*
Vierhoff Van Geison	Vessel wall connective tissue	VOD, Budd-Chiari syndrome	Helpful in the identification of obliterated vessels not readily seen by standard stains
Rhodanine	Copper in cytoplasm and lysosomes of hepatocytes	Wilson disease	Most useful in late stages of Wilson disease; uneven distribution in the liver so that a negative stain does not rule out the possibility of Wilson disease
		Chronic cholestasis	Granular reactivity in zone 1 or periseptal hepatocytes
Orcein	Copper-associated protein	Wilson disease, chronic cholestasis	Less sensitive than rhodanine for copper
	Elastic fibers	Recent necrosis, collapse Scar tissue formation	Passive septa: no elastic fibers detected Active septa: elastic fibers present
	Hepatitis B virus (HBV) surface antigen	Eccentric cytoplasmic reactivity corresponds with the ground-glass change seen by hematoxylin and eosin; indicates the presence of viral components in hepatocytes	Less sensitive than immunohistochemical stain for HBV surface antigen
Oil Red O	Red globules correspond to fat droplets	Diseases in which microvesicular steatosis occurs in hepatocytes	Confirms the presence of microvesicular steatosis
Congo Red Crystal Violet Thioflavin-T	Confirmation of amyloid protein deposition in the space of Disse or hepatic arterioles	Amyloid infiltration	Immunohistochemical stains for protein A or immunoglobulin light chain will distinguish secondary (AA) from primary/plasma cell dyscrasia-related (AL) amyloidosis
Immunostains	*Antigen*	*Reactivity in liver tissue*	*Diagnostic utility*
HBV surface antigen	HBsAg	Cytoplasmic reactivity: diffuse or inclusion; membrane reactivity	Confirmatory of the presence of HBV surface antigen in hepatocytes
HBV core antigen	HBcAg	Nuclear reactivity; may see cytoplasmic reactivity in occasional hepatocytes	Confirmatory of HBV core antigen in hepatocytes; indicates active replication of the virus
A_1AT	α_1-Antitrypsin protein	Immunoreactive globules or diffuse cytoplasmic blush	Reactivity with globules may be positive or negative with a positive rim; this is more specific for A_1AT in the secretory apparatus than diffuse cytoplasmic reactivity
Other viral antigens HSV	Herpes simplex, I and II	Immunoreactivity localizes to infected cells	Confirmatory of HSV in intranuclear inclusions
CMV	Cytomegalovirus	As above	Confirmatory of CMV in intranuclear and intracytoplasmic inclusions
Cytokeratins	CK 8, 18	Hepatocyte cytokeratin	May be useful in confirming the hepatocellular origin of the tumor
	CK 8, 18, 7, 19	Biliary epithelium	Useful in delineating biliary differentiation in tumors; helpful in identifying bile duct epithelium in ductopenic conditions
Note: Immunohistochemical markers for other viral hepatitis markers, hepatitis δ agent, hepatitis C antigen, and hepatitis A antigen are available in research facilities. VOD, veno-occlusive disease; A_1AT, α_1-antitrypsin deficiency; HSV, herpes simplex virus; CMV, cytomegalovirus.			

Table 7.3 Histochemical and immunohistochemical stains.

Liver biopsy assessment begins with an initial impression of overall pattern of injury (inflammatory or not) or neoplastic growth; in non-neoplastic liver disease, this is broadly categorized as predominantly hepatitic, cholestatic, mixed, or vascular. Microscopic regions of greatest involvement, commonly sub-divided as portal-based or lobular, are useful distinctions. Lobular, or more correctly, acinar, involvement is subdivided into zone 3 (or perivenular) or zone 1 (or periportal). These categorizations reflect differing pathophysiologic mechanisms in liver disease and are useful for diagnostic algorithms. Within acini and portal

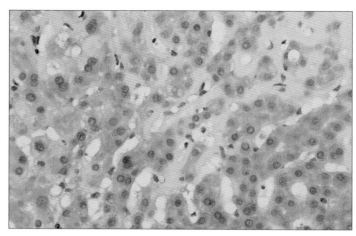

Figure 7.2 Amyloidosis. Accumulation of amyloid is in the space of Disse, with consequent compression of hepatocytes within the cords (hematoxylin and eosin).

Clues to etiology of acute and chronic hepatitis in liver biopsies	
Histologic features	*Etiology*
Zone 1 necrosis, predominantly plasma cell infiltrates, cholestasis, and iron-laden Kupffer cells	Hepatitis A
Cytoplasmic ground-glass change (demonstrates HBsAg by orcein or immunostain), sanded nuclei (demonstrate HBcAg by immunostain)	Hepatitis B (chronic)
Portal lymphoid follicles, bile duct injury, mild macrovesicular steatosis, scattered acidophil bodies (immunostains for HCV, PCR utilized in research)	Hepatitis C (chronic)
Severe hepatitis with massive or submassive necrosis, with HBsAg immunostaining	Hepatitis D (δ virus)
Predominantly plasma cell infiltrates, hepatocellular rosettes, giant cell transformation of hepatocytes, confluent acinar necrosis, collapse, or scar	Autoimmune hepatitis
Cholestasis, eosinophils, granulomas, steatosis Acute hepatitis Chronic hepatitis Granulomatous hepatitis Submassive or massive necrosis	Drug-induced hepatitis e.g. isoniazid e.g. α-methyldopa e.g. aspirin, valium e.g. acetaminophen, halothane
Atypical lymphocytes in portal areas and sinusoids	Epstein-Barr virus
Focal granulomatous necrosis; microabscesses, nuclear and cytoplasmic viral inclusions in immunocompromised patients	Cytomegalovirus
Steatosis, glycogen nuclei, anisocytosis, copper demonstrated by rhodanine or orcein stains, Mallory hyaline	Wilson disease
Eosinophilic PAS-d-positive globules in zone 1 hepatocytes PAS, periodic acid-Schiff	α_1-Antitrypsin deficiency

Table 7.4 Clues to etiology of acute and chronic hepatitis in liver biopsies.

tracts vascular structures are evaluated for location and structural integrity; biliary structures are assessed for inflammation and cellular or architectural alterations. Hepatocytes are noted for inclusions and structural alterations. Sinusoids are evaluated for infiltrates; **Figure 7.2** is an example of amyloidosis infiltrating the sinusoids. The cells of the sinusoids, collectively referred to as sinusoidal lining cells, are assessed. **Table 7.4** lists examples of common histologic features and associated disease processes. As will be noted in the following sections, few microscopic diagnoses can be made based on single histologic features.

HEPATITIS

Hepatitis is microscopically characterized by chronic inflammation, varying degrees of hepatocellular degeneration, apoptosis and/or necrosis, and concurrent hepatocellular regeneration. Bile stasis, damage to bile ducts and inflammation of vessels may variably be present. This pattern of liver injury is commonly attributed to hepatotropic viruses; other processes include drugs, autoimmune hepatitis (AIH) and some metabolic liver diseases, discussed below. Fibrosis indicates chronicity.

Acute hepatitis

Histologic changes of acute hepatitis are commonly accentuated in the lobules compared with portal tracts; often, this accentuation is in zone 3, or perivenular areas. Disarray, or 'lobular unrest', is due to concomitant hepatocellular necrosis, dropout and regeneration (**Fig. 7.3**). Mononuclear cell inflammation and sinusoidal lining cell 'activation' are panlobular; ballooning hepatocellular degeneration is most often in perivenular hepatocytes; acidophilic (apoptotic) degeneration of hepatocytes is non-zonal and seen as single eosinophilic fragments. Kupffer cell hypertrophy, PAS-d (+/− iron) pigmentation and foci of reticulin condensation are common.

Confluent necrosis [zone 3 in hepatitis B virus (HBV), AIH, or zone 1 in hepatitis A virus (HAV), pre-eclampsia], bridging necrosis and reticulin collapse (submassive necrosis) or panacinar collapse (massive necrosis) characterize severe injury. Acinar collapse is noted on reticulin stain (**Fig. 7.4**); distinguishing recent and remote collapse requires evaluation by orcein stain

(Table 7.3). Features of recovery include regenerative hepatocellular changes, increased lipofuschin pigment in zone 3 hepatocytes, and mild portal inflammation. Pigmented Kupffer cells denote phagocytosed necrotic hepatocytes or apoptotic hepatocytes (**Fig. 7.5**).

Chronic hepatitis

Chronic hepatitis may show lesions described above for acute hepatitis. Interface hepatitis and portal involvement predominant to lobular activity are characteristic. Fibrosis and

Chronic cholestatic syndromes			
Morphology	*PBC/AIC*	*PSC*	*IAD*
Portal tracts/bile ducts			
Ductopenia	+ +	+	+
· With lymphoid aggregates	+ +	–	–
· With residual fibrosis	– –	+	–
Lymphoid aggregates	+ +	–	–
Granulomatous inflammation	+ +	–	–
Florid duct lesion	+ +	–	–
Concentric periductal fibrosis	– –	+	–
Interface activity	+ +	+	±

PBC, primary biliary cirrhosis; AIC, autoimmune cholangiopathy; PSC, primary sclerosing cholangitis; IAD, idiopathic adulthood ductopenia.

Table 7.8 Chronic cholestatic syndromes.

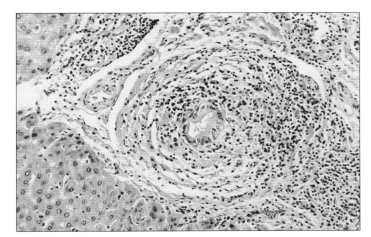

Figure 7.17 Primary biliary cirrhosis. A periductal granuloma is present; the florid duct lesion of primary biliary cirrhosis is characterized by lymphocytic infiltration around and into the interlobular bile duct (hematoxylin and eosin).

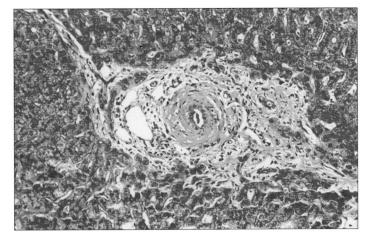

Figure 7.18 Primary sclerosing cholangitis. The interlobular bile duct in the center of the photomicrograph appears to be enlarged when compared with the hepatic artery branch nearby. This is due to the concentric, 'onion-skin' fibrosis investing the duct. This fibro-obliterative lesion is characteristic of primary sclerosing cholangitis, but the diagnosis requires cholangiographically demonstrated ductal changes (Masson trichrome).

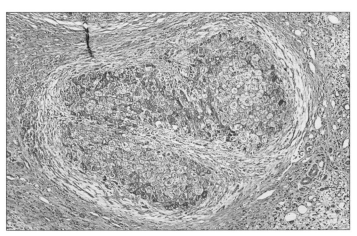

Figure 7.19 Primary sclerosing cholangitis. The cirrhotic nodule in biliary cirrhosis is irregular and surrounded not only by scar tissue but also by the loose, edematous stroma shown in this photomicrograph. This latter change is known as cholate stasis (Masson trichrome).

the association of a particular drug with histologic alterations is well-known. Examples of the latter include zone 3 'bland' necrosis (acetaminophen), submassive necrosis (halothane), bile duct inflammation (amoxicillin-clavulanic acid), hepatic adenoma (oral contraceptives), Budd-Chiari syndrome (oral contraceptives).

VASCULAR LESIONS

Primary vascular disorders of the liver are uncommon. Vascular changes due to systemic circulatory disease processes are more common; these include congestive heart failure and/or circulatory collapse. In these conditions, liver biopsy for elevated liver tests is uncommon. An exception is the consideration of amiodarone toxicity in patients with refractory arrhythmias.

Disease processes of the hepatic outflow veins are broadly divided into occlusion of large outflow veins, as in severe right-sided cardiac failure and Budd-Chiari syndrome, and damage to the smallest terminal hepatic venules, as noted in **Table 7.9**. The latter has been referred to as 'veno-occlusive' disease in the past, but based on recent work, is currently referred to as 'sinusoidal obstruction syndrome'. **Figure 7.20** illustrates lesions of acute large vein outflow obstruction. Without relief from the obstruction, perisinusoidal fibrosis and bridging fibrosis can be documented. The red cell extravasation lesion can also still be recognized. **Figure 7.21** illustrates the perivenular necrosis and dropout, and terminal hepatic venule intraluminal fibrosis associated with sinusoidal obstruction syndrome.

Decreased afferent blood flow to the liver, such as in systemic shock, may result in ischemic 'hepatitis'. The histologic changes are those of pauci-inflammatory zone 3 coagulative necrosis (**Fig. 7.22**). When severe, there may be zone 3–3 bridging. True infarction of the liver is rare because of the dual blood supply; however, in the non-allograft liver, damage to arterial branches may occur in processes such as polyarteritis nodosa, or as an 'innocent bystander' in primary biliary cirrhosis; resultant parenchymal changes may be subtle and include nodular regenerative hyperplasia. Acute arterial obstruction, such as inadvertent surgical ligation, rarely results in infarction, but may result in biliary strictures. Thrombosis of portal vein branches leads to

Causes of hepatic venous outflow obstruction	
Obstruction of large veins	Budd-Chiari syndrome
	Hematologic abnormalities, hypercoagulable states, myeloproliferative disorders, such as polycythemia vera
	Membranous obstruction, often associated with hepatocellular carcinoma
	Chemotherapy
	Radiation therapy
	Neoplasms, primary and metastatic
	Oral contraceptives
	Trauma
	Pregnancy
	Abscess
Damage to small veins	Hepatic sinusoidal obstruction syndrome (veno-occlusive disease)
	Chemotherapy, including thioguanine and 6-mercaptopurine
	Azathioprine
	Ingestion of toxic pyrrolizidine alkaloids (bush tea)
	Radiation
	After bone marrow transplantation

Table 7.9 Causes of hepatic venous outflow obstruction.

sharply demarcated albeit subtle cord atrophy, known as the 'infarcts' of Zahn.

Hepatoportal sclerosis may manifest clinically as non-cirrhotic portal hypertension and is characterized by eccentric scarring, and luminal narrowing of portal tract portal vein branches (**Fig. 7.23**). Biopsy samples may or may not contain the affected portal vein branches, but may be useful in either confirming or excluding the fibrosis and nodularity of cirrhosis.

Nodular regenerative hyperplasia (NRH) results from altered regional blood flow and encompasses lesions of the smallest acini to complex acini. The lesions of NRH are subtle on liver biopsy and consist of nodules formed by alternating groups of atrophic and hypertrophic cords without surrounding fibrosis. Reticulin stain may be useful for documentation (**Fig. 7.24**).

METABOLIC LIVER DISEASE

Most metabolic liver diseases are encountered in pediatric patients. Common findings may be chronic hepatitis, fibrosis and storage of abnormal products in hepatocytes or Kupffer cells. Histochemical stains, polarizing light and ultrastructural evaluation are useful techniques in categorizing some metabolic disorders while other metabolic defects may require enzymatic or molecular analyses in fresh tissue specimens in order to provide an accurate diagnosis. Primary metabolic disorders of concern in Western adults are hereditary hemochromatosis and α_1-antitrypsin deficiency; Wilson disease and the porphyrias are much less common, albeit clinically significant disorders.

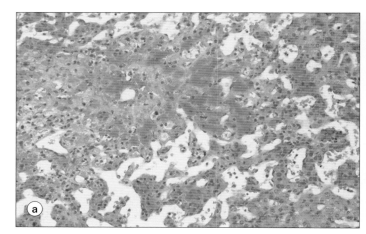
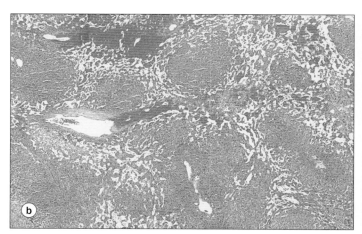

Figure 7.20 Budd-Chiari syndrome. (a) The lesions of acute Budd-Chiari syndrome are characterized by the striking sinusoidal dilatation and red blood cell extravasation into hepatic cords (hematoxylin and eosin). (b) This low-power photomicrograph illustrates 'reverse lobulation' with the illusion that outflow veins and portal triads have altered relationships and the latter occupy the 'center' of the acinus (hematoxylin and eosin).

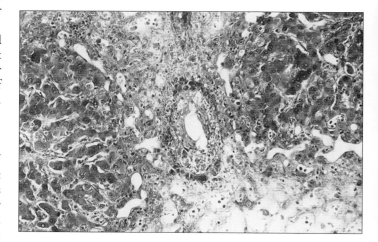

Figure 7.21 Veno-occlusive disease. The obliterative lesion of small, terminal hepatic venules characteristic of veno-occlusive disease is well documented on a connective tissue stain, such as the trichrome stain (Masson trichrome).

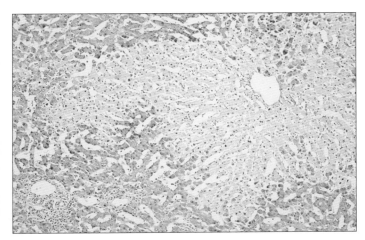

Figure 7.22 Ischemia. Zone 3 coagulative necrosis, as illustrated in this photomicrograph, is characteristic of ischemic liver disease and is usually associated with profound hypotension or shock (hematoxylin and eosin).

Hereditary hemochromatosis (HH)

Currently, indications for liver biopsy are limited to assessment for fibrosis. Iron pigment is visible by routine hematoxylin and eosin stain as a granular, slightly chunky golden-brown refractile pigment within hepatocytes, but is best semiquantitated by iron stain. Initial deposits are in the periportal (zone 1) hepatocytes. The iron stain highlights the distinct pericanalicular location of iron as well as gradient of decreasing deposition from zones 1 to 3; in later stages, iron granules are seen in bile duct epithelia, sinusoidal lining cells (Kupffer cells and endothelial cells) and endothelia of portal and/or terminal hepatic venules (**Fig. 7.25**). 'Grading' iron depends on the use of an iron stain; published systems vary in complexity, but are relatively reproducible among pathologists and correlate with chemically-determined quantitation. When necessary, exact quantitation can be accomplished utilizing paraffin-embedded tissue by chemical analysis. In the setting of HH, foci of non-iron-reactive hepatocytes, 'iron-free foci' are considered preneoplastic lesions (**Fig. 7.26**). Secondary

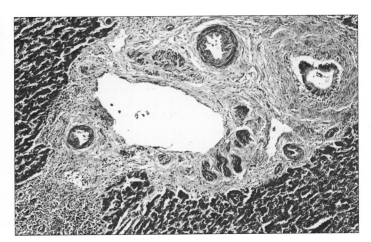

Figure 7.23 Hepatoportal sclerosis. The abnormalities of the portal tract and the portal vein branch within it are characteristic; numerous muscle bundles are absent (Masson trichrome).

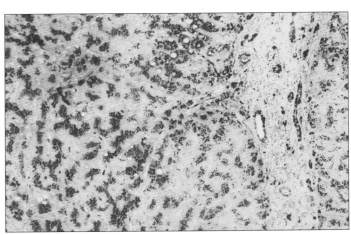

Figure 7.25 The Prussian blue stain highlights the pericanalicular location in hepatocytes, as well as iron in Kupffer cells and ductular epithelium. (Prussian blue).

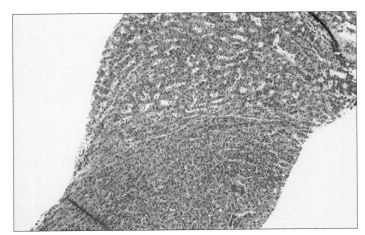

Figure 7.24 Nodular regenerative hyperplasia. The architecture of the hepatic parenchyma in this biopsy is very distorted; compressed cords of hepatocytes noted centrally, are separated from the hypertrophic cords above. This case of nodular regenerative hyperplasia was secondary to azathioprine (Masson trichrome).

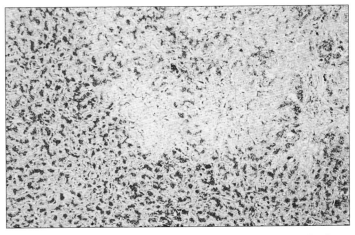

Figure 7.26 Non-reactive hepatocytes in a cluster in an otherwise iron-loaded liver. This is an example of an 'iron-free focus'. There was hepatocellular carcinoma elsewhere in the liver (Prussian blue).

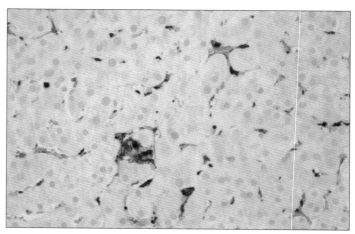

Figure 7.27 Iron overload, secondary to blood transfusion. This Prussian blue-stained liver biopsy shows the early lesions of secondary iron overload: Sinusoidal lining cell reactivity is highlighted by the stain. The hepatocytes are non-reactive (Prussian blue).

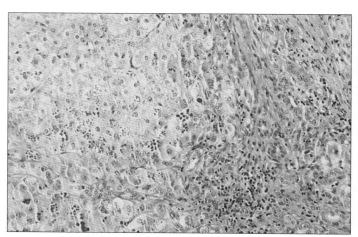

Figure 7.28 α_1-Antitrypsin deficiency. In the adult α_1-antitrypsin may show changes similar to chronic hepatitis of other causes including cirrhosis and interface hepatitis. The diastase pretreated periodic acid-Schiff (PAS-d) stain shows the characteristic intracytoplasmic globules of varying sizes located in hepatocytes adjacent to a fibrous septum (PAS-d).

iron overload is characterized by preferential Kupffer cell iron deposition (**Fig. 7.27**). Other conditions that result in excess iron accumulation are listed in **Table 7.10**; some may or may not be histologically distinguishable from HH by light microscopic evaluation. Genetic testing is required for a definitive diagnosis.

α_1-Antitrypsin deficiency

This protein storage disorder is histologically apparent by varying-sized round eosinophilic 1–30 μm cytoplasmic inclusions within zone 1 or periseptal hepatocytes. The globules may be noted by routine hematoxylin and eosin stains, but the strong PAS-d positivity readily brings them to the pathologist's attention (**Fig. 7.28**). Immunohistochemical confirmation is not commonly required, but the halo-like peripheral reactivity is characteristic. Biliary cirrhosis may occur in affected children; in neonates, the globules may not be present prior to 12 weeks of age. Clinical evaluation is required for differentiating the variety of processes that result in neonatal cholestatic liver disease.

Wilson disease

The liver biopsy in Wilson disease typically exhibits various histologic findings, none of which are diagnostic. Copper or copper-binding protein stains may or may not be positive, and diagnosis relies on a high index of clinical and/or pathologic suspicion; ultimately, the diagnosis rests with tissue copper quantitation. Microscopic findings include non-zonal macrovesicular steatosis, glycogenated nuclei, anisonucleosis, abundant and 'chunky' lipofuschin deposits; iron deposits and canalicular cholestasis may also be present. Portal and lobular inflammatory lesions of chronic hepatitis may be noted; alternatively, bridging fibrosis and features of submassive necrosis may or may not be present. Mallory hyaline may be present in periportal hepatocytes (**Fig. 7.29**). Ultrastructural changes include 'fishmouth' canaliculi and mitochondrial alterations, but are not sufficient to be considered diagnostic (**Fig. 7.30**).

Distribution of hepatic iron* in clinical conditions with iron overload			
Clinical condition	*Hepatocellular iron*	*Kupffer cell iron*	*Bile duct iron*
Hereditary hemochromatosis	1+–4+, zone 1> zone 3	Large aggregates, only with 4+ hepatocellular iron	+
After portacaval shunt	1+–4+, zone 1> zone 3	Only with 4+ hepatocellular iron	+
Alcoholic liver disease	1+–2+, non-zonal	+, panacinar	−
Porphyria cutanea tarda	1+–2+, non-zonal	+, panacinar	−
Transfusions, hemolytic anemias	1+–2+, up to 4+ with massive Kupffer iron	+, panacinar	±
Ineffective erythropoiesis (sideroblastic and chronic disease anemias, myelofibrosis)	1+–2+	+, panacinar	−
*The Prussian blue histochemical stain is necessary when evaluating increased iron deposition in liver parenchyma.			

Table 7.10 Distribution of hepatic iron in clinical conditions with iron overload.

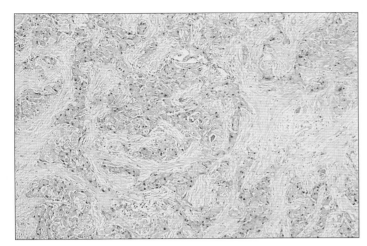

Figure 7.42 Fibrolamellar variant of hepatocellular carcinoma. The lamellar pattern of fibrosis is apparent in this photomicrograph. Clusters of fairly uniform, large eosinophilic tumor cells are separated by the fibrosis (hematoxylin and eosin).

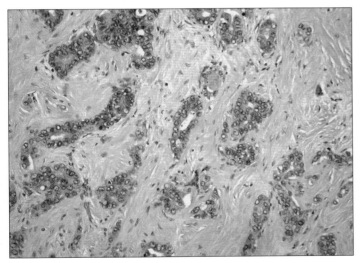

Figure 7.43 Cholangiocarcinoma. The tumor grows in glandular structures in abundant desmoplastic stroma (hematoxylin and eosin).

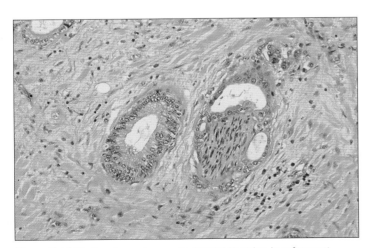

Figure 7.44 Cholangiocarcinoma. Perineural invasion is a frequent finding (hematoxylin and eosin).

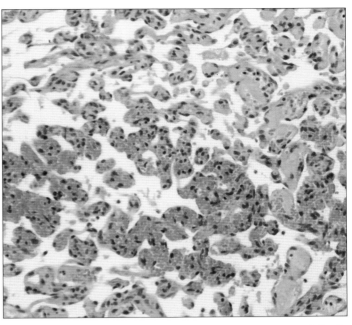

Figure 7.45 Angiosarcoma. The malignant nature of the endothelial cells is apparent in this tumor (hematoxylin and eosin).

Epithelioid hemangioendothelioma

Eosinophilic or 'dendritic' tumor cells, positive for factor VIII, Ulex endothelial cell markers by immunohistochemistry, insinuate into the cords and may be in fibrous or hyalinized stroma. Intracytoplasmic vacuoles, some of which contain red blood cells, may be seen. Tumor infiltrates may obliterate veins (**Fig. 7.46**).

Miscellaneous sarcomas

Usually metastatic but, rarely, primary sarcomas of the liver, malignant fibrous histiocytoma, leiomyosarcoma and undifferentiated (embryonal) sarcoma may occur. Characterization requires a battery of immunohistochemical stains with or without ultrastructural evaluation.

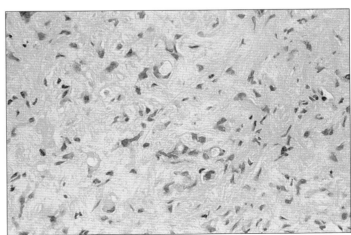

Figure 7.46 Epithelioid hemangioendothelioma. This unusual neoplasm consists of dendritic-type cells, some of which contain intracellular lumina. The tumor is embedded in a hyalinized stroma (hematoxylin and eosin).

Lymphoma

When primary in the liver, lymphoma may present as a mass lesion, or as portal-based nodules of tumor cells. Some lymphomas are associated with chronic HCV. Hodgkin cells may involve the liver; Hodgkin's is also a rare but known cause of duct paucity and hepatic granulomas.

Extrahepatic malignancy with presentation as liver disease

Non-tumor lesions in liver biopsy may be paraneoplastic; some are suggestive of extrahepatic malignancy. Hemophagocytosis is commonly associated with lymphoma. The varieties of lesions that may be associated with Hodgkin disease are discussed above.

TRANSPLANT PATHOLOGY

Orthotopic liver transplantation

Biopsy of the donor liver before the transplant procedure may be indicated for pretransplant evaluation of the donor organ and for prediction of post-transplant function. In the case of the former, the evaluation is most commonly a frozen section request for evaluation of donor disease or steatosis. Necrotizing granulomas, malignancy, or evidence of chronic liver disease are criteria for exclusion in some centers; the presence of more than 30% steatosis has been correlated with subsequent dysfunction or non-function of the allograft.

Liver biopsy remains the 'gold standard' for post-transplant evaluation as biochemical assays do not adequately discriminate immune-mediated, technical (biliary and vascular), or systemic complications that may cause allograft dysfunction. Post-transplant biopsies done at predetermined protocol intervals may be useful in detecting clinically inapparent graft injury. Rejection remains a leading cause of allograft dysfunction. Terminology currently in use for rejection reflects both pathogenesis and potential reversibility. Acute rejection, a cell-mediated entity, is characterized by mixed portal infiltrates with lymphocytes and eosinophils, bile duct injury, and endothelial inflammation (endotheliitis) of terminal hepatic and portal veins (**Fig. 7.47**). Acute rejection is potentially responsive to increased immuno-suppression. Ductopenic rejection usually evolves from acute rejection and may include a component of secondary ischemia from immune injury of the biliary vascular supply. The portal tracts become devoid of bile ducts and inflammation, and features of chronic cholestasis and ischemia may be seen in the lobules (**Fig. 7.48**). Hyperacute rejection, a rare complication in liver transplantation, is caused by preformed antibodies usually in the ABO blood group system and is not responsive to medical intervention.

Table 7.11 shows the common causes of allograft dysfunction and their respective histologic lesions. **Figures 7.49** and **7.50** are illustrations of the most common opportunistic infections of allograft patients: cytomegalovirus and herpes virus. Recurrent disease and post-transplant lymphoproliferative disorder (**Fig. 7.51**) are important considerations in the later time period. At any time post-transplant, acute rejection, pathologic

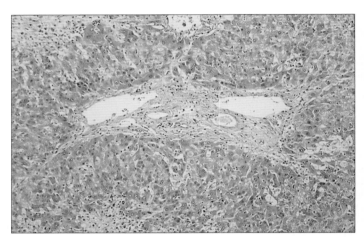

Figure 7.48 Chronic allograft rejection. In ductopenic rejection, the portal tracts are nearly devoid of inflammation. Absence of the interlobular bile duct is apparent in this portal tract in which only the hepatic artery and portal vein branches are seen (hematoxylin and eosin).

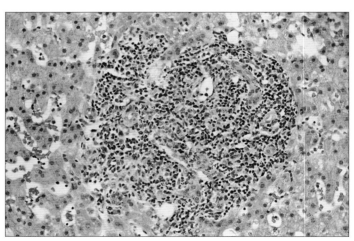

Figure 7.47 Acute allograft rejection. On high power, the triad of acute rejection is seen: mixed chronic inflammation with eosinophils and occasional polymorphonuclear leukocytes, bile duct infiltration and damage, and subendothelial inflammation of the portal vein, endotheliitis (hematoxylin and eosin).

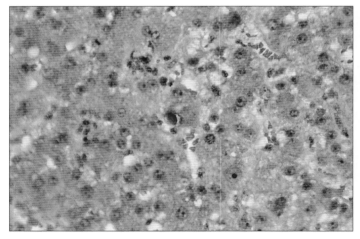

Figure 7.49 Post-transplant opportunistic infection. Cytomegalovirus infection, a common post-transplant opportunistic infection, may involve the allograft liver as well as other organs. The enlarged infected cells contain the characteristic intranuclear inclusion; frequently, a small cluster of acute inflammatory cells is present in adjacent parenchyma (hematoxylin and eosin).

Liver transplant pathology	
Diagnostic considerations	*Morphologic findings*
Rejection	
Hyperacute	Hemorrhagic necrosis or polymorphonuclear infiltrates; IgM, complement in vessel walls
Acute	Triad: mixed chronic inflammation with eosinophils in portal tracts; bile duct infiltration, injury; portal or central endotheliitis; zone 3 necrosis, dropout in severe rejection
Early chronic rejection	Degenerative changes in a majority of interlobular bile ducts or loss of bile ducts in less than 50% of portal tracts; foam cells in the sinusoids; zone 3 necrosis, dropout common
Late chronic rejection	Loss of interlobular bile ducts in ≥50% of portal tracts; zone 3 ballooning, cholestasis, or dropout; foam cells in the sinusoids; foam cell arteriopathy
Preservation-related changes	Zone 3 hepatocellular ballooning ± canalicular cholestasis; subcapsular necrosis
Vascular thrombosis	
Outflow compromise	Zone 3 congestion or red blood cell extravasation into cords
Venous or arterial inflow compromise	Zone 3 hepatocellular ballooning; less commonly, ischemic infarct
Arterial thrombosis	As above ± bile duct ischemic change or necrosis
Biliary obstruction	Acute cholestasis with portal edema, proliferating ductules, and polymorphonuclear leukocytes
Transmission of donor disease	Excess iron pigment (hemochromatosis); zone 1 PAS-d globules (α_1-antitrypsin globules); chronic hepatitis (HCV); malignancy
Recurrence of original disease	Viral hepatitis; HBV surface and core antigens, HDV antigens may be demonstrated with immunohistochemistry; HBV and HCV recurrences may be seen as fibrosing cholestatic hepatitis
	Malignancy: hepatocellular carcinoma; cholangiocarcinoma
	Primary biliary cirrhosis, Autoimmune hepatitis
	Steatohepatitis, alcoholic or nonalcoholic
Post-transplant lymphoproliferative disorder	Atypical lymphoid infiltrate, monoclonal B- or T- cell proliferation demonstrated by flow cytometry, DNA gene rearrangement studies on fresh tissue
Opportunistic infections	
CMV	Microabscesses; intranuclear and intracytoplasmic inclusions in hepatocytes, biliary epithelium, or sinusoidal lining cells
HSV	Non-zonal 'punched-out' necrosis; ground-glass viral inclusions at the periphery of the necrotic foci
EBV	Sinusoidal and portal atypical lymphocytic inflammation
Fungal	Necrosis with organisms demonstrated by GMS or other fungal stains
Drug-induced hepatoxicity	As in non-transplant liver pathology
CMV, cytomegalovirus; EBV; Epstein-Barr virus; HBV, hepatitis B virus; HCV, hepatitis C virus; HDV, hepatitis D virus; HSV, herpes simplex virus; IgM, immunoglobulin M; PAS-d, diastase-treated periodic acid-Schiff; GMS, Gomori methenamine silver.	

Table 7.11 Liver transplant pathology.

findings related to surgical complications, the transmission of clinically unknown donor disease, drug hepatotoxicity, and hepatic manifestations of sepsis may be seen. Finally, because the vascular supply to the biliary ductal system derives entirely from the hepatic artery, bile duct injury and related morphologic changes may be related to either the biliary anastomosis or to hepatic artery insufficiency from occlusion or immune-mediated injury. This change is more common in the later post-transplant period.

Recurrence of viral hepatitis
A major challenge occurs in distinguishing allograft injury caused by a recurrence of viral hepatitis B or hepatitis C infection from rejection. In some cases, there may be an overlap of findings and more than one process may be present. Ground-glass change in hepatocytes and immunohistochemical stains for HBV antigens are helpful in documenting the presence of HBV. Infiltration of bile ducts by lymphocytes may be seen in either acute rejection or infection with HCV; portal inflammation greater than acinar inflammation and endotheliitis favors the former, whereas ballooning of hepatocytes, steatosis, acidophil bodies and lymphoid aggregates are more indicative of the latter. Eosinophils may be seen in both processes. In some cases, serial biopsies are necessary for determining the causes of allograft dysfunction.

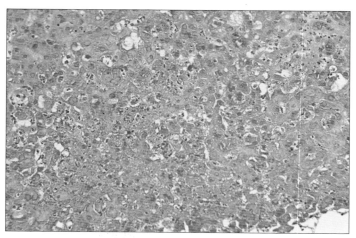

Figure 7.50 Post-transplant opportunistic infection. Herpes virus infection of the allograft liver shows similar histologic features as seen in the non-allograft liver: non-zonal 'punched-out' necrosis of hepatic parenchyma. On the borders of these foci, hepatocytes with the ground-glass nuclear features of herpes simplex virus inclusions are present (hematoxylin and eosin).

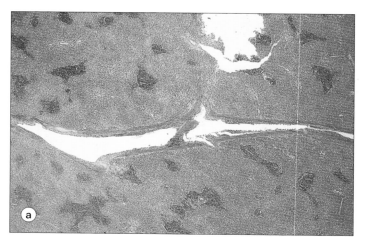

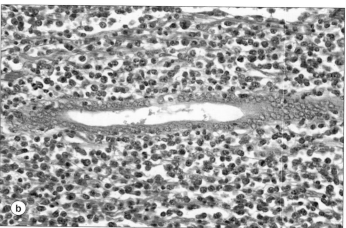

Figure 7.51 Post-transplant lymphoproliferative disorder. (a) Post-transplant lymphoproliferative disorder is a process that may also lead to marked cellular expansion of portal tracts (hematoxylin and eosin). (b) High-power examination of the involved portal tracts shows that the infiltrate consists of atypical, monomorphic lymphoid cells. The bile duct is surrounded but not destroyed by the infiltrate. Further phenotypic and genotypic characterization of the infiltrate is necessary to determine the clonality of the process (hematoxylin and eosin).

In addition, both recurrent HBV and HCV may cause severe graft dysfunction in the form of fibrosing cholestatic hepatitis, characterized by clinical jaundice and graft deterioration. The histopathologic features include hepatocellular ballooning, marked ductular proliferation, periportal fibrosis and cholestasis. Abundant intracytoplasmic viral antigens are readily demonstrated in HBV fibrosing cholestatic hepatitis (**Fig. 7.52**).

LIVER BIOPSY IN BONE MARROW TRANSPLANTATION

Liver dysfunction following bone marrow transplantation (BMT) may be attributable to processes that occur in the non-BMT setting, such as infection and drug toxicity, to processes that are unique to the post-BMT clinical setting, or to a combination of problems. Veno-occlusive disease is a serious, often fatal complication, with characteristic clinical findings. Rarely is

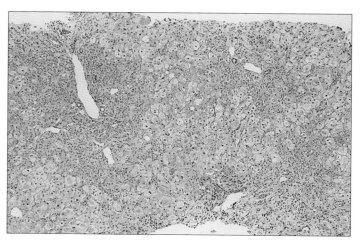

Figure 7.52 Recurrent hepatitis B. This biopsy is an example of a variant of recurrent hepatitis B infection known as fibrosing cholestatic hepatitis. There is panacinar hepatocyte ballooning; the portal tracts are expanded by chronic inflammation and ductular proliferation. In these cases, diffuse immunoreactivity with hepatitis B virus surface and core antigens will be present (hematoxylin and eosin).

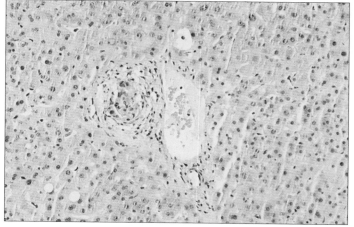

Figure 7.53 Graft versus host disease. Acute graft versus host disease may show significant damage to the interlobular bile ducts. As illustrated, the changes in the ductal epithelium include loss of nuclear polarity and cytoplasmic vacuolization. Inflammation is relatively mild (hematoxylin and eosin).

follow-up of patients with chronic liver disease, a combination of ultrasound, CT and α-fetoprotein levels have been shown to have a moderate sensitivity of approximately 84% in detecting small HCC; however, a significant number of individual nodules can be missed. Other studies have been shown to have fairly low sensitivity of CT in the identification of HCC. The addition of arterial phase images on CT and MRI protocols has allowed detection of additional lesions that would not be visible on the portal venous phase and conventional MR pulse sequences. MRI may provide further information when differentiating HCC from regenerating nodules.

In patients who are being evaluated for hepatectomy or transplantation, identification of individual lesions is critical; therefore, the most sensitive techniques should be used. CT and MRI are commonly used to diagnose and stage HCC in patients with cirrhosis. A commonly used system for non-invasive diagnosis of HCC has been proposed by a group of experts under the auspices of the European Association for the Study of the Liver (EASL). Under these criteria, HCC can be reliably diagnosed in a cirrhotic individual if there are two consecutive imaging studies of the liver which show a hypervascular lesion >2 cm in diameter or one imaging technique with a hypervascular lesion >2 cm combined with a serum α-fetoprotein level >400 ng/mL. The choice of CT or MRI appears to be based on local institutional expertise.

Cavernous hemangioma

Hemangiomata are exceedingly common and are present in 15–20% of the adult population. These lesions are commonly found on imaging of the liver. When these lesions are detected in an individual with a malignancy, they may mimic metastases. Because of the frequency of this dilemma, several studies have been done to evaluate the sensitivity and specificity of CT, MRI and tagged red blood cells in differentiating hemangiomas from metastases.

The imaging features of hemangioma reflect the histology and hemodynamics of the tumor, which is characterized by a cavernous collection of blood spaces. Blood flow is very slow and almost undetected, except for peripheral sites of entry. With intravenous contrast administration, hemangiomas demonstrate a classic pattern of peripheral nodular enhancement, centripetal filling and uniform enhancement with retention of the blood pool product (**Fig. 8.8**).

Using the aforementioned criteria, CT has a sensitivity and specificity of 80% and almost 100%, respectively. The appearance of hemangioma on MRI is that of a well-defined lesion with a very strong signal (equivalent to fluid) on heavily T_2-weighted images (**Fig. 8.9**). Enhancement with gadolinium is similar to that seen on a CT scan. Using these criteria, the specificity is similar to tagged red blood cell scans and is higher than 95%. MRI, although more expensive than tagged red blood cell scans in the confirmation of hemangioma, does offer some advantages. MRI can detect smaller lesions that are slightly less than 1 cm, whereas tagged red blood cell scans using SPECT techniques can only detect lesions on the order of 1–1.5 cm. MRI offers improved visualization of lesions near larger vessels, which may be subtle on tagged red blood cell scans because of the blood pool activity within the vessel. MRI also allows identification of other unsuspected lesions that would be missed by performing tagged red blood cell scans.

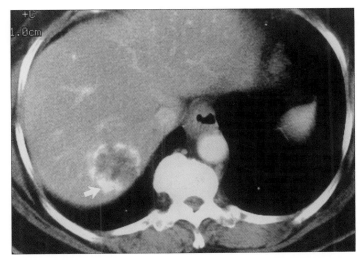

Figure 8.8 Hemangioma. Computed tomography demonstration of the classic early enhancement appearance showing nodular discontinuous peripheral enhancement (arrow).

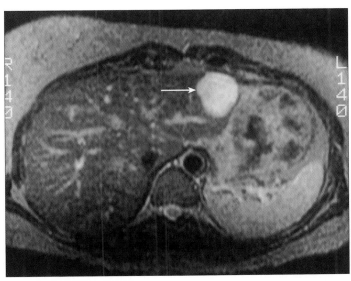

Figure 8.9 Hemangioma. Magnetic resonance imaging appearance of a hemangioma consists of a well-defined high signal intensity mass on T_2 imaging (arrow).

Miscellaneous tumors

The sensitivity of CT in detecting other primary tumors of the liver is quite high; however, many of the features are non-specific and do not allow definitive characterization. Certain tumors may have features that can suggest the diagnosis. For example, hepatic adenomas may contain areas of fat, necrosis and hemorrhage. The presence of a central scar suggests the diagnosis of FNH (**Fig. 8.10**) although this feature can sometimes be seen in fibrolamellar HCC and hepatic adenomas.

VASCULAR ABNORMALITIES

Ultrasound can provide exquisitely sensitive information regarding the hemodynamics of the liver, such as vascular patency, velocity and directional flow, and should be the initial study of

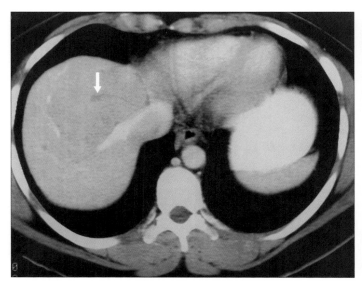

Figure 8.10 Focal nodular hyperplasia. An enhanced computed tomography scan demonstrates an isodense mass in the dome of the liver with a central scar, which is characteristic of focal nodular hyperplasia.

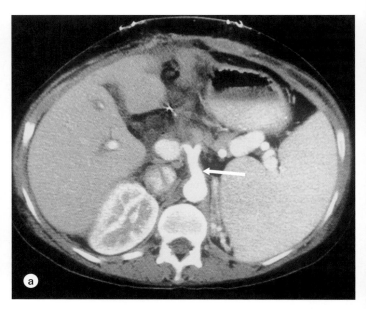

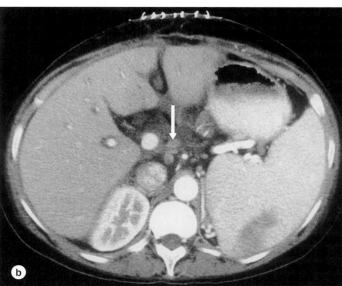

Figure 8.11 Hepatic artery thrombosis. The hepatic artery was unable to be identified by ultrasound in this patient who is status post-liver transplant. Axial images from a computed tomography angiogram show the celiac axis (a, arrow) and a thrombus (b) within the proximal hepatic artery (arrow).

choice when evaluating suspected vascular abnormalities. Ultrasound has a sensitivity of approximately 87% in the diagnosis of Budd-Chiari syndrome. Characteristic findings include the absence of the normal hepatic veins with areas of stenoses, webs, or thrombus. Abnormal Doppler wave forms may consist of absent or reversed flow in hepatic vein tributaries or the inferior vena cava, turbulent flow, or continuous flow. Ultrasound is 100% sensitive and 93% specific for the diagnosis of main portal vein thrombus and has been shown to be 97% sensitive for the diagnosis of significant arterial vascular disease in post-liver transplant patients.

MRI, with its ability to image flowing blood and determine the direction and velocity of flow, is generally complementary to ultrasound in the evaluation of hepatic vessels. However, MR should be used in select cases in which ultrasound is non-diagnostic or confusing. Because of its expanded field of view, MRI also shows associated collateral vessels throughout the abdomen.

With the rapid, high-resolution images obtained with helical CT, intravenous enhanced spiral CT scans can exquisitely demonstrate vascular anatomy and patency, especially of the arterial system (**Figs 8.11** and **8.12**). Delayed images during the portal venous phase can evaluate the venous structures; however, occasionally flow defects within these vessels can mimic thrombus.

BILIARY ABNORMALITIES

Gallstones

The primary modality that should be used to confirm the presence of cholelithiasis is ultrasound. Sonography has a sensitivity of greater than 95% in the diagnosis of cholelithiasis and can detect approximately 70–80% of choledocholithiasis. Gallstones within the distal part of the common bile duct are slightly more difficult to detect secondary to overlying bowel gas. On ultrasound, gallstones appear as echogenic structures with posterior acoustic shadowing. Because of the numerous possible pitfalls in diagnosis, meticulous technique and knowledge of these drawbacks are a necessity. To allow distention of the gallbladder and improve detection of gallstones, patients should be asked to fast for at least 4 to 6 h before the examination.

When using a high-resolution technique, CT can detect a significant number of calcified or dense gallstones because of the contrast between the calcium and bile. However, many gallstones demonstrate similar attenuation to bile, thus decreasing their rate of detection. Intravenous contrast agents that are excreted in the bile have been found to increase contrast between the stone and surrounding bile and improve detection; however, because of numerous side-effects, these agents are not widely

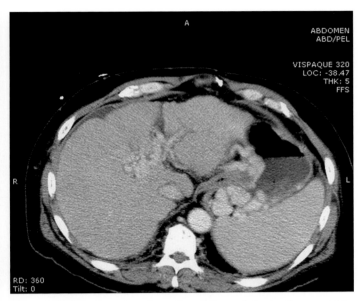

Figure 8.12 Cavernous transformation of the portal vein. Severe portal hypertension or occlusion of the portal vein may result in the development of large adjacent collaterals, evidenced by cavernous transformation of large veins in the upper abdomen related to the spleen and portal vein.

used in clinical practice. MRC has been shown to be useful in the diagnosis of gallstones with a sensitivity for detecting choledocholithiasis of 70–100% (**Fig. 8.13**).

Acute cholecystitis

In patients with suspected acute cholecystitis, sonography or hepatobiliary scintigraphy should be the initial imaging study performed. An advantage of ultrasound over scintigraphy is that ultrasound allows a generalized screening of the right upper quadrant, which may detect other abnormalities that mimic

acute cholecystitis. Findings of acute cholecystitis on ultrasound include the presence of gallstones with focal tenderness over the gallbladder (sonographic Murphy sign), gallbladder distention, gallbladder wall thickening, and air within the wall or lumen of the gallbladder, internal membranes and pericholecystic fluid. The most reliable sign is the presence of gallstones and the positive sonographic Murphy sign with a positive predictive value of 92% and a negative predictive value of 95%.

In acute cholecystitis, hepatobiliary scintigraphy (technetium-labeled iminodiacetic acid scans) demonstrates lack of visualization of the gallbladder secondary to obstruction of the cystic duct. Hepatobiliary scintigraphy has a high sensitivity and specificity of more than 95%. Occasionally, patients with acute cholecystitis may have non-specific clinical findings and be referred for CT examination. The CT findings are similar to those found on ultrasound, including gallbladder wall thickening, pericholecystic stranding, gallbladder distention, pericholecystic fluid, subserosal edema, high attenuation bile and sloughed membranes (**Fig. 8.14**). In one study CT allowed detection of approximately 50% of cases of acute cholecystitis; however, the absence of findings does not exclude the diagnosis, and further imaging with ultrasound or scintigraphy should be performed.

Biliary obstruction

Biliary obstruction can be caused by many conditions, including extrinsic or intrinsic masses, inflammation and strictures. The evaluation of individuals with suspected biliary obstruction should begin with right upper quadrant sonography. Ultrasound allows detection of bile duct dilatation and can usually determine the site of obstruction in more than 90% of the cases and the cause in more than 70% of the cases. CT may provide useful information when the ultrasound is inconclusive or incompletely evaluates or stages the abnormality detected. MRC is a non-invasive technique to obtain cholangiographic images and the detection of bile duct strictures.

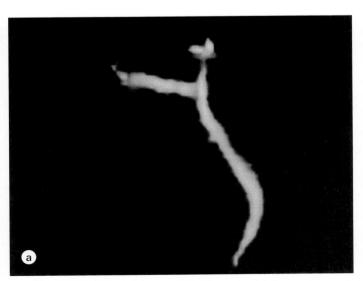
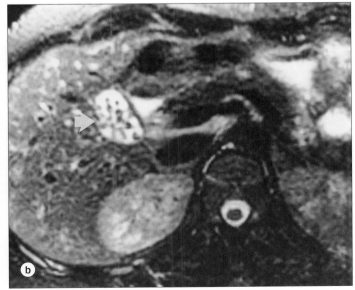

Figure 8.13 Magnetic resonance cholangiography. (a) A normal-appearing magnetic resonance imaging (MRI) cholangiogram. (b) Cholelithiasis. Note the appearance of gallstones on the MRI. The typical gallstone is a low signal intensity structure seen within the high-intensity bile, such as in the gallbladder (arrow).

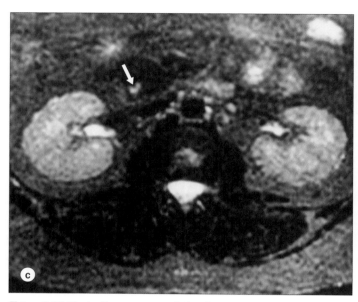

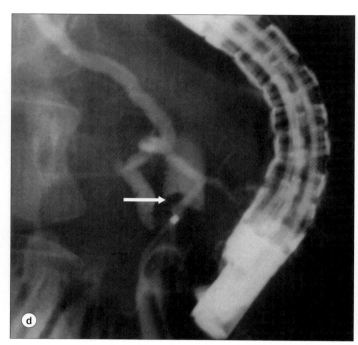

Figure 8.13 Magnetic resonance cholangiography. (*Cont'd*) (c) Choledocholithiasis. A tiny, 2–3 mm, low-signal intensity structure is seen on the axial images from a magnetic resonance cholangiogram in the distal common bile duct (arrow). (d) Gallstone. This tiny gallstone was confirmed on subsequent endoscopic retrograde cholangiopancreatography.

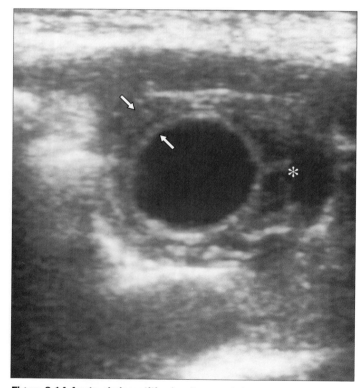

Figure 8.14 Acute cholecystitis. An ultrasound demonstrates a greatly thickened gallbladder wall (arrows) with intramural fluid (asterisk). These findings combined with a positive 'sonographic Murphy sign' are diagnostic of acute cholecystitis.

OTHER IMAGING TECHNIQUES

Conventional arteriography of the liver was previously done in preparation for surgery but is now more frequently done as part of a therapeutic intervention, such as with chemoembolization, to assess arterial stenoses after liver transplantation or to embolize sources of hemorrhage within the liver. Angiography has also been used to enhance the sensitivity of CT. Because of the wide variation of tumor enhancement and the less than satisfactory results for individual lesion identification utilizing dynamic bolus techniques, other methods to administer contrast at angiography with selected cannulation of the hepatic artery [CT arteriography (CTA)] or by the superior mesenteric artery and splenic artery (CTAP) are commonly performed. These techniques offer improved contrast and sensitivity in individual lesion detection; however, due to variations in the portal venous perfusion, they are plagued by the problem of perfusion defects that can cause false-positive diagnoses of lesions.

Lipiodol CT is a technique in which an oily contrast medium derived from poppy seed oil is infused into the hepatic artery by using angiographic techniques. This oily material is retained selectively by HCC tissues which can be more readily seen when a CT scan of the liver is performed some days after the lipiodol is infused.

^{18}F-fluorodeoxyglucose (FDG) uptake allows estimation of glucose metabolism of cells using positron emission tomography (PET). Normal liver contains a relative abundance of glucose 6-phosphatase (G6P) and lower levels of hexokinase (HK) while tumor cells tend to have increased HK activity but little, if any, G6P. This difference in metabolism results in increased accumulation of FDG in cholangiocarcinoma, HCC and metastatic liver tumors, potentially allowing differentiation between normal tissue and tumor on PET images. While PET of extra-hepatic

CHAPTER
9

Portal Hypertension and Gastrointestinal Hemorrhage

Anastasios A. Mihas and Arun J. Sanyal

INTRODUCTION

Variceal bleeding, a direct consequence of portal hypertension, is the most lethal complication of cirrhosis and accounts for approximately one-third of all deaths among patients with chronic liver disease and cirrhosis. Optimal management of portal hypertension and variceal hemorrhage requires a clear understanding of the pathophysiology of portal hypertension, its pathogenesis and the natural history of varices as well as the risk factors associated with their bleeding.

Portal hypertension is defined as the elevation of hepatic venous pressure gradient (HVPG) to greater than 5 mmHg. Portal hypertension is caused by a combination of two hemodynamic processes:

- increased intrahepatic resistance to the passage of blood flow through the liver, and
- increased splanchnic blood flow secondary to vasodilatation within the splanchnic vascular bed.

Hence, numerous vasoconstrictors and vasodilators can have an impact on portal pressure and act therapeutically by decreasing both portal hypertension and intravariceal pressure.

Portal hypertension is responsible for the two major complications of cirrhosis – variceal bleeding and ascites. These two complications account for a large proportion of the 32 000 deaths and 20 million days of work loss related to cirrhosis annually in the USA. Of these complications, variceal hemorrhage is more immediately life threatening and is associated with a 20–30% mortality with each episode of bleeding.

PATHOPHYSIOLOGY OF PORTAL HYPERTENSION

Portal venous anatomy

The portal venous system normally drains blood from the stomach, intestines, spleen, pancreas and gallbladder. The portal vein is formed by the confluence of the superior mesenteric and splenic veins (**Fig. 9.1**). The superior mesenteric vein drains deoxygenated blood from the small bowel, the head of the pancreas, the ascending colon and part of the transverse colon whereas the splenic vein drains the spleen and the pancreas and is joined by the inferior mesenteric vein, which brings blood from the transverse and descending colon as well as the superior two-thirds of the rectum. Thus, the portal vein normally receives blood from almost the entire gastrointestinal tract.

Classification of portal hypertension

The causes of portal hypertension are usually classified into prehepatic, intrahepatic and posthepatic. Prehepatic causes are those affecting the venous system before it enters the liver, such

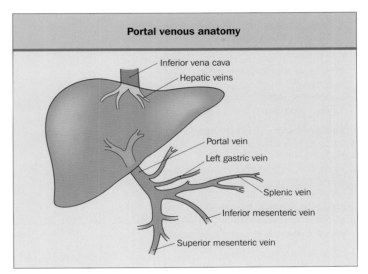

Figure 9.1 Portal venous anatomy.

as thrombosis of the portal vein. Intrahepatic causes represent the main group, with cirrhosis accounting for the vast majority of cases. Posthepatic causes encompass those affecting the hepatic veins and venous drainage to the heart. (e.g. Budd-Chiari syndrome).

A more precise classification emerges when the intrahepatic anatomy of the venous connections is taken into account. The portal vein divides and branches throughout the liver, eventually forming portal venules at the lobular level. These connect to the central veins via the hepatic sinusoids. The pressure in the portal venules is the same as that in the systemic venous circulation. There is a normal gradient of approximately 3 mmHg across the liver from portal (7 mmHg) to hepatic (4 mmHg) venous systems.

In cases of portal hypertension, a high wedged hepatic venous pressure (WHVP) suggests an intrahepatic block at the level of the sinusoids (flow being obstructed between a portal venule and central vein, with a resulting high pressure in the venule), whereas a normal WHVP reflects normal pressure in the portal venule and thus a presinusoidal cause of portal hypertension, such as disease around the portal tracts or outside the liver. Thus, portal hypertension can be reclassified as presinusoidal (both prehepatic and intrahepatic), sinusoidal (intrahepatic) and postsinusoidal (intrahepatic and posthepatic) (**Table 9.1**).

This classification has immediate clinical implications: for example, in presinusoidal portal hypertension (both pre- and intrahepatic) where the liver function is well preserved and liver

Causes of portal hypertension
Presinusoidal portal hypertension
Extrahepatic causes
Portal vein thrombosis
Cavernous transformation of the portal vein
Extrinsic compression of the portal vein
Arterioportal fistula
Massive splenomegaly
Intrahepatic causes
Schistosomiasis
Sarcoidosis
Primary biliary cirrhosis
Idiopathic portal hypertension (non-cirrhotic portal hypertension)
Sinusoidal portal hypertension
Cirrhosis
Alcoholic hepatitis
Vitamin A toxicity
Postsinusoidal portal hypertension
Veno-occlusive disease
Budd-Chiari syndrome
Hepatic venous or inferior vena cava web
Restrictive heart disease
Constrictive pericarditis
Severe congestive heart failure

Table 9.1 Causes of portal hypertension.

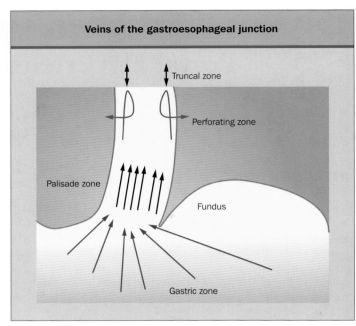

Figure 9.2 Veins of the gastroesophageal junction. The venous anatomy allows subdivision of the region into four zones: the gastric, palisade, perforating and truncal zones. Modified from Vianna in McIntyre et al (91) by permission of Oxford University Press.

failure and hepatic encephalopathy are infrequent following variceal hemorrhage. Nevertheless, many hepatic causes of portal hypertension produce pathologic changes that cause a block at both the presinusoidal and sinusoidal levels and often, therefore, the distinction is academic. In contrast, there are clear therapeutic implications for differentiating hepatic venous outflow obstruction (posthepatic) from other causes of portal hypertension.

Anatomy and classification of gastroesophageal varices

The tributaries of the portal vein also communicate with veins draining the systemic venous circulation. Such portosystemic communications exist primarily in five locations:

- at the cardia via the intrinsic and extrinsic veins of the region,
- in the anal canal via anastomoses between the superior and middle hemorrhoidal veins,
- in the falciform ligament via recanalization of the para-umbilical veins draining the abdominal wall,
- the splenic venous bed and the left renal vein, and
- the retroperitoneum.

Of these, the gastroesophageal collaterals have the greatest clinical significance and allow portal blood flow to return to the heart when flow through the portal system is obstructed.

The veins draining the esophagus may be classified as intrinsic, extrinsic and venae comitantes of the vagal verve. The intrinsic veins are comprised of a subepithelial and submucosal plexus, which run along the length of the esophagus. These drain via perforating veins into an extrinsic plexus of veins surrounding the esophagus. In the cervical region and superior mediastinum, they drain into the inferior thyroid and brachiocephalic veins, whereas in the posterior mediastinum they drain into the

azygous vein. The extrinsic venous plexus around the abdominal part of the esophagus drains into the left gastric vein.

The intrinsic veins of the gastroesophageal junction are divided into four well-defined zones (**Fig. 9.2**):

- The *gastric zone* is a 2–3 cm zone with its upper border at the gastroesophageal junction and consists of veins arranged radially, in the submucosa and lamina propria.
- The *palisade zone* commences at the gastroesophageal junction and extends cranially for 2–3 cm and is a direct extension of the veins of the gastric zone, which runs in 'palisades' or packs of longitudinally arrayed veins in the lamina propria. When portal pressures rise and impede drainage of the veins in the gastric zone into the left gastric vein, flow is directed via the veins of the palisade zone into the esophagus and eventually into the azygous vein.
- The intrinsic veins drain into the extrinsic veins primarily in the *perforating zone* via the valved perforating veins that normally allow only unidirectional flow. However, flow through these veins increases in subjects with portal hypertension, the valves become incompetent and allow bidirectional flow. The perforating zone extends 2–3 cm cranially from the palisade zone.
- The *truncal zone* is an 8–10 cm zone extending upward from the perforating zone. The intrinsic veins consist of three or four large venous trunks in the submucosa, which communicate with an irregular polygonal venous plexus in the submucosa. Blood in these veins flows from a cranial to a caudal direction and drains via the perforating veins into the extrinsic veins.

When portal hypertension occurs, the impediment to portal flow is partly compensated for by an increase in flow through portosystemic communications, especially the intrinsic veins around the gastroesophageal junction, which dilate and become varicose veins. Such gastroesophageal varices occur in four basic patterns:

- varices in the fundus of the stomach,
- gastric and palisade zone varices,
- varices in the perforating zone, and
- paraesophageal varices that involve the extrinsic esophageal veins.

Clinically, varices are classified by their location as esophageal or gastric varices. Esophageal varices are graded by their size (**Table 9.2**).

In contrast, gastric varices are classified primarily by their location (**Fig. 9.3**). As agreed at the Baveno Consensus Conference, they are classified as follows: gastroesophageal varices (GOV, gastric varices in continuity with esophageal varices) or isolated gastric varices (IGV) (Table 9.2).

GOV1 are formed by a communication between the deep submucosal veins in the gastric zone with a branch of the left gastric vein. These varices allow blood from the left gastric vein to drain via palisade zone veins into the systemic circulation. GOV1 varices are invariably associated with large esophageal varices. In contrast, only 50% of GOV2 are associated with large esophageal varices. IGV1 are usually associated with either segmental portal hypertension (splenic vein thrombosis) or the presence of spontaneous collaterals from the splenic vein to the renal vein, which feed these varices. Approximately 50% of cases of ectopic varices, including IGV2, are associated with portal hypertension. The mechanism underlying the predilection for varices to develop at sites away from the gastroesophageal junction when the portal vein is occluded remains unknown.

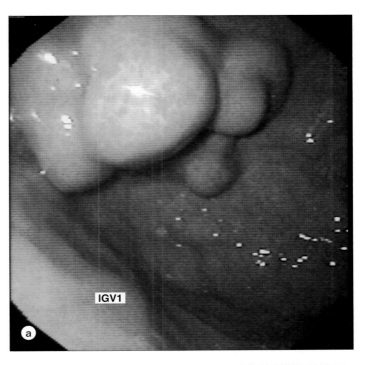

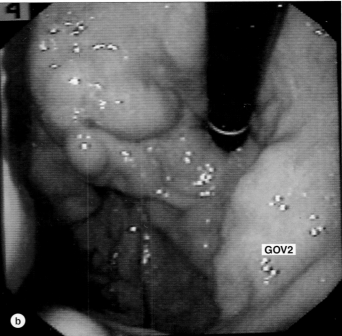

Figure 9.3 Type I isolated gastric varices (IGV1) as a cluster of varices in the fundus (a) and cardia (b) of the stomach.

Gastrointestinal manifestations of portal hypertension	
Manifestation	*Comments*
Varices	
1. Esophageal	
F1	Small, straight
F2	Enlarged, tortuous, <1/3 of lumen
F3	Large, coil-shaped, >1/3 of lumen
2. Gastroesophageal (GEV)	
GEV-1	Along lesser curve, 2–5 cm
GEV-2	Along greater curve and fundus
3. Isolated gastric (IGV)	
IGV-1	Isolated in the fundus
IGV-2	Limited in the corpus, antrum, pylorus
4. Ectopic varices	Duodenum, small bowel, colorectum
Portal hypertensive gastropathy	
PHG	Fundus and corpus of the stomach
GAVE	Limited to the antrum
GAVE, gastric antral vascular ectasia; PHG, portal hypertensive gastropathy	

Table 9.2 Gastrointestinal manifestations of portal hypertension

The pressure in the portal vein is a direct product of portal inflow and outflow resistance. Thus:

$$\text{portal pressure} = \text{portal venous inflow} \times \text{outflow resistance} \qquad \text{(eq. 1)}$$

Portal pressure is determined by hepatic venous catheterization and measurement of the free hepatic venous pressure (FHVP) and WHVP and calculation of the HVPG:

$$HVPG = WHVP - FHVP \qquad \text{(eq. 2)}$$

WHVPs reflect sinusoidal pressures and, in the absence of portal vein thrombosis, reflect portal vein pressures. The free hepatic venous pressure corrects for the effects of intra-abdominal pressures. Portal hypertension usually occurs when the resistance to flow through the portal venous bed is increased. As mentioned earlier, this may result from an obstruction to portal venous flow before it enters the hepatic sinusoids (presinusoidal portal hypertension, e.g. portal vein thrombosis), in the hepatic sinusoids (sinusoidal portal hypertension, e.g. cirrhosis), or beyond the hepatic sinusoids (postsinusoidal portal hypertension, e.g. hepatic vein thrombosis). In patients with cirrhosis, the increase in portal pressures is further compounded by a secondary increase in portal flow that results from splanchnic arteriolar dilatation.

A principal hemodynamic consequence of portal hypertension is diversion of portal flow to the systemic circulation via porto-systemic communications that dilate to form varices. These varices, especially in the intrinsic veins around the gastro-esophageal junction, are likely to rupture bringing them to clinical attention.

The likelihood of variceal rupture is determined by its wall tension, which may be defined as:

wall tension = (transmural pressure gradient) ×
radius of varix/width of variceal wall (w)   (eq. 3)

The transmural pressure gradient is the product of flow and resistance through the varix and is defined as:

$$P_1 - P_2 = Q \times R \qquad \text{(eq. 4)}$$

where P_1 and P_2 are the pressure within and outside the varix respectively, Q is the blood flow per unit time, and R is the resistance to flow through the varix. The resistance to flow may be calculated by Poiseuille formula and expressed as:

$$R = 8\acute{\eta}l/pr^4 \qquad \text{(eq. 5)}$$

where l is the length of the varix, $\acute{\eta}$ is related to blood viscosity (Reynold number), and r is the radius of the vessel. Interposing equations 4 and 5 in equation 3, variceal tension may be redifined as:

Wall tension = $Q \times (8\acute{\eta}lkpr^4) \times \acute{\eta}w$ (eq. 6)

Consequently, based on equation 6 above, long, large varices with high flow rates and a thin wall are most likely to rupture and bleed. Conversely, decreasing collateral flow, resistance to flow, or increasing wall thickness should decrease the risk of variceal rupture. Variceal flow is decreased primarily by decreasing portal pressures. This is accomplished in most cases by inducing splanchnic arteriolar constriction, which reduces portal inflow (see equation 1) and forms the physiologic basis for most forms of pharmacologic treatment of portal hypertension. Whereas decreasing resistance to flow through the varices should decrease wall tension also, the results are less predictable due to an associated increase in collateral flow that negates the beneficial effects of decreased collateral resistance. This may explain some of the interindividual variability in hemodynamic response to pharmacologic treatment.

NATURAL HISTORY AND CLINICAL FEATURES OF PORTAL HYPERTENSION

The three primary features of portal hypertension are gastro-esophageal varices, ascites and hypersplenism. The latter two topics are dealt with elsewhere.

Esophageal varices

Endoscopic screening among cirrhotics has shown that approximately one-third have varices. An additional 5–15% of those with cirrhosis without varices develop varices de novo each year. It is estimated that most cirrhotic individuals (~75%) will develop varices during their lifetime and that about one-third of all patients with esophageal varices will experience variceal hemorrhage. Several factors predict the risk of bleeding from esophageal varices (**Table 9.3**)

It is both intuitively as well as clinically obvious that varices cannot bleed if they do not develop. Several studies have now shown that at HVPG values less than 12 mmHg, varices do not form and therefore do not bleed. Varix formation as identified by endoscopy is invariably associated with a HVPG greater than 12 mmHg. However, the precise level of portal pressure above 12 mmHg does not correlate well with the likelihood of bleeding. An important implication of these observations is that if the HVPG is maintained below 12 mmHg, the risk of variceal hemorrhage can be minimized. Another corollary of these findings is that occurrence of varices may be prevented by decreasing the portal pressure below 12 mmHg before the development of varices. Clinical trials designed to test this hypothesis are currently under way.

The portal pressure determines the degree of portosystemic shunting and is an indirect marker of variceal flow and trans-mural pressure gradient. Traditionally, intravariceal measure-

Predictive factors for variceal bleeding
Child class
HVPG >12 mmHg
Intravariceal pressure
Size of varix
Location of varix
Endoscopic stigmata (various color signs)
Red wales
Hematocystic spots
Diffuse erythema
Bluish color
Cherry-red spots
White nipple
Alcohol consumption (in alcoholic cirrhosis)
Tense ascites
HVPG, hepatic venous pressure gradient.

Table 9.3 Predictive factors for variceal bleeding

an option only for patients ready for transplantation at a recognized transplant center. Many patients with variceal hemorrhage, such as unreformed alcoholics, are not suitable candidates for liver transplantation. The use of orthotopic liver transplantation (OLT) is limited further by the paucity of available donor livers and the high procedure costs.

THERAPEUTIC OPPORTUNITIES

Primary prevention of variceal bleeding

According to the recent Veterans Affairs (VA) Hepatitis Resource Centers' recommendations, three major factors identify accurately patients at high risk of bleeding from varices: large variceal size, red wale markings on the varices, and severe liver failure, as defined by the Baveno III Consensus conference. Thus, patients with these features can be considered targets for strategies to prevent the first episode of bleeding.

Pharmacologic measures

Pharmacologic therapy with non-selective β blockade remains the treatment of choice for primary prevention of variceal hemorrhage. A total of 10 placebo-controlled clinical trials of propranolol or nadolol have been reported and reviewed extensively. Comparisons across trials are confounded by the differences in patient populations studied as well as treatment regimens used. Despite the heterogeneity between trials, several general observations can be made. In the first year of follow-up (the period of greatest risk of bleeding), those treated with β blockers had a lower risk of variceal hemorrhage than did those treated with placebo (0–18% versus 12–30%) (**Fig. 9.5**). These effects were even more pronounced after 2 years of follow-up. Also, there was a decrease in variceal hemorrhage-related mortality. However, these beneficial effects translated into an overall survival advantage in only one study.

Meta-analyses of the data suggest that non-selective β blockade reduces the risks of initial variceal hemorrhage by 45% and bleeding-related deaths by 50%. The factors associated with failure of treatment included younger age, large variceal size, advanced liver failure and lower doses of propranolol. On the other hand, good compliance with treatment was an important predictor of a good outcome. It has also been shown that an important predictor of a favorable outcome is the degree of portal decompression achieved. Those patients who are able to sustain a drop in hepatic venous pressure gradient by 25% or to levels below 12 mmHg over time did not bleed and had a significantly prolonged survival. It has been suggested, therefore, that repeated measurements of HVPG be used to guide pharmacologic therapy of portal hypertension. However, the cost effectiveness of such an approach remains to be demonstrated and routine measurement of HVPG is not available at most community hospitals.

An important study prospectively randomized 118 patients to receive either ISMN (20 mg t.i.d.) or propranolol (to the maximum tolerated dose). Although no differences were noted during initial analysis 29 months after entry into the study, an increased mortality especially in those older than 51 years of age (72 versus 48%) was noted in those receiving ISMN after 7 years of follow-up (**Fig. 9.6**).

Potential explanations for the increased mortality in those receiving nitrates include worsening of the hyperdynamic circulatory state and a decrease in effective circulating volume, increased sodium retention and tissue hypoxia with increased lactate levels in cirrhotic individuals. At this time, the data do not support a role for nitrates as monotherapy for the primary prophylaxis of variceal hemorrhage. It has been shown that a combination of nitrates and β blockers is more effective than β blockers alone for the prevention of variceal hemorrhage (**Fig. 9.7**). However, this does not translate to a survival advantage.

Endoscopic therapy

In recent years, various endoscopic therapeutic modalities have been proposed for the prevention of the initial variceal hemorrhage in patients with cirrhosis. The observation that EIS is an effective therapeutic modality for bleeding esophageal varices has led to a large number of randomized controlled trials

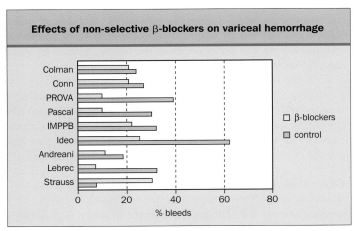

Figure 9.5 Effects of non-selective β-blockers on variceal hemorrhage. Effects on rates of variceal hemorrhage in clinical trials of β blockers for primary prophylaxis of variceal hemorrhage. Modified from Sanyal et al (97).

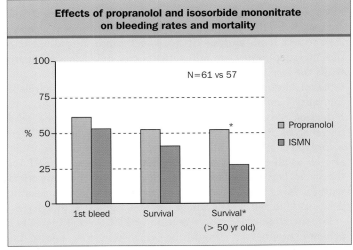

Figure 9.6 Effects of propranolol and isosorbide mononitrate on bleeding rates and mortality. Used for primary prophylaxis of variceal hemorrhage. Modified from Angelico et al (97).

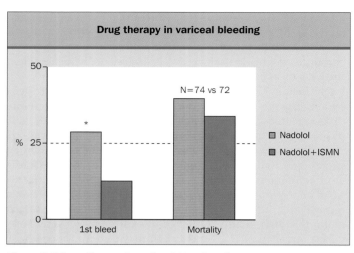

Figure 9.7 Drug therapy in variceal bleeding. β blockers versus a combination of β blocker plus nitrates for the primary prevention of (first) variceal bleeding.

evaluating its role in primary prophylaxis. Unfortunately, the efficacy of prophylactic sclerotherapy remains unclear because most of the published studies have produced conflicting results. These clinical trials are characterized by significant heterogeneity in the patient population, the use of sclerotherapy for acute bleeding, and particularly, the baseline bleeding risk ranging from 0 to 75%. Although some earlier studies found sclerotherapy beneficial for both preventing first bleeding and reducing mortality, more recent studies have failed to confirm these observations. In fact, a VA cooperative multicenter study, one of the largest trials (n = 81) of prophylactic sclerotherapy, was terminated prematurely due to the higher mortality in the sclerotherapy arm than the sham therapy arm (32 versus 17.4%). Thus, EIS either alone or in combination with β blockers is not recommended because of its high complication rates and the availability of other less invasive and more cost-effective therapeutic modalities.

In recent years, the observation that EVL obliterates and eradicates esophageal varices as effectively as EIS but with fewer complications, has led to an explosion of clinical trials comparing EVL in the primary prophylaxis of variceal bleeding.

A recent meta-analysis of five randomized controlled trials that included more than 600 patients concluded that compared with the no treatment arm, prophylactic EVL significantly reduced the risk of first variceal bleeding, bleeding-related mortality, and all-cause mortality. More interestingly, the reduction in the risk of the initial bleeding remained when the analysis included only the four trials in which EVL was compared to β blockade. In contrast, bleeding-related mortality as well as all-cause mortality did not differ between EVL and the β-blocker arms. The results clearly show that in patients with cirrhosis, EVL is as effective and as safe as non-selective β blockade in the prevention of the first variceal hemorrhage.

For the time being, the selection of EVL over β blockers in primary prophylaxis should be very judicious, taking into account the cost, inconvenience and risks associated with variceal band ligation. Furthermore, EVL may not be a permanent solution and varices may recur after initial eradication.

Several studies have shown a significant rate of variceal recurrence, following the initial EVL, thus necessitating continued patient surveillance.

Other measures

Currently, neither TIPS nor surgery have a role for primary prevention of variceal bleeding.

Treatment of active bleeding

Acute variceal hemorrhage is the most ominous complication of cirrhosis with portal hypertension and accounts for about one-third of all deaths related to cirrhosis. The outcome of an episode of active hemorrhage depends upon the control of active bleeding and avoidance of major complications associated with bleeding and its treatment. Establishing the correct diagnosis is also important. Other causes of upper gastrointestinal bleeding in patients with liver disease include peptic ulcer disease, Mallory-Weiss tear, PHG and GAVE, esophagitis and gastroduodenitis. Moreover, any of these lesions is more likely to bleed in the presence of portal hypertension and may indeed bleed briskly. The frequency with which varices account for upper gastrointestinal (UGI) bleeding in patients with cirrhosis is uncertain. Varices appeared to be the source of bleeding in 50–90% of cirrhotic patients with UGI bleeding in various reports, although a variety of other causes may also be responsible. In a recent multicenter prospective study among 465 cirrhotics with acute UGI bleeding, 72% percent bled from varices.

There are two distinct phases in the course of variceal hemorrhage: an acute phase; and a later phase in which there is a high risk of recurrent bleeding. The acute phase starts with the onset of active hemorrhage. Only 50% of patients with variceal hemorrhage stop bleeding spontaneously; this is quite different from the more than 90% spontaneous cessation rate in patients with other forms of UGI hemorrhage. Patients with Child class C cirrhosis and large, actively spurting varices are less likely to achieve spontaneous hemostasis.

Following cessation of active hemorrhage, there is a period of approximately 6 weeks in which there is a high risk of recurrent hemorrhage. The greatest risk is within the first 48–72 h, and over 50% of all early rebleeding episodes occur within the first 10 days. Risk factors for early rebleeding include age greater than 60 years, renal failure, large varices, and severe initial bleeding as defined by hemoglobin below 8 g/dL at admission. Survival during this period mirrors the risk of rebleeding and is directly related to the outcome of bleeding.

The risk of bleeding and of death in patients who survive 6 weeks is similar to that in cirrhotic patients of equivalent severity who have never bled. Approximately 52% of those who survive 2 weeks after a variceal bleed reach 1-year survival. Survival appears to have increased slightly in the past two decades largely due to a decrease in short-term mortality.

General principles of management

Acute variceal hemorrhage can be torrential, constituting a medical emergency that may culminate in death if bleeding is not controlled promptly. Hence, adequate resuscitation remains the single most important step in the management of these patients, before diagnostic or therapeutic interventions (**Table 9.4**).

General medical management of variceal hemorrhage
Volume resuscitation: – keep hemoglobin 9–10 g/dL – maintain urine output of at least 50 cc/h Correct hematologic status: – packed red cells to replace blood loss – platelet transfusions if platelet counts ≤50 000/mm³ – fresh frozen plasma for severe coagulopathy (consider recombinant factor VII) Sepsis: – blood cultures and diagnostic paracentesis of acites – prophylactic intravenous antibiotics (switch to oral when feasible) Electrolytes: – monitor for hypercalcemia, hypomagnesemia and hypophosphatemia (in alcoholics) – monitor for hypocalcemia if large amounts of EDTA-containing blood are used Management of encephalopathy and mental status changes: – thiamine for alcoholic patients – monitor for and manage alcohol withdrawal – clear the gastrointestinal tract of blood and control bleeding Maintain cardiopulmonary functions: – protect airway (particularly with severe bleeding or mental status changes) – optimize volume status Renal function: – monitor urine output and serum creatinine levels – aseptic technique for urinary bladder catheterization
EDTA, ethylenediaminetetraacetic acid

Table 9.4 General medical management of variceal hemorrhage

Pharmacologic measures

Drug therapy has inherent advantages because it is readily available and its administration does not require specially trained personnel. Pharmacologic treatment is usually employed to stop or decrease variceal bleeding, pending further endoscopic treatment, although drug monotherapy has been reported to be effective in active variceal bleeding. The rationale for pharmacologic therapy is to lower the increased portal pressure and thereby the intravariceal pressure. This is achieved by either decreasing portal venous blood flow or by decreasing intrahepatic or portosystemic resistance.

Vasopressin has been used in the management of acute variceal hemorrhage for the last three decades. Pooled data from a number of studies have shown significant beneficial effect of vasopressin in reducing failure to control bleeding. Vasopressin can achieve initial hemostasis in 60–80% of patients, but has only marginal effects on early rebleeding episodes and does not improve survival from active variceal hemorrhage. The benefit of bleeding cessation may be counterbalanced by enhanced mortality due to extrasplanchnic vasoconstrictive properties and resultant myocardial, cerebral and bowel ischemia.

The systemic vasodilator NTG has been concurrently administered in an attempt to avoid the adverse effects related to vasopressin-induced systemic vasoconstriction. It is recommended that, when used, intravenous vasopressin should be combined with intravenous NTG. Several clinical trials have shown that glypressin (terlipressin) is at least as effective as somatostatin and more effective than placebo.

A number of clinical trials have compared somatostatin or octreotide to either vasopressin or placebo in the management of active bleeding. Most of these studies have demonstrated that somatostatin is more effective for controlling bleeding than placebo or vasopressin and has fewer side-effects than vasopressin. Although the role of octreotide is less well established, it is the current drug of choice in the USA because of its easy availability compared to somatostatin. Interestingly, despite their widespread use, neither drug has a clearly established benefit on mortality. The current view of most hepatologists is that octreotide should only be used as an adjunctive therapy to endoscopic variceal sclerotherapy or band ligation in the control of acute variceal hemorrhage.

Endoscopic treatment is currently the intervention of choice for acute variceal bleeding. Furthermore, endoscopy can provide valuable diagnostic information. Several trials have shown that EIS is highly effective in the control of acute bleeding and prevention of early rebleeding in more that 85–90% of patients. Both esophageal as well as GOV1 and GOV2 are amenable to treatment by sclerotherapy. However, gastric varices do not lend themselves to this modality of treatment. Clinical trials have shown sclerotherapy to be superior to balloon tamponade alone, vasopressin alone, and a combination of vasopressin and balloon tamponade for control of active hemorrhage, prevention of early rebleeding, reduction of complication rates, and improved survival.

During the past decade, EVL has emerged as an alternative endoscopic modality to sclerotherapy because of the relatively high rate of complications associated with EIS. A number of controlled trials have shown that EVL controls bleeding in approximately 85–100% of patients.

Emergency endoscopic therapy fails to control bleeding in 10–20% of patients. In case of failure to control bleeding or early rebleeding, a prompt decision for rescue therapy should be made (i.e. no more than two sessions of endoscopic therapy) as these patients are at high risk of both exsanguination and other complications related to active bleeding. Most patients will have already received a trial of pharmacologic treatment by the time a diagnosis of failed endoscopic treatment is established. In such patients, a second attempt at endoscopic hemostasis may be made (e.g. band ligation for failed sclerotherapy). However, if bleeding is not quickly and effectively stopped, more definitive therapy must be instituted immediately with balloon tamponade or some type of portosystemic shunt. Once the patient is stabilized by whatever means, a more definitive therapy such as TIPS or surgery should be instituted immediately. Factors affecting risk of continued bleeding or recurrent bleeding are shown in **Table 9.5**.

Transjugular intrahepatic portosystemic shunt and emergency surgery

In the early clinical TIPS studies, hemostasis was achieved in the vast majority of patients with refractory variceal hemorrhage despite endoscopic treatment. TIPS could be performed in a reasonable period of time in most patients with low procedure-related morbidity or mortality. However, interpretation of the efficacy of TIPS in the setting of active hemorrhage was confounded by the heterogeneous patient populations and failure to define the nature of active bleeding.

Factors affecting risk of continued bleeding or recurrent bleeding
Factors associated with failure to control acute variceal hemorrhage
– Spurting varices
– Child-Pugh score
– Hepatic venous pressure gradient
– Infection
– Portal vein thrombosis
Factors associated with early rebleeding
– Severity of initial bleeding
– Overly aggressive volume resuscitation
– Infection
– Hepatic venous pressure gradient
– Complications of endoscopic treatment
– Renal failure
Factors associated with late rebleeding
– Child-Pugh score
– Variceal size
– Continued alcohol use
– Hepatocellular carcinoma

Table 9.5 Factors affecting risk of continued bleeding or recurrent bleeding

The data are difficult to combine due to heterogeneity of patients studied, different types of operations used, and varying protocols used for supportive management. However, the following general conclusions can be made:

- Both portal decompressive surgery and esophageal transection are highly effective in achieving hemostasis.
- Emergency portacaval shunts are more likely to thrombose than elective shunts. In addition, portacaval shunts alter vascular anatomy, complicate future liver transplant surgery and are associated with an approximately 40–50% incidence of encephalopathy.

Large-scale, randomized prospective trials are needed to establish the roles of surgery and TIPS in average risk subjects with active hemorrhage who have failed endoscopic and medical treatment. At present, TIPS is the procedure of choice in such patients who are poor risks for surgery; the relative roles of TIPS and surgery in those who are good candidates are uncertain. The ideal patient for surgical therapy is one with well-preserved liver function who fails emergent endoscopic treatment and has no complications from the bleeding or endoscopy. The choice of surgery is usually dependent on the training and expertise of the surgeon.

Acute bleeding from gastric varices

Bleeding gastric varices can be technically difficult to treat. They frequently rebleed despite initially successful endoscopic therapy; as a result, endoscopic treatment should not be used outside of randomized studies. Successful hemostasis and obliteration of gastric varices has been reported with intravariceal injection of sclerosants, absolute alcohol, thrombin and cyanoacrylate. Cyanoacrylate injection appears to be more effective and safer than band ligation or alcohol injection.

At present, patients with bleeding intragastric varices should be treated with octreotide (or somatostatin) and balloon tamponade followed by either TIPS or surgery. Emergency TIPS appears to be as effective for short-term control of bleeding gastric varices as esophageal varices. However, TIPS may be less effective than surgery in patients with bleeding gastric varices who have spontaneous splenorenal collaterals.

Prevention and treatment of recurrent variceal bleeding

The probability of recurrent variceal bleeding, following control of the acute hemorrhage, is approximately 30% at 6 weeks and ultimately close to 75%. The corresponding mortality rate is about 33%. The causes of death include recurrent variceal bleeding, liver failure, hepatic encephalopathy and progressive ascites and infections. These points underscore the importance of preventing recurrent hemorrhage, sustaining liver function, maintaining an ascites-free state, and avoiding infections to achieve prolonged survival. At this time, OLT is the only treatment which achieves all of these objectives and prolongs long-term survival with any degree of certainty.

Currently, there are two main areas of intervention for the prevention of recurrent variceal bleeding:

- at the 'local' level, i.e. the obliteration of the target organ (varices), which can be achieved either by EIS or EVL, and rarely by surgical devascularization procedures; and
- at the 'central' level, i.e. by lowering the portal pressure below the threshold (12 mmHg) that is known to be associated with variceal bleeding.

The latter can be accomplished either pharmacologically (β blockers) or by mechanical intervention with creation of a portosystemic shunt radiologically (TIPS) or surgically.

Pharmacological therapy

Studies on the pharmacological prevention of recurrent variceal hemorrhage have focused on the use of β blockers and, to a lesser extent, nitrates. Several clinical trials have compared β blockers and placebo for the prevention of recurrent variceal hemorrhage. With a few exceptions, an overall improvement in rebleeding rate was noted, but a survival advantage was shown in only one study. Meta-analysis of these data suggests that the risk of bleeding is decreased by approximately 40% while the risk of death is decreased by 20%. Propranolol has also decreased recurrent bleeding (35 versus 62% at 1 year) from portal hypertensive gastropathy.

The presence of HCC, poor compliance and continued alcohol use are risk factors for recurrence of variceal hemorrhage in patients treated with propranolol. Although acute hemodynamic changes after initiation of propranolol do not predict long-term outcome, the presence of a sustained portal hypotensive effect at 1 month after initiation of therapy appears to be an important predictive factor. Thus, measurement of portal hemodynamics may be an important prognostic element of treatment. However, facilities for routine measurement of portal pressures are not widely available and the cost-effectiveness of these measurements for guidance of medical therapy remains to be established. As a general rule, the optimal candidate for management with β blockers is one with well-compensated alcoholic liver disease who is likely to be compliant with therapy.

Several studies have suggested that the combination of β blockers and nitrates improves the hemodynamic response

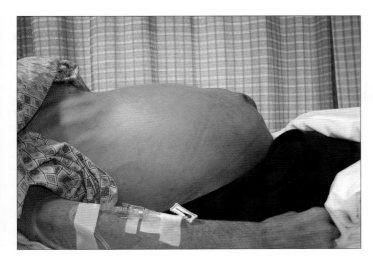

Figure 10.2 Patient with advanced cirrhosis and tense ascites. Note the decreased muscle mass in the patient's arms and chest.

of 5–10%. The effusion is usually mild or moderate and more frequent on the right side. In some cases, pleural effusions recur after therapy with diuretics and constitute the main manifestation of the disease. These cases are usually caused by the existence of anatomic defects in the diaphragm that create a communication between the peritoneal and pleural cavities.

Diagnostic approach to the patient with ascites
General evaluation (Table 10.3)

The general evaluation of the patient with cirrhosis is dealt with in Section II but the issues pertinent to patients with ascites are outlined in Table 10.3. The abdominal ultrasound is important to screen for hepatocellular carcinoma and evaluate patency of the portal venous system. Upper gastrointestinal endoscopy is performed to assess the presence of esophageal or gastric varices or portal hypertensive gastropathy. Percutaneous liver biopsy, if needed, can be performed after resolution of ascites because its presence increases the risk of complications. In patients with coagulation disturbances or intractable ascites, liver biopsy may be performed using a transjugular approach.

Evaluation of ascitic fluid

A diagnostic paracentesis of approximately 30–40 mL of fluid is required in all patients presenting with ascites de novo, requiring hospitalization, and those with any evidence of clinical deterioration such as fever, abdominal pain, gastrointestinal bleeding, or hepatic encephalopathy. Basic parameters to be determined in ascitic fluid are cell count, culture in blood culture bottles (10 mL of fluid injected at the bedside), albumin and total protein. The protein concentration of ascitic fluid is usually low in cirrhotic patients, with 60% of patients having an ascitic fluid protein concentration lower than 10 g/L. The difference between serum and ascites albumin is greater than 1.1 g/dL; values lower than 1.1 g/dL suggest a cause of ascites other than cirrhosis. The protein concentration of ascitic fluid is an important predictive factor in cirrhosis, because patients with ascitic protein concentrations lower than 10 g/L have a higher probability of developing spontaneous bacterial peritonitis and shorter survival expectancy than do patients with protein concentrations higher than 10 g/L (**Fig. 10.3**). The ascitic fluid red blood cell count is usually low

Evaluation of patients with cirrhosis and ascites
General evaluation
Complete history and physical examination
Arterial blood pressure, heart rate and pulse oxymetry
Standard hematology, coagulation, liver tests and α-fetoprotein
Abdominal ultrasonography and Doppler flow (including the kidneys)
Upper gastrointestinal endoscopy
Liver biopsy (selected cases)
Evaluation of ascitic fluid
Total protein and albumin measurement
Cell count
Culture in blood culture bottles
Evaluation of renal function*
24 h urine sodium
Diuresis after water load (5% dextrose i.v., 20 mL/kg)†
Serum electrolytes, serum blood urea nitrogen and serum creatinine
Urine sediment and protein excretion
Evaluation of circulatory function*
Arterial pressure
Plasma renin activity and plasma norepinephrine concentration†
*Renal and circulatory function should preferably be assessed with the patient maintained on a low-sodium diet without diuretic therapy. †May provide important information when an accurate estimate of prognosis is required. ‡In clinical research setting.

Table 10.3 Evaluation of patients with cirrhosis and ascites.

(<1000 cells/mm^3), although bloody ascites ($>50\,000$ red blood cells/mm^3) may be seen in some patients. In bloody ascites a correction factor of 1 polymorphonuclear (PMN) cell/250 red blood cells is recommended. A superimposed hepatocellular carcinoma should be excluded in the latter patients. The ascitic fluid white blood cell count is less than 500/mm^3 in most patients, and mononuclear cells predominate ($>75\%$). As discussed later, a high number of polymorphonuclear cells (>250 cells mm^3) in the ascitic fluid indicates infection of the ascitic fluid, particularly spontaneous bacterial peritonitis (SBP).

Evaluation of renal function

The evaluation of renal function in patients with cirrhosis and ascites is important in the assessment of prognosis and response to therapy. The evaluation should be performed while on low-sodium diets and at least 4 days after withdrawal of diuretics. Parameters of interest include 24 h urine volume and sodium excretion, urine volume after a water load of 5% dextrose (20 mL/kg), serum electrolytes and serum creatinine. A strong prognostic marker of cirrhotic patients with ascites is the ability to handle water by means of a water load test. In this test a

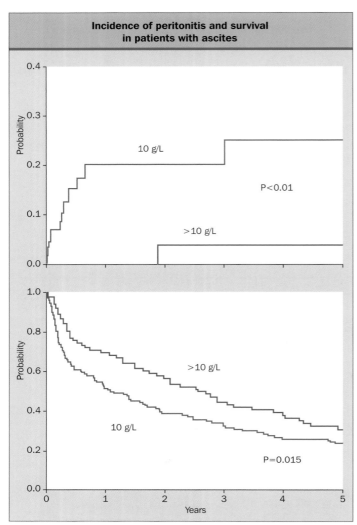

Figure 10.3 Incidence of spontaneous bacterial peritonitis and survival in cirrhotic patients. Probability of developing spontaneous bacterial peritonitis (top) and survival (bottom) in cirrhotic patients with ascites according to the protein concentration in ascitic fluid. Modified from Llach et al (92) by permission of Wiley-Liss, Inc.

patient receives 20 mL/kg of intravenous 5% dextrose and following this, the renal excretion of water is measured. An impaired ability to excrete the water load (urine volume of <8 mL/min) is associated with a poor prognosis. In patients with renal failure (serum creatinine >1.5 mg/dL), tests of urine sediment, 24 h urine protein, and a renal ultrasound should also be performed.

Evaluation of circulatory function

Evaluation of circulatory function provides prognostic information in patients with cirrhosis and ascites. The evaluation of circulatory function should include the measurement of arterial pressure in conditions of bed rest, low-sodium diet, and without diuretic therapy. Measurement of plasma renin activity and plasma norepinephrine concentration as an index of the activity of the renin–angiotensin system and sympathetic nervous system, respectively, also provide important prognostic information but are only used in a clinical research setting.

Treatment

All patients should be evaluated for liver transplantation. Early referral is advocated due to the short survival expectancy patients have once they develop this complication. The objective of the treatment of ascites or edema in cirrhosis is to reduce the patient's discomfort due to abdominal or leg swelling. Besides, the decrease in the amount of fluid in the peritoneal cavity reduces the risk of complications related to abdominal hernias, such as incarceration or rupture. Consequently, therapeutic measures in these patients should be oriented to reduce the amount of ascites and edema and to prevent their reaccumulation after therapy.

The initial step in the management of cirrhotic patients with ascites or edema is sodium restriction, because the amount of extracellular fluid retained within the body depends on the balance between the sodium ingested in the diet and the sodium excreted in the urine. As long as the sodium excreted is lower than that ingested, patients will accumulate ascites or edema. Conversely, when sodium excretion is greater than intake, ascites or edema will decrease. The reduction of sodium content in the diet to 70–90 mEq/day (approx. 1.5 g of salt) causes a negative sodium balance and loss of ascites and edema in patients with mild sodium retention (5–20% of the whole population of patients with ascites). In patients with moderate or marked sodium retention, such dietary sodium restriction is not sufficient by itself to achieve a negative sodium balance, but it may slow the accumulation of fluid. These patients need diuretic therapy.

Patients with *moderate ascites* (grade 2 ascites) should be treated with sodium restriction and diuretics. As plasma aldosterone concentration is usually increased in patients with ascites and plays an important role in the increased tubular sodium reabsorption, spironolactone, a drug that competes with aldosterone for the binding to the mineralocorticoid receptor in the collecting tubular epithelial cells of the kidney, is the diuretic of choice in these patients. Other diuretics acting in the distal tubules, such as amiloride or triamterene, are less effective. Spironolactone is initially given at a dose of 50–100 mg/day and increased as needed every 7 days up to a maximum dose of 400 mg/day. Loop diuretics, especially furosemide (20 mg/day initially and increased up to 160 mg/day) which acts by inhibiting the Na^+-K^+-$2Cl^-$ cotransporter in the loop of Henle, may be given in combination with spironolactone to increase the natriuretic efficacy. Loop diuretics should not be used as single therapy in patients with cirrhosis, because they may put the patients with mild sodium retention at risk for volume depletion and prerenal failure and are less effective than spironolactone in patients with marked sodium retention. The combination of starting furosemide 20–40 mg/day and spironolactone 100 mg is another option and doses may be increased in a stepwise fashion every 7–10 days by doubling doses (ratio of 40 mg:100 mg); furosemide up to 160 mg/day and spironolactone up to 400 mg/day. The response to diuretic therapy in cirrhotic patients should be evaluated regularly by measuring body weight, urine volume and sodium excretion. Diuretics should be given at the minimum effective dose to achieve a maximum weight loss of approximately 0.5 kg/day in patients with ascites without edema and 1 kg/day in patients with ascites and edema. An inadequate sodium restriction is a common cause of failure of diuretic therapy, especially in non-hospitalized patients who usually eat more salt than inpatients. This situation should be

HEPATORENAL SYNDROME

Definition

Hepatorenal syndrome (HRS) is a unique form of functional renal failure without identifiable renal pathology that occurs in approximately 10% of patients with advanced cirrhosis or acute liver failure. HRS is characterized by impaired renal function and marked disturbances in the arterial circulation and activity of vasoactive systems. In the renal circulation there is a marked increase in vascular resistance, whereas total systemic vascular resistance is reduced and leads to arterial hypotension. This reduction in systemic vascular resistance is mainly caused by an arterial vasodilatation of the splanchnic circulation.

Pathophysiology

The pathophysiologic hallmark of HRS is renal vasoconstriction. The kidneys are structurally intact. The mechanism of this vasoconstriction is poorly understood and possibly multifactorial, involving increased vasoconstrictor and reduced vasodilator factors that act on the renal circulation. The most accepted theory on the pathogenesis of HRS (*Arterial Vasodilation Theory*) proposes that renal hypoperfusion represents the extreme manifestation of an underfilling of the arterial circulation secondary to a marked vasodilatation of the splanchnic area (**Fig. 10.9**). This arterial underfilling would result in a progressive baroreceptor-mediated activation of vasoconstrictor systems (i.e. renin-angiotensin and sympathetic nervous systems) that would cause vasoconstriction not only in the renal circulation but also in other vascular beds (lower and upper extremities). The splanchnic area would escape the effect of vasoconstrictors and a marked vasodilation would persist, probably because of the existence of very potent local vasodilator stimuli. In early phases following the development of ascites, renal perfusion would be maintained within normal or near-normal levels despite the overactivity of vasoconstrictor systems by an increased synthesis/activity of renal vasodilator factors. The development of renal hypoperfusion leading to HRS would occur either as a result of a maximal activation of vasoconstrictor systems that could not be counteracted by vasodilator factors, decreased

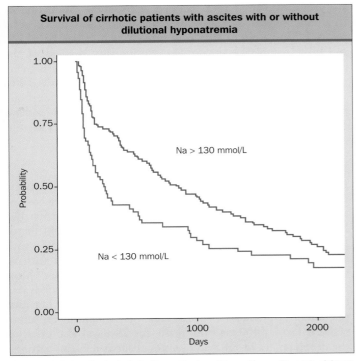

Figure 10.8 Survival of cirrhotic patients with ascites with and without dilutional hyponatremia.

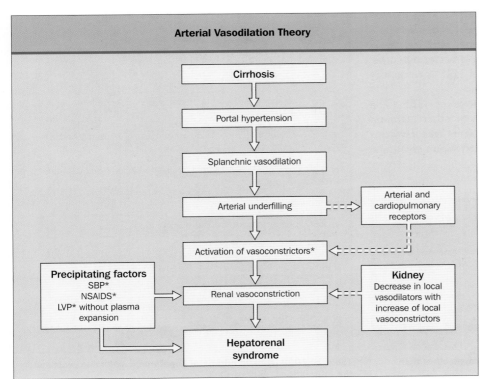

Figure 10.9 Arterial vasodilation theory.
Pathogenesis of hepatorenal syndrome as proposed by the Arterial Vasodilation Theory.
*Renin–angiotensin–aldosterone system (RAAS), sympathetic nervous system (SNS), and arginine vasopressin. SBP, spontaneous bacterial peritonitis; NSAIDS, non-steroidal anti-inflammatory drugs; LVP, large volume paracentesis.

activity of vasodilator factors, and/or increased production of intrarenal vasoconstrictor factors. An alternative theory proposes that renal vasoconstriction is the result of a direct relationship between the liver and the kidney, without any relationship with disturbances in systemic hemodynamics. The link between the liver and the kidney would be either a liver vasodilator factor, the synthesis of which would be reduced as a consequence of liver failure, or a hepatorenal reflex causing renal vasoconstriction. However, there is little or no evidence supporting this latter sequence of events in humans with cirrhosis.

Clinical features and diagnosis

Two different types of HRS, which likely represent distinct expressions of the same pathogenic mechanism, exist. *Type 1 HRS* is characterized by rapid and progressive impairment of renal function as defined by a doubling of the initial serum creatinine to a level higher than 2.5 mg/dL or a 50% reduction of the initial 24 h creatinine clearance to a level lower than 20 mL/min in less than 2 weeks. Renal failure in these patients is often associated with progressive oliguria, marked sodium retention and dilutional hyponatremia. Serum creatinine levels in HRS are usually lower than values observed in patients with acute renal failure without liver disease due to a reduced muscle mass and low endogenous production of creatinine in cirrhosis. Patients with type 1 HRS are usually in a very severe clinical condition and show signs of advanced liver failure. In approximately half of the cases, this type of HRS develops spontaneously without any identifiable precipitating factor, whereas in the remaining patients it occurs in close chronologic relationship with some complications or therapeutic interventions [e.g. bacterial infections, particularly spontaneous bacterial peritonitis, administration of non-steroidal anti-inflammatory drugs (NSAIDs), large-volume paracentesis without plasma expansion]. *Type 2 HRS* is characterized by moderate and stable reduction of GFR with serum creatinine levels around 1.5–2.5 mg/dL that does not meet the criteria proposed for type 1. Unlike type 1 HRS, type 2 HRS usually occurs in patients with relatively preserved hepatic function and patients have a better outcome. The main clinical consequence of this type of HRS is refractory ascites.

There is no specific test for the diagnosis of HRS. The diagnosis of HRS is based on the exclusion of other common causes of renal failure that may occur in patients with cirrhosis (**Table 10.9**) and demonstration of an increased serum creatinine

(>1.5 mg/dL in the absence of diuretic therapy). Criteria for the diagnosis of HRS are shown in **Table 10.10**. Although a cut-off value of serum creatinine of 1.5 mg/dL may seem low, cirrhotic patients with ascites with serum creatinine above 1.5 mg/dL have a GFR below 30 mL/min, which represents only a quarter of the normal GFR for healthy subjects of the same age. The low serum creatinine values relative to the reduction in GFR are probably related to a reduced endogenous production of creatinine caused by the poor nutritional status of cirrhotic patients. Most cases of HRS have urine sodium below 10 mEq/L and urine osmolality above plasma osmolality because of the preservation of tubular function. Nevertheless, some patients may have high urine sodium and low urine osmolality, similar to what occurs in acute tubular necrosis. Conversely, cirrhotic patients with acute tubular necrosis may have low urine sodium and high osmolality. For these reasons, urinary indices are not considered major criteria for the diagnosis of HRS.

Prevention

HRS can be prevented in two clinical settings. First, in patients with SBP the administration of albumin (1.5 g/kg at diagnosis of infection and 1 g/kg 48 h later) prevents the circulatory dysfunction and subsequent development of HRS. The incidence of HRS in patients with SBP receiving albumin together with antibiotic therapy is in the order of 10%, compared with an incidence of 30% in patients not receiving albumin. Most importantly, the administration of albumin improves survival in these patients. Second, in patients with acute alcoholic hepatitis the administration of pentoxifylline, an inhibitor of tumor necrosis factor (400 mg t.i.d. orally for 28 days) also prevents the development of HRS and improves survival in this setting.

Common causes of renal failure in cirrhosis other than hepatorenal syndrome
Prerenal failure due to volume depletion (diuretics, vomiting, diarrhea)
Acute tubular necrosis after hypovolemic shock
Glomerulonephritis associated with hepatitis B and C
Nephrotoxicity (non-steroidal anti-inflammatory drugs, aminoglycosides)

Table 10.9 Common causes of renal failure in cirrhosis other than hepatorenal syndrome.

Diagnostic criteria of hepatorenal syndrome proposed by the International Ascites Club
*Major criteria**
Serum creatinine greater than 1.5 mg/dL
Exclusion of shock, ongoing bacterial infection, volume depletion and use of nephrotoxic drugs
No improvement in creatinine despite stopping diuretics and volume repletion with 1.5 L of saline
No proteinuria or ultrasonographic evidence of obstructive uropathy or parenchymal renal disease
Minor criteria
1. Urine volume lower than 500 mL/day
2. Urine sodium lower than 10 mEq/L
3. Urine osmolality greater than plasma osmolality
4. Urine red blood cells less than 50 per high power field
5. Serum sodium concentration lower than 130 mEq/L
(*) Only major criteria are necessary for the diagnosis of hepatorenal syndrome.

Table 10.10 Diagnostic criteria of hepatorenal syndrome proposed by the International Ascites Club.

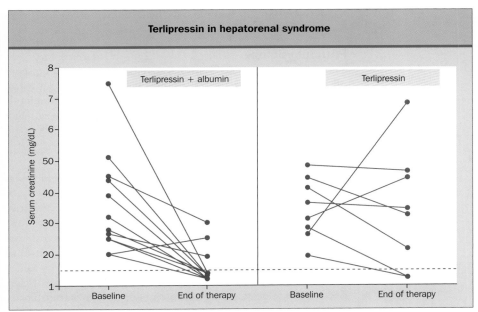

Figure 10.10 Terlipressin in hepatorenal syndrome. The effects of terlipressin and albumin compared to terlipressin alone in the treatment of type 1 hepatorenal syndrome. Reproduced from Ortega et al (02) by permission of Wiley-Liss, Inc.

Treatment

Effective therapies for HRS include liver transplantation, vasoconstrictors with plasma expansion and TIPS. Liver transplantation is the best treatment for suitable candidates with HRS because it offers a cure to the diseased liver and the HRS. However, a significant proportion of patients die before transplantation can be done because of their extremely short survival time. Therefore, liver transplantation should be indicated whenever possible, before the development of HRS. The presence of HRS is associated with increased morbidity and early mortality after transplantation. Patients with ascites who are more likely to develop HRS are those with greatly reduced urine sodium (<10 mmol/L or mEq/L), dilutional hyponatremia, arterial hypotension and marked activation of renin-angiotensin and sympathetic nervous systems.

Renal vasodilator drugs such as dopamine and prostaglandin analogs were used in the past to treat HRS. However, this approach has been largely abandoned due to poor results, side-effects and lack of data confirming benefit. In contrast, systemic vasoconstrictors such as intravenous vasopressin analogs (terlipressin), α-adrenergic agonists (midodrine) plus octreotide, or intravenous noradrenaline, and all of them in association with intravenous albumin, are effective in the treatment of HRS.

Intravenous terlipressin along with albumin as a plasma expander is associated with a significant improvement of renal function and normalization of serum creatinine in approximately 75% of patients treated for at least 5 days (**Fig. 10.10**). Administration of midodrine, an α-adrenergic agonist in association with octreotide, a glucagon inhibitor, and albumin has also proved efficacious in HRS. Finally, noradrenaline in combination with albumin expansion also improves renal function in HRS. After stopping therapy, which typically lasts between 5 and 15 days, recurrence is uncommon. Due to limited information and the possibility of ischemic side-effects, treatment with vasoconstrictors should probably be restricted to patients with type 1 HRS. The main end point of therapy is a reduction of serum creatinine below 1.5 mg/dL. This ensures

that suitable transplant candidates can undergo transplantation without renal failure. Successful therapy probably improves the outcome after transplantation. Patients that successfully respond to treatment before transplantation have the same outcome as those that did not have HRS at the time of transplantation. Non-transplant candidates may also benefit by reducing readmissions, morbidity and mortality but this remains to be proved. The recommended doses and duration of vasoconstrictor therapy are summarized in **Table 10.11**.

Recommendations for using vasoconstrictors in type 1 hepatorenal syndrome
1. Treat for a maximum of 15 days
2. End point of treatment is reduction of serum creatinine below 1.5 mg/dL
3. Recommended medications and doses are:
A. Terlipressin 0.5–1 mg i.v. every 4 h; increase dose every 2–3 days up to 2 mg/4 h when there is no decrease in creatinine
B. Midodrine 7.5 mg orally three times daily with an increase to 12.5 mg three times daily and octreotide 100 µg subcutaneously three times daily with an increase to 200 µg three times daily if creatinine not decreasing
C. Noradrelanine 0.5–3 mg/h continuous i.v. infusion
4. Intravenous albumin infusion (20–40 g daily)
5. Monitor for side-effects such as chest pain, distal ischemia, abdominal pain
6. Avoid in patients with cardiac disease, peripheral vascular disease, and/or cerebrovascular disease, due to the potential risk of ischemic events

Table 10.11 Recommendations for using vasoconstrictors in type 1 hepatorenal syndrome.

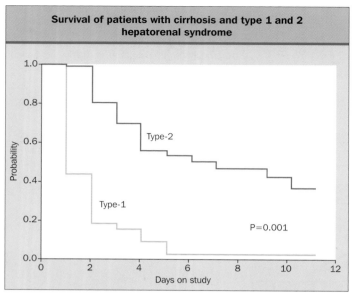

Figure 10.11 Survival of patients with cirrhosis and type 1 and 2 hepatorenal syndrome. Reproduced from Ginés P et al (03) by permission of Elsevier.

TIPS may improve renal function in type 1 HRS. Although the use of vasoconstrictors and albumin followed by TIPS is effective in a subset of patients, experience is limited and most patients with HRS have advanced cirrhosis that would preclude them from receiving a TIPS. Although uncontrolled studies suggest that TIPS improves prognosis in types 1 and 2 HRS, the real impact on survival remains to be assessed. Conventional hemodialysis is not routinely recommended in HRS unless there is volume overload, severe hyperkalemia or severe metabolic acidosis. Albumin dialysis [molecular adsorbent recirculating system (MARS)] has shown efficacy in one study, but its possible beneficial effects need to be confirmed in further studies.

Prognosis

The prognosis of patients with HRS is very poor. Type 1 HRS is the complication with the worst prognosis for cirrhotic patients. The median survival time of these patients with HRS without therapy is less than 2 weeks, which is a survival time shorter than that of patients with acute renal failure of other etiologies. The combination of several factors, including renal failure, advanced liver failure, and, in some cases, associated infections, accounts probably for this extremely poor outcome. The median survival of patients with type 2 HRS is usually several months, which is a longer survival time than those with type 1 but shorter than patients with ascites without renal failure (**Fig. 10.11**).

SPONTANEOUS BACTERIAL PERITONITIS (SBP)

Definition

SBP is a common and severe complication of cirrhotic patients with ascites characterized by spontaneous infection of ascitic fluid without an intra-abdominal infection. The prevalence of SBP in hospitalized patients with ascites ranges from 10 to 30%. Cirrhotic patients with hydrothorax may also develop a sponta-

neous infection of the pleural fluid, known as spontaneous bacterial empyema.

Pathophysiology

The isolation of aerobic Gram-negative bacteria in most episodes of SBP suggests that the gastrointestinal tract is the source of bacteria. Although the pathogenesis of SBP is not completely understood, it is generally accepted that it involves three major steps:

- passage of bacteria from the intestinal lumen to the systemic circulation;
- bacteremia secondary to the impairment of reticuloendothelial system (RES) phagocytic activity, and
- infection of ascites caused by poor opsonization and defective bactericidal activity of the ascitic fluid.

Studies in experimental animals with cirrhosis suggest that bacterial translocation (i.e. passage of bacteria from the intestinal lumen to mesenteric lymph nodes) is the mechanism by which bacteria from the intestinal lumen reach the systemic circulation. Bacterial translocation may increase under several circumstances, such as gastrointestinal bleeding and hemorrhagic shock. This may explain, at least in part, the high incidence of infections caused by enteric bacteria in cirrhotic patients with gastrointestinal hemorrhage. The reduced phagocytic activity of the RES (a system that removes bacteria from the circulation) is another important pathogenic factor in the development of SBP. Cirrhotic patients with reduced activity of the RES are highly predisposed to develop SBP, whereas this infection is rarely seen in patients with normal activity of the RES. Finally, a reduced antimicrobial activity of the ascitic fluid also plays a very important role in the development of SBP. Patients with reduced antimicrobial activity of ascitic fluid have a greater risk of developing ascitic fluid infection than those with normal antimicrobial activity of the ascitic fluid. As the antimicrobial activity of ascites correlates with total ascitic fluid protein concentration, patients with low ascites protein content (<10 g/L) have a greater risk of developing SBP compared with patients with higher ascites protein concentration (Fig. 10.3, top).

The most plausible theory on the pathogenesis of SBP is shown in **Figure 10.12**. The initial step involves translocation of bacteria from the gut flora to mesenteric lymph nodes. This translocation would occur either spontaneously or as a consequence of some precipitating events (i.e. gastrointestinal hemorrhage). An increased permeability related to gut edema, intestinal bacterial overgrowth, or increased transit time may facilitate bacterial translocation. The bacteria then reach the systemic circulation through the lymphatic system. In cases of SBP that are not caused by bacteria from enteric origin, the bacteria would reach the systemic circulation from other areas (i.e. respiratory or urinary tracts or skin). In patients with normal activity of the RES, bacteria are efficiently removed from the circulation, but persistent bacteremia develops in patients with impaired activity of the RES. Subsequently, bacteria may reach the ascitic fluid through a hematogenous route. The development of SBP depends on the opsonic and bactericidal activity of ascitic fluid. Infection of ascites does not usually occur in patients with good antimicrobial activity of the ascitic fluid. In contrast, patients with reduced antimicrobial activity of the ascitic fluid are at high risk of developing SBP. A similar mechanism may explain the development of spontaneous bacterial empyema.

CHAPTER
11
Hepatic Encephalopathy

Andres T. Blei

Hepatic encephalopathy can be broadly defined as the alterations in mental state and cognitive function that occur in liver failure. The course of both acute and chronic liver failure can be complicated by the development of neurologic dysfunction. In acute liver injury, encephalopathy portends a poor prognosis and death can occur as a result of neurologic complications. In patients with cirrhosis, encephalopathy is a cause of major morbidity, and when chronic, can be an incapacitating condition. The latter is especially problematic in subjects awaiting liver transplantation, in whom chronic hepatic encephalopathy is increasingly noted.

CLASSIFICATION

A classification of hepatic encephalopathy should encompass the clinical setting in which symptoms occur. A recent consensus has been published which addresses three main clinical situations: acute liver failure, portal-systemic bypass and chronic liver failure (**Table 11.1**). Additional divisions within chronic liver failure in different clinical situations are also included.

Cases with isolated portal-systemic shunting are rare and are mainly due to congenital alterations of the portal circulation. A survey from Japan revealed more than 100 such cases, with variable clinical presentation, including some, where symptoms become manifest after the age of 50. A case of a portal vein–

hepatic vein connection is illustrated in **Figure 11.1**, in whom neuropsychologic testing and magnetic resonance (MR) spectroscopy of the brain shared the same features with the

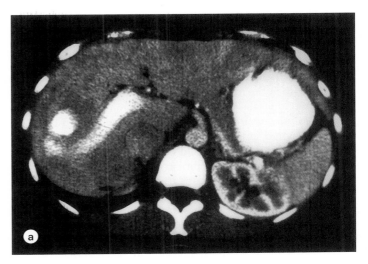

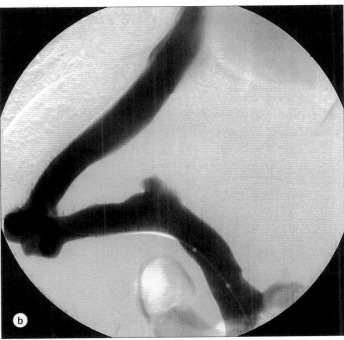

Figure 11.1 A case of "endogenous TIPS". (a) Spiral abdominal computed tomography image demonstrating a massively enlarged portal vein (PV) running toward the hepatic vein (HV). (b) Portal venous system injection performed from the right transjugular approach. Portal venogram showing a direct connection from the PV and the HV. Reproduced from Crespin et al (2000) by permission of Blackwell.

Proposed nomenclature of hepatic encephalopathy			
HE type	Nomenclature	Subcategory	Subdivisions
A	Encephalopathy associated with acute liver failure		
B	Encephalopathy associated with portal-systemic bypass and no intrinsic liver disease		
C	Encephalopathy associated with cirrhosis and portal hypertension/or portal-systemic shunts	Episodic HE	Precipitated Spontaneous Recurrent
		Persistent HE	Mild Severe Treatment dependent
		Minimal HE	

Table 11.1 Proposed nomenclature of hepatic encephalopathy.

brain of chronic liver disease. These cases highlight an important concept: development of portal-systemic shunts as a result of portal hypertension is a major contributor to encephalopathy in chronic liver disease.

While a decrease in functional hepatic mass also contributes to the process of encephalopathy, the term 'portal-systemic encephalopathy' is commonly used as a synonym for 'hepatic encephalopathy'. However, it should be best reserved for the variable disturbance of consciousness and impairment of intellectual function that result from extensive portal-systemic shunting or after a decompressive procedure for portal hypertension.

NEUROPATHOLOGY

A striking feature of the examination of the brain of patients dying in hepatic coma is the paucity of anatomic findings. Microscopic studies show hyperplasia of astrocytes of the cerebral cortex, lenticular and dentate, diencephalic and other brainstem nuclei. Morphometric studies demonstrate enlargement in size and increase in the number of astrocyte nuclei. The presence of Alzheimer type II astrocytes is a common and characteristic feature of the neuropathologic examination (**Fig. 11.2**). The change is noted in brains fixed by immersion. In experimental models, where the brain is fixed via perfusion, astrocyte swelling can be seen. Loss of glial fibrillary acidic protein, a key component of intermediate filaments in astrocytes, accompanies such astrocyte swelling.

Astrocytes comprise approximately a third of the brain's cellular mass. They have small cellular bodies and extend their foot processes to contact adjacent neurons, capillaries and axonal processes. Viewed for some time as a simple anatomical support for the other structures, their varied physiologic importance has been increasingly recognized. They are involved in the control of the extracellular concentration of ions and neurotransmitters, providing a stable milieu for neuronal function. They are the

sole brain cell that contains glutamine synthetase, which under normal conditions catalyzes the use of ammonia to amidate glutamate for the formation of glutamine. The marked increase in brain glutamine seen in hepatic encephalopathy highlights the functional importance of astrocytes in the process that leads to alterations in mental state.

Neuronal involvement is rare. Cortical atrophy may represent the effects of other insults, including chronic alcohol consumption. A patchy laminar necrosis of the cerebral cortex can be seen in hepatocerebral degeneration, a condition that arises from long-standing portal-systemic shunting. However, the main pathology in this condition is centered on the striatum, where polymicrocavitation can be seen. This lesion is similar to the one observed in Wilson disease, and hence the term 'acquired hepatolenticular degeneration' that has also been coined for this condition. Demyelination is exceptional; long-standing portal-systemic shunting can be associated with spinal demyelination and the development of spastic paraparesis. In addition, patients with hepatic encephalopathy are at increased risk for central pontine myelinolysis.

PATHOGENESIS

An explanation for the mechanisms responsible for hepatic encephalopathy has been sought for many decades. Studies in humans are limited by the difficulties in studying brain neurochemistry, though newer techniques such as MR spectroscopy and positron-emission tomography have provided new insights. Work in experimental models of acute liver failure and portal-systemic shunting have also provided valuable insights.

The search for the pathogenesis of hepatic encephalopathy has focused on deleterious neurotoxins that escape hepatic removal and then access the brain. Clinical clues point at the nature of such toxins: of intestinal origin, as witnessed by the aggravation of encephalopathy with constipation and the presence of portal-systemic shunts; nitrogenous in origin, as a large protein load can precipitate encephalopathy. Intestinal bacteria are related to the development of encephalopathy, as changes in the intestinal flora can improve an abnormal mental state in chronic liver disease. Finally, the toxin(s) must be metabolized by the liver and have a high first-pass extraction; its concentration in the hepatic effluent should be tightly regulated to prevent an altered mental function.

Ammonia meets all the above-mentioned criteria. In the splanchnic territory, ammonia originates from the action of glutaminase on glutamine in the mucosa of the small bowel, from the degradation of luminal protein and from the urease-containing activity of intestinal bacteria. In the liver, it is utilized for urea synthesis in periportal hepatocytes and for the formation of glutamine in last rim of perivenous hepatocytes. The dual metabolizing capacity of the liver allows for tight control of ammonia efflux. Indeed, portal venous ammonia levels are 10-fold higher than levels seen in the hepatic vein effluent.

Administration of ^{13}N-labeled ammonia has allowed examination of the disposition of ammonia in humans. Conversion to glutamine in peripheral muscle accounts for approximately 50% of ammonia metabolism, followed by liver, kidney and to a much lesser extent (7%) brain. In the latter, uptake is a linear function of its arterial concentration and is highest in the cerebral cortex.

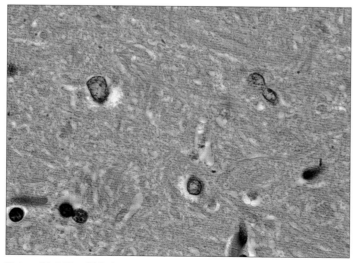

Figure 11.2 The Alzheimer type II astrocyte. This is characterized by an enlarged pale nucleus and is seen in patients with cirrhosis who die in hepatic coma. (Courtesy of Dr Ellen Bigio, Dept of Pathology, Northwestern University Feinberg School of Medicine.)

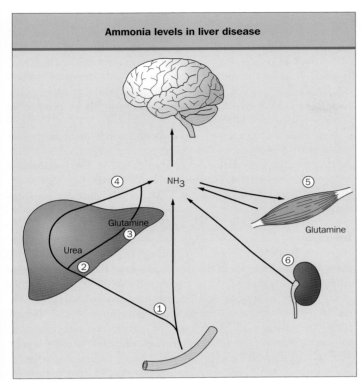

Figure 11.3 Ammonia levels in liver disease. Several factors combine to raise ammonia levels in liver disease. As the hepatic extraction of ammonia is high, > 0.9, portal-systemic shunting (1) will be a major factor. Hepatic metabolism of ammonia, via the formation of urea [periportal area (2)] or glutamine [perivenular hepatocyte (3)], may be impaired. Intrahepatic shunts (4) are present in cirrhosis. Metabolism of ammonia in muscle (5) becomes an important alternative pathway; loss of muscle mass may reduce the formation of glutamine. Renal vein ammonia (6) rises as a consequence of primary respiratory alkalosis. Reproduced from Kaplowitz (92) by permission of Lippincott, Williams & Wilkins.

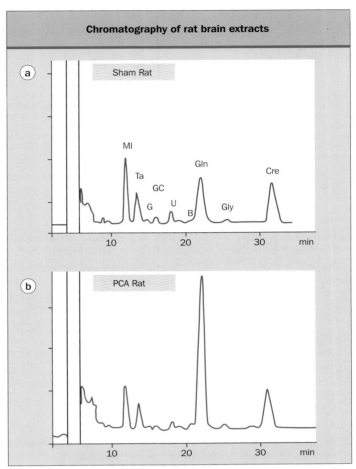

Figure 11.4 Chromatography of rat brain extracts. High performance liquid chromatography chromatograms of brain extracts from (a) a sham-operated rat and (b) a rat that underwent portacaval anastomosis (PCA). MI, myo-inositol; Ta, taurine; G, glycerophosphoroethanolamine; U, urea; B, betaine; Gln, glutamine; Gly, glycine; Cre, creatine. Note the marked increase in the glutamine peak in the PCA animal. The sum of organic osmolytes is similar in both groups. Reproduced from Cordoba et al (96) by permission of Wiley-Liss, Inc.

In liver disease, the disposition of ammonia is affected at multiple levels (**Fig. 11.3**):

- Bowel motility is slower in established cirrhosis, a situation that favors the generation of ammonia in both the small and large bowel.
- Portal hypertension results in the development of extrahepatic and intrahepatic collaterals, shunting higher portal ammonia into the systemic circulation. A decrease in functional liver mass also results in a higher output of splanchnic ammonia to the systemic circulation, as seen in acute liver failure and in the later stages of the course of chronic liver disease. Portal-systemic shunting can by itself cause hepatic atrophy, a phenomenon well documented in the experimental animal but also present in human disease.
- In liver disease, muscle becomes an important site for ammonia detoxification, especially in acute liver failure. An increase in the activity of muscle glutamine synthetase can be seen in experimental models. As a result of this uptake, arterial levels are higher than corresponding venous samples, especially in acute liver failure. In cirrhosis, however, the arteriovenous difference in plasma ammonia is less predictable. Loss of muscle mass, seen with malnutrition and especially in patients with ascites, can adversely affect the ability to remove ammonia.

- Ammonia is generated in the kidney for the production of titerable acidity. While it can be eliminated in the urine, the effectiveness of this route is limited in view of its reabsoption, favored in liver disease by the presence of respiratory alkalosis.
- Entry of gaseous ammonia (NH_3) into the brain is thought to occur by diffusion, as the blood–brain barrier is viewed as impermeable to ionized NH_4^+. Recent studies suggest the presence of specialized NH_4^+ channels. Brain glutamine levels markedly increase, as seen with MR spectroscopy. Multiple functional consequences arise within brain:
  - Swelling of astrocytes, driven by the osmotic effects of glutamine, affects their function at multiple levels, including the re-uptake of ions and neurotransmitters. Osmotic compensation is demonstrated by the reduction in the level of myoinositol, as seen in MR spectroscopy in humans and by direct measurements in the experimental animal (**Fig. 11.4**). Ammonia induces the mitochondrial permeability transition in isolated astrocytes; oxidative and nitrosative stress can also be detected in animal models.

– Increased transport of neutral amino acids across the blood–brain barrier, a process that allows extrusion of some of the increased glutamine from brain. In the case of tryptophan, this amino acid is a precursor of serotonin; an increased serotoninergic tone may contribute to the symptomatology of hepatic encephalopathy.

– Inhibition of the activity of the Krebs cycle by decreasing the activity of α-ketoglutarate dehydrogenase. This alteration can result in anaerobic glycolysis with an accumulation of brain lactate.

– Variable effects on cerebral perfusion.

– In neurons, ammonia can inhibit chloride extrusion from cortical neurons, affecting thus postsynaptic inhibitory potentials.

A wide range of disorders that affect mental state are associated with hyperammonemia, including diseases with hepatic microvesicular steatosis, such as Reye syndrome and sodium valproate toxicity, urea cycle enzyme defects and breakdown of urea by urease-producing bacteria colonizing intestinal urinary conduits. All share clinical features with the hyperammonemia of liver disease.

Synergism

In the early 1970s, a number of other compounds arising from bacterial metabolism in the colon were shown to induce encephalopathy in experimental animals. Fatty acids (especially octanoic acid), phenols and mercaptans (derivatives of methionine) potentiate the neurotoxicity of ammonia. The mechanisms by which these toxins may induce encephalopathy is unclear; among proposed pathways are inhibition of mitochondrial electron transfer (mercaptans) and $Na^+–K^+$ ATPase activity (octanoic acid).

False neurotransmitter hypothesis

This theory was proposed in the late 1970s. Weak neurotransmitters, such as octopamine and phenylethanolamine, would replace established neurotransmitters such as dopamine and noradrenaline. The source of these neurotransmitters could be twofold:

• Octopamine can be generated from the activity of intestinal bacteria on protein. Increased plasma levels and facilitated entry into the brain would increase cerebral levels of this false neurotransmitter.

• They could also be generated within the brain from aromatic amino acid precursors. An abnormal plasma amino acid pattern is seen in liver disease, with elevated plasma aromatic amino acids (as a result of decreased hepatic uptake) and a reduction in branched-chain amino acids (the consequence, in part, of peripheral insulin resistance). Entry of aromatic amino acids into the brain is favored via exchange with brain glutamine.

The importance of this mechanism in the development of encephalopathy appears to have lessened in light of the overall lack of significant benefit from the use of therapeutic branched-chain amino acid solutions.

GABAergic neurotransmission

GABA (γ-aminobutyric acid), generated in the brain from the decarboxylation of glutamate, is the main brain inhibitory neurotransmitter. Ligation of GABA to its receptor increases the permeability to chloride, resulting in hyperpolarization and a decrease in neurotransmission. In 1982, intestinally generated GABA was proposed as a mediator of encephalopathy. In view of the lack of conclusive evidence for an effect of GABA itself, 6 years later emphasis was made on a role for endogenous benzodiazepine ligands. Binding of benzodiazepine to its receptor facilitates GABA effects on its own receptor, hence promoting GABAergic neurotransmission.

Now, the importance of this hypothesis has decreased. The nature of the endogenous benzodiazepine ligand remains obscure. A therapeutic experience with flumazenil, a benzodiazepine receptor antagonist, has not been clinically convincing. Moreover, direct effects of ammonia on GABAergic neurotransmission may exist.

Infection

Increasingly, evidence is mounting that the presence of infection plays an important role in the development of hepatic encephalopathy. In acute liver failure, the development of the systemic inflammatory response and/or the presence of infection via positive cultures is associated with worsening of the mental state. In patients with cirrhosis, resolution of infection will improve cognitive function in spite of similar ammonia levels. The role of circulating cytokines may be of special importance, as they can result in intracerebral signals via different pathways. This is an area of active research at this time.

Manganese

Neuropathologic changes in the basal ganglia of patients with cirrhosis have been highlighted. Radiologically, a hyper-resonant globus pallidus is a frequent finding in patients with cirrhosis and portal-systemic shunting (**Fig. 11.5**). Measurements in human brain tissue have shown elevated manganese levels in basal ganglia.

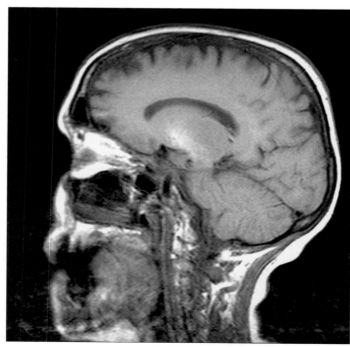

Figure 11.5 Sagittal plane: T_1-weighted image (500/18). The image shows increased intensity in the globus pallidus. Reproduced from Crespin et al (00) by permission of Blackwell.

Manganese intoxication can result in loss of dopamine receptors in this area and development of Parkinsonian features. In liver disease, manganese accumulates as a result of both portal-systemic shunting and decreased biliary excretion. An explanation for the selective deposition of manganese in subcortical nuclei is not forthcoming at this time. The impact of its removal has not been assessed clinically, in view of the lack of a specific chelator.

CLINICAL MANIFESTATIONS

Encephalopathy in acute liver failure

Patients with acute liver failure may develop changes in mental state within 1 week (hyperacute), 1 month (acute) or up to 6 months after the development of jaundice (subacute). Although patients can quickly evolve from a state of somnolence to coma, excitation and mania can be seen in the early stages of evolution, a symptom seldom seen in chronic encephalopathy. The Glasgow Coma Scale may be useful to monitor the evolution of patients with severe encephalopathy.

Brain edema is a unique complication seen in patients with acute liver failure and severe encephalopathy. It is not the result of a generalized breakdown of the blood–brain barrier, as seen in vasogenic edema. Rather, cytotoxic mechanisms predominate, with predominant swelling of the gray matter. Brain edema can be reproduced in animal models of acute liver failure, where a complex pathogenesis has emerged. It includes osmotic alterations in the brain, triggered by the accumulation of glutamine in astrocytes, a metabolic effect, with an increase in brain lactate, as well as hemodynamic changes, namely cerebral hyperemia. The increase in cerebral blood flow, also seen in humans with the disease, may be the result of intracerebral vasodilatory signals, whose nature has not been yet identified.

Brain edema can also be reproduced in the experimental animal after the administration of ammonia. Clinically, arterial ammonia levels above 200 μmol/L have been associated with cerebral herniation. Such hyperammonemia in urea cycle enzyme defects is also associated with brain edema and when uncontrolled, can result in death from cerebral herniation. Rather than ammonia itself, it is the product of its metabolism, glutamine, which has emerged as the key factor in the pathogenic sequence that leads to brain swelling.

A rise in intracranial pressure can be clinically silent or result in changes in oculovestibular reflexes and decerebrate posturing. Myoclonic seizures have been reported. Abnormalities in pupillary reflexes may herald the development of temporal lobe herniation.

Precipitant-induced encephalopathy in cirrhosis

This presentation is the most commonly seen form of encephalopathy in clinical practice. A wide range of precipitating events may be seen (**Table 11.2**). Many of them result in an increased ammonia load. However, other factors do not implicate such a load. For example, the mechanisms by which infection triggers encephalopathy are complex, and include hemodynamic and metabolic effects. The brain in liver disease is more susceptible to the effects of sedatives and caution should be exercised in their use.

Early stages of encephalopathy may be subtle. Family members note a change in personality, with dull speech and a sullen

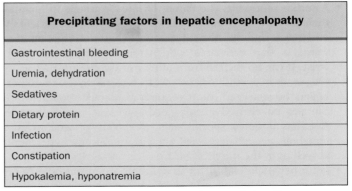

Precipitating factors in hepatic encephalopathy
Gastrointestinal bleeding
Uremia, dehydration
Sedatives
Dietary protein
Infection
Constipation
Hypokalemia, hyponatremia

Table 11.2 Precipitating factors in hepatic encephalopathy.

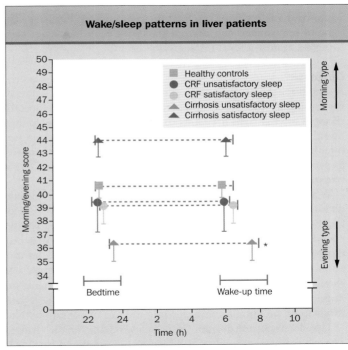

Figure 11.6 Wake/sleep patterns in liver patients. Bedtime and wake-up time of patients with cirrhosis, chronic renal failure (CRF) (grouped by sleep complaints), and healthy controls are plotted against the values of Horne-Osberg questionnaire (chronotypology profile). Results expressed as means ± SE. *Cirrhotic patients with unsatisfactory sleep show a delayed bedtime, a delayed wake-up time, and a lower score (evening type) in this questionnaire compared with their satisfactory sleep counterparts ($P<0.05$). Reproduced from Cordoba et al (98) by permission of Wiley-Liss, Inc.

attitude. The ability to perform mental and physical tasks decreases and assessment by a close relative provides better information than the one offered by the patient. Errors in motor activity reflect difficulties in recognizing the shape and position of objects. Altered sleep–wake patterns are characterized by difficult or late onset of sleep at night with sleepiness during the day (**Fig. 11.6**).

Overt encephalopathy has been classified in four stages: I, subtle changes; II, lethargy, confusion; III, stupor; IV, coma. Several physical signs can be detected during this evolution.

- Asterixis represents the failure of muscle groups to maintain their posture. It is traditionally elicited by asking patients to outstretch and fix their forearms while retroflexing their wrists; a 'flap' reflects a sudden forward movement of the wrist. It can be elicited from other muscle groups, such as the tongue, or in debilitated patients by requesting the examiner's fingers be squeezed. As it requires voluntary cooperation, it can not be elicited in advanced stages of encephalopathy. Asterixis is not a specific sign, as it can be seen in other metabolic encephalopathies, such as uremia and hypercapnia, as well as in the intoxication from certain drugs.
- Fetor hepaticus is difficult to describe: a pungent odor can be detected in the exhaled breath of such patients. Volatile sulfur-containing compounds, such as mercaptans, may account for this finding.
- Long-tract neurologic signs can be confusing, especially at the time of the first encounter. Unilateral hyper-reflexia, Babinski sign and ankle clonus can lead to an erroneous diagnosis. The rapid appearance and disappearance of such long-tract signs argues against a focal intracerebral event.

Diagnosis

A search for the precipitating event should be initiated. Evidence for blood in the stool, infected ascitic fluid or orthostatic changes in vital signs are clues to the nature of the precipitant. Standard laboratory testing is critical to detect uremia and hypokalemia. Respiratory alkalosis is common, with patients hyperventilating as a result of toxin-induced stimulation of the respiratory center.

While measurement of plasma ammonia is preferentially obtained from arterial blood, venous samples can also provide the needed information: a clue to the origin of an unknown encephalopathy. Once the diagnosis has been established, repeat measurements of ammonia do not provide additional information to that furnished by an evaluation of mental state and should be discouraged. Technical aspects of measurement are important Samples should be promptly assayed and the laboratory should be familiar with possible sources of contamination.

The electroencephalogram (EEG) shows characteristic changes. The normal background of 9–12 cycles/s is replaced by slower waves, including theta waves (seen in earlier stages of encephalopathy), triphasic waves and δ waves (two to three cycles/s). Frequency analysis may provide an integrated assessment of EEG abnormalities. Other neurophysiologically-based tests include visual and auditory evoked potentials. Recently, the critical flicker frequency test has been shown to discriminate patients with lesser degrees of encephalopathy.

A differential diagnosis arises in patients with alcoholic cirrhosis. Alcohol withdrawal is characterized by agitation and tremor, but not asterixis. Wernicke encephalopathy is suggested by the presence of a disconjugate gaze in the setting of a confusional state. Exclusion of chronic meningeal infection (tuberculosis, fungi) and subdural hematomas may require lumbar puncture and radiologic examination of the brain. Brain atrophy is common in cirrhosis, but this is a non-specific finding.

Persistent encephalopathy

This can be mild, severe or treatment-dependent, as noted in Table 11.1. It carries a poor prognosis, as recognized in the classic Child criteria. It may be the result of poor hepatic function, in which case appropriate candidates should be considered for liver transplantation. Severe encephalopathy may also be seen in patients with acute-on-chronic liver failure, where short-term prognosis is poor and transplantation can be problematic due to the presence of multi-organ failure.

Chronic encephalopathy may also reflect, in part, the presence of a large spontaneous portal-systemic collateral, most often a splenorenal communication. A clinical clue to the latter is a patient with chronic encephalopathy and relative preservation of liver function. Encephalopathy can also arise from the construction of a portal-systemic shunt, either radiologically [in the case of transjugular intrahepatic portal-systemic shunt (TIPS)] or surgically. The latter is less frequently performed nowadays, but performance of a selective distal splenorenal shunt may reduce the incidence of post-surgical encephalopathy. TIPS, which represents non-selective portal decompression, results in encephalopathy in 30–40% of individuals, with severe symptoms in <5% of subjects. Such patients may require radiologic occlusion of the shunt.

Hepatocerebral degeneration describes an entity appearing many years after a surgical portacaval anastomosis or extensive spontaneous shunting in which varying degrees of tremor, ataxia, choreoathetosis and disturbances of gait are noted. The mood can become jovial, inappropriate to the limitations of lifestyle imposed by the neurologic picture. Varying degrees of dementia may be observed. Spastic paraparesis has also been described.

Minimal encephalopathy

Patients with cirrhosis may appear intellectually appropriate, exhibit a normal neurologic examination and yet have evidence of cognitive defects elicited by neuropsychologic testing. Patients likely to have such changes exhibit some degree of hepatic functional impairment (Child class B) and have esophageal varices. An elaborate psychologic evaluation indicates a predominant alteration in attention. A psychometric hepatic encephalopathy score has been proposed using five tests, including the Reitan trail-making test parts A and B, digit symbol test, line drawing test and serial dotting test.

The impact of minimal encephalopathy on daily activities has been shown to affect selected areas of function: sleep, work capacity and recreation. A recent study describes impairment in the ability to drive an automobile. In the absence of clear guidelines on the matter, it may be prudent to have patients at risk, especially those with a prior history of encephalopathy, to undergo a neuropsychologic evaluation and therapy instituted if results are abnormal.

THERAPY OF HEPATIC ENCEPHALOPATHY

There are basically three strategies for therapy:

- control of precipitating factors;
- changes in the nature of dietary protein;
- removal of nitrogenous products, mainly through effects on the intestine.

Control of precipitating factors

Control of the precipitating factor may be the single most important therapeutic measure in patients with acceptable liver function. Correction of diuretic-induced hypokalemia and/or dehydration will improve the encephalopathic picture. Systemic treatment of infection with antibiotics may also affect the gut flora. Reversal of encephalopathy due to narcotics and sedatives may be possible with specific antagonists. Prevention of encephalopathy after upper gastrointestinal bleeding can be accomplished with vigorous bowel cleansing.

Diet

While animal-based protein is implicated in the precipitation of encephalopathy, dietary protein restriction should be abandoned. Patients with cirrhosis are hypercatabolic and require a higher dietary protein content (1–1.5 g/kg). Vegetable-based protein will have a cathartic effect and result in decreased ammoniagenesis. A casein-based diet is also beneficial.

Many studies have examined potential benefits of oral and intravenous formulations of branched-chain amino acids. Normalization of the abnormal ratio of aromatic/branched-chain amino acids is difficult to achieve. Numerous trials in different clinical situations have yielded variable results; meta-analysis has been complicated by marked differences in study design. The product is expensive and the benefit over standard measures may only be marginal. It is reserved for patients intolerant to the minimum amount of required protein.

Removal of nitrogenous products from the intestine
Use of non-absorbable carbohydrates

Non-absorbable disaccharides, lactulose and lactitol, reach the colon as they are not metabolized in the small bowel. Once in the colon, these disaccharides are metabolized, mainly by anaerobic bacteria, to acetic and lactic acid, resulting in colonic acidification. Such changes in pH favor the passage of ammonia into the intestinal lumen where it is used by bacteria as an energy source. A cathartic effect ensues, contributing to the elimination of nitrogenous products.

A recent analysis of the evidence supporting the use of such disaccharides has pointed at the weak support for their use. However, fault may also lie in the design of the original studies, as precipitant-induced encephalopathy was included and mental state in this situation may improve simply by removing the precipitating factor. There is a body of evidence indicating several mechanisms by which such drugs may help encephalopathy, supporting their continued use, especially in chronic encephalopathy.

Doses of lactulose range from 15 to 30 mL, two to four times a day. The goal is to obtain two to three soft bowel movements a day. Improvement of encephalopathy is not immediate; patients may require 48–72 h before a marked change occurs. Administration of lactulose enemas (300 mL in a total of 1 L volume) may be useful to hasten the process in comatose patients. In areas of the world with a high prevalence of lactose malabsorption, this disaccharide may be used for oral treatment, at a considerably lower cost.

If diarrhea develops, the drug should be stopped to be re-initiated later. Patients may complain of flatulence and cramping and the sweet syrupy taste of lactulose may not be palatable to all patients. Persistence of diarrhea may result in excessive loss of hypotonic colonic water. This leads to hypernatremia, with changes in mental state associated with hyperosmolarity. Lack of awareness of this possibility may result in an inappropriate increase in lactulose dosage.

Lactitol, a more palatable non-absorbable disaccharide, has been tested with success in Europe; another benefit over lactulose appears to be its quicker onset of action.

Antibiotics

A reduction of aerobic, urease-splitting bacterial flora is the rationale for the use of neomycin. Such treatment has also been recently criticized for the lack of supportive evidence in clinical trials, in consonance with criticisms on non-absorbable disaccharides. Clinical experience suggests that 2–4 g/day in divided doses may be effective. A minimal amount is absorbed, and long-term use requires monitoring of renal and auditory function. The combination of lactulose and neomycin is effective in reducing ammonia levels; although neomycin reduces the aerobic intestinal flora, lactulose is mainly split by *Bacteroides fragilis* and other anaerobes.

In patients with renal dysfunction, other oral antibiotics such as vancomycin may be used; metronidazole has been postulated to be as effective as neomycin. As hepatic metabolism of metronidazole is impaired, doses should be reduced and started at 250 mg twice daily. A recent study compared the effects of rifaximin, a non-absorbable antibiotic, and lactulose in the management of precipitant-induced encephalopathy. Similar efficacy was seen in both groups.

Removal of nitrogenous products by other organs

In children with urea cycle enzyme deficiencies, alternative pathways for hepatic nitrogen excretion have been delineated. These consist of the administration of a drug (sodium benzoate or sodium phenylbutyrate), conjugation with an aminoacid (glycine or glutamine) and excretion in the urine (as hippurate or phenylacetylglutamine). A trial with sodium benzoate in cirrhosis showed equivalence with lactulose in precipitant-induced encephalopathy.

Ornithine-aspartate has been used outside the USA to treat hepatic encephalopathy. Transamination of these amino acids can increase the availability of glutamate and enhance the production of glutamine in muscle. Provision of ornithine can also improve rates of urea synthesis. Zinc, a cofactor of all five enzymatic reactions in the urea cycle, can also be administered (as acetate or sulfate). Improvement in encephalopathy is especially noted in patients with malnutrition.

Treatment of chronic intractable encephalopathy

Patients with chronic encephalopathy pose major problems in management. Once the previously discussed measures have been exhausted, four therapeutic possibilities arise:

- Use of bromocriptine, a dopamine antagonist, has yielded conflicting results in patients with chronic encephalopathy. Rationale for its use centers on the 'false neurotransmitter' hypothesis, with correction of supposed deficiency of dopaminergic neurotransmission. Doses of up to 15 mg/day may be tried before attempting other alternatives.
- A portacaval shunt may be either occluded with the use of a balloon technique or closed at surgery, with a simultaneous esophageal transection to prevent variceal rebleeding. Radiologic occlusion of a TIPS catheter may improve intractable encephalopathy.

- In a suitable candidate, liver transplantation may offer a radical solution. Recent reports document clear improvement in a few patients with hepatocerebral degeneration after this procedure, patients who had a short duration of their chronic symptomatology. However, poor outcomes may also be possible and more definitive data are needed.
- An abdominal colectomy, a measure of last resort, may provide relief in patients in whom other treatments are not possible. This procedure is rarely employed, as major abdominal surgery is by itself riskier in patients with liver failure.

FURTHER READING

First descriptions
Adams RD, Foley JM. The neurological disorder associated with liver disease. Proc Ass Res Nerv Dis 1953; 32:198–237.
Sherlock S, Summerskill WHJ, White LP, et al. Portal-systemic encephalopathy; neurological complications of liver disease. Lancet 1954; 2:453–456. *Classic descriptions of the syndrome, noting astrocyte pathology at autopsy as well as coining the term 'portal-systemic encephalopathy'.*

General reviews
Blei AT, Cordoba J. Hepatic encephalopathy. Am J Gastroentrol 2001; 96:1968–1976.
Ferenci P, Lockwood A, Mullen K, et al. Hepatic encephalopathy-definition, nomenclature, diagnosis, and quantification: final report of the working party at the 11th World Congresses of Gastroenterology, Vienna, 1998.

Pathogenesis
Butterworth RF. Pathogenesis of hepatic encephalopathy: new insights from neuroimaging and molecular studies. J Hepatol 2003; 39:278–285.
Cordoba J, Gottstein J, Blei AT. Glutamine, myo-inositol and organic brain osmolytes after portocaval anastomosis in the rat: implications for ammonia-induced brain edema. Hepatology 1996; 24:919–923.
Crespin J, Nemark A, Rehkemper et al. Intrahepatic portal-hepatic venous anastomosis: a portal-systemic shunt with neurological repercussions. Am J Gastroenterol 2000; 95:1568–1571.
Kaplowitz N. Liver and biliary disorders. Baltimore: Williams & Wilkins; 1992:557.
Rama Rao KV, Jayakumar AR, Norenberg DM. Ammonia neurotoxicity: role of the mitochondrial permeability transition. Metab Brain Dis 2003; 18:113–127.
Vaquero J, Chung C, Cahill ME, et al. Pathogenesis of hepatic encephalopathy in acute liver failure. Semin Liver Dis 2003; 23:259–269. *Ammonia-induced oxidative stress and mitochondrial alterations in astrocytes has emerged as an important pathogenic mechanism, especially in the encephalopathy of acute liver failure.*

Clinical features
Bustamante J, Rimola A, Ventura PJ, et al. Prognostic significance of hepatic encephalopathy in patients with cirrhosis. J Hepatol 1999; 30:890–895. *Deleterious impact on survival in all forms of presentation of hepatic encephalopathy.*

Clemmesen Jo, Larsen FS, Kondrup J, et al. Cerebral herniation in patients with acute liver failure is correlated with arterial ammonia concentration. Hepatology 1999; 29:648–653.
Cordoba J, Cabrera J, Lataif L, et al. High prevalence of sleep disturbance in cirrhosis. Hepatology 1998; 27:339–345.
Haussinger D, Laubenberger J, vom Dahl S, et al. Proton magnetic resonance spectroscopy studies on human brain myo-inositol in hypo-osmolarity and hepatic encephalopathy. Gastroenterology 1994; 107:1475–1480.
Krieger D, Krieger S, Jansen O, et al. Manganese and chronic hepatic encephalopathy. Lancet 1995; 346:270–274.

Minimal hepatic encephalopathy
Conn HO. Trailmaking and number-connection tests in the assessment of mental state in portal systemic encephalopathy. Am J Dig Dis 1977; 22:541–550.
Wein C, Koch H, Popp B, et al. Minimal hepatic encephalopathy impairs fitness to drive. Hepatology 2004; 39:599–601.
Weissenborn K, Ennen JC, Schomerus H, et al. Neuropsychological characterization of hepatic encephalopathy. J Hepatol 2001; 34:768–773.

Therapy
Als-Nielsen B, Gluud LL, Gluud C. Non-absorbable disaccharides for hepatic encephalopathy: systemic review of randomized trials. BMJ 2004;328:1046–1050. *A review of the evidence for the use of these medications indicates insufficient evidence for the effectiveness of these agents based on the quality of the studies performed.*
Cordoba J, Lopez-Hellin J, Planas M, et al. Normal protein diet for episodic hepatic encephalopathy: results of a randomized study. J Hepatol 2004; 41:38–43.
Jalan R, Kapoor D. Reversal of diuretic-induced hepatic encephalopathy with infusion of albumin but not colloid. Clin Sci (Lond) 2004; 106:467–474.
Liu Q, Duan ZP, Hada K, et al. Synbiotic modulation of gut flora: effect on minimal hepatic encephalopathy in patients with cirrhosis. Hepatology 2004; 39:1441–1449.
Riordan SM, Williams R. Treatment of hepatic encephalopathy. N Engl J Med 1997; 337:473–479. *A general review of available medications.*
Weissenborn K, Tietge UJ, Bokemeyer M, et al. Liver transplantation improves hepatic myelopathy: evidence by three cases. Gastroenterology 2003; 124:346–351.

CONCLUSION

Hepatic encephalopathy develops in patients with liver failure. It carries a poor prognosis in both acute and chronic liver disease. Recognition of precipitating events is critical for its management. There is a lack of specific medications directed at the abnormal brain neurochemistry. Rather, most of the current available therapies are directed at improving ammonia removal in the gut, muscle, kidney and/or liver.

Guidelines for nutritional therapy					
	Protein (g/kg/day)	Energy (kcal/kg/day)	Energy substrate %CHO	%fat	Nutritional goal
1. Hepatitis (acute or chronic*)	1.0–1.5	30–40	67–80	20–33	Prevent malnutrition Enhance regeneration
2. Cirrhosis (uncomplicated)	1.0–1.2	30–40	67–80	20–33	Same as 1.
3. Cirrhosis (complicated)[†] a. Malnutrition	1.2–1.8	40–50	72	28	Restore normal nutritional status
b. Cholestasis	1.0–1.5	30–40	73–80	20–27	Prevent malnutrition Treat fat malabsorption[†]
c. Encephalopathy[§] Grade 1 or 2	0.5–1.2	25–40	75	25	Provide nutritional needs without precipitating encephalopathy
Grade 3 or 4	0.5	25–40	75	25	
4. Liver transplant a. Peritransplant	1.2–1.8 1.0	30–50	70-80	20–30	Restore normal nutritional status
b. Post-transplant		30–35	>70	≤30	Retain and maintain ideal body weight

*There are no convincing data indicating any extraordinary vitamin or trace metal requirements in liver disease. A typical substitution solution for parenteral feeding is provided. Vitamins: (10 cc/L) – ascorbic acid (20 mg/mL), vitamin A (660 IU/mL), vitamin D (40 IU/mL), thiamine HCL (0.6 mg/mL), riboflavin phosphate (0.72 mg/mL), pyridoxine HCl (0.8 mg/mL), niacinamide (8 mg/mL), D-pantothenic acid (3 mg/mL), vitamin E (2 IU/mL), biotin (12 mcq/m), folic acid (0.08 mg/5 mL), vitamin B_{12} (1 mcq/5 mL). Trace metals: (1 mL/L) – zinc chloride (10.42 mq/5 mL, copper chloride (2.68 mq/5 mL), manganese (1.44 mq/5 mL), chromium chloride (0.012 mq/5 mL)

[†]Ascites and sepsis are two complications which are not listed but which should be treated aggressively as part of nutritional therapy (see text).

[†]Medium chain triglycerides may be necessary if fat malabsorption is present. Pancreatic enzymes are necessary if pancreatic insufficiency is present; especially in alcoholic cirrhosis and primary sclerosing cholangitis.

[§]Branched-chain amino acid (BCAA) formulations may be necessary. Available hepatic enteral formulations are 45% BCAA enriched and parenteral formulations are 36% BCAA enriched. This compares to standard formulations for preparations which contain 26% BCAA. For outpatients, diets high in vegetable protein or casein hydrolysates may be better tolerated than standard dietary protein in the protein-intolerant patient with cirrhosis.

Table 12.6 Guidelines for nutritional therapy.

often self-select a higher proportion of their dietary intake at breakfast, a full day's calorie count is required to obtain an accurate assessment.

Physical examination

During physical examination one should look for signs of decompensation, such as mental status changes, asterixis, jaundice, ascites, leg edema and bruising. Weight should be recorded with specific attention to fluid overload. Signs of specific nutritional deficiency, such as acrodermatitis from zinc deficiency or pellagra from niacin deficiency, should be sought. Patients with cholestatic liver disease and steatorrhea may have skin excoriations related to pruritus, xanthomas due to hyperlipidemia, or dermatitis from essential fatty acid deficiency.

Evaluation of the oral mucosa, skin and hair are particularly important. In the oral mucosa, glossitis (raw tongue), atrophic tongue (slick tongue) and angular stomatitis are common findings and result from deficiencies in the B vitamins, iron and folate. Less common are gingivitis (vitamin C deficiency) and altered taste/smell (zinc deficiency).

On the skin, petechiae (vitamin C deficiency) and purpura (vitamin A and zinc deficiency) may be present. Hair may demonstrate sparseness (protein, zinc and biotin deficiencies),

follicular hyperkeratosis (vitamins A and C deficiency) or be corkscrewed and coiled (vitamin C deficiency).

NUTRITIONAL REQUIREMENTS

Nitrogen

In stable cirrhotics, the average protein requirement to maintain positive nitrogen balance is 0.8 g/kg/day, which is similar to that required in the normal population. Because the range of protein required is larger in cirrhotics than in controls, compensated cirrhotics should receive at least 1.2 g/kg/day. Although nitrogen balance is achieved at this amount, nitrogen retention continues to improve up to 1.8 g/kg/day. Even stable cirrhotics are protein deficient and this is an important management consideration. Cirrhotic patients undergoing surgery should receive protein doses between 1.2 and 1.5 g/kg/day (**Table 12.6**).

Energy

Abnormalities in extracellular fluid levels in fat and non-fat body compartments, portosystemic shunting, and variability in energy expenditure between different body requirements make the prediction of energy requirements quantitatively unreliable in cirrhosis. Therefore, with knowledge that hypermetabolism

Vitamins in liver disease
• Many complications associated with liver disease are manifestations of vitamin deficiencies. These include: macrocytic anemia (folate and vitamin B_{12} deficiency); neuropathy (pyridoxine, thiamine or vitamin B_{12}); confusion, ataxia and ocular disturbances (thiamine) and impaired adaptation to dark (vitamin A)
• Pyridoxine phosphate (the major active form of pyridoxine) rather than pyridoxine itself may be required to correct pyridoxine deficiency; especially in alcoholics
• The clinical response to thiamine is usually rapid and effective. However, the neuropathy may be irreversible and abnormalities in red cell transketolase may not improve
• Deficiencies in vitamin B_{12} and folic acid may develop faster in cirrhotic patients due to diminished hepatic storage
• In the presence of active hepatic inflammation, fatty liver or hepatocellular cancer, normal or elevated levels of vitamin B_{12} levels do not exclude a deficiency of this vitamin
• Decreased serum levels of vitamin A do not necessarily reflect vitamin A deficiency. Zinc deficiency may be causing decreased transport out of the liver
• In non-cholestatic liver disease, abnormal serum levels of fat-soluble vitamins should not be sought or treated in the absence of clinical or laboratory abnormalities, which indicate a functional vitamin deficiency. In cholestatic liver diseases, abnormal serum levels of the fat soluble vitamins may be treated even in the absence of clinical symptoms or laboratory abnormalities
• Suggestions for use of vitamin supplements: (a) Water-soluble vitamins may be supplied with a multivitamin preparation; (b) fat-soluble vitamins should be used in a water-soluble form whenever possible. Vitamin A, Aquasol 1 capsule daily (50 000 IU), vitamin K, Synkayvite, 1 tablet daily (15 mg). Vitamin D treatment should be individualized by monitoring plasma 25-hydroxy vitamin D levels and serum and urinary calcium levels. Vitamin D_2 (ergocalciferol), 1.25 mg (50 000) U, 1 tablet three to four times a day, may be adequate. Vitamin E (D-α-tocopheryl polyethelene glycol 1000 succinate (TPGS) 23 IU kg/day)

Table 12.7 Vitamins in liver disease.

Nutritional considerations for specific alterations in liver disease	
Specific alterations	Implications for nutritional management
1. Accelerated starvation	1. Frequent feedings with night-time snack
2. Hepatic encephalopathy	2. Routine or prophylactic protein restriction should be discouraged
3. Hepatic metabolism of non-essential amino acids	3. Cysteine and tyrosine may become essential amino acids in cirrhosis
4. Salt restriction	4. Salt restriction should be balanced against palatability of the diet
5. Alcohol toxicity	5. Abstinence needs to be continually reinforced
6. Obesity	6. Gradual weight loss should be instituted

Table 12.8 Nutritional considerations for specific alterations in liver disease.

Vitamins

Approximately 40% of patients with non-alcoholic liver disease have fat soluble vitamin deficiencies (vitamin A and E); 8–10% have deficiencies in the B complex vitamins (nicotinic acid, thiamine, vitamin B_{12}, riboflavin and pyridoxine) and 17% have folate deficiency. These abnormalities are related more to disordered hepatic function and diminished reserve rather than deficient dietary intake or malabsorption. However, in severe advanced cirrhosis, malabsorption may play a role in both fat soluble vitamins and the B complex vitamins. These vitamin deficiencies are more prevalent and severe in alcoholic than non-alcoholic liver disease. Specific issues regarding vitamins in liver disease are provided in **Table 12.7**.

SPECIFIC ALTERATIONS IN LIVER DISEASE (Table 12.8)

Accelerated starvation

Cirrhosis is a disease of accelerated starvation with early recruitment of alternative fuels. Cirrhotic patients should avoid any extended period of time without feeding. The advantage of a frequent feeding approach has been confirmed by nitrogen balance and indirect calorimetry measurements in cirrhotic patients.

Hepatic encephalopathy

Advanced acute or chronic liver failure often presents with a constellation of neuropsychiatric abnormalities known as hepatic encephalopathy. These mental status alterations may range from mild behavioral changes to deep coma. Subclinical hepatic encephalopathy is present in up to 70% of patients with cirrhosis and currently does not require any specific nutritional therapy. Overt encephalopathy is almost always associated with some precipitating event such as gastrointestinal bleeding, infection/sepsis, fluid and electrolyte imbalances, constipation, acid–base

may have adverse clinical sequelae, energy expenditure should be measured with indirect calorimetry, especially in hospitalized patients undergoing liver transplantation. If indirect calorimetry is not available, the daily resting energy expenditure for cirrhosis should be assumed as 25–30 kcal/kg body weight (based on ideal body weight if ascites and/or edema is present) for decisions regarding restorative or maintenance needs.

Energy is proportionally provided by carbohydrates and fat (Table 12.6). Two points are important:

• Insulin resistance is universal in cirrhosis irrespective of the type or severity of the disease. Glucose intolerance is not typically an important management issue, except hypoglycemia, which develops in up to 50% of cirrhotic patients during sepsis.

• Lipid formulations are very useful in cirrhosis because of their low water content and high caloric density. Initial concerns that lipids might precipitate encephalopathy have not been confirmed.

abnormalities or the use of sedating drugs. In a minority of cirrhotic patients, hepatic encephalopathy may be precipitated by protein intake (especially animal protein) without any other precipitating factor. These patients are considered protein intolerant. More than 95% of cirrhotic patients can tolerate diets containing as much as 1.5 g/kg/day of mixed proteins. Therefore, true protein intolerance is rare except for fulminant hepatic failure, or the occasional patient with 'endogenous' chronic encephalopathy.

In those few cirrhotic patients with endogenous protein intolerance, branched-chain amino acid formulations are better tolerated than standard amino acid supplements and can achieve positive nitrogen balance. It should be emphasized, however, that there is no clearly proven benefit of branched-chain amino acids. Thus, standard amino acid formulations are suitable for the majority of patients with chronic liver disease.

Protein restriction

There is no justification for the routine use of protein restriction as prophylaxis against precipitating hepatic encephalopathy. Available data indicate that the vast majority of cirrhotic patients and even patients with severe alcoholic hepatitis can tolerate large quantities of protein feeding (up to 1.75 g/kg/day).

Non-essential amino acids

Administration of standard or specialized total parenteral nutrition solutions devoid of the non-essential amino acids tyrosine and cysteine may not achieve positive nitrogen balance in cirrhosis despite provisions of adequate amounts of essential amino acids. This observation emphasizes the observation that certain intrinsic liver functions may be rate limiting in cirrhosis such as the ability to synthesize cysteine from methionine and tyrosine from phenylalanine.

Salt restriction

Although frequently necessary, sodium and consequently salt restriction significantly decreases the palatability of the diet and consequently may diminish food intake. In the hospitalized patient, very low 250–500 mg sodium (0.63–1.3 g salt) diets may be appropriate. In the non-hospitalized patient, every effort should be made to avoid salt restriction. In those patients with fluid overload who otherwise cannot be managed effectively, the least sodium restriction that is effective should be employed. A 2.5 g sodium (6.3 g salt) intake approximates a no added salt diet. This restriction can be tolerated by the motivated patient and is usually effective for fluid management in most patients and does not significantly limit calorie or protein intake.

Alcohol related alterations

Alcohol has direct deleterious effects on muscle protein status independent from associated liver injury. Alcohol is known to inhibit meal stimulated hepatic protein production which is an important contributor to skeletal muscle and whole body protein synthesis in humans. In addition alcohol increases intestinal permeability which in turn initiates endotoxin/cytokine induced muscle proteolysis. Alcohol also has a caloric density of seven but produces less efficient energy per gram of nutrient than both carbohydrates and lipids. Further, it replaces the amount of other caloric sources.

Obesity

Obesity is associated with hepatic steatosis which not only causes cirrhosis per se, but also is a risk factor in the development of cirrhosis in patients with alcohol and hepatitis C associated liver disease. It is also associated with multiorgan failure post-liver transplant.

NUTRITIONAL MANAGEMENT

Goals

Although early studies used survival as the primary outcome measure for determining the efficacy of nutritional therapy, more recently, improvement in nutritional status, infection rates, immune function, nitrogen balance and perioperative morbidity have been shown to improve with nutritional therapy in cirrhotic patients. Nutritional therapy is most effective when used for longer periods or in certain subgroups such as in those with severe malnutrition, chronic hepatic encephalopathy and decompensated liver disease. No reliable information is available regarding the cost-effectiveness of nutritional therapy or its effect on the quality of life of cirrhotic patients.

Regarding goals specific for liver disease, nutritional therapy needs to correct pre-existing PEM while simultaneously providing sufficient amino acids to encourage hepatic regeneration and normalization of function without precipitating encephalopathy. The clinical emphasis should be placed on supplying the basic requirements of nitrogen and calories. Overall recommendations are provided in **Table 12.9**.

Specific patient populations
Cirrhosis
Enteral feeding improves liver function, encephalopathy and perhaps survival in severely malnourished cirrhotics and in patients with decompensated alcoholic liver disease. Nutrient intake is increased by enteral nutrition in all published studies to date and may in part be responsible for these benefits. Providing nutritional supplements (1000 cal and 34 g of protein – casein based) for 1 year to patients with complicated alcoholic cirrhosis resulted in higher protein and caloric intake to levels which simply met their required needs.

Alcoholic hepatitis
There have been eight published trials on the use of standard intravenous amino acid formulations as primary therapy for alcoholic hepatitis. The results are conflicting, but six of the eight studies showed improvement in either liver histology or function. One of these studies additionally showed a strong trend toward an improvement in mortality. Two of the studies concluded that supplemental amino acids were of no benefit. In one of these negative studies, the mortality was 3.3% in the 30 patients in whom positive nitrogen balance was achieved, but was 58% in those patients who remained in negative nitrogen balance despite nutritional therapy. A recent trial also reported enteral feedings to be equally as effective as corticosteroids.

Fulminant hepatic failure
Fulminant hepatic failure defined as the development of hepatic encephalopathy within 8 weeks of the onset of liver disease is a life-threatening illness associated with a rapid development of protein calorie malnutrition; even when what is calculated to be

Overall guidelines for the nutritional management of patients with liver disease
· Assume protein calorie malnutrition is present in all patients
· Assume an inadequate dietary intake, even in hospitalized patients
· Qualitative stool fat should be done intermittently, especially in patients with alcoholic or cholestatic cirrhosis. If malabsorption is present; determine the cause and treat
· Treatment with either neomycin or lactulose for hepatic encephalopathy may exacerbate malabsorption, which should be considered in nutritional management
· Treat ascites aggressively to decrease energy expenditure
· Diuretic therapy is preferred over large volume paracentesis for the management of ascites in order to minimize protein loss
· Balance the need for sodium restriction with nutritional considerations and diet palatability
· Nutritional assessment is useful in all types of cirrhotic patients
· A composite score (emphasizing anthropometry and creatinine height index) combined with overall clinical judgment should be employed
· The clinician should remember that all the methods for nutritional assessment in cirrhosis are influenced or potentially influenced by the presence of liver disease alone as well as abnormalities associated with liver disease such as renal failure, alcohol ingestion and expansion of the extracellular water compartment
· Determine energy expenditure requirements with indirect calorimetry (if possible) in hospitalized patients or patients listed for liver transplantation. If energy expenditure requirements are estimated from prediction equations, calculate energy need based on ideal weight rather than actual weight if extracellular water (ascites/edema) is present
· Multiple (five to six) small feedings with a carbohydrate-rich evening snack, which consists of approximately 10–15% of caloric needs, should be given. The need for breakfast feeding must also be stressed to the patient
· For calories, complex rather than simple carbohydrates should be used. Lipids should supply 20–40% of caloric needs
· Nutritional requirements may vary according to the specific type of patient and/or clinical situation as listed in Table 12.6
· Severely malnourished or decompensated cirrhotics should be given oral or enteral supplements as recommended in Table 12.6
· Long-term nutritional supplements may be necessary to provide recommended protein and caloric supplements
· Patients with severe alcoholic hepatitis should be given supplemental standard protein 1.0 g/kg via an enteral or peripheral parenteral route
· Perioperative nutritional therapy should be given to those cirrhotic patients with significant malnutrition as defined by weight loss of more than 10% or for anthropometry or creatinine height index less than 5% of predicted values
· Post-liver transplant, patients need higher amounts of protein and energy (see Table 12.6)
· Pediatric patients undergoing liver transplant may benefit from branched-chain amino acids
· Cirrhotics should never be treated prophylactically with protein restriction to prevent hepatic encephalopathy.
· Standard protein or amino acid mixtures should be supplied to meet the measured estimated nitrogen needs (as provided in Table 12.6)
· Protein restriction should be implemented only if protein intolerance as manifested by encephalopathy occurs in the absence of precipitating factors is found
· Protein restriction below the required amounts should not be continued for more than 3–4 days
· Branched-chain amino acids should be given only if the required amount of standard feedings cannot be tolerated without precipitating hepatic encephalopathy
· Monitor for hypoglycemia and treat aggressively with concentrated glucose solutions which may also decrease serum ammonia levels
· Enteral feeding is the preferred route of feeding patients with insufficient oral intake. Enteral feeding tubes may be used even if non-bleeding varices are present.
· Do not use any nutritional product devoid of cysteine or tyrosine as the only nitrogen source for any prolonged period of time. Be aware of clinically important issues related to vitamins listed in Table 12.7.

Table 12.9 Overall guidelines for the nutritional management of patients with liver disease.

adequate amounts of calories and nitrogen are supplied. Up to four times the normal rate of protein breakdown accompanied by decreased hepatic amino acid oxidation leads to the accumulation of potentially toxic levels of certain amino acids (e.g. tyrosine, phenylalanine and methionine).

Hypoglycemia occurs commonly, and serum glucose levels must be maintained with concentrated glucose infused (20–40%) to avoid the risks of exacerbating cerebral edema. Lipid emulsions may be particularly useful in this setting.

Recent work suggests that administering at least 40–60 g of protein diminishes the rapid depletion of protein stores in patients with stages 1 and 2 encephalopathy. If necessary, the use of branched-chain amino acids may be necessary to achieve this goal in patients with more advanced stages of encephalopathy. However, the efficacy of branched-chain amino acids in this situation remains unproven. If encephalopathy should develop or worsen with protein feeding, the use of specialized formulations of branched-chain amino acids seems indicated.

Weight loss

Serum aminotransferases almost always improve with weight loss in the obese patient (with as little at 5–10% decrease in body weight), but they are poor predictors of histology which does not always improve and may, in fact, worsen if weight loss occurs too rapidly. Gradual weight loss (1–2 lbs/week) with an overall goal of 10% weight loss over 6 months is recommended as a safe and effective clinical strategy especially in patients who are 30% overweight.

With success, further weight loss can be attempted, if indicated. Multiple interventions and strategies, including diet modifications, physical activity, behavioral therapy and pharmacotherapy with Orlistat, or a combination of these treatment modalities is recommended. The particular treatment modality should be individualized taking into consideration the BMI and presence of concomitant risk factors and other diseases. Given the lack of clinical trials in this area, these overall recommendations are a useful and safe first step for obese patients with NAFLD. The only prospective study using restrictive bariatric surgery in NAFLD patients was very effective in diminishing hepatic injury.

Liver transplantation

There is no uniform approach among transplant centers regarding the management of nutrition in transplant patients. There is general agreement that malnutrition reflects the severity of chronic liver disease and should not be considered, in general, as an exclusion for patients receiving liver transplant. Most centers administer post-operative nutrition in a fashion similar to that given other patients after major gastrointestinal surgery. Therefore the recognition that malnutrition is a significant problem has been gaining momentum.

In the pretransplant patient, there are insufficient data upon which any specific recommendations can be based. Consequently, general principles of nutritional management as outlined in Tables 12.6 and 12.9 should be followed.

In the post-transplant patient, a number of benefits to nutritional therapy have been shown as demonstrated in **Table 12.10**. As compared to conventional therapy, early enteral feeding was shown to decrease the number of viral infections and obtain better nitrogen retention post-operatively. Both nasogastric and jejunostomy tubes have been used successfully in these patients post-operatively. The available information also indicates that both enteral and parenteral nutrition are equivalent in their ability to deliver nutrients and improve nutritional status at the tenth postoperative day.

In contrast to these positive results, 1 year after follow-up, protein breakdown and lipolysis in these patients improved, but did not normalize, with improvement in total body water and total body fat but no change in body cell mass. An increasingly important nutritional problem which develops in the first 1–2 years after liver transplant is obesity which has been reported to occur in 30–70% of patients. Therefore, it is important to follow the nutritional status of these patients postoperatively and treat obesity aggressively if it develops.

PRINCIPLES AND PRACTICAL IMPLEMENTATION

The nutritional support for patients with liver disease follows the general principles applicable to any other type of patient. However, there are a number of principles particularly relevant to liver disease patients with guidelines provided in Tables 12.6 and 12.9.

Glucose requirement

Although insulin resistance and hyperglycemia are commonly observed in cirrhosis, hypoglycemia (<50 mg/dL) occurs in up to 50% of cirrhotic patients during episodes of stress. Therefore, serum glucose must be closely monitored in patients with fulminant or decompensated chronic liver disease.

Route of nutrient administration

The least invasive route for nutritional supplementation is oral which should be tried first. If attempts at oral supplementation fail, enteral feedings can be administered via a small caliber nasogastric or nasojejunal tube. The presence of non-bleeding esophageal varices is not a contraindication to the use of enteral feeding tubes in these patients. However, feeding tubes should not be used if there is active esophageal variceal bleeding.

The placement of a gastrostomy or a jejunostomy tube in cirrhotics with ascites is not recommended due to the possible complications of peritonitis or ascitic fluid leakage. Unfortunately, this limits the potential of long-term enteral feeding in many of these patients.

Parenteral nutrition should be initiated only if nutritional requirements cannot be supplied orally or enterally in situations such as gastrointestinal bleeding, ileus, or after abdominal surgery. Because of its relatively low caloric density, peripheral parenteral

Benefits of nutritional therapy post-transplant
Improved nitrogen balance
Less time in the ICU (trend)
Lower hospital cost (trend)
Fewer viral infections with early enteral feeding which is equivalent to parenteral feeding
Both nasogastric and jejunostomy tubes have been used successfully

Table 12.10 Benefits of nutritional therapy post-transplant.

Use of nutritional supplements and medications in NAFLD			
Possibly harmful		**Possibly helpful**	
Supplements	*Medications*	*Supplements*	*Medications*
St John's wort	Acetaminophen[4]	Vitamin E[8]	Betaine[11]
Ephedrine containing compounds	Tamoxifen[5]	MVI[9]	Ursodeoxycholic acid[11]
Excessive vitamin A[1]	Amiodarone[5]	SAMe[10,11]	Metformin[11,12]
Glucosamine[2]	Iron[6]	Milk thistle[11]	Statins[11,13]
Others[3]	Estrogen[7]		Thiazolidinediones[11,12]

1. Vitamin A should not be used in excess of that contained in a daily multivitamin (MVI) which is 5000 IU.
2. Since hexosamines in general cause insulin resistance, glucosamine should be used with some caution.
3. All other herbs should be considered as possible causes of injury and should be avoided.
4. Acetaminophen should be restricted to less than 2–3 g daily. Repeated or ongoing use of acetaminophen for longer than 3 days with daily doses above 1.5 g should be discouraged. Many over the counter (OTC) medications contain acetaminophen. Therefore the amount of acetaminophen in the OTC medications should be carefully sought.
5. These drugs may cause hepatic injury that histologically looks similar to non-alcoholic fatty liver disease (NAFLD)/non-alcoholic steatohepatitis (NASH). Therefore, the benefit risk of using these drugs in NAFLD/NASH should be carefully considered.
6. Since iron may cause oxidative stress in the liver, iron supplements should only be used as per standard management for anemia. Transferrin saturation should not exceed 50%.
7. Estrogens used as oral contraception pills (OCP) or as hormonal replacement therapy (HRT) do not have to be discontinued.
8. Vitamin E should not be used at doses less than 400 IU daily.
9. A daily multivitamin (MVI) with iron content <20 mg should be used.
10. SAMe = S-Adenosylmethionine.
11. The use of these supplements or medications should not be encouraged. However, there are uncontrolled studies suggesting their benefit in NAFLD.
12. This agent is approved for use in patients with type II diabetes.
13. The use of the statins used as cholesterol lowering agents is not contraindicated (and in fact, may be beneficial) in NAFLD. However, baseline and interval measurements of liver tests should be performed.

Table 12.11 Use of nutritional supplements and medications in NAFLD.

nutrition cannot supply total nutritional requirements and is usually not a good choice in cirrhotic patients with sodium and water retention. Peripheral parenteral nutrition may be useful in supplementing enteral or oral feeding; especially for providing amino acids in severe alcoholic hepatitis. Central parenteral nutrition is preferred in most cirrhotic patients despite the risk of central vein catheter replacement in patients with coagulopathy and thrombocytopenia.

The amount of protein recommended for different types of liver disease patients in various situations is provided in Table 12.6. If these amounts of protein cannot be provided without precipitating hepatic encephalopathy, formulations enriched with branched-chain amino acids should be substituted for standard formulations. There are oral or enteral feedings (Nutrihep; – 50% branched-chain amino acid enriched and Hepatic Aid II – 46% branched-chain amino acid enriched) as well as intravenous formulations (Hepatamine and Hepatasol; both 36% branched-chain amino acid enriched) available. In addition to these formulations which have been tried in liver patients, there are also stress formulations (Freamine HBC and Aminosyn-HBC) both of which are approximately 45% branched-chain amino acid enriched. However, these stress formulations have not been evaluated in patients with liver disease.

Dietary supplements

Many patients seek advice regarding the efficacy and safety of vitamins, herbs or other nutritional supplements. Unfortunately, there is insufficient information in this area to make sound recommendations. General recommendations are provided in **Table 12.11**.

Obesity

A number of different diets have been suggested, including: the American Heart Association healthy heart diet, the Diabetic Diet as recommended by the American Diabetes Association, a low glycemic diet, and diets enriched with omega 3 polyunsaturated fatty acids. However, the effect of these diets in NAFLD is unproven. Diets used to produce weight loss must always be individualized and related to the overall health status of the patient.

In general, patients should follow a well-balanced diet. One such diet is recommended by the National Cholesterol Education Program (www.nhlbi.nih.gov/about/ncep). This diet makes specific recommendations regarding total caloric intake, as well as the amount and type of fat and carbohydrate for patients who do not have to lose weight. If the patient has diabetes, specific recommendations have been made by the American Diabetes Association.

Overweight patients (BMI >25 kg/m^2 based on dry weight) should be given a diet with a goal of losing and sustaining an initial weight loss of 10% of body weight. The weight loss should be gradual and should not exceed 2 lbs/week. The National Heart, Lung and Blood Institute (NHLBI) guidelines for weight loss are provided in **Table 12.12** as one typical diet that might be employed.

hemopoiesis must be interpreted cautiously in the setting of acute or chronic liver disease. True iron deficiency occurs in chronic liver disease most often due to blood loss from the gastrointestinal tract and patients may bleed from either portal hypertensive sources or non-liver related gastrointestinal disorders.

Interpretation of serum ferritin levels in defining iron status is problematic in patients with liver disease. Elevated ferritin levels are commonly seen in patients with acute hepatic necrosis when levels may be massively elevated (10–50-fold increase from normal) due to release from damaged hepatocytes. In addition, ferritin is an acute phase protein and may be elevated in a number of inflammatory liver conditions. Interpretation of serum iron levels are inaccurate for similar reasons and use of the total iron binding capacity may be unhelpful since decreased synthesis of transferrin by the liver can lead to artificially high levels of transferrin saturation even in the context of iron deficiency. Therefore, it may be necessary to treat anemia on grounds of clinical suspicion following appropriate assessment and appraise the response to iron supplementation.

Commonly, patients with chronic liver disease due to alcohol misuse display abnormalities of folate metabolism due to decreased levels of absorption from the small intestine. Similarly, alcohol can interfere with the absorption of vitamin B_{12}, fat, nitrogen, sodium, water, thiamine, and D-xylose all of which contribute to the malnutrition observed in such patients.

Hemolysis and changes in red cell morphology and membrane

Hemolysis is a frequent complication of liver disease. Its presentation may be a life-threatening event such as that seen during an acute presentation of Wilson disease, or it may be related to the underlying disorder such as an autoimmune hemolysis complicating autoimmune liver disease. In many patients, a decreased red cell life span can be demonstrated, regardless of the etiology of the liver disease. The commonest site for the destruction of red cells is the spleen and hypersplenism accelerates this process, making the presence of hypersplenism a risk factor for hemolysis in its own right. In addition, chronic liver disease can cause changes in the phospholipid component of the red cell membrane, inducing changes in their shape, flexibility and osmotic fragility and therefore increasing the likelihood of destruction within the spleen.

Macrocytosis is the commonest abnormality of red cell morphology seen in patients with chronic liver disease. It is identified in up to 90% of patients with alcohol related liver disease, but is not specific for this diagnosis as it occurs in up to 70% of cirrhotic patients of any etiology. The etiology of this macrocytosis is unclear and is often multifactorial. Increases in the mean corpuscular volume (MCV) may be related to reticulocytosis consequent upon anemia, hemolysis and bleeding. It can also be due in part to abnormal (usually increased) cholesterol and phospholipids within the cell membrane or it may be contributed to by deficiency of vitamin B_{12} and folic acid seen in both alcoholic cirrhotics and malnourished cirrhotic patients independent of etiology.

Other abnormalities of red cell morphology that can be observed within the blood film of patients with chronic liver disease include the presence of target cells and echinocytes. Target cells result from increased levels of cholesterol and phospholipids within the cell membrane. This causes alteration of the surface area of the cells and thus the characteristic target appearance on microscopy. Echinocytes are 'spiky' red cells that may be seen in the blood film, although are best appreciated on electron microscopy. Their presence may be related to changes in high density lipoprotein (HDL) within the serum of patients with liver disease. The HDL fraction from affected individuals is able to turn normal red cells into echinocytes. The presence of echinocytes does not seem to carry any pathologic or prognostic significance, as opposed to the more severe red cell abnormality acanthocytosis. Acanthocytes are bizarrely shaped red cell forms that can be appreciated in the blood films of patents with severe advanced (usually) alcoholic liver disease. They can be associated with a hemolytic anemia, this combination being known as spur cell anemia. The presence of acanthocytes implies advanced liver disease and carries a worse prognosis. It has been proposed that the hemolysis arises from the destruction of acanthocytes by the spleen but this is unlikely given that acanthocytes are observed in abetalipoproteinemia, yet, hemolysis does not occur.

Hemolysis has also been described in the setting of alcoholic liver disease in association with jaundice and hypertriglyceridemia. This combination, termed Zieve syndrome, is differentiated from alcoholic hepatitis by the presence of hemolysis. Considerable debate has occurred as to the prevalence and incidence of the syndrome because the components of the syndrome are frequently observed independently in liver disease.

Thrombocytopenia and platelet function

Thrombocytopenia is very common and has been dealt with in the section above relating to coagulation disorders. Prolongation of bleeding time in patients with liver disease, despite adequate circulating platelet numbers, is suggestive of abnormal platelet function. Impaired aggregation to factors such as ADP and arachidonic acid can be demonstrated in patients with liver disease. Local factors related to the vessel wall such as increased production of NO are also important in disease pathogenesis.

Neutropenia and neutrophil dysfunction in liver disease

Patients with cirrhosis are often neutropenic and therefore have a high incidence and prevalence of bacterial infections. Apart from a reduction in absolute neutrophil numbers, abnormalities of neutrophil function have been described in patients with advanced liver disease. A number of investigators have demonstrated increased apoptosis of neutrophils. The exact cause for this is unknown, but patients with neutropenia secondary to chronic schistosomiasis have had reversal of this apoptosis by splenectomy. Neutrophils of patients with cirrhosis also display deficient phagocytosis. Although increased adhesion of neutrophils to endothelium has been demonstrated, there is reduced transendothelial migration of neutrophils. Deficiency of the tetrapeptide called tuftsin has been demonstrated in patients with advanced liver disease. Tuftsin is a necessary cofactor for efficient neutrophil function, and the addition of tuftsin to neutrophils from cirrhotic patients reversed the abnormalities in their function. Tuftsin is activated within the spleen, and it has been proposed that the impaired tuftsin activity seen in cirrhosis results from decreased splenic function.

HEPATOGENOUS DIABETES

The association between diabetes and hepatic cirrhosis was first observed in 1906 when the syndrome hepatogenous diabetes was coined. The prevalence of diabetes amongst cirrhotic patients is reported at between 10 and 70%, with the majority of the remainder displaying some degree of impaired glucose tolerance. The onset of diabetes following a diagnosis of cirrhosis appears to be rapid with up to 20% of patients displaying diabetes within 5 years of diagnosis. Interestingly, the presence of hepatogenous diabetes does not affect the short-term prognosis of patients with cirrhosis but does increase the risk of decompensation and therefore negatively impacts upon the long-term prognosis.

Despite similarities with non-insulin dependent diabetes mellitus (NIDDM), there are clear differences between hepatogenous diabetes and NIDDM. First, there is a family history of diabetes in only 20% of affected individuals and second, obesity has a less important role in pathogenesis. Finally, the incidence of both macro- and microvascular complications appears to occur at a significantly lower frequency than that seen in patients with NIDDM.

The pathogenesis of hepatogenous diabetes is complex and incompletely understood, but it is clear that both insulin resistance and hyperinsulinemia have an important role. Almost all cirrhotics that display insulin resistance have hyperinsulinemia and it is proposed that hyperinsulinemia is the first step in the development of hepatogenous diabetes. The cause of the hyperinsulinemia is unclear although decreased hepatic clearance of insulin and portosystemic shunting are thought to be important. Chronically elevated insulin levels in the serum, as occur in cirrhosis, cause inhibition of muscle glucose utilization primarily due to inhibition of glycogen formation. The molecular mechanism underpinning this effect is unknown, but the end point of this process is peripheral insulin resistance. The point at which this insulin resistance and impaired glucose tolerance develops into diabetes is determined by the capacity of the β cells of the pancreas to respond to the increased need of insulin. **Figure 13.3** summarizes the putative mechanisms in the development of hepatogenous diabetes.

The reversal of hepatogenous diabetes after liver transplantation supports its status as an acquired metabolic syndrome. Although liver transplantation is associated with a deterioration of glucose tolerance and a worsening of diabetes in the initial postoperative period, up to 67% of diabetic cirrhotic patients can be cured by transplantation. This improvement occurs irrespective of the etiology of the liver disease, immunosuppressive regimen, age and body mass index. For patients who continue to have ongoing diabetes post-transplant, a markedly low insulin response during oral glucose tolerance testing pretransplant predicts ongoing diabetes. This is consistent with the persistence of reduced β-cell function post-transplant and suggests that islet cell transplant may be useful for this patient group. Beyond transplantation, the treatment of hepatogenous diabetes mirrors that of NIDDM. Weight loss in the obese patient, regular exercise and compliance with a diabetic diet are cornerstones of management. Where oral hypoglycemic agents are needed, metformin should be avoided. Although the incidence of both macro- and microvascular complications in patients with hepatogenous diabetes is reported to be less than 10%, patients should be screened for retinopathy, renal disease and cardiovascular complications. Current data from natural history studies suggest that just over half of patients die within 10 years of the diagnosis of cirrhosis, mainly of complications of the cirrhosis and end-stage liver disease.

ACQUIRED HEPATOCEREBRAL DEGENERATION AND HEPATIC MYELOPATHY

Acquired (non-Wilsonian) hepatocerebral degeneration (AHCD) is a syndrome of brain dysfunction associated with a variety of liver diseases. Clinically and pathologically, the condition is similar to Wilson disease. Clinical features of this chronic syndrome are intention tremor, dysarthria, dementia, ataxia of gait, and choreoathetotic movements. The neuropathologic findings include patchy cortical laminar neuronal necrosis, diffuse proliferation of Alzheimer type II glial cells and neuronal dropout in the cerebral cortex, basal ganglia and cerebellum. Multiple bouts of hepatic coma appear to be the only risk factor to

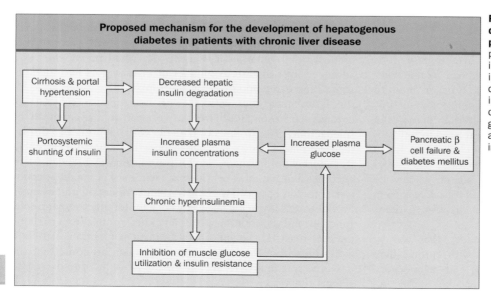

Proposed mechanism for the development of hepatogenous diabetes in patients with chronic liver disease

Figure 13.3 Proposed mechanism for the development of hepatogenous diabetes in patients with chronic liver disease. The presence of cirrhosis results in both decreased insulin breakdown and portosystemic shunting of insulin which results in increased levels of circulating insulin. Chronic insulinemia results in inhibition of glucose utilization within muscle and ongoing insulin resistance. Increased plasma glucose concentrations result in β cell failure and a vicious cycle of hyperinsulinemia and worsening insulin resistance.

trigger this condition, although Wilson disease must be considered. Liver transplantation has been reported as successfully treating this condition and reduction of lucencies noted within the basal ganglia on magnetic resonance imaging has also been described.

The second syndrome referred to by the term hepatic myelopathy or alternatively, post-shunt myelopathy, is characterized by the presence of progressive spastic paraplegia and hyperreflexia with preservation of normal sensation. Described in patients who have developed spontaneous portosystemic shunts and following surgical shunt creation, the cause of this syndrome is uncertain. Postmortem examinations have revealed demyelination of the lateral column of the spinal cord in some cases.

Although shunting of various toxins such as ammonia have been proposed as a cause of this entity, the majority of patients with significant shunting do not develop this syndrome. In addition, the syndrome of myelopathy has been described in patients without evidence of portosystemic shunts suggesting alternative etiologies. Moreover, conventional therapies directed at reducing intestinal uptake of potential toxins fail to improve symptoms. Spastic paraparesis following portosystemic shunting has been reversed by liver transplantation and current thinking suggests that the efficacy of transplant is optimal when spastic paraparesis has been present for less than 1 year, although an exact threshold has yet to be defined.

FURTHER READING

Metabolic bone disease

Ascott-Evans BH, Guanabens N, Kivinen S, et al. Alendronate prevents loss of bone density associated with discontinuation of hormone replacement therapy: a randomized controlled trial. Arch Intern Med 2003; 163:789–794. *Primary data demonstrating the effect of alendronate therapy in patients who stop hormone replacement therapy.*

Isoniemi H, Appelberg J, Nilsson CG, et al. Transdermal oestrogen therapy protects postmenopausal liver transplant women from osteoporosis. A 2-year follow-up study. J Hepatol 2001; 34:299–305.

Cirrhotic cardiomyopathy

Wong F, Girgrah N, Graba J, et al. The cardiac response to exercise in cirrhosis. Gut 2001; 49:268–275.

Hepatogenous diabetes

Holstein A, Hinze S, Thiessen E, et al. Clinical implications of hepatogenous diabetes in liver cirrhosis. J Gastroenterol Hepatol 2002; 17:677–681.

Perseghin G, Mazzaferro V, Sereni LP, et al. Contribution of reduced insulin sensitivity and secretion to the pathogenesis of hepatogenous diabetes: effect of liver transplantation. Hepatology 2000; 31:694–703. *Seminal report describing the effects of liver transplantation on insulin resistance.*

Hematology

Caldwell SH, Chang C, Macik BG. Recombinant activated Factor VII (rFVII) as a hemostatic agent in liver disease: a break from convention in need of controlled trials. Hepatology 2004; 39:592–598.

Hepatic myelopathy

Weissenborn K, Tietge UJ, Bokemeyer M, et al. Liver transplantation improves hepatic myelopathy: evidence by three cases. Gastroenterology 2003; 124:346–351. *Original report describing the features of hepatic myelopathy and its improvement with liver transplantation.*

Hepatopulmonary and portopulmonary syndrome

Krowka MJ, Mandell MS, Ramsay MA, et al. Hepatopulmonary syndrome and portopulmonary hypertension: a report of the multicenter liver transplant database. Liver Transpl 2004; 10:174–182. *A report from 10 centers on the outcome of hepatopulmonary syndrome, portopulmonary hypertension with and without liver transplantation.*

Schenk P, Schoniger-Hekele M, Fuhrmann V, et al. Prognostic significance of the hepatopulmonary syndrome in patients with cirrhosis. Gastroenterology 2003; 125:1042–1052. *Original data that demonstrates conclusively the effect of Child Pugh grade on prognosis in patients with hepatopulmonary syndrome.*

Recommended schedule for hepatitis A vaccines						
Vaccine	Age group (years)	HAV Ag dose	HBsAg dose (µg)	Volume	No. of doses	Schedule (Months)
Havrix[1]	2–18	720 EL U	N/A	0.5 mL	2	0, 6–12
	19 or older	1440 EL U	N/A	1.0 mL	2	0, 6 –12
Vaqta[2]	2–18	25 units	N/A	0.5 mL	2	0, 6–18
	19 or older	50 units	N/A	1.0 mL	2	0, 6–12
Twinrix[3]	1–15	360 EL U	10	0.5 mL	3	0, 1, 6
	16 or older	720 EL U	20	1.0 mL	3	0, 1, 6

HAV Ag, hepatitis A virus antigen; HBsAg, hepatitis B surface antigen
EL U=enzyme-linked immunosorbent assay (ELISA) units
[1]Hepatitis A vaccine, inactivated, GlaxoSmithKline
[2]Hepatitis A vaccine, inactivated, Merck & Co., Inc.
[3]Combined hepatitis A and hepatitis B vaccine, GlaxoSmithKline
Modified from Lemon in Schiff et al by permission of Lippincott, Williams & Wilkins

Table 14.1 Recommended schedule for hepatitis A vaccines

two-dose schedule. Indications for vaccination include: travelers who are 2 years of age or older to areas of intermediate or high prevalence of HAV infection, men who have sex with men, users of illicit drugs, persons with chronic liver disease of any etiology, recipients of liver transplants and laboratory personnel who work with HAV. Protective levels of specific humoral antibodies are detectable in 80–98% of adult recipients 15 days after the first dose and in 96% after 1 month. Estimates of antibody persistence derived from kinetic models of antibody decline indicate that protective levels of anti-HAV could be present for ≥ 20 years. On the other hand, in some studies, administration of hepatitis A vaccine to persons with HIV infection resulted in lower seroprotection rates and antibody concentrations, and this phenomenon may be directly related to the degree of CD4+ cell depletion. The most frequently reported side-effects occurring within 3 days after the 1440 EL U dose were pain at the injection site, headache and malaise. Reviews of data from multiple sources for >5 years regarding adverse events did not identify any serious side-effects among children or adults that could be definitively attributed to hepatitis A vaccine.

A combined hepatitis A and B vaccine (Twinrix®) has been released for use in persons aged >18 years in the USA and elsewhere. Twinrix is manufactured and distributed by GlaxoSmithKline Biologicals (Rixensart, Belgium) and is made of the antigenic components used in Havrix and Engerix-B (GlaxoSmithKline). The antigenic components in Twinrix have been used routinely in separate single antigen vaccines in the USA since 1995 and 1989 as hepatitis A and B vaccines, respectively. The efficacy of Twinrix is expected to be comparable with existing single antigen hepatitis vaccines. The persistence of anti-HAV and anti-HBV following Twinrix administration is similar to that following single antigen hepatitis A and B vaccine administration at 4-year follow-up (GlaxoSmithKline Biologicals, unpublished data, 2001).

HEPATITIS E

Introduction

Hepatitis E is an enterically transmitted form of viral hepatitis that appears to be common in tropical and subtropical areas and epidemics have been reported in Asia, Africa, the Middle East and Central America. An extensive outbreak of water-borne hepatitis was reported in India in 1955. In further retrospective analysis 25 years later, all stored serum samples were found to have IgG anti-HAV but not IgM anti-HAV, evidence against the assumption that the etiologic agent responsible for this outbreak was HAV. This was the first of many documented outbreaks of water-borne non-A, non-B hepatitis. Subsequently, similar outbreaks were reported especially associated with a high fatality rate among pregnant women in South East Asia. In 1990 the genome of the virus was cloned and named hepatitis E virus (HEV), which allowed the development of specific diagnostic tests and expanded the knowledge about this agent. It is a distinct agent which has been associated with fulminant hepatic failure among pregnant women, but, similarly to hepatitis A, has no known chronic sequelae. HEV has not yet been classified taxonomically. Immunoelectron microscopy permitted the identification of HEV particles measuring around 32 nm, spheric shaped, non-enveloped and very similar to those of the *Caliciviridae* family. The virus exhibits spikes and indentations in the particle surface, that give it a feathery aspect. It is disintegrated by exposure to cesium chloride and storage at –20ºC. The genome of HEV consists of 7.5 kb and has three separate, partially overlapping ORFs which encode structural and nonstructural proteins (**Fig. 14.4**). Eight different genotypes of HEV have been identified to date: Burma (type 1), Mexican (type 2), North American (type 3), Chinese (type 4), European (types 5, 6 and 7), and the recently discovered Argentinean type (type 8). The existence of many more genotypes is a possibility, as suggested by Austrian investigators who recently isolated the

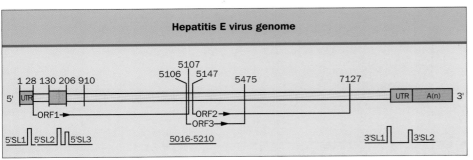

Figure 14.4 Hepatitis E virus genome. ORF, open reading frame. Reproduced from Surgit et al by permission of The American Society for Microbiology Journals Department.

variant HEV-Au1. Despite differences in genotypes, there is only one serotype explaining cross-reactivity for the main viral epitopes, allowing serologic diagnosis with commercially available kits.

Epidemiology and pathogenesis

Epidemics of HEV infection have been described throughout Asia, large parts of northeastern and eastern Africa and Mexico (**Fig. 14.5**). Hepatitis E is implicated in about 50% of sporadic cases of acute viral hepatitis in developing countries. North America and Europe have been considered non-endemic for HEV, although seroprevalence ranges from 1 to 5%. In the last few years some HEV strains associated with sporadic acute hepatitis have been isolated from human serum samples in North America. Spanish investigators analyzed the excreted virus in the urban sewage of Barcelona (Spain) and other countries like USA (Washington DC area), Greece, France and Sweden. Around 84% of sewage samples from Barcelona tested positive for HEV RNA. One of five samples from Washington DC and one of four samples tested from France were positive. HEV RNA was not detected in any of the samples from Greece or Sweden. These data suggest that HEV strains are more widespread than previously thought and endemic HEV infections are likely to be present in Europe and the USA. Recently, seroprevalence studies have demonstrated the endemic nature of HEV in some regions of South America. HEV attacks mostly young adults and is rarely seen in children <15 years of age, in contrast to HAV infection, which is a rare event in adults due to the longstanding immunity against the virus acquired in childhood (see section on hepatitis A in this chapter). In Egypt, the seroprevalence of anti-HEV exceeds 60% in the first decade of life, peaks at 76% in the second decade and remains above 60% until the eighth decade. This is the highest prevalence reported in the world for HEV. Seroconversion to anti-HEV was documented in 4 of 211 travelers from the USA to Thailand, Russia, China and Peru. None of the individuals reported any symptoms of hepatitis before, during or after travel, implying that exposure to HEV resulted in subclinical infections.

It has been proposed that animal reservoirs of HEV may exist in some regions and that human infections may represent a zoonosis. HEV has been isolated in 22% of pooled stool samples from 115 swine farms in the Netherlands. It was found that 90% of wild rats from Hawaii, 77% from Maryland and 44% from Louisiana were seropositive for HEV. In Vietnam, where hepatitis E is endemic, anti-HEV has been detected in 44% of chickens, 36% of pigs, 27% of dogs and 9% of rats. Swine veterinarians in eight different states of the USA were 1.5 times more likely to be anti-HEV positive than healthy volunteer blood donors.

Person-to-person transmission is a potential route of infection, as suggested by the epidemiologic pattern seen in the Mexican outbreak. Pregnant women in the third trimester are at very high risk of developing fulminant hepatitis and this is probably the most prominent epidemiologic feature of this disease. Possible parenteral transmission of HEV can occur as suggested by a report of a hospital outbreak of hepatitis E.

HEV replicates in the liver and is excreted in the feces via the biliary tract. This has been extensively studied in non-human primates, after inoculation with fecal samples obtained from patients with established HEV infection. Pathologic changes in the liver during acute HEV infection can vary from canalicular cholestasis to ballooning degeneration of the hepatocytes and acute portal inflammatory infiltrates. HEV particles appear in

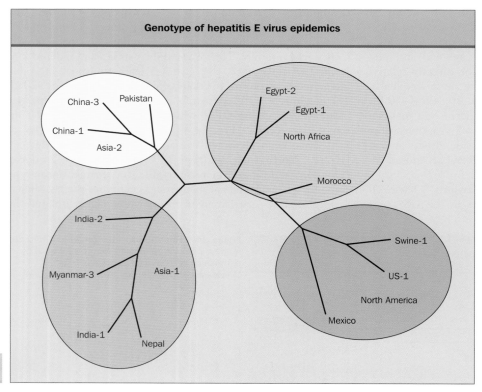

Genotype of hepatitis E virus epidemics

Figure 14.5 Genotype of hepatitis E virus epidemics. Reproduced from Jameel, Shabid. Molecular biology and pathogenesis of hepatitis E virus. Expert Reviews in Molecular Medicine, 1999. By permission of Cambridge University Press.

feces during prodromal symptoms of hepatitis E, which can be associated with a viremic phase. Several weeks after exposure, HEV antigen appears in blood and antibody responses start to develop approximately 1 month later, coincident with the ALT peak. The first antibody to be detected is IgM, which declines during the convalescent phase. Simultaneously IgG anti-HEV appears and reaches peak levels later, although the duration of detectable antibody is unknown. The pathogenesis of hepatitis E may be a combination of direct cytotoxicity and immunologic mechanisms.

Clinical manifestations

The incubation period of hepatitis E is approximately 40 days (2–8 weeks). It is a self-limited disease and cannot be distinguished from other forms of viral hepatitis based on clinical features alone. However, it should be suspected in any person with acute hepatitis with a history of recent travel to underdeveloped areas and negative serologies for hepatitis A, B and C.

Anicteric forms of hepatitis E are very frequent, making the diagnosis in acute phase very puzzling. Fever, arthralgias, general malaise and nausea are common prodromal manifestations. Jaundice and dark urine start shortly after as it occurs in hepatitis A. Anorexia, abdominal discomfort, diarrhea, pale stools, arthralgia, pruritus, rash, hepatomegaly and splenomegaly are described. These symptoms resolve within 6 weeks in most patients. There have been no case reports of chronic hepatitis E infection to date. Severe disease typically occurs in pregnant women during the third trimester with a mortality rate of about 20%. All nine pregnant women in an outbreak in Algeria died of fulminant hepatic failure. This predilection for fulminant forms in pregnant women is not seen in other forms of viral hepatitis, and there is no clear pathophysiologic explanation for this catastrophic occurrence. Sera from 22 patients with fulminant hepatitis in Bangladesh showed anti-HEV IgM in 63.6%, HEV being the most common cause of fulminant viral hepatitis in that series.

Asymptomatic or subclinical infection may occur but the magnitude of this is not known due to the lack of epidemiologic and serologic studies.

Diagnosis

The serologic diagnosis of infection with HEV is made by the determination of the anti-HEV antibodies (IgG and IgM) (**Fig. 14.6**). IgM anti-HEV has been identified in most patients and as early as 4 days after the onset of symptoms of the infection. IgM anti-HEV peak titers are coincidental with the serum aminotransferase elevation, and it is usually undetectable within 6 months after the onset of the infection. Essentially IgM anti-HEV is analogous to IgM anti-HAV, and is a reliable marker of recent infection. IgG is a serologic marker of convalescent phase or past exposure to the virus. The serum aminotransferases and serum bilirubin tend to normalize over a 1–6-week period. Due to the possibility of a false-positive reaction, anti-HEV could be confirmed by immunoblot assays. There is controversy regarding the existence of prolonged immunity in cases of infection with HEV. There is some evidence that anti-HEV titers decrease progressively raising the possibility of infection post re-exposure. However, some other authors have documented prolonged immune reaction post acute infection, suggesting the role of immunologic memory. The polymerase chain reaction (PCR) technique has been used to detect HEV in stools, serum and liver of acutely infected patients, but it is still considered experimental. In 1995 HEV infection was identified in a group of United Nations Bangladeshi peace keepers in Haiti by direct fecal HEV RNA determination, allowing infection control within the group and avoiding dissemination of the disease.

Treatment and prognosis

There is no specific treatment for acute hepatitis E, and the above-mentioned general support measures for hepatitis A apply (see section on treatment for hepatitis A). In acute,

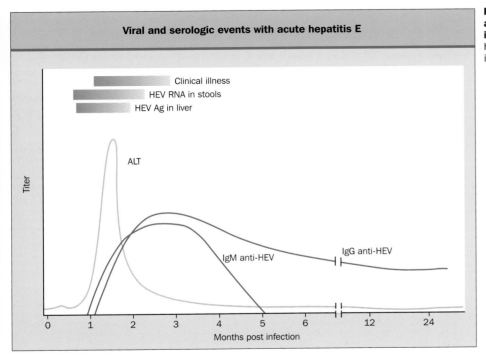

Viral and serologic events with acute hepatitis E

Clinical illness
HEV RNA in stools
HEV Ag in liver

ALT

IgM anti-HEV

IgG anti-HEV

Titer

Months post infection

0 1 2 3 4 5 6 12 24

Figure 14.6 Viral and serologic events associated with acute hepatitis E virus infection. ALT, alanine aminotransferase; HAV, hepatitis A virus; IgG, immunoglobulin G; IgM, immunoglobulin M.

uncomplicated hepatitis E complete recovery is the rule. The case fatality rate is around 0.5–4.0% and is higher than for hepatitis A. Pregnant women are considered to have the highest mortality, especially during the second and third trimesters. The reported mortality rates range from 20 to 25% in India. No convincing explanation for the pregnancy-related morbidity has been proposed.

A study performed in India among over 400 patients with fulminant hepatitis, where 38% were infected with HEV, revealed that age >40 years, prolongation of prothrombin time >25 s and total bilirubin >15 mg/dL were associated with a poor outcome. Not surprisingly, pregnant women were found to be more prone to develop acute liver failure.

Prevention

Improvement in the general hygiene conditions and access to clean drinkable water are ideal measures to prevent hepatitis E.

Consumption of raw fish, shellfish and other seafood products should be avoided especially in areas with poor sanitary conditions. The use of immunoglobulins extracted from individuals of endemic areas seems to have some role in attenuating the severity of infection in exposed persons. However, these are only preliminary experimental data and there is no commercially available immunoglobulin preparation. A vaccine for hepatitis E is in the early stages of development and, based on animal studies, looks promising. Purdy et al (1993) immunized two cynomolgus macaques with trpE-C2 protein that represents the carboxy-two-thirds of the HEV capsid protein. After challenge with wild-type HEV from stool isolates, neither of the vaccinated animals developed elevation in the ALT levels, in contrast to the control macaques. The preliminary findings of this animal study are encouraging and there is ongoing research directed towards the development of an effective vaccine against HEV infection in humans.

FURTHER READING

Hepatitis A

Alter MJ, Mast EE. The epidemiology of viral hepatitis in the United States. Gastroenterol Clin N Am 1994; 23:437–455. *A very detailed and comprehensive analysis on the outbreaks and epidemiologic behavior of the different viral hepatitides in the United States, showing changes in patterns over the years.*

Bell BP, Shapiro CN, Alter MJ, et al. The diverse patterns of hepatitis A epidemiology in the United States. Implications for vaccination strategies. J Infect Dis 1998; 178:1579–1584.

Center for Disease Control. Notice to readers: FDA approval for a combined hepatitis A and B vaccine. MMWR 2001; 50:806–807.

Center for Disease Control. Prevention of hepatitis A through active or passive immunization: Recommendations of the Advisory Committee on Immunization Practices (ACIP). MMWR 1999; 48:1–37.

Center for Disease Control. Licensure of inactivated hepatitis A vaccine and recommendations for use among international travelers. MMWR 1995; 44:559.

Center for Disease Control. Foodborne transmission of hepatitis A – Massachusetts 2001. MMWR Morb Mortal Wkly Rep 2003; 52:565–567.

Costa-Mattioli M, Di Napoli A, Ferre V, et al. Genetic variability of hepatitis A virus. J Gen Virol 2003; 84:3191–3201.

Craig AS, Schaffner W. Prevention of hepatitis A with the hepatitis A vaccine. N Engl J Med 2004; 350:476–481.

Dan M, Yaniv R. Cholestatic hepatitis, cutaneous vasculitis, and vascular deposits of immunoglobulin M and complement associated with hepatitis A virus infection. Am J Med 1990; 89:103–104.

Gordon SC, Reddy KR, Schiff L, et al. Prolonged intrahepatic cholestasis secondary to acute hepatitis A. Ann Int Med 1984; 101:635–637. *Case reports illustrating an atypical (though not rare) clinical course of acute hepatitis A.*

Katz MH, Hsu L, Wong E, et al. Seroprevalence of and risk factors for hepatitis A infection among young homosexual and bisexual men. J Infect Dis 1997; 175:1225–1229.

Koziel MJ: Immunology of viral hepatitis. Am J Med 1996; 100:98–109.

Hepatitis E

Bradley DW. Hepatitis E virus: a brief review of the biology, molecular virology, and immunology of a novel virus. J Hepatol 1995; 22:140–145.

This article reviews the main virologic and immunologic features of this relatively recently discovered hepatitis virus.

Clemente-Casares P, Pina S, Buti M, et al. Hepatitis E virus epidemiology in industrializad countries. Emerg Infect Dis 2003; 9:448–454.

Drabick JJ, Gambel JM, Gouvea VS, et al. A cluster of acute hepatitis E infection in United Nations Bangladeshi peace keepers in Haiti. Am J Trop Med Hyg 1997; 57:449–454.

Favorov MO, Fields HA, Purdy MA, et al. Serologic identification of hepatitis E virus infections in epidemic and endemic settings. J Med Virol 1992; 36:246–250. *This study helped to establish the serologic course of acute and convalescent titers of anti-HEV IgM and IgG.*

Fix AD, Abdel-Hamid M, Purcell RH, et al. Prevalence of antibodies to hepatitis E in two rural Egyptian communities. Am J Trop Med Hyg 2000; 62:519–523.

Jameel S. Molecular and pathogenesis of hepatitis E virus. Exp Rev Mol Med 1999. Online. Available: http://www-erm.cbcu.cam.ac.uk/99001271h.htm. 6 Dec 1999.

Kabrane-Lazizi Y, Fine JB, Elm J, et al. Evidence for widespread infection of wild rats with hepatitis E virus in the United States. Am J Trop Med Hyg 1999; 61:331–335. *Wild rats (from urban and rural areas in the U.S.) are an important reservoir for HEV infection, another piece of evidence suggesting HEV can be a zoonotic disease.*

Meng J, Pillot J, Dai X, et al. Neutralization of different geographic strains of the hepatitis E virus with anti-hepatitis E virus positive serum samples obtained from different sources. Virology 1998; 249:316–324.

Meng XJ, Wiseman B, Elvinger F, et al. Prevalence of antibodies to hepatitis E virus in veterinarians working with swine and in normal blood donors in the United States and other countries. J Clin Microbiol 2002; 40:117–122.

Ooi WW, Gawoski JM, Yarbough PO, et al. Hepatitis E seroconversion in United States travelers abroad. Am J Trop Med Hyg 1999; 61:822–824.

Purdy MA, McCaustland KA, Krawczynski K, et al: Preliminary evidence that a trpE-HEV fusion protein protects cynomolgus macaques against challenge with wild-type hepatitis E virus (HEV). J Med Virol 1993; 41:90–94.

Surgit M, Jameel S, Lal SKI. The ORF2 protein of hepatitis E virus binds the 5' region of viral RNA. J Virol 2004; 78:320–328.

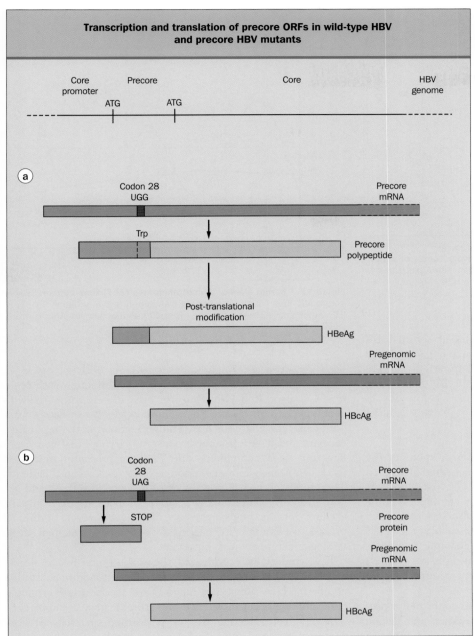

Transcription and translation of precore ORFs in wild-type HBV and precore HBV mutants

Figure 15.5 Transcription and translation of precore and core open reading frames in wild-type hepatitis B virus (HBV) and precore HBV mutants. (a) Transcription of precore and core regions of wild-type HBV produces the precore polypeptide which undergoes post-translational modification to hepatitis B e antigen (HBeAg). (b) Precore mutant with premature stop codon at codon 28 prevents the production of HBeAg, but the translation of pregenomic RNA is not affected.

restricted to specific HBV genotypes. Other mutations that can decrease HBeAg production include changes in the core promoter region, most commonly A–T and G–A changes at nucleotides 1762 and 1764, respectively, which downregulates transcription of the precore messenger RNA.

Serum HBV DNA assays

Sensitive quantitative assays for HBV DNA in serum have been developed to assess the level of HBV replication. The branched DNA (bDNA) assay can detect HBV DNA levels down to 2000 copies/mL. Polymerase chain reaction (PCR) assays are even more sensitive with detection limits of 50 copies/mL. In patients with acute hepatitis B, serum HBV DNA appears early and may precede the detection of HBsAg. In patients with HBeAg-positive chronic hepatitis, serum HBV DNA levels are usually much higher than 100 000 copies/mL (median level is 10^9, ranging from 10^6 to 10^{11}) (**Fig. 15.6**). In patients with HBeAg-negative chronic hepatitis B, serum HBV DNA levels are usually lower (median level is 10^7, ranging from 10^4 to 10^8) and fluctuating with the possibility of periods with very low levels (below 10^4). In inactive HBsAg carriers, serum HBV DNA levels are typically low (median 10^3, ranging from undetectable to 10^5). Therefore, it is important to perform serial measurements of serum HBV DNA and ALT levels in order to distinguish true inactive HBsAg carriers from patients with fluctuating HBeAg-negative chronic hepatitis B (**Fig. 15.7**).

Measurement of the serum HBV DNA level is necessary for the diagnosis [in case of chronic hepatitis with increased ALT levels and persistently low levels of HBV DNA (less than 10^4 copies/mL), another cause must be looked for]; for the

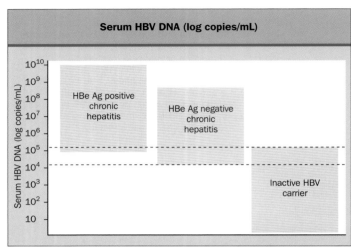

Figure 15.6 Serum hepatitis B virus (HBV) DNA levels. Range of serum HBV DNA levels in patients with hepatitis B e antigen (HBeAg)-positive and HBeAg-negative chronic hepatitis B and inactive HBV carriers.

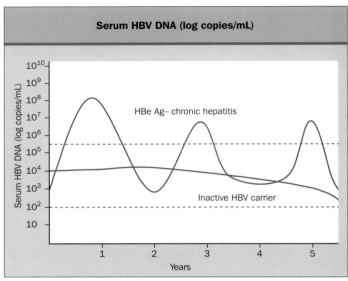

Figure 15.7 Serum alanine aminotransferase (ALT) time course. Typical serum ALT time course in a patient with hepatitis B e antigen (HBeAg)-negative chronic hepatitis B and in an inactive hepatitis B virus (HBV) carrier.

indication for therapy (treatment is indicated if serum HBV DNA level is higher than 10^4 in HBeAg chronic hepatitis B and higher than 10^5 in HBeAg-positive chronic hepatitis B); and to assess response to antiviral therapy (serum HBV DNA level below 10^4 in HBeAg chronic hepatitis B and below 10^5 in HBeAg-positive chronic hepatitis B).

HBV genotypes

Based upon an intergroup divergence of 8% or more in the complete nucleotide sequence, HBV can be classified into seven unique HBV genotypes, designated A to G. The first reports of classification of HBV genotypes were based on complete genome sequences. However, HBV genotypes can also be determined from a partial sequence of the entire genome such as the pre-S or S gene without determining the entire genomic sequence. Currently, restriction fragment length polymorphisms (RFLP) and the line probe assay (LiPA) are the most commonly used genotyping methods.

Data from multinational clinical trials have confirmed a preponderance of HBV genotypes B and C in Asian and Pacific Islander patients, while genotypes A and D are more common in patients from Western European countries. HBV genotypes B and C are most prevalent in highly endemic areas where vertical transmission is the primary means of transmission. In contrast, HBV genotypes A, D, E, F and G are found in areas where horizontal or sexual transmission of HBV is more common. Data from adefovir clinical trials also demonstrate marked differences in HBV genotypes and subject race with 93% of Asians having genotype B or C and 93% of white patients having either genotype A or D.

All of the cross-sectional studies from endemic areas in Asia demonstrate that genotype C is associated with more advanced liver disease than genotype B. Consistently higher levels of serum HBV DNA and aminotransferase levels have been reported as well as more advanced histology and a greater likelihood of cirrhosis. The prevalence of detectable HBeAg is also higher in patients with genotype C than B. In addition, spontaneous HBeAg seroconversion occurred nearly 10 years earlier in patients

with genotype B compared with patients with genotype C. Taken together, these findings suggest that infection with genotype C is associated with more aggressive disease compared with genotype B. The reasons for a more aggressive disease course with genotype C are unclear. Studies comparing the replicative capacity and host immune response to varying HBV genotypes have not been completed. The TA core promoter mutations were significantly more common in genotype C than B patients. Therefore, the higher prevalence of detectable HBeAg and TA core promoter mutations in genotype C patients may, in part, account for the more aggressive disease. However, additional prospective studies are needed to determine which of these virologic factors is most important.

Few studies have evaluated the role of non-B and non-C genotypes on the outcome of infection. Clearly, additional studies comparing HBV genotypes A and D are needed to determine if clinically significant differences in natural history are apparent.

Several retrospective studies performed on trials of conventional or pegylated interferon (peginterferon) showed that the rate of HBeAg seroconversion was higher among patients with genotype A and B than in those with genotype C or D. These data suggest that HBV genotype may be an important predictor of response to interferon, but larger studies are needed in different geographic regions of the world and particularly in patients with HBeAg-negative chronic hepatitis B. In HBeAg-positive chronic HBV patients treated with lamivudine, no significant difference in HBeAg seroconversion was seen in patients with HBV genotype B or C. Finally, a recent study of 694 chronic HBV patients treated with adefovir dipivoxil showed no difference in viral load reduction or HBeAg seroconversion after 48 weeks of treatment among patients with genotype A to G.

Liver histology

Liver biopsy is seldom indicated in acute hepatitis B. Histologic changes include lobular disarray, acidophilic degeneration of

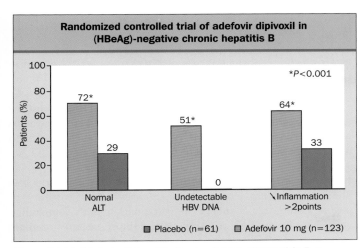

Figure 15.14 Adefovir dipivoxil in the treatment of hepatitis B e antigen (HBeAg)-negative chronic hepatitis B. In this randomized controlled trial, at 48 weeks of therapy, the rates of normal alanine aminotransferase, undetectable hepatitis B virus DNA and histologic improvement were higher in the group of patients receiving adefovir, at the dose of 10 mg daily, as compared with the group receiving a placebo. ALT, alanine aminotransferase. Data from Hadziyannis et al (03).

liver transplantation (128 and 196 patients, respectively) with lamivudine-resistant HBV received adefovir dipivoxil for varying lengths of time up to a maximum of 72 weeks (pre-liver transplantation) and 129 weeks (post-liver transplantation), respectively. Serum HBV DNA was reduced by approximately 4 $\log_{10}$ copies/mL in both groups, and ALT level normalized in 76% and 49% of patients in the two groups, respectively. Patients also had significant improvement of liver function. Kaplan-Meier survival curves estimates by week 48 were 84% and 93% in the pre- and post-transplantation groups, respectively. These 1-year survival rates are significantly better than survival rates observed in historical groups of patients with no treatment. Noteworthy, in a significant number of patients who improved, the liver transplantation was postponed.

Although many of the patients, all of whom had lamivudine-resistant HBV, were medically compromised as a result of advanced liver disease and co-morbidities, there was a low rate of adverse events leading to drug discontinuation in pre- and post-liver transplantation patients (5% and 6%, respectively). A total of 42 deaths (11%) were reported in pre- and post-transplantation patients (24 and 18 patients, respectively). The deaths were considered to be due to complications of progressive liver disease or liver transplantation surgery. There may be some concern about the long-term administration of adefovir in these patients with common concomitant renal dysfunction and therefore dose reduction, according to the package insert, based on creatinine clearance is advised.

In an open-label pilot study conducted in 35 HIV–HBV co-infected patients with lamivudine-resistant HBV and controlled HIV infection, adefovir therapy, at the dose of 10 mg, induced a 4 log decrease in serum HBV DNA levels at 48 weeks. Two patients underwent HBe seroconversion. A transient increase in serum ALT levels was observed in 15 patients without consequence on liver function. The explanation for this observation is unclear. No HBV DNA breakthrough and no viral resistance

were observed through week 48. In addition no significant changes in either HIV RNA or CD4 cell count were observed.

New agents
Entecavir
Entecavir, a cyclopentyl guanosine analog, is a potent inhibitor of HBV DNA polymerase, inhibiting both the priming and elongation steps of viral DNA replication. Entecavir is phosphorylated to its triphosphate, the active compound, by cellular kinases. It is a selective inhibitor of HBV DNA and is less effective against lamivudine-resistant mutants than against wild-type HBV.

Two large randomized controlled trials showed that entecavir is effective in patients with HBeAg-positive or -negative chronic hepatitis B. In HBeAg-positive chronic hepatitis B, entecavir induced a marked decrease in HBV DNA levels (7 logs) with undetectable HBV DNA in 91% of patients and histologic improvement in 72%. In HBeAg-negative chronic hepatitis B, entecavir induced also a marked decrease in HBV DNA levels (5 logs) with undetectable HBV DNA in 91% of patients and histologic improvement in 70%. These results were significantly better than those observed in the lamivudine control arms. Interestingly, no resistance was observed at 1 year of therapy in the 432 nucleoside naive patients; however, resistance (mutations rt184, rt202 and rt250) was observed in 5.8% of the patients who had received previous treatment with lamivudine. These results indicate that entecavir is a potent antiviral against HBV.

Emtricitabine
Emtricitabine (FTC) is a cytosine nucleoside analog with antiviral activity against both HBV and HIV. It is structurally similar to lamivudine: it only differs from by a fluorine at the 5-position of the nucleic acid.

A randomized controlled trial of emtricitabine at the dose of 200 mg versus placebo showed undetectable HBV DNA in 56% of the patients treated and histologic improvement in 62%. However, the rate of HBe seroconversion was low (12%) and no different from that observed in the placebo group. In addition, a relatively high rate of resistance (12.6%) (same YMDD mutations as those associated with lamivudine) was observed. Therefore, the role of emtricitabine as a monotherapy may be limited by its structural similarity to lamivudine with the risk of development of drug resistance. Emtricitabine is available in a combination pill with tenoforin.

Telbivudine
The natural nucleosides in the β-L-configuration [β-L-thymidine (LdT), β-L-2-deoxycytidine (L-dC) and β-L-2-deoxyadenosine (L-dA)] represent a newly discovered class of compounds with potent, *selective and specific activity against* hepadnavirus. 'In vitro' studies have shown that these compounds have marked effects on HBV replication. Telbivudine (LdT) is at the most developed stage of clinical investigation.

A phase II study including 104 HBeAg-positive patients showed that telbivudine administered at the dose of 600 mg daily, for 1 year induced a mean HBV DNA reduction of 6 logs with undetectable HBV DNA by PCR in 61% and HBeAg loss in 33%. YMDD HBV mutants were found in 4.4% of the patients. The safety profile of telbivudine appeared similar to placebo. Thus, this study confirms the marked antiviral effect of

227

telbivudine with a safe profile with however a non-negligible 1-year resistance rate (4.4%). On the basis of these data, phase III studies have been initiated.

Another promising β-L-nucleoside compound is val-LdC (valtorcitabine). It is in phase II testing and preliminary results indicate interesting antiviral activity with a good safety profile. A combination of these two compounds which act at different levels of HBV replication could be of interest.

Clevudine

Clevudine (1-2-fluoro-5-methyl-β-L-arabinosyl uracil, L-FMAU) is a pyrimidine analog with marked 'in vitro' activity against HBV but not HIV. The active triphosphate inhibits HBV DNA polymerase but is not an obligate chain terminator.

Phase II studies showed that clevudine at the dose of 100 mg administered for 4 weeks induced a rapid decrease of HBV DNA (3.5 logs) with interestingly a lasting effect with a slow reincrease of HBV DNA after withdrawal of treatment without rebound. Further studies are in progress to assess the long-term efficacy and safety of this drug.

Combinations

Combination of pegylated interferon with lamivudine

Previous studies on the combination of interferon and lamivudine suggested that this combination could be more effective than lamivudine monotherapy. However, the results of different studies were discordant which could be due to different treatment regimens which could not be optimal.

HBeAg-positive chronic hepatitis In a large randomized controlled study, 307 patients with HBeAg-positive chronic hepatitis B were randomized to receive either the combination of peginterferon α2b 100 μg per week for 32 weeks then 50 μg for 20 weeks and lamivudine 100 mg per day or peginterferon α2b at the same dose with placebo. At the end of the 26-week post-treatment follow-up, there was no difference in response rates between the two treatment groups: serum HBV DNA was undetectable by PCR (below 400 copies/mL) in 7% and 9%; HBeAg loss was observed in 36% and 35%; normal ALT was obtained in 32% and 35% in the peginterferon monotherapy and the peginterferon with lamivudine combination therapy groups, respectively. Interestingly, a relatively high rate of HBsAg loss was observed (7% in both groups).

Main predictors of response were HBV genotype and pre-treatment ALT level. Response was 34% for those with ALT levels under three times the upper limit of normal and 50% for those with ALT levels above five times the upper limit of normal. Response was 60% for genotype A versus 42% for genotype B, 32% for genotype C and 28% for genotype D.

Another large randomized controlled trial compared the efficacy of the combination of peginterferon α2a with or without lamivudine versus lamivudine alone. Patients were randomized to one of the following treatments: peginterferon α2a, 180 μg once weekly plus oral placebo once daily for 48 weeks; peginterferon α2a, 180 μg once weekly plus lamivudine 100 mg once daily for 48 weeks; lamivudine 100 mg once daily for 48 weeks. At the end of the 24-week post-treatment follow-up, the two peginterferon treatment arms (with or without lamivudine) showed the same efficacy which was superior to that observed in the lamivudine treatment arm: a virologic response (serum

HBV DNA below 100 000 copies/mL by quantitative PCR) in 32%, 34% and 22% of the patients, respectively. HBeAg seroconversion was observed in 32%, 27% and 19%, respectively. Interestingly, a substantial rate of HBsAg loss was observed in this study in patients who received peginterferon α2a (3% and 4% versus <1% in the lamivudine group).

These studies show that in patients with HBeAg-positive chronic hepatitis B, 6 months after therapy, the combination of peginterferon with lamivudine (with the simultaneous regimen used) is not superior to peginterferon used in monotherapy.

HBeAg-negative chronic hepatitis A phase III, partially double-blinded study has evaluated the efficacy and the safety of peginterferon α2a alone or in combination with lamivudine versus lamivudine in patients with HBeAg-negative chronic hepatitis B.

Patients were randomized to one of the following treatments: peginterferon α2a, 180 μg once weekly plus oral placebo once daily for 48 weeks; peginterferon α2a, 180 μg once weekly plus lamivudine 100 mg once daily for 48 weeks; lamivudine 100 mg once daily for 48 weeks. In total, 552 patients were enrolled in the study. At the end of the 24-week post treatment follow-up, the two peginterferon treatment arms (with or without lamivudine) showed the same efficacy which was superior to that observed in the lamivudine treatment arm: a biochemical response (normal ALT) was observed in 59%, 60% and 44% of the patients, respectively and a virologic response (serum HBV DNA below 20 000 copies/mL by quantitative PCR) in 43%, 44% and 29% of the patients, respectively (**Fig. 15.15**). Interestingly, taking into account that HBsAg loss is rarely

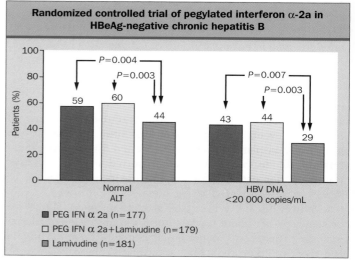

Figure 15.15 Pegylated (PEG)-interferon α2a in patients with hepatitis B e antigen (HBeAg)-negative chronic hepatitis B. In this randomized controlled trial, 24 weeks after therapy, the rates of response (normal alanine aminotransferase level and serum hepatitis B virus DNA below 20 000 copies/mL) were higher in the two groups which received peginterferon α2a (with or without lamivudine) as compared with the group which received lamivudine. There was no difference in response rates between the group which received peginterferon α2a alone and the group which received the peginterferon α2a plus lamivudine combination. ALT, alanine aminotransferase. Reproduced from Marcellin et al by permission of the Massachusetts Medical Society.

observed in HBeAg-negative patients, a substantial rate of HBsAg loss was observed in this study in patients who received peginterferon α2a (4% and 3% versus 0% in the lamivudine group).

Of note, at the end of the 48-week treatment period, there was a higher incidence of lamivudine resistance in the lamivudine monotherapy group when compared with the peginterferon α2a plus lamivudine combination group, which confirms previous studies suggesting that interferon decreases the risk of lamivudine resistance.

The adverse events associated with peginterferon α2a therapy were similar to those observed in previous trials in patients with chronic hepatitis C. Interestingly, the frequency of the adverse events was lower than that observed in patients with chronic hepatitis C. In particular, the frequency of depression was much lower: 3–4% as compared with 16–20% in patients with chronic hepatitis C.

This study shows that in patients with HBeAg-negative chronic hepatitis B, first, the efficacy, as assessed at 24 weeks post-treatment, of peginterferon α2a monotherapy is superior to lamivudine monotherapy and, second, the combination of peginterferon α2a with lamivudine (with the simultaneous regimen used) is not superior to peginterferon α2a used in monotherapy. However, longer follow-up is needed to confirm this conclusion and to assess the rate of possible late reactivations which are common after treatment in this population of patients.

Combination of adefovir with lamivudine

The concept of improving the efficacy by combining two analogs is based on the hypothesis that the combination would maximize the viral suppression and would decrease the occurrence of viral resistance.

One randomized study evaluated the efficacy of the combination of adefovir with lamivudine as compared to lamivudine alone or adefovir alone in 59 patients with HBeAg-positive chronic hepatitis B with lamivudine resistant HBV. There was no significant difference in median serum HBV DNA reduction (–3.59 and –4.04 log copies/mL), rates of ALT normalization (53% and 47%) and HBeAg loss (three patients in each group) between the adefovir–lamivudine combination group and the adefovir monotherapy group. Of note, serum HBV DNA level remained stable and there was no significant biochemical or serologic change during the study in the patients who remained under lamivudine monotherapy. Therefore, the clinical benefit of continuing lamivudine therapy once resistance develops appears to be questionable. However, it seems reasonable, at least in patients with bridging fibrosis or cirrhosis, to continue lamivudine administration after initiation of adefovir until a significant decrease of serum HBV DNA and serum ALT has been obtained. This is based on the observation that a significant number of patients will have an ALT flare after withdrawal of lamivudine which is probably due to rapid emergence of wild type HBV. In one study in which lamivudine-resistant patients received adefovir monotherapy, 37% of patients had an ALT flare soon after discontinuing lamivudine. Such flares have not been observed when patients are maintained on adefovir in combination with ongoing lamivudine maintenance.

Another study compared the efficacy of the combination of adefovir with lamivudine versus lamivudine used in mono-

therapy in 112 treatment-naive patients (107 HBeAg-positive). There was no significant difference in median serum HBV DNA reduction (–5.41 and –4.80 log copies/mL), rates of undetectable HBV DNA with PCR (39% and 41%) and HBeAg loss (19% and 20%) between the adefovir–lamivudine combination group and the adefovir monotherapy group. Interestingly, there was a lower incidence of lamivudine resistance in the combination group (2%) than in the lamivudine monotherapy group (20%)(*P*<0.003).

These two studies do not answer the question of the benefit of the long-term treatment with the combination of adefovir and lamivudine as compared to adefovir monotherapy. Large randomized controlled trials with a long follow-up are needed to address this issue.

Future treatment strategies

Based on current experience, monotherapy with interferon or an antiviral drug is unlikely to achieve sustained responses in most patients with chronic hepatitis B. Combination therapy as in the case of treatment of HIV infection is the logical next step. However, which agents to combine is unclear. Ideally, the two agents should have synergistic, long-lasting effects on HBV clearance; no added toxicity and potential to decrease resistance. Finally, different therapies may have to be designed for different patient populations. Several practice guidelines on treatment of hepatitis B have recently been published, including those by the American Association for the Study of Liver Disease (AASLD) and the European Association for the Study of the Liver (EASL). The former are summarized in **Tables 15.3** and **15.4**.

Liver transplantation

The early results with OLT for chronic hepatitis B were disappointing, with more than 80% of patients experiencing HBV reinfection. Most importantly, in many patients, reinfection was associated with severe and rapidly progressive liver disease. However the prognosis has been substantially improved with the use of hyperimmune B immunoglobulin and lamivudine or adefovir (see O'Grady 2000, Ch. 37).

Association for the Study of Liver Disease (AASLD) practice guideline on treatment of chronic hepatitis B

HBeAg	HBV DNA (copies/mL)	ALT	Strategy
+	>10⁵	<2 × ULN	Observe
+	>10⁵	>2 × ULN	IFN, lam or adefovir
–	>10⁵	>2 × ULN	IFN, or adefovir
–	<10⁵	<2 × ULN	Observe

× ULN, times upper limit of normal; IFN, interferon; lam, lamivudine; adefovir, adefovir dipivoxil; ALT, alanine aminotransferase; HBeAg, hepatitis B e antigen; HBV, hepatitis B virus.

Table 15.3 Association for the Study of Liver Disease (AASLD) practice guideline on treatment of chronic hepatitis B.

Association for the Study of Liver Disease (AASLD) practice guidelines for patients with cirrhosis due to hepatitis B			
HBeAg	HBV DNA (copies/mL)	Cirrhosis	Strategy
+/–	>10^5	Compensated	Lam or adefovir
+/–	>10^5	Decompensated	Lam or adefovir; OLT
+/–	<10^5	Compensated	Observe
+/–	<10^5	Decompensated	OLT

adefovir, adefovir dipivoxil; IFN, interferon; lam, lamivudine; OLT, orthotopic liver transplantation; ALT, alanine aminotransferase; HBeAg, hepatitis B e antigen; HBV, hepatitis B virus.

Table 15.4 Association for the Study of Liver Disease (AASLD) practice guidelines for patients with cirrhosis due to hepatitis B.

Vaccination against HBV

Safe and effective hepatitis B vaccines have been available for the prevention of HBV infection in the past 15 years.

Vaccine formulations

Hepatitis B vaccines that are currently available in most countries are genetically engineered and consist of recombinant HBV small S protein (HBsAg) only. Although it has been suggested that incorporation of pre-S antigens into hepatitis B vaccines may increase the immunogenicity, this hypothesis remains to be confirmed.

Administration and efficacy

Hepatitis B vaccine is given intramuscularly, usually in three doses at 0, 1 and 6 months. The dose recommended for adults is 10–20 μg and for children 2.5–10 μg. Immune response defined as anti-HBs titers >10 IU/L is as high as 90–95% in immunocompetent persons, but is lower in older individuals (60% above age 60 years) and in immunocompromised patients such as dialysis patients (40%) and organ transplant recipients (80%). An additional one to three doses are recommended for nonresponders. Individuals who fail to respond after receiving two complete courses are unlikely to benefit from a third course. Although the anti-HBs titer decreases with time, the duration of protection is probably life-long, because most responders can mount an amnestic anti-HBs response on rechallenge. In addition, clinical infection is rarely observed during long-term follow-up of responders.

The implementation of universal vaccination of all newborns in endemic areas such as Taiwan and Senegal has been shown to dramatically reduce not only the carrier rate among children but also the incidence of childhood HCC.

Indications

Vaccination is most important for infants, particularly newborns of HBsAg carrier mothers, because of the high risk of progression to chronic infection after perinatal infection. Universal vaccination of all newborns with incorporation of hepatitis B vaccines into the Expanded Program for Immunization in Children is now recommended in most countries. In infants born to carrier mothers, an additional dose of HBIg is administered at birth to provide immediate protection. Catch-up vaccination is also recommended for all children and adolescents who have not been previously immunized.

Adults at increased risk of HBV infection such as healthcare workers, spouses of hepatitis B carriers, patients with chronic liver disease, dialysis patients, male homosexuals and intravenous drug abusers should also be vaccinated.

Postexposure prophylaxis should consist of the administration of a single dose of HBIg and the simultaneous initiation of a course of vaccination.

Adverse reactions

Adverse reactions to hepatitis B vaccine are uncommon. Approximately 20% of vaccinees may experience mild reactions at the injection site and a minority may have transient flu-like symptoms. Particular concern has been raised by the observation of cases of multiple sclerosis occuring after vaccination. However several large studies did not show a significant difference in the rates of incidence of multiple sclerosis in vaccinated subjects as compared with comparable control populations.

Vaccine-escape mutant

Mutations in the HBV S gene have been described in infants born to carrier mothers despite adequate anti-HBs response after vaccination. The commonest mutation is a glycine to arginine substitution at codon 145 (G145R) in the 'a' determinant of HBsAg. This mutation has been shown to decrease the binding of HBsAg to anti-HBs, accounting for the breakthrough infection. The exact incidence of this mutant among vaccinees is not clear but is likely to be <5%. There is no evidence to suggest that the efficacy of current vaccines is diminishing. In addition, there is no evidence to suggest that these mutants are transmitted to other family members or the community.

HEPATITIS D

Introduction

Hepatitis D is caused by a defective virus: the hepatitis D virus (HDV). Infection with HDV is closely associated with HBV infection. Although HDV can replicate autonomously, the simultaneous presence of HBV is required for complete virion assembly and secretion. As a result, individuals with hepatitis D are always dually infected with HDV and HBV.

The hepatitis D virion or δ agent comprises a single stranded RNA genome, the hepatitis D antigen (HDAg), and an envelope consisting of HBV envelope proteins (**Fig. 15.17**). Hepatitis D virus replicates via its complementary or antigenomic RNA.

Epidemiology

It is estimated that approximately 5% of the HBV carriers worldwide may be infected with HDV, leading to a total of 15 million persons infected with HDV worldwide. However, the geographic distribution of HDV infection does not parallel that of HBV.

The Mediterranean Basin

Infection with HDV is endemic in these countries. Infection tends to occur early, affecting mainly children and young adults.

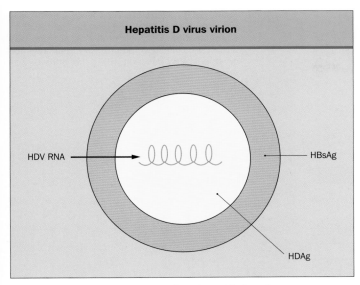

Figure 15.16 Hepatitis D virion. HDAg, hepatitis D antigen.

The main route of transmission is inapparent permucosal or percutaneous spread. Intrafamilial transmission has also been reported.

The Far East
Despite the high prevalence of HBV infection, the prevalence of HDV infection in these countries is, in general, low. Transmission occurs sexually or amongst intravenous drug users.

Western countries
Infection with HDV is uncommon and predominantly confined to intravenous drug users.

Changes in epidemiology
Evidence accrued in the last decade, however, is suggestive of a changing trend in the epidemiology of HDV. A decline in HDV prevalence in both acute and chronic hepatitis has been observed in the Mediterranean area, most likely due to universal HBV vaccination, measures to control HIV and socioeconomic improvements, whereas new foci of HDV infection are emerging in other parts of the world. South America, especially the subtropical area, remains an important potential reservoir for new outbreaks of HDV infection.

Natural history
The natural history of chronic HDV infection is characterized by a wide spectrum of clinical expressions. Since the earliest studies, HDV turned out to be a highly pathogenic virus causing a severe and rapidly progressive disease, with very infrequent spontaneous resolutions. Cirrhosis was shown to develop in up to 70% of the cases. Although HDV cirrhosis, once established, may be a stable disease for many years, co-infection with HDV was shown to significantly increase the risk of HCC and death in patients with compensated HBV cirrhosis. The link between HDV and severe and progressive liver disease has been found at all ages, as suggested by the detection of markers of HDV infection in up to 40% of children with HBsAg-positive cirrhosis.

Most patients with chronic HDV infection are HBeAg-negative. Low levels of HBV DNA replication occur due to the inhibition of HBV replication by HDV.

Clinical features
Due to its dependence on HBV, HDV infection always occurs in association with HBV infection. The clinical manifestations of HDV infection vary from benign acute hepatitis to fulminant hepatitis (**Fig. 15.16**), and from an asymptomatic carrier state to rapidly progressive chronic liver disease. In most cases of chronic HDV infection, HBV replication is suppressed to very low levels by HDV. Liver damage in these patients is essentially due to HDV only.

Co-infection
Co-infection of HBV and HDV in an individual susceptible to HBV infection results in an acute hepatitis. The clinical picture is indistinguishable from that of classic acute hepatitis B and is usually transient and self-limited (Fig. 15.16). However, a high incidence of acute liver failure has been reported among drug addicts. The rate of progression to chronic HDV infection is no different from that observed after classic acute hepatitis B because the persistence of HDV infection is dependent on the persistence of HBV infection.

Hepatitis D virus superinfection
Hepatitis D virus superinfection of an HBsAg carrier may present as unusually severe acute hepatitis in a previously unrecognized HBV carrier or an exacerbation of pre-existing chronic hepatitis B. Progression to chronic HDV infection is almost invariable.

Latent infection
This was initially described in the liver transplantation setting. In this situation, the allograft is reinfected with HDV but not HBV. The hepatitis D antigen (HDAg) can be detected in the liver, but HDV RNA cannot be detected in the serum. During this phase, there is usually no evidence of liver disease. Infection with HDV is abortive unless the graft is later reinfected with HBV.

Diagnosis
The serum biochemical profiles associated with HDV and HBV infections are given in **Figure 15.18**.

Hepatitis D virus antibody assays
Total (IgM and IgG) anti-HDV can be detected by enzyme-linked or radioimmune assays. These are the only commercially available tests for HDV infection in many countries. Anti-HDV-IgG appears late in acute hepatitis D. Thus, its clinical value is limited unless repeated testing is performed. Nonetheless, a well-documented anti-HDV seroconversion may be the only way to diagnose acute HDV infection. High-titer IgG anti-HDV is present in chronic HDV infection. It correlates well with ongoing HDV replication.

IgM anti-HDV is transient and delayed if the course of acute hepatitis D is self-limited. In patients who progress to chronic HDV infection, IgM anti-HDV is long-lasting and present in high titer. The IgM anti-HDV titer tends to correlate with the level of HDV replication and severity of liver disease.

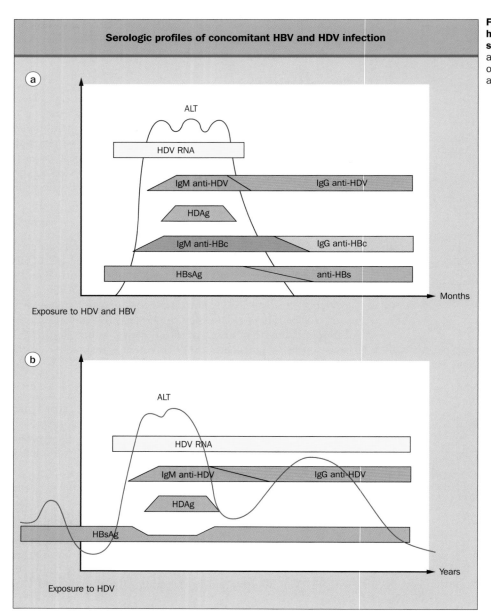

Serologic profiles of concomitant HBV and HDV infection

(a)

ALT

HDV RNA

IgM anti-HDV   IgG anti-HDV

HDAg

IgM anti-HBc   IgG anti-HBc

HBsAg   anti-HBs

Months

Exposure to HDV and HBV

(b)

ALT

HDV RNA

IgM anti-HDV   IgG anti-HDV

HDAg

HBsAg

Years

Exposure to HDV

Figure 15.17 Acute hepatitis B virus (HBV) and hepatitis D virus (HDV) co-infection and HDV superinfection. Serologic profile of (a) acute HBV and HDV co-infection, and (b) HDV superinfection on chronic HBV infection. HDAg, hepatitis D antigen.

Detection of serum hepatitis D antigen

In acute HDV infection, serum hepatitis D antigen appears early but is very short-lived and may escape detection if repeated testing is not performed. In chronic HDV infection, hepatitis D antigen is usually undetectable because of the formation of immune complexes with anti-HDV.

Detection of serum hepatitis D virus RNA

Serum HDV RNA is an early and sensitive marker of HDV infection in acute hepatitis D. In chronic HDV infection, only 70–80% of patients have detectable serum HDV RNA when tested by hybridization assays but most are positive by PCR assays.

Tissue markers of HDV infection

The antigen HDAg can be detected by immunohistochemical staining of liver tissues. The detection of intrahepatic HDAg has been proposed to be the 'gold' standard for the diagnosis of ongoing HDV infection. Hepatic HDV RNA can be detected by in situ hybridization.

Detection of serum HBV markers

Due to the dependence of HDV on HBV, the presence of HBsAg is necessary for the diagnosis of HDV infection. Documentation of the presence of HDV infection relies largely on the detection of anti-HDV. In patients with acute HBV/HDV co-infection, IgM anti-HBc is also present. Tests for serum HDAg and/or HDV RNA should also be performed if available. In patients with HDV superinfection, anti-HDV is usually present in high titers along with serum HDV RNA, while markers of HBV replication may be suppressed and IgM anti-HBC absent.

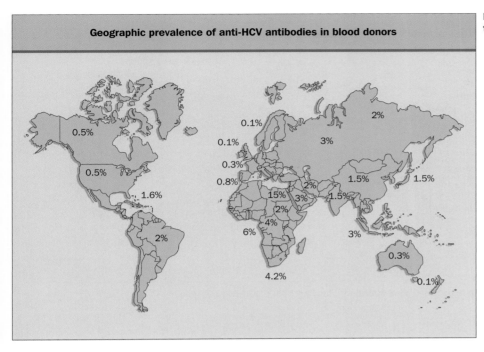

Geographic prevalence of anti-HCV antibodies in blood donors

0.1%
0.1%
0.3%
0.8%
0.5%
0.5%
1.6%
2%
2%
3%
15%
3%
2%
4%
6%
1.5%
1.5%
1.5%
3%
0.3%
0.1%
4.2%

Figure 16.3 Geographic prevalence of antibodies to hepatitis C virus antibodies in blood donors.

mice with HCV in the doubly homozygous animals and transient replication of HCV in the hemizygous animals using human hepatocytes.

PATHOGENETIC MECHANISMS

HCV is thought to be a non-cytopathic virus and liver damage is probably immune mediated. The large majority of infected individuals exposed to HCV become chronically infected although the mechanisms underlying this high rate of chronicity are not known. Neutralizing antibodies to HCV can be detected in serum and T-helper (CD4) lymphocytes responsive to both structural and non-structural HCV proteins can often be detected in patients with chronic HCV infection. Cytotoxic T lymphocytes (CTLs) are thought to be particularly important in viral pathogenesis as they recognize viral antigens on cell surfaces in conjunction with major histocompatibility complex (MHC) class I proteins and lyse infected target cells.

Progression of liver disease due to HCV is marked by progressive increases in hepatic fibrosis associated with activation of hepatic stellate cells, presumably through cytokine mediators produced as part of the immune response to HCV.

EPIDEMIOLOGY

HCV is transmitted by parenteral contact with blood or blood products. Recognized routes of infection include transfusion of blood or blood products, injection drug use, needlestick or other forms of contaminated injury among healthcare workers, maternal–infant transmission and sexual spread. In most developed countries post-transfusion HCV has been virtually eliminated by screening of donated blood, but chronic infection remains prevalent as demonstrated in studies of volunteer blood donors (**Fig. 16.3**). Injection drug use appears to be the most common remaining risk factor for HCV infection (**Fig. 16.4**).

Maternal–infant transmission may occur if a mother is seropositive for HCV RNA. This occurs in approximately 5% of infants, although the risk appears to be increased by the presence of co-infection with the human immunodeficiecy virus (HIV) in the mother, presumably because the serum levels of HCV RNA are higher in mothers with HIV co-infection.

Although occupational exposure to HCV may occur, the risk of acquiring HCV though needlestick injury appears very slight. Sexual transmission of HCV has been well documented to occur but the exact frequency of this occurrence is debated. Studies from the Centers for Disease Control and Prevention (CDC) have shown an increased risk of HCV infection in those individuals with multiple sexual partners or partners known to have HCV infection. However, studies of stable monogamous couples have shown very little evidence of sexual spread of HCV. Furthermore, the risk of HCV infection among men having sex with men is only about 5%, lower than what might be expected if HCV was readily spread by sexual contact.

Recent reports from the CDC have shown a dramatic decrease in the number of new cases of HCV infection in the USA from nearly 300 000 in the early 1990s to only 25 000 in 2001 (**Fig. 16.5**). Most of this decrease seems to have occurred among injection drug users and can be attributed to various public health measures.

Although the exact incidence and prevalence of HCV infection are not known in the USA accurate estimates of these figures have been possible by the use of sampling methods. Information on HCV incidence is derived from the Sentinel Counties Study while information on the prevalence of HCV is derived from the National Health and Nutrition Evaluation Survey (N-HANES) which is based on a random sample of the adult, non-institutionalized population of the USA. Based on these studies, it is estimated that 1.8% of the population is seropositive for anti-HCV, of whom about 75% have HCV RNA detectable in serum. Thus there are approximately 2.7 million

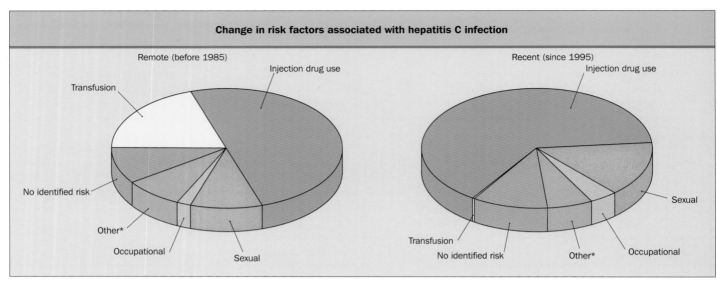

Figure 16.4 Change in risk factors associated with hepatitis C viral infection. Modified from CDC (www.cdc.gov).

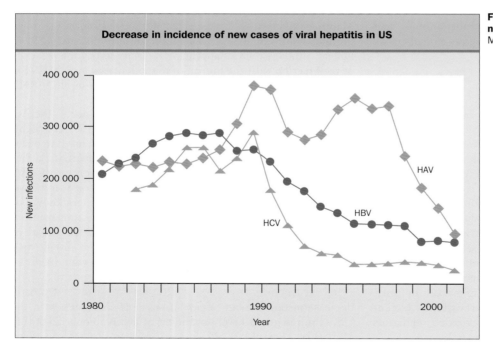

Figure 16.5 Decrease in annual incidence of new cases of viral hepatitis in the USA. Modified from CDC (www.cdc.gov).

HCV-infected individuals in the USA, a figure that is perhaps underestimated because individuals in institutions, such as prisons and nursing homes, were not sampled.

Given this frequency of HCV in the USA, the impact of this condition is not surprising. In addition to 8000–10 000 deaths each year attributed to HCV, it leads to more than one-third of liver transplants and is associated with expenditures of more than $1 billion annually.

DIAGNOSIS OF HEPATITIS C

The diagnosis of hepatitis C is relatively simple and is based on detection of anti-HCV through enzyme-linked immunoassays (EIA) that are both sensitive and specific. The EIA now in use represents a third generation of this assay and consists of recombinant viral protein cores, NS3 and NS5 regions of the viral genome in a solid phase assay. The presence of anti-HCV

Centers for Disease Control and Prevention (CDC) recommendations for HCV testing
Persons who should be tested routinely for HCV infection based on their risk of infection
Persons who ever injected illegal drugs
Persons with selected medical conditions, including:
• Persons who received clotting factor concentrates before 1987
• Persons who were ever on chronic hemodialysis
• Persons with persistently abnormal alanine aminotransferase levels
• Prior recipients of transfusions or organ transplants
Persons notified that they received blood from a donor who later tested positive for HCV
Persons who received a transfusion of blood or blood components before July 1992
Persons who received an organ transplant before 1992
Persons who should be tested routinely for HCV infection based on a recognized exposure
Healthcare, emergency medical and public safety workers after exposure to HCV-positive blood
Children born to HCV-positive women

Table 16.1 Centers for Disease Control and Prevention (CDC) recommendations for HCV testing.

Diagnosis of hepatitis C virus (HCV)				
	Anti-HCV (EIA)	Anti-HCV (RIBA)	HCV RNA	ALT
Acute or chronic hepatitis C	Positive	Positive	Positive	Elevated or normal
Recovered HCV	Positive	Positive	Negative	Normal
False-positive anti-HCV	Positive	Negative	Negative	Normal
ALT, alanine aminotransferase; EIA, enzyme-linked immunoassays; RIBA, recombinant immunoblot assay.				

Table 16.2 Diagnosis of hepatitis C virus (HCV).

can be confirmed using the recombinant immunoblot assay (RIBA), another immunoassay using a different, Western blot-like format. Anti-HCV may persist for years after HCV infection and clearance.

Testing for anti-HCV should be routinely offered to all persons identified as being at risk (**Table 16.1**).

Individuals who are currently infected with HCV have HCV RNA detectable in their serum. The levels of HCV RNA typically found with human infection are not easily detected using standard hybridization assays and require amplification of either the target (by PCR) or signal. As few as 50 copies of viral RNA per ml of serum can be detected with some modern assays.

The amount of HCV RNA in the circulation is readily quantifiable and is on average 2 to 3 million copies per ml. The level of HCV RNA may however vary considerably from patient to patient but is generally consistent over time in individual patients. The level of HCV RNA in serum does not appear to correlate with the severity of liver disease assessed either by serum aminotransferase activities or liver histopathology. Finally, the serum level of HCV RNA appears to be a good predictor of response to antiviral therapy. Assays to determine HCV genotype are now widely available although they lack standardization. Commonly used assays are based on amplification and sequencing or a line probe hybridization assay.

The duration of infection with HCV is difficult to estimate (**Table 16.2**). Patient histories are often unreliable and serologic tests do not accurately distinguish acute from chronic HCV infection. Jaundice is uncommon with acute hepatitis C. The

appearance of anti-HCV may be delayed a few weeks after HCV RNA following acute infection. A liver biopsy would show features of acute rather than chronic hepatitis but is not routinely recommended. The diagnosis of acute hepatitis C cannot be made with certainty unless the patient was known to be HCV negative previously and then developed HCV RNA in serum with or without clinical features of acute hepatitis.

LIVER HISTOPATHOLOGY

Liver biopsy plays a major role in the management of chronic hepatitis C. The histologic features of chronic hepatitis C commonly include an infiltrate of chronic inflammatory cells within portal areas, interface hepatitis, lobular hepatocellular injury and hepatic steatosis. Less commonly, the portal infiltrates take on the form of lymphoid aggregates or sometimes even lymphoid follicles. Progression of chronic hepatitis C is marked by progressive increases in hepatic fibrosis, consisting largely of collagen. Hepatic fibrosis due to HCV infection begins within the portal triads but may form bridges between portal areas or with terminal hepatic venules (bridging fibrosis). Cirrhosis represents the most advanced form of hepatic fibrosis.

Several systems for scoring the severity of chronic hepatitis C have been developed. They have in common assigning a grade to the degree of necrosis and inflammation and a stage to the degree of fibrosis. These scoring systems have proved to be very useful in clinical trials as a means of measuring improvement in liver histopathology as a result of antiviral therapy, but are also valuable in clinical practice as a means of assessing and following the severity and possible prognosis of liver disease. Commonly used systems include those described by Knodell and colleagues, Scheuer, Ishak and a French collaborative group (METAVIR) (**Table 16.3**) Brunt (01)).

CLINICAL FEATURES

The clinical features of acute and chronic hepatitis C are not specific for this form of hepatitis. Many patients with either acute or chronic hepatitis C are asymptomatic. Acute hepatitis C may sometimes result in jaundice, nausea, vomiting and general malaise. Fulminant hepatic failure is an extremely rare complication of acute HCV infection. The symptoms of chronic hepatitis C are non-specific and include fatigue and right upper

The Scheuer scoring systems for liver histopathology in chronic hepatitis		
Grade	Portal/periportal activity	Lobular activity
0	None/minimal	None
1	Portal inflammation	Inflammation but no necrosis
2	Mild piecemeal necrosis	Focal necrosis
3	Moderate piecemeal necrosis	Severe focal cell damage
4	Severe piecemeal necrosis	Damage includes bridging necrosis
Stage	Fibrosis	
0	None	
1	Enlarged, fibrotic portal tracts	
2	Periportal or portal–portal septa but intact architecture	
3	Fibrosis with architectural distortion but no obvious cirrhosis	
4	Probable or definite cirrhosis	

Table 16.3 The Scheuer scoring system for liver histopathology in chronic hepatitis. This is a simple scoring system that can be readily adapted to clinical practice.

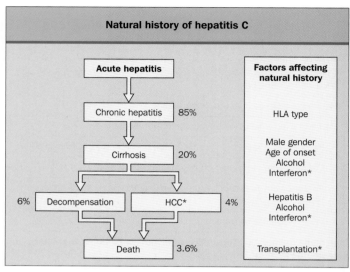

Figure 16.6 Natural history of hepatitis C. Natural history and factors affecting its outcome. Reproduced from Di Bisceglie (2000) by permission of Wiley-Liss, Inc. *, these factors improve outcome while others worsen it.

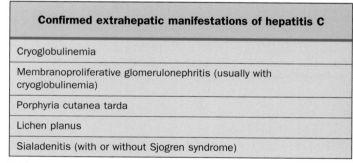

Table 16.4 Confirmed extrahepatic manifestations of hepatitis C.

Confirmed extrahepatic manifestations of hepatitis C
Cryoglobulinemia
Membranoproliferative glomerulonephritis (usually with cryoglobulinemia)
Porphyria cutanea tarda
Lichen planus
Sialadenitis (with or without Sjogren syndrome)

quadrant pain. Pruritus may sometimes be a presenting symptom for hepatitis C, probably related to cholestatic liver injury. Patients may sometimes present with features of extrahepatic manifestations of chronic hepatitis C such as porphyria cutanea tarda or cryogobulinemia (see below) or advanced liver disease with cirrhosis and liver failure. Asymptomatic patients with chronic hepatitis C may be detected at the time of routine health evaluations, insurance physicals or at the time of blood donation.

NATURAL HISTORY AND PROGNOSIS

The natural history of HCV infection is quite variable but is notable for a strong propensity to become chronic. Thus, as many as 85% of those individuals infected with HCV develop persistent infection marked by the ongoing presence of HCV RNA in serum for more than 6 months after the onset, although the rate of chronicity appears to be lower among younger individuals (**Fig. 16.6**). Among those with chronic infection, there is also considerable variability with regard to rates of progression of hepatic fibrosis. Some patients appear to have very rapidly progressive liver disease and may develop cirrhosis in less than 5 years. On the other hand there are others who do not have significant fibrosis even after 20 years or more of infection.

Some of the factors thought to contribute to severity of chronic hepatitis C include older age at infection, male gender and alcohol consumption. Once cirrhosis has developed, further progression may result in hepatic decompensation or the development of HCC.

COMPLICATIONS AND EXTRAHEPATIC MANIFESTATIONS

Hepatic decompensation in cirrhosis due to hepatitis C is very similar to liver failure associated with other forms of chronic liver disease. Features of decompensation such as ascites, jaundice and bleeding from esophageal varices occur in about 30% of patients with cirrhosis over a period of 10 years. Once features of hepatic decompensation have occurred, the mortality rate from liver disease increases to approximately 10% per year. For this reason, hepatic decompensation due to hepatitis C represents an indication for liver transplantation.

Some of the well known extrahepatic manifestations of chronic hepatitis C are listed in **Table 16.4**. Cryoglobulinemia is defined by the presence of cryoglobulins in serum. These are abnormal immunoglobulins that characteristically precipitate out in the cold and can redissolve when warmed. Low levels of cryoglobulins can be detected in as many as 40–50% of patients with chronic hepatitis C but are associated with symptoms only rarely, presumably when high levels are present. Symptoms of cryoglobulinemia include joint aches and skin rashes. The presence of palpable purpura on the lower legs is a characteristic

therapy. The dosing of interferon is not well established in patients with very advanced liver disease, but in general should be lower than in otherwise healthy individuals.

Recurrence of HCV infection is almost universal after liver transplantation and may result in recurrence of severe liver disease and cirrhosis in a proportion of patients within a few years. There is growing evidence of benefit from antiviral therapy in these patients with recurrent hepatitis C. In this setting, ribavirin should be used with extreme caution because of the typical renal insufficiency associated with use of calcineurin inhibitors to prevent rejection. Furthermore, the rate of SVR is substantially lower than in pretransplant patients with mild liver disease (no more than 10% using current treatment regimens). However it appears that the use of interferon after transplant may be associated with some histologic benefit.

PREVENTION OF HCV INFECTION

Substantial progress has already been made in preventing the spread of HCV infection. HCV has been virtually eliminated from the blood supply and the number of new cases is decreasing. Further decreases in the incidence of hepatitis C would require a reduction in cases associated with injection drug use. This would require either the primary prevention of illegal drug injecting or, possibly, secondary prevention among drug users by methods such as needle exchange programs.

Another approach to preventing the spread of HCV involves development and use of vaccines against HCV. There is currently no vaccine in clinical use or even undergoing clinical trial in large numbers of patients. Development of a vaccine has been hampered by the lack of a clear understanding of what constitutes a sterilizing immune response to HCV and by the considerable variability of the HCV genome. Vaccines based on recombinant forms of HCV envelope proteins have been tested in chimpanzees with at least partial success.

FUTURE OUTLOOK

Further studies are still needed to clarify the use of existing therapies. Thus, while the optimal dose of ribavirin has been established by these recent studies, the optimal dosing of peginterferon deserves further study. It is not clear if lower doses of peginterferon can perhaps be used for some patients – perhaps those infected with non-1 genotypes, or those with low levels of HCV RNA in serum. Because body weight has proven to be a factor influencing the response to antiviral therapy, further study of weight-based dosing may be appropriate, particularly for those patients at the extremes of high or low body weight. Studies such as the HALT-C trial and follow-up of patients achieving SVR in other clinical trials will hopefully clarify whether antiviral therapy against hepatitis C is effective in achieving the goals of slowing or preventing the progression of liver disease.

Considerable efforts have gone into developing new approaches to therapy of hepatitis C, largely based on the design of specific antiviral agents aimed at inhibiting various viral enzymes or functions, such as the HCV polymerase, HCV protease or the ribosomal docking function of the IRES. Several antiviral agents are in the process of development based on this progress. Preliminary data were recently reported on the antiviral effect of a novel protease inhibitor, showing very potent antiviral effect in the short term. Issues that are likely to arise with the use of specific antiviral agents include the risks of unexpected toxicity, development of viral resistance due to mutations and possibly the need for continuous or long-term therapy. It is likely that peginterferons will continue to play a major role in therapy of HCV for some time to come, at least until the widespread availability of other antivirals. Given that peginterferon and ribavirin are effective in eliminating HCV infection in nearly 80% of patients infected with genotypes 2 or 3 when given for a relatively short period of time, this combination of drugs may remain the mainstay of therapy in this subgroup of patients.

FURTHER READING

Epidemiology, pathogenesis and natural history

Alter MJ. Epidemiology of hepatitis C. In, Liang TJ, Hoofnagle JH, eds. Hepatitis C. San Diego: Academic Press; 2000:169–184. *A recent review of the epidemiology of HCV infection in the USA.*

Benvegnu L, Gios M, Boccato S, et al. Natural history of compensated viral cirrhosis: a prospective study on the incidence and hierarchy of major complications. Gut 2004; 53:744–749. *An excellent study of the natural history of hepatitis* C.

Brunt EM. Grading and staging the histopathological lesions of chronic hepatitis: the Knodell histology activity index and beyond. Hepatology 2001; 31:241–246. *A thorough description and comparison of the various systems for grading and staging of liver histology in hepatitis* C.

Di Bisceglie AM. Natural history of hepatitis C: its impact on clinical management. Hepatology 2000; 31:1014–1018.

Mercer P, Schiller D, Elliot J, et al. Hepatitis C virus replication in mice with chimeric human livers. Nature Medicine 2001; 7:727–733.

National Institutes of Health Consensus Development Conference Statement: Management of Hepatitis C, June 10–12, 2002. Hepatology 2002; 36S(suppl):S3–S20.

Shakil AO and Di Bisceglie AM. Images in medicine: a patient with cryoglobulinemia and hepatitis C. N Engl J Med 1994; 331:1624.

Thomas DL. Hepatitis C and human immunodeficiency virus infection. Hepatology 2002; 36 (suppl):S201–S209. *A review of issues affecting hepatitis C in patients with HIV infection.*

Thomson M, Liang TJ. Molecular biology of hepatitis C virus. In, Liang TJ, Hoofnagle JH, eds. Hepatitis C. San Diego: Academic Press; 2000:1–24.

Treatment

Davis GL. Monitoring of viral levels during therapy of hepatitis C. Hepatology 2002; 36(Suppl. 1):5145–5151.

Fried MW, Shiffmann ML, Reddy R, et al. Peginterferon α2a plus ribavirin for chronic hepatitis C virus infection. N Engl J Med 2002; 347:975–982. *One of two pivotal trials showing the superior value of pegylated interferon in combination with ribavirin in therapy of hepatitis* C.

Hadziyannis SJ, Sette H Jr, Morgan TR, et al. Peginterferon-α2a and ribavirin combination therapy in chronic hepatitis C: a randomized study of treatment duration and ribavirin dose. Ann Intern Med 2004; 140:346–355. *A randomized controlled trial stratifying for HCV genotype.*

Maddrey WC. Safety of combination interferon α2b/ribavirin therapy in chronic hepatitis C-relapsed and treatment naive patients. Semin Liver Dis 1999; 19(suppl 1):67–76.

Manns MP, McHutchison JG, Gordon SC, et al. Peginterferon α2b plus ribavirin compared with interferon α2b plus ribavirin for initial treatment of chronic hepatitis C: a randomized trial. Lancet 2001; 358:958–965. *One of two pivotal trials showing the superior value of pegylated interferon in combination with ribavirin in therapy of hepatitis* C.

Poynard T, McHutchison J, Manns M, et al for the PEG-FIBROSIS project group. Impact of pegylated interferon α2b and ribavirin on liver fibrosis in patients with chronic hepatitis C. Gastroenterology 2002; 122:1303–1313.

Zeuzem S, Feinman SV, Rasenack J, et al. Peginterferon α2a in patients with chronic hepatitis C. N Engl J Med 2000, 343:1666–1672.

Miscellaneous Infections of the Liver

Rachel Baden Herman and Margaret James Koziel

INTRODUCTION

Infections frequently involve the liver, either as part of a disseminated infection or due to a specific tropism of the infectious agent for the liver and biliary tree. The liver is at particular risk of infection due to the large vascular supply and in particular the close relationship to the venous drainage system of the gut, by which many infectious agents gain access to the body. Given that many infections will present non-specifically, with elevations in serum aminotransferases or alkaline phosphatase as the only clue to involvement of the liver, the clinician needs to be aware of what infections to which a particular host may be susceptible, as well as the best means to achieve diagnosis of a particular pathogen. In this chapter, we will describe infections other than classic viral hepatitis (A, B, C, D and E) with respect to their presentations as hepatic diseases.

HEPATIC MANIFESTATIONS OF SYSTEMIC DISEASE

Hepatosplenic candidiasis
Epidemiology

Hepatosplenic candidiasis (HSC; otherwise known as chronic disseminated candidiasis) is a form of invasive fungal infection that primarily affects the liver, kidneys and spleen. Most often the disease is caused by *Candida albicans*, but rare cases of *Candida tropicalis*, and *Candida glabrata* as well as other species have been described. It most often occurs in the setting of hematologic malignancies. It has been recognized as a distinct form of invasive fungal disease in this setting for the last two to three decades, although the incidence of HSC is rising because of more widespread use of cytotoxic agents. One large retrospective study in Taiwan reported an incidence of up to 8% in 500 patients with acute leukemia receiving chemotherapy. Patients with these conditions are at risk secondary to a combination of mucotoxic chemotherapeutic regimens and periods of neutropenia. Other potential risk factors are intravascular catheters and use of broad-spectrum antibiotics. However, hepatosplenic candidiasis in non-leukemic patients is rare. The most likely pathophysiology is that the mucosal damage caused by chemotherapeutic agents causes invasion of the bloodstream and hematologic spread of *Candida*, which is a part of the normal gastrointestinal flora. Given that the portal system would then be the first site of dissemination, its location puts the liver and spleen at particular risk of infection. Coupled with periods of neutropenia, this places patients with hematologic malignancies at extreme risk of hepatosplenic candidiasis.

Clinical signs, symptoms and diagnosis

The presentation of hepatosplenic candidiasis is usually subacute, lasting weeks to months. The most common presenting sign of hepatosplenic candidiasis may only be a persistent fever despite appropriate broad-spectrum antimicrobial therapy. Patients may also present with abdominal pain, nausea, vomiting and an elevated serum alkaline phosphatase. Blood cultures are positive in less than 50% of patients. Hepatic lesions can usually be identified on magnetic resonance imaging (MRI), computed tomography (CT) scan and ultrasound. However, these lesions may disappear in periods of neutropenia or only become visible after neutropenia has resolved. One series described serial sonography as a means of increasing sensitivity. Typically, the lesions associated with hepatosplenic candidiasis appear irregularly-shaped and hypoechoic on ultrasound. A definitive diagnosis usually requires a biopsy of these lesions demonstrating budding yeast or pseudohyphae. Given the focality of these lesions, ultrasound-guided or laparoscopic biopsies are recommended. Histologically, early lesions consist of a mixture of polymorphonuclear inflammatory cells and mononuclear cells that surround a center of viable yeast. After treatment, these lesions then become a center of necrotic fungal elements surrounded by lymphocytes, macrophages and giant cells. The periphery is made up of fibrotic tissue.

Treatment and prophylaxis

There is wide variation in treatment protocols for hepatosplenic candidiasis, and to date no definitive regimen is agreed upon. Amphotericin is the drug of choice, and most sources recommend amphotericin B in combination with 5-flucytosine. Amphotericin can cause significant renal toxicity and electrolyte abnormalities. If the patient has underlying renal impairment, liposomal formulations of amphotericin can be used. Once stable, the patient can be switched to fluconazole. Most sources recommend continuing therapy until radiographic evidence of disease has disappeared or a total of 4 g of amphotericin has been given. Fluconazole has also been used successfully in non-neutropenic patients as primary treatment, providing the *Candida* isolate is susceptible to fluconazole; some species, such as *Candida kruseii*, are intrinsically resistant to fluconazole. Other azole formulations and caspofungin have activity against *Candida* species, but there is too little information about their use in this setting to recommend them as initial treatment.

The overall incidence of disease had declined significantly in the last decade, attributed largely to institution of fluconazole prophylaxis as standard of care for patients with prolonged neutropenia in most large cancer centers. This has been confirmed in several studies, including one large autopsy study in which there were fewer cases of candidal liver infections in patients on fluconazole prophylaxis.

Histoplasmosis
Epidemiology
Histoplasmosis is endemic in certain areas in North, Central and South America. In the USA it is the most common cause of fungal infection in the Ohio and Mississippi River valleys, although it is present in most of the USA. Cases reported in residents of areas that are not endemic usually represent re-activation of disease acquired during previous travel to endemic zones. Disseminated histoplasmosis occurs in patients with impaired cellular immunity as in patients with acquired immunodeficiency syndrome (AIDS), advanced age, malignancy and diabetes or even in immunocompetent patients if the yeast burden is high enough. Disseminated disease occurs in approximately 1/2000 exposed individuals. While disease normally starts in the lungs, as it occurs when infectious microconidia are inhaled and then transform into pathogenic yeast-phase organisms, liver involvement is extremely common in disseminated histoplasmosis. Rarely, histoplasmosis may occur in the liver without any evidence of disseminated disease.

Clinical signs and symptoms
Most people who are infected with histoplasmosis remain asymptomatic or experience a self-limited course that consists of fever, cough and fatigue. The symptoms of disseminated disease uniformly include fever, weight loss and malaise. Patients may also present with hepatomegaly and lymphadenopathy. Alkaline phosphatase, alanine aminotransferase (ALT) and aspartate aminotransferase (AST) are usually elevated to twice the upper limit of normal. Patients can also have a markedly elevated lactate dehydrogenase (LDH). Patients may present with shock, multiorgan failure and disseminated intravascular coagulation (DIC). In cases that are not disseminated and only hepatic involvement is reported, patients usually present with right upper quadrant pain and a hepatic mass.

Diagnosis
Diagnosis of disseminated disease can be made by biopsy of the lung, lymph node or liver. Oval, budding yeast are seen on methenamine silver stain. On hepatic biopsy, granulomatous hepatitis will be present with or without necrosis. Blood cultures and smears may also be useful. Urinary histoplasmosis antigen can be obtained if disseminated disease is suspected. It has a sensitivity of 90% in patients with disseminated disease.

Treatment
In patients with severe pulmonary, hepatic or disseminated disease, treatment should be initiated with amphotericin B. In patients who are to be treated as outpatients or in whom amphotericin B is initially used with good clinical response, itraconazole can be used as it has good activity against histoplasmosis. Itraconazole can also be used in AIDS patients as secondary prophylaxis.

SYSTEMIC DISEASE – BACTERIAL

Listeriosis
Background
Hepatic involvement in the course of any serious bacterial infection is common. Like many other bacteria, *Listeria* has a propensity for invading the liver. This has been well documented in both human and animal studies. In fact, before *Listeria* was given the name *Listeria monocytogenes* it was first called *Listeria hepatolytica* because of the common finding of focal necrosis in the liver during animal studies.

Epidemiology
Listeria is a motile, Gram-positive organism. Infection is commonly associated with pregnancy, extremes of age, chronic disease states and immunosuppression. Transmission of *Listeria* is usually through contaminated food. Outbreaks have been associated particularly with meat or dairy products, such as undercooked hotdogs, which incur 12 times the risk, or undercooked chicken, which is associated with a 20-fold increase in risk. Recent outbreaks of listeriosis have also been associated with chocolate milk, delicatessen meats, unpasteurized diary products, soft cheeses, blue-veined cheeses and Mexican-style cheese products.

Clinical presentation
The most common presentation of listeriosis, especially in the elderly, pregnant and newborn populations, is meningitis or a meningoencephalitis. However, there are three distinct entities comprising the hepatic involvement of *Listeria*: hepatitis, single liver abscess and multiple liver abscesses. In the case of hepatitis, the diagnosis is often mistaken initially for acute viral hepatitis. It is often not until other more common signs of listeriosis, such as meningeal signs, develop that *Listeria* is considered in the differential diagnosis of acute hepatitis. Patients may initially present with fever and right upper quadrant tenderness. Physical examination may reveal hypotension and hepatomegaly. Laboratory tests will usually demonstrate markedly elevated AST and ALT, with peak aminotransferase levels as high as in the 5000–6000 U/L range. Patients may also initially present with a febrile gastroenteritis. Diarrhea is likely to be non-bloody and last for a median of 40 h. Median duration of fever with this presentation is approximately 1 day.

Solitary abscesses have mostly been described in patients with diabetes. They rarely have associated meningitis or bacteremia. Patients may present with fever and right upper quadrant pain. They have an excellent prognosis with proper treatment. Multiple liver abscesses caused by *Listeria* carry a worse prognosis. In one study, only 13% of patients survived. Given the likelihood of many extrahepatic sites of *Listeria*, it is likely that multiple abscesses are a sign of disseminated disease.

Diagnosis
The diagnosis is usually confirmed when *L. monocytogenes* is isolated from blood cultures. In culture, the organism possesses flagellae and exhibits a tumbling motility at 25°C. It is commonly misidentified as a diphtheroid, and reports of diphtheroids in blood in a patient with a compatible clinical syndrome should prompt the clinician to query the laboratory about the possibility of *Listeria* and consider empiric antibiotic treatment. A diagnostic clue that might help distinguish *Listeria* from acute viral hepatitis is the presence of high temperatures (≥39° C) and shaking chills, which is atypical for viral hepatitis but common in *Listeria* infection.

Treatment

Intravenous ampicillin is usually effective in the treatment of hepatitis. Single abscesses usually require drainage and may require addition of an aminoglycoside. However, in the case of multiple abscesses and disseminated disease, high-dose ampicillin in combination with gentamicin is recommended.

Melioidosis
Background

Melioidosis is caused by a Gram-negative, motile bacillus called *Burkholderia pseudomallei*. Until 1992, the organism was known as *Pseudomonas pseudomallei*. Before the return of troops from endemic areas during the Vietnam War, melioidosis was virtually unheard of in the USA and Western Europe, but with increasing global travel and appreciation of the disease more cases have been identified.

Epidemiology

The organism is an environmental saprophyte in soil and fresh water in endemic regions. It is endemic to Southeast Asia, northern Australia, southern Asia and China, with most cases being reported from northern Thailand and northern Australia. In endemic areas, melioidosis is a disease of the rainy season. The primary mode of acquisition is now thought to be percutaneous, with subsequent dissemination of organisms to distant sites such as the lungs, skin, joints and liver. It normally affects individuals with diabetes, chronic renal failure, alcoholic liver disease or any degree of immunosuppression. Up to 50% of patients with melioidosis have diabetes associated with poor glucose control. The peak incidence is in the fourth and fifth decades of life.

Presentation

Disease usually occurs by inoculation or inhalation rather than ingestion. The incubation period following inoculation ranges from 1 to 21 days (mean 9 days) in those with symptomatic disease, with shorter periods seen in those with heavy exposure to the organism. Most infections are asymptomatic, but when symptoms are present they may be either acute or chronic in nature. Disease can present many years after initial exposure, with a reactivation syndrome similar to what occurs with tuberculosis, although such cases appear to be rare. The presenting signs and symptoms depend on the organ(s) involved, and range from a full-blown sepsis syndrome to non-specific fever. In the liver, the disease is characterized by abscess formation, which may be accompanied by other abscesses, particularly in the spleen, or radiologic evidence of pulmonary involvement.

Diagnosis

Abdominal ultrasound is helpful in identifying the hepatic abscess of melioidosis, although no ultrasonographic features of melioidosis are specific for this infection. If there are also splenic abscesses this can help in establishing the diagnosis in endemic areas, as other causes of liver abscess in these areas are less likely to cause a concomitant splenic lesion. While serologies may be helpful, definitive diagnosis is made by culturing the organism from the abscess site or blood. If the diagnosis is suspected based on residence or travel in an endemic area, the microbiology laboratory should be notified to enhance recovery of the organism, although *B. pseudomallei* grows on a wide range of commercially available media. On examination, the Gram-negative organisms have a characteristic 'safety pin' appearance. Direct immunofluorescence microscopy from sputum, urine or purulent drainage is 98% specific. It is only 70% sensitive, but can make the diagnosis in 30 minutes or less.

Treatment

Melioidosis can be a difficult disease to treat. *B. pseudomallei* is inherently resistant to many antibiotics, including first and second generation penicillins and cephalosporins, as well as the aminoglycosides. It should be treated with either ceftazidime or a carbapenem such as meropenem, although sulfa agents may be used as adjunctive therapy in severe infections. If hepatic abscesses are large, they need to be drained. Patients may be slow to respond to antibiotics, but resistance to either ceftazidime or carbapenems is rare so physicians should keep these drugs patiently on board as the first-line regimen. Patients are usually treated with at least 2 weeks of intravenous therapy, followed by a prolonged period of oral therapy for a minimum of 3 months, usually with high dose trimethoprim-sulfamethoxazole (TMP-SMX)

Brucellosis
Background and epidemiology

Brucella is a small, non-motile, Gram-negative coccobacillus. Worldwide, it is a significant cause of disease in domesticated animals with humans as an incidental host. Brucellosis can be an occupational hazard for livestock workers and anyone in the meatpacking industry. There are several possible routes of exposure, including direct inoculation through breaks in the skin, via the conjunctiva, inhalation and ingestion of contaminated food. It can be transmitted to humans through ingestion of unpasteurized dairy products or by handling meat or blood samples from infected animals. There are four species that are pathogenic to humans (*Brucella melitensis*, *Brucella abortus*, *Brucella suis* and *Brucella canis*). Hepatic involvement has been widely reported, primarily from *abortus*, which is found in cattle and *B. melitensis*, which is found in goats.

Clinical presentation

Brucellosis is a well-documented cause of fever of unknown origin with varied and often non-specific symptoms, the most prominent of which is fever, thus earning the sobriquets of undulant, Mediterranean or Malta fever. Patients will present with fatigue, fever, night sweats, weight loss and headache, which may be either acute or subacute in onset. Patients may develop these symptoms acutely, or the disease may also lay dormant for many years in which case patients will present with a more indolent course that is only episodically symptomatic. Physical findings, if present, will be limited to minimal lymphadenopathy or hepatosplenomegaly. In the acute phase, up to 10% of patients will have hepatitis. Laboratory values will reveal an elevation in AST, ALT and alkaline phosphatase. Patients may also present in either the acute or the chronic phases of the disease with hepatic abscess formation, but this is much less common than a clinical hepatitis. Other common manifestations of localized infection are osteoarticular involvement, epididymoorchitis, meningitis and endocarditis.

Diagnosis

Risk factors for this disease, such as contact with animal tissues or ingestion of unpasteurized milk or cheeses, should prompt specific microbiologic testing. The organism can be isolated from blood cultures, which are relatively insensitive and may need to be held for prolonged periods (7–21 days) to reveal growth of the organism. Routine techniques used for culturing of blood are not optimal for recovery of the organisms, and so the microbiology laboratory should be alerted to perform special techniques to enhance recovery. Given the difficulty involved in culturing the organism, serologic testing is often used to establish the diagnosis. Biopsy of the liver usually demonstrates non-caseating granuloma formation.

Treatment

In adults and children over 8 years old, treatment is doxycycline and rifampin (rifampicin) for 6 weeks, or doxycycline for 6 weeks plus streptomycin intramuscularly daily for 14–21 days. Other agents, such as fluoroquinolones, have some activity against *Brucella* but should not be used as monotherapy. In children less than 8 years of age, treatment consists of TMP-SMX for 45 days plus rifampin (rifampicin) for 6 weeks; alternatively, gentamicin may be used.

SYSTEMIC DISEASE – VIRAL

Cytomegalovirus
Background

Cytomegalovirus, CMV, is a member of the Herpesviridae family. Infection is common early in life, but is usually asymptomatic. It can be acquired transplacentally, through saliva, blood and urine; and may be associated with congenital abnormalities. In the adult population, disease can represent primary infection or reactivation. Symptomatic infection in immunocompetent patients is rare, but can occur. In all states that compromise T-cell immunity symptomatic infection is frequent, putting patients who are post-transplant and patients with HIV infection at particular risk. In these patients, infection can be severe and life threatening.

Clinical presentation

The clinical spectrum associated with active CMV disease is vast. It can cause pneumonia, gastrointestinal findings, hepatitis, central nervous system involvement, retinitis and nephritis. In one review analyzing the presentation in the immunocompetent population, abnormal liver specific tests were the most common clinical finding along with the less common fever, malaise and night sweats. In this 'mononucleosis-like syndrome', patients may also present with lymphadenopathy and lymphocytosis with greater than 10% atypical lymphocytes. In primary hepatitis, hepatomegaly is a common presenting feature. In the transplant population, CMV infection is most likely to occur within the first 18 months post-transplant. Patients who are seronegative prior to transplant but receive a graft from a seropositive donor are particularly at risk. However, reactivation disease in a previously seropositive patient can also occur and be quite severe. In transplant patients, the allograft is a particular target for CMV disease thus making CMV infection a risk for graft failure. Additionally, CMV has a number of host proteins that interact with the host immune response, and thus may independently increase the risk of other opportunistic infections.

In patients with HIV infection, CMV disease typically occurs when the CD4 count is less than 100. The most common presentations in this population are retinitis, esophagitis and colitis. Liver enzyme abnormalities are common in these patients and active replication in the liver can be documented in 30–50% of patients with evidence of disease elsewhere. Active replication in the liver can also cause an acalculous cholecystitis and even a sclerosing cholangitis in these patients. A markedly disproportionately elevated alkaline phosphatase may be a sign of biliary disease in patients with CMV.

Diagnosis

CMV infection is defined as the isolation of CMV virus or the detection of viral proteins or nucleic acid in any body fluid or tissue specimen. The diagnosis can be established using viral culture detection of viral antigens, or CMV DNA by polymerase chain reaction (PCR)-based techniques. PCR can be used in both a qualitative and quantitative modality.

Treatment and prophylaxis

CMV in the immunocompetent host is usually self-limiting and generally no antiviral therapy is warranted. The recommendations for treatment of CMV in the immunocompromised host are varied. In AIDS patients and in transplant recipients with active CMV, the consensus is that an induction period with intravenous ganciclovir for at least 2–3 weeks is considered gold standard for treatment. However, for the maintenance therapy that follows the induction period, there is no general agreement about optimal therapy. Oral ganciclovir is often implemented in the maintenance period. In HIV patients, it is usually continued lifelong or until immune reconstitution has occurred. Oral valganciclovir, which is a pro-drug of ganciclovir, has been approved by the Food and Drug Administration (FDA) for both the induction and maintenance periods.

Prophylaxis in the transplant population is a complicated topic. The recommendations vary based on the organ allograft. However, the general principle is that patients who are seronegative for CMV and receive a transplant from a seropositive donor are at highest risk of CMV disease. Aggressive monitoring for CMV antigenemia is often implemented post-transplantation, including use of leukocyte depleted red cells. Typically, high-risk patients undergo an induction period of IV ganciclovir for the first 2 weeks post-transplant. Immunoglobulin is also often administered post-transplant as additional prophylaxis in donor CMV positive/recipient CMV negative cases. A recent study demonstrated that after this initial 2 weeks of therapy, the patient could then be switched to oral ganciclovir. However, there is also some data to support use of oral agents for the entire period of prophylaxis. There is no consensus on duration of therapy, but patients usually remain on prophylaxis in the first 1–3 months post-transplant. The issue of prophylaxis should be addressed on an individual patient basis taking into account the immunosuppressive medical regimen and risk of renal toxicity.

Epstein-Barr virus
Background

Epstein-Barr virus (EBV) is a widely disseminated herpesvirus which is spread by intimate contact between susceptible persons and those shedding EBV. It is a member of the γ herpesvirus family and infects B lymphocytes. This typically results in a latent infection in which there is persistence of the viral genome

antigen detection in the stool, *E. histolytica*-specific DNA by PCR, or isoenzyme analysis of stool culture. Stool culture, though more sensitive than microscopy, can take up to 1 week; so antigen testing, which usually takes 2–3 h, and PCR, which may take 2–3 days, may prove to be more useful in establishing a diagnosis of *E. histolytica*.

Treatment

Commonly, treatment for amebic liver abscess is metronidazole (500–750 mg orally three times daily for 7–10 days). This therapy is effective in about 90% of patients. If patients are slow to respond or relapse following therapy, aspiration and/or a prolonged course of metronidazole should be considered. Intraluminal infection should also be treated even if stool studies are negative. Either Paromomycin or Iodoquinol can be used to treat intraluminal disease.

PARASITIC INFECTIONS OF THE LIVER AND BILIARY TREE

Schistosomiasis
Background
In the mid-19th century Theodor Bilharz first described a parasitic infection called bilharzia that would later become known as schistosomiasis. It is caused by a trematode blood fluke from the genus *Schistosoma*. The species that infect humans are *Schistosoma hematobium*, *Schistosoma mansoni*, *Schistosoma japonicum*, *Schistosoma intercalatum* and *Schistosoma mekongi*. *S. mansoni* and *S. japonicum* are the two species that most commonly infect the liver and biliary tree, while *S. hematobium* infects the bladder and urinary tract. There are over 70 countries in tropical and subtropical areas of Asia, South America, Africa and the Caribbean that are endemic for schistosomiasis. It is estimated that over 200 million people have this infection, and that 120 million are symptomatic.

Life cycle
Infection is caused by direct contact with water that contains free-swimming larvae. These larvae penetrate the skin of humans or other hosts. The larvae shed their tails and the resulting schistosomula penetrate the capillaries and lymphatic vessels and enter the lungs mostly through the venous system. They then enter the circulation in the left heart and travel to the liver through the portal system. The worms mature in the portal system. From the systemic circulation they may then travel to either the liver or the urinary tract where they produce eggs. Eggs are shed in the urine or feces. If the eggs are retained in tissue, chronic schistosomiasis occurs. The eggs can hatch in freshwater and infect snails where the life cycle commences again.

Clinical presentation
At the site of inoculation with the larvae, a local response may occur. In primary infection, it usually consists of a maculopapular eruption. In sensitized individuals, 'swimmer's itch', a more severe dermatitis may occur at the site if infection. Acute schistosomiasis, otherwise known as Katayama fever, usually occurs within 2–3 weeks of freshwater exposure in endemic areas. Symptoms include fever, myalgias, right upper quadrant pain and bloody diarrhea. Respiratory symptoms are also reported. Tender hepatomegaly is present as is splenomegaly in certain cases. Patients will usually have a peripheral eosinophilia.

In chronic liver involvement, patients develop granulomatous disease. The granuloma formation and inflammation from the retained eggs cause presinusoidal inflammation and periportal fibrosis (**Fig. 17.3**). This condition is referred to as clay-pipe-stem fibrosis. It is a major cause of portal hypertension in endemic areas. In certain areas, such as Egypt, this problem is compounded by co-infection with hepatitis C; the two infections together result in a very rapid progression to advanced fibrosis compared to either infection alone.

Diagnosis
Definitive diagnosis can be made by detecting the eggs in the feces or urine. Antibody testing can be helpful in ruling out infection, but it does not distinguish between past or present disease. Recently, an antigen test has been developed. Two parasite proteins, circulating anodic antigen (CAA) and circulating cathodic antigen (CCA), are present in the blood during infection. These proteins may be detected by ELISA in active infection.

Treatment and prophylaxis
Treatment of schistosomiasis consists of praziquantel with a single dose of 40 mg/kg. If infection with *S. japonicum* is confirmed or even suspected a higher dose of 60 mg/kg should be implemented. Feces or urine should be re-examined after 1 month to confirm cure. If praziquantel is ineffective, oxamniquine can be used as an alternative. In acute infection, if there is cerebral involvement, coricosteroids may prove to be helpful in reducing cerebral edema. Artemisinin in combination with praziquantel can be used for chemoprophylaxis. However, the best form of prevention is avoidance of contaminated water sources. Travelers should avoid swimming in fresh-water in endemic

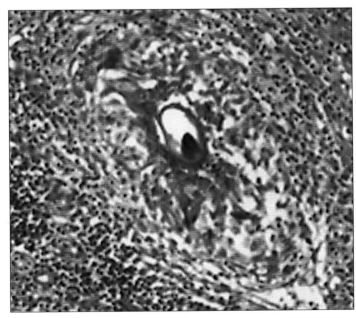

Figure 17.3 Liver biopsy schistosomiasis egg causing granulomatous hepatitis. (Courtesy of Dr Sanaa Kamal.)

areas. In these areas, bathing water should be heated for 5 min prior to use and pretreated with chlorine or iodine. Some sources also suggest allowing bath water to stand for 3 days prior to use as the larvae only survive for 48 h.

Ascariasis
Background
Ascariasis is a helminthic infection caused by the nematode *Ascaris lumbricoides*. *A. lumbricoides* is both the most prevalent and largest of human helminths. Adult worms can be up to 50 cm in length and 6 mm in width. Ascariasis is most commonly seen in crowded rural areas. It is related to the density of population, dietary habits, sanitation and agricultural customs. It is estimated that 1.4 billion people are infected with *Ascaris*. Ascariasis is a global problem as it is endemic in parts of Southeast Asia, China, India, Africa and Latin America. In the USA, it is estimated that over 4 million people are infected. A large percentage of those infected in the USA are thought to be immigrants from endemic areas.

Life cycle
Infection with *Ascaris* usually occurs after ingestion of embryonated eggs that exist in the hospitable environment of moist soil. These eggs can commonly infect water and food supplies. After ingestion, the outer layer of the egg is digested by gastric juices. The larvae emerge in the duodenum. In the small intestine, the larvae can penetrate the intestinal mucosa and enter the portal system thereby entering the liver and then freely move either through the bloodstream or the lymphatic system throughout the body. Once the larvae reach the bronchial tree and upper respiratory tract, they are then swallowed and re-enter the digestive system. At this point, they undergo a sexual maturation in the small intestine that takes approximately 3 months. The adult worm then is able to exist in the lumen of the human intestine through the use of its muscles. Its lifespan may be anywhere from 6 months to up to 2 years during which time the female adult will release millions of egg into the feces.

Clinical signs and symptoms
The clinical presentation of ascariasis is very much related to the organism's life cycle. In most hosts, the infection is asymptomatic. However, if the organism burden is high enough, clinical disease will be present. Hepatobiliary ascariasis is one of the most common manifestations of this disease. Not only can the larvae infect the liver, but the worm itself can enter the hepatic ductal system from the ampulla of Vater in the small intestines. Therefore, the spectrum of disease ranges from hepatic abscess to biliary disease. In the liver, live larvae do not cause an inflammatory response. However, if the organism dies in the liver, or in any organ for that matter, a granulomatous reaction occurs. In some areas ascariasis is as common as gallstones as a cause of biliary disease. Given the range of pathophysiology, the symptoms can be anything from simple biliary colic to vague weight loss and epigastric discomfort to fever and intense right upper quadrant pain. Protein malnutrition, especially in children, is a common manifestation of ascariasis. Depending on the degree of liver involvement and/or biliary disease accounting for any obstruction, liver enzyme tests may be abnormal. While the worm is present in the bloodstream of the patient a peripheral eosinophilia will also be present.

Diagnosis
Ascariasis can be diagnosed by finding the worms, larvae or eggs in the feces. If the infection is only with male worms, no eggs will be detected in the stool. Diagnosis of hepatobiliary ascariasis is usually made with ultrasound and/or endoscopic retrograde cholangiopancreatography (ERCP). Ultrasound is useful in detecting worms in the biliary tree and hepatic abscesses. On ERCP, ductal ascariasis will present as smooth linear filling defects. ERCP allows the added benefit of then removing the worms from the ductal system and, if present, in the duodenum. Liver abscesses caused by *Ascaris* have no distinct clinical features and percutaneous needle aspiration is often needed for both therapeutic and diagnostic purposes. Examination of the fluid will reveal broken or collapsed eggs. The necrotic focus in the liver is usually surrounded by granulomatous hepatitis.

Treatment
Treatment of hepatobiliary ascariasis usually consists of supportive care for the cholangitis/pancreatitis that may be present as well as oral administration of antihelminthic agents to paralyze the worms in the intestine. Antihelminthic agents that are commonly used include pyrantel pamoate, mebendazole and albendazole, all administered as single doses. Parasite paralysis and death with clearance from the intestine can take up to 3 days. Endoscopic intervention with worm extraction is performed if patients do not respond to treatment within a few days or if after 3 weeks the worms in the ducts have not migrated out into the intestine.

Liver flukes
Life cycle and epidemiology
The groups of parasitic trematodes commonly referred to as the liver flukes include the *Opisthorchis* and *Clonorchis* species as well as *Fasciola hepatica*. These organisms asexually reproduce in their intermediate host, which is usually the snail. They then multiply into thousands of free-swimming cercariae which penetrate freshwater fish and are then infective to humans when eaten raw, as in the case of *Opisthorchis* and *Clonorchis*, or encyst on plants like watercress, as is the case with *Fasciola*. In the human, they undergo sexual reproduction. As adults, they are flat, hermaphroditic worms that range in size from a few millimeters to several centimeters. They pass directly into the bile ducts through the ampulla of Vater. *F. hepatica* can actually penetrate the intestinal mucosa into the peritoneum and then enter the liver and the biliary tree from there. They then excrete their eggs into feces. The adult worm can survive for decades in the bile ducts.

Epidemiologically, *Opisthorchis* and *Clonorchis* are very similar. They are found primarily in Eastern Europe and Asia. *Clonorchis* is endemic in China, Hong Kong, Japan, Taiwan and Vietnam, where dogs and cats can serve as reservoirs. *Fasciola*, however, is quite distinct epidemiologically from *Clonorchis* and *Opisthorchis*. It primarily affects sheep and cattle and can be found where they are raised worldwide.

Clinical course

Most people infected with liver flukes are asymptomatic. However, in acute infection, if the worm burden is high enough, patients will be symptomatic. Patients will present with fever, right upper quadrant pain, anorexia, and diarrhea 10–26 days after ingestion of the larvae that may last a few days to weeks during the migrating stage of the larvae. Liver tests and imaging are likely to be normal, but patients will have a peripheral eosinophilia. Over time the flukes can cause mechanical injury to the bile ducts. They are also thought to secrete substances that are toxic and immunogenic in the biliary tree. This inflammation results in periductal fibrosis, bile duct dilatation and epithelial hyperplasia. This pathology places patients at risk for cholangitis, cholangiohepatitis and even cholangiocarcinoma.

Diagnosis and treatment

Diagnosis of liver fluke infection can be accomplished by demonstrating eggs in the stool, bile or ascitic fluid. However, stool studies may be negative as eggs may only be produced intermittently. An ELISA test for antiparasitic antibodies and antigens can then be performed. *Opisthorchis* and *Clonorchis* can be successfully treated with one single oral dose of praziquantel. *Fasciola*, however, is best treated with bithionol which can be obtained in the USA from the Centers for Disease Control and Prevention (CDC). *Fasciola* is relatively resistant to praziquantel, and it has not been shown to be effective in eradicating infection.

FURTHER READING

Syphilis
Agrawal NM, Sassaris M, Brooks B, et al. The liver in secondary syphilis. South Med J 1982; 75(9):1136–1138.

Maincent G, Labadie H, Fabre M, et al. Tertiary hepatic syphilis. A treatable cause of multinodular liver. Dig Dis Sci 1997; 42(2):447–450.

Schlossberg D. Syphilitic hepatitis: a case report and review of the literature. Am J Gastroenterol 1987; 82(6):552–553.

Echinoccoccus
Akhan O, Ozmen MN. Percutaneous treatment of liver hydatid cysts. Eur J Radiol 1999; 32(1):76–85.

Gottstein B. Molecular and immunological diagnosis of echinococcosis. Clin Microbiol Rev 1992; 5(3):248–261.

Smego RA, Jr, Bhatti S, Khaliq AA, et al. Percutaneous aspiration-injection-reaspiration drainage plus albendazole or mebendazole for hepatic cystic echinococcosis: a meta-analysis. Clin Infect Dis 2003; 37(8):1073–1083.

Candidiasis
Bjerke JW, Meyers JD, Bowden RA. Hepatosplenic candidiasis – a contraindication to marrow. Blood 1994; 84(8):2811–2814. *Observational study of 15 patients followed prospectively after marrow transplantation.*

Karthaus M, Huebner G, Elser C, et al. Early detection of chronic disseminated *Candida* infection in leukemia patients with febrile neutropenia: value of computer-assisted serial ultrasound documentation. Ann Hematol 1998; 77(1–2):41–45.

Pappas PG, Rex JH, Sobel JD, et al. Guidelines for treatment of candidiasis. Clin Infect Dis 2004; 38(2):161–189.

Listeriosis
Braun TI, Travis D, Dee RR, et al. Liver abscess due to *Listeria monocytogenes*: case report and review. Clin Infect Dis 1993; 17(2):267–269.

Hof H, Nichterlein T, Kretschmar M. Management of listeriosis. Clin Microbiol Rev 1997; 10(2):345–357.

Leptospirosis
Levett PN. Leptospirosis. Clin Microbiol Rev 2001; 14(2):296–326. *Excellent review of pathogenesis, clinical presentation and diagnosis.*

Panaphut T, Domrongkitchaiporn S, Vibhagool A, et al. Ceftriaxone compared with sodium penicillin g for treatment of severe leptospirosis. Clin Infect Dis 2003; 36(12):1507–1513.

Cytomegalovirus
Ljungman P, Griffiths P, Paya C. Definitions of cytomegalovirus infection and disease in transplant recipients. Clin Infect Dis 2002; 34(8):1094–1097.

Oldakowska-Jedynak U, Niewczas M, Ziolkowski J, et al. Cytomegalovirus infection as a common complication following liver transplantation. Transplant Proc 2003; 35(6):2295–2297.

Wreghitt TG, Teare EL, Sule O, et al. Cytomegalovirus infection in immunocompetent patients. Clin Infect Dis 2003; 37(12):1603–1606.

Miscellaneous
Bonacini M. Hepatobiliary complications in patients with human immunodeficiency virus infection. Am J Med 1992; 92(4):404–411.

Haque R, Huston CD, Hughes M, et al. Amebiasis. N Engl J Med 2003; 348(16):1565–1573. *Excellent review of amebiasis, everything from pathogenesis to treatment.*

Khuroo MS. Ascariasis. Gastroenterol Clin North Am 1996; 25(3):553–577.

Klioze AM, Ramos-Caro FA. Visceral leprosy. Int J Dermatol 2000; 39(9):641–658.

Liu LX, Harinasuta KT. Liver and intestinal flukes. Gastroenterol Clin North Am 1996; 25(3):627–636.

Markin RS. Manifestations of Epstein-Barr virus-associated disorders in liver. Liver 1994; 14(1):1–13. *Examination of broad clinical presentations of EBV.*

Piggott JA, Hochholzer L. Human melioidosis. A histopathologic study of acute and chronic melioidosis. Arch Pathol 1970; 90(2):101–111.

Rahmatulla RH, al-Mofleh IA, al-Rashed RS. Tuberculous liver abscess: a case report and review of literature. Eur J Gastroenterol Hepatol 2001; 13(4):437–440.

Ross AG, Bartley PB, Sleigh AC, et al. Schistosomiasis. N Engl J Med 2002; 346(16):1212–1220.

Salles JM, Moraes LA, Salles MC. Hepatic amebiasis. Braz J Infect Dis 2003; 7(2):96–110.

White NJ. Melioidosis. Lancet 2003; 361(9370):1715–1722. *Comprehensive historical and clinical review.*

Williams RK, Crossley K. Acute and chronic hepatic involvement of brucellosis. Gastroenterology 1982; 83(2):455–458.

SECTION IV: SPECIFIC DISEASES OF LIVER AND BILIARY TREE

CHAPTER 18
Autoimmune Hepatitis

Christian P. Strassburg, Arndt Vogel and Michael P. Manns

INTRODUCTION

Autoimmune hepatitis (AIH) is a chronic inflammatory disease of the liver, characterized by a loss of tolerance against hepatic tissue. Historically, AIH was first defined by Waldenström in 1950 when he described a form of chronic hepatitis in young women showing jaundice, elevated γ-globulins and amenorrhea, which eventually led to liver cirrhosis. This form of chronic hepatitis was later also noticed in combination with other extrahepatic autoimmune syndromes. Mainly due to similarities with systemic lupus erythematosus and in particular the presence of antinuclear antibodies (ANA) it was initially termed lupoid hepatitis by Mackay (56). Systematic evaluation of the cellular and molecular immunopathology, of the clinical symptoms and of laboratory features has subsequently led to the establishment of autoimmune hepatitis as a separate clinical entity which has been subclassified based on serology, and is treated by a specific therapeutic strategy (**Table 18.1**). A recently established and meanwhile revised scoring system allows for a reproducible and standardized approach to diagnosing and consequently treating AIH in a scientific context (**Table 18.2**). The use and interpretation of seroimmunological and molecular biological tests together with the exclusion of other etiologies and the scoring system permits a precise discrimination of autoimmune hepatitis from other etiologies of chronic hepatitis, in particular from chronic viral infection as the most common cause of chronic hepatitis worldwide.

Differential diagnosis of autoimmune hepatitis and diagnostic tests	
Suspected differential diagnosis	*Test performed to exclude*
Hepatitis C infection (HCV)	Anti-HCV (HCV RNA)
Hepatitis B and D (HBV, HDV)	HBsAg, anti-HBc (HBV DNA) Anti-HDV, HDV DNA only when HBsAg positive
Hepatitis A virus	Antibodies, serology: IgG, IgM
Hepatitis E virus	Only if suspected
Epstein-Barr virus	Only if suspected
Herpes simplex virus	Only if suspected
Cytomegalovirus	Only if suspected
Varicella zoster virus	Only if suspected
Drug induced hepatitis	History, if applicable withdrawal of drug. LKM-2, LM autoantibody in selected cases
Primary biliary cirrhosis	Antimitochondrial antibodies specificity of reactivity: PDH-E2, BCKD-E2 Liver histology: copper deposition in bile ducts Unresponsive to steroids
Primary sclerosing cholangitis	Cholangiography
Wilson disease	Ceruloplasmin, urine copper, eye examination, quantitative copper in liver biopsy
Hemochromatosis	Serum ferritin, serum iron, transferrin saturation, liver histology: iron staining, quantitative iron in biopsy Genetic testing: *C282Y, H63D* mutation of *HFE* gene in Caucasoids
α_1-Antitrypsin deficiency	Phenotype testing: PiZZ/PiSS/PiMZ/PiSZ

HBc, hepatitis B core; HBsAg, hepatitis B surface antigen; IgG, immunoglobulin G; IgM, immunoglobulin M; LKM, liver–kidney microsomal autoantibodies; LM, liver microsomal.

Table 18.1 Differential diagnosis of autoimmune hepatitis and diagnostic tests.

International diagnostic criteria for the diagnosis of autoimmune hepatitis	
Parameter	*Score*
Gender	
Female	+ 2
Male	0
Serum biochemistry	
Ratio of elevation of serum alkaline phosphatase versus aminotransferase	
>3.0	− 2
1.5–3	0
<1.5	+ 2
Total serum globulin, γ-globulin or IgG	
Times upper normal limit	
>2.0	+ 3
1.5-2.0	+ 2
1.0-1.5	+ 1
<1.0	0
Autoantibodies (titers by immunofluorescence on rodent tissues)	
Adults	
ANA, SMA or LKM-1	+ 3
>1:80	+ 2
1:80	+ 1
1:40	0
<1:40	
Antimitochondrial antibody	
Positive	− 4
Negative	0
Hepatitis viral markers	
Negative	+ 3
Positive	− 3
Other etiological factors	
History of drug usage	
Yes	− 4
No	+ 1
Alcohol (average consumption)	
<25 g/day	+ 2
>60 g/day	− 2
Genetic factors: HLA DR3 or DR4	+ 1
Other autoimmune diseases	+ 2
Response to therapy	
Complete	+ 2
Relapse	+ 3
Liver histology	
Interface hepatitis	+ 3
Predominant lymphoplasmacytic infiltrate	+ 1
Rosetting of liver cells	+ 1
None of the above	− 5
Biliary changes	− 3
Other changes	− 3
Seropositivity for other defined autoantibodies	+ 2

ANA, antinuclear antibodies; IgG, immunoglobulin G, LKM-1, liver–kidney microsomal autoantibodies; SMA, smooth muscle antibodies. Interpretation of aggregate scores: definite autoimmune hepatitis (AIH), >15 before treatment and >17 after treatment; probable AIH, 10–15 before treatment and 12–17 after treatment. Reproduced from Alvarez et al (99) by permission of Wiley-Liss, Inc.

Table 18.2 International diagnostic criteria for the diagnosis of autoimmune hepatitis.

fixed neutrophils. The target antigen in AIH is unknown, but, apart from myeloperoxidase, proteinase 3 and elastase have been ruled out as candidates. The role of ANCA in AIH is unclear, but routine determination might be useful to identify patients formerly classified as having cryptogenic hepatitis.

ETIOLOGY OF AIH

Conclusive evidence of a single etiology of AIH has not yet been presented. Many findings have pointed towards a viral etiology which has been investigated by numerous studies. However, a viral etiology of AIH remains a matter of controversy. In anecdotal reports the relationship of the hepatitis A virus, hepatitis B virus, EBV and herpes simplex virus (HSV) with autoimmune hepatitis has been implicated. As a potential mechanism molecular mimicry between viral and body proteins has been suggested. In this respect, it was shown that the B-cell epitope of CYP2D6, which is targeted by LKM-1 autoantibodies, displays homology with the immediate early antigen IE175 of HSV. A case has been reported in which the only difference in HLA identical twins with discordant manifestation of AIH was HSV exposure.

HCV infection is associated with a broad array of serological markers of autoimmunity and immune-mediated syndromes. LKM autoantibodies are present in 3–5%. However, this serological autoimmunity differs with respect to recognition of antigen targets (CYP2D6 and CYP2A6), recognition of epitopes (AIH mainly 257–269, HCV more diverse and also more conformation dependent epitopes) and the clinical presentation. From these considerations it is unlikely that HCV is etiologically responsible for AIH.

Apart from viral agents a genetic predisposition must be regarded as a mandatory prerequisite of AIH. However, the genetic background of AIH does not follow a Mendelian pattern and a conclusive role of a single genetic locus capable of explaining the etiology of AIH has not yet been identified. AIH is therefore considered as a complex trait like most other human diseases, which means that there are numerous genes acting alone or in concert to reduce or increase the risk of that trait. The inheritable component of AIH is currently regarded as small. However, the absence of evidence does not mean evidence of absence and these data have yet to be established.

The most conclusive association with AIH is related to the major histocompatibility complex (MHC) alleles. The significance of HLA polymorphisms in terms of disease susceptibility and severity lies in the observation that most autoimmune reactions are T-cell dependent and all T-cell mediated responses are MHC restricted. In European patients several studies identified a strong genetic association with the HLA haplotype A1-B8-DRB1*0301 and DRB*0401 (**Table 18.4**). Patients with the HLA A1-B8-DRB1*0301 haplotype were found to be younger at disease onset, relapse more frequently under immunosuppressive treatment and more frequently require liver transplantation. Subsequent investigations of the encoding HLA alleles identified that genetic susceptibility to AIH is related to the six amino acid sequence LLEQKR at position 67–72 of the DRB1 polypeptide. Within these six amino acids the critical amino acid appears to be that found on position 71 – namely, lysine or arginine on susceptibility alleles and alanine on resistance alleles. Polymorphisms within this region may affect the predisposition to autoimmune diseases by several mechanisms. This

Classification of autoimmune hepatitis based on genetic markers		
HLA	*DR3*	*DR4*
Genotype	DR B1*0301	DR B1*0401 (DR B1*0405 in Japanese)
Age at onset	<30	>40
Disease activity	+++	+
Treatment response	++	++++
Relapse after treatment	+++	+
Liver transplantation	+++	+
DR β chain amino acid as risk factor	Lysine at AA71	?

Table 18.4 Classification of autoimmune hepatitis based on genetic markers.

includes shaping of the T-cell repertoire, peptide selection and presentation as well as peptide transport. However, exactly how particular HLA alleles contribute to autoimmunity is still poorly understood. Analysis of MHC genes in different populations of AIH patients revealed that the immunogenetic associations with AIH vary regionally. Along this line an alternative model based on valine/glycine dimorphism at position –86 pf the DR β-polypeptide has been proposed, which better represents the key HLA associations in patients from Argentina and Brazil. These findings are likely to be influenced by genetic heterogeneity that exists in evolutionary divergent populations. On the other hand they may reflect different underlying etiologies in terms of initiating events such as different viral triggers. Regardless of the mechanisms, it is apparent that the MHC locus per se is insufficient for the development of autoimmune diseases, as shown by the decrease of the autoimmune disease concordance rate of siblings in comparison to that of monozygotic twins. Therefore several studies have focused on other non-MHC genes and variations in a number of genes that are important in the regulation of immune responses have been associated with the development of AIH.

Tumor necrosis factor-α (TNF-α) has diverse effects on immune responses and inflammatory cells. In some contexts, TNF-α promotes self-tolerance and T-cell deletion, whereas in others TNF-α promotes T-cell activation and autoimmune diseases. Two polymorphisms in the TNF promoter have been identified: one at position 308 (TNF2) and another at position 238 (TNFA). Some studies have shown that TNF2 and TNFA lead to increased constitutive and inducible expression compared with the wild type TNF, although this remains a matter of debate. TNF2 has been associated with an increased risk of developing AIH of a type with an unfavorable clinical course. However, TNF-α exhibits a strong linkage disequilibrium with the HLA A1-B8-DR3 haplotype and stratification analysis indicates that the association with the TNF2 promoter polymorphism is interdependent with DRB1*0301. This is further confirmed by findings in a population where the disease is not primarily associated with HLA-DRB1*03. AIH in Brazilian patients is obviously not linked to TNF-α polymorphisms at position −308. Polymorphisms of other candidate genes encoding proinflammatory and immunoregulatory cytokines such the IL-1B, IL-1RN and IL-10 genes are not associated with AIH.

Cytotoxic T-lymphocyte antigen 4 (CTLA4) and CD28 are important regulators of T-lymphocyte activation and polymorphisms of *CTLA4* have been linked to a variety of autoimmune diseases. A single nucleotide polymorphism at position −318 of the CTLA4 gene is located in the promoter region. Another polymorphism, an A/G variation at position +49 in the first exon of the gene leads to a threonine to alanine change in the leader peptide and was found to correlate with a reduced inhibitory function of CTLA4. A similar effect on CTLA4 function has been suggested for the third polymorphism, a microsatellite AT repeat, which is located in the 3′ untranslated region of the last exon and has at least 20 alleles. All three polymorphisms are in strong linkage disequilibrium, which makes it difficult to distinguish which variations actually cause the functional difference. In addition, an increased transmission of the 49A alleles and *CTLA4 (AT)$_n$* has been reported in children with type 1 AIH, but interestingly no deviation in transmission was found in AIH type 2. This genetic heterogeneity might indicate genetic differences between type 1 and type 2 AIH.

In a recent analysis a lack of genetic association between idiopathic autoimmune liver diseases and hepatitis as part of APECED has been demonstrated. APECED is a rare autosomal recessive disorder which is characterized by an immune-mediated destruction of endocrine tissues, chronic candidiasis and additional ectodermal disorders. Typically, the disease presentation includes candidiasis, hypoparathyroidism and adrenocortical failure. The spectrum of associated clinical disease components includes insulin-dependent diabetes mellitus, autoimmune thyroid disease, pernicious anemia and chronic active hepatitis. While the phenotype of the syndrome is largely heterogeneous, APECED is viewed as a genetically homogenous syndrome caused by mutations in a recently identified gene, the autoimmune regulator, *AIRE*. The expression pattern and the predicted protein function suggest that *AIRE* plays a role in the induction and maintenance of immune tolerance. Interestingly, the recently created *AIRE* knock out mice present like human APECED patients with a variable combination of endocrine and non-endocrine autoimmune components with a variable age of onset. The variety of autoimmune diseases seen in APECED patients suggested that *AIRE* might contribute to the etiology of other autoimmune disorders. However, recent findings indicate that common mutations in the *AIRE* gene do not play a major role in sporadic autoimmune diseases such as autoimmune thyroid disease, diabetes mellitus type 1, Addison disease and autoimmune liver diseases, and are therefore a unique feature of APECED. Similar to AIH type 2, hepatitis in APECED is associated with autoantibodies directed against cytochrome P450 proteins. In patients with APECED, autoantibodies to CYP1A2 and CYP2A6 have been described as markers of an autoimmune liver disease. However, recent data indicate that only antibodies to CYP1A2 are specific for hepatitis in APECED, albeit with a low sensitivity. Furthermore, it has been demonstrated that there is no overlap between the different molecular targets of microsomal autoantibodies in AIH and APECED patients.

CLINICAL FEATURES AND SUBCLASSIFICATION

Clinical features

Systematically, AIH is part of the syndrome of chronic hepatitis, which is characterized by sustained hepatocellular inflammation of at least 6 months duration and elevation of alanine aminotransferase (ALT) and aspartate aminotransferase (AST) of 1.5 times the upper normal limit. In about half of AIH patients an acute onset of AIH is observed and rare cases of fulminant AIH have been reported. In the remainder, the clinical presentation is not spectacular and characterized by fatigue, right upper quadrant pain, jaundice and occasionally also by palmar erythema and spider nevi. In later stages, the consequences of portal hypertension dominate, including ascites, bleeding esophageal varices and encephalopathy. A specific feature of AIH is the association of extrahepatic immune-mediated syndromes including autoimmune thyroiditis, vitiligo, alopecia, nail dystrophy, ulcerative colitis, rheumatoid arthritis, diabetes mellitus and glomerulonephritis (**Table 18.5**).

Subclassification

Immunoserological parameters assume a central role in the subclassification of AIH and allow the discrimination of clinically differing groups of patients. The International Autoimmune Hepatitis Group (IAIHG) has not recommended these subdivisions for other than research purposes, because autoantibodies do not define distinct therapeutic groups. However, they noted that the distinction between AIH type 1 and type 2 has already been widely adopted in clinical practice.

AIH type 1 is characterized by ANA and in most cases also SMA autoantibodies. In 97% of patients hypergammaglobulinemia with elevated immunoglobulin G (IgG) is present. Representing 80% of the cases of AIH, this form is the most prevalent subclass, which was historically described as lupoid, classical or idiopathic AIH. Of these patients, 70% are female with a peak incidence between the ages of 16 and 30 years. However, 50% are older than 30 years. An association with other immune syndromes is observed in 48%, with autoimmune thyroid disease, synovitis and ulcerative colitis being the most prevalent. The

Extrahepatic associations of autoimmune hepatitis are present in 10–50% of patients	
Frequent	Autoimmune thyroid disease Ulcerative colitis Synovitis
Rare or individual reports	Rheumatoid arthritis Lichen planus Diabetes mellitus CREST syndrome Autoimmune thrombocytopenic purpura Vitiligo Nail dystrophy Alopecia
CREST, calcinosis cutis, Raynaud phenomenon, esophageal hypomobility, sclerodactyly, telangiectasia.	

Table 18.5 Extrahepatic associations of autoimmune hepatitis are present in 10–50% of patients.

clinical course is often unspectacular and acute onset is rare. About 25% have cirrhosis at the time of diagnosis.

Autoimmune hepatitis type 2 is characterized by the presence of LKM-1 autoantibodies. In 10% LKM-3 autoantibodies are also present. In contrast to AIH type 1, additional organ-specific autoantibodies are present such as antithyroid, antiparietal cell and anti-Langerhans cell autoantibodies. Extrahepatic immune syndromes such as diabetes, vitiligo and autoimmune thyroid disease are also more prevalent. Serum immunoglobulin levels are moderately elevated with a reduction of immunoglobulin A (IgA). AIH type 2 affects 20% of AIH patients in Europe but only 4% in the USA. There is again a female predominance. The peak age at presentation is around 10 years but AIH type 2 is also observed in adults, especially in Europe. AIH type 2 carries a higher risk of acute presentation and progression to cirrhosis.

Autoimmune hepatitis type 3 is characterized by SLA/LP autoantibodies, but 74% also have other serological markers of autoimmunity, including SMA and AMA. AIH type 3 has a lower prevalence than AIH type 2. 90% of affected patients are female with a peak in age between 20 and 40 years. AIH type 3 is a matter of debate and further evaluations will have to determine whether it represents an entity in itself or is a variation of AIH type 1. However, it is important to diagnose anti-SLA/LP-positive AIH, which occurs in 10% of AIH cases as the only serological markers. This may therefore decrease the likelihood of misclassification.

Differentiation of cryptogenic hepatitis and overlap syndromes

Cryptogenic hepatitis is an etiologically undefined chronic hepatitis. It is unclear how many of these patients in fact suffer from AIH without the presence of serum autoantibodies detectable with the available state-of-the-art techniques. In about 13% of these patients, who had initially been tested by indirect immunofluorescence for ANA, SMA and LKM, it was possible to detect SLA autoantibodies and contribute to their diagnostic clarification. Clinically this group of cryptogenic hepatitis resembles AIH type 1 with respect to age and sex distribution, HLA antigen types, inflammatory activity and response to therapy.

Overlap syndromes are conditions in which there are leading symptoms of AIH, but with additional markers or symptoms pointing to other diseases within the differential diagnosis of AIH. Among these are PBC in 8% with serum AMA and histologic signs of cholangitis, PSC in 6% with typical changes of the cholangiography, and autoimmune cholangitis in 10% with ANA, SMA and histologic inflammation of the biliary system. However, a concise and universally accepted definition of an overlap syndrome is currently lacking. In addition the frequency of this condition is a matter of controversy.

A clinically significant association is virus-associated autoimmunity, which describes the coexistence of autoantibodies and virus infection. The most important associations are HCV infection and HDV infection in which LKM autoantibodies can be detected in 2–5% and 6–12%, respectively. AIH type 2 and HCV infection with LKM autoantibodies are clinically distinct entities (**Table 18.6**). LKM autoantibodies in virus infection are present at lower titers and recognize more conformational and diverse epitopes than in genuine AIH. This discrimination is relevant since it forms the basis for mutually exclusive thera-

Comparison between genuine and virus-induced autoimmunity		
	Autoimmune hepatitis	Viral hepatitis
Autoantibody titer	↑↑↑	↑
Linear autoepitopes	+ + +	+
Conformational epitopes	+	+ + + +
Inhibitory antibodies	+ +	+ +
Autoimmune response	Homogenous	Heterogeneous
Treatment	Immunosuppression	(Antiviral)

Table 18.6 Comparison between genuine and virus-induced autoimmunity.

peutic strategies: immunosuppresssion in AIH and interferon in chronic virus hepatitis.

NATURAL HISTORY AND PROGNOSIS

Data describing the natural history of AIH are scarce. The last placebo-controlled immunosuppressive treatment trial was published in 1980. The value of these studies is limited considering that these patients were only screened for epidemiological risk factors for viral hepatitis and had not been characterized by standardized diagnostic criteria. Nevertheless these studies revealed that untreated AIH had a very poor prognosis and 5- and 10-year survival rates of 50% and 10% have been reported. They furthermore demonstrated that immunosuppressive treatment significantly improved survival.

Recent data revealed that up to 30% of adult patients had histologic features of cirrhosis at diagnosis. In 17% of patients with periportal hepatitis cirrhosis developed within 5 years, but cirrhosis develops in 82% when bridging necrosis or necrosis of multiple lobules is present. The frequency of remission (86%) and treatment failure (14%) are comparable in patients with and without cirrhosis at presentation. Importantly, the presence of cirrhosis does not influence the 10-year survival rate (90%) and these patients require a similarly aggressive treatment strategy.

Almost half of the children with AIH already have cirrhosis at the time of diagnosis. Long-term follow-up revealed that only a few children can completely stop all treatment and about 70% of children receive long-term treatment. Most of these patients relapse when treatment is discontinued, or if the dose of immunosuppressive drug is reduced. About 15% of patients develop chronic liver failure and are transplanted before the age of 18 years.

In elderly patients, a more severe initial histologic grade has been reported, but the frequency of definite cirrhosis seems not to differ from that of younger patients. At follow-up, about 30% of patients develop cirrhosis. Response to immunosuppression is similar in old and young patients and up to 90% of the older patients reach complete remission. However, in a study from the UK, 41% of the elderly patients with AIH received no immunosuppressive therapy and the prognosis did not appear to be worse than that for younger patients who usually receive

Treatment regimen* and follow-up examinations of autoimmune hepatitis regardless of autoantibody type		
	Monotherapy	*Combination therapy*
Prednis(ol)one	60 mg	30 mg
	Reduce within 4 weeks to maintenance dose 20 mg or lower	Reduce within 4 weeks to maintenance dose 10 mg or lower
Azathioprine	n.a. (consider maintenance with azathioprine: monotherapy: 2 mg/kg body weight)	50–150 mg
After remission is reached (treatment length 12–24 months) monitor, consider repeat biopsy, avoid premature treatment reduction		
Prednis(ol)one	Reduction of daily dose by 2.5 mg/week	Reduction of daily dose by 2.5 mg/week
Azathioprine	n.a.	Reduction: 25 mg every 3 weeks to 50 mg per day

Examination	*Before therapy*	*During therapy before remission – 4 weeks*	*Remission under therapy – 3–6 months*	*Cessation of therapy – 3 weeks*	*Remission post-therapy – 3–6 months (x 4)*	*Evaluation of relapse*
Physical	+		+	+	+	+
Liver biopsy	+		(+/−)			+
Blood count	+	+	+	+	+	
Aminotransferases	+	+	+	+	+	+
γ-glutamyltransferase	+	+	+			
γ-globulin	+	+	+	+	+	+
Bilirubin	+	+	+	+	+	+
Coagulation studies	+	+	+	+	+	
Autoantibodies	+	+/−				+
Thyroid function tests	+	+/−				+

n.a. – not applicable. In the elderly patient with low inflammatory activity the indication to treat must be weighed against side-effects and some of these patients may best remain untreated. *The table reflects the Mayo Clinic approach. In our own experience, monotherapy with prednisolone beginning with 50 mg and tapered by 10 mg every 10 days to a maintenance dose of 15–20 mg is equally effective as combination therapy with 1 mg/kg body weight of azathioprine for 3 weeks and tapering to 50 mg daily combined with prednisolone therapy tapered to 10 mg daily. There is no published evidence of an advantage of an individual tapering regimen and different tapering and dosing regimens are employed by different centers. In the individual young patient without severe symptoms and with low inflammatory activity [inactive biopsy, alanine aminotransferase (ALT) <5 × upper limit of normal] treatment can be initiated with maintenance doses.

Table 18.7 Treatment regimen* and follow-up examinations of autoimmune hepatitis regardless of autoantibody type.

treatment. Hepatocellular carcinoma can complicate AIH cirrhosis, although with a lower frequency than in other etiologies of cirrhosis.

TREATMENT

Medical treatment

The indication for treatment of AIH is based on inflammatory activity and not so much on the presence of cirrhosis. In the absence of inflammatory activity immunosuppressive treatment has only limited effects. Independent of AIH type, treatment is initiated with prednis(ol)one alone or in combination with azathioprine. Both strategies are equally effective. The use of prednisone or its metabolite prednisolone is equally effective since chronic liver disease does not seem to have an effect on the synthesis of prednisolone from prednisone. It is important

to differentiate between virus infection and autoimmune hepatitis prior to starting therapy as corticosteroids induce viral replication while interferon can lead to dramatic disease exacerbations in AIH.

An indication for treatment is present when aminotransferases are elevated twofold, γ-globulin levels are elevated and histology shows moderate to severe periportal hepatitis. Symptoms of severe fatigue are also an indication for treatment. An absolute indication exists in cases with a 10-fold or higher elevation of aminotransferase levels, histologic signs of severe inflammation and necrosis, and with disease progression.

The treatment regimen and suggested follow-up examinations are summarized in **Table 18.7**. Therapy is usually administered over the course of 2–3 years. The decision between monotherapy and combination therapy is guided by the balance between efficacy and toxicity. Long-term corticosteroid therapy leads to

Side-effects of prednis(ol)one and azathioprine	
Side-effects of prednis(ol)one	Acne
	Moon-shaped face
	Striae rubrae
	Dorsal hump
	Obesity
	Weight gain
	Osteoporosis
	Aseptic bone necrosis
	Psychiatric symptoms (euphoria, psychosis, depression)
	Diabetes mellitus
	Cataract
	Hypertension
Side-effects of azathioprine	Nausea
	Vomiting
	Abdominal discomfort
	Hepatotoxicity
	Rash
	Leucocytopenia
	Teratogenicity?
	Oncogenicity?

Table 18.8 Side-effects of prednis(ol)one and azathioprine.

cushingoid side-effects that may reduce patient compliance considerably (**Table 18.8**). Serious complications such as diabetes, osteopenia, aseptic bone necrosis, psychiatric symptoms, hypertension and cataract formation also have to be anticipated in long-term treatment. Side-effects are present in 44% of patients after 12 months and in 80% of patients after 24 months of treatment. Predniso(lo)ne monotherapy is possible in pregnant patients. Azathioprine reduces reliance on corticosteroids, especially in maintenance therapy. It bears a theoretical risk of teratogenicity but this fear has not been borne out in clinical experience. In addition, abdominal discomfort, nausea, cholestatic hepatitis, rashes and leucopenia can be encountered. These side-effects are seen in 10% of patients receiving a dose of 50 mg/day. From a general point of view, a postmenopausal woman with osteoporosis, hypertension and elevated blood glucose would be a candidate for combination therapy. In young women, pregnant women or patients with hematological abnormalities, prednis(ol)one monotherapy may be the treatment of choice.

Treatment is initiated according to the regimen in Table 18.8. Continuous administration is essential since most cases of relapse are the result of erratic changes of medication and/or dosage. Dose reduction is aimed at finding the optimal maintenance regimen for each individual patient. Since histology lags 3–6 months behind the normalization of serum parameters, therapy has to be continued beyond the normalization of aminotransferase levels. Usually, maintenance doses of prednis(ol)one range between 2.5 and 10 mg. After 12–24 months of therapy prednis(ol)one can be tapered over the course of 4–6 weeks to test whether a sustained remission has been achieved. Tapering regimens should be attempted with great caution and only after obtaining a liver biopsy that demonstrates a complete resolution of inflammatory activity. Relapse of AIH, and the risk of progression of fibrosis,

is almost universal when immunosuppression is tapered in the presence of residual histologic inflammation.

Outcomes can be classified into four categories: remission, relapse, stabilization and treatment failure.

- Remission is a complete normalization of all inflammatory parameters including histology. This is achieved in 65% of patients after 24 months of treatment. Remission can be sustained with azathioprine monotherapy with doses up to 2 mg/kg body weight. This prevents cushingoid side-effects. However, side-effects such as arthralgia (53%), myalgia (14%), lymphopenia (57%) and myelosuppression (6%) have been observed.

- Relapse is characterized by a threefold increase of aminotransferase levels and the reoccurrence of clinical symptoms. Relapse is present in 50% of patients within 6 months of treatment withdrawal and in 80% after 3 years. Relapse is associated with progression to cirrhosis in 38% and liver failure in 14%. Occurrence of a relapse calls for re-initiation of standard therapy and perhaps long-term maintenance with prednis(ol)one or azathioprine monotherapy.

- Stabilization is the achievement of a partial remission not fulfilling the definition of remission. Since 90% of patients are expected to attain remission within 3 years, the therapeutic strategy should be re-evaluated in this subgroup of patients, particularly with regard to the use of the newer immunosuppressive agents. Ultimately, liver transplantation may be required.

- Treatment failure characterizes a progression of clinical, serologic and histologic parameters during standard therapy. This is seen in about 10% of patients. In these cases the diagnosis of AIH has to be carefully reconsidered to exclude other etiologies of chronic hepatitis. In these patients, new or experimental regimens can be administered but, again, liver transplantation may become necessary.

When standard treatment fails or drug intolerance occurs, alternative therapies such as cyclosporin, tacrolimus, cyclophosphamide, mycophenolate mofetil, rapamycin, ursodeoxycholic acid (UDCA) and budesonide can be considered. The efficacy of these options has not yet been definitively established.

Budesonide is a synthetic steroid with high first-pass metabolism in the liver, which should limit systemic side-effects compared to conventional steroids. A small study showed that the drug was well tolerated and aminotransferase levels were normalized, but a contradictory study found that budesonide therapy was associated with a low frequency of remission and a high occurrence of side-effects. It is not clear whether budesonide offers an advantage over conventional corticosteroids when cirrhosis and portosystemic shunts are present. The main advantage of budesonide for the future treatment of AIH may be to replace prednisone in long-term maintenance therapy to reduce corticosteroid side-effects. The long-term role of second generation corticosteroids, to sustain remission in AIH patients with reduced treatment related side-effects, requires further controlled studies.

Cyclosporin is a lipophylic cyclic peptide of 11 residues produced by *Tolypocladium inflatum* that acts on calcium dependent signaling and inhibits T-cell function via the interleukin 2 gene. Of all the alternative agents, the greatest experience to date has been with cyclosporin and it is undoubtedly effective and well tolerated in the short to medium term. However, the principal difficulty in advocating widespread use of the drug as first-line therapy relates to its toxicity profile, particularly with long-term use (increased risk of hypertension, renal insufficiency, hyperlipidemia, hirsutism, infection and malignancy).

Tacrolimus is a macrolide lactone compound with immunosuppressive capabilities exceeding those of cyclosporin. The mechanism of action is similar to that of cyclosporin but it binds to a different immunophilin. The application of tacrolimus in a small study led to an improvement of aminotransferase and bilirubin levels with a minor increase in serum blood urea nitrogen (BUN) and creatinine levels over a 1-year period. Although tacrolimus represents a promising immunosuppressive candidate drug, larger randomized trials are required to assess its role in the therapy of AIH.

Mycophenolate is a non-competitive inhibitor of inosine monophosphate dehydrogenase, which blocks the rate-limiting enzymatic step in de novo purine synthesis. Mycophenolate has a selective action on lymphocyte activation, with marked reduction of both T- and B-lymphocyte proliferation. A pilot study of patients with AIH type 1 who were unresponsive to standard therapy demonstrated normalization of aminotransferase levels within 3 months in the majority of patients. These preliminary data suggest that mycophenolate may represent another promising treatment strategy for AIH.

Cyclophosphamide can induce remission with 1–1.5 mg/kg/day in combination with corticosteroids. However, cyclophosphamide with its potentially severe hematologic side-effects should be considered an experimental treatment option.

UDCA is a hydrophilic bile acid with putative immunomodulatory capabilities. It is presumed to alter HLA class I antigen expression on cellular surfaces and to suppress immunoglobulin production. Uncontrolled trials have shown a reduction in histologic abnormalities, as well as clinical and biochemical improvement, but not a reduction in fibrosis AIH type 1. However, its role in AIH therapy or in combination with immunosuppressive therapy remains uncertain.

LIVER TRANSPLANTATION

In approximately 10% of AIH patients liver transplantation remains the only life-saving option. The indication for liver transplantation in AIH is similar to that in other chronic liver diseases and includes clinical deterioration, development of cirrhosis, bleeding esophageal varices and coagulation abnormalities despite adequate immunosuppressive therapy. There is no single indicator or predictor for the necessity of liver transplantation. Candidates for liver transplantation are usually patients who do not reach remission within 4 years of continuous therapy. Indicators of a high mortality associated with liver failure are histologic evidence of multilobular necrosis and progressive hyperbilirubinemia. The long-term results of liver transplantation for AIH are excellent and well within the range of other indications for liver transplantation.

The potential for AIH to recur after liver transplantation has been a matter of controversial debate. The first case of recurrent AIH after liver transplantation was reported in 1984, and was based upon serum biochemistry, biopsy findings and steroid reduction. Studies published during the past years indicate that the rate of recurrence of AIH ranges between 10 and 35%, and that the risk of AIH recurrence is perhaps as high as 68% after 5 years of follow-up. It is important to consider the criteria upon which the diagnosis of recurrent AIH is based. When transaminitis is chosen as a practical selection parameter many patients with mild histologic evidence of recurrent AIH may be missed. It is therefore suggested that all patients with suspected recurrence of AIH receive a liver biopsy, biochemical analyses of aminotransferases as well as a determination of immunoglobulins and autoantibody titers. Significant risk factors for the recurrence of AIH have not yet been identified although it appears that presentation with acute liver failure before transplantation protects against the development of recurrent disease. A risk factor for the development of recurrent AIH is the presence of specific HLA antigens that may predispose toward a more severe immunoreactivity. In two studies recurrence of AIH appeared to occur more frequently in HLA DR3-positive patients receiving HLA DR3-negative grafts. However, this association was not confirmed in all studies. Interestingly, there have been no conclusive data to support the hypothesis that a specific immunosuppressive regimen represents a risk factor for the development of recurrent AIH. However, data indicate that patients transplanted for AIH require continued steroid treatment in 64% versus 17% of patients receiving liver transplants for other conditions. Based on these results and other studies it would appear that maintenance of steroid medication in AIH patients is indicated to prevent not only cellular rejection but also graft-threatening recurrence of AIH. Corticosteroid withdrawal should therefore be performed with great caution in this setting.

Autoantibody prevalence and titers have been studied in patients receiving liver transplantations for AIH and PBC. In general, autoantibody types persist in the majority of patients after transplantation. In PBC AMA persisted, albeit at lower titers in almost 100% of the patients. In AIH, autoantibodies of the specific subtype present before transplantation were detected at lower titers in 77% of post-transplant patients in one study and were found in 82% of those patients who did not develop recurrence of AIH. A recent study has suggested that an increase in titer exceeding levels detected prior to transplantation may be indicative of AIH recurrence. The majority of published data presently do not support a prognostic role for autoantibodies in AIH and liver transplantation.

FURTHER READING

Clinical reviews

Mackay IR, Taft LI, Cowling DC. Lupoid hepatitis. Lancet 1956; 2:1323–1326.

Manns MP, Strassburg CP. Autoimmune hepatitis: clinical challenges. Gastroenterology 2001; 120:1502–1517.

Mieli-Vergani G, Mieli-Vergani D. Autoimmune hepatitis. Arch Dis Child 1996; 74:2–5.

Waldenström J. Leber, Blutproteine und Nahrunseiweiss. Deutsche Z Verd Stoffwechselkr 1950; 15:113–121. *From a historical point of view the very interesting first description of a disease we now call autoimmune hepatitis.*

Diagnosis

Alvarez F, Berg PA, Bianchi FB, et al. International Autoimmune Hepatitis Group Report: review of criteria for diagnosis of autoimmune hepatitis. J Hepatol 1999; 31:929–938. *Describes the efforts to devise an internationally versatile definition of autoimmune hepatitis based upon biochemical, histologic, clinical and seroimmunological criteria. It is important to appreciate that a score cannot substitute for a clinical approach in defining patients requiring therapy. It also shows that most of the criteria employed are not unique to autoimmune hepatitis but occur in many chronic liver diseases. The optimization of a scoring system is currently ongoing.*

Czaja AJ, Carpenter HA. Validation of a scoring system for the diagnosis of autoimmune hepatitis. Dig Dis Sci 1996; 41:305–314.

Homberg JC, Abuaf N, Bernard O, et al. Chronic active hepatitis associated with anti liver/kidney microsome antibody type 1: a second type of 'autoimmune' hepatitis. Hepatology 1987; 7:1333–1339.

Johnson PJ, MacFarlane IG, Alvarez F, et al. Meeting report: International Autoimmune Hepatitis Group. Hepatology 1993; 18:998–1005.

Pathogenesis

Agarwal K, Czaja AJ, Jones DE, et al. Cytotoxic T lymphocyte antigen-4 (CTLA-4) gene polymorphisms and susceptibility to type 1 autoimmune hepatitis. Hepatology 2000; 31:49–53.

Beaune PH, Dansette PM, Mansuy D, et al. Human antiendoplasmatic reticulum autoantibodies appearing in a drug induced hepatitis directed against a human liver cytochrome P450 that hydroxylates the drug. Proc Natl Acad Sci USA 1987; 84:551–555. *The mechanism(s) of autoimmune hepatitis are unclear. Drug induced hepatitis offers an attractive model by which immunological mechanisms leading to hepatic damage are studied and characterized. This is particularly interesting in view of the fact that the epitopes recognized by anti-CYP autoantibodies in drug-induced hepatitis and autoimmune hepatitis are located in similar CYP domains.*

Czaja AJ, Carpenter HA, Santrach PJ, et al. Significance of HLA DR4 in type 1 autoimmune hepatitis. Gastroenterology 1993; 105:1502–1507.

Gelpi C, Southeimer EJ, Rodriguez-Sanchez JL. Autoantibodies against a serine t-RNA-protein complex implicated in cotranslational selenocysteine insertion. Proc Natl Acad Sci (USA) 1992; 89:9739–9743.

Lapierre P, Hajoui O, Homberg J-C, et al. Fomiminotransferase cyclodeaminase is an organ specific autoantigen recognized by sera of patients with autoimmune hepatitis. Gastroenterology 1999; 116:643–649.

Manns MP, Gerken G, Kyriatsoulis A, et al. Characterization of a new subgroup of autoimmune chronic active hepatitis by autoantibodies against soluble liver antigen. Lancet 1987; 1:292–294.

Manns MP, Griffin KJ, Quattrochi LC, et al. Identification of cytochrome P450 1A2 as a human autoantigen. Arch Biochem Biophys 1990; 280:229–232.

Manns MP, Griffin KJ, Sullivan KJ, et al. LKM-1 autoantibodies recognize a short linear sequence in P4502D6, a cytochrome P450 monoxygenase. J Clin Invest 1991; 88:1370–1378. *Characterization of LKM-1 autoantibodies against CYP2D6 which highlights one of the hypotheses regarding molecular mimicry and herpes virus infection. Although conformation dependent epitopes have also been characterized in the meantime the epitope described is also relevant in regard to LKM-1 autoantibodies occurring in autoimmune hepatitis and hepatitis C virus infection.*

Manns MP, Krüger M. Immunogenetics of chronic liver disease. Gastroenterology 1994; 106:1676–1697. *The immunogenetic associations of autoimmune liver diseases are complex. More and more a picture emerges, that individual markers confer only a very small risk and that patterns of genetic traits need to be identified to define risk. The mode of inheritance is not Mendelian and the number of candidate genes is high. This review gives an overview of some of the immunogenetic hypothesis and associations and should be viewed in the context of recent publications of individual genes in this field.*

Philipp T, Durazzo M, Straub P, et al. Recognition of uridine diphosphate glucuronosyltransferase by LKM-3 autoantibodies in chronic hepatitis D. Lancet 1994; 344:578–581.

Rizzetto M, Swana G, Doniach D. Microsomal antibodies in active chronic hepatitis and other disorders. Clin Exp Immunol 1973; 14:331–334.

Strassburg CP, Obermayer-Straub P, Alex B, et al. Autoantibodies against glucuronosyltransferases differ between viral hepatitis and autoimmune hepatitis. Gastroenterology 1996; 111:1576–1586.

Vogel A, Liermann H, Harms A, et al. Autoimmune regulator AIRE: Evidence for genetic differences between autoimmune hepatitis and hepatitis as part of the autoimmune polyglandular syndrome type 1. Hepatology 2001; 33:1047–1052. *Among a large body of literature this paper analyzes the relationship of an inheritable form of autoimmune hepatitis as part of the APECED syndrome, which has a monogenetic association with common autoimmune hepatitis. Although CYP antibodies are detectable in both entities the pathophysiology appears to be different based on the association with mutations in the AIRE gene.*

Volkmann M, Bäurle A, Heid H, et al. Soluble liver antigen: Isolation of a 35 kDa recombinant protein (SLA-P35) specifically recognizing sera from patients with autoimmune hepatitis type 3. Hepatology 2001; 33:591–596.

Wies I, Brunner S, Henninger J, et al. Identification of target antigen for SLA/LP autoantibodies in autoimmune hepatitis. Lancet 2000; 355:1510–1515.

Zanger UM, Hauri HP, Loeper J, et al. Antibodies against human cytochrome P450 dbl in autoimmune hepatitis type 2. Proc Natl Acad Sci USA 1988; 27:8256–8260.

Treatment

Heneghan MA, McFarlane IG. Current and novel immunosuppressive therapy for autoimmune hepatitis. Hepatology 2002; 35:7–13.

Johnson PJ, McFarlane IG, Williams R. Azathioprine for long-term maintenance of remission in autoimmune hepatitis. N Engl J Med 1995; 333:958–963.

Reich DJ, Fiel I, Guarrera JV, et al. Liver transplantation for autoimmune hepatitis. Hepatology 2000; 32:693–700.

Vogel A, Heinrich E, Bahr MJ, et al. Long term outcome of liver transplantation for autoimmune hepatitis. Clin Transpl 2004; 18:62–69.

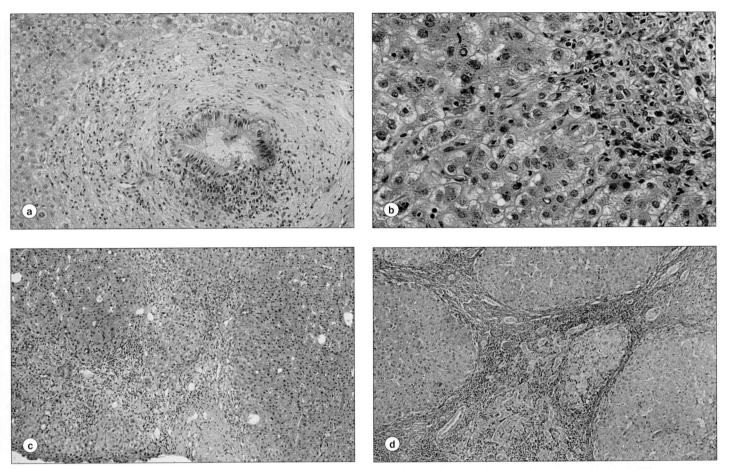

Figure 19.4 Histological staging. (a) Stage I. Non-suppurative destructive cholangitis affecting a medium-sized interlobular bile duct. Biliary epithelium is partly destroyed. Original magnification × 50. (b) Stage II. Proliferating ductules with rupture of limiting plate. Original magnification × 100. (c) Stage III. Inflammatory fibrous septa with aggregates of lymphoid cells. Original magnification × 25. (d) Stage IV. Cirrhosis. Several regenerative nodules are seen. Original magnification × 25.

In addition to aiding in diagnosis, histologic stage and some individual liver histologic features, such as the degree of severity of the lymphocytic piecemeal necrosis and of ductopenia, are valuable prognostic indicators in addition to serum bilirubin.

The diagnosis of primary biliary cirrhosis is sometimes very difficult for the following reasons: the typical histological lesions of primary biliary cirrhosis or primary sclerosing cholangitis are not present in the liver specimen, the classic stricturing lesions are not obvious particularly in the intrahepatic form of primary sclerosing cholangitis especially when MRI is used to visualize the biliary tree.

In approximately 5–10% of the patients, M2 antibodies are absent or present at a low titer, when immunofluorescent techniques are used. In some patients, antinuclear antibodies, anti-gp210 and/or anti-Sp100 are present; in some of them antibodies against the major M2 components (PDC-E2) are present using enzyme-linked immunosorbent assay (ELISA) or Western blotting techniques and finally elevated IgM levels are usually observed. Thus, in the absence of M2 antibodies, the diagnosis of primary biliary cirrhosis can still be made if gp210 or Sp100 antibodies or frank elevation of IgM coexists with biochemical cholestasis and histopathologic evidence of bile duct lesions.

Differential diagnosis

Up to 10% of patients have characteristics of both primary biliary cirrhosis and autoimmune hepatitis. In those patients, the following features are found: strikingly elevated aminotransferase activity, moderate to severe piecemeal necrosis lesions, marked

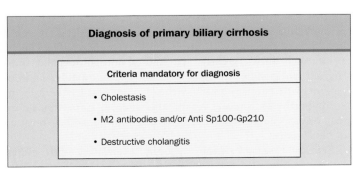

Figure 19.5 Diagnosis of primary biliary cirrhosis.

increase in IgG levels, and sometimes antiactin or antinuclear antibodies with homogeneous pattern by immunofluorescence. Patients who present the characteristics of both diseases have been diagnosed with so-called 'overlap syndrome' or 'autoimmune cholangiopathy'. In some patients, features of autoimmune hepatitis occur in those who initially had typical primary biliary cirrhosis. This mixed form must be identified, because in addition to UDCA treatment, they have to be treated with corticosteroids or even with cyclosporine.

Several drugs have been reported to induce cholestasis, cholangitis and ductopenia. The most frequently incriminated drugs are phenothiazines, haloperidol, imipramine, amoxicillin and clavulanic acid, and Cox-2 inhibitors. Acute onset of cholestasis (sometimes associated with pruritus) is usually observed and resolves completely after several weeks or months after the medication is discontinued. AMAs are absent. Ductopenia, fibrosis or even cirrhosis may occur.

Primary sclerosing cholangitis is characterized by chronic inflammation and fibrosis of intra- or extrabiliary ducts. In this setting, AMAs are absent. Cholangiography shows the classic stricturing and beading of the extra- and intrahepatic bile ducts. Liver biopsy shows the concentric periductular fibrosis that leads to progressive atrophy or even to the disappearance of the bile ducts.

Sarcoidosis can cause considerable diagnostic difficulty. Characteristics of these two diseases are compared in **Table 19.2**. Sarcoidosis and primary biliary cirrhosis usually have typical characteristics that allow clear distinction between the entities. However, sarcoidosis may be complicated by severe chronic cholestasis and portal hypertension, a clinical form that can mimic primary biliary cirrhosis. Finally, sarcoidosis and primary biliary cirrhosis may coexist in a single patient.

Causes of chronic cholestasis in adulthood
• Primary biliary cirrhosis
• Autoimmune hepatitis – overlap syndrome
• Primary sclerosing cholangitis   – intrahepatic   – intra- and extrahepatic
• Drug-induced cholestasis
• Low phospholipid associated cholelithiasis (LPAC) syndrome (*ABCB4/MDR3* gene defect)
• Sarcoidosis
• Idiopathic ductopenia
• Lymphoma
• Stenosis, strictures and developmental abnormalities of the biliary tree (Caroli disease, congenital hepatic fibrosis)
• Allograft rejection, graft versus host disease
• Parenteral nutrition

Table 19.3 Causes of chronic cholestasis in adulthood

MDR3 or *ABCB4* gene mutations may induce type 3 familial intrahepatic cholestasis in infancy. In young adults, the *MDR3* gene defect is associated with a peculiar form of cholestasis associated with symptomatic intrahepatic and gallbladder cholelithiasis.

Idiopathic adulthood ductopenia is a term proposed to describe a form of chronic cholestasis of unknown origin with clinical onset in adulthood, associated with loss of intrahepatic bile ducts. In these patients, AMAs are absent; there is no drug history; and cholangiographic findings show a normal biliary tree.

Other causes of chronic cholestasis are listed in **Table 19.3**.

ASSOCIATED DISORDERS

Scleroderma, especially minor forms such as the CREST syndrome, may be observed in approximately 10% of patients. Systemic forms of scleroderma are often limited to a minor esophageal motor disorder or to a reduction in carbon dioxide diffusion capacity. Raynaud phenomenon is usually observed in 10–20% of the patients. Anticentromere antibodies, characteristic of CREST syndrome, are found in 10–20% of the patients. Sjögren syndrome, most often in its minor form, is frequent in primary biliary cirrhosis. Arthropathies and arthralgias are noted in 5–50% of patients with primary biliary cirrhosis. The clinical significance varies greatly. Thyroid abnormalities and antithyroid antibodies are observed in approximately 15% of patients with primary biliary cirrhosis. The most frequent forms are hyperthyroidism and Hashimoto disease. Hyperthyroidism may be associated with a rise in serum bilirubin and aggravation of cholestasis.

Several cases of villous atrophy associated with gluten intolerance have been reported in patients with primary biliary cirrhosis. The number of cases reported indicates more than a

Cholestatic sarcoidosis compared with primary biliary cirrhosis		
	Sarcoidosis	*Primary biliary cirrhosis*
Gender	Equal	80% female
Age of onset	Young	Middle age
Pruritus	Yes (rare)	Yes (frequent)
Erythema nodosum	Yes	No
Respiratory symptoms	Yes (frequent)	Yes (rare)
Hepatosplenomegaly	Yes	Yes
Hilar adenopathy	Usual	Rare
Pulmonary infiltrate	Yes	Rare
Positive mitochondrial antibody	No	90%
Elevation of serum angiotensin converting enzyme	50%	10%
Positive Kveim-Siltzbach test	70%	No

Table 19.2 Cholestatic sarcoidosis compared with primary biliary cirrhosis

random association. Primary biliary cirrhosis should be suspected in a patient in whom celiac disease is discovered and liver test results are abnormal. A similar association has been reported in patients with sclerosing cholangitis. In this setting, in contrast to primary biliary cirrhosis, a gluten-free diet led to an improvement in liver test results. Villous atrophy is sometimes asymptomatic.

The frequency of gallstones can reach 30–50% according to the duration and severity of the disease. It is higher in patients with cirrhosis. Migration of stones through the bile ducts can aggravate cholestasis. Treatment of hypercholesterolemia with fibrates can lead to the formation of gallstones, which disappear when the drug is withdrawn. Supersaturation of the bile by calcium has been reported during long-term treatment with cholestyramine.

Pancreatic abnormalities, particularly involving the tail and detected by pancreatography have been reported in primary biliary cirrhosis. Severe pancreatic insufficiency is however rare and does not generally explain steatorrhea observed in patients with marked cholestasis.

Lung involvement is frequent in primary biliary cirrhosis but is generally subclinical. Pulmonary fibrosis occurs most frequently in patients with CREST syndrome or Sjögren syndrome. The hepatopulmonary syndrome, characterized by hypoxemia, and intrapulmonary vascular dilatation can also be observed in patients with advanced primary biliary cirrhosis. Pulmonary hypertension can occur in primary biliary cirrhosis, as in other forms of cirrhosis.

Renal tubular acidosis is frequent but usually subclinical. An increased susceptibility to urinary tract infections has been reported but has not been confirmed in other studies. Neuropsychiatric problems (e.g. anxiety, fatigue, depression) are frequent in women with primary biliary cirrhosis, especially those with Sjögren syndrome.

The incidence of breast cancer appears to be higher in women with primary biliary cirrhosis. In contrast, the incidence of other cancers is not different from expected rates.

The onset of pregnancy in patients with primary biliary cirrhosis is rare because the disease usually occurs after menopause or causes amenorrhea itself. Pregnancy, especially in the last few weeks, induces subclinical cholestasis. Pregnancy in patients with primary biliary cirrhosis generally leads to an aggravation in cholestasis. In contrast, in UDCA-treated women with primary biliary cirrhosis, pregnancy produces further improvement of liver biochemistries but after delivery, frank relapse usually occurs.

COMPLICATIONS OF PRIMARY BILIARY CIRRHOSIS

Pruritus is present in approximately 70–80% of patients with primary biliary cirrhosis. It is usually moderate, but can be severe in approximately 5–10% of cases. The pathogenesis of pruritus is unknown. Opiate antagonists (naloxone and nalmefene) modulate the perception of pruritus and induces an opiate withdrawal syndrome, suggesting a possible role of endorphins.

Fatigue is reported by patients as a symptom that often dramatically impairs their quality of life. Three studies focused on the impact of fatigue score using specific questionnaires. The prevalence of fatigue varied greatly between these studies (8–80%) and might be related to patient selection criteria. Scores of fatigue were augmented in patients with primary biliary cirrhosis but no relationships were found between these scores and any parameter of disease severity. As the pathogenesis of fatigue in primary biliary cirrhosis still remains to be defined, no specific treatments are available.

In primary biliary cirrhosis, osteopenia is mainly caused by osteoporosis, whereas osteomalacia is rare. Osteopenia is present in 10–35% of the patients at the time of diagnosis. This frequency does not differ from that observed in other chronic liver diseases, such as sclerosing cholangitis, hemochromatosis or chronic hepatitis.

Deficiencies of fat-soluble vitamins (A, D, E and K) can occur in primary biliary cirrhosis, especially in advanced or severe forms. This deficiency is mainly due to malabsorption but rarely results in clinical manifestations. Vitamin A deficiency must be corrected with care, because overdosage can lead to liver damage, particularly fibrosis. Vitamin D deficiency should be corrected, given the risk of osteopenia.

Portal hypertension is frequent in the course of primary biliary cirrhosis, generally developing after the onset of cirrhosis. In fewer than 5% of cases, portal hypertension or gastrointestinal bleeding may be the first manifestation of the disease. Portal hypertension can occur in the absence of cirrhosis and may be caused by portal inflammation, compression of small portal venules, and regenerative nodular hyperplasia. Patients with primary biliary cirrhosis and portal hypertension complicated by gastrointestinal bleeding should first be treated with β blockers and, in case of failure, with sclerosis or ligation of varices. If these treatments fail, liver transplantation should be preferred to portacaval shunt surgery.

Hepatocellular carcinoma appears to be a rare complication of primary biliary cirrhosis. When hepatocellular carcinoma occurs, the liver is cirrhotic. The low incidence of hepatocellular carcinoma may be explained by the relatively late formation of regenerative nodules in the course of the disease.

PROGNOSIS AND TREATMENT

Most of the patients in whom primary biliary cirrhosis was diagnosed when asymptomatic will develop symptoms in the following years (**Fig. 19.6**). In a 40-month period, 10–30% of asymptomatic patients become symptomatic. The mean duration of the asymptomatic phase is extremely variable but is on the order of 6 years. The 5-year survival rate of asymptomatic patients is approximately 90%. After 5 years of progression, the proportion of survivors is significantly lower than in a paired control population. The duration of the symptomatic phase varies greatly but can last for 10 years. The mean 5-year survival rate among symptomatic patients is 50%, with a range of 30–70%. In terms of histologic progression, the median time to progress from histologic stage II to stage IV, i.e. cirrhosis, is 4 years. The terminal phase of the disease is defined when serum bilirubin level is higher than 100 μmol/L (6 mg/dL), with or without signs of portal hypertension (gastrointestinal bleeding, ascites or encephalopathy). The disease progression is summarized in **Table 19.4**.

Shapiro et al (1979) showed the importance of serum bilirubin as a factor prognostic for survival in primary biliary cirrhosis. They noted that, after a relatively stable phase, serum

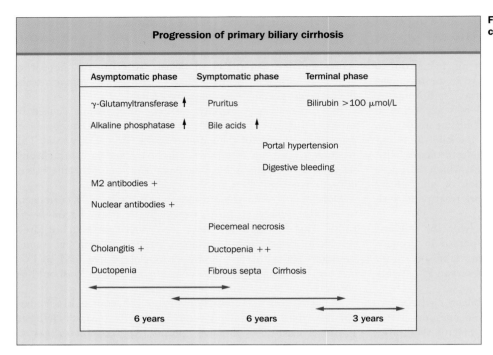

Figure 19.6 Progression of primary biliary cirrhosis.

Progression of primary biliary cirrhosis with time	
Feature	%
Hepatomegaly	+30
Splenomegaly	+28
Ascites	+25
Gastrointestinal bleeding	+22
Cirrhosis	+50
Bilirubin >105 μmol/L (>6.2 mg/dL)	+25
Albumin <29 g/L	+35
Reproduced from Christense 1980 et al (80) by permission of The American Gastroenterological Association.	

Table 19.4 Progression of primary biliary cirrhosis with time. Cumulative percentage of patients with each feature after 4 years of follow-up

Calculation and interpretation of the Mayo risk score for primary biliary cirrhosis.

Step 1: Calculate R

R = 0.871 × log (bilirubin in mg/dL) + (−2.53 $\log_e$ [albumin in g/dL]) + 0.039 age in years + 2.38 $\log_c$ prothrombin time in s) = 0.859 (if edema is present).

Step 2: To obtain the probability of survival for at least t more years, one reads $S_0(t)$ from the table below and computes $S(t) = [S_0(t)]^{\exp(R-0.57)}$

t (years)	1	2	3	4	5	6	7
$S_0(t)$	0.970	0.941	0.883	0.833	0.774	0.721	0.651

Table 19.5 Calculation and interpretation of the Mayo risk score for primary biliary cirrhosis

bilirubin increased sharply in the months preceding death. In patients with serum bilirubin levels above 34 μmol/L (2 mg/dL), the mean survival was 4 years; in those with values above 102 μmol/L (60 mg/dL) 2 years, and in those with values above 170 μmol/L (10 mg/dL) 1.4 years. The extraordinary importance of bilirubin for short-term and long-term survival was confirmed in all later studies. Several prognostic models have been proposed to improve the prognostic value of serum bilirubin. These models are complex or are not highly superior to serum bilirubin alone. The Mayo risk score has been used as a prognostic index in patients with primary biliary cirrhosis (**Table 19.5**).

It is important to emphasize that the prognostic value of serum bilirubin level for survival free of liver transplantation is similar in UDCA-treated patients as in non-treated patients.

Medical treatments

As with all chronic diseases, the most difficult choice for assessing efficacy is the endpoint(s). Survival is clearly a valid criterion of efficacy, but creates a number of problems; for example:

- the need for long-term follow-up of a large number of patients; and
- ethical considerations if the treatment is ineffective or carries a high risk of side-effects.

One way of shortening the study period is to use surrogate markers. Given the lack of validated surrogate markers in primary biliary cirrhosis, survival free of liver transplantation appears to be one of the best endpoints. Finally, with long-term treatment, the balance between benefit and adverse effects is of crucial importance.

As primary biliary cirrhosis is known to be an autoimmune disease, most drugs used for its treatment have been selected on

CHAPTER
20

Primary Sclerosing Cholangitis

K. V. Narayanan Menon and Russell H. Wiesner

INTRODUCTION

Primary sclerosing cholangitis (PSC) is a chronic cholestatic syndrome of unknown etiology that is characterized by chronic cholestasis and diffuse inflammation and fibrosis that involve the entire biliary tree. The pathologic process obliterates intrahepatic and extrahepatic bile ducts, which ultimately leads to biliary cirrhosis, portal hypertension and liver failure.

The syndrome, PSC, was first described by Delbet in 1924, and as of 1980 only 100 cases were documented in the English literature. It was therefore considered a rare disease before the widespread application of endoscopic retrograde and percutaneous transhepatic cholangiography in the late 1970s, which allowed the diagnosis of PSC to be made without surgery (**Fig. 20.1**). The recognition of the association between PSC and inflammatory bowel disease coupled with the use of screening biochemical liver tests as part of routine general examination has further increased the frequency with which PSC is diagnosed. Today, the detection of abnormal liver tests in patients with inflammatory bowel disease leads to an earlier diagnosis of PSC, frequently when the patient has minimal or no symptoms related to liver disease. These advances in the diagnosis of PSC have led to a better understanding of this previously seldom diagnosed syndrome; in particular, its clinical features and natural history.

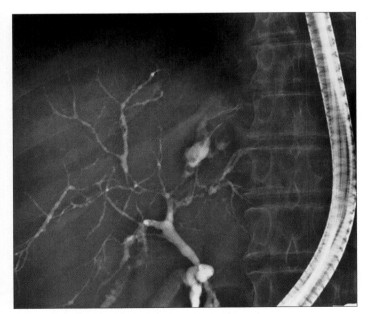

Figure 20.1 Cholangiogram. Classic cholangiographic findings in the setting of PSC are noted including strictures, beading and irregularities of the intrahepatic and extrahepatic biliary system.

Despite these advances, the etiology remains unknown and no curative therapy has been identified. Immunopathogenic mechanisms seem likely to play a major etiologic role based on the strong association of PSC with certain human leukocyte antigens (HLA haplotype), the presence of autoantibodies, a close relationship with other autoimmune diseases and the presence of multiple immunologic abnormalities. However, to date, target antigens have not been identified and, importantly, immuno-suppressive therapy has had minimal impact on disease progression.

EPIDEMIOLOGY

Although the prevalence of PSC in the USA is unknown, it can be estimated because of its frequent association with chronic ulcerative colitis (CUC). Studies have shown a 2.4–7.5% prevalence of PSC in patients with CUC. Because the incidence of CUC ranges from 40 to 225 cases/100 000 population, the incidence of PSC in the USA is estimated to be between two and seven cases/100 000 population. The prevalence of PSC in one midwestern community in the USA was 20.9/100 000 men and 6.3/100 000 women. These estimates are supported by the results of epidemiologic studies from Sweden and Norway, where the incidence of CUC and PSC was noted to be 171 and 6.3 cases/100 000 population, respectively. These results, however, probably underestimate the actual incidence of PSC because the disease can occur in patients with normal serum levels of alkaline phosphatase, and 20–30% of patients with PSC do not have associated inflammatory bowel disease. Therefore PSC seems to be more common than previously suspected, and may have a frequency similar to that reported for primary biliary cirrhosis (PBC).

PATHOPHYSIOLOGY

The cause of PSC remains unknown despite extensive investigation into various mechanisms related to bacteria, viral infections, toxins, genetic predisposition and immunologic mechanisms, all of which have been postulated to contribute to the pathogenesis and progression of this syndrome (**Table 20.1**).

Bacteria toxin theory

The close association of inflammatory bowel diseases, especially CUC, with PSC has been intriguing and led several investigators to postulate that portal bacteremia or absorption of toxins or toxic bile acids from the inflamed colon may play a major role in the pathogenesis of PSC. It was postulated that the primary event in PSC was a chronic, low-grade portal vein bacteremia that caused chronic biliary tract inflammation and fibrosis. However,

Pathophysiology of PSC		
Causal factor	*Supportive features*	*Contradicting aspects*
Colonic bacteria or toxins	Association with UC Bacterial peptides induce changes seen in PSC	Portal bacteremia not a feature of severe PSC Clinical association with quiescent PSC
Viral	Some viruses (e.g. CMV) can cause bile duct damage	No direct link between any virus and PSC has been established
Genetic	Strong HLA associations reported	Associations are not totally consistent
Immunologic	Hypergammaglobulinemia Autoantibodies Circulating immune complexes Complement activation Abnormal cell mediated immunity	No clinical response to immunosuppressive therapy

Table 20.1 Pathophysiology of primary sclerosing cholangitis (PSC). The pathophysiology is probably multifactorial involving some or all of these proposed causative factors. UC, ulcerative colitis; CMV, cytomegalovirus; HLA, human leukocyte antigen.

investigators were unable to demonstrate a significant incidence of portal vein bacteremia in patients undergoing surgery for severe, uncontrolled CUC. Furthermore, detailed hepatic histologic analysis revealed that portal phlebitis, the hallmark of portal vein bacteremia, was mild or absent in most patients with PSC. Thus, little evidence supports the hypothesis that portal bacteremia plays a major pathogenic role in this syndrome.

It has been postulated that PSC is caused by a reaction to toxic bile acids, such as lithocholic acid, formed by the bacterial action in the diseased colon that allows absorption of the toxin directly into the portal blood. This hypothesis has also been refuted as multiple studies have been unable to demonstrate major abnormalities in bile acid metabolism in patients with PSC or CUC.

Proinflammatory bacterial peptides synthesized by colonic bacteria in a rat model caused portal inflammation and neutrophilic cholangitis similar to the histopathologic lesion seen in early PSC. Animals that had experimentally induced colitis experienced an eightfold increase in biliary excretion of these proinflammatory bacterial peptides. In another study, investigators demonstrated that intestinal bacterial overgrowth in rats was associated with hepatic inflammation similar to that seen in PSC. Thus, further investigation into the potential pathogenic role that proinflammatory bacterial peptides may play in PSC seems warranted. However, other evidence suggests that increased absorption of toxins by way of an inflamed colon does not play a major part in the pathophysiology of PSC. For example, the severity of CUC does not appear to predict the likelihood of PSC developing, since most patients with PSC have mild or quiescent inflammatory bowel disease. Moveover, PSC has been known to develop years before the onset of CUC and may develop years after proctocolectomy for CUC. In addition, PSC

is diagnosed in a substantial number of patients who have no past or present clinical or histologic evidence of CUC. These findings suggest that colonic disease leading to increased absorption of bacterial products or toxins is not a major factor in the pathogenesis of this syndrome.

The remaining 'toxin' worth mentioning in relation to the pathophysiology of PSC is copper. It has been shown that PSC leads to an accumulation of hepatic copper. This probably represents an epiphenomenon related to cholestasis since it has now been well demonstrated that increased hepatic copper levels are found in patients with all causes of chronic cholestasis. Furthermore, D-penicillamine therapy, which is known to reduce in hepatic copper levels, was not shown to be beneficial in PSC patients in a controlled clinical trial. Therefore, there is little evidence to support hepatic copper toxicity being a major factor in the pathophysiology or disease progression of PSC.

Viral infection

Infection of biliary epithelial cells by viral agents has been postulated by some to be involved in the pathogenesis of PSC. Previous studies have excluded hepatitis A, B and C viruses as causative factors in PSC. Cytomegalovirus has been implicated in the pathophysiology of PSC. It can cause intralobular bile duct destruction and has been implicated in causing a decrease in the number of intralobular bile ducts. However, fibrosis and the destruction of large ducts have never been shown to be associated with cytomegalovirus infection. More importantly, inclusion bodies, typical of cytomegalovirus infection, have never been demonstrated histologically in bile duct epithelial cells or hepatocytes from patients with PSC.

Other reports suggesting that reovirus type 3 can induce cholangitis and biliary atresia in weanling mice and primates raised the possibility that this virus may also play a causative role in PSC. However, more recent data have shown that neither the prevalence nor the titers of antibodies to reovirus type 3 differ between patients with PSC and normal adult controls. Thus, there is no evidence to support the hypothesis that the pathophysiology of PSC is related to a viral infection.

Genetic predisposition

Genetic factors have been proposed to contribute to the pathogenesis of PSC. Familial clustering of PSC has been reported. In addition multiple studies have shown a strong association between PSC and certain HLA haplotypes suggesting genetic susceptibility. The first HLA haplotypes shown to be associated with PSC were B8, DR3, DR2, and A1, B8, DR3. In 1990, investigators reported a 100% association of PSC with the HLA-DRw52a (or DRB3*0101). Subsequent studies failed to confirm this observation but demonstrated that only 52–55% of PSC patients are positive for the HLA-DRw52a haplotype. Later, HLA haplotypes DR3 and DR6 were also found to be highly associated with PSC. Finally, a strong association of PSC with the DRB1*1301, DQA1*1301, and DQB1*0603 alleles was demonstrated.

Meanwhile, investigators began to examine the relationship between HLA genotype and prognosis. One study revealed that HLA-DRw52a-positive PSC patients had a significantly diminished estimated median survival compared with the HLA-DRw52a-negative group. Other studies also reported that PSC patients with HLA-DR4 haplotype and DR3, DQ2 heterozygosity experienced relatively rapid disease progression. In contrast, another report concluded that HLA-DR and HLA-DQ haplotypes do not represent markers for a more rapid disease progression. Detailed analysis of the characteristics of each study population and additional studies are needed to clarify this issue.

Immunologic cause

To date, the most attractive hypothesis for the pathogenesis of PSC is immune-mediated damage of bile ducts. For example, the HLA haplotypes associated with PSC (i.e. HLA-B8, HLA-DR3) are also associated with known autoimmune disorders. In addition, abnormal humoral and cellular immune profiles have been described in PSC patients, which although inconclusive, support the hypothesis. Finally, a shared and specific epitope has been detected on human colonic and biliary epithelium. Circulating autoantibodies against this specific epitope were detected in the serum of two-thirds of PSC patients.

The immunohumoral abnormalities reported in PSC patients include

- hypergammaglobulinemia, often with a disproportionate elevation of serum IgM levels;
- increased titers of antismooth muscle, antinuclear, anticolonic, antiportal tract, perinuclear antineutrophilic cytoplasmic (pANCA) and antiendothelial cell antibodies;
- increased levels of circulating immune complexes in serum and bile; and
- activation of the complement system and abnormal clearance of immune complexes from the circulation.

Recent interest has focused on the high prevalence of pANCA in PSC patients with or without CUC. Currently, pANCA is considered a marker of PSC despite the variation in its specificity and sensitivity reported in studies due to methodologic differences. Nevertheless, pANCA is not suggested for screening of PSC since it is not pathognomonic and its titer widely fluctuates during the course of the disease. The pattern of pANCA staining in PSC has been characterized as atypical perinuclear and is distinct from that seen in Wegener granulomatosis, possibly reflecting a difference in the target antigen. The antigen(s) that reacts with pANCA in PSC remain unknown. Proposed antigens include cathepsin G, a chymotrypsin-like protease, and the bactericidal/permeability increasing protein, an endotoxin-binding protein of polymorphonuclear granulocytes. A number of studies have investigated the prognostic significance of pANCA in PSC. These reports demonstrated that the titer of pANCA in PSC patients does not correlate with liver histology, clinical activity and biochemical profiles, but has been associated with more extensive biliary disease. Of interest, pANCA titers can persist after liver transplantation and proctocolectomy. Further studies are needed to identify the antigenic determinants of pANCA in PSC and to better understand the role of these antibodies in PSC.

In an early study, the inhibition of leukocyte migration by biliary antigens in PSC patients suggested the presence of a cellular-mediated immune mechanism in its pathogenesis. The cellular immune abnormalities described in PSC patients include the following:

- a significant decline in the total number of circulating T cells due to a disproportionate decrease in CD8 (suppressor/cytotoxic) cells leading to an increase in the ratio of CD4+ to CD8+ cells;

- a significantly increased ratio of CD4+ to CD8+ T cells in the blood of those with cirrhosis compared with non-cirrhotics;
- an increase in the absolute number and percentage of peripheral B cells;
- an increase in the absolute number and percent of γ δ-T cells in the peripheral blood and portal areas; and
- a dominant usage of the V β 3 gene segment of the T-cell receptor in the T lymphocytes infiltrating the liver.

These findings suggest altered immunoregulation in PSC. Further studies to characterize the activated T lymphocytes infiltrating the liver are necessary to elucidate their role in the pathogenesis of PSC.

The enhanced expression of HLA class II antigens on the biliary epithelial cells of patients during the early stages of PSC and after extrahepatic biliary obstruction has been reported. Although this finding may suggest an autoimmune activation of host lymphocytes by the bile duct epithelia that become capable of presenting self or foreign antigens, it most likely reflects an epiphenomenon of the disease since it is not specific for PSC.

Adhesion molecules such as the intercellular adhesion molecule (ICAM)-1, a ligand for the leukocyte adhesion receptor lymphocyte function-associated antigen (LFA)-1, are involved in the communication between T lymphocytes and antigen-presenting cells (APCs). ICAM-1 has been detected on bile duct epithelia in cirrhotic-stage PSC; increased serum levels of circulating ICAM-1 have also been found in PSC. The fact that the expression of HLA-DR predates the expression of ICAM-1 in bile ducts of PSC patients suggests minimal participation of the latter in the initiation of PSC. Nevertheless, LFA-1 is over-expressed in intrahepatic lymphocytes, implying that additional unidentified adhesion molecules may exist in the bile ducts of patients with PSC. Proinflammatory cytokines induce the expression of ICAM-1, and HLA class I and II molecules on human bile duct epithelia. However, the importance of cytokines in the pathogenesis of PSC remains unclear and further studies are needed.

Finally it has been proposed that PSC is the consequence of an environmental insult that leads to the autoimmune destruction of biliary epithelia in a genetically predisposed individual. Understanding the molecular basis of the genetic and autoimmune milieu involved in PSC is a prerequisite to clarifying the pathogenesis of PSC and devising rational and effective medical therapies.

CLINICAL FEATURES

The syndrome of PSC can affect any age group and any race, but it appears to occur predominantly in young Caucasian males. In the Mayo Clinic series of 174 adult PSC patients, two-thirds were male and the mean age at the time of diagnosis was 39 years. The clinical presentation of PSC can range from the finding of an increased serum alkaline phosphatase level in an asymptomatic patient to a complication of portal hypertension, such as the onset of ascites, variceal bleeding or portosystemic encephalopathy. With increasing frequency, PSC is being diagnosed in patients with established inflammatory bowel disease who develop abnormal biochemical liver function tests. However, even patients with advanced-stage PSC can have normal liver tests.

Frequency of symptoms and signs of PSC	
Symptom/sign	Frequency (%)
Fatigue	66
Pruritis	59
Jaundice	59
Hepatomegaly	48
Weight loss	34
Splenomegaly	34
Cholangitis	28
Hyperpigmentation	14
Ascites	7
Variceal bleed	6
Xanthoma	4
Hepatic encephalopathy	2

Table 20.2 Frequency of symptoms and signs of primary sclerosing cholangitis (PSC). Profile of the signs and symptoms present at the time of diagnosis.

Symptoms and signs

Many patients are asymptomatic at the time of presentation and diagnosis; however, most of them have a cholestatic biochemical profile that is characterized by an increased serum alkaline phosphatase level. Of the 75% of patients who are symptomatic, presentation can be with a variety of symptoms including fatigue, pruritus or jaundice. Ascending cholangitis secondary to bacterial infection of the biliary tree, characterized by pain, fever and jaundice, is an unusual presenting feature unless the biliary tree has a stricture or has been previously surgically or endoscopically manipulated. Other signs and symptoms are similar to those that occur in patients with other chronic liver diseases such as weight loss, ascites variceal bleeding from an esophageal or stomal source, and hepatic encephalopathy (**Table 20.2**). On physical examination, nearly 50% of PSC patients will have hepatomegaly or jaundice at the time of diagnosis. Other common signs include splenomegaly, hyperpigmentation and xanthomas.

DIAGNOSIS

Criteria used to diagnose PSC have evolved with time. Originally, the diagnosis of PSC was established only at laparotomy, by palpation of a fibrotic common bile duct, and a biopsy of the common bile duct which excluded bile duct cancer. Later, operative cholangiography revealed beading and irregularity of the extrahepatic and intrahepatic bile ducts, which today are the characteristic radiologic findings and are diagnostic of PSC in the appropriate clinical setting. The development of endoscopic retrograde cholangiopancreatography (ERCP) and transhepatic cholangiography (THC), both of which became technically feasible in the late 1970s, have had the greatest impact on the diagnosis of PSC. With ERCP, the spectrum of PSC rapidly expanded to include patients with isolated intrahepatic disease alone, and the number of cases of PSC diagnosed per year

increased two to threefold at most centers. In addition, the important relationship between PSC and the development of cholangiocarcinoma was confirmed using serial cholangiograms in patients with PSC. Therefore, cholangiocarcinoma, once considered an exclusionary criterion for the diagnosis of PSC, was shown to be within the spectrum of complications that developed during the course of PSC. More recently, non-invasive techniques such as magnetic resonance imaging (MRI) and magnetic resonance cholangiography (MRC) may allow for the diagnosis of PSC, and also can be useful in the diagnosis of cholangiocarcinoma.

Currently, the diagnostic criteria for PSC are centered on characteristic cholangiographic findings, which are by no means entirely specific for PSC; however, in the appropriate clinical setting these findings are useful in establishing the diagnosis of PSC. Cholangiographic changes similar to those found in PSC can be seen in other conditions and can cause difficulty in making the correct diagnosis. In general, these conditions also can be readily diagnosed by obtaining a detailed history and by carefully evaluating the cholangiographic and histologic findings, which are frequently helpful in excluding causes of secondary sclerosing cholangitis.

The diagnostic inclusion and exclusion criteria for PSC are outlined in **Table 20.3**.

These include:

- a cholestatic biochemical profile (alkaline phosphatase level of more than 1.5 times the upper limits of normal for 6 months or more). PSC can be diagnosed with a normal alkaline phosphase level;
- a cholangiogram showing strictures in the intrahepatic, or extrahepatic biliary tree, or both (Fig. 20.1);
- a liver biopsy showing inflammatory fibrosis of interlobular and septal bile ducts, as well as early evidence of obliteration in the absence of evidence of other causes of chronic liver disease; and
- exclusion of causes of secondary sclerosing cholangitis (see Table 20.3).

Biochemical and immunologic testing

Biochemical abnormalities are not specific for the diagnosis of PSC. However, a cholestatic profile of 6 or more months' duration is the hallmark of PSC, and most patients have at least a twofold increase in serum levels of alkaline phosphatase activity. Nevertheless, patients with cholangiographically documented PSC in whom alkaline phosphatase levels were normal have been described and a number of these patients had advanced histologic-stage disease on liver biopsy.

Serum aminotransferase levels are increased in 92% of patients, but are usually less than five times the upper limits of normal, except in children, and the mean increase is about three times the upper limits of normal. In patients with the highest aminotransferase levels, histologic features of autoimmune hepatitis have been noted, and an overlap syndrome including histologic and clinical features of both PSC and autoimmune hepatitis has been described.

While serum bilirubin levels are typically elevated in patients with advanced PSC, they tend to fluctuate widely during the course of the disease. At the time of diagnosis, serum albumin levels are decreased and prothrombin times prolonged in 17 and 16% of patients, respectively. Hypergammaglobulinemia is present

(Table 20.7). Overall, this approach does not appear to be of major benefit to patients with cholestatic-induced osteoporosis. Other treatments such as the use of calcitonin, which inhibits bone reabsorption, and the use of sodium fluoride, which can enhance spine density and increase bone formation, have been shown to be of limited benefit in a small number of PSC patients.

The use of estrogen therapy, which has been shown to be of benefit in the treatment of postmenopausal osteoporosis, has also been shown to be of benefit in patients with osteoporosis associated with cholestasis. However, bisphosphonate compounds such as etidronate and alendronate have been shown to be of much greater value than any of the previously listed therapies for the treatment of osteopenia associated with both chronic cholestatic liver disease and post-transplant bone disease. They can be particularly useful in patients prior to liver transplantation as they can raise the bone density to levels above the fracture threshold and thus help prevent spine fractures in the early post-transplant period. However, caution should be exercised with the use of oral bisphosphates in patients with portal hypertension because of the potential for esophageal ulceration with these drugs.

Following liver transplantation for PSC, the rate of bone loss is accelerated in the PSC patient. This is probably due to a combination of factors, including immobilization, the use of high doses of corticosteroids and increased circulating levels of certain cytokines. Recent studies from the Mayo Clinic have shown that bone mineral density of the lumbar spine decreases for the first 3–6 months post-transplant, during which time there is an increase in pathologic fractures (**Fig. 20.5**). However, bone mineral density subsequently increases to levels above baseline by 1-year post-transplantation, and generally by 2 years post-transplantation, bone density has been shown to be well above pretransplantation levels. The use of antireabsorptive drugs, such as bisphosphonates, has been shown to be effective in preventing the early bone loss after liver transplantation.

A high incidence of avascular necrosis in PSC patients post-transplant, which frequently requires joint replacement, has also been reported. Avascular necrosis is most likely related to the

Treatment of osteopenia associated with PSC
Avoid alchohol
Avoid smoking
Increase ambulation
Vitamin D (maintain serum hydroxyvitamin D levels)
Calcium
Estrogen
Calcitonin
Fluoride
Bisphosphonates
Liver transplantation

Table 20.7 Treatment of osteopenia associated with primary sclerosing cholangitis (PSC). Factors that may improve bone density in patients with PSC.

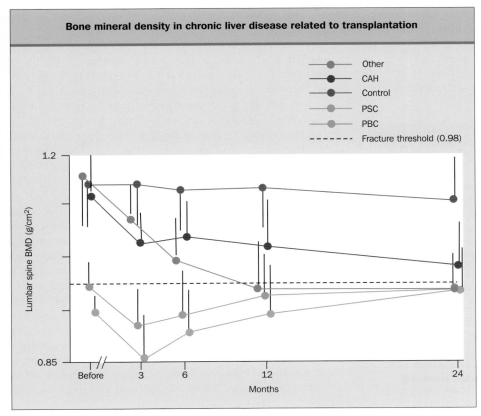

Figure 20.5 Bone mineral density in chronic liver disease related to transplantation. Measurements (mean ± SD) of the lumbar spine using dual photon absorptiometry pretransplantation, at 3 months, 6 months, 12 months and 24 months after liver transplantation in patients with chronic liver disease and in an age- and sex-matched control population. CAH, chronic active hepatitis. Reproduced from Porayko et al (91) by permission of Elsevier.

use of high-dose corticosteroids, but the advent of new and more powerful immunosuppressive agents and the trend toward early steroid withdrawal should reduce the incidence of both pathologic fractures and avascular necrosis in the early post-transplant period.

Complications characteristic of primary sclerosing cholangitis

These are included in Table 20.5. Bacterial cholangitis is an unusual presenting symptom of PSC, but frequently occurs in patients who have had previous bile duct surgery or in whom intervention with radiologic or endoscopic dilatation has been carried out for an obstructing dominant stricture of the large bile ducts. Back pressure resulting from extensive biliary stricturing and the presence of concurrent debris or stones in the large bile ducts is believed to be partially responsible for the deterioration in liver function and is frequently associated with bacterial cholangitis. Progression of the disease to cirrhosis and liver failure may be delayed if obstruction is relieved during the early stages of the disease. In managing such cases, endoscopic decompression is an attractive, temporary therapeutic alternative because it can be performed with relative ease, can facilitate dilatation of multiple strictures at the same time the procedure is performed, and eliminates surgical therapy that might ultimately complicate the liver transplant procedure. The results of trials suggest that balloon dilatation and stenting can alter the usually protracted course of PSC and may delay the timing of, or even the necessity for, liver transplantation (**Table 20.8**). Patients undergoing endoscopic decompression, or who have severe intrahepatic disease associated with bacterial cholangitis, should receive prophylactic broad-spectrum antibiotic therapy to prevent recurrent bouts of bacterial cholangitis. Preference is for quinolone antibiotics because of their high biliary concentration and broad-spectrum action against both Gram-positive and Gram-negative bacteria. In addition, one study has suggested that the combination of ciprofloxacin and ursodeoxycholic acid may be beneficial in preventing sludge formation in those patients undergoing biliary dilatation with stent placement.

Cholelithiasis and choledocholithiasis occur in up to 30% of patients with PSC. Chronic cholestasis predisposes to the formation of cholesterol gallstones and bacterial cholangitis, causing bile stasis, predisposes to the formation of pigment stones. Indeed, diagnosing choledocholithiasis can be extremely difficult in patients with PSC. Therefore, a cholangiogram is essential for eliciting the cause of new onset jaundice or bacterial cholangitis. If choledocholithiasis is documented, stone extraction or surgical intervention is indicated.

Approximately 20% of patients with PSC develop a dominant stricture of the biliary tree. Frequently, the site of the stricture is in the biliary hilum, but strictures can also occur in the common bile duct and the common hepatic duct. This complication is often associated with the acute onset of jaundice, pruritus and/or fever related to bacterial cholangitis. If a dominant stricture is found on cholangiography, cytologic specimens should be obtained in order to exclude bile duct carcinoma, and balloon dilatation should be performed with the use of either a transhepatic or endoscopic retrograde approach, depending on the site of the stricture. In general, balloon dilatation of dominant strictures and removal of biliary sludge, while the patient is receiving antibiotics, is an effective treatment in alleviating the recent onset of jaundice or pruritus related to this complication. Approximately 50% of patients with PSC who undergo balloon dilatation of dominant strictures will have improvement for up to 2 years. Although some centers have advocated a surgical approach for biliary strictures related to PSC, the absence of prospective controlled data makes it difficult to assess the effect of the surgical treatment on the natural history of PSC. Because PSC is generally a progressive disease, surgical intervention should be considered only as a palliative measure aimed at relieving symptoms and excluding a concomitant diagnosis of cholangiocarcinoma. Surgical intervention has little or no value for PSC patients with cirrhosis or for those who have severe intrahepatic bile duct disease on cholangiography. Biliary tract surgery also seems to increase the difficulty and risk of liver transplantation.

Several recent series of PSC patients followed long term reported that cholangiocarcinoma may develop in 6–30% of patients with PSC over a period of 10–30 years (**Fig. 20.6**). PSC should therefore be considered a premalignant condition of the biliary tree just as CUC is considered a premalignant condition of the colon. Cholangiocarcinoma in the setting of PSC is difficult to diagnose because of the lack of serologic markers and the fact that biliary cytologic and histologic studies for the most part have been insensitive in diagnosing cholangiocarcinoma. This is illustrated by the fact that 10% of patients with PSC undergoing liver transplantation are found to have an unsuspected cholangiocarcinoma. A persistent increase in serum bilirubin levels in patients with PSC may be an indication of the development of cholangiocarcinoma. Newer techniques examining cellular detail may be useful in the diagnosis of biliary tract malignancies. Examining bile duct cells obtained by brushing at ERCP for high cellular DNA content by techniques such as DIA has improved the diagnosis of cholangiocarcinoma when compared with routine cytology. Other investigators have used flow cytometry to detect DNA aneuploidy in cholangiocarcinoma from patients with PSC. In one study, these tumors displayed DNA aneuploidy significantly more often when compared to benign strictures. However further studies are needed before these newer techniques can be incorporated into routine clinical practice.

Summary of endoscopic therapy for PSC				
Year	n	Procedure	Follow-up (months)	Result
1997	23	Balloon dilation and ursodiol	45	Improved survival
1996	25	Dilation and stenting	29	Improved symptoms 57%
1995	53	Dilation and stenting	31	Improved symptoms 77%
1993	42	Dilation and stenting	52	Improved symptoms 70%
1991	35	Dilation and stenting	35	Improved symptoms 85%

Table 20.8 Summary of endoscopic therapy in primary sclerosing cholangitis (PSC). Summary of the outcome of five studies reported between 1991–97.

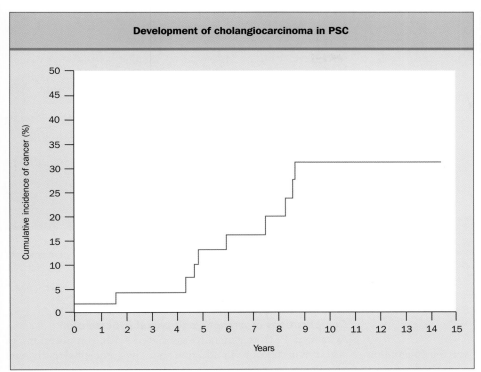

Figure 20.6 Development of cholangiocarcinoma in PSC. Cumulative actuarial incidence of cholangiocarcinoma from the time of onset of PSC. Reproduced from Farges et al (95) by permission of Mosby.

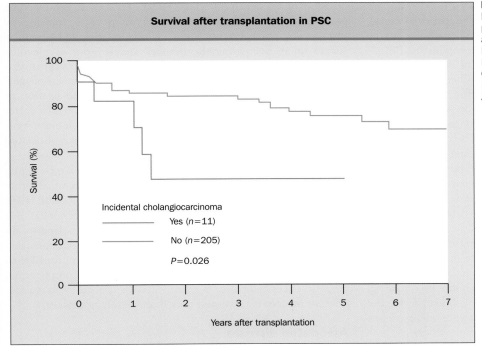

Figure 20.7 Survival after transplantation in PSC. Kaplan-Meier survival plot after transplantation in patients with PSC with and without detection of an incidental cholangiocarcinoma in the excised liver. The difference was statistically significant. Five-year survival rates 0.47 ± 0.17 and 0.75 ± 0.04, respectively. Reproduced from Abu-Elmagd KM et al (93) by permission of the American College of Surgeons.

Patients with PSC and cholangiocarcinoma that was diagnosed before transplantation have very poor prognosis with liver transplantation with less than 10% surviving for more than 2 years. Even patients in whom an incidental cholangiocarcinoma is found at the time of transplantation have a 2-year survival rate of only a 40%, which is far below that of PSC patients who do not have a concurrent cholangiocarcinoma (**Fig. 20.7**). Thus, most liver transplant centers consider a diagnosis of cholangiocarcinoma at least a relative and often an absolute contraindication to liver transplantation. However, a few centers are employing multi-modal adjuvant therapeutic protocols (i.e. radiation and chemotherapy) to improve the results of liver transplantation for this complication and preliminary results have been encouraging. In a study from the Mayo Clinic, highly select patients with

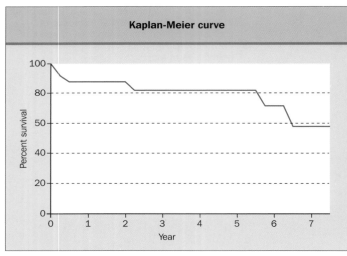

Figure 20.8 Kaplan-Meier curve. A Kaplan-Meier curve showing survival rate after liver transplantation in select patients with unresectable hilar cholangiocarcinoma.

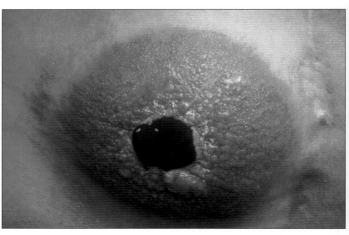

Figure 20.9 Peristomal varix. A peristomal varix surrounding the abdominal ileostoma in a patient with PSC. Reproduced by permission of the Mayo Foundation for Medical Education and Research.

cholangiocarcinoma undergoing orthotopic liver transplantation after neoadjuvant chemotherapy and radiotherapy had a 1-year actuarial survival of 88% and 5-year actuarial survival of 82% (**Fig. 20.8**). This compares favorably with 86% 1-year survival and 72% 5-year survival among deceased donor liver transplant recipients in the USA. Operative management (hepatic resection), chemotherapy and radiotherapy have not been shown to be useful in the treatment of bile duct cancer complicating PSC.

Because of the serious implications of a concomitant cholangiocarcinoma in the PSC patient, it has been important to identify which patients are at a high risk for developing this complication. There are conflicting data on the correlation between the duration of CUC or cirrhotic-stage PSC and the risk of developing cholangiocarcinoma. The use of tumor markers, such as CA 19-9, and cytologic techniques are helpful in diagnosing an existing cholangiocarcinoma, but have not been shown to date to be helpful in the early diagnosis or in screening for cholangiocarcinoma in PSC patients. Clearly, further studies will be needed to better identify those PSC patients at high risk for developing cholangiocarcinoma.

Hepatocellular carcinoma can also develop during the course of PSC. The patients at risk appear to be those who have advanced-stage PSC with extensive fibrosis, cirrhosis and diffuse nodular regeneration of the liver. The question of screening PSC patients for hepatocellular cancer has arisen; however, in the absence of well-established advanced cirrhosis, screening cannot be recommended at this time.

Finally, gallbladder cancer can also arise in patients with PSC. In a retrospective study of 102 patients with PSC who underwent a cholecystectomy, 57% of patients with a mass lesion in the gallbladder had adenocarcinoma and 33% of patients with benign lesions also had associated epithelial cell dysplasia. The presence of dysplasia may therefore indicate a dysplasia–carcinoma sequence in PSC similar to that seen in ulcerative colitis. Patients with PSC and gallbladder polyps should be considered for cholecystectomy. If a cholecystectomy is not performed, careful interim follow-up is warranted.

Complications of cirrhosis and portal hypertension

Advanced PSC is generally associated with complications of portal hypertension. In addition to ascites, encephalopathy and bleeding from esophageal or gastric varices, one special complication is the development and bleeding from peristomal varices in patients who have undergone proctocolectomy with the creation of an ileostomy (**Fig. 20.9**). Treatment for bleeding peristomal varices has been the creation of a transjugular intrahepatic portosystemic shunt, which has usually been quite successful in decreasing the number and severity of bleeding episodes. Non-selective β blockade may also be useful in this situation. As in other forms of chronic liver disease, esophageal variceal bleeding is best managed by variceal band ligation or sclerotherapy. Another option is the use of a transjugular intrahepatic portosystemic shunt. If possible, surgical shunting procedures should not be performed to avoid the risks associated with a subsequent liver transplant if indicated.

Ascites is best treated with sodium restriction, large-volume paracentesis and diuretic therapy. Administration of albumin should be considered in patients who have serum albumin levels below 2.6 g/L. In PSC, spontaneous bacterial peritonitis is a complication often related to biliary sepsis and cholangitis. In this situation, the use of oral selective bowel decontamination solution or chronic antibiotic therapy is especially appropriate to prevent recurrence of this severe life-threatening complication. Hepatic encephalopathy is managed with the use of lactulose. Dietary protein is restricted only if absolutely necessary.

Associated diseases

The syndrome of PSC is associated with a variety of autoimmune-type diseases (**Table 20.9**). These include inflammatory bowel disease, celiac disease, retroperitoneal fibrosis, rheumatoid arthritis, thyroiditis and a host of other diseases that are thought to be of autoimmune origin. Of importance, inflammatory bowel disease occurs in up to 80% of patients with PSC. The majority of these patients have CUC and a minority has Crohn colitis. In general, inflammatory bowel disease is diagnosed several years before PSC. However, inflammatory bowel disease can be diagnosed simultaneously with PSC or years after the diagnosis of

University, Philadelphia, PA), 426 PSC patients with a mean follow-up of 3 years were studied. In this study, serum bilirubin level, histologic stage, patient age and splenomegaly were identified as independent prognostic variables. With these variables, a severity risk score was determined and translated into a survival function so that survival of any PSC patient at any point in the disease process could be estimated. Subgroup analysis from these various liver transplant centers indicates that this model is generalizable to a wide spectrum of patients who have PSC. However, the new model also requires the need for a liver biopsy, which often limits the utility of the model as a clinical tool.

This deficit was addressed in a study from the Cleveland Clinic where the authors evaluated the Child-Pugh classification as a prognostic indicator for survival in PSC. The authors further compared the Child-Pugh model with the Mayo disease-specific PSC model. The Child-Pugh model utilizes the following clinical factors:

- serum bilirubin level;
- serum albumin level;
- prothrombin time;
- presence or absence of ascites; and
- grade of portosystemic encephalopathy.

The study demonstrated that the age-adjusted Child-Pugh model predicted survival before liver transplantation with accuracy similar to that of the Mayo PSC model. It also had the advantage of not requiring a liver biopsy and avoided complex mathematical computations. Furthermore, it is ideal for use in formulating minimal listing criteria for liver transplantation for the United Network for Organ Sharing (UNOS). This essentially places PSC patients on a level playing field with all chronic liver disease patients in whom the Child-Pugh classification is utilized for liver transplantation listing purposes and avoids having different criteria for each disease.

However, there are obvious shortcomings with regard to all of these models in that none of them has been prospectively evaluated, they all use historic data, and they do not take into account certain risk factors that are important in determining the timing for liver transplantation in the PSC patient, such as variceal bleeding, quality of life and the possibility of developing a hepatobiliary malignancy. Nevertheless, these models have been useful in counseling patients and have been important in advising the appropriate timing for liver transplantation for patients with this disease. Additional ongoing studies will be needed to assess prospectively the models and their applications toward further optimizing the timing of liver transplantation. In addition, the challenge remains to refine further these models so that they might be applied to monitoring the effect of experimental therapy on disease progression.

MANAGEMENT

Primary therapy for PSC aimed at interrupting the disease process can be subdivided into medical, radiologic, and surgical approaches (**Table 20.11**).

Medical therapy

Over the past 20 years, various medical treatments have been used in PSC patients in the hope of improving survival. The diversity of medical therapies includes the use of cupruretic, immunosuppressive, antifibrogenic and choleretic agents, which suggests their ineffectiveness and reveals a lack of complete understanding of the pathophysiology of the disease.

Cupruretic therapy

The evidence of increased hepatic copper in PSC provided the main rationale for evaluating D-penicillamine as a therapeutic agent for PSC. In a prospective randomized, double-blind, placebo-controlled trial, D-penicillamine had no favorable effect on PSC progression and patient survival. This was determined after 36 months of follow-up based on careful analysis of clinical and biochemical profiles, radiologic findings, liver histology and survival data between the two groups of PSC patients. Furthermore, major adverse effects of D-penicillamine including proteinuria and thrombocytopenia, led to the discontinuation of the drug in 20% of treated patients.

Immunosuppressive therapy

The use of immunosuppressive agents in the therapy of PSC was based on the concept that PSC is an autoimmune disease. In uncontrolled observations, oral corticosteroids have been shown

Treatment of PSC
Medical
Cupruretic:
D-penicillamine
Immunosuppressive:
Prednisone
Azathioprine
Cyclosporin
Methotrexate
Tacrolimus
Mycophenolate mofetil
Antifibrotic:
Colchicine
Etanercept pentoxifylline
Choleretic:
Ursodeoxycholic acid
Radiological
Cholangioplasty
Biliary infusion therapy
Surgical
Reconstructive surgery
Proctocolectomy
Liver transplantation

Table 20.11 Treatment of (PSC). The treatments include drugs, radiologic and surgical approaches. All are aimed at retarding disease progression.

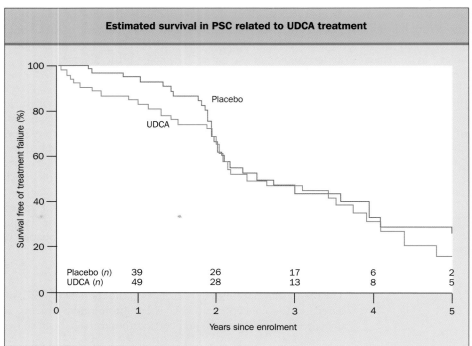

Figure 20.15 Estimated survival in PSC related to UDCA treatment. Kaplan-Meier analysis of survival free of treatment failure among study patients. Treatment failure was defined as one or more of the following: death, liver transplantation, histologic progression by two stages, progression to cirrhosis, development of esophageal varices, development of ascites or encephalopathy, sustained quadrupling of the serum bilirubin concentration, marked worsening of fatigue or pruritus, inability to tolerate the drug and voluntary withdrawal from the study. UDCA, ursodeoxycholic acid. Reproduced from Lindor et al (97) by permission of the Massachusetts Medical Society.

to improve the biochemical profile in PSC patients; however, long-term or controlled studies of corticosteroids are lacking. In a small, controlled study in PSC patients, topical corticosteroid application in the biliary tree via nasobiliary lavage provided no advantage over placebo. Other immunosuppressive agents that have been employed in the treatment of PSC include:

- azathioprine – the experience has been mostly anecdotal;
- cyclosporin – the results were negative;
- methotrexate – a randomized, double-blind, placebo-controlled trial showed no benefit in the treatment group; and
- tacrolimus – a small open-label study showed only improvement in liver enzymes.

These attempts at immunosuppressive therapy lead to the conclusion that further studies are needed to define the immunosuppressive effects in PSC patients. In addition, an open trial of prednisone and colchicine in PSC patients demonstrated no benefit on progression of hepatic histology and liver biochemical tests over a 2-year period. A pilot study combining ursodeoxycholic acid and methotrexate for the treatment of PSC was associated with toxicity and without improvement in liver tests compared with ursodeoxycholic acid therapy alone.

Antifibrotic therapy

Due to the fact that PSC leads to liver cirrhosis, antifibrotic agents, such as colchicine, were suggested as a therapeutic option for PSC. Recently, in a prospective, double-blind study, 84 PSC patients were randomized to receive 1 mg of colchicine versus placebo daily for a period of 3 years. The results of this multicenter study revealed that colchicine had no beneficial effect on patient symptoms, liver biochemistry, hepatic histology or survival.

Choleretic therapy

The enthusiasm for the use of ursodeoxycholic acid, a hydrophilic bile acid, in the treatment of PSC emerged from favorable

data on its use for PBC and from promising clinical and biochemical improvement reported in PSC patients receiving ursodeoxycholic acid in small uncontrolled studies. Subsequently, a prospective, randomized, double-blind, placebo-controlled trial involving 14 PSC patients was performed to examine further the efficacy of ursodeoxycholic acid. The authors of that study concluded that PSC patients treated with ursodeoxycholic acid at 13–15 mg/kg of body weight per day for 1 year demonstrated marked improvement in serum liver tests and histology on liver biopsy. The proposed benefit of orally administered ursodeoxycholic acid in cholestatic patients is thought to be related to:

- its accumulation in the endogenous bile pool which leads to replacement of endogenous potentially toxic bile acids in the cholestatic liver;
- its protective effect at the cellular and subcellular levels of the hepatocyte and cholangiocyte;
- its hypercholeretic activity; and
- its immunomodulatory effect.

However, in the recently published largest randomized, double-blind, placebo-controlled trial of ursodeoxycholic acid treatment for PSC, no clinical benefit was found. The study included 105 patients with well-established PSC given ursodeoxycholic acid 13–15 mg/kg of body weight/day compared with placebo. The mean follow-up was 2.2 years. In this study, ursodeoxycholic acid, but not placebo, demonstrated improvement in liver tests at 1 and 2 years of treatment. Nevertheless, the primary outcome (time to treatment failure), as defined by the authors, and survival were not significantly different in the two groups of PSC patients (**Fig. 20.15**). However, in a randomized, placebo-controlled study of 26 patients followed over 2 years, the use of high dose ursodeoxycholic acid (20 mg/kg/day) was found to result in improved liver biochemistries, cholangiographic appearances and fibrosis. Another pilot study of high dose ursodeoxycholic acid (25–30 mg/kg/day) in 30 patients with PSC also demonstrated improved biochemistries and the Mayo risk score, translating into a significantly better survival compared to patients on a placebo or low dose ursodeoxycholic acid. These promising results need to be explored further in patients with PSC.

In summary, to date, effective pharmacologic treatment for the underlying hepatobiliary disease in PSC is lacking. The data do not support the use of any mentioned agent except in the context of well-designed experimental studies. Future therapeutic trials for PSC must be centered on the asymptomatic patient because, when ductopenia occurs, the disease appears to be irreversible since bile duct epithelial cells are unable to regenerate.

Surgical therapy

Until the advent of liver transplantation, surgical therapy for PSC was focused on alleviation of pruritus and jaundice, exclusion of cholangiocarcinoma, and the prevention of colonic adenocarcinoma by performing a proctocolectomy in patients with concurrent PSC and CUC.

Biliary surgery

Since PSC is a progressive disease, biliary surgery was introduced primarily to improve symptoms. Biliary enteric anastomoses with biliary stenting and reconstruction of the hepatic duct bifurcation with long-term transhepatic stents have been performed. In two retrospective studies evaluating biliary tract reconstructive surgery, cirrhotic PSC patients showed a significantly higher mortality rate compared to the non-cirrhotic patients. Thus, it is now widely accepted that biliary surgery should be avoided in PSC patients with cirrhosis or severe, diffuse intrahepatic disease. Instead, these patients should be considered for liver transplantation.

Although biliary reconstruction may benefit non-cirrhotic PSC patients with extrahepatic disease, the lack of prospective, controlled data makes it impossible to assess the long-term effects of this procedure on the natural history of PSC and the subsequent risk of developing cholangiocarcinoma. In our view, the value of biliary surgery is limited to selected PSC patients without cirrhosis who are not candidates for liver transplantation when extrahepatic dominant strictures are not amenable to endoscopic or transhepatic dilatation.

Proctocolectomy

In patients with both PSC and CUC, proctocolectomy is frequently performed due to indications relevant to inflammatory bowel disease. The possible effect of proctocolectomy on the natural history of PSC was examined in a retrospective analysis involving 45 patients with coexisting PSC and CUC, of whom almost half had undergone proctocolectomy and the rest had not. This study revealed that the clinical signs, biochemical profile, histologic progression on liver biopsy, and survival were not different in the two groups. Moreover, the fact that PSC can occur years after proctocolectomy argues against any beneficial effect of this procedure on the progression of PSC. Nonetheless, patients with both PSC and CUC remain at high risk for the development of adenocarcinoma of the colon; thus, an annual surveillance colonoscopy is strongly indicated, particularly in patients with PSC who have undergone liver transplantation. Proctocolectomy should be performed for intractable symptoms of inflammatory bowel disease that are not amenable to medical treatment and for colonic dysplasia and malignancy. In patients with PSC and CUC, if proctocolectomy is indicated, an IPAA is the procedure of choice since this procedure prevents the development of peristomal varices. Of note, a complication of the IPAA is pouchitis, a non-specific inflammation of the ileal reservoir that occurs more frequently in patients with coexisting PSC and CUC than in CUC patients alone. Frequently, treatment with metronidazole or other antibiotics will effectively control this condition.

Orthotopic liver transplantation

Currently, the only suitable life-saving treatment for patients with end-stage PSC is orthotopic liver transplantation. Over the past decade, the outcome of liver transplantation in PSC patients with end-stage disease has improved significantly, and liver transplantation has emerged as the treatment of choice for these patients. Indeed, retrospective analysis of PSC patients using the Mayo PSC natural history model has shown that liver transplantation significantly improves the survival rate at all risk stratifications compared with the estimated survival and the absence of liver transplantation. Recently, the 1-year and 5-year patient survival after liver transplantation for PSC have been reported to be 90–97% and 85–88%, respectively (**Fig. 20.16**), based on independent studies from three major liver transplant centers. In patients with end-stage PSC, one of the major clinical challenges is selecting the ideal time for liver transplantation. It is known that patients with high Mayo PSC risk scores have an increased risk of death after orthotopic liver transplantation compared with patients with low Mayo risk scores. In addition, risk factors specific to PSC that affect the outcome of liver transplantation have been recognized. Recently, a prognostic model to predict the post-liver transplant morbidity in PSC and PBC has been described. In PSC patients, the guidelines for liver transplantation should include intractability of symptoms, signs and complications of portal hypertension. However, careful consideration of each patient's needs and quality of life remain important in this disease.

Despite a favorable outcome, liver transplantation for PSC is associated with specific complications. Post-liver transplant complications include an increased incidence of acute and chronic rejection frequently leading to graft loss, biliary strictures and leakage, hepatic artery thrombosis and lymphoproliferative disease. Recurrence of PSC after liver transplantation has been controversial primarily due to the lack of gold standard criteria for the diagnosis of recurrent PSC. When a cohort of patients was evaluated for recurrent disease based on biochemical, cholangiographic and histologic criteria, 20% were found to have evidence of recurrent disease at a mean of 55 months after liver transplantation. A number of these patients have required retransplantation, and the impact of the recurrence of PSC is yet to be determined.

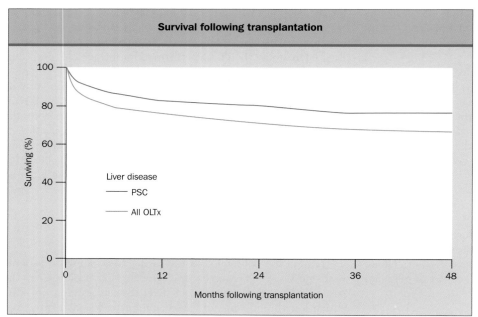

Figure 20.16 Survival following transplantation.
Survival in patients undergoing liver transplantation for PSC in comparison with overall survival for all indications for orthotopic liver transplantation. Patients undergoing liver transplantation for PSC had significantly improved survival ($P<0.01$) on the basis of 1992 data from UNOS. Patients with PSC (n = 499); other indications (n = 4332). Reproduced with permission from Aegean communications (94) Contemp Internal Med.

FURTHER READING

Diagnosis

Bhamba K, Kim WR, Talwalkar J, et al. Incidence, clinical spectrum, and outcomes of primary sclerosing cholangitis in a United States community. Gastroenterology 2003; 125(5):1364–1369.

Craig DA, MacCarty RL, Wiesner RH, et al. Primary sclerosing cholangitis: value of cholangiography in determining the prognosis. Am J Roentgenology 1991; 157:959–964.

Devrroede G. Colorectal cancer. In: Winawer S, Schottenfeld D, Sherlock P, eds. Prevention, epidemiology, screening. New York: Raven Press; 1980.

Graziadei IW, Wiesner RH, Batts, et al. Recurrence of primary sclerosing cholangitis following liver transplantation. Hepatology 1999; 29:1050–1056. *A large group of patients with well-characterized PSC developed non-anastomic biliary strictures following liver transplantation highly suggestive of recurrence of disease. These findings were not seen in a control group of patients who underwent a Roux-en-Y anastomosis for indications other than PSC.*

Wiesner RH. Current concepts in primary sclerosing cholangitis. Mayo Clin Proc 1994; 69:969–982.

Wilschanski M, Chait P, Wade JA, et al. Primary sclerosing cholangitis in 32 children: clinical, laboratory, and radiographic features with survival analysis. Hepatology 1995; 22:1415–1420.

Pathophysiology

Bansi DS, Fleming KA, Chapman RW. Importance of antineutrophil cytoplasmic antibodies in primary sclerosing cholangitis and ulcerative colitis: prevalence, titer, and IgG subclass. Gut 1996; 38:384–389.

Ben-Ari Z, Czaja AJ. Autoimmune hepatitis and its variant syndromes. Gut 2001; 49:589–594.

Boberg KM, Fausa O, Haaland T, et al. Features of autoimmune hepatitis in primary sclerosing cholangitis: an evaluation of 114 primary sclerosing cholangitis patients according to a scoring system for the diagnosis of autoimmune hepatitis. Hepatology 1996; 23:1369–1376.

Lee YM, Kaplan MM. Primary sclerosing cholangitis. N Engl J Med 1995; 332:924–933. *An excellent overall review of PSC with regard to diagnosis, treatment, epidemiology and overall outcome.*

Ludwig J. Small duct primary sclerosing cholangitis. Semin Liv Dis 1991; 11:1791–1796.

Ludwig J, Barham SS, LaRusso NF, et al. Morphologic features of chronic hepatitis associated with primary sclerosing cholangitis and chronic ulcerative colitis. Hepatology 1981; 1:632–640.

Treatment

Abu-Elmagd KM, Malinchoc M, Dickson ER, et al. Efficacy of hepatic transplantation in patients with primary sclerosing cholangitis. Surg Gynecol Obstet 1993; 177:335–344.

Aegean communications. Contemp Internal Med 1994; 6:37–46.

Ahrendt SA, Pitt HA, Kalloo AN, et al. Primary sclerosing cholangitis: resect, dilate, or transplant? Ann Surg 1998; 227:412–423.

Bjornsson E, Lindqvist-Ottosson J, Asztely M, et al. Dominant strictures in patients with primary sclerosing cholangitis. Am J Gastroenterol 2004; 99(3):502–508.

Brandsaeter B, Isonjemi H, Broome U, et al. Liver transplantation for primary schlerosing cholangitis; predictors and consequences of hepatobiliary malignancy. J Hepatol 2004; 40:815–822.

Farges O, Malassagne B, Sebagh M, et al. Primary sclerosing cholangitis, liver transplantation, or biliary surgery. Surgery 1995; 22:451–457.

Heimbach JK, Gores GJ, Haddock MG, et al. Liver transplantation for unresectable perihilar cholangiocarcinoma. Semin Liver Dis 2004; 24:201–207.

Lindor KD. Ursodiol for primary sclerosing cholangitis. N Eng J Med 1997; 336:691–695.

Mayo PSC Study Group. Ursodiol for primary sclerosing cholangitis. N Engl J Med 1997; 336:691–695. *A prospective randomized trial evaluating Ursodiol in the treatment of PSC, indicating that Ursodiol is of little benefit in preventing progression of disease.*

Stiehl A, Rudolph G, Sauer P, et al. Efficacy of ursodeoxycholic acid treatment and endoscopic dilation of major duct stenoses in primary sclerosing cholangitis. An 8-year prospective study. J Hepatol 1997; 26:560–566.

Complications

Bergquist A, Glauman H, Persson B, et al. Risk factors and clinical presentation of hepatobiliary carcinoma in patients with primary sclerosing cholangitis: a case-control study. Hepatology 1998; 27:311–316. *An assessment of*

are TGF-β 1, platelet derived growth factor, FGF, hepatocyte growth factor, platelet activating factor, and endothelin-1. With resolution of inflammation, activated HSC undergo apoptosis, leaving scar tissue. With time, scar tissue may resolve or the hepatic lobule may remodel, leaving nodules with altered blood flow surrounded by bands of scar tissue.

CLINICAL: HISTORY, PHYSICAL EXAMINATION AND DIAGNOSIS

Alcohol use and abuse
The CAGE (*c*utback, *a*nnoyed, *g*uilty, *e*ye-opener) questions can be used to screen for alcohol abuse (**Table 21.4**).Two positive answers indicate alcohol dependency, with a sensitivity of 70% and a specificity of 90%. Estimating the amount of alcohol consumed can be difficult. It may be helpful to ask about the amount of alcohol purchased per week rather than the amount consumed. In some instances family and friends may provide useful information. When in doubt, it is often wise to assume the patient may have an alcohol problem and to refer the patient to an alcohol treatment program.

When abnormal, serum γ-glutamyltransferase and mean corpuscular volume have a sensitivity of 30–40% in determining excessive alcohol use. Carbohydrate deficient transferrin is a specific, although not necessarily a sensitive, marker of excess alcohol use. It is not routinely available and is relatively costly. In practice, it is rarely used as a screening test for alcohol use.

Fatty liver
Fatty liver is present in 80–90% of patients drinking more than 60 g of ethanol per day. Most patients are asymptomatic or have non-specific complaints such as mild nausea, fatigue or right upper quadrant discomfort. Patients with fatty liver disease often present to healthcare providers for treatment of alcoholism or trauma, or for routine medical care, and are incidentally found to have liver disease.

Approximately two-thirds of patients with fatty liver have hepatomegaly. The remainder of the physical examination is usually unremarkable. Aspartate aminotransferase (AST) may be raised, although rarely more than five times the upper limit of normal. As a rule alanine aminotransferase (ALT) is normal. Total bilirubin is frequently normal, but occasionally may be as high as 5 mg/dL. Typically, albumin is normal, as are the white blood cell (WBC) count, hemoglobin and prothrombin time. A reliable diagnosis of fatty liver is best made by liver biopsy, but in practice liver biopsy is not often obtained unless there is a suggestion of more advanced disease.

Foamy degeneration (microvesicular fatty liver disease)
Patients with foamy degeneration can present with jaundice, hepatic encephalopathy and marked elevation of AST and alkaline phosphatase. In general, the WBC count is not elevated and prothrombin time is normal. Liver biopsy is required to make the definitive diagnosis of microvesicular fatty liver disease. Patients with foamy degeneration usually recover quickly if they remain abstinent.

Alcoholic hepatitis
Typically, patients with alcoholic hepatitis have consumed large amounts of alcohol for decades, although patients may have stopped drinking several weeks prior to admission to hospital, possibly because of the ill effects of the liver disease. Patients hospitalized for alcoholic hepatitis may have a variety of symptoms related to their inflammatory liver disease, including fever, nausea, anorexia, fatigue, pruritus, weakness, right upper quadrant pain and confusion (**Table 21.5**).

Physical examination is markedly abnormal in patients hospitalized with alcoholic hepatitis. Jaundice is the cardinal sign in alcoholic hepatitis and is present in all patients. Fever is frequently present (without infection). Common cutaneous signs include telangectasias, spider angiomas and palmar erythema. Scratch marks, whitening of the nails and prominent venous collaterals in the periumbilical area are less common. Malnutrition, measured as decreased muscle mass, decreased serum proteins and decreased muscle strength, is present in more than 90% of hospitalized patients with alcoholic hepatitis. A minority have overt hepatic encephalopathy (i.e. asterixis), but most have subclinical hepatic encephalopathy. More than 75% of patients with severe alcoholic hepatitis have ascites and peripheral edema. Up to one-third have a hepatic bruit, heard over the liver either anteriorly or posteriorly, which is thought to be caused by increased blood flow through the hepatic artery. Splenomegaly is often present, but may not be detected by physical examination because of ascites.

Total serum bilirubin and conjugated bilirubin are elevated in all patients with alcoholic hepatitis and can exceed 30 mg/dL in patients with renal insufficiency. The WBC count is frequently elevated, with an increase in PMN and as well as increase in premature neutrophils ('bands'). Hemoglobin is mildly decreased (often to 11–12 g/L) due to dilution effect of increased plasma volume, decreased red blood cell (RBC) production, and increased RBC destruction. Variceal hemorrhage may contribute to decreased hemoglobin levels. AST (serum glutamic-oxaloacetic transaminase; SGOT) is elevated, although rarely more than five times the upper limit of normal. ALT (serum glutamic-pyruvic transaminase; SGPT) is often normal, but may be elevated above normal if the AST is more than threefold elevated. The AST/ALT ratio is greater than 1 in virtually all patients, and is generally close to 3. Alkaline phosphatase is moderately elevated, but is not a sensitive, specific or prognostic test in alcoholic hepatitis. Prothrombin time is elevated in most patients. Platelet count is decreased, but is generally >75 000/mm³. More often than not serum sodium is decreased (often less than 130 mEq/L) due to the reduced ability of the kidney to excrete free water. More often than not serum

CAGE questions
1. Have you ever felt like you should cut down on your drinking?
2. Have people annoyed you by criticizing your drinking?
3. Have you ever felt bad or guilty about your drinking?
4. Have you ever had a drink first thing in the morning (eye-opener) to steady your nerves or get rid of a hangover?
Answering 'yes' to two or more questions is suggestive of alcohol dependency.

Table 21.4 CAGE questions

Relative frequency of various symptoms, physical findings and laboratory tests in patients admitted to hospital with alcoholic hepatitis	
Symptom	*Frequency of abnormal finding (+, ++ or +++)*
Weakness	+++
Anorexia	++
Fever	++
Confusion	+
Abdominal pain	+
Physical finding	
Fever	++
Jaundice	+++
Malnutrition, muscle wasting	+++
Telangiectasia, palmar erythema	+++
Hepatomegaly	++
Ascites	+++
Hepatic encephalopathy	+
Hepatic bruit	+
Abnormal laboratory test	
Bilirubin	+++
AST (usually <200 IU/mL)	+++
ALT (usually normal)	+
Albumin	+++
Creatinine	+
WBC, PMN	++
Hemoglobin	++
Platelet	+++
INR (prothrombin time)	++
Serum sodium (low)	++
Urine sodium (low)	+++
ALT, alanine aminotransferase; AST, aspartate aminotransferase; INR, international normalized ratio; PMN, polymorphonuclear leukocytes; WBC, white blood cell count.	

Table 21.5 Relative frequency of various symptoms, physical findings and laboratory tests in patients admitted to hospital with alcoholic hepatitis

creatinine is normal, although creatinine clearance may be modestly reduced (60–80 mL/min). Elevated serum creatinine is a sign of hepatorenal syndrome and carries an ominous short-term prognosis. Urinalysis is unremarkable except for elevated bilirubin and urobilinogen. As a rule, urine sodium is low, often <10 mEq/L, even in patients without hepatorenal syndrome. The urine osmolality is higher than would be expected from the low serum osmolality. Excess protein is not present in the urine.

Up to 25% of patients are infected on admission to hospital, either in the ascites (spontaneous bacterial peritonitis), urine or blood. Cultures of ascites are recommended on admission to hospital and if the patient's hospital course deteriorates. If the patient is febrile, blood and urine cultures should be considered.

The diagnosis of alcoholic hepatitis is usually made on clinical grounds based on the presence of three or more of the following:
- serum total bilirubin >10 mg/dL,
- WBC count >10 000/ mm^3,
- fever,
- ascites, and
- AST elevation in the appropriate range [i.e. AST:ALT ratio >1 (usually approximately 3), AST <10 upper limits of normal (ULN) (usually <5 × ULN)].

Transjugular liver biopsy is useful to confirm the diagnosis but is not available in many hospitals. A PMN count greater than 5500/mm^3 has an acceptable specificity and can be used to confirm the diagnosis of alcoholic hepatitis if a liver biopsy cannot be performed.

Patients may have milder forms of alcoholic hepatitis. In these patients, the symptoms, physical examination, and laboratory tests are less severely affected than those with severe alcoholic hepatitis although all patients have an elevated serum bilirubin level.

Cirrhosis

Cirrhosis covers a broad spectrum of disease, from patients with 'early' cirrhosis to patients with decompensated cirrhosis, diagnosed by the presence of ascites, jaundice, encephalopathy or variceal bleeding. Patients with 'early' cirrhosis may be asymptomatic or complain of non-specific symptoms such as fatigue or weakness. As cirrhosis progresses, and especially in decompensated disease, patients are more likely to be symptomatic, often with fatigue, malaise and impotence.

The liver is firm and may be enlarged, especially the left lobe, or small and not palpable. The spleen is often, but not invariably, enlarged. The remainder of the physical examination may be normal in patients with early cirrhosis. Cutaneous signs of cirrhosis include palmar erythema and spider telangiectasias. Ascites is the most common form of decompensation in cirrhosis and is usually accompanied by peripheral edema. Overt hepatic encephalopathy (e.g. asterixis) is infrequent, although subclinical hepatic encephalopathy is common in decompensated cirrhosis. Muscle wasting and decreased muscle strength are universal in advanced alcoholic cirrhosis.

All routine laboratory tests may be normal in 'early' cirrhosis. However, one or more laboratory tests are usually abnormal, with the degree of abnormality increasing in advanced cirrhosis. Albumin and hemoglobin levels may be decreased, in part because of the dilutional effect of increased plasma volume as well as decreased production. Typically, serum total bilirubin is normal, but it may be elevated several fold in advanced cirrhosis. Direct bilirubin is frequently mildly elevated in patients with normal total bilirubin, and is a sign of hepatic dysfunction. Prothrombin time may be elevated. Platelet count is decreased although usually not to the level in patients with hepatitis C cirrhosis. The serum AST is elevated if the patient is drinking alcohol, but may be normal in abstinent patients. Serum ALT is usually normal. Serum sodium is normal unless the patient has ascites. The WBC count may be decreased due to

Treatment of patients hospitalized with alcoholic hepatitis		
Accepted treatment		
Corticosteroids	Prednisolone 40 mg p.o. QAM, 28 days	Indicated if DF >32 or hepatic encephalopathy Contraindicated if sepsis, bleeding, renal failure
Nutritional supplementation	Oral or enteral Calories: 35 kcal/kg/day Protein: 1.5 g/kg/day Sodium: 2 g/day (88 mEq)	Does not improve survival Unlikely to worsen hepatic encephalopathy
Possibly effective treatment		
Anticytokine	Pentoxifylline 400 mg p.o. t.i.d.	Single study Reduced hepatorenal syndrome
Not accepted treatment		
Anti-TNF	Infliximab Etanercept	Possibly effective in small, uncontrolled trials Increased mortality with infliximab in RCT
Anabolic steroids	Oxandralone Testosterone	May improve nutritional status, does not improve survival
Anti-thyroid	Propylthiouracil	Does not improve survival
Antioxidants	Vitamins, selenium, *N*-acetylcysteine, etc.	Does not improve survival
Hepatic mitogens	Insulin and glucagon	Several deaths from hypoglycemia
Other treatment	Colchicine, verapamil, penicillamine	Do not improve survival
QAM; quality addiction management; RCT, randomized controlled trial; TNF, tumor necrosis factor		

Table 21.9 Treatment of patients hospitalized with alcoholic hepatitis.

recommended by the American College of Gastroenterology in patients with severe alcoholic hepatitis (DF >32). Specific treatments are reviewed below (**Table 21.9**).

Corticosteroids
Corticosteroids inhibit the inflammatory response, in part by inhibiting activation of NF-κB, a transcription factor that activates TNF-α and other proinflammatory cytokines. Corticosteroids have been evaluated in at least 17 clinical trials enrolling more than 900 patients. Two randomized controlled trials published in the 1990s, one from France and the other from the USA, demonstrated improved 1-month survival with corticosteroid treatment. These authors combined their primary data with data from a third, negative study, to evaluate survival in a total of 215 patients (102 placebo and 113 corticosteroid). Survival at day 28 was 85% in patients receiving corticosteroids and 65% in placebo patients (*p* <0.001). Survival was significantly higher in the corticosteroid treated group at 6 and 12 months, but not at 24 months. Patients with a decrease in serum total bilirubin 7 days after starting corticosteroid treatment have an 82% survival at 6 months compared with a 23% survival in patients whose total bilirubin increases during the first 7 days of corticosteroid treatment. The latter group, which represents 28% of patients, and which cannot be determined from pretreatment assessment, is the group of patients in whom other forms of treatment are needed.

The recommended treatment is prednisolone 40 mg orally every morning (or methylprednisolone 32 mg/day intravenously in patients unable to tolerate oral medications). Treatment is restricted to patients with a DF >32 or those with overt hepatic encephalopathy (e.g. asterixis). It is important to exclude infection prior to starting treatment, during treatment, and after treatment has stopped. Despite the theoretical risk for infection, only one study reported increased mortality from infection, and that occurred in the 11 months after corticosteroids were stopped. It seems reasonable to start corticosteroids if patients have received adequate antibiotic treatment for at least 48 h. Recent (past 2 weeks) upper gastrointestinal bleeding is commonly listed as a contraindication to starting corticosteroid treatment based on the (now incorrect) belief that corticosteroids cause duodenal ulcers. In practice corticosteroids may be started when patients have not bled for at least 48 h. Corticosteroids are not recommended if the serum creatinine is >2.0 mg/dL since these patients are likely to die from hepatorenal syndrome, a condition that is not improved by corticosteroid use.

Despite these recommendations, there continues to be controversy about the use of corticosteroids in alcoholic hepatitis. Only 7 of the 17 studies were randomized controlled trials that were evaluated on an intention to treat basis. In these seven studies, the relative risk of death with steroids was 1.06 (95% confidence interval of 0.87–1.31). The clinical trials have been the subject of three meta-analyses, two of which found corticosteroid treatment to be beneficial while the third meta-analysis performed using a different approach, found corticosteroids to not be beneficial. In addition, there may be a publication bias towards studies with positive results, especially trials with a small number of patients. Finally, one of the concerns with corticosteroids is the exclusion of patients with infection, upper gastrointestinal bleeding, or renal insufficiency.

Up to 40% of patients with alcoholic hepatitis might be excluded from treatment using these criteria. Additional studies with corticosteroids would be desirable, but are unlikely to be performed.

Pentoxifylline

Pentoxifylline (PTX) is an oral phosphodiesterase inhibitor which decreases expression of TNF-α (and other proinflammatory cytokines) and which may inhibit apoptosis. Based on its anti-cytokine activity, a placebo controlled trial was undertaken in 103 patients with alcoholic hepatitis and a DF >32. Pentoxifylline 400 mg p.o. t.i.d. for 28 days decreased mortality during the index hospitalization from 46.1% in the placebo patients to 24.5% in the PTX group (p <0.05). The reduction in mortality was due to a decrease in the number of patients dying with hepatorenal syndrome. No significant side-effects were reported in patients receiving PTX. This study needs to be confirmed, preferably in comparison with corticosteroids, before use of PTX can be recommended in patients with alcoholic hepatitis. Nevertheless, experts frequently use PTX, especially if there are contraindications to corticosteroid use since PTX has minimal side-effects and few other treatments are available.

Nutritional therapy

The universal presence of malnutrition, as well as the prior belief that alcoholic liver disease was a consequence of malnutrition rather than alcohol, prompted multiple studies of nutritional therapy for alcoholic hepatitis. The earliest studies, performed more than 20 years ago, involved parenteral feeding and demonstrated an improvement in nitrogen balance or serum albumin, but no improvement in survival. Five randomized controlled trials of oral/enteral feeding have confirmed improvement in nutritional status but have failed to show improved survival. A recent trial suggests enteral feeding decreases mortality from infections. This study compared corticosteroid treatment (with 2000 kcal standard hospital diet) to enteral feeding with a 2000 kcal diet (without corticosteroid treatment) in 71 patients with DF >32. Mortality at 28 days was similar in the corticosteroid group (25%) and in the enteral feeding group (31%). Mortality during the next 11 months was higher in the corticosteroid group (37%) than in the enteral feeding group (8%) primarily due to fewer infections in patients receiving enteral feeding. Overall survival at 12 months was similar in both groups (39% in corticosteroid versus 62% in enteral feeding, p=0.26). Although this study suggests that enteral feeding may be superior to corticosteroid treatment, especially after the first month of treatment, the overall survival in the corticosteroid group (39% at 12 months) was considerably worse than the survival rate in other randomized controlled studies with corticosteroids. Overall, enteral nutrition during the initial hospitalization with severe alcoholic hepatitis improves markers of nutritional status but has not been shown convincingly to improve survival.

Anti-tumor necrosis factor

TNF-α plasma levels are increased in patients with alcoholic hepatitis and correlate with disease severity. TNF-α stimulates the proinflammatory cytokines IL-6 and the neutrophil chemotactic cytokine IL-8. In animal studies, knocking out the TNF receptor, or administration of TNF antibodies, reduces alcoholic liver damage. Given the effectiveness of anti-TNF treatment of rheumatoid arthritis and Crohn disease, these agents have been evaluated in several small studies in patients with alcoholic hepatitis. Two small, non-randomized studies of infliximab (chimeric human-mouse monoclonal antibody against TNF-α) treatment and one study of Etanercept (a TNF receptor: Fc fusion protein that binds to TNF-α) reported no significant adverse events with anti-TNF treatment. Survival could not be evaluated since the studies were not randomized. There has been one prospective, randomized, controlled trial of anti-TNF treatment in alcoholic hepatitis. Patients with a DF >32 received treatment with prednisolone for 28 days. Patients were randomized with respect to additional treatment with infliximab (10 mg/kg at day 0, 14 and 28) or placebo. The study was discontinued prematurely because of increased mortality in patients receiving infliximab (39%) as compared with patients receiving placebo (18%) at 2 months (p = not significant). Furthermore, the rate of serious bacterial infections was significantly higher in patients receiving infliximab (13 patients) than in placebo patients (three patients, p<0.002). Further studies of these agents are planned; their use is not recommended outside of clinical trials.

Anabolic steroids

Anabolic steroids improve nitrogen balance and were studied because of the universal malnutrition in patients with severe alcoholic hepatitis. In the largest study to date, 273 patients were randomized with respect to treatment for 3 months with both oxandralone and a branched chain amino acid supplement or placebo (oxandralone and a low-calorie, low-protein food supplement). Overall survival was similar at 28 days, although survival was higher in patients receiving oxandralone after 6 months of follow-up. Subsequent analysis suggested the improved survival was due to better nutritional intake in patients receiving oxandralone, rather than to the effects of oxandralone itself. Anabolic steroids have not been compared with corticosteroid treatment. A Cochrane review did not demonstrate significant beneficial outcome with anabolic steroid use in patients with alcoholic liver disease. Anabolic steroids are not currently used to treat alcoholic hepatitis.

Propylthiouracil

Alcohol induces a hypermetabolic state in the liver similar to the hypermetabolic state found in hyperthyroidism. Propylthiouracil (PTU) has been used as a treatment for alcoholic hepatitis based on its ability to reduce hepatic oxygen consumption. Several randomized, placebo-controlled clinical trials have evaluated PTU treatment in hospitalized patients, although patients were not selected on the basis of their DF score. In one study PTU treatment led to a more rapid improvement in liver tests, but no study demonstrated an improvement in survival with PTU. Based on these negative studies, and rare hepatotoxicity, PTU is not recommended for alcoholic hepatitis.

Antioxidants

There is increased oxidative stress and reduced levels of several antioxidants in alcoholic hepatitis. A clinical trial compared corticosteroids to an antioxidant cocktail (vitamins A, C, E, selenium, allopurinol, desferrioxamine and N-acetylcysteine) in

101 hospitalized patients with alcoholic hepatitis. The study was terminated prematurely because of increased mortality in patients receiving antioxidant treatment. A second study evaluated antioxidant treatment (*N*-acetylcysteine intravenously for 1 week, followed by vitamins A–E, biotin, selenium, zinc, manganese, copper, magnesium folic acid and Coenzyme Q daily for 6 months) in patients with advanced alcoholic hepatitis. Corticosteroids were used if prescribed by the attending gastroenterologist. Antioxidant treatment showed no benefit and did not improve 6-month survival, either alone or in combination with corticosteroid treatment. Based on these studies, currently available antioxidant treatments do not improve survival and are not recommended in alcoholic hepatitis.

Hepatic mitogens

Insulin and glucagon stimulate hepatic regeneration following partial hepatectomy in rats and improved survival in a mouse model of fulminant hepatitis. In an effort to stimulate hepatic regeneration, five randomized controlled trials have evaluated intravenous insulin and glucagon treatment in alcoholic hepatitis. Two studies reported improved short-term survival while three found no difference in survival. Hypoglycemia occurred in several patients receiving insulin and glucagon, with two deaths due to hypoglycemia. Insulin and glucagon are not recommended for patients with alcoholic hepatitis.

Other treatments

Colchicine, penicillamine and the calcium channel blocker, verapamil, have been used but are ineffective in alcoholic hepatitis.

Cirrhosis

The natural history of cirrhosis is influenced by abstinence and the severity of the liver disease. Five-year survival is greater than 90% in non-decompensated patients who are abstinent but drops to less than 70% if patients continue to consume alcohol. In various studies, mean survival after the development of a complication of cirrhosis varies from 24 to 48 months. Established alcoholic cirrhosis is rarely, if ever, reversible to a state of minimal liver fibrosis, even if patients are abstinent for many years.

Several treatments have been evaluated in patients with alcoholic cirrhosis, although none is recommended for routine use at the current time.

S-adenosylmethionine (SAMe) is a high-energy compound formed from methionine and ATP by the enzyme methionine adenosyltransferase (MAT). SAMe is the primary methyl donor for biochemical reactions involving DNA methylation, and is a precursor of glutathione, a major intracellular antioxidant. Hepatic levels of MAT are decreased in cirrhosis, probably due to oxidative damage, leading to decreased SAMe synthesis. Because of the known abnormalities in SAMe metabolism, oral SAMe has been studied as a treatment for alcoholic cirrhosis. A total of 123 patients with alcoholic cirrhosis (25% of whom also had viral hepatitis) were entered into a randomized controlled trial of SAMe 1200 mg/day versus placebo. Survival at 24 months was higher in patients receiving SAMe, although this did not reach statistical significance unless the eight patients with Pugh C cirrhosis were excluded from analysis (88% versus 71%, *p*<0.025) (**Fig. 21.7**). Side-effects of SAMe treatment were minimal (nausea, diarrhea). SAMe is moderately expensive

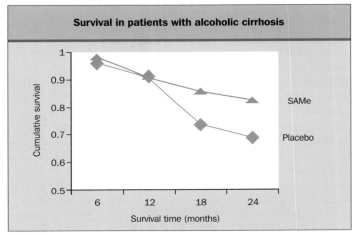

Figure 21.7 Survival in patients with alcoholic cirrhosis. Patients received either placebo or S-adenosylmethionine (SAMe) 1200 mg/day orally for 24 months. Modified from Mato et al (99).

(approximately $0.50 to 1.00/400 mg tablet) and would have to be taken for at least 2 years in order to obtain survival benefit. Although there are few side-effects of SAMe treatment, it is premature to recommend SAMe treatment until a confirmatory study has been conducted.

Colchicine treatment prolonged survival and reversed cirrhosis in a study of 100 patients with cirrhosis of various etiologies (45% had alcoholic cirrhosis) conducted in the 1970s and 1980s. However, a recent randomized, controlled trial of 549 VA (Veterans' Affairs) patients with Pugh B or C alcoholic cirrhosis found no improvement in survival with colchicine treatment. A Cochrane review conducted prior to the recent VA study did not recommend colchicine use in patients with alcoholic liver disease. Based on the negative results of the large VA clinical trial, colchicine treatment cannot be recommended for alcoholic cirrhosis.

Polyenoyl phosphatidylcholine (PPC), an extract of soy beans containing high amounts of dilinoleoyl phosphatidylcholine, prevented liver disease in alcohol-fed baboons and stimulates collagenase activity in isolated stellate cells. A placebo-controlled trial of 789 patients with alcoholic fibrosis, but not cirrhosis, was undertaken to determine whether oral PPC improved liver histology in humans with alcoholic fibrosis. In the 412 patients who had a repeat liver biopsy after 24 months of treatment, PPC was not more effective than the placebo in reducing the progression of liver disease. Thus, PPC treatment has not been shown to be effective in preventing progression of fibrosis in humans with alcoholic liver disease although the clinical trial was limited by the large number of dropouts and the low alcohol consumption in patients remaining in the study.

Nutritional therapy may be beneficial in hospitalized patients with alcoholic cirrhosis. A randomized, controlled trial compared an enteral diet containing 2115 kcal with an isocaloric hospital diet in 35 patients hospitalized with cirrhosis. The enteral diet contained branched-chain amino acids, medium-chain triglycerides (with adequate amounts of long-chain triglycerides) and maltodextrin. The in-hospital mortality rate was significantly lower in patients receiving enteral nutrition (12%) than in patients receiving standard hospital diet (47%). However, several other studies have failed to show a survival benefit with nutritional therapy in patients hospitalized with cirrhosis, although nutritional therapy did improve nutritional status in several of these studies. At the present time routine enteral feeding is not recommended in patients hospitalized with cirrhosis.

Nutritional therapy of outpatients with alcoholic cirrhosis may reduce complications and hospitalizations. Two randomized, controlled clinical trials in patients with cirrhosis of various etiologies reported fewer complications of liver disease in patients receiving nutritional supplementation in addition to a standard diet. Similar to the findings of nutritional treatment in alcoholic hepatitis, mortality was not improved with dietary supplementation of outpatients with cirrhosis. A late evening snack has a positive effect on nitrogen balance on patients with cirrhosis when compared with an equicaloric diet without a late-evening meal. These studies suggest that oral nutritional support, when added to a regular diet, may improve nutritional status and reduce complications of liver disease in outpatients with advanced alcoholic cirrhosis. Due to differences in study design and diet used, no recommendations can be made regarding routine nutritional supplementation for outpatients with alcoholic cirrhosis. Further studies are needed to determine which nutritional supplementation is ideal and whether nutritional therapy is cost effective and improves survival.

A randomized, placebo controlled trial compared propylthiouracil (PTU) treatment with placebo in 310 outpatients with alcoholic liver disease. Overall, PTU reduced 2-year mortality from 25 to 13% ($p<0.05$). In patients with more advanced liver disease, mortality declined from 55 to 25% with PTU treatment. PTU was not effective if patients continued to drink alcohol. Despite this positive study, PTU has not gained acceptance as a treatment for alcoholic liver disease, and is not currently used by the authors of this study. A Cochrane review of six randomized controlled trials failed to demonstrate an improvement in survival, liver-related mortality, complications of liver disease, or liver histology with PTU treatment.

Silymarin is an antioxidant derived from milk thistle and is a commonly used complementary and alternative medicine in the USA. Two long-term studies of silymarin have been performed in Europe. The first study randomized 140 patients with cirrhosis with respect to treatment with placebo or silymarin (140 mg three times/day) for 24 months, with continued follow-up for up to 6 years. Silymarin improved survival in the subgroup of patients with Pugh A cirrhosis although mortality in the placebo patients (50%) was much higher than would be expected in patients with Pugh A cirrhosis. Survival was not improved in a subsequent 5-year study of silymarin (150 mg t.i.d.) of 200 patients with alcoholic cirrhosis.

Treatment of ascites, esophageal varices, spontaneous bacterial peritonitis and hepatorenal syndrome associated with alcoholic liver disease can be found in other chapters.

LIVER TRANSPLANTATION

Liver transplantation is now widely accepted as treatment for end-stage liver disease due to alcohol and alcoholic liver disease is the second most common indication for liver transplantation in adults in the USA, and the most common indication for liver transplantation in Europe. All transplant centers require a 6-month period of pretransplant sobriety, usually with participation in a substance abuse program and random testing for alcohol use. Indications for liver transplant are the same in alcoholic liver disease as in other liver diseases. Most transplant centers do not require additional cardiac evaluation to exclude alcoholic cardiomyopathy unless patients have clinical signs of heart failure. Several studies have shown that the 5–10 year survival of patients transplanted for alcoholic liver disease is similar, if not slightly better, than the survival for patients transplanted for hepatitis C (**Fig. 21.8**). The rate of recidivism after liver transplant is up to 30% at 5 years post-transplant, but alcohol leads to graft dysfunction in less than 15% of patients and to mortality in less than 5%. Nevertheless, post-transplant care by a specialist in addiction as well as strict abstinence is recommended in all patients receiving a liver transplant for alcoholic liver disease. At the current time, acute alcoholic hepatitis is not an indication for liver transplant because of the high risk of recidivism.

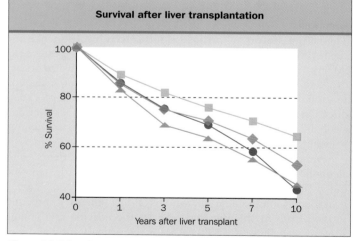

Figure 21.8 Survival after liver transplantation. Long-term survival for patients receiving liver transplant for alcoholic cirrhosis (blue diamonds) is similar to survival for patients receiving transplant for hepatitis C (green squares) or for hepatitis B (yellow triangles). Survival is best for patients receiving transplant for cholestatic liver disease/autoimmune liver disease (pink X). Modified from Jain et al (03).

FURTHER READING

Pathogenesis

Bellentani S, Saccoccio G, Costa G, et al. Drinking habits as cofactors of risk for alcohol induced liver disease. Gut 1997; 41:845–850.

Best CH, Hartroft WS, Lucas CC, et al. Liver damage produced by feeding alcohol or sugar and its prevention by choline. Br J Med 1949; 2:1001–1006.

Bhattachayra R, Shuhart MC. Hepatitis C and alcohol: interactions, outcomes and implications. J Clin Gastroenterol 2003; 36:242–252. *Hepatitis C infection occurs commonly together with alcoholic liver disease and may contribute substantially to the liver injury.*

Corrao G, Arico S. Independent and combined action of hepatitis C virus infection and alcohol consumption on the risk of symptomatic liver cirrhosis. Hepatology 1998; 27:914–919.

Donato F, Tagger A, Gelatti U, et al. Alcohol and hepatocellular carcinoma: effects of lifetime intake and hepatitis virus infections in men and women. Am J Epidemiol 2002; 155:323–331.

El Serag HB, Mason AC. Risk factors for rising rates of primary liver cancer in the United States. Arch Intern Med 2000; 160:3227–3230.

Jain AB, Fung JJ. Alcoholic liver disease and transplantation. Transplant Proc 2003; 35:358–360.

Lelbach WK. Epidemiology of alcoholic liver disease. In: Hall P, ed. Alcoholic liver disease. New York: Wiley; 1985:130–166.

Mato JM, Camara J, Fernandez de Paz J. S-adenosylmethionine in alcoholic liver cirrhosis: a randomized, placebo-controlled, double-blind, multicenter clinical trial. J Hepatol 1999; 30:1081–1089.

Morgan TR, Mandayam S, Jamal MM. Alcohol and hepatocellular carcinoma. Gastrenterology 2004; (in press)

Stickel F, Hoehn B, Schuppan D, et al. Review article: nutritional therapy in alcoholic liver disease. Aliment Pharmacol Ther 2003; 18:357–373.

Tilg H, Diehl AM. Cytokines in alcoholic and nonalcoholic steatohepatitis. N Engl J Med 2004; 343(20):1467–1476.

Alcoholic hepatitis

Akriviadis E, Rotla R, Briggs W, et al. Pentoxifylline improves short-term survival in severe acute alcoholic hepatitis: a double-blind, placebo-controlled trial. Gastroenterology 2000; 119:1673–1648. *The only study of pentoxifylline in alcoholic hepatitis. Pentoxifylline treatment reduced the incidence of hepatorenal syndrome and improved survival.*

Mathurin P, Abdelnour M, Ramond M-J, et al. Early changes in bilirubin levels is an important prognostic factor in severe alcoholic hepatitis treated with prednisolone. Hepatology 2003; 38:1363–1369. *Patients with a decrease in bilirubin during the first week in hospital have high survival rate. Mortality is high in patients with rising bilirubin during first week in hospital.*

Mathurin P, Mendenhall CL, Carithers RL, et al. Corticosteroids improve short-term survival in patients with severe alcoholic hepatitis (AH): individual data analysis of the last three randomized placebo controlled double blind trials of corticosteroids in severe AH. J Hepatol 2002; 36:480–487. *Meta-analysis of three prior randomized controlled trials performed by combining the data from the individual studies demonstrates improved survival in patients receiving corticosteroid treatment.*

McCullough AJ, O'Connor JFB. Alcoholic liver disease: proposed recommendations for the American College of Gastroenterology. Am J Gastroenterol 1998; 93:20220–20236.

Naveau S, Chollet-Martin S, Dharancy S, et al. A double-blind randomized controlled trial of infliximab associated with prednisolone in acute alcoholic hepatitis. Hepatology 2004; 39:1390–1397.

CHAPTER
22

Fatty Liver, Non-alcoholic Steatohepatitis

Brent A. Neuschwander-Tetri

The accumulation of fat in hepatocytes, or hepatic steatosis, is a common histologic finding. As specific causes of liver disease have been identified and characterized, more attention has focused on the causes and consequences of non-alcoholic fatty liver disease (NAFLD), and especially non-alcoholic steatohepatitis (NASH), because these syndromes remain relatively enigmatic.

This chapter reviews the current knowledge about NAFLD and its worrisome subset, NASH. Most patients with NAFLD have insulin resistance as the primary cause of triglyceride accumulation in hepatocytes. Because the inciting factors that cause some patients to develop NASH in the setting of NAFLD are not presently known, the cumulative clinical knowledge is necessarily descriptive. As specific causes of these disorders such as insulin resistance are identified, we will begin to recognize NAFLD and NASH as histologic manifestations of specific metabolic defects, nutritional deficiencies, or possibly even unrecognized infections.

EPIDEMIOLOGY

Benign steatosis

Body habitus is the primary predictor of the presence of benign hepatic steatosis. Whereas hepatic steatosis is found in 21% of lean healthy males, almost all morbidly obese individuals will have hepatic steatosis. In the less obese, including those with body mass higher than 10% above lean body weight, about 75% have some degree of hepatic steatosis. How fat is distributed on the body predicts the presence of hepatic steatosis. Analogous to coronary artery disease risk, body fat distributed about the hips is probably not a risk factor; however, a high ratio of abdominal fat to hip fat is a significant risk factor for hepatic steatosis. Youth is not protective; hepatic steatosis is found in obese children and just as frequently as in adults.

Non-alcoholic steatohepatitis

The risks factors for developing NASH are similar to the risks for benign steatosis. Because little is known of the underlying causes of NASH, efforts have been directed towards characterizing the recognizable risk factors for developing NASH. Although patients with NASH were once characterized as being obese, diabetic, female, and hyperlipidemic, not all patients fit this description. In fact, recent surveys have underscored the relatively high prevalence of NASH in patients without these 'classic' risk factors (**Table 22.1**).

Obesity

Obesity is clearly the most significant risk factor for the development of NASH. The overall prevalence of NASH in obese patients has been estimated in both surgical series and autopsy studies. *Lobular hepatitis* (which in retrospect probably rep-

Risk factors for hepatic steatosis and non-alcoholic steatohepatitis			
	Steatosis	*NASH*	*Cirrhosis*
Obesity (centripetal)	+++	++	++
Type 2 diabetes	++	+	+
Drugs	++	++	+/−
Female gender	+	−	−
Hypertriglyceridemia	+/−	+/−	−
Hypercholesterolemia	−	−	−
NASH, non-alcoholic steatohepatitis; +, minor risk factor; ++, moderate risk factor; +++, major risk factor; −, no risk			

Table 22.1 Risk factors for hepatic steatosis and non-alcoholic steatohepatitis

resents NASH) was found in 8.7% of patients in a large series of morbidly obese individuals about to undergo surgical small bowel bypass as a treatment for obesity; however, at autopsy, NASH was found in 18.5% of obese patients. Careful exclusion of coexisting risks (e.g. alcohol use, diabetes, protein malnutrition and drug toxicity) has confirmed that obesity alone is a major risk for the development of this syndrome.

Diabetes

Diabetes mellitus is also frequently associated with hepatic steatosis. Steatosis is found in about one-third of non-obese persons with type 2 diabetes at autopsy. As a group, patients found to have hepatic steatosis by ultrasound examination are more likely to have glucose intolerance and elevated baseline insulin levels than patients without ultrasonographic evidence of hepatic steatosis. Chronically elevated circulating insulin levels typically found in type 2 diabetic patients may be at least partly responsible for the accumulation of fat in the liver because of insulin's role in regulating intrahepatic fat synthesis and metabolism. In contrast, hepatic steatosis is relatively uncommon in type 1 diabetes, a condition characterized by primary loss of insulin-secreting β cells in pancreatic islets and manifested by episodes of hyperglycemia and low to normal insulin levels. When steatosis is present in patients with type 1 diabetes, it seems to correlate with poor glycemic control.

Hyperlipidemia and lipodystrophies

Hyperlipidemia, a condition that broadly includes elevations of serum cholesterol, serum triglycerides, or both, has been thought to be a risk factor or clinical marker for the development of hepatic steatosis and NASH. In reality, this association lacks solid epidemiologic evidence because establishing hyper-triglyceridemia as a risk for the development of NASH has been confounded by the dominant effects of obesity and dietary habits. Nonetheless, genetic disorders of serum lipid metabolism are often characterized by hepatic steatosis. Additionally, the lipodystrophies are definitely associated with the development of NASH and the progression to end-stage liver disease. These rare diseases are characterized by the abnormal mobilization of fat from peripheral stores, which greatly increases the flux of fatty acids through the liver. Whether the liver demonstrates abnormal fat metabolism in the lipodystrophies or is a passive target of the unusually high traffic of fatty acids is not known.

Gender

Of the risk factors for NASH identified in early surveys, female gender was overemphasized and has been refuted. The prevalence of NASH is equal among men and women at autopsy and the prevalence of hepatic steatosis found by computed tomography (CT) imaging is equal among men and women. Recent surveys of patients with NASH have accordingly demonstrated an equal gender distribution.

Drugs

Several drugs have been implicated in the development of benign steatosis and NASH (**Table 22.2**). The most common drugs implicated have been corticosteroids, estrogens and tamoxifen. Estrogens increase hepatic triglyceride synthesis, possibly outpacing the secretory capacity. Seemingly paradoxic

Causes of macrovesicular steatosis

Insulin resistance and hyperinsulinemia
   Obesity (especially centripetal)
   Type 2 diabetes

Drugs
   Corticosteroids
   Estrogens
   Tamoxifen (acting as a weak estrogen agonist)
   Amiodarone
   Chloroquine
   Nifedipine and dilitiazem (case reports)

Metabolic   Wilson disease

Nutritional
   Starvation
   Protein deficit (kwashiorkor, eating disorders)
   Choline deficiency
   Excess carbohydrate

Infections   Chronic hepatitis C (especially genotype 3)

Miscellaneous
   Indian childhood cirrhosis
   Jejunoileal bypass

Table 22.2 Causes of macrovesicular steatosis

is the association between the use of tamoxifen and the development of NASH. Well-characterized cases have been described in women using it as an estrogen antagonist and as adjuvant therapy for breast cancer. This is explained by the observation that, although tamoxifen is used as an estrogen receptor antagonist, it can display weak estrogenic activity depending on the target tissue. This activity may be responsible for its association with NASH.

PATHOPHYSIOLOGY

Hepatic steatosis is caused by an imbalance between the delivery or synthesis of fat in the liver and its subsequent secretion or metabolism. In other words, fat accumulates when the delivery of fatty acids to the liver, either from the circulation or by de novo synthesis within the liver, exceeds that capacity of the liver to metabolize the fat by β-oxidation or secrete it as very low-density lipoprotein (VLDL). These are the two major mechanisms of fat delivery and two major mechanisms of fat disposal. Derangements in any of these pathways alone or in combination cause fat to accumulate in the liver and are discussed later in detail. **Figure 22.1** shows how fat cycles between the liver and peripheral stores and the influence of major regulatory factors in governing the flux between the liver and the peripheral sites.

Delivery of fatty acids from peripheral stores to the liver

Triglycerides, or triacylglycerol (TAG), are stored in adipose tissue and released as free fatty acids into the circulation through the actions of lipoprotein lipases. The hydrolysis of TAG in adipocytes is controlled by intracellular cyclic adenosine monophosphate (cAMP) levels. Therefore, hormonal and pharmacologic stimuli that increase adipocyte cAMP cause the release of free fatty acids from peripheral stores and increase the delivery of fat to the liver. Epinephrine, norepinephrine, adrenocorticotropic hormone (ACTH), glucagon, corticosteroids, and methylxanthines (e.g. caffeine) are agents that stimulate adenyl cyclase and potently increase adipocyte lipolysis via a hormone-sensitive lipase. The increased lipolysis brought about by corticosteroids may reflect a protective response to prolonged starvation.

In the fed state, insulin exerts the opposite effect by increasing phosphodiesterase activity, thus depleting intracellular cAMP and preventing peripheral lipolysis. Insulin is also required for the reincorporation of fatty acids into triglyceride in both the liver and peripheral stores. Thus, after feeding, fat release from peripheral stores is normally inhibited and fat release from the liver is promoted. In states of insulin resistance, the normal post-prandial inhibition of lipolysis can be impaired leading to inappropriate release of free fatty acids from adipose tissues in the fed state.

Free fatty acids released from peripheral stores are hydrophobic and are strongly bound to circulating albumin. They are transported by albumin to tissues capable of taking up fatty acids and using them as metabolic substrates. The liver is the major site of fatty acid uptake, but the heart and skeletal muscle are also highly dependent on free fatty acids as a metabolic fuel and thus remove a fraction from the circulation.

Whereas the cAMP-mediated release of free fatty acids from the peripheral stores is highly regulated, the uptake of fatty

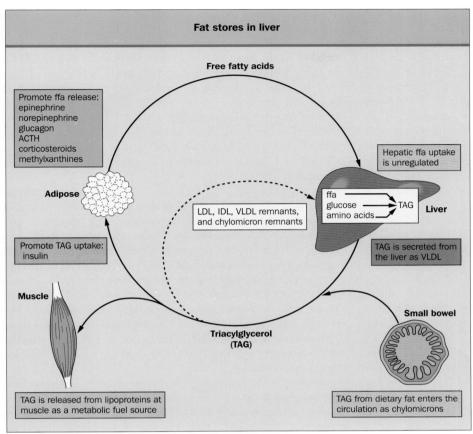

Fat stores in liver

Free fatty acids

Promote ffa release:
epinephrine
norepinephrine
glucagon
ACTH
corticosteroids
methylxanthines

Adipose

Promote TAG uptake:
insulin

Muscle

LDL, IDL, VLDL remnants,
and chylomicron remnants

Hepatic ffa uptake
is unregulated

ffa
glucose → TAG
amino acids

Liver

TAG is secreted from
the liver as VLDL

Small bowel

Triacylglycerol
(TAG)

TAG is released from lipoproteins at
muscle as a metabolic fuel source

TAG from dietary fat enters the
circulation as chylomicrons

Figure 22.1 Fat stores in the liver. Fat cycles from peripheral stores to the liver as free fatty acids (ffa) bound to albumin and back to peripheral stores as triacylglycerol (TAG) as a component of very low-density lipoprotein (VLDL). TAG is also synthesized within the liver from excess glucose and amino acids and a small fraction of the total is taken up by hepatocytes in the form of lipoprotein remnants. Dietary fat is converted to free fatty acids within the bowel lumen. Whereas short chain fatty acids (<11 carbons) can be delivered directly to the blood, longer chain fatty acids are re-esterified into TAG, incorporated into chylomicrons, and delivered to the circulation via the lymphatics. Fatty acids are removed from the TAG in circulating VLDL and chylomicrons by vascular lipoprotein lipases. In energy-requiring tissues such as muscle, the released fatty acids serve as a source of fuel whereas adipose tissue resynthesizes TAG for storage.

The flux of fat through this cycle is highly dependent on the feeding state. During fasting, glucagon facilitates the release of TAG from peripheral fat stores. After a meal, insulin promotes the incorporation of fat into adipose tissue by locally upregulating vascular lipoprotein lipase activity. Insulin also promotes the formation of TAG from glucose within the liver and switches the trafficking of fatty acids from β-oxidation to TAG formation. ACTH, adrenocorticotropic hormone; IDL, intermediate-density lipoprotein; LDL, low-density lipoprotein.

acids by the liver is passive and unregulated. In the absence of feedback regulation, the liver cannot decrease fatty acid uptake even when the capacity to catabolize fatty acids or re-esterify them and secrete them back into the circulation as VLDL is overwhelmed. Derangements in peripheral lipolysis thus have a direct impact on the flux of fat through the liver.

Fatty acid synthesis within the liver

TAG is the most compact form of energy storage. Conversion of most excess dietary carbohydrate and protein to fatty acids and then to TAG is a primary responsibility of the liver. Excess glucose is converted to fat by both the liver and adipocytes. In the liver, the backbone of most amino acids can be converted to pyruvate and then to acetyl-coenzyme A (acetyl-CoA), which feeds directly into cytosolic fatty acid synthesis. For this reason, a recommendation for patients to adhere to a low fat diet when the calories are simply replaced by carbohydrate may not have the desired effect on reducing fat accumulation in the liver.

Fate of fatty acids in the liver
β-Oxidation

In the fasting state, adipocyte TAG is hydrolyzed to release free fatty acids, which are transported to the liver where they can serve as substrates for mitochondrial β-oxidation. β-Oxidation of fatty acids is a major source of energy needed to maintain liver viability during fasting. It is also the source of the ketone bodies, acetoacetate, acetone, and D-3-hydroxybutyrate. These are released into the blood and are essential fuel sources for

peripheral tissues, especially neurons, muscle and brain when glucose is in short supply because of the inability of neural tissues to use free fatty acids as fuel. Defects in hepatic β-oxidation cause microvesicular steatosis of the liver, intolerance to fasting, and in some cases a myopathy because of the muscle's normal requirement for fatty acids as an energy source.

The first step in any pathway that metabolizes fatty acids is the formation of esters with coenzyme A, also called acyl coenzyme A (acyl-CoA). Because acyl-CoA cannot enter the mitochondria directly, the fat moiety is transferred to carnitine and the acyl conjugates with carnitine are selectively transported into the mitochondria. This carnitine shuttle requires three enzymes:

- carnitine palmitoyl transferase I (CPTI), which forms the acyl carnitines;
- a translocase, and
- CPTII, which reverses the first step to form acyl-CoA from acylcarnitine within the mitochondria.

Once inside the mitochondria, acyl-CoA undergoes progressive shortening, two carbons at a time, to generate nicotinamide adenine dinucleotide in reduced form (NADH) and acetyl-CoA. This is the process of β-oxidation. The electrons carried by the NADH drive the production of adenosine triphosphate (ATP) and the acetyl-CoA produced is further catabolized by the Krebs cycle to form more ATP and other key metabolic intermediates, such as the ketone bodies. Different enzymes required for the chain shortening have relative preferences for the newly delivered long chain fatty acids, the partly processed medium chain fatty acids, and the almost completely processed short chain fatty acids.

Defects in the function of the enzymes responsible for β-oxidation are increasingly recognized and associated with liver disorders that commonly present with some degree of microvesicular steatosis. Severe defects, such as CPTI deficiency, typically present during early childhood with fatty liver and intolerance to fasting. A defect in medium chain acyl-CoA dehydrogenase (MCHAD) has been found in some infants with sudden infant death syndrome. Other defects may manifest themselves during adulthood. One example is the association between acute fatty liver of pregnancy and a maternal partial defect in long chain hydroxyacyl-CoA dehydrogenase (LCHAD).

Certain drugs and toxins are known to impair mitochondrial β-oxidation and cause microvesicular steatosis. Valproic acid can undergo β-oxidation to intermediates that are toxic to mitochondria. Methylenecyclopropylalanine (hypoglycin) is a natural product found in unripe ackee fruit (*Blighia sapida*), which potently inhibits β-oxidation. Ackee is a popular fruit in Jamaica, and several deaths characterized by prodromal vomiting and hypoglycemia have been reported after the ingestion of unripe ackee.

The reason why impaired mitochondrial β-oxidation causes microvesicular steatosis has not been established. In general, the conditions under which β-oxidation is required (i.e. the non-fed state) are the same circumstances under which peripheral mobilization of fat is increased. Thus, there may be increased delivery of fatty acids to a liver which is relatively energy deprived with respect to its ability to generate ATP. Potentially, the impaired mitochondrial function per se with the attendant ATP deficiency and other resulting metabolic abnormalities may impair the complex process of packaging and secreting TAG as VLDL.

An oxidation pathway of secondary importance in the flux of fatty acids through the liver is the peroxisomal pathway. Peroxisomes oxidize very long chain fatty acids (>22 carbons) and dicarboxylic acids to shorter chain lengths, which can then be managed by mitochondrial β-oxidation. Importantly, peroxisomal oxidation of fatty acids generates hydrogen peroxide and thus peroxisomes may be an important source of oxidant stress in hepatocytes overburdened by a high flux of free fatty acids.

Formation and secretion of VLDL

In the fed state, β-oxidation of fatty acids is not required as an energy source, and fatty acids delivered to the liver are mainly converted to TAG. Insulin regulates the metabolic path that fatty acids take in the liver. Without insulin, CPTI commits fatty acids to mitochondrial β-oxidation; when insulin levels are high, glycerol-3-phosphate acyltransferase commits fatty acids to the formation of TAG. Whether this partitioning is altered in states of insulin resistance has not been established.

In the fed state, the liver also efficiently converts excess glucose and the backbone of many amino acids to TAG. Energy storage as TAG is probably preferred because of its compactness; TAG energy density is 9 kcal/g and can be stored as a relatively dehydrated mass. Carbohydrates and amino acids are inherently less energy dense (3 and 4 kcal/g dry weight, respectively) and require solvation with a substantial amount of water,

which only further reduces the energy density on a per weight basis.

Although delivery of fatty acids to the liver and fatty acid synthesis in the liver are the major contributors to liver TAG, not all liver TAG is derived from fatty acids. A fraction of liver TAG is taken up directly by endocytosis of lipoproteins and lipoprotein remnants such as low-density lipoprotein (LDL), intermediate-density lipoprotein (IDL), VLDL remnants and chylomicron remnants. After binding to the LDL receptor and endocytosis, the TAG contained within these particles is released in a lysosomal compartment and mixed with newly synthesized TAG.

The secretion of TAG into the circulation in the form of VLDL is the only mechanism of disposing of TAG from the hepatocyte. Because of its complexity, the synthesis and secretion of VLDL from the liver is the rate-limiting step in the cycling of fat between the liver and peripheral stores. Through a process of combining TAG with apolipoprotein B-100, phosphatidylcholine, cholesterol, and cholesterol esters, functional VLDL is formed and secreted by exocytosis (**Fig. 22.2**). Much can go awry in the complex process of VLDL secretion. The result is TAG accumulation and its common clinical correlate, hepatic steatosis (**Table 22.3**). This simple fact explains why the many seemingly unrelated causes of steatosis have but this one clinical manifestation.

Although VLDL may acquire minor amounts of other lipoproteins once it enters the circulation, when it is secreted from the liver apolipoprotein B-100 (apoB-100) is the only protein component. ApoB-100 is coded by a single gene on chromosome 2, and the gene structure is defined by 29 exons (expressed sequences) and 28 introns (intervening sequences). The product of mRNA translation is a 4536 amino acid protein with a molecular weight of 512 kDa and an amino terminus LDL receptor-binding domain. Post-translational processing includes N-glycosylation, acylation, and phosphorylation to achieve the functional protein. The synthesis of apoB-100 is rapid; protein synthesis requires less than 15 min and incorporation into VLDL followed by secretion requires another 30 min. Incorporation of TAG into nascent VLDL also requires microsomal triglyceride transfer protein (MTTP) and genetic defects in MTTP are associated with fatty liver and NASH. Much newly synthesized apoB-100 never reaches the circulation and is instead subject to intracellular degradation. This excess synthesis may occur when the supply of TAG is inadequate to form VLDL. Conversely, the constitutive rate of apoB-100 synthesis can be outpaced by excessive free fatty acid delivery to the liver and hepatocellular TAG accumulation develops.

Defects in apoB-100 synthesis and function cause TAG to accumulate in the liver. A simple deficiency of amino acids can prevent adequate apoB-100 synthesis, which may explain the steatosis commonly found in protein malnutrition (kwashiorkor). ApoB-100 is rich in threonine, and its synthesis is thus particularly sensitive to a deficiency of this amino acid. Certain apoB-100 gene mutations result in partial or complete loss of functional protein synthesis. Complete absence of functional protein (abetalipoproteinemia) presents in infancy with severe fat malabsorption and can lead to cirrhosis. The fat malabsorption associated with abetalipoproteinemia is probably due to the obligate deficiency of apoB-48, the intestinal lipoprotein analog of apoB-100 that is required for chylomicron assembly. ApoB-48 is

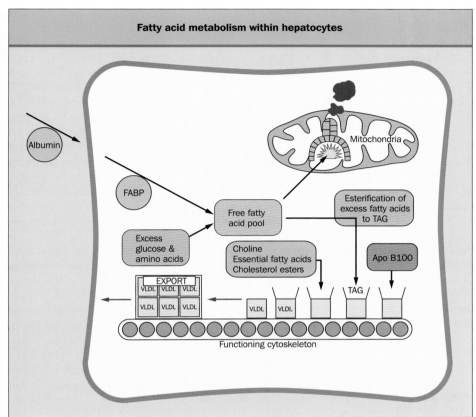

Fatty acid metabolism within hepatocytes

Figure 22.2 Fatty acid metabolism within hepatocytes. In hepatocytes, free fatty acids are primarily delivered from peripheral stores bound to albumin or synthesized from excess carbohydrate or amino acids. Fatty acids within hepatocytes are bound to the carrier protein, fatty acid-binding protein (FABP) and they are either shuttled to the mitochondria to generate energy [adenosine triphosphate (ATP)] and ketone bodies or esterified into triacylglycerol (TAG) and packaged in very low-density lipoprotein (VLDL) for secretion back into the blood. The packaging of TAG and the export of VLDL requires multiple cellular functions. An adequate supply of precursor amino acids and unimpaired protein synthesis are needed to make apolipoprotein B-100 (apoB-100) and microsomal triglyceride transfer protein (MTTP); choline, essential fatty acids, and cholesterol esters are required to assemble VLDL. Finally, a functioning cytoskeletal network is then needed to export vesicles containing the VLDL particles from the hepatocyte. Defects or deficiencies in any one of these components can impair VLDL secretion and lead to fat accumulation within the cell.

Defects in very low-density lipoprotein (VLDL) synthesis	
Defect	*Comments*
ApoB gene defect	Homozygous abetalipoproteinemia is a severe disease of infancy; heterozygous hypobetalipoproteinemia varies in its phenotypic expression
MTP polymorphisms	MTP is required for lipidation of apolipoprotein B-100 during the formation of VLDL and polymorphisms of its gene have been associated with NAFLD
Dietary protein deficiency	VLDL synthesis is especially sensitive to threonine deficiency
Choline deficiency	Required to form phosphatidylcholine, an essential component of VLDL Methionine may be able to replace choline as a methyl donor May be a cause of TPN-induced steatosis
Essential fatty acid deficiency	Essential fatty acids are required for phosphatidylcholine synthesis
Cholesterol esterification defect	Cholesterol esters are required for VLDL assembly
Altered cytoskeleton	Impairs exocytosis
ApoB, apolipoprotein B; MTP, microsomal triglyceride transfer protein; NAFLD, non-alcoholic fatty liver disease; TPN, total parenteral nutrition; VLDL, very low-density lipoprotein	

Table 22.3 Defects in very low-density lipoprotein (VLDL) synthesis.

required for intestinal fat absorption and is coded by the same gene as apoB-100 (see later). Partial loss of functional apoB-100, or hypobetalipoproteinemia, has a more diverse phenotypic expression depending on the degree of protein absence, but deficiencies have been identified in adults with NASH.

Sources of plasma triacylglycerol

In the fasted state, most plasma triglyceride is found within VLDL secreted from the liver, whereas the small remaining fraction is distributed among various VLDL degradation products (see later). In contrast, in the fed state, the majority of triglyceride is found within chylomicrons. There are two reasons for the dominance of chylomicron TAG over VLDL TAG in the fed state. The most obvious is that dietary fat absorbed from the small intestine is wholly incorporated into chylomicrons. In addition to the postprandial increase in circulating chylomicrons, there is a decrease in hepatic VLDL secretion because of the inhibitory effects of insulin on VLDL synthesis and secretion. States of insulin resistance are associated with compensatory hyperinsulinemia, an abnormality which may impair secretion of VLDL from the liver.

Chylomicron synthesis in the small bowel epithelial cells is analogous to hepatic VLDL synthesis and secretion in most respects. However, in humans, the predominant lipoprotein incorporated into nascent chylomicrons in enterocytes is apoB-48, whereas the liver incorporates apoB-100 into VLDL. Interestingly, apoB-48 is a protein with 2152 amino acids with a final molecular weight of 248 kDa coded by the amino terminus of the apoB-100 gene; the 2153rd codon of the apoB-48 gene is a stop codon that leads to the smaller protein product. During the final assembly of chylomicrons, smaller amounts of the A lipoproteins are also incorporated, and the final product is secreted into the lymphatics. Short chain fatty acids less than 10 carbons can bypass this route of absorption and pass directly into the circulation.

Fate of plasma triacylglycerol
Lipoprotein modification
Circulating lipoprotein complexes undergo several modifications before they release TAG at peripheral sites. Both VLDL and chylomicrons acquire C lipoproteins and apoE from circulating high-density lipoprotein (HDL). Neither VLDL nor chylomicrons lose apoB-100 or apoB-48 respectively to other lipoproteins, presumably because of the extensive hydrophobic interactions between these two lipoproteins and the lipid cores of the entire particles.

Release of fatty acids
Very little of the TAG in the circulation is absorbed by the liver. Depending on the levels of circulating insulin, circulating TAG is consumed either by adipose tissue or by energy-requiring tissues such as muscle. In the fed state, high insulin levels favor uptake by adipose tissue. In the fasted state, lower insulin levels favor utilization by muscle and other tissues able to release fatty acids from lipoprotein-bound TAG. The lack of direct uptake of TAG or fatty acids from VLDL or chylomicrons may explain the paradoxic lack of a strong correlation between hyperlipidemic states and hepatic steatosis.

The uptake of fat from lipoproteins requires release of free fatty acids from TAG by lipoprotein lipase (LPL) at the vascular endothelium. LPL is an enzyme that belongs to a multigene family that includes pancreatic lipase. Although it is synthesized by many tissues, LPL is found predominantly in muscle and adipose tissue, which correlates with the major sites of TAG consumption. The enzyme attaches to vascular endothelial cells by its interaction with the glycoprotein heparan sulfate. The enzyme is not produced by vascular endothelial cells but instead is synthesized by adipocytes and myocytes. Because of their disparate roles in fat metabolism, fat and muscle express LPL under different conditions. LPL expression by the adipocyte is increased in the fed state by insulin, whereas expression in muscle is constitutively high and increases modestly with fasting.

Through the action of LPL, TAG is removed from VLDL and chylomicrons. Removal of TAG from VLDL sequentially generates VLDL remnants, IDL, and finally LDL in an increasing order of density. The increasing density reflects the progressively decreasing TAG content. The removal of TAG from VLDL is relatively rapid; after 15–60 min, most TAG is removed from circulating VLDL. About half of VLDL is processed to LDL, whereas the other half is less fully defatted and generates VLDL remnants and IDL. Chylomicrons are depleted of their TAG even more rapidly, with a substantial fraction of TAG removed within 5 to 10 min after entering the circulation. As a result, chylomicron remnants contain 10–20% of their original TAG and all of the dietary cholesterol originally incorporated into this gut-derived lipoprotein.

The end products after TAG is removed from VLDL and chylomicrons (namely VLDL remnants, IDL, LDL and chylomicron remnants) are taken up by the liver. How much this uptake of these relatively dense lipoproteins containing residual TAG contributes to the triglyceride pool in the liver is unknown but is probably minor compared with the intrahepatic synthesis of fatty acids and the delivery of fatty acids to the liver from peripheral stores. Uptake of lipoproteins is carried out by the hepatic LDL receptor. The receptor usually interacts with the apoE component of VLDL remnants, but in the more TAG-depleted and apoE-depleted LDL, the interaction is with apolipoprotein B-100. The LDL receptor has a relatively low affinity for LDL, and this weak interaction is probably one reason why LDL has a long circulating half-life of 3 days compared with its precursor VLDL. The role of defects in LDL clearance as a cause of vascular disease remains controversial. ApoB-100 and apoE polymorphisms have been identified and these decrease binding of LDL to the hepatic receptor and its subsequent clearance from the circulation. Although these genetic abnormalities are associated with hypercholesterolemia and vascular disease, the relative importance of defects in each of the lipoproteins has not been resolved, and their role in contributing to hepatic steatosis is uncertain.

Other forms of hepatic steatosis
Microvesicular steatosis
Microvesicular steatosis is distinguished from macrovesicular steatosis on well-defined morphologic grounds and also by pathophysiologic mechanisms. Whereas macrovesicular steatosis is caused by an imbalance in the hepatic synthesis and export of TAG, all causes of microvesicular steatosis are related to defects in mitochondrial function (**Table 22.4**). The reason why the accumulated TAG of microvesicular steatosis is retained in smaller vesicles distributed pancellularly rather than coalescing into large droplets characteristic of macrovesicular steatosis is unknown.

Alcoholic steatosis
The pathogenesis of alcoholic liver disease is reviewed in Chapter 21. The accumulation of TAG in the liver caused by alcohol, even in normal individuals with modest alcohol consumption, has not been fully explained. Hepatic TAG synthesis is increased after the consumption of alcohol. Fat may accumulate simply as a result of excessive TAG synthesis, or there may be a concomitant defect in the secretion of VLDL that contributes synergistically to the accumulation of fat in the liver.

Causes of microvesicular steatosis	
Cause	*Mechanism*
Drugs	
Valproic acid	Depletion of mitochondrial CoA; β-oxidation and blockade of β-oxidation enzymes by P-450 drug metabolites
Tetracycline (high dose)	Inhibited β-oxidation; impaired hepatic triglyceride secretion
Aspirin	Uncoupling oxidative phosphorylation; depletion of extramitochondrial acetyl-CoA, which prevents transport of fatty acids into the mitochondria
2-Arylpropionate NSAID (pirprofen, naproxen, ibuprofen, ketoprofen)	Inhibit β-oxidation of medium- and short-chain fatty acids
Amineptine	Inhibit β-oxidation of medium- and short-chain fatty acids
Nucleoside analogs (zidovudine, didanosine, zalcitabine, fialuridine)	Inhibition of mitochondrial DNA replication
Toxins	
Ethanol	Diminished mitochondrial NAD^+ impairs β-oxidation; mitochondrial oxidant stress damages mtDNA
Hypoglycin (unripe ackee)	Impaired β-oxidation
Bacillus cereus emetic toxin	Impaired β-oxidation
Toxic shock syndrome	Unknown bacterial toxins
Genetic defects	
Acute fatty liver of pregnancy	Defects in the β-oxidation; LCHAD defect in a subset of patients
β-Oxidation defects:	
CPT I	Inadequate substrate for β-oxidation
CPT II	Inadequate substrate for β-oxidation
Others	Inadequate substrate for β-oxidation
Ornithine transcarbamylase deficiency	Inhibition of long- and medium-chain fatty acid β-oxidation by ammonium
Alpers disease	Unknown mitochondrial defect
Other	
Reye syndrome	Combined acquired and genetic defects in β-oxidation or ureagenesis
Cholestasis (foamy degeneration)	Impaired mitochondrial function by bile acids
CoA, coenzyme A; CPT, carnitine palmitoyl transferase; NSAID, non-steroidal anti-inflammatory drugs; LCHAD, long-chain hydroxyacyl-CoA dehydrogenase	

Table 22.4 Causes of microvesicular steatosis.

Alcohol is also a major mitochondrial toxin, which explains features seen in severe alcoholic hepatitis such as megamitochondria and microvesicular fat. Hepatic lipid peroxidation occurs during alcohol metabolism by the liver, and oxidant stress may play a key role in the development of hepatic steatosis and the development of the inflammatory response characteristic of alcoholic hepatitis.

Phospholipidoses
Phospholipid accumulation in the liver causes steatohepatitis and can cause a histologic picture similar to the steatosis caused by TAG accumulation. The phospholipidosis syndromes are caused by the accumulation of phospholipids in lysosomes. The expansion of membranes by excess phospholipids results in the development of enlarged lysosomes with a redundant membrane that is folded over repeatedly to form 'lamellar bodies'. These laminar bodies can be identified by electron microscopy because of their characteristic membranous whirl appearance.

The phospholipidoses are caused by impaired breakdown of phospholipids within lysosomes, leading to the accumulation of these amphipathic lipids in the lysosomal membranes. Genetic deficiencies of enzymes that metabolize phospholipids can cause a lethal accumulation of phospholipids within lysosomes. Wolman disease occurs in childhood and is caused by the absence of lysosomal acid lipase. Cholesterol ester storage disease is caused by defective expression of the same enzyme, yet small residual activity can allow survival past childhood. Lysosomal sphingomyelinase is deficient in patients with Niemann-Pick disease.

Drugs that impair the lysosomal enzymes that metabolize phospholipids or diminish the lateral mobility of phospholipids within membranes are the major causes of the phospholipidoses (**Table 22.5**). Generally, drugs that cause phospholipidosis are polycationic (meaning that they have more than one positive charge) and amphipathic (meaning that in addition to a polar charged region of the molecule, much of the drug is non-polar or hydrophobic). These properties allow such drugs to bind phospholipids within membranes and prevent their normal mobility and enzymatic degradation. The lysosomes are probably a target for such amphipathic drug accumulation because of their lower intraorganelle pH, which favors compartmental accumulation. The same mechanism is also responsible for

Hepatic phospholipidoses
Metabolic diseases
Niemann-Pick disease
Wolman disease
Cholesterol ester storage disease
Drugs (after long-term use)
Amantadine
Amiodarone
Amitriptyline
Chloroquine
Chlorphenteramine
Chlorpromazine
Diltiazem
Fenfluramine
Imipramine
Nifedipine
Oral contraceptives
Propranolol
Thioridazine
Gentamicin

Table 22.5 Hepatic phospholipidoses.

mitochondrial accumulation of similar drugs where they can be concentrated and impair mitochondrial function.

Because of the slow accumulation rate in the lysosomal membrane compartment, drugs that cause clinically apparent phospholipidosis are typically administered for prolonged periods before a significant amount of phospholipid accumulates. Thus, antibiotics such as gentamicin, ketoconazole and azithromycin, which cause phospholipidosis after chronic administration experimentally, are not major causes of clinically evident phospholipidosis, because of their typically short treatment regimens. By contrast, the now abandoned antianginal drug perhexiline maleate and the antiarrhythmic drug amiodarone cause clinically relevant phospholipidosis because of their need for prolonged use.

The relationship between phospholipidosis and injury to the liver is unclear. Although there are reports of idiosyncratic-type reactions to amiodarone with clinically evident liver injury, this occurs only in a minority of cases compared with the frequent development of phospholipidosis. Steatohepatitis, as distinguished from phospholipidosis, can be found following amiodarone treatment but does not appear to be a direct consequence of phospholipidosis.

Steatosis and inflammation

The inflammatory response characteristic of NASH appears to develop only in the setting of pre-existing steatosis. The converse – the development of the characteristic mixed cellular infiltrate throughout the acinus without steatosis – is not a known histopathologic condition. One hypothesis is that the fat within the steatotic liver serves as a readily available target for lipid peroxidation. Lipid peroxidation produces highly toxic intermediates that promote inflammation and directly compromise cellular integrity. This hypothesis is supported primarily by animal data. Evidence in humans has been less convincing. Alternative explanations include hepatocellular toxicity of excess free fatty acids, mitochondrial dysfunction

and hepatocellular ATP deficiency, and injury mediated by hepatic Kupffer cells and circulating endotoxin.

CLINICAL FEATURES

Symptoms

Hepatic steatosis is usually asymptomatic. The most common complaint in patients with benign steatosis or NASH, particularly in the obese, is dull right upper quadrant pain, which may be caused by a distended liver capsule. A minority of patients may have quite severe pain. A variety of less common non-specific constitutional symptoms such as weakness, fatigue and malaise are offered by patients with NASH. The prevalence and severity of these same constitutional symptoms is much greater in patients with alcoholic hepatitis, despite the similarity of biopsy findings and aminotransferase elevations.

Physical examination

Palpable hepatomegaly can signify a liver enlarged by benign steatosis or NASH. However, hepatomegaly can be difficult to detect by palpation in many patients because of the coexistent obesity. There are no other specific physical findings that would suggest hepatic steatosis. Findings such as jaundice, spider angiomas, muscle wasting, ascites, and palmar erythema point to the development of cirrhosis. Many patients with NAFLD have underlying insulin resistance and two findings characteristic of the metabolic syndrome, hypertension and acanthosis nigricans, can be found in patients with NAFLD.

Laboratory evaluation

Most patients who come to medical attention for the evaluation of subclinical liver disease do so because of incidental laboratory abnormalities. This fact biases all clinical surveys that attempt to establish the sensitivity of laboratory testing for identifying patients with NASH. Progression of NASH can occur with normal laboratory testing; this has been shown in reports of the preoperative evaluation of patients undergoing surgical treatment for obesity. Nonetheless, among the laboratory tests available, the aminotransferases are the most likely to be abnormal. Other biochemical abnormalities that are common in alcoholic hepatitis (e.g. hypoalbuminemia, hyperbilirubinemia and prothrombin time elevations) are not observed in NASH unless the disease has progressed to cirrhosis.

Aminotransferases

Patients with NASH typically have serum aminotransferases that range from normal to a maximum of four times the upper limit of normal (**Table 22.6**). The prevalence of elevated aminotransferases in patients with NASH is unknown. This is mainly because the presence of liver disease is not routinely pursued in patients with normal aminotransferases, even when imaging studies suggest hepatic steatosis. The presence of elevated aminotransferases cannot be used to distinguish benign steatosis from NASH.

One way in which aminotransferase elevations can be useful in identifying patients with NASH is the ratio of alanine aminotransferase (ALT) to aspartate aminotransferase (AST) activities. Whereas patients with alcoholic hepatitis typically have serum AST levels that exceed the ALT, patients with NASH often have an ALT that is greater than the AST level in the absence

Laboratory findings of steatosis and NASH	
Aminotransferases (ALT and AST)	Normal values do not exclude steatosis or NASH Typically normal to 250 U/L. ALT is greater than AST in most patients (helpful in distinguishing from alcoholic steatosis/steatohepatitis; AST is usually greater than the ALT in alcoholic liver disease and cirrhosis from any cause)
Alkaline phosphatase	Typically normal but can be up to two times the upper limit of normal
γ-Glutamyltranspeptidase (GGT)	Can be elevated
Triglycerides	Frequently elevated in children with steatosis and NASH but not consistently elevated in adults
Cholesterol	No correlation; abnormally low cholesterol may indicate hypobetalipoproteinemia as a cause of steatosis/NASH
Total bilirubin, prothrombin time, albumin	Normal in the absence of cirrhosis
ALT, alanine aminotransferase; AST, aspartate aminotransferase; NASH, non-alcoholic steatohepatitis	

Table 22.6 Laboratory findings of steatosis and NASH.

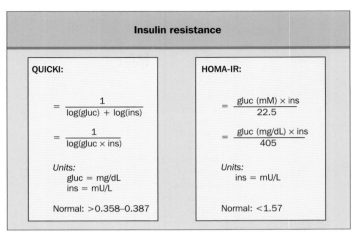

Figure 22.3 Insulin resistance. Insulin resistance can be estimated by calculating the product of the fasting insulin times the fasting glucose. Two commonly used formulas, the QUICKI and the HOMA-IR, are based on this product. The cutoffs for normal ranges of these values may depend on the method used to measure insulin; the values given are derived from published studies and may not apply to every laboratory.

of cirrhosis. Identification of the intracellular origin of serum aminotransferases has not proved helpful in distinguishing NASH from alcoholic hepatitis. In both diseases, the ratio of mitochondrial AST to total AST is elevated, possibly reflecting a shared pathogenetic mechanism of mitochondrial injury. Patients with cirrhosis from any cause, including NASH, typically have serum AST levels that exceed ALT levels. For this reason, using the AST/ALT ratio is only helpful in patients without cirrhosis.

Other biochemical markers

γ-Glutamyltranspeptidase (GGT) elevations may correlate with increases in hepatic fat content, yet elevations of this enzyme are rarely isolated when substantial and are rarely worth pursuing further when trivial. Serum triglyceride elevations are found in only a few adults with NASH but are common in children.

Estimating insulin resistance

Insulin resistance, and its resulting state of hyperinsulinemia, may be a primary underlying disorder in most patients with NAFLD. Insulin resistance is best measured by rigorous techniques such as the euglycemic insulin clamp method. Because performing this test is difficult in the routine clinical environment, simpler tests have been sought. Several generally accepted methods of approximating insulin sensitivity have been developed that are based on the product of the fasting insulin multiplied by the fasting glucose. Two of the most commonly used, the homeostasis model (HOMA-IR) and quantitative

insulin sensitivity check index (QUICKI), rely on this product and are mathematically related (**Fig. 22.3**). An even simpler method is that a product of fasting insulin (mU/L) × fasting insulin (mg/dL) >700 may indicate insulin resistance. Unfortunately, lack of standardization of insulin assays makes these values approximate and creates difficulties in comparing values from different laboratories. The value of estimating insulin resistance in patients with NAFLD is that it may provide patients with an additional incentive to adopt lifestyle modifications that include increased physical activity and caloric restriction.

Imaging

The major abdominal imaging modalities – ultrasound, CT, magnetic resonance imaging (MRI) and radionuclide techniques – can each contribute to the identification of focal or diffusely distributed hepatic steatosis (**Table 22.7**). Each has the ability to indicate the presence of hepatic steatosis, yet none of these techniques has the ability to distinguish benign hepatic steatosis from NASH. Generally, NASH is non-focal, and thus areas of focal fat or areas of focal sparing in a fatty liver can create difficulties in distinguishing these lesions from malignancy. Several circumstances responsible for focal involvement or sparing have been described. Patients with diabetes and renal failure who receive insulin in their peritoneal dialysis fluid can develop subcapsular steatosis, which can progress to NASH that is confined to the periphery of the liver exposed to high concentrations of insulin. Additionally, a minority of patients has pancreatic venous drainage into a localized area of the liver and focal NAFLD can sometimes be found in this region. The opposite anatomic anomaly can also exist; some patients have gastric venous drainage, which contains less insulin than the portal blood flow, directed into a localized hilar region. If the remainder of the liver is fatty in such patients, the region spared of insulin is also spared of fatty infiltration. Such observations may provide important insights into the role of insulin in

Imaging findings of steatosis and NASH		
	Ultrasonography	*Computed tomography*
Diffuse steatosis and NASH	Echogenic liver parenchyma Loss of contrast between the bile duct wall and liver parenchyma Hemangiomas may appear hypoechoic compared with the surrounding liver parenchyma	Low-density liver parenchyma compared with the spleen
Focal steatosis	Often a geometrically shaped echogenic area No mass effect Can be transient, absent on follow-up studies	Single or multiple low-density areas (often with the appearance of metastatic disease)
Focal sparing	Area of decreased echogenicity Often in caudate lobe or adjacent to the gallbladder	Regions of normal density in an otherwise low-density liver
NASH, non-alcoholic steatohepatitis		

Table 22.7 Imaging findings of steatosis and NASH.

the accumulation of hepatic fat and the importance of fat as a precursor lesion to NASH.

Ultrasonography

Compared with the normal liver, the fatty liver is diffusely echogenic or 'bright' (**Fig. 22.4**). However, ultrasonography of the liver is a reliable technique for the detection of hepatic steatosis only when the degree of steatosis is substantial. Thus, when biopsy results are compared with ultrasonographic findings, a significant amount of fat must be present for the liver to appear sonographically dense. The finding of a diffusely echogenic liver is also not entirely specific for steatosis because cirrhosis can cause a similar appearance albeit with a subjectively coarser texture.

Computed tomography

CT scanning of the fatty liver typically reveals an abnormally low-density liver parenchyma compared with the spleen (**Fig. 22.5**). A low-density liver is a relatively common finding, occurring in up to 10% of all abdominal CT scans. Most commonly, the low attenuation is diffuse. However, in up to one-third of the patients, the involvement is focal and appears as one or more low-density lesions in an otherwise normal liver. Focal fat can be found anywhere in the parenchyma or can be localized only to the periportal region. Focal sparing in an otherwise fatty liver can also be seen, and it has the appearance of a high-density lesion that can be confused with a malignancy. A comparison of the density of the focal area of sparing with its surrounding liver and with the spleen is helpful to identify its nature.

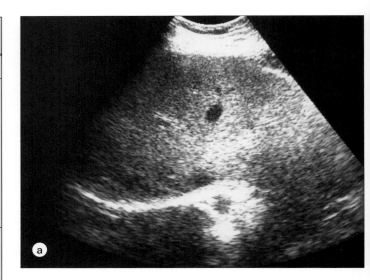

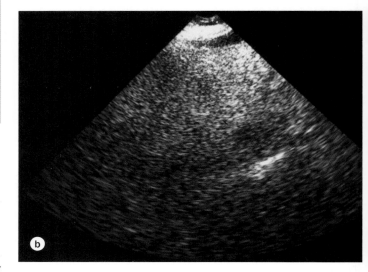

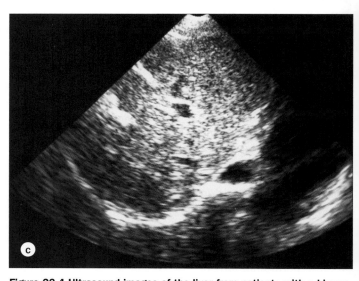

Figure 22.4 Ultrasound images of the liver from patients with a biopsy proven normal liver (a), severe steatosis (b), and cirrhosis caused by primary sclerosing cholangitis (c). Increased echogenicity is evident in both the steatotic and cirrhotic liver images compared with the normal liver.

FURTHER READING

General reviews

Andrews NC. Disorders of iron metabolism. N Engl J Med 1999; 341:1986–1995.

Bacon BR, Powell LW, Adams PC, et al. Molecular medicine and hemochromatosis: At the crossroads. Gastroenterology 1999; 116:193–207.

Bottomley SS. Secondary iron overload disorders. Semin Hematol 1998; 35:77–86.

Gordeuk VR. African iron overload. Semin Hematol 2002; 39:263–269.

Harrison SA, Bacon BR. Hereditary hemochromatosis: Update for 2003. J Hepatol 2003; 38:S14–S23.

Knisely AS, Mieli-Vergani G, Whitington PF. Neonatal hemochromatosis. Gastroenterol Clin North Am 2003; 32:877–889.

Pietrangelo A. Non-HFE hemochromatosis. Hepatology 2004; 39:21–29.

Pietrangelo A. Hereditary hemochromatosis: A new look at an old disease. N Engl J Med 2004; 350:2383–2397.

Powell LW. Hereditary hemochromatosis. Pathology 2000; 32:24–36.

Genetics of HH

Burke W, Thomson E, Khoury MJ, et al. Hereditary hemochromatosis: Gene discovery and its implications for population-based screening. JAMA 1998; 280:172–178.

Camaschella C, Roetto A, Cali A, et al. The gene TFR2 is mutated in a new type of hemochromatosis mapping to 7q22. Nat Genet 2000; 25:14–15.

Feder JN, Gnirke A, Thomas W, et al. A novel MHC class 1-like gene is mutated in patients with hereditary hemochromatosis. Nat Genet 1996; 13:399–409. *The first description of the mutations found in HFE and represents a seminal work describing the hemochromatosis gene.*

Gordeuk VR, Caleffi A, Corradini E, et al. Iron overload in Africans and African-Americans and a common mutation in the SCL40A1 (ferroportin 1) gene. Blood Cells Mol Dis 2003; 31:299–304.

Papanikolaou G, Samuels ME, Ludwig EH, et al. Mutations in HFE2 cause iron overload in chromosome 1q-linked juvenile hemochromatosis. Nat Genet 2004; 36:77–82.

Pathophysiology of HH

Bridle KR, Frazer DM, Wilkins SJ, et al. Disrupted hepcidin regulation in HFE-associated hemochromatosis and the liver as a regulator of body iron homoeostasis. Lancet 2003; 361:669–673.

Feder JN, Tsuchihashi Z, Irrinki A, et al. The hemochromatosis founder mutation in HLA-H disrupts β(2)-microglobulin interaction and cell surface expression. J Biol Chem 1997; 272:14025–14028.

Fleming RE, Britton RS, Waheed A, et al. Pathogenesis of hereditary hemochromatosis. Clin Liver Dis (in press), 2004.

Lebron JA, Bennett MJ, Vaughn DE, et al. Crystal structure of the hemochromatosis protein HFE and characterization of its interaction with transferrin receptor. Cell 1998; 93:111–123.

Nicolas G, Viatte L, Bennoun M, et al. Hepcidin, a new iron regulatory peptide. Blood Cells Mol Dis 2002; 29:327–335.

Parkkila S, Waheed A, Britton RS, et al. Immunohistochemistry of HLA-H, the protein defective in patients with hereditary hemochromatosis, reveals unique pattern of expression in gastrointestinal tract. Proc Natl Acad Sci USA 1997; 94:2534–2539.

Parkkila S, Waheed A, Britton RS, et al. Association of the transferrin receptor in human placenta with HFE, the protein defective in hereditary hemochromatosis. Proc Natl Acad Sci USA 1997; 94:13198–13202.

Roetto A, Papanikolaou G, Politou M, et al. Mutant antimicrobial peptide hepcidin is associated with severe juvenile hemochromatosis. Nat Genet 2003; 33:21–22.

Santos M, Schilham MW, Rademahers LHPM, et al. Defective iron homeostasis in β2-microglobulin knockout mice recapitulates hereditary hemochromatosis in man. J Exp Med 1996; 184:1975–1985.

Waheed A, Parkkila S, Zhou XY, et al. Hereditary hemochromatosis: Effects of C282Y and H63D mutations on association with β2-microglobulin, intracellular processing, and cell surface expression of the HFE protein in COS-7 cells. Proc Natl Acad Sci USA 1997; 94:12384–12389.

Waheed A, Parkkila S, Saarnio J, et al. Association of HFE protein with transferrin receptor in crypt enterocytes of human duodenum. Proc Natl Acad Sci USA 1999; 96:1579–1584.

Zhou XY, Tomatsu S, Fleming RE, et al. HFE gene knockout produces mouse model of hereditary hemochromatosis. Proc Natl Acad Sci USA 1998; 95:2492–2497.

Diagnosis of HH

Adams PC, Kertesz AE, Valberg LS. Clinical presentation of hemochromatosis: A changing scene. Am J Med 1991; 90:445–449.

Adams PC, Deugnier Y, Moirand R, et al. The relationship between iron overload, clinical symptoms, and age in 410 patients with genetic hemochromatosis. Hepatology 1997; 25:162–166.

Bacon BR, Sadiq S. Hereditary hemochromatosis: Diagnosis in the 1990s. Am J Gastroenterol 1997; 92:784–789.

Bassett ML, Halliday JW, Powell LW. Value of hepatic iron measurements in early hemochromatosis and determination of the critical iron level associated with fibrosis. Hepatology 1986; 6:24–29. *Describes the value of the hepatic iron index which is less frequently used currently with the advent of genetic testing.*

Beutler E, Felitti VJ, Koziol JA, et al. Penetrance of 845G → A (C282Y) HFE hereditary hemochromatosis mutation in the USA. Lancet 2002; 359:211–218.

Brunt EM, Olynyk JK, Britton RS, et al. Histological evaluation of iron in liver biopsies: Relationship to HFE mutations. Am J Gastroenterol 2000; 95:1788–1793.

Olynyk JK, O'Neill R, Britton RS, et al. Determination of hepatic iron concentration in fresh and paraffin-embedded tissue: Diagnostic implications. Gastroenterology 1994; 106:674–677.

Olynyk JK, Hagan SE, Cullen DJ, et al. Evolution of untreated hereditary hemochromatosis in the Busselton population: A 17-year study. Mayo Clin Proc 2004; 79:309–313.

Iron and HFE in liver disease

Bacon BR, Faravesh MJ, Janney CG, et al. Nonalcoholic steatohepatitis: An expanded clinical entity. Gastroenterology 1994; 107:1103–1109.

Bacon BR, Olynyk JK, Brunt EM, et al. HFE genotype in patients with hemochromatosis and other liver diseases. Ann Intern Med 1999; 130:953–962. *HFE genotype in a large series of patients with a variety of liver diseases is described in this carefully written manuscript.*

Bonkovsky HL, Banner BF, Rothman AL. Iron and chronic viral hepatitis. Hepatology 1997; 25:759–768.

Bonkovsky HL, Poh-Fitzpatrick M, Pimstone N, et al. Porphyria cutanea tarda, hepatitis C, and HFE gene mutations in North America. Hepatology 1998; 27:1661–1669.

Chapman RW, Morgan MY, Laulicht M, et al. Hepatic iron stores and markers of iron overload in alcoholics and patients with idiopathic hemochromatosis. Dig Dis Sci 1982; 27:909–916.

Di Bisceglie AM, Axiotis CA, Hoofnagle JH, et al. Measurement of iron status in patients with chronic hepatitis. Gastroenterology 1992; 102:2108–2113. *This paper points out that serum indices of iron are very often abnormal in chronic viral hepatitis and estimation of hepatic iron concentration is the most accurate way of diagnosing iron overload.*

Smith BC, Grove J, Guzail MA, et al. Heterozygosity for hereditary hemochromatosis is associated with more fibrosis in chronic hepatitis C. Hepatology 1998; 27:1695–1699.

CHAPTER
24

Wilson Disease

Peter Ferenci

DEFINITION

Wilson disease is an autosomal recessive inherited disorder of copper metabolism resulting in pathologic accumulation of copper in many organs and tissues. The hallmarks of the disease are the presence of liver disease, neurologic symptoms and Kayser-Fleischer corneal rings. The familial nature of Wilson disease was recognized in the original description of this disease by Samuel Alexander Kinnier Wilson.

EPIDEMIOLOGY

Until very recently, Wilson disease was believed to be very rare. By a population-based approach, the incidence of Wilson disease was estimated to be at least 1:30 000–50 000 (Ireland: $17/10^6$ live births, former East-Germany: 29) with a gene frequency of 1:90 to 1:150. However, these estimations were mostly based on adolescents or adults presenting with neurologic symptoms. More recent data however indicate that neurologic symptoms occur only in about half of Wilson disease patients. Thus, the incidence of Wilson disease was underestimated by these studies. Furthermore, in selected populations (Jews from Uzbekistan, China) Wilson disease seems to be even more common. Among selected groups of patients Wilson disease is certainly more frequent. About 3–6% of patients transplanted for fulminant hepatic failure and 16% of young adults with chronic active hepatitis of unknown origin have Wilson disease.

PATHOGENESIS

The basic defect in Wilson disease is the impaired biliary excretion of copper resulting in the accumulation of copper in various organs including the liver, the cornea and the brain. The consequence of copper accumulation is the development of severe hepatic and neurological disease. Copper's unique electron structure allows these cuproenzymes to catalyze redox reactions, but causes ionic copper to be very toxic, readily participating in reactions that promote the synthesis of damaging reactive oxygen species. Copper overload particularly affects mitochondrial respiration and causes a decrease in cytochrome C activity. Damage to mitochondria is an early pathologic effect in the liver. Damage to the liver has been shown to result in increased lipid peroxidation and abnormal mitochondrial respiration both in copper loaded dogs and in patients with Wilson disease. The mechanism(s) triggering copper-induced lipid peroxidation are unknown. However, it is conceivable that, due to hepatic copper accumulation, patients with Wilson disease are particularly sensitive to any oxidative stress.

The pathogenesis of neurologic disease is less clear. Neuronal damage is mediated by copper deposition in the brain. Copper may be directly toxic to neurons or may exert its effects by selective inhibition of brain monoamine oxidase A (MAO-A). Copper accumulation in the brain may be secondary to liver damage, but this hypothesis is inconsistent with the clinical observation that many patients with neurologic disease have only mild liver disease, and that conversely patients with advanced liver failure have no neurologic symptoms. Furthermore the preferential affection of basal ganglia cannot be explained. The discovery of the Wilson disease gene may help to better understand the pathophysiology of copper metabolism. ATP7B is also expressed in the brain, but its function is unknown. It is conceivable that increased copper uptake into the brain is a direct result of a certain mutation resulting in specific functional alterations of cerebral ATP7B.

The Wilson disease gene

The Wilson disease gene was localized to human chromosome 13 by cosegregation of the disease with the red cell enzyme marker, esterase D, in several large Middle Eastern kindred. Further linkage analysis of additional families, using more polymorphic DNA markers defined a region close to the retinoblastoma locus as the candidate region for the Wilson disease gene. By positional cloning strategies, the Wilson disease gene was identified by three independent groups in 1993. Final identification was established with the use of conserved regions of the previously discovered Menkes disease (another disease with impaired copper metabolism) gene. The Wilson disease gene codes for a copper transporting P-type adenosine triphosphatase (ATPase), ATP7B.

Wilson disease protein contains the following functional domains and is thought to form an ion channel: six copper binding regions [Cu] containing Cys-X-X-Cys motifs at the amino terminal end; and adenosine triphosphate (ATP) binding, aspartyl kinase and phosphorylation domains. Alternatively spliced forms of Wilson disease protein lacking transmembrane sequences 3 and 4 (exon 8) are expressed in brain.

The functionally important regions of the Wilson disease gene are six copper binding domains, a transduction domain (amino acid residues 837–864; containing a Thr-Gly-Glu motif) involved in the transduction of the energy of ATP hydrolysis to cation transport, a cation channel and phosphorylation domain (amino acid residues 971–1035; containing the highly conserved Asp-Lys-Thr-Gly-Thr motif), an ATP-binding domain (amino acid residues 1240–1291) and eight hydrophobic transmembrane sequences (1–8), in one of which (region 6) is the Cys-pro-Cys sequence found in all P-type ATPases.

Common mutations of the Wilson disease gene in various populations		
	Most common mutation (exon)	*Other common mutations*
Central-, eastern-, northwestern Europe*	H1069Q	3400delC, exon 8 (multiple), P969Q
Sardinia	-441/-421 del (5' UTR)	2463delC, V1146M
Canary Islands	L708P	
Turkey	R969Q, A1003T	Exon 8, H1069Q,
Brazil	3400delC	
Saudi Arabia	Q1399R	
Far East	R778L	
* Russia, Bjelorus, Poland, Bulgaria, former Yugoslavia, Czech Republic, Slovakia, Hungary, Germany, Benelux, Greece (Ferenci P, unpublished data)		

Table 24.1 Common mutations of the Wilson disease gene in various populations.

Phenotype-genotype correlation in 474 patients with both mutations of the Wilson disease gene identified			
Mutation	*n*	*Percentage with liver disease*	*Mean age at onset*
H1069Q/H1069Q	215	46	21.5 (liver:19.8; neuro: 24.6)
H1069Q/2299insC	24	70	17.4
H1069Q/3400delC	22	30	18.8
H1069Q/R969Q	14	92	24.1
H1069Q/Q1351X	11	37	18.9
H1069Q/W779X	10	60	19.5
G710S/G710S	8	50	17.9
H1069Q/G710S	6	82	22.2
H1069Q/K844Kfs	7	60	19.4

Table 24.2 Phenotype-genotype correlation in 474 patients with both mutations of the Wilson disease gene identified. (Ferenci, unpublished data.)

Molecular genetic analysis of affected patients reveals over 200 distinct mutations (database maintained at the University of Alberta -http://www.medgen.med.ualberta.ca). Mutations include missense and nonsense mutations, deletions and insertions. Some mutations are associated with a severe impairment of copper transport resulting in severe liver disease very early in life; other mutations appear to be less severe with disease appearance in mid adulthood. While most reported mutations occur in single families, a few are more common. The His1069Gln (H1069Q) missense mutation occurs in 30–60% of patients of eastern-, northern- and central-European origin. It is less frequent in patients of Mediterranean descent and only rarely seen in patients of non-European origin. About 10% of patients of French or British extraction have a Gly1266Lys mutation in the ATP hinge domain. The 2299insC mutation can be detected in some patients of European and Japanese descent. The Arg778Leu mutation is present in 27% of Taiwanese patients, but is not found in non-Asian patients. In Sardinia two frameshift mutations (1515insT and 2464delC) are found in about 20% of patients. These mutations were not found in other populations (**Table 24.1**).

The study of genotype–phenotype correlations is hampered by the lack of clinical data, the rarity of some mutations and the high frequency of the presence of two different mutations in individual patients (compound heterozygotes) (**Table 24.2**). In an ongoing study involving 820 patients with Wilson disease mostly from Europe, mutations on both chromosomes were identified in 58% of the patients (Table 24.2), with at least one mutation in 30%. Sufficient information is available only for the H1069Q mutation. Homozygosity for H1069Q is associated with late onset neurologic disease. In contrast, patients with mutations in exon 8 commonly present with liver disease.

Hepatic copper metabolism and the role of ATP7B

Copper is an essential nutrient needed for such diverse processes as mitochondrial respiration (cytochrome C), melanin biosynthesis (tyrosinase), dopamine metabolism (DOPA-β-mono-oxygenase), iron homeostasis (ceruloplasmin), antioxidant defense (superoxide dismutase), connective tissue formation (lysyl oxidase) and peptide amidation.

Dietary copper intake is approximately 1–2 mg/day. Quoted copper contents of foods are unreliable. While some foods, such as meats and shellfish, have consistently high copper concentrations, others such as dairy produce are consistently low in copper. However, the copper content of cereals and fruits varies greatly with soil copper content and the method of food preparation. Estimates of copper intake should include water copper content, the permitted upper concentration for copper in drinking water being 2 mg/L. The recommended intake in the first 6 months of life is 80 mg/kg/day. Thus, dietary copper intake far exceeds the trace amounts required. Approximately 10% of dietary copper is absorbed in the upper intestine and binds loosely to albumin, certain amino acids (histidine, cysteine and threonine) and peptides. Most of the ingested copper is taken up by the liver. The hepatic uptake of diet-derived copper appears to be an unsaturable, carrier-mediated, energy independent mechanism.

Specific pathways allow the intracellular trafficking and compartmentalization of copper, ensuring adequate cuproprotein synthesis while avoiding cellular toxicity (**Fig. 24.1**). After uptake by hepatocytes, copper is bound to metallothionein, a cytosolic, low molecular weight, cysteine-rich, metal binding protein. The copper stored in metallothionein can be donated to other proteins, either following degradation in lysosomes or by exchange via a glutathione (GSH) complex. Biliary excretion is the only mechanism for copper elimination, and the amount of copper excreted in the bile is directly proportional to the size of the hepatic copper pool. Trafficking of copper in hepatocytes is complex and involves several transport proteins: the copper transporter 1 (Ctr1) transports copper with high affinity in a metal-specific, saturable fashion at the hepatocyte plasma

Zinc

Zinc interferes with the intestinal absorption of copper by two mechanisms. Both metals share the same carrier in enterocytes and pretreatment with zinc blocks this carrier for copper transport (with a half-life of about 11 days). The impact of zinc-induced blockade of copper transport by other carriers into the enterocyte was not studied. Second, zinc induces metallothionein in enterocytes, which acts as an intracellular ligand, binding metals which are then excreted in the feces with desquamated epithelial cells. Indeed, fecal excretion of copper is increased in patients with Wilson disease on treatment with zinc. Furthermore, zinc also induces metallothionein in the liver, protecting hepatocytes against copper toxicity.

Data on zinc in the treatment of Wilson disease are derived from uncontrolled studies using different zinc preparations (zinc sulfate, zinc acetate) at different doses (75–250 mg/day). The efficacy of zinc was assessed by four different approaches. First, patients successfully decoppered by D-penicillamine were switched to zinc and the maintenance of their asymptomatic condition was monitored. Most patients maintained a negative copper balance and no symptomatic recurrences occurred. Some patients, however, died of liver failure after treatment was switched to zinc. Stremmel et al (1991) observed the occurrence of severe neurologic symptoms in a 25-year-old asymptomatic sibling 4 months after switching from D-penicillamine to zinc.

A second group of symptomatic patients switched to zinc as an alternate treatment due to intolerance to D-penicillamine. Sixteen case histories have been published so far. Liver function and neurologic symptoms improved in three and five patients, respectively. One patient further deteriorated neurologically and improved on retreatment with D-penicillamine. The remaining patients remained in a stable condition. Follow-up studies in 141 patients demonstrated that zinc is effective as sole therapy in the long-term maintenance treatment of Wilson disease. In a third group zinc was used as first line therapy. About one-third were asymptomatic siblings and two-thirds presented with neurologic or hepatic symptoms. Most patients remained free of symptoms or improved. In 15% neurologic symptoms worsened and improved on D-penicillamine treatment. Three patients died of progressive liver disease. Finally, in a prospective study in 67 newly diagnosed cases, the efficacy of D-penicillamine and zinc was similar. This was not a randomized study; every other patient was treated with zinc. Zinc was better tolerated than D-penicillamine. However, two zinc-treated patients died of progressive liver disease.

It is unknown whether a combination of zinc with chelation therapy is useful or not. Theoretically these drugs may have antagonistic effects. Interactions in the maintenance phase of zinc therapy with penicillamine and trientine were investigated by copper balance studies and absorption of orally administered ^{64}Cu as endpoints. The result on copper balance was about the same with zinc alone as it is with zinc plus one of the other agents. Thus, there appears to be no advantage to concomitant administration.

Antioxidants

As discussed before, the main mechanism of hepatocellular injury by excess copper is the formation of free radicals resulting in lipid peroxidation and impaired mitochondrial respiration.

Thus, antioxidants such as α-tocopherol may be important adjuncts in the treatment of Wilson disease. There are no large experiences with α-tocopherol. A few observations indicate that this therapeutic adjunct may be useful in severe liver disease.

Monitoring therapy

If a decoppering agent is used for treatment, compliance can be tested by repeated measurement of the 24 h urinary copper excretion. This approach is not useful if patients are treated with zinc. If in a compliant patient urinary copper excretion decreases over time and stabilizes at <500 μg/day the dose of D-penicillamine can be lowered.

Efficacy of treatment can be monitored by the determination of 'free' copper in serum, depending on the presenting symptoms. Liver disease can be assessed by routine liver tests. Repeated liver biopsies with measurement of hepatic copper content are not helpful. Improvement of neurologic symptoms can be documented by clinical examination. In addition, some of the MRI abnormalities are fully reversible on treatment. Auditory evoked brainstem potentials are also helpful to document improvement by decoppering treatment.

Liver transplantation

Liver transplantation is the treatment of choice in patients with fulminant Wilson disease and in patients with decompensated cirrhosis. Besides improving survival, liver transplantation also corrects the biochemical defect underlying Wilson disease. However, the role of this procedure in the management of patients with neurologic Wilson disease in the absence of hepatic insufficiency is still uncertain.

Schilsky et al (1994) analyzed 55 transplants performed in 33 patients with decompensated cirrhosis and 21 with Wilsonian fulminant hepatitis in the USA and Europe. The median survival after orthotopic liver transplantation was 2.5 years, the longest survival time after transplantation was 20 years. Survival at 1 year was 79%. Non-fatal complications occurred in five patients. At the University of Pittsburgh 51 orthotopic liver transplants (OLT) were performed on 39 patients (16 pediatric, 23 adults). The rate of primary graft survival was 73% and patient survival was 79.4%. Survival was better for those with chronic advanced liver disease (90%) than it was for those with fulminant hepatic failure (73%). In the Mayo Clinic series 1-year survival ranged from 79 to 87%, with an excellent chance of long-term survival. The outcome of neurologic disease following OLT is uncertain. In a retrospective survey, four of seven patients with neurologic or psychiatric symptoms due to Wilson disease improved after OLT. Anecdotal reports document a dramatic improvement in neurologic function within 3 to 4 months after OLT. In contrast, central pontine and extrapontine myelinolysis and new extrapyramidal symptoms developed in a patient 19 months after OLT. Some patients transplanted for decompensated cirrhosis have had psychiatric or neurologic symptoms, which improved following OLT.

PREGNANCY IN PATIENTS WITH WILSON DISEASE

Prior to the introduction of penicillamine, successful pregnancies in patients with Wilson disease were rare due to reduced

Outcome of pregnancy in different series						
	USA	UK	UK	USA	India	Austria*
Number of patients	18	10	7	19	16	11
Number on treatment (DPEN/Zn/TRI)	18 (+/−/−)	9 (+/−/−)	7 (−/+/+)	19 (−/+/−)	6 (+/+/−)	10 (+/−/+)
Mean duration of treatment (years)	6.6	11.7	5	5.1	5.2	5
Number of successful conceptions	29	15	11	26	59	19
Number of abortions (spontaneous/elective)	-	5 (3/2)	1 (1/−)	-	26 (24/2)	4 (4/−)
Type of delivery	NA	13/2	8/1	26/-	30/-	NA
Full-term normal/Premature						

DPEN: D-Penicillamine, Zn: zinc, TRI: trientine NA: not assessed;* currently we have followed two additional pregnant patients with an uneventful course; one of them had a successful in vitro fertilization.
Of the 120 life births, 117 were normal, one with isochromosome X was born prematurely, 1 required surgery for a heart defect at 6 months, 1 microcephalic baby died 1 h postpartum.
The condition of all mothers remained unchanged during and after pregnancy. One patient was transplanted for deteriorating liver disease 2 years after delivery.

Table 24.8 Outcome of pregnancy in different series. (In addition there are several case reports on successful pregnancies in patients with Wilson disease.)

fertility, menstrual irregularities and consequences of severe liver dysfunction. Since then, many case reports and series reported successful pregnancies in more than 100 patients with Wilson disease (**Table 24.8**). In general, the outcome both for mother and child is excellent. During pregnancy, serum copper and ceruloplasmin levels rise until 24 weeks and decline thereafter possibly due to copper uptake by the fetus.

Assessment prior to pregnancy

Patients with Wilson disease wishing to become pregnant should be seen prior to conception for assessment of their hepatic function and copper status. Patients who are copper overloaded or who have esophageal varices should possibly avoid or delay pregnancy. Patients on well-established therapy should continue with this treatment through the pregnancy and compliance with treatment must be emphasized to the patient. If the patient has been decoppered, it is prudent to reduce the dose of penicillamine to 500 mg daily. Reducing the dose of penicillamine amongst patients who are not decoppered, however, places the patient at risk of neurologic and hepatic compromise and trientine should be considered as an alternative treatment.

Drug therapy during pregnancy

Controversy over prescribing penicillamine in pregnant patients exists due to its possible teratogenic effects. Rare cases of birth defects including hydrocephalus and cerebral palsy have been reported in patients treated with penicillamine for a variety of diseases. However, the overall teratogenic risk of penicillamine is low and there is general support for continuing treatment throughout pregnancy to avoid the risk of relapse in the mother, although the optimal dosage of penicillamine is not known. Trientine appears to be an alternative to penicillamine with no

reported teratogenic effects, but the experience with this drug is limited. The use of zinc in pregnancy has not been associated with any fetal abnormality and possibly has a protective effect from some birth defects. The limited experience with zinc or trientine in pregnancy does not justify a change in drug therapy during pregnancy.

PROGNOSIS

Untreated, symptomatic Wilson disease progresses to death in all patients. The majority of patients will die of complications of advanced liver failure, some of progressive neurologic disease. The overall mortality from Wilson disease treated medically (in most cases by D-penicillamine) has not been assessed prospectively. The mortality in 33 patients followed for 21 years by Scheinberg & Sternlieb (1987) was approximately 20%. This figure is close to the cumulative mortality in 69 Austrian patients (**Fig. 24.10**). In this group there was a substantial early mortality due to liver failure within the first 2 months after diagnosis. Only two patients died during the follow-up, one of them developed liver failure after a 2-year period of non-compliance. About an equal number of patients with severe liver failure survived following orthotopic liver transplantation. In a German study in 51 patients the cumulative survival was slightly reduced during the early period of follow-up but was not different from an age- and sex matched control population after 15 years of observation (96%).

Liver disease

In general, prognosis depends on the severity of liver disease at diagnosis. In patients without cirrhosis or with compensated cirrhosis, liver disease does not progress after initiation of decoppering therapy. Liver function improves gradually (**Fig.**

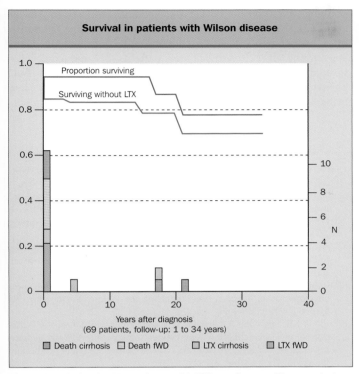

Figure 24.10 Survival in patients with Wilson disease. The cumulative survival of 60 Austrian patients was followed. The broken lines indicate 'survival rates' if death or liver transplantation (LTX) are chosen as endpoints. The bars refer to the number of patients dying from or transplanted for fulminant Wilson disease (fWD) or decompensated cirrhosis.

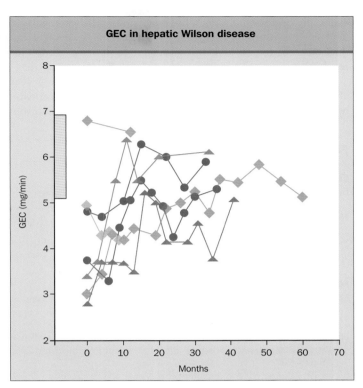

Figure 24.11 GEC in patients with hepatic Wilson disease. Serial determination of galactose elimination capacity (GEC) in seven patients with hepatic Wilson disease.

Prognostic index in Wilson disease					
	0*	1*	2*	3*	4*
Serum bilirubin (μmol/L)	<100	100–150	151–200	201–300	>301
AST (x ULN)	<2.5	2.6–3.5	3.6–5	5.1–7.5	>7.5
PTT (sec over control)	<4	4–8	9–12	13–20	>21

Modified from Nazer et al (77).
*= score points; AST, aspartate aminotransferase; PTT, partial thromboplastin time; ULN, upper limit of normal
A score = 7 is associated with high probability of death

Table 24.9 Prognostic index in Wilson disease.

24.11) and liver function parameters (serum albumin, prothrombin time) will become normal in most patients within 1 to 2 years. In compliant patients treated with D-penicillamine or trientine, liver function remains stable and no progressive liver disease is observed.

Schilsky et al (1991) followed 20 patients with Wilsonian chronic active hepatitis. Treatment with D-penicillamine was promptly initiated in 19 patients. One refused treatment and died 4 months later. Treated patients received D-penicillamine or trientine for a total of 264 patient-years (median: 14). In 18 patients, symptomatic improvement and virtually normal levels of serum albumin, bilirubin, aspartate aminotransferase and alanine aminotransferase followed within 1 year. One woman died after 9 months of treatment. Two patients, who became non-compliant after 9 and 17 years of successful pharmacologic treatment, required liver transplants.

In patients presenting with fulminant Wilson disease, medical treatment is rarely effective. Without emergency liver transplantation, mortality is very high. In a group of 34 patients, a prognostic index based on serum bilirubin levels, aspartate aminotransferase activity, and prothrombin time (Table 24.9) was developed. A score >7 was always associated with death. However, this prognostic score has not been validated prospectively. Nevertheless, it is a useful guide to assess short-term mortality in the setting of liver transplantation.

Hemolytic anemia

If diagnosed and treated early, hemolysis subsides within a few days after initiation of D-penicillamine therapy. Spontaneous remissions may occur even without treatment but relapse usually within few months. Hemolysis associated with active liver disease may progress rapidly to fulminant Wilson disease.

Neurologic disease

Patients presenting with neurologic symptoms have a better prognosis than those presenting with liver disease. None of our patients died; two required liver transplantation. In Brewer's series (Brewer et al 1992), 2 out of 54 patients died due to complications which were attributed to their impaired neurologic function. Neurologic symptoms are partly reversible. Improvement of neurologic symptoms occurs gradually over several months. Initially, neurologic symptoms may worsen, especially on treatment with D-penicillamine. In some patients neurologic symptoms disappear completely, and abnormalities documented by evoked responses or MRI may completely resolve within 18–24 months.

Ten of our patients were followed prospectively for 5 years after diagnosis. Brain function was assessed by repeated recording of short latency sensory potentials, auditory brainstem potentials and cognitive P300 evoked potentials. Electrophysiologic and clinical improvement was observed as early as 3 months after initiation of chelation therapy and continued until final assessment after 5 years. Three patients became completely normal but residual symptoms were detectable in seven. Such permanent deficits are unlikely to be improved by liver transplantation.

FURTHER READING

Overviews

Brewer GJ, Yuzbasiyan-Gurkan V. Wilson disease. Medicine 1992; 71:139–164.

Hoogenraad TU. Wilson's disease. London: Saunders; 1996. *A recent authoritative review of Wilson disease.*

Scheinberg IH, Sternlieb I. Wilson's disease, vol 23. Major problems in internal medicine. Philadelphia: Saunders; 1984.

Hepatic copper transport

Hamza I, Schaefer M, Klomp LW, et al. Interaction of the copper chaperone HAH1 with the Wilson disease protein is essential for copper homeostasis. Proc Natl Acad Sci USA 1999; 96:13363–13368.

Huffman DL, O'Halloran TV. Function, structure, and mechanism of intracellular copper trafficking proteins. Annu Rev Biochem 2002; 70:677–701.

Kelley EJ, Palmiter RJ. A murine model of Menkes disease reveals a physiological function of metallothionein. Nat Genet 1996; 13:219–222.

Klomp AE, Tops BB, Van Denberg IE, et al. Biochemical characterization and subcellular localization of human copper transporter 1 (hCTR1). Biochem J 2002; 364:497–505.

Larin D, Mekios C, Das K, et al. Characterization of the interaction between the Wilson and Menkes disease proteins and the cytoplasmic copper chaperone, HAH1p. J Biol Chem 1999; 274:28497–28504.

Lee J, Pena MM, Nose Y, et al. Biochemical characterization of the human copper transporter Ctr1. J Biol Chem 2001; 277:4380–4387.

Lutsenko S, Petris MJ. Function and regulation of the mammalian copper-transporting ATPases: Insights from biochemical and cell biological approaches. J Membr Biol 2003; 191:1–12.

Palmiter RD. The elusive function of metallothioneins. Proc Natl Acad Sci USA 1998; 95:8428–8430.

Rae T, Schmidt P, Pufahl R, et al. Undetectable intracellular free copper: the requirement of a copper chaperone for superoxide dismutase. Science 1999; 284:805–808.

Tao YT, Gitlin JD. Hepatic copper metabolism: Insights from genetic disease. Hepatology 2003; 37:1241–1247. *An excellent review of hepatic copper metabolism.*

Walker JM, Tsivkovskii R, Lutsenko S. Metallochaperone Atox1 transfers copper to the NH2-terminal domain of the Wilson's disease protein and regulates its catalytic activity. J Biol Chem 2002; 277:27953–27959.

Wernimont AK, Huffman DL, Lamb AL, et al. Structural basis for copper transfer by the metallochaperone for Menkes/Wilson disease proteins. Nat Struct Biol 2000; 7:766–771.

Mutations of the Wilson disease gene

Caca K, Ferenci P, Kuhn HJ, et al. High prevalence of the H1069Q mutation in East German patients with Wilson disease: rapid detection of mutations by limited sequencing and phenotype–genotype analysis. J Hepatol 2001; 35:575–581.

Cox DW. Molecular advances in Wilson disease. In: Progress in liver disease, vol X. 1996:245–263.

Deguti MM, Genschel J, Cancado EL, et al. Wilson disease: novel mutations in the ATP7B gene and clinical correlation in Brazilian patients. Hum Mutat 2004; 398:1–8.

Figus A, Angius A, Loudianos O, et al. Molecular pathology and haplotype analysis of Wilson disease in Mediterranean populations. Am J Hum Genet 1995; 57:1318–1324.

Firneisz G, Lakatos PL, Szalay F, et al. Common mutations of ATP7B in Wilson disease patients from Hungary. Am J Med Genet 2002; 108:23–28.

Garcia-Villareal L, Daniels S, Shaw SH, et al. High prevalence of the very rare Wilson disease gene mutation Leu708Pro in the Island of Gran Canaria (Canary Islands, Spain): a genetic and clinical study. Hepatology 2000; 32:1329–1336.

Maier-Dobersberger Th, Ferenci P, Polli C, et al. The His1069Gln mutation in Wilson's disease: Detection by a rapid PCR-test, clinical course and liver biopsy findings. Ann Intern Med 1997; 127:21–26.

Petrukhin K, Fischer SG, Pirastu M, et al. Mapping, cloning and genetic characterization of the region containing the Wilson disease gene. Nat Genet 1993; 5:338–343.

Petrukhin KE, Lutsenko S, Chernov I, et al. Characterization of the Wilson disease gene encoding a P-type copper transporting ATPase: genomic organization, alternative splicing, and structure/function predictions. Hum Mol Genet 1994; 3:1647–1656.

Tanzi RE, Petrukhin K, Chernov I, et al. The Wilson disease gene is a copper transporting ATPase with homology to the Menkes disease gene. Nat Genet 1993; 5:344–350.

Thomas GJ, Forbes JR, Roberts EA, et al. The Wilson disease gene: spectrum of mutations and their consequences. Nat Genet 1995; 9:210–217.

Diagnosis

Ferenci P, Caca K, Loudianos G, et al. Diagnosis and phenotypic classification of Wilson disease. Final report of the proceedings of the working party at the 8th International Meeting on Wilson disease and Menkes disease, Leipzig/Germany, 2001. Liver Int 2003; 23:139–142. *A comprehensive overview of the diagnosis of Wilson disease.*

Ferenci P, Steindl-Munda P, Vogel W, et al. Diagnostic value of quantitative hepatic copper determination in patients with Wilson disease. Clinical Gastroenterol Hepatol 2005.

Grimm G, Madl Ch, Katzenschlager R, et al. Detailed evaluation of brain dysfunction in patients with Wilson's disease. Electroencephalogr Clin Neurophysiol 1992; 82:119–124.

Maier-Dobersberger Th, Rack S, Granditsch G, et al. Diagnosis of Wilson's disease in an asymptomatic sibling by DNA linkage analysis. Gastroenterology 1995; 109:2015–2018.

Oder W, Grimm G, Kollegger H, et al. Neurological and neuropsychiatric spectrum of Wilson's disease. A prospective study in 45 cases. J Neurol 1991; 238:281–287.

Scheinberg IH, Sternlieb I. Wilson's disease, vol 23. Major problems in internal medicine. Philadelphia: Saunders; 1984.

Scott J, Gollan JL, Samourian S et al. Wilson's disease, presenting as chronic active hepatitis. Gastroenterology 1978; 74:645–651.

Sternlieb I, Scheinberg IH. The role of radiocopper in the diagnosis of Wilson's disease. Gastroenterology 1979; 77:138–142.

van Wassenaer-van Hall HN, van den Heuvel AG, Algra A, et al. Wilson disease: findings at MR imaging and CT of the brain with clinical correlation. Radiology 1996; 198: 531–536.

Wiebers DO, Wilson DM, McLeod RA, et al. Renal stones in Wilson's disease. Am J Med 1979; 67:249–254.

Treatment

Brewer GJ, Dick RD, Johnson V et al. Treatment of Wilson's disease with ammonium tetrathiomolybdate: I. Initial therapy in 17 neurologically affected patients. Arch Neurol 1994; 51:545–554.

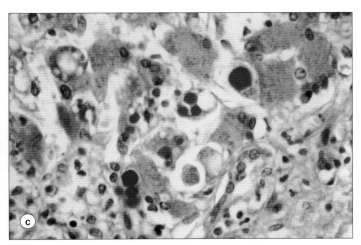
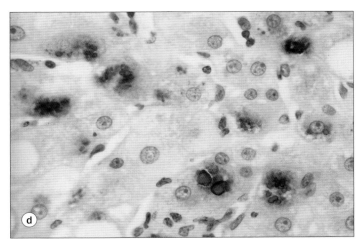

Figure 25.8 α₁-Antitrypsin deficiency: liver pathology. (*Cont'd*) (c) Photomicrograph showing that the cytoplasmic globules are periodic acid-Schiff (PAS)-positive and diastase-resistant (PAS-diastase, × 250). (d) Liver biopsy immunostained using α₁-antitrypsin as primary antibody. A positive reaction is indicated by the brown color (ABC immunostain technique × 400). (Courtesy of Barbara Banner, University of Massachusetts Medical Center.)

phoresis. Although both P₁ZZ and P₁SZ patients are predisposed to hepatic disease, specific genotyping may be important for genetic counseling. Quantitative serum α₁-AT may be helpful in determining heterozygosity in such patients, although parental phenotyping may be necessary. Prenatal diagnosis and phenotyping are possible by amniotic fluid analysis. Genetic testing is also possible now, especially if a causative mutation has already been uncovered in the kindred.

Treatment

Several established and experimental therapies exist for pulmonary disease, including cessation of tobacco use and avoidance of other potentially toxic inhalants, and infusion or inhalation of purified plasma α₁-AT. Some studies suggest that breast-feeding is beneficial for newborns with the disease during the first year of life, as functional antitrypsin is provided by maternal macrophages within the breast milk. Surgical shunting has been used to maintain patients with moderate histologic liver disease complicated by severe portal hypertension, and transjugular intrahepatic portosystemic shunts (TIPS) may serve as a bridge to transplant. Orthotopic liver transplantation has remained the definitive intervention for patients with progressive liver failure and portal hypertension. Hepatic decline may proceed slowly, however, and patients may be maintained for years with conservative measures before surgical intervention is warranted. Survival of subjects with α₁-AT deficiency who have undergone orthotopic liver transplantation may be similar to that of patients with other liver diseases, with 1- and 5-year survival rates of approximately 80–70%, respectively. Recent retrospective reviews suggest survival rates at five years and beyond may surpass 90% in children requiring transplantation. The donor liver synthesizes normal protein and, therefore, the disease does not recur in the new liver, and serum levels of α₁-AT become normal.

With the understanding that liver pathology in α₁-AT results from polymerization of abnormal protein attempts have been made to either interfere with the formation of these aggregates using competitive molecules, or induce rapid clearance of the aggregates using chemical 'chaperones'. These novel therapies may become useful in the treatment of α₁-AT deficiency and other conformational diseases.

At this time, gene therapy does not seem promising for the treatment of hepatic disease in α₁-AT deficiency. Such therapy aims for the re-expression of a normal α₁-AT protein but will not prevent the accumulation of mutant protein within hepatocytes. Moreover, expression of the normal gene may be associated with up regulation of the synthesis of mutant protein, possibly promoting and accelerating the development of liver disease. By stimulating expression of abnormal protein, gene therapy of *pulmonary* disease might also promote the development of hepatic disease, as may treatment of pulmonary disease with purified plasma α₁-AT. It appears that successful gene therapy of hepatic disease will mandate prevention of mutant protein expression while normal protein synthesis is promoted.

Interestingly, a recent analysis of transgenic P₁ZZ mouse liver showed a proliferative advantage of hepatic cells without intracellular α₁-AT aggregates over those encumbered with these aggregates. This suggests that the accumulation of defective α₁-AT aggregates leads to a functional disadvantage at the cellular level. Such a selective functional and proliferative advantage of non-affected hepatocytes over those affected by abnormal α₁-AT aggregates is intriguing as it may someday provide an opportunity to promote repletion and replacement of α₁-AT encumbered cells with viable unaffected cells. Studies in a murine model of another metabolic liver disease, hereditary tyrosinemia type 1, have suggested a possible strategy for gene therapy providing adequate synthesis of normal protein and suppression of mutant protein. By conferring a genetic, selective advantage upon retrovirally corrected cells, in vivo propagation of corrected cells (producing normal protein) to the exclusion of mutant cells might be accomplished for α₁-AT deficiency. Such strategies are discussed further in this chapter in the section on hereditary tyrosinemia type 1.

CYSTIC FIBROSIS

Cystic fibrosis (CF) is a chronic disease of deficient chloride conductance manifested by tenacious, often obstructive epithelial secretions that result in clinical disease in several organ systems. Although pulmonary disease is frequently the most visible consequence of the disease (**Fig. 25.9**), CF is the most common cause of pancreatic insufficiency in young adults in the USA and is associated as well with hepatobiliary disease. Because of improved management, life expectancy for most patients with CF is greater than 30 years, and it is increasingly likely that the hepatic manifestations of this disease will be encountered. Indeed, liver disease is the second leading cause of death in patients with CF.

Epidemiology and pathophysiology

CF is inherited as an autosomal recessive trait, affecting more than 1 in 2000 white births, making it the most common autosomal recessive disease expressed clinically in white children. The disease is associated with a defect of the CF transmembrane conductance regulator (CFTR), a cyclic adenosine monophosphate (cAMP)-activated chloride channel that is predicted to be a protein of 1480 amino acids coded for by a gene located on chromosome 7q31. The CFTR has 12 membrane-spanning segments clustered into two regions, two nucleotide binding folds, and a regulatory region. Nearly 1000

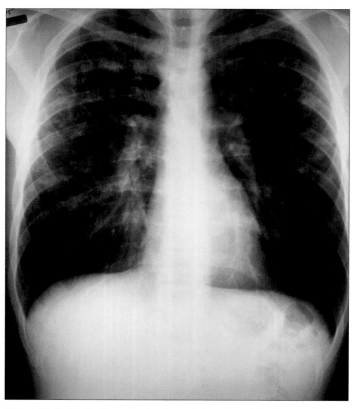

Figure 25.9 Cystic fibrosis: chest roentgenogram. Twenty-year-old man with cystic fibrosis showing early cystic changes as well as 'train tracking', parallel lines representing thickened, dilated bronchi. Patchy densities are evident in the upper lung fields, consistent with bronchiectasis. (Courtesy of the Department of Radiology, University of Massachusetts Medical Center.)

mutations of the CFTR gene have been described. Mutations causing clinical disease are chiefly found in the nucleotide binding folds, and more than 70% of North American and northern European CFTR mutations involve a deletion of a single phenylalanine, at position 508 (Delta F508) of the first nucleotide binding fold (**Fig. 25.10**).

Within the liver, the CFTR is located along the apical membrane of biliary epithelial cells. Defective CFTR results in severely diminished chloride conductance, insufficient luminal fluid and, consequently, viscous, inspissated bile. Bile flow is reduced; secretion of protective mucin is decreased; and the concentrations of bile acids in bile are increased. Pancreatic insufficiency is associated with changes in bile acid absorption, and the intraluminal bile acid pool is shifted from hydrophilic, taurine-conjugated bile acids to hydrophobic, glycoconjugated bile acids, which are hepatotoxic. The result is ductal obstruction and oxidative ductal injury, leading to disease of the intra- and extrahepatic biliary system.

Clinical features

Hepatobiliary complications of CF may present as disease of the liver, biliary tract, or gallbladder (**Table 25.3**).

Liver

More than half of patients with CF may have hepatic involvement, but only about 10% of patients with hepatic disease are symptomatic. Fatty liver is common, particularly in infancy. Chronic ductal obstruction is eventually accompanied by ductal proliferation, inflammatory infiltrate, and periportal fibrosis, known as biliary fibrosis (**Fig. 25.11**a). Hepatocytes are spared at this point, and the architecture of the liver is mostly preserved. Involved portal tracts may be unevenly distributed, such that liver biopsy is subject to sampling error. With persistent insult, fibrosis progresses and multilobular biliary cirrhosis develops, initially leaving spared foci of structurally uninvolved hepatic tissue, but ultimately leading to a hard and nodular cirrhotic liver. Approximately 2–5% of patients, during their lifetimes, will develop cirrhosis as a complication of CF.

Although hepatic involvement in CF more typically presents in children with concurrent respiratory and pancreatic insufficiency, liver disease may be the first clinical feature, particularly in infants. More commonly, hepatomegaly is noted in an otherwise asymptomatic adolescents or young adults. Fatty liver is the most common cause of hepatomegaly in CF, but hepatomegaly may also be falsely suggested if the liver is displaced inferiorly by pulmonary hyperinflation. Alternatively, hepatomegaly may be caused by passive congestion secondary to pulmonary hypertension in CF. A hard, nodular liver is suggestive of cirrhosis. Associated splenomegaly may be present and may cause left upper quadrant pain. Peripheral stigmata of liver disease are not frequently seen, and the first presenting sign of portal hypertension may be variceal hemorrhage. The risk of developing portal hypertension increases with age and, interestingly, shows familial clustering.

Biliary tract and gallbladder

Biliary tract involvement is common and may present independently of hepatic disease. In infants, CF may be manifested as jaundice because of obstructive liver disease, presenting similarly to biliary atresia. It is intriguing that neonatal jaundice

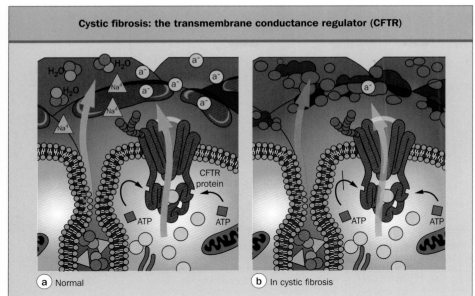

Cystic fibrosis: the transmembrane conductance regulator (CFTR)

(a) Normal   (b) In cystic fibrosis

Figure 25.10 Cystic fibrosis: the transmembrane conductance regulator (CFTR). Schematic showing (left) normal transmembrane transport of chloride, mediated by active transport, requiring binding of adenosine triphosphate (ATP) at the nucleotide binding region of the CFTR. Water molecules follow chloride conductance. Deletion (right) of a single phenylalanine at position 508 (Delta F508) of the nucleotide binding site of the CFTR results in inadequate ATP binding and diminished chloride conductance. As a result, little water follows and secretions are inspissated.

Hepatobiliary features of cystic fibrosis		
Liver	Biliary tract	Gallbladder
Only 10% symptomatic although > half affected	May present independently of hepatic disease	Most disease asymptomatic
Fatty liver	Common duct stricture	Microgallbladder
Common in infancy and adulthood, most common cause of hepatomegaly	Caused by pancreatic fibrosis	Gallbladder atrophied and collapsed
Biliary fibrosis	Choledocholithiasis	Cholecystic dyskinesia
Hepatocytes spared; architecture preserved		Gallbladder filled with thick bile
Multilobular cirrhosis	Sclerosing cholangitis	Cholelithiasis
2–5% of patients, may be accompanied by portal hypertension and splenomegaly	1% of patients, ?chronic inflammation causative	10–25% of patients, most asymptomatic, calcium bilirubinate
Neonatal jaundice		
Not predictive of adult disease		
Comments:	Comments:	Comments:
Liver chemistries neither sensitive nor specific	Alkaline phosphatase likely most sensitive test but must be fractionated; ultrasound may be helpful	Ultrasound helpful
Uneven distribution of disease → sampling error on liver biopsy		

Table 25.3 Hepatobiliary features of cystic fibrosis.

does not seem to be predictive of future hepatic disease for patients with CF. As patients age, pancreatic fibrosis (Fig. 25.11b) can result in common bile duct stricture. Approximately 10–25% of patients with CF have gallstones, most of which remain asymptomatic. Although they were thought in the past to be composed of cholesterol, the stones are believed now to consist chiefly of calcium bilirubinate. The gallbladder may be dyskinetic and filled with thick, mucoid bile or may be atrophied and collapsed ('microgallbladder'). Almost a third of patients may have such a gallbladder. About 1% of patients with CF develop sclerosing cholangitis, possibly because of chronic inflammatory changes within the biliary system.

Diagnosis

The laboratory detection of early liver disease in CF may be difficult. More than 85% of patients with hepatomegaly will

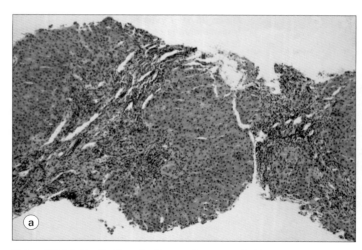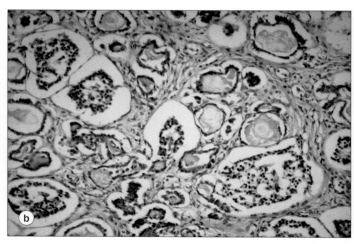

Figure 25.11 Cystic fibrosis: liver and pancreatic histopathology. (a) Photomicrograph of a liver needle biopsy from a patient with cystic fibrosis showing portal triads greatly expanded as bands that extend across the biopsy and delineate nodules of residual parenchyma. These changes are typical of secondary biliary cirrhosis in cystic fibrosis (hematoxylin and eosin, × 40). (b) Photomicrograph of a pancreas from a child with cystic fibrosis. The pancreatic acini have been replaced by fibrosis. Dilated ducts are filled with inspissated eosinophilic secretions. The islets remain untouched but are closer together than normal because of the loss of parenchyma between them (hematoxylin and eosin, × 100). (Courtesy Barbara Banner, University of Massachusetts Medical Center.)

have abnormal liver chemistry test results, but the remainder may have entirely normal tests. Conversely, approximately 13% of patients with CF *without* histologic liver disease will have abnormal liver chemistries. Liver chemistry tests, therefore, are neither highly sensitive nor specific for underlying hepatic disease in CF. Serum alkaline phosphatase is probably the most sensitive chemistry for underlying cholestasis but must be fractionated because non-hepatic alkaline phosphatase may also be elevated in CF.

Underlying biliary disease may be revealed by diagnostic imaging. Ultrasound or oral cholecystography may demonstrate cholelithiasis, cholecystitis or microgallbladder. Ultrasound may be particularly useful and has a high specificity and sensitivity for detecting CF-related liver fibrosis at an early stage. Endoscopic retrograde cholangiopancreatography (ERCP) can additionally reveal common duct stricture or sclerosing cholangitis. Hepatic scintigraphy may be helpful in detecting early liver involvement, even when ultrasound has been unrevealing. Liver biopsy serves as an important method for staging intrahepatic disease and for following progression, despite the recognized possibility of sampling error due to uneven hepatic involvement, even when multilobular cirrhosis has developed. Sweat testing in the young adult or adolescent with unexplained cholestatic disease or portal hypertension may reveal CF and should always be performed in young patients with hepatobiliary disease of unclear origin.

Attempts to identify patients with CF at risk for developing liver disease have identified some predisposing factors. Foremost, hepatobiliary complications occur almost exclusively in patients with pancreatic insufficiency, although the degree of pancreatic insufficiency seems to have little significance. The prevalence of hepatobiliary disease is higher among males than females. Although a history of meconium ileus carries an increased risk, neonatal jaundice does not. Some studies have suggested a possible association between hepatobiliary disease in CF and certain human lymphocyte antigen (HLA) types (e.g. DQ6), but no characteristic genotype has been identified. While

severe genotype is a likely risk factor for liver disease, non-CF genes and exogenous factors may serve as important determinants in whether liver disease will develop and how severe it will be. The familial clustering of portal hypertension in CF-related liver disease suggests such factors may play a key role in its pathogenesis. Despite the potential severity of liver disease in CF, prospective studies of patients with CF-related liver disease have failed to show that liver disease confers a higher mortality, highlighting the difficulty in predicting clinical outcomes in this phenotypically heterogeneous disease.

Treatment

The primary care for patients with CF is supportive. Avoidance and prompt, vigorous treatment of infection are continual challenges in patients with CF. Maintaining nutrition is of fundamental importance, with high-calorie, vitamin-enriched (particularly fat-soluble vitamins D, E and K), elemental dietary supplementation as well as pancreatic enzyme administration. Vitamin A may be toxic to the liver in CF and should be supplemented with caution.

UDCA has emerged as an important therapy in patients with CF with hepatobiliary disease. UDCA is the major component of bear bile, found in much lower concentrations in human bile as a derivative of chenodeoxycholic acid. It is hydrophilic and may have a cytoprotective effect on biliary epithelium by displacing more toxic hydrophobic bile acids. In addition, micelles of UDCA are smaller and facilitate choleresis. Administration of UDCA in CF has been associated with improved liver chemistries, suggesting reduced hepatotoxicity and diminished cholestasis; the latter is further supported by studies of biliary scintigraphy. Improvement in nutritional status is observed, perhaps by way of increasing fat absorption. UDCA has been associated with delayed progression of other cholestatic liver diseases such as primary biliary cirrhosis, and long-term prospective trials seem to confirm that the benefits of UDCA outlined above may well impart an improved prognosis. Ultrasonographic study of patients receiving UDCA has shown dramatic arrest of nodular biliary cirrhosis, as well as halting and possibly reversal of focal biliary cirrhosis. Patients receiving UDCA are given taurine supplementation, because therapy with UDCA exacerbates chronic CF-associated taurine deficiency. Taurine administration has also been associated with augmented fat absorption in patients with CF.

In patients who have developed advanced liver disease, management of portal hypertension becomes critical. TIPS may help manage portal hypertension for several years, or serve as a bridge to transplant. Orthotopic liver transplantation (OLT) in CF presents particular challenges because of the multiorgan, systemic nature of CF. In such patients, pulmonary disease and nutritional deficiency may affect outcome, and subsequent immunosuppressive therapy must be managed especially carefully to balance the risk of infection with that of graft rejection. One- and 5-year survival rates of patients with CF who have undergone OLT have been approximately 85 and 70%, respectively.

There are promising potential therapeutic advances under development. Because heterozygosity for defective CFTR function is not associated with clinical hepatobiliary disease, it has been postulated that fewer than half of functional CFTR receptors are needed for normal hepatobiliary phenotype and that homozygous disease might thus be amenable to gene therapy. Unlike gene therapy for other genetic diseases of the liver, gene therapy for CF must target not hepatocytes primarily, but the biliary epithelial cells, which divide infrequently. Recombinantly attenuated adenoviral vectors can infect non-dividing cells and have been used successfully for gene transfer to biliary epithelial cells in human cell lines and are promising for future application in CF therapy. Endoscopic retrograde biliary access might be used to distribute adenoviral or similar vectors of normal CFTR genes to biliary epithelial cells. The study of CFTR conformation and genetics seems likely to afford a plethora of potential therapies for the future treatment of CF-related liver disease.

HEREDITARY TYROSINEMIA TYPE 1

Tyrosine is an essential aromatic amino acid, required for the synthesis of catecholamines, melanin and thyroid hormones. Impaired catabolism of tyrosine occurs in several genetic or acquired disorders that may result in elevated plasma concentrations (>200 μM) of tyrosine (tyrosinemia). Four autosomal recessive inborn errors result from deficiencies in enzymes of the catabolic pathway of tyrosine: hereditary tyrosinemia (HT) types 1, 2 and 3, and alkaptonuria (see the Online Mendelian Inheritance in Man at [http://www.ncbi.nlm.nih.gov/entrez/query.fcgi?db=OMIM]). Tyrosinemia is suspected in otherwise unexplained neurological abnormalities (seizures, developmental delay) or liver disease. If the latter is present, testing for HT1 is urgent. HT1 is associated with severe liver disease. It is due to an autosomal recessive deficiency of the enzyme fumaryl acetoacetate hydrolase. There is a very high risk of development of hepatocellular carcinoma and, although the disease is rare worldwide, there are populations in which the gene is common and where complications of HT1 account for almost one in three liver transplantations. Until recently, treatment has been limited to variably effective conservative measures such as dietary changes and liver transplantation.

Now, directed enzyme repression may serve as an important modality of non-surgical intervention and promising advances in gene therapy are being examined.

Epidemiology and pathophysiology

HT1 presents early in life as either an acute disease of infants, which results in fatal liver failure within several months if left untreated, or as a chronic syndrome marked by progressive cirrhosis, renal tubular dysfunction, severe neurologic symptoms, and failure to thrive. Due to founder effects, the disease is geographically clustered and is notably prevalent in the Netherlands and French Canada. In the Saguenay-Lac St Jean region of Quebec more than 4% of individuals carry the defective gene, and the disease occurs in 1 in 1846 live births.

Several autosomal recessive mutations result in defective fumaryl acetoacetate (FAA) hydrolase activity, promoting the accumulation of toxic metabolites in hepatocytes and renal tubular cells. The defective enzyme's substrate, FAA, and the precursor maleyl acetoacetate increase in plasma concentration as do tyrosine, methionine, and sometimes phenylalanine (**Fig. 25.12**). Urinary concentrations of succinylacetone (SA, 4,6-dioxoheptanoic acid) are increased by the shunted metabolism of FAA and maleyl acetoacetate. Several different mutations of FAA hydrolase have been identified. For unclear reasons, affected members of the same family may have either the acute or chronic form, such that individuals with the same mutation may have different clinical diseases. This variable phenotypic expression suggests that other factors – environmental influences or the influences of other genes – may affect the severity and course of the illness.

An accumulation of ALA occurs as enzymatic shunting results in increased succinylacetone, which is a potent inhibitor of 5-aminolevulinic acid dehydratase. Increased 5-aminolevulinic acid is likely responsible for marked neuropathy resembling that seen with elevated 5-aminolevulinic acid in the hepatic porphyrias (vide supra).

Clinical features

The acute form of HT1 results in hepatic failure over the first several months of life. The chronic form presents with more gradually progressive disease. Failure to thrive may be followed by more focal findings, such as hepatomegaly and, as cirrhosis develops, splenomegaly, ascites, jaundice, easy bruisability, and peripheral edema may ensue. Vitamin D-resistant, hypophosphatemic rickets may develop, and peripheral neuropathy may occur. The risk of hepatocellular carcinoma increases monthly such that, by 2 years of age, the risk of hepatocellular carcinoma is approximately 40%.

Diagnosis

Type 1 HT may be anticipated from a family history or genetic screening, or the diagnosis may be made prenatally. Postgestationally, the diagnosis is typically made by the detection of biochemical abnormalities, including elevated urinary succinyl acetone and increased serum and urinary tyrosine, phenylalanine and methionine. Decreased FAA hydrolase activity may also be detected in cultured skin fibroblasts. α-Fetoprotein elevation may reflect development of hepatocellular carcinoma, and more moderate elevations may also precede the development of neurologic disease.

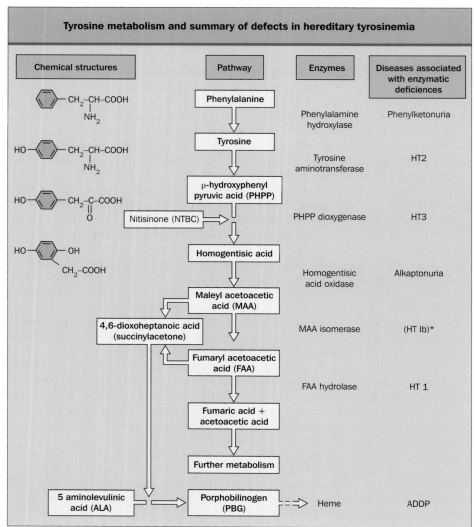

Figure 25.12 Tyrosine metabolism and summary of defects in hereditary tyrosinemia. The pathway of phenylalanine and tyrosine metabolism is outlined, and the enzymes responsible and diseases associated with defects in enzyme activities are shown. The effects of nitisinone (NTBC) to inhibit PHPP dioxygenase and 4,6-dioxoheptanoic acid (succinyl acetone) to inhibit ALA dehydratase, the second enzyme of the heme biosynthetic pathway (cf Fig. 25.1), are also shown. The most severe of the hereditary disorders of tyrosine metabolism is hereditary tyrosinemia type 1. Its treatment with nitisinone has led to much improvement. Adequate therapy with nitisinone converts hereditary tyrosinemia type 1 (HT1) into an HT2-type phenotype, which is not associated with excesses of the highly toxic mutagenic maleyl acetoacetate, FAA, or 4,6-dioxoheptanoic acid (succinyl acetone). *Tentative designation. Abbreviations used: ALA, 5-aminolevulinic acid; FAA, fumaryl acetoacetic acid; MAA, maleyl acetoacetic acid; NTBC, nitisinone [2-(2-nitro-4-trifluoro-methylbenzoyl)-1,3-cyclohexanedione] ; PBG, porphobilinogen; PHPP, *para*-hydroxy phenyl pyruvic acid.

Treatment

Traditionally, HT1 has been treated by eliminating dietary intake of tyrosine or related precursors so as to prevent the production of toxic metabolites. By this means, variable control of the disease is obtained, and some patients may not respond. Until recently, early OLT has been the only means for more definitive treatment. Because of the progressive risk for hepatoma, transplantation in the first 2 years of life has been recommended to avoid progression to metastatic disease. The new liver has no defect in tyrosine metabolism, and hepatic manifestations thus do not recur. Although, the renal defect in FAA hydrolase persists as does renal tubular dysfunction, renal tubular defects persisting after hepatic transplantation do not appear to be clinically significant. Neurologic sequellae of HT1 may resolve gradually but entirely after successful liver transplantation.

The treatment of choice is nitisinone, formerly known as NTBC [2-(2-nitro-4-trifluoro-methylbenzoyl)-1,3-cyclohexanedione]. Nitisinone selectively inhibits 4-hydroxyphenylpyruvate dioxygenase, diminishing the formation of toxic metabolites (FAA and SA) and reducing hepato- and nephrotoxicity (see Fig. 25.12). It has improved and ultimately eliminated peripheral neuropathy, reduced the need for liver transplantation, and reduced significantly the risk of hepatocellular carcinoma. The typical starting dose is 1 mg/kg/day, divided in two doses and given orally. Therapy is monitored by measuring plasma amino acids, blood and urinary SA, liver tests, complete blood cell count (CBC), and serum α-fetoprotein. Goals include normalization of SA levels, which may require 3 months, and plasma tyrosine levels <500 μM.

Promising possibilities for new, effective modes of gene therapy are being investigated and may have important implications for the treatment of hereditary tyrosinemia and other diseases subject to hepatic gene therapy. It has been observed that the resected livers of patients with HT1 are often a mosaic of cells, with cells expressing normal FAA hydrolase existing in regenerative nodules alongside mutant cells. It was postulated that this apparent spontaneous reversion to a normal allele might confer a selective advantage to these cells and promote their repopulation of the liver. The possibility of initiating and accelerating the repopulation of normal liver cells became a focus of attention.

In a murine model of HT1, transplantation of normal hepatocytes resulted in their seeding and repopulation of the liver, to the exclusion of mutant cells. Similarly, repeated portal vein infusion of retroviruses carrying the normal FAA hydrolase gene afforded complete repopulation of the liver with normally functioning, retrovirally transduced cells. In this model, it appears that normal differentiated hepatocytes preferentially multiply and replace cells carrying the mutant enzyme. By improving the efficiency of gene transfer, similar manipulations may become possible for repopulating mutant human liver with genotypically normal cells. By combining within the retroviral vector both the gene for transfer and also a second gene that affords a selective advantage for hepatocytes, it eventually may be feasible both to initiate and promote the repopulation of human liver with functional hepatocytes and overcome or eliminate the enzymatic defect without the need for liver transplantation.

ACID LIPASE DEFICIENCY (WOLMAN DISEASE AND CHOLESTEROL ESTER STORAGE DISEASE)

Epidemiology and pathophysiology
Deficiency of acid lipase results in two phenotypically distinct syndromes, Wolman disease and cholesterol ester storage disease (CESD), each inherited as an autosomal recessive disorder. They are marked by diffuse deposition of cholesterol esters, resulting in hepatic and multiorgan disease. Wolman disease presents with severe acute decline in early infancy, whereas CESD has a more benign course throughout adulthood **(Table 25.4)**.

The gene coding for acid lipase has been localized to chromosome 10 and has recently been cloned. Acid lipase is a widely distributed lysosomal enzyme that normally hydrolyzes cholesterol esters of low-density lipoproteins (LDL). While other lysosomal enzymes metabolize the protein component of LDL to peptides and amino acids, acid lipase frees LDL cholesterol from esterification, making it available for cellular metabolism and for feedback repression of extrahepatic cholesterol synthesis. Therefore, deficiency of the enzyme results

in an accumulation of cholesterol esters as well as increased cellular cholesterol synthesis. The liver, spleen, lymph nodes and intestine are typically laden with cholesterol esters and triglycerides. In Wolman disease, the adrenal glands are invariably affected as well.

Clinical features
For unclear reasons, Wolman disease and CESD have different clinical courses despite an apparently similar enzyme deficiency. Wolman disease is characterized in early infancy by abdominal pain and distention, vomiting and diarrhea, and hepatosplenomegaly. Growth and neurologic development are retarded. Progressive hepatosplenomegaly and distention are accompanied by profound malabsorption, and death usually occurs within the first year of life. CESD has a more benign course and usually presents in childhood, although some patients present as young adults. The patient may be asymptomatic, but hepatomegaly is universal and typically progressive, with hepatic fibrosis leading ultimately to cirrhosis and complications of portal hypertension. Premature atherosclerosis accompanies hyperlipoproteinemia.

Liver chemistries (conjugated bilirubin and serum aminotransferases) are typically elevated in Wolman disease but are usually normal in CESD. Plasma cholesterol and triglycerides are normal in Wolman disease but usually elevated in CESD. Serum LDL may be elevated in CESD, whereas low hepatic synthesis in Wolman disease likely accounts for low LDL levels. Without exception, patients with Wolman disease have distinctive granular calcification diffusely involving enlarged adrenal glands, which is easily seen on abdominal roentgenograms. The adrenal glands are enlarged but not calcified in CESD.

Liver biopsy demonstrates steatosis with cholesterol ester-laden Kupffer cells that are swollen and vacuolated. Hepatic fibrosis and, ultimately, cirrhosis may occur. In CESD, hepatocytes show birefringent lipid globules. Kupffer cells do not show birefringence, probably owing to peroxidation of the Kupffer cell cholesterol esters.

Diagnosis and treatment
A diagnosis is made from the characteristic clinical findings and from the demonstration of lysosomal acid lipase deficiency in cultured leukocytes or skin fibroblasts. Traditionally, intervention has been limited to supportive care. Inhibitors of 3-hydroxy-3-methylglutaryl-CoA reductase (e.g. atorvastatin, lovastatin) may be used to diminish intracellular cholesterol synthesis. Recently, bone marrow transplantation has shown promise for patients with Wolman disease, and cloning of the gene for acid lipase has engendered hope for eventual recombinant enzyme replacement therapy and gene therapy.

HEREDITARY FRUCTOSE INTOLERANCE

Hereditary fructose intolerance (HFI) is an autosomal recessive defect of aldolase B, an isozyme of fructose bisphosphate aldolase. The enzyme is found in liver, intestine and kidney, where it normally cleaves fructose-1-phosphate into dihydroxyacetone phosphate and glyceraldehyde. Deficiency results in cytoplasmic accumulation of fructose-1-phosphate **(Fig. 25.13)**.

The gene for aldolase B (ALDOB) is located on chromosome 9q; many mutations associated with the HFI phenotype have been described. More than half of North American and European

Acid lipase deficiency – Wolman disease and cholesterol ester storage disease	
Enzyme defect	Lysosomal acid lipase
Clinical features	Wolman disease: infant with abdominal pain and distention, vomiting, diarrhea, hepatosplenomegaly, mental retardation, adrenal calcification, and enlargement. CESD: may be asymptomatic; child/adult with hepatomegaly, cirrhosis, premature atherosclerosis, adrenal enlargement
Diagnosis	Acid lipase deficiency in cultured leukocytes or skin fibroblasts. Liver biopsy with cholesterol ester–laden Kupffer cells, fibrosis, cirrhosis. Birefringent hepatocytes in CESD
Treatment	Wolman disease: supportive care, death by age one. Bone marrow transplant under investigation. CESD: 3-hydroxy-3-methylglutaryl-CoA (HMG-CoA) reductase inhibitors, supportive care of liver disease
CESD, cholesterol ester storage disease.	

Table 25.4 Acid lipase deficiency – Wolman disease and cholesterol ester storage disease.

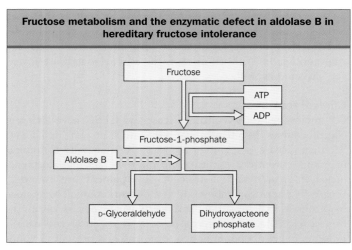

Fructose metabolism and the enzymatic defect in aldolase B in hereditary fructose intolerance

Figure 25.13 Hereditary fructose intolerance – enzymatic defect.

Hereditary fructose intolerance

Enzyme defect	Aldolase B (fructose-1-phosphate aldolase)
Inheritance	Autosomal recessive
Clinical features	Hypoglycemia, abdominal pain, vomiting, hepatomegaly, renal tubular damage, hypophosphatemia, growth retardation
Diagnosis	Intravenous fructose challenge, liver biopsy, molecular diagnosis (DNA analysis)
Treatment	Avoidance of fructose-containing sugars; normal lifespan if treated

Table 25.5 Hereditary fructose intolerance.

allelic defects are accounted for by the A149P mutation. A strong founder effect is shown by linkage studies, suggesting that the distribution of the A149P mutation was likely by way of genetic drift, rather than by recurrent de novo mutation. HFI is most prevalent among northern Europeans.

Clinical findings include marked abdominal pain and vomiting after the ingestion of fructose, sucrose or sorbitol (**Table 25.5**). Hypoglycemia may follow and can be fatal. Chronic effects include growth retardation, hepatomegaly, renal tubular damage and hypophosphatemia. The diagnosis has traditionally been made by intravenous fructose challenge or by liver biopsy. However, as most enzymatic defects are coded for by just a few mutations, molecular diagnostic methods are leading to less invasive diagnosis. Genetic screening of affected kindred may be accomplished by similar means. Treatment involves the avoidance of fructose or sugars metabolized to fructose, and patients typically develop a strong distaste for sweet foods. Patients without chronic fructose exposure may anticipate a normal life span.

HEPATIC GLYCOGENOSES (GLYCOGEN STORAGE DISEASES)

Epidemiology and pathophysiology

The glycogenoses, or glycogen storage diseases (GSD), are caused by defects of glycogen metabolism, resulting in tissue accumulation of normal or abnormal glycogen molecules and impaired conversion of glycogen stores to glucose. In most types, hypoglycemia ensues and may be severe or even fatal. Their inheritance is autosomal recessive, except for type VI, which is sex-linked. We limit our discussion to those affecting the liver (**Table 25.6**), which includes all but type V, which affects muscle, and type VII, which affects erythrocytes.

Type I glycogen storage disease

Type 1, or GSD 1 (von Gierke disease), affects the liver and kidney. There are three subtypes. Type 1a is caused by deficiency of hepatic microsomal glucose-6-phosphatase. The gene coding for glucose-6-phosphatase has been cloned and is located on chromosome 17. Type 1b is caused by a defective translocase required for glucose-6-phosphatase activity at the endoplasmic reticulum, and type 1c by defective microsomal phosphate/pyrophosphate translocase T-2 (**Fig. 25.14**).

Clinical features

Clinical findings in infants include difficulty feeding and hypoglycemic seizures. Children have short stature and adiposity. Marked hepatomegaly is universal (**Fig. 25.15a**), but the absence of splenomegaly is a distinguishing feature from other storage diseases. Adults are short, often anemic, with proteinuria, microalbuminuria, renal calcifications and chronic renal failure. Osteopenia and related fractures are not uncommon. Hyperlipidemia may be manifest as xanthomata, and hyperuricemia as gout. Liver findings in adults commonly include adenomas (as many as 75% of patients), and there is an increased incidence of hepatocellular carcinoma. In contrast to hepatic adenomas in the general population, there is a strong male predominance in GSD 1. Notably, cirrhosis does not occur.

Type 1a (as well as types III, VI and IX) is associated with the polycystic ovary syndrome, which is found in almost all female patients older than 5 years of age and is likely a consequence of hyperinsulinemia. Type 1b is associated with defective neutrophil glucose-6-phosphatase transport and, as a result, bacterial infections and gingivitis are frequent problems. Platelet dysfunction can be seen in all subtypes. Hypoglycemia is evident on laboratory testing, as is metabolic acidosis. Serum aminotransferases are usually normal, but alkaline phosphatase and γ-glutamyltranspeptides (GGTP) may be elevated. Increased serum cholesterol, triglycerides and uric acid levels are typical.

Diagnosis

Glucagon challenge and liver biopsy have traditionally been used to make the diagnosis. Administration of glucagon intramuscularly results in poor blood glucose response and elevated lactate levels. Liver biopsy shows hepatocytes filled with glycogen (see **Fig. 25.15b**), and special care must be taken to forward the sample to a specialized center for glycogen and specific enzyme measurement. Interestingly, Mallory bodies are found in adenomas of GSD 1 patients, in contrast with most other adenomas.

The gene for glucose-6-phosphatase, the enzyme deficient in type 1a, has been cloned. Although many different mutations have been identified, they are clustered by ethnic background. Through DNA-based analysis, type 1a may be diagnosed noninvasively, and prenatal diagnosis is being developed as well.

The hepatic glycogen storage diseases – enzyme defects, clinical features		
Glycogenosis	*Enzyme defect*	*Clinical features*
Type I (von Gierke) Type Ia Type Ib Type Ic	Glucose-6-phosphatase Translocase Phosphate/pyrophosphate translocase T-2	Hypoglycemia, acidosis, seizures, short stature, adiposity, hepatomegaly without cirrhosis and without splenomegaly. Adults with renal failure, anemia, osteopenia, hyperlipidemia, hepatic adenoma/adenocarcinoma, platelet dysfunction, gout, polycystic ovaries – type Ia, bacterial infection – type Ib
Type II (Pompe)	Lysosomal acid maltase	No hypoglycemia, macroglossia, cardiomegaly, hepatomegaly without cirrhosis and without splenomegaly
Type III (Cori)	Amylo-1,6 glucosidase	Hypoglycemia, myopathy, cardiomyopathy, hepatomegaly without cirrhosis or splenomegaly, polycystic ovaries
Type IV (Andersen)	Amylo-1,4→1,6 transglucosidase	Cirrhosis, death from liver failure
Type VI (Her)	Hepatic phosphorylase	Polycystic ovaries
Type IX	Hepatic phosphorylase-β-kinase	Mild course, growth retardation, hepatomegaly, polycystic ovaries

Table 25.6 The hepatic glycogen storage diseases – enzyme defects, clinical features.

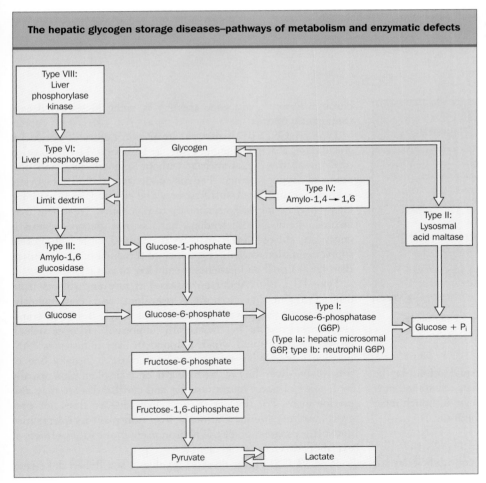

Figure 25.14 The hepatic glycogen storage diseases – pathways of metabolism and enzymatic defects.

Similar non-invasive molecular diagnosis will likely follow for the other glycogenoses.

Treatment

Management focuses on maintaining adequate blood glucose levels (**Table 25.7**). Continuous nocturnal high-carbohydrate enteral feeding and frequent daytime feedings of a diet rich in carbohydrates are the mainstays of therapy. Raw cornstarch serves as a delayed-release source of glucose and may supplement feedings. Medical treatment is given as warranted for hyperlipidemia, gout, infections and osteopenia. Granulocyte colony-stimulating factor has been used to boost neutrophil

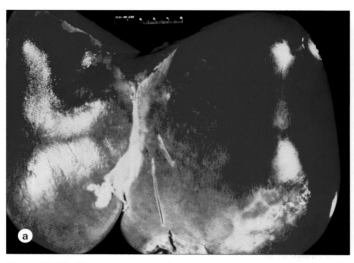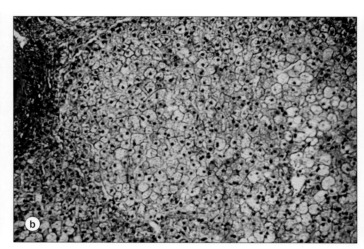

Figure 25.15 Glycogen storage disease Ia (von Gierke disease): liver pathology. (a) Capsular surface of a liver from a patient with glycogen storage disease Ia (von Gierke disease). The liver is enlarged, and the capsule appears smooth and shiny, with the liver edges rounded rather than sharp. (b) Photomicrograph of a liver from a patient with glycogen storage disease type Ia. All of the hepatocytes are expanded and pale due to glycogen-laden cytoplasm. Unlike fatty liver, in which the nucleus is pushed to the side by a single large cytoplasmic vacuole, glycogen storage is more diffuse within the cytoplasm and the nucleus remains in the center of the cell. The cells appear pale because much of the glycogen dissolves during processing (hematoxylin and eosin, × 40). (Courtesy of Joseph Alroy, Tufts University School of Veterinary Medicine, and Barbara Banner, University of Massachusetts Medical Center.)

Hereditary fructose intolerance The hepatic glycogen storage diseases – inheritance, diagnosis, treatment	
Inheritance	Autosomal recessive, except type IV, which is sex-linked, and type IX, which has sex-linked forms
Diagnosis	Glucagon challenge → low blood glucose, high lactate Liver biopsy → glycogen-laden hepatocytes Molecular diagnosis becoming available
Treatment	Continuous nocturnal high-carbohydrate feeds, raw corn starch; supportive care of hyperlipidemia, gout, infection, osteopenia; potential gene therapy

Table 25.7 The hepatic glycogen storage diseases – inheritance, diagnosis, treatment.

number and function in GSD 1b. Liver transplantation may be required for treatment of adenomas, although adenomas may regress upon commencement of enteral feedings. Although most patients survive to adulthood, many die as children.

Types II–IX GSD (see Table 25.6, 25.7 and Fig. 25.14)
Type II GSD (Pompe disease) results from deficiency of lysosomal acid maltase (α-1,4 glucosidase). Glycogen accumulates within lysosomes of all tissues in this generalized glycogenosis, but hypoglycemia does not occur. Onset may be in infancy or adulthood, the former typically more severe. Patients have hepatomegaly without splenomegaly, macroglossia and cardiomegaly. Hyperlipidemia is evident and liver biopsy shows vacuolated lysosomes, packed with glycogen, as do all organs. The gene for lysosomal acid maltase has also been localized to

chromosome 17, and gene therapy is being investigated as a therapeutic option.

Type III GSD (Cori disease) involves a defect of amylo-1,6 glucosidase, a debranching enzyme, and is marked by myopathy, cardiomyopathy, hepatomegaly without splenomegaly, and pronounced hypoglycemia. Female patients develop polycystic ovaries. Serum aminotransferases may be elevated, and creatinine kinase may be increased secondary to myopathy. Treatment may involve enteral glucose feedings but, because gluconeogenesis is enhanced, glucose levels may be maintained with high-protein supplementation as well. The course of the disease is less virulent than GSD I or II and patients usually live to adulthood.

Type IV GSD (Andersen disease) is rare and differs from other GSD in that cirrhosis is prevalent, and, consequently, splenomegaly is as well. Deficiency of amylo-1,4→1,6 transglucosidase results in structurally abnormal glycogen which affects all tissues and which is found in liver biopsies as PAS-positive intracellular aggregates. The course is usually one of progressive liver failure with death or transplantation usually by 5 years of age. Neuromuscular and cardiac disease may also predominate. For unclear reasons, liver disease does not progress in some patients. Curiously, liver transplant recipients may not suffer progression of the neuromuscular or cardiac effects of extrahepatic enzyme deficiency.

Type VI GSD (Her disease) involves a sex-linked deficiency of phosphorylase and causes isolated hepatic disease marked by hepatomegaly without splenomegaly, hypoglycemia and subsequent acidosis. Polycystic ovaries are commonly found. Type VIII is caused by deficient phosphorylase activation and presents similarly. Type IX involves deficiency of phosphorylase kinase as detected in erythrocytes. Its course is typically mild, with some growth retardation, hepatomegaly and polycystic ovaries. Sex-linked forms exist.

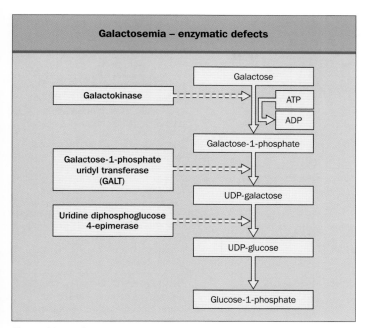

Figure 25.16 Galactosemia – enzymatic defects.

GALACTOSEMIA

There are three key enzymes in the metabolism of galactose: galactokinase, galactose-1-phosphate uridyl transferase (GALT), and uridine diphospho-glucose 4-epimerase (**Fig. 25.16**). Classic galactosemia involves hepatic and erythrocytic deficiency of GALT, inherited as an autosomal recessive trait. Galactose accumulation ensues and is toxic to tissues throughout the body, although the mechanism of toxicity remains unclear. The disease may be severe and result in childhood death or have a more moderate course, such that patients may survive to adulthood. This may depend on the severity of the enzyme deficiency (**Table 25.8**).

Accumulation of galactose is found within the fetus by 10–20 weeks' gestation, and toxic effects in utero are evidenced by early cataract development, low birth weight, and probable prenatal liver pathology. Newborns have difficulty feeding, with vomiting and diarrhea, malnutrition and growth retardation. Hepatosplenomegaly is followed by development of macro-nodular cirrhosis, portal hypertension and ascites. Mental development is poor, with retardation and speech deficits. Ovarian failure is seen in most girls surviving to puberty. Patients with partial enzyme deficiency may survive well into adulthood, and the diagnosis should be considered in young cirrhotic patients as well as adult cirrhotic patients with other characteristic findings.

Screening tests will detect the presence of galactose as a glucose-oxidase negative urinary reducing agent; diagnosis is made definitively by measuring erythrocytic GALT activities. Prenatal diagnosis can be made by culturing cells from amniotic fluid and measuring GALT activity. Liver biopsy reveals fatty deposition in newborns and later shows regeneration, giant cells and cirrhotic changes.

Dietary intervention is the mainstay of treatment. Avoidance of galactose or lactose products can result in significant improvement and even recovery. For unclear reasons, however, dietary-independent deficits may persist and progress. These can include mental deficits, speech pathology and growth retardation. Ovarian failure almost invariably occurs in women and may be treated with exogenous estrogen and progesterone to promote the development of secondary sex characteristics and manage postmenopausal sequellae.

Deficiencies of the other key enzymes of galactose metabolism are rare. Galactokinase deficiency is mild and results in cataract formation; uridine diphosphoglucose 4-epimerase deficiency is severe and presents like classic galactosemia. Dietary intervention is the pillar of treatment.

THE MUCOPOLYSACCHARIDOSES

Epidemiology and pathophysiology

The mucopolysaccharidoses (MPS) are a group of lysosomal storage disorders leading to the lysosomal accumulation of mucopolysaccharides (glycosaminoglycans), resulting in a variety of mental and physical abnormalities. With one exception, their inheritance is autosomal recessive (type II is X-linked recessive). Ten known enzymatic deficiencies account for six distinct syndromes that are classified by clinical features, urinary mucopolysaccharide analysis, and are identified by historical eponyms. Enzyme deficiencies result in defective metabolism of heparan sulfate, dermatan sulfate, chondroitin sulfate, or keratan sulfate (**Table 25.9**).

Galactosemia			
Enzyme defect	*Clinical features*	*Diagnosis*	*Treatment*
Galactose-1-phosphate uridyltransferase (GALT)	*Prenatal*: cataract-like corneal changes, liver disease *Newborns*: vomiting, malnutrition, hepatosplenomegaly, macronodular cirrhosis, portal hypertension, mental and growth retardation, death *Adults*: ovarian failure, cirrhosis	*Screening*: glucose-oxidase negative urinary reducing agent *Confirmation*: erythrocyte GALT deficiency *Prenatal*: GALT levels in cultured amniotic cells	Avoidance of galactose and lactose Estrogen replacement therapy for ovarian failure
Galactokinase	Cataracts, mild course	Erythrocyte enzyme deficiency	Avoidance of galactose/lactose
Uridine diphosphoglucose 4-epimerase	Clinical picture similar to GALT deficiency (above), severe course	Erythrocyte enzyme deficiency	Avoidance of galactose/lactose

Table 25.8 Galactosemia.

The mucopolysaccharidoses			
Type of MPS	*Enzyme defect→ stored MPS*	*Inheritance*	*Clinical features*
Type IH (Hurler)	α-L-Iduronidase→ dermatan sulfate	Autosomal recessive	Hepatosplenomegaly, coarse facial features, skeletal defects (gibbus, clawhand), mental retardation, cardiac disease, corneal disease
Type IS (Scheie)	α-L-Iduronidase → heparan sulfate	Autosomal recessive	Same as type 1H, but no mental retardation
Type II (Hunter)	Iduronosulfate sulfatase → dermatan and heparan sulfate	Sex-linked recessive	Similar to type 1, but mental retardation less severe, retinal degeneration, no corneal disease
Type III (Sanfilippo)	(Four subtypes) → heparan sulfate	Autosomal recessive	Severe mental retardation, coarse facial features, little hepatosplenomegaly, moderate skeletal disease, eyes uninvolved
Type IV (Morquio)	N-acetylgalactosamine-6-sulfate sulfatase → keratan sulfate	Autosomal recessive	Severe skeletal deformity, corneal disease, cardiac disease, little hepatosplenomegaly, mental status unaffected
Type VI (Maroteaux-Lamy)	N-acetylhexosamine-4-sulfate sulfatase → dermatan sulfate	Autosomal recessive	Corneal disease, cardiac disease, coarse facial features, mental status unaffected
MPS, mucopolysaccharidoses			

Table 25.9 The mucopolysaccharidoses.

Clinical features and diagnosis

Although specific enzyme deficiencies may produce characteristic phenotypic presentations in MPS, there are many similarities among the several forms of MPS. Hepatosplenomegaly is a prominent feature, as are coarse facial features, skeletal defects, mental retardation, corneal clouding, joint stiffness and cardiac disease.

Type IH (Hurler syndrome) is most frequently encountered and involves a deficiency of L-iduronidase, with an accumulation of dermatan sulfate and heparan sulfate. Its inheritance is autosomal recessive, and it is marked by dwarfism as well as the findings described earlier. Skeletal disease includes lumbar gibbus (hunchback) and clawhand. The adult Scheie variant, type IS, presents without mental retardation.

Type II, Hunter syndrome, involves deficiency of iduronosulfate sulfatase with an accumulation of dermatan sulfate and heparan sulfate. It is sex-linked recessive and seen only in males. Less severe than type I, patients typically survive well into adulthood. The remaining MPS have autosomal recessive inheritance, including type III (Sanfilippo syndrome). There are four enzymatic deficiencies classified as Sanfilippo variants, each resulting in accumulation of heparan sulfate. They all cause severe mental retardation and moderate skeletal deformity. Skeletal abnormalities (**Fig. 25.17**) are most severe in type IV, Morquio syndrome, in which keratan sulfate aggregates are found because of N-acetylgalactosamine-6-sulfate sulfatase deficiency. Corneal clouding is typical. In both types III and IV, there is less liver or spleen enlargement than types I and II. In the Maroteaux-Lamy variant, type VI, N-acetylhexosamine-4-sulfate sulfatase causes an accumulation of dermatan and presents with the characteristic MPS findings already described.

Hepatosplenomegaly is a characteristic finding on examination in all types, and liver biopsy may demonstrate fibrosis or cirrhosis. Vacuolation of hepatocytes and Kupffer cells is

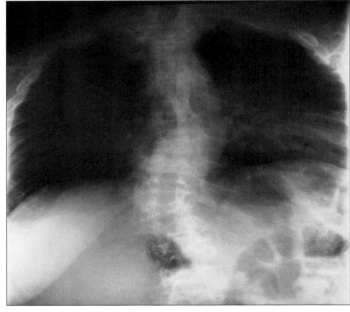

Figure 25.17 Mucopolysaccharidosis (MPS) type IV (Morquio syndrome): chest roentgenogram. This 59-year-old woman has several findings typical of MPS IV, including spinal shortening, marked kyphoscoliosis (together contributing to dwarfism), and widening of the ribs anteriorly but narrowing posteriorly. (Courtesy of the Department of Radiology, University of Massachusetts Medical Center.)

produced by glycosaminoglycan-laden lysosomes, most evident on colloidal iron staining. Electron microscopy shows membrane-bound inclusions within hepatocytes, Kupffer cells and hepatic stellate cells.

Treatment

Until recently, treatment has been supportive. However, animal models of enzyme replacement therapy seem promising, and bone marrow transplantation has been successfully carried out with halting of disease progression and improvement in skin, joint, heart and liver manifestations. Models for gene therapy are now being explored. Presently, life expectancy for type IH is less than 10 years, normal for type IS, and nearly normal for types II and IV. Patients with type III disease live into the second or third decade. For reasons as yet unclear, there is a great variation in the penetrance of each MPS and, therefore, in life expectancies.

GAUCHER DISEASE

Epidemiology and pathophysiology

The most common lysosomal storage disease and most frequent inborn error of lipid metabolism, Gaucher disease, is a paramount example of the profound implications of genetic mutation and the tangible benefits of advances in molecular medicine. The disease is caused by a defect in β-glucocerebrosidase (glucosylceramidase), which catalyzes the cleavage of glucocerebroside (glucosylceramide) to glucose and ceramide (**Fig. 25.18**). The gene of this enzyme has been cloned and localized to chromosome 1q21. Deficiency results in the accumulation of glucocerebroside in tissue macrophages, known as Gaucher cells (**Fig. 25.19**b), with subsequent toxicity to these tissues. Affected macrophages are present in the liver as Kupffer cells, in bone as osteoclasts, and are present in the spleen and lung as well.

Clinical features

The clinical syndrome was first described by Charles Earnest Gaucher in 1882, although he erroneously believed an unidentified malignancy caused this multiorgan disease. As

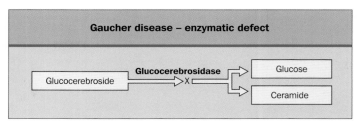

Figure 25.18 Gaucher disease – enzymatic defect.

would be predicted from the distribution of tissue macrophages, the primary syndrome is of hepatosplenomegaly, bone pain and fractures, hematopoietic disease, and pulmonary compromise. Three clinical syndromes are described (**Table 25.10**), classified by whether the nervous system is affected and by the age and rate of the onset of nervous system disease. Type I (non-neuronopathic) is without central nervous system (CNS) involvement. Type II is marked by early and rapid CNS affliction (acute neuronopathic), and type III (subacute neuronopathic) by CNS involvement that is delayed and more slowly progressive.

Type I is the most common. Its inheritance is autosomal recessive, with a particularly high prevalence (1 in 500–1 in 1000) among the Ashkenazi Jewish population. The incidence among all Jews is about 1 in 60 000 and is 1 in 100 000 among the general population of the USA. Onset is in childhood or adulthood, and disease severity is variable. In children, growth retardation may be subtle or severe. In advanced disease, hepatomegaly may be massive, with the sinusoidal sequestration of glucocerebroside-laden Kupffer cells (Fig. 25.19). Fibrosis is not unusual, but hepatocytes are not involved. Similarly, marked splenomegaly may develop, with Gaucher cell aggregation and fibrosis. Although spleen enlargement is usually asymptomatic, infarction may cause pain. Pulmonary disease is rare and suggests poor prognosis. The degree of bone involvement may vary widely; osteoporosis, cortical rarefaction, erosions and even avascular necrosis and collapse are all possible. Painful infarcts, known as pseudo-osteomyelitis or 'bone crises', are common.

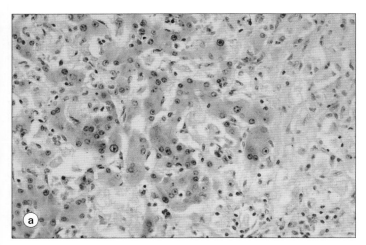
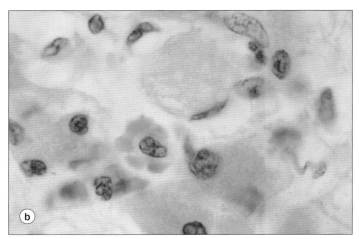

Figure 25.19 Gaucher disease: liver histopathology. (a) Photomicrograph of a liver biopsy from a patient with Gaucher disease showing infiltration of the sinusoids and compression of the hepatic cords by glucocerebroside-laden Kupffer cells, known as Gaucher cells (hematoxylin and eosin, ×200). (b) High-power photomicrograph of a liver biopsy from a patient with Gaucher disease. A Gaucher cell with the characteristic 'wrinkled tissue paper' cytoplasmic appearance is seen in a sinusoid, adjacent to hepatocytes (hematoxylin and eosin, × 1000). (Courtesy of Barbara Banner, University of Massachusetts Medical Center.)

Gaucher disease – inheritance, incidence, clinical features and treatment			
Disease type	*Inheritance and incidence*	*Clinical features*	*Treatment*
Type I	• Autosomal recessive • 1/500–1/1000 Ashkenazi Jewish • 1/60,000 general Jewish • 1/100,000 general United States	• Onset as a child or an adult • Hepatosplenomegaly • No neurologic disease • Growth retardation • Bone involvement • Pulmonary disease (poor prognosis)	• Hydration, analgesia • Enzyme replacement therapy • Calcium, vitamin D, bisphosphonates, orthopedic repair • Splenectomy if symptomatic • Bone marrow transplantation
Type II	• Autosomal dominant • Less than 1/100 000 • No ethnic predisposition	• Onset in infancy • Rapidly progressive neurologic decline • Hepatosplenomegaly • Growth retardation • Pulmonary involvement	• As for type I disease
Type III	• Autosomal dominant • Incidence unclear,? 1/50 000 • No ethnic predisposition	• Onset in childhood • Slowly progressive neurologic disease	• As for type I disease

Table 25.10 Gaucher disease – inheritance, incidence, clinical features and treatment.

The head and shaft of the femur are commonly affected with characteristic 'Erlenmeyer flask' deformity, and the humerus, vertebrae and pelvis may be involved (**Fig. 25.20**).

Thrombocytopenia and anemia secondary to splenic sequestration are common, and patients may have a history of easy bruising or bleeding. By definition, type I disease spares the CNS.

Type II is much less prevalent, likely less than 1 in 100 000. The incidence of type III may be as high as 1 in 50 000 live births, but no clear estimates are available. The inheritance of both types II and III is autosomal dominant, and there is no ethnic predilection. Rapidly progressive CNS disease in infancy is the hallmark of type II, which is also associated with poor growth, hepatosplenomegaly and pulmonary disease. Death may occur early, with an average life span of just 2 years. In type III disease, neurologic disease progresses slowly; hepatosplenomegaly is prominent. Onset is in childhood, with the expected life span varying from infancy to adulthood.

Diagnosis

Diagnosis should be suspected in anyone with the features described above. A careful family history may further suggest the diagnosis. Marrow, liver, spleen or lung may demonstrate glucocerebroside-packed Gaucher macrophages. These are seen in other diseases, however, such as hematopoietic malignancies, and definitive diagnosis is made by demonstration of deficient β-glucocerebrosidase activity in leukocytes. Increased glucocerebroside levels are found but are not specific. Prenatal testing in gestations at risk can be carried out via amniocentesis or chorionic villus sampling.

With the localization and cloning of the gene for Gaucher disease, mutations have been identified which may be prognostic of the type and severity of disease. Although many mutations have been characterized, a small number constitute the majority, and a few presently have specific prognostic value. Hence, more than 95% of Ashkenazi heterozygotes can be identified by screening for just five mutations. Indeed, a single alanine to guanine point mutation at nucleotide 1226, which

codes for an asparagine to serine substitution at amino acid 370, is responsible for almost 75% of affected Ashkenazis. Homozygosity predicts moderate type I disease, but compound heterozygosity with another Gaucher allele causes type I disease with more severe enzymatic deficiency and a more severe course.

Treatment

Traditional conservative therapy for symptomatic disease involves hydration, analgesia and surgery as warranted for bone disease. Calcium, vitamin D and bisphosphonates are helpful in delaying bone afflictions. Splenectomy is sometimes carried out but is of little benefit for the asymptomatic patient. Bone marrow transplantation has been successful but carries significant risk.

Recent advances in the therapy of Gaucher disease have, at once, begotten hope and controversy. Enzyme replacement therapy, first proposed decades ago, has become a reality in recent years and provides remarkable benefit. By targeting a mannose receptor on the plasma membrane surface of macrophages, exogenous β-glucocerebrosidase, which has been modified to expose mannose residues, is directed selectively to macrophages. In type I disease, this therapy has been shown to halt the progression of and actually reverse hepatosplenomegaly, hypersplenism and pulmonary disease. Marrow composition, osteoporosis and other bone lesions may improve. The therapy has not been shown effective for neurologic involvement in types II and III disease.

By targeting macrophages, replacement therapy has been made more efficient but is still very expensive. One year of therapy can cost more than $200 000. Controversy has therefore arisen over the dose and duration of therapy necessary to evoke and maintain an adequate response, and dose-response clinical trials continue. Development of methods for mass production of the enzyme by cells containing its cDNA, to replace placenta-derived enzyme, is not expected to dramatically decrease cost. Of note, animal models of gene therapy have been promising in vivo as have been in vitro studies with human cells, and human trials of gene therapy for Gaucher disease are now underway.

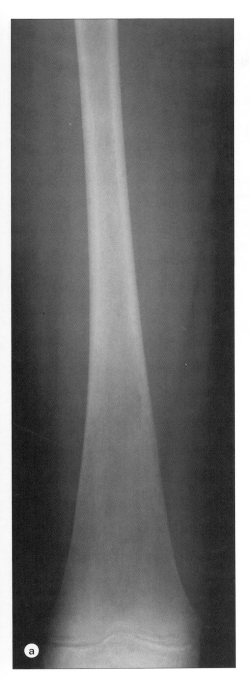

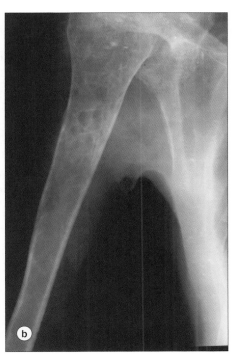

Figure 25.20 Gaucher disease: extremity roentgenograms. (a) Femur of a 12-year-old male who presented with dull bone pain and splenomegaly and was found to have Gaucher disease type I. The distal end of the femur has lost its normal concavity, resulting in the characteristic 'Erlenmeyer flask' deformity. (b) Humerus of a 26-year-old woman with Gaucher disease type I. There is marked osteopenia with cortical rarefaction and erosions. Painful infarcts, known as pseudo-osteomyelitis, may accompany advanced disease. (Courtesy of the Department of Radiology, University of Massachusetts Medical Center.)

FURTHER READING

General

Ghishan FK, Greene HL. Inborn errors of metabolism that lead to permanent liver injury. In: Scriver C, Sly WS, Barton Childs AL, et al (eds). The metabolic and molecular bases of inherited disease. New York: McGraw Hill; 1995:1084–1137.

The porphyrias

Anderson KE. The porphyrias. In: Zakim D, Boyer TD (eds). Hepatology, 4th ed. Philadelphia: WB Saunders; 2003:291–346. *An excellent overview of the porphyrias.*

Bonkovsky HL. Porphyria cutanea tarda and hepatitis C. Viral Hepatitis Rev 1998; 4:75–95.

Bonkovsky HL, Healey JF, Lourie AN, et al. Intravenous heme-albumin in acute intermittent porphyria: Evidence for repletion of hepatic hemoproteins and regulatory heme pools. Am J Gastroenterol 1991; 86:1050–1056.

Bonkovsky HL, Banner BF, Lambrecht RW, et al. Iron in liver diseases other than hemochromatosis. Annals Int Med 2005; 16:65–82.

Do KD, Banner BF, Katz E, et al. Benefits of chronic plasmapheresis and intravenous heme-albumin in erythropoietic protoporphyria after orthotopic liver transplantation. Transplantation 2002; 73: 469–472.

Gouya L, Puy H, Robreau AM, et al. The penetrance of dominant erythropoietic protoporphyria is modulated by expression of wild type FECH. Nat Genet 2002; 30:27–28.

Hahn M, Bonkovsky HL. Disorders of porphyrin metabolism. In: Wu G, Israel J (eds). Diseases of the liver and bile ducts: a practical guide to diagnosis and treatment. Totowa: Humana; 1998:249–272.

Reichheld JH, Katz E, Banner BF, et al. The value of intravenous heme-albumin and plasmapheresis in reducing postoperative complications of orthotopic liver transplantation for erythropoietic protoporphyria. Transplantation 1999; 67:922–928.

Waldenström J. Neurological symptoms caused by so-called acute porphyria. Acute Psychiatr Neurol 1939; 14: 375.

α₁-Antitrypsin deficiency

Askari FK. Molecular mechanism of hepatocellular injury in α-1-antitrypsin deficiency. Hepatology 1995; 21:1745–1747.

Carrell RW, Lomas DA. α-1-Antitrypsin deficiency – a model for conformational diseases. N Engl J Med 2002; 346:45–53. *This is a complete and intriguing review of the disease, in the context of clinically diverse but etiologically similar diseases.*

Carrell RW, Whisstock J, Lomas DA. Conformational changes in serpins and the mechanism of α-1-antitrypsin deficiency. Am J Respir Crit Care Med 1994; 150:S171–175. (Published erratum appears in Am J Respir Crit Care Med 1995; 151:926.)

Francavilla R, Castellaneta SP, Hadzic N, et al. Prognosis of α-1-antitrypsin deficiency-related liver disease in the era of paediatric liver transplantation. J Hepatol 2000; 32:986–992.

Perlmutter DH. Clinical manifestations of α-1-antitrypsin deficiency. Gastroenterol Clin North Am 1995; 24:27–43.

Perlmutter DH. Liver injury in α-1-antitrypsin deficiency: an aggregated protein induces mitochondrial injury. J Clin Invest 2002; 110:1579–1583.

Rudnick DA, Liao Y, An JK, et al. Analyses of hepatocellular proliferation in a mouse model of α-1-antitrypsin deficiency. Hepatology 2004; 39:1048–1055.

Cystic fibrosis

Colombo C, Crosignani A, Assaisso M, et al: Ursodeoxycholic acid therapy in cystic fibrosis-associated liver disease: a dose-response study. Hepatology 1992; 16:924–930.

Colombo C, Battezzati PM, Crosignani A, et al. Liver disease in cystic fibrosis: a prospective study on incidence, risk factors, and outcome. Hepatology 2002; 36:1374–1382.

Feranchak AP, Sokol RJ. Cholangiocyte biology and cystic fibrosis liver disease. Semin Liver Dis 2001; 21:471–488. *A detailed and updated review of the molecular biology of cystic fibrosis and its liver-specific histopathology, clinical features, diagnosis and management.*

Nousia-Arvanitakis S, Fotoulaki M, Economou H, et al. Long-term prospective study of the effect of ursodeoxycholic acid on cystic fibrosis-related liver disease. J Clin Gastroenterol 2001; 32:324–328.

Slieker MG, Deckers-Kocken JM, Uiterwaal CS, et al. Risk factors for the development of cystic fibrosis related liver disease. Hepatology 2003; 38:775–776; author reply 776–777.

Tanner MS, Taylor CJ. Liver disease in cystic fibrosis. Arch Dis Child 1995; 72:281–284.

Yang Y, Raper SE, Cohn JA, et al. An approach for treating the hepatobiliary disease of cystic fibrosis by somatic gene transfer. Proc Natl Acad Sci USA 1993; 90:4601–4605.

Hereditary tyrosinemia type I

Gibbs TC, Payan J, Brett EM, et al. Peripheral neuropathy as the presenting feature of tyrosinaemia type I and effectively treated with an inhibitor of 4-hydroxyphenylpyruvate dioxygenase. J Neurol Neurosurg Psychiatry 1993; 56:1129–1132.

Holme E, Lindstedt S. Tyrosinaemia type I and NTBC (2-(2-nitro-4-trifluoromethylbenzoyl)-1,3-cyclohexanedione). J Inherit Metab Dis 1998; 21:507–517.

Kvittingen EA, Rootwelt H, Berger R, et al. Self-induced correction of the genetic defect in tyrosinemia type I. J Clin Invest 1994; 94:1657–1661.

Laine J, Salo MK, Krogerus L, et al. The nephropathy of type I tyrosinemia after liver transplantation. Pediatr Res 1995; 37:640–645.

Mohan N, McKiernan P, Preece MA, et al. Indications and outcome of liver transplantation in tyrosinaemia type 1. Eur J Pediatr 1999; 158: S49–S54.

Overturf K, Al-Dhalimy M, Tanguay R, et al. Hepatocytes corrected by gene therapy are selected in vivo in a murine model of hereditary tyrosinaemia type I. Nat Genet 1996; 12:266–273.

Poudrier J, Lettre F, Scriver CR, et al. Different clinical forms of hereditary tyrosinemia (type I) in patients with identical genotypes. Mol Genet Metab 1998; 64:119–125.

Russo PA, Mitchell GA, Tanguay RM. Tyrosinemia: a review. Pediatr Dev Pathol 2001; 4:212–221. *An excellent, recent review on tyrosinemia.*

Acid lipase deficiency (Wolman disease and cholesterol ester storage disease)

Krivit W, Freese D, Chan KW, et al. Wolman's disease: a review of treatment with bone marrow transplantation and considerations for the future. Bone Marrow Transplant 1992; 10 (suppl 1):97–101.

Leone L, Ippoliti PF, Antonicelli R. Use of simvastatin plus cholestyramine in the treatment of lysosomal acid lipase deficiency. J Pediatr 1991; 119:1008–1009.

Wolman M. Wolman disease and its treatment. Clin Pediatr 1995; 34:207–212.

Hereditary fructose intolerance

Cox TM. Aldolase B and fructose intolerance. FASEB J 1994; 8:62–71.

Tolan DR. Molecular basis of hereditary fructose intolerance: mutations and polymorphisms in the human aldolase B gene. Hum Mutat 1995; 6:210–218.

Hepatic glycogen storage diseases

Bianchi L. Glycogen storage disease I and hepatocellular tumours. Eur J Pediatr 1993; 152(suppl 1):S63–S70.

Lei KJ, Chen YT, Chen H, et al. Genetic basis of glycogen storage disease type 1a: Prevalent mutations at the glucose-6-phosphatase locus. Am J Hum Genet 1995; 57:766–771.

Talente GM, Coleman RA, Alter C, et al. Glycogen storage disease in adults. Ann Intern Med 1994; 120:218–226.

Galactosemia

Beutler E: Galactosemia. Screening and diagnosis. Clin Biochem 1991; 24:293–300.

Holton JB. Effects of galactosemia in utero. Eur J Pediatr 1995; 154:S77–S81.

Sardharwalla IB, Wraith JE. Galactosaemia. Nutr Health 1987; 5:175–188.

Mucopolysaccharidoses

Resnick JM, Whitley CB, Leonard AS, et al. Light and electron microscopic features of the liver in mucopolysaccharidosis. Hum Pathol 1994; 25:276–286.

Wraith JE. The mucopolysaccharidoses: a clinical review and guide to management. Arch Dis Child 1995; 72:263–267.

Gaucher disease

Balicki D, Beutler E. Gaucher disease. Medicine 1995; 74:305–323. A thorough review on Gaucher disease.

Brady RO, Murray GJ, Barton NW. Modifying exogenous gluco-cerebrosidase for effective replacement therapy in Gaucher disease. J Inherit Metab Dis 1994; 17:510–519.

Gaucher disease. Current issues in diagnosis and treatment. NIH Technology Assessment Panel on Gaucher Disease. JAMA 1996; 275:548–553.

Rosenthal DI, Doppelt SH, Mankin HJ, et al. Enzyme replacement therapy for Gaucher disease: skeletal responses to macrophage-targeted glucocerebrosidase. Pediatrics 1995; 96:629–637.

CHAPTER

26 Pediatric Liver Disease

Deirdre A. Kelly

NEONATAL LIVER DISEASE

Jaundiced baby

Two-thirds of children with liver disease present in the neonatal period with persistent jaundice. Although physiologic jaundice is common in neonates (**Table 26.1**), infants who develop severe or persistent jaundice should be investigated to exclude hemolysis, sepsis or underlying liver disease. Neonatal jaundice that persists beyond 14 or 21 days should always be investigated, even in breast-fed babies.

Clinical features suggesting liver disease include pale stools and dark urine, dysmorphic features, bruising, petechiae or bleeding, hepatomegaly and/or splenomegaly, slow weight gain or failure to thrive, and previous family history or consanguinity. The differential diagnosis is between extrahepatic biliary disease, the neonatal hepatitis syndrome, and intrahepatic biliary hypoplasia.

Unconjugated hyperbilirubinemia

The most common causes of unconjugated hyperbilirubinemia are physiologic jaundice or breast-milk jaundice (**Tables 26.1** and **26.2**), although systemic disease or hemolysis from any cause must be excluded. It is important to screen for Coomb positivity, and glucose-6-phosphate dehydrogenase deficiency, and to exclude red cell membrane defects such as spherocytosis. Systemic sepsis is an important cause of unconjugated hyperbilirubinemia in the early neonatal period and requires prompt treatment with antibiotics, fluids, phototherapy and/or exchange transfusion.

Inherited disorders: Crigler-Najjar type I and II

This autosomal recessive disease is secondary to mutations in two genes *B-UGT1* and *B-UGT2* which lead to a deficiency of the hepatic enzyme, bilirubin diglucuronide transferase, which causes high levels of unconjugated hyperbilirubinemia in the perinatal period. In Crigler-Najjar type I peak serum bilirubin levels vary between 15 and 50 mg/dL (250–850 μmol/L), whereas in Crigler-Najjar type II peak bilirubin levels are 12–18 mg/dL (200–300 μmol/L).

Diagnosis

The diagnosis of Crigler-Najjar type I is suspected by the high level of unconjugated hyperbilirubinemia in the absence of other clinical causes. Confirmation may be obtained by aspiration of bile from the duodenum in infants over 3 months old as bilirubin diglucuronides are not present in Crigler-Najjar type I, but small amounts are detected in type II. Liver biopsy to measure enzyme levels is not necessary.

Physiologic neonatal jaundice
Peak 2–5 days after birth
Normal stools and urine
More severe in premature babies
Clears within 2 weeks
May persist for 4 weeks in breast-fed infants
Can rarely lead to kernicterus
Diagnosis: 80% total bilirubin is unconjugated
Treatment includes phototherapy, fluids, reassurance

Table 26.1 Physiologic neonatal jaundice.

Causes of unconjugated hyperbilirubinemia
Physiologic/breast-milk jaundice

Hemolysis
    Immune
    Red blood cell membrane abnormality

Metabolic disorders
    Crigler-Najjar types I and II
    Gilbert syndrome
    Galactosemia
    Fructosemia

Hypothyroidism
Sepsis
Hypoxia

Table 26.2 Causes of unconjugated hyperbilirubinemia.

Management

Prompt treatment is required for Crigler-Najjar type I with exchange transfusion and phototherapy to prevent kernicterus. Infants do not respond to phenobarbital. Long-term phototherapy is essential, but becomes difficult when 12–16 h per day are required for school-going children. Auxiliary liver transplantation or hepatocyte transplantation effectively reduces bilirubin levels while retaining native liver for future gene therapy. Treatment for Crigler-Najjar type II is not required except for cosmetic reasons, but bilirubin levels reduce on phenobarbital 5–15 mg/kg.

Extrahepatic biliary disease

Biliary atresia occurs in 1:14 000 live births worldwide. There is a slight female predominance. The etiology is unknown although the association of biliary atresia with other extrahepatic anomalies suggests an abnormality of the embryologic development of the biliary tree. There is no clear genetic basis despite the association of biliary atresia with trisomy 18 and human leukocyte antigen (HLA)-B12 subtype. Although isolated cases of biliary atresia are associated with proven viral infection (cytomegalovirus), numerous studies have not indicated an association with any hepatotropic RNA viruses such as reovirus or rotavirus.

Pathogenesis

Biliary atresia affects all parts of the biliary tree. There is gradual fibrosis and destruction of the extra- and intrahepatic biliary ducts with progressive cholestasis. The lumen of the extrahepatic duct may be obliterated at different levels leading to three main types: type I in which the common bile duct is obstructed; type II in which the common hepatic duct is obstructed; and type III in which there is fibrosis at the level of the porta hepatis – this occurs in 85% of cases.

Clinical features

Infants who have biliary atresia are usually born at term with a normal birth weight. Jaundice is apparent on the second day of life, but is mistaken for physiologic jaundice. Biliary obstruction, as evidenced by pale stools and yellow urine, gradually develops over the next 2–4 weeks, and is associated with a gradual increase in liver size and failure to gain weight adequately despite a good appetite. Approximately 25% of babies have associated anomalies: dextracardia, ventricular or atrial septal defects, polysplenia, and the hypovascular syndrome (HVS) (**Table 26.3**).

The spleen is not enlarged unless there is significant hepatic fibrosis. Ascites may occasionally be present.

Diagnosis

All children who have persistent neonatal jaundice need thorough investigation (**Fig. 26.1**).

A diagnosis of biliary atresia is dependent on:
- conjugated hyperbilirubinemia;
- liver biochemistry which indicates raised alkaline phosphatase (>600 IU/L) and γ-glutamyltranspeptidase (γ-GT) (>100 IU/L), and moderate elevation of alanine and aspartate aminotransferases (100–200 IU/L);
- abdominal ultrasound performed after a 4-h fast will either not demonstrate a gallbladder or indicate a small contracted gallbladder;
- radionuclide hepatobiliary imaging will not demonstrate biliary excretion from the liver into the gut after 24 h (**Fig. 26.2**); and
- histology that demonstrates the characteristic findings of expansion of portal tracts, proliferation of bile ducts and ductules with bile plugs, portal fibrosis, and portal edema – there may be an increase in inflammatory reaction at the porta hepatitis and variable giant cell transformation of hepatocytes (**Fig. 26.3**).

As none of these tests are pathognomonic for biliary atresia, the diagnosis should be confirmed by operative cholangiography with progression to a Kasai portoenterostomy if required.

Congenital abnormalities in biliary atresia	
Anomaly	*Comment*
Cardiac	
Dextrocardia	+/– situs inversus
VSD	
ASD	
Left atrial isomerism	With HVS
Vascular	
Preduodenal portal vein	HVS
Absent inferior vena cava	Azygous drainage
Splenic	
Polysplenia	+/– HVS
Double spleen	
Asplenia	
Malrotation	
Situs inversus	+/– HVS, NHP
Annular pancreas	
Immobile cilia syndrome	Bronchiectasis
ASD, atrial septal defect; HVS, hypovascular syndrome; VSD, ventricular septal defect; NHP, normal heart position.	

Table 26.3 Congenital anomalies in biliary atresia.

Endoscopic retrograde cholangiography (ERCP) in this age group is now possible using prototype pediatric duodenoscopes. Biliary atresia can be confidently excluded if the biliary tree is visualized, but a failure to do so may either be due to technical failure or biliary atresia and progression to operative cholangiography and laparotomy is then required.

Management

The Kasai portoenterostomy involves resection of the obliterated biliary tract and formation of a Roux loop which is anastomosed to the porta hepatis. Between 50 and 60% of cases achieve biliary drainage which may be improved by administration of a short course of corticosteroids at the end of the first postoperative week. Revised Kasai operations are not indicated because of the poor success rate, and because of increased technical difficulties at subsequent liver transplantation.

The success of the Kasai portoenterostomy operation depends on a number of factors, which include the timing of the operation, the expertise of the surgeon, the degree of hepatic fibrosis at operation, and the presence or absence of other congenital abnormalities. Operations should be performed before 8 weeks of age, although there is no clear effect of age on survival unless the operation takes place after 100 days of age. Surgery is not recommended if there is evidence of advanced hepatic fibrosis with splenomegaly, ascites or varices.

Cholangitis is most common in the immediate postoperative period. The incidence is reduced by prophylactic antibiotics, either intravenously for 10–14 days or orally for 3–6 months.

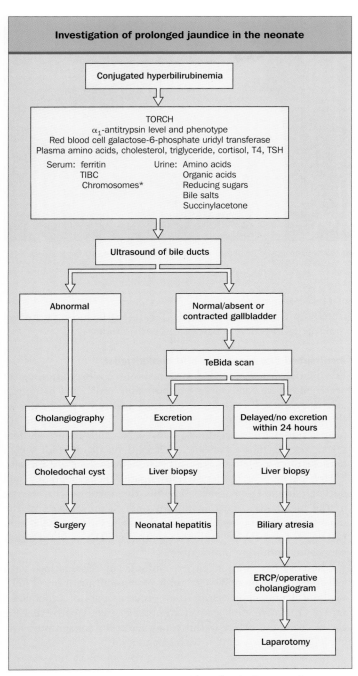

Figure 26.1 Investigation of prolonged jaundice in the neonate.
T4, thyroxine; TIBC, total iron-binding capacity; TSH, thyroid-stimulating hormone; TORCH, serology for toxoplasma, other, rubella, cytomegalovirus, and herpes simplex viruses; TeBida, 99 technetium trimethyl-1-bromoimino diacetic acid. *Chromosomes for 18, 21, Alagille syndrome.

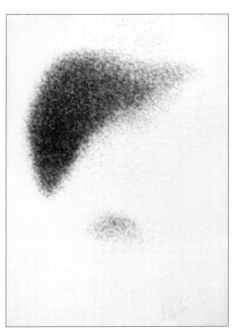

Figure 26.2 Radioisotope scanning demonstrating excellent uptake of radioisotope but no excretion at 24 h. This represents either severe intrahepatic cholestasis, but more likely the diagnosis of extrahepatic biliary atresia.

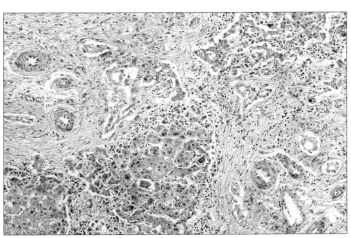

Figure 26.3 Biopsy showing features suggestive of biliary obstruction. These are portal fibrosis, biliary ductular proliferation with bile plugs, and portal edema. There may be considerable histologic overlap between biliary atresia and the neonatal hepatitis syndrome.

The clinical signs include an increase in jaundice, pyrexia, acholic stools, and tenderness over the liver. Broad spectrum antibiotics are usually effective.

Malabsorption is usually associated with a partially successful Kasai portoenterostomy and is an important factor in the development of malnutrition in neonatal liver disease. The development of cirrhosis and portal hypertension is inevitable even in those children who have had a successful Kasai portoenterostomy, although the need for transplantation varies with the rate of progression of liver disease and complications. Unsuccessful Kasai portoenterostomy is an immediate indication for liver transplantation and these children should be referred early to specialized centers for follow-up.

Choledocal cyst

Choledocal cysts are localized cystic dilatation of all or part of the common bile duct. Cysts are more common in Japan (1:100 000 live births) and in females (4:1). Choledocal cysts may be congenital or acquired. There may be a structural weakness with subsequent dilatation in the wall of the biliary tree or alternatively the biliary dilatation may be secondary to pancreatitis associated with a common pancreaticobiliary channel or repeated cholangitis.

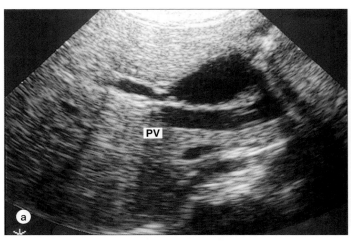
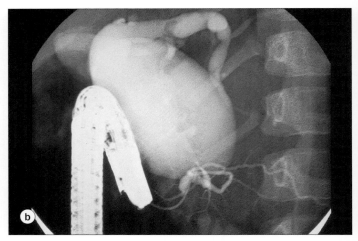

Figure 26.4 Abdominal ultrasound demonstrating a large cystic swelling. (a) Shows the cystic swelling, which was **(b)** confirmed to be a choledochal cyst on endoscopic retrograde cholangiopancreatography (ERCP).

The cyst may present in infancy with prolonged jaundice and must be differentiated from biliary atresia or the neonatal hepatitis syndrome. In older children a history of abdominal pain, jaundice and abdominal mass is classic, but is a rare presentation in childhood. Jaundice may be intermittent and associated with ascending cholangitis and recurrent pancreatitis.

Diagnosis

Choledocal cysts are diagnosed by abdominal ultrasound which may detect the cysts antenatal. Confirmation of the anatomy is obtained by radioisotope scan, percutaneous transhepatic cholangiogram, or endoscopically by an endoscopic retrograde cholangiopancreatography (**Fig. 26.4**). Histology of the liver usually indicates biliary fibrosis, cholestasis and bile plugs in the portal tract. The histologic features are completely reversible following successful surgery.

Management

Surgical treatment includes excision of all the affected ducts and re-establishment of biliary drainage by forming a hepatico-jejunostomy. Drainage of the cyst into adjacent duodenum or jejunum is now contraindicated, because of the potential malignant transformation. The results of surgery are excellent, cholangitis is an occasional complication, and there is a 2.5% risk of malignancy in the residual biliary tree in adult life.

Spontaneous perforation of the bile ducts

This is a rare complication in which perforation occurs at the junction of the cystic and common hepatic ducts, perhaps due to a congenital weakness, inspissated bile, or gallstones. Infants may present at any age from 2 to 24 weeks of age with abdominal distention, ascites, jaundice and acholic stools. Biliary peritonitis, with bile in hydroceles, hernial sacs and the umbilicus may be obvious.

The diagnosis may be confirmed by abdominal ultrasound, which may show free intraperitoneal fluid and dilated intrahepatic ducts. Biochemical liver tests may be abnormal, with conjugated hyperbilirubinemia and raised alkaline phosphatase and γ-GT. If the biliary leak is large, liver tests may be virtually normal. Hepatobiliary scanning will demonstrate isotope in the peritoneal cavity. Treatment includes peritoneal drainage followed by repair of the perforation.

Inspissated bile syndrome and cholelithiasis

Bile duct obstruction secondary to inspissated bile syndrome may be secondary to total parenteral nutrition, prolonged hemolysis and dehydration. It is more common in premature babies or those undergoing major surgery. The clinical picture is of biliary obstruction with pale stools, dark urine and abnormal liver tests. The diagnosis may be confirmed by ultrasound, which demonstrates a dilated intra- and extrahepatic duct system with biliary sludge. Percutaneous transhepatic cholangiography will outline the anatomy and may be therapeutic with lavage of the biliary tree, but laparatomy and decompression of the biliary tree may be required. The use of ursodeoxycholic acid (20 mg/kg) and cholecystokinin may prevent the need for either surgical or radiologic intervention.

Cholecystitis may occur in infants in association with gallstones from hemolysis or total parenteral nutrition (TPN), while acalculus cholecystitis may occur as part of generalized sepsis. Operative cholecystectomy (rather than laparoscopic) is the treatment of choice in this young age group for symptomatic cholecystitis in association with gallstones.

Neonatal hepatitis syndrome

The neonatal hepatitis syndrome includes many different causes of neonatal liver disease (**Table 26.4**), which may have a similar presentation (see Fig. 26.1). The commonest causes are intra-uterine infections or inherited metabolic diseases.

In contrast to children who have extrahepatic biliary disease, babies who have a neonatal hepatitis syndrome may have the following characteristics:

- small for dates or have intrauterine growth retardation (**Fig. 26.5**);
- pigment is usually present in the stools although the urine will be yellow;
- dysmorphic features characteristic of Alagille syndrome or Zellweger syndrome may be present; and
- hepatosplenomegaly is usually present.

Biochemical features include:

Neonatal hepatitis syndrome and diagnostic approach

Disease	Diagnosis	Treatment
Intrauterine infection		
Cytomegalovirus	Urine for viral culture	Ganciclovir
Toxoplasmosis	IgM antibodies	Spiramycin
Rubella	IgM antibodies	Supportive
Herpes simplex	EM/viral culture of vesicle	Aciclovir
Syphilis	VDRL test	Penicillin
Metabolic		
AAT deficiency	AAT level and phenotype	Supportive
Cystic fibrosis	Sweat chloride, immunoreactive trypsin, AFO8 mutation	Supportive
Galactosemia	Galactose-1-6-phosphate uridyltransferase	Galactose-free diet
Tyrosinemia	Urine succinylacetone, serum amino acids, α-fetoprotein	NTBC
Hereditary fructosemia	Enzymes in liver	Fructose-free diet
Niemann-Pick type A	Sphingomyelinase	Supportive
Niemann-Pick type C	Storage cells in bone marrow aspirate and liver biopsy; fibroblast culture	Supportive
Wolman disease	Abdominal radiograph of adrenal glands	Supportive
Primary disorders of bile acid synthesis	Urinary bile acids by FAB-MS	Bile acids
Zellweger syndrome	Very-long-chain fatty acids	Supportive
Endocrine		
Hypopituitarism (septo-optic dysplasia)	Cortisol TSH, T4	Hormone replacement
Hypothyroidism	TSH, T4, free T4, T3	Hormone replacement

AAT, α_1-antitrypsin; EM, electron microscopy; FAB-MS, fast atom bombardment ionization mass spectrometry; NTBC, 2(2-nitro-trifluoromethylbenzoyl)-1, 3-cyclonescanedione; T3, triiodothyronine; T4, thyroxine; TSH, thyroid-stimulating hormone; VDRL, venereal disease research laboratory

Table 26.4 Neonatal hepatitis syndrome and diagnostic approach.

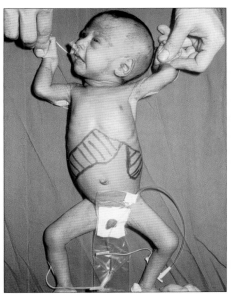

Figure 26.5 Neonatal hepatitis. This baby was born at 37 weeks' gestation, with obvious intrauterine retardation. He was jaundiced with hepatosplenomegaly, and malnourished with loss of fat and muscle stores. The most likely differential diagnosis is neonatal hepatitis secondary to a uterine infection or inborn error of metabolism.

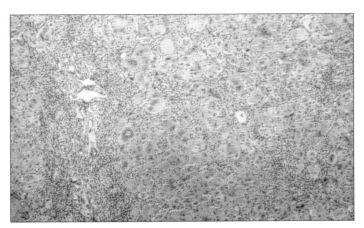

Figure 26.6 Most babies who have neonatal hepatitis have giant cell hepatitis with extramedullary hemopoiesis and a rosette formation of hepatocytes. This is a non-specific finding and may represent many different causes of neonatal liver disease.

- conjugated bilirubin 6 mg/L ($>100\,\mu$mol/L);
- alkaline phosphatase 600–800 IU/L;
- aspartate aminotransferase (AST) and alanine aminotransferase (ALT) 200–300 IU/L; and
- hypoglycemia (depending on etiology).

Liver histology is non-specific and demonstrates giant cell hepatitis with fibrosis of the portal tracts, extramedullary hemopoiesis, cholestasis and biliary ductule proliferation. There may be histologic overlap with biliary atresia (**Fig. 26.6**).

Intrauterine infection

The most common cause of intrauterine infection causing neonatal hepatitis is cytomegalovirus (CMV) infection. Infants are small for dates with hepatosplenomegaly and may have thrombocytopenia, choreoretinitis, or microcephaly. A diagnosis (see Table 26.4), is based on identification of immunoglobulin (Ig)M antibodies, virus culture or a positive polymerase chain reaction (PCR) for CMV DNA. The outcome is variable. In most babies the hepatitis resolves completely within 3–6 months, but neurologic involvement with spasticity or sensorineural deafness and developmental delay may be present. Treatment with ganciclovir or oral valaciclovir is rarely necessary.

Rubella hepatitis is almost unknown now following universal vaccination, but may present with neonatal hepatitis, cataracts, congenital heart disease and deafness. Progressive liver disease has been reported.

401

Toxoplasmosis is prevalent in parts of France and Germany, but is unusual in the UK. It is associated with persistent neonatal jaundice, failure to thrive, hepatosplenomegaly, central nervous system involvement with choreoretinitis, hydrocephaly, microcephaly and intracranial calcification. Treatment with spiramycin may be helpful for liver disease. The long-term outcome is related to the neurologic disease, as by the time of diagnosis many children are blind or severely handicapped.

Herpes simplex in the newborn usually causes a multisystem disorder with encephalitis and acute liver failure. Antiviral treatment with acyclovir is successful if started early enough.

Congenital syphilis is now rare, but may also cause a multisystem disease with intrauterine retardation, anemia, thrombocytopenia, nephrotic syndrome, skin rash, diffuse lymphadenopathy and hepatomegaly. Diagnosis is based on serologic testing (see Table 26.4). Treatment with penicillin is usually curative.

Hepatitis A, B and C viruses and human immunodeficiency virus (HIV) are rare causes of persistent neonatal jaundice. Vertical transmission of hepatitis B virus (HBV) and hepatitis C virus (HCV) leads to an asymptomatic carrier state.

Endocrine disorders

The neonatal hepatitis syndrome is associated with pituitary or adrenal dysfunction in approximately 30% of patients. Hypopituitarism may be due to hypothalamic dysfunction and is associated with septo-optic dysplasia, which includes absence of the septum pelucidum or malformation of the forebrain and hypoplasia of one or both optic nerves.

Hypoglycemia is a prominent symptom that is not associated with the severity of liver disease. Other signs of hypopituitarism include microgenitalia in boys, midline facial abnormalities, or nystagmus. A number of children may have severe cholestasis with acholic stools and dark urine and differentiation from biliary atresia may be difficult.

The diagnosis is established by demonstrating hypothyroidism and a low random or 9.00 am cortisol. A synacten test is rarely required for confirmation. Treatment is with hormone replacement with thyroxine, hydrocortisone and growth hormone. If diagnosed early enough, liver disease will completely resolve, but hormone replacement is required lifelong.

Inborn errors of metabolism

The commonest inborn error of metabolism to present with persistent neonatal jaundice is α_1-antitrypsin deficiency, which is an autosomal recessive disorder with an incidence of 1:7000 live births worldwide. Infants may present with intrauterine growth retardation, cholestasis, failure to thrive, hepatomegaly, or a vitamin K responsive coagulopathy which is more likely in those infants who are not given prophylactic vitamin K at birth and who are being breast-fed. The coagulopathy may be obvious with bruising and bleeding from the umbilicus, but the initial symptom may be intraventricular hemorrhage which may result in neurologic disability.

Diagnosis

Liver biochemistry demonstrates a mixed hepatic/obstructive picture with elevated aminotransferases, alkaline phosphatase, and γ-GT. Radiologic investigations may indicate severe intrahepatic cholestasis with a contracted gallbladder on a fasting

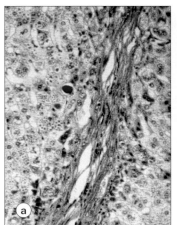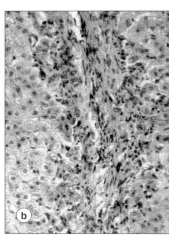

Figure 26.7 α_1-Antitrypsin deficiency is the commonest inherited liver disease. The diagnosis is made on histology, demonstrating granules in hepatocytes either by a periodic acid-Schiff (PAS)-stain **(a)**, or by immunoperoxidase staining **(b)**, which may be detected as early as 6–8 weeks.

ultrasound, and delayed or absent excretion of radioisotope on hepatobiliary scanning. In homozygotes the diagnosis is easily confirmed by detection of a low level of α_1-antitrypsin (<0.9 g/L). Liver disease is usually associated with phenotype protease inhibitor P$_i$ZZ but may occur with P$_i$MZ heterozygotes or other variants. Liver histology demonstrates giant cell hepatitis with characteristic periodic acid-Schiff (PAS), diastase resistant, positive granules of α_1-antitrypsin in hepatocytes which may be detected by 6–8 weeks of age (**Fig. 26.7**).

Management

This consists of nutritional support, fat-soluble vitamin supplementation, and treatment of pruritus and cholestasis (**Table 26.5**).

The prognosis is varied. Jaundice disappears in most infants, of whom approximately one-third regain normal function, one-third develop an inactive fibrosis and/or cirrhosis, and one-third develop chronic liver failure requiring transplantation. Respiratory disease is rare in childhood but long-term follow-up is essential to monitor growth, development and the need for liver transplantation. Antenatal diagnosis by chorionic villus sampling is now available using synthetic oligonucleotide probes specific for the *M* and *Z* genes, or by restriction fragment length polymorphism.

Intrahepatic biliary hypoplasia

The term intrahepatic biliary hypoplasia refers to an absence or reduction of a number of interlobular bile ducts or ductules seen in portal tracts in association with normal-sized branches of the portal vein and hepatic arteries. Biliary hypoplasia may occur in a wide spectrum of liver diseases, such as α_1-antitrypsin deficiency, chromosomal abnormality such as Down syndrome, or intrauterine infection (CMV). However, this term is conventionally used with syndromic biliary hypoplasia or Alagille syndrome, or non-syndromic biliary hypoplasia which includes Byler disease and progressive familial intrahepatic cholestasis.

Management of neonatal liver disease	
Nutritional support	
Modular feed	Energy intake 150–200 cal/kg
Carbohydrate	Glucose polymer (8–10 g/kg/day)
Protein	Whey protein (2.5–3.5 g/kg/day)
Fat	50/50 MCT/LCT (8 g/kg/day)
Fat soluble vitamins	
A: 5–10 000 U/day	
E: 50–100 mg/day	
K: 1–2 mg/day	
D: 50 mg/kg/day	
Pruritus/cholestasis	
Phenobarbital 5–15 mg/kg	
Ursodeoxycholic acid 20 mg/kg	
Rifampin (rifampicin) 3 mg/kg	
Colestyramine 1–2 g/day	
Topical skin care	
MCT, medium-chain triglyceride; LCT, long-chain triglyceride	

Table 26.5 Management of neonatal liver disease.

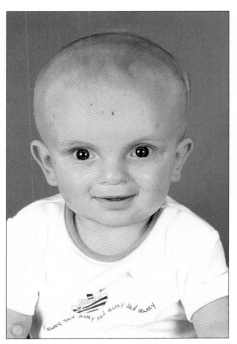

Figure 26.8 Alagille syndrome. This is an autosomal dominant disorder in which the typical facies may be less obvious in infants. This baby demonstrates hypertelorism, widely spaced eyes, depressed nasal bridge, and a pointed chin. He also has curving of the second metacarpal on his little finger, which is characteristic of this syndrome.

Alagille syndrome

This is an autosomal dominant condition with an incidence of 1:100 000 live births worldwide. It is a multisystem disorder which is associated with cardiac, facial, renal, occular and skeletal abnormalities. Mutations in the *Jag 1* gene on chromosome 20p have been identified in 60% of patients. Infants may present with persistent cholestasis, severe pruritus, hepatomegaly and failure to thrive. The characteristic facial features are very difficult to identify in infancy, but become more prominent later in childhood. They include a triangular face with high forehead and frontal bossing, deep widely spaced eyes, saddle-shaped nasal bridge, and pointed chin (**Fig. 26.8**).

Cardiac abnormalities include peripheral pulmonary stenosis, pulmonary and aortic valve stenosis and Fallot tetralogy.

Skeletal abnormalities are widespread and include abnormal thoracic vertebrae, 'butterfly' vertebrae, and curving of the proximal digits of the third and fourth finger. Posterior embryotoxin, which is detected on the inner aspects of the cornea near the junction of the iris, is demonstrated in 90% of patients by slit-lamp examination. Retinal pigmentation on fundoscopy and calcific deposits (optic drusen) in the optic nerve may be detected by ultrasound. Renal disease varies in severity from mild renal tubular acidosis to severe glomerular nephritis. One of the most difficult management problems is severe failure to thrive, which is complicated by gastrointestinal reflux and severe steatorrhea secondary to fat malabsorption or pancreatic insufficiency.

Diagnosis

Liver biochemistry indicates severe cholestasis with:

- conjugated bilirubin 6 mg/dL (>100 μmol/L);
- raised alkaline phosphatase >600 IU/L;
- γ-GT >200 IU/L;
- raised aminotransferases; and
- plasma cholesterol >6 mmol/L with normal triglycerides (0.4–2 mmol/L).

Tests of hepatic function such as albumin and coagulation are usually normal. Renal dysfunction may be identified by the presence of aminoaciduria or estimating urinary protein/creatinine ratio (normal <20).

The skeletal abnormalities are easily identified by radiologic examination of the chest and hands. Electrocardiography may demonstrate right bundle branch block or right ventricular hypertrophy in children who have peripheral pulmonary stenosis. Echocardiography may be normal but if cardiac abnormalities are suggested clinically, then cardiac catheterization should be performed for confirmation.

Liver histology may be non-specific. The reduction in interlobular bile ducts is often difficult to identify in the neonatal period, particularly if cholestasis and giant cell hepatitis are also present. The histologic appearance differs from extrahepatic biliary atresia because of the absence of portal fibrosis and biliary ductular proliferation.

Management

Intensive nutritional support is essential (see Table 26.5) and pancreatic supplements may be required. Pruritus may be intractable and an indication for liver transplantation, although recent experience with a molecular reabsorbent recirculating system (MARS) has produced relief for 6–12 months. Prognosis is varied and depends on the extent of liver, cardiac or renal disease. Approximately 50% of children may regain normal liver function by adolescence while others require liver transplantation in childhood. The indications for liver transplantation are

Inherited disorders of bile acid synthesis		
Enzyme	*Features*	*Treatment*
3 β-hydroxy-δ+^{5}-C$_{27}$-steroid dehydrogenase/isomerase	Neonatal hepatitis; normal γ-GT; low bile acid concentration; no pruritus	CDCA or UDCA
δ^4-3-oxosteroid 5 β-reductase	Jaundice, coagulopathy; elevated bile acid concentrations	UDCA + cholic acid
24,25-dihydroxy-cholanoic cleavage enzyme	Giant cell hepatitis; normal γ-GT; elevated serum cholesterol; low bile acid concentrations	CDCA + cholic acid
CDCA, chenodeoxycholic acid; γ-GT, γ-glutamyltranspeptidase; UDCA, ursodeoxycholic acid		

Table 26.6 Inherited disorders of bile acid synthesis.

the development of cirrhosis and portal hypertension, intractable pruritus or severe growth failure. Pretransplant cardiac surgery or balloon dilatation may be indicated for severe pulmonary stenosis.

Progressive familial intrahepatic cholestasis

Progressive familial intrahepatic cholestasis (PFIC) is the term given to a number of conditions in which there is persistent jaundice, cholestasis, hepatomegaly, pruritus and failure to thrive. The genetic mutations underlying a number of these have been identified (PFIC-1, 2, 3) and they are now known to be disorders of bile salt transport.

Byler disease (PFIC-I)

This severe form of familial idiopathic cholestasis was first described in an Amish family. It is now known that it is due to mutation in the *FIC1* gene which encodes a P type ATPase which is expressed in many tissues including the liver, gut, pancreas and lung. In contrast to children who have intrahepatic cholestasis of other causes, this group of children had normal serum γ-GT and low or normal serum cholesterol. The clinical presentation is with persistent conjugated hyperbilirubinemia, severe pruritus, diarrhea and growth retardation. Histology shows a lack of hepatic inflammation but paucity of bile ducts and canalicular bile plugs. Cirrhosis develops in early childhood requiring liver transplantation.

The management consists of nutritional support (see Table 26.5) and treatment of pruritus which includes biliary diversion, an operative technique in which bile is diverted externally by an enterostomy. Most children have progressive fibrosis with the development of cirrhosis and portal hypertension requiring liver transplantation in childhood. The gut defect is not reversed by transplantation, and diarrhea continues.

PFIC-2

PFIC-2 is due to a defect on chromosome 2q24 which encodes for a human bile salt transport pump (BSEP). The clinical phenotype is milder and children do not have diarrhea.

PFIC-3

Mutations in the *MDR-3* gene affect the bile canalicular membrane translocator of phospholipids leading to this disorder in which there is severe pruritus, features of biliary obstruction and a high γ-GT. Most children require transplantation.

Arthrogryposis, cholestasis, renal tubular dysfunction (ARC)

This rare autosomal disorder presents with cholestasis, biliary hypoplasia, renal dysfunction and a low γ-GT. It is usually fatal and infants die of liver and renal failure within 12 months. The genetic defect is now known to be a disorder in a soluble N-ethylmaleimide-sensitive fusion protein attachment protein (SNARE) protein (Vps33b) involved in the regulation of vesicle and membrane fusion. It is the first human disorder associated with mutations in a gene involved in regulation of the SNARE-mediated mechanism of membrane tether and fusion and may lead to further understanding of the pathophysiology of biliary disorders.

Inherited disorders of bile salt metabolism

The development of fast atom bombardment ionization mass spectrometry (FABMS) has allowed many defects in primary bile acid synthesis to be identified (**Table 26.6**).

Infants present with cholestasis, hepatomegaly, failure to thrive, and possible pruritus (Table 26.6). Biochemistry indicates non-specific abnormalities of aminotransferases and elevated alkaline phosphatase and/or γ-GT. Liver histology indicates a giant cell transformation with cholestasis and rapid development of fibrosis and cirrhosis. The diagnosis is confirmed by identifying the specific abnormal bile acid metabolites in urine. These diseases are fatal without liver transplantation, but treatment with a combination of cholic acid, chenodeoxycholic acid or ursodeoxycholic acid may prevent progression to cirrhosis and portal hypertension if started sufficiently early.

Zellweger syndrome (cerebrohepatorenal syndrome)

This is an autosomal recessive syndrome with multisystem disease. It is associated with absent or dysfunctional peroxisome biogenesis leading to secondary defects of bile acid synthesis and abnormal β-oxidation of fatty acids. The incidence is 1:100 000 live births. The initial presentation is with severe hypotonia, feeding difficulties and failure to thrive. Jaundice is only present in 50% of babies, but dysmorphic features which include epicanthic folds, brush field spots and a high forehead are common in association with psychomotor retardation. There is multisystem involvement involving the brain, heart, liver and kidneys.

The diagnosis is confirmed by demonstrating abnormal bile salt metabolites using FABMS or the detection of very-long-chain fatty acids in serum. Initially hepatic pathology may appear normal, but there is excessive hepatic iron in the first few months with the subsequent development of fibrosis and micronodular cirrhosis. Ultra-electron microscopy may indicate abnormal mitochondria and the absence of peroxisomes.

Treatment is supportive as death is inevitable. Liver transplantation is not indicated because of the progression of multisystem disease. Initial attempts to induce peroxisomes with hypolipemic drugs were unsuccessful. Primary bile acid therapy with cholic and chenodeoxycholic acid may produce some histologic improvement, but has no effect on survival.

Cystic fibrosis

Cystic fibrosis is an unusual cause of neonatal cholestasis accounting for <1% of children who have persistent jaundice. It is an autosomal recessive disorder with an incidence of 1:2000 live births. The genetic defect has been localized to the long arm of chromosome 7, and more than 300 mutations have been identified in the gene coding for the cystic fibrosis transmembrane conductance regulator (CFTR). The commonest mutation is Delta 508, but no mutation is specific for liver disease. The prominent clinical symptoms include persistent cholestasis, meconium ileus, hepatomegaly, failure to thrive and recurrent respiratory infections. If cholestasis is complete with acholic stools, differentiation from biliary atresia may be difficult.

Diagnosis

Biochemical liver tests reveal raised aminotransferases, alkaline phosphatase, and γ-GT. Immunoreactive trypsin may be higher than normal for age [1300 ng/dL (>130 ng/mL)]. Serum cholesterol and triglycerides are usually normal. Although a sweat test is thought to be pathognomonic for this diagnosis, it is not usually worth doing this in babies under 4–6 weeks of age [values of 5 mg/dL (<50 mmol/L) for children <5 years]. Liver histology is varied, but usually demonstrates diffuse cholestasis with bile duct proliferation, focal biliary cirrhosis, and portal fibrosis.

Management

The efficacy of ursodeoxycholic acid (20–50 mg/kg/day) in the treatment of neonatal cholestasis secondary to cystic fibrosis is unknown, but clinical studies in older children indicate that it induces a biochemical and histologic improvement. It is usual to treat children with cholestasis secondary to cystic fibrosis with ursodeoxycholic acid and fat-soluble vitamin supplementation and appropriate nutritional support (see Table 26.5). In most children who have neonatal cystic fibrosis, jaundice resolves, although persistence has been reported with the development of cirrhosis, portal hypertension and liver failure. Ongoing malnutrition and respiratory disease may contribute to death in infancy.

Niemann-Pick disease type C

This is a rare autosomal recessive disorder in which there is a defect in cholesterol esterification that results in a neurovisceral lipid storage disorder with an extremely varied spectrum of clinical findings. About 60% of children will present with prolonged cholestasis and hepatosplenomegaly in infancy, some of whom may present with fetal ascites. A number of children present later (3–5 years of age) with isolated splenomegaly and/or neurologic signs and symptoms.

Diagnosis

Liver histology may indicate giant cell hepatitis. The diagnosis is determined by detecting PAS diastase-resistant storage in Kupffer cells and hepatocytes. If there is active hepatitis, it is easier to detect these characteristic foamy storage cells in bone marrow aspirate. Neuronal storage indicating central nervous system involvement is present at birth and is demonstrable in the ganglion cells of a rectal biopsy. Skin fibroblast cultures will define the enzyme defect and enable antenatal diagnosis.

Management

Jaundice subsides in most children although hepatosplenomegaly may persist with abnormal biochemical liver tests. Hepatic fibrosis with progression to cirrhosis and portal hypertension is a rare occurrence. Sadly, all children develop neurologic complications at a median age of 5 years, which include ataxia, convulsions, developmental delay and dementia. Supranuclear ophthalmoplegia is considered pathognomonic for this condition. Most children die in late childhood or early adolescence from respiratory infections. There is no specific treatment, although a low cholesterol diet has been suggested. Liver and bone marrow transplantation are not curative. Genetic counseling is essential, and antenatal diagnosis may be performed by chorionic villus biopsy.

LIVER DISEASE IN OLDER CHILDREN

Liver disease in children older than 6 months may be acute or chronic. As in infancy, there is a predominance of inherited disorders (**Table 26.7**) and multisystem involvement (**Fig. 26.9**).

Liver diseases in older children	
Disease	*Diagnostic investigations*
Chronic hepatitis	Portal inflammatory infiltrate on biopsy
Hepatitis B, C, D, EBV, CMV	Serology
Autoimmune hepatitis	IgG >2 g/dL (>20 g/L) C3, C4, LKM, ANA, SMA
Wilson disease	Serum Cu, ceruloplasmin, urinary Cu
α_1-Antitrypsin deficiency	α_1-Antitrypsin level and phenotype
Cystic fibrosis	Sweat test, liver biopsy
Cryptogenic cirrhosis	Liver biopsy
Primary sclerosing cholangitis	ERCP and liver biopsy
Tyrosinemia type 1	Urinary succinylacetone
Hereditary fructose intolerance	Fructose 1-6-phosphate aldolase in liver
ANA, antinuclear antibodies; C3 and C4, complement; ERCP, endoscopic retrograde cholangiopancreatography; LKM, liver, kidney microsomal antibodies; SMA, smooth muscle antibodies; Cu, copper	

Table 26.7 Liver diseases in older children.

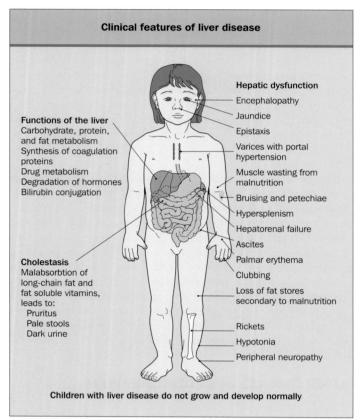

Clinical features of liver disease

Functions of the liver
Carbohydrate, protein, and fat metabolism
Synthesis of coagulation proteins
Drug metabolism
Degradation of hormones
Bilirubin conjugation

Cholestasis
Malabsorbtion of long-chain fat and fat soluble vitamins, leads to:
  Pruritus
  Pale stools
  Dark urine

Hepatic dysfunction
Encephalopathy
Jaundice
Epistaxis
Varices with portal hypertension
Muscle wasting from malnutrition
Bruising and petechiae
Hypersplenism
Hepatorenal failure
Ascites
Palmar erythema
Clubbing
Loss of fat stores secondary to malnutrition
Rickets
Hypotonia
Peripheral neuropathy

Children with liver disease do not grow and develop normally

Figure 26.9 Clinical features of liver disease. Chronic liver disease affects every organ in the growing child and leads to significant growth failure and psychosocial delay, which are indications for liver transplantation.

Acute liver disease
Acute viral hepatitis
All forms of acute viral hepatitis occur in children and include hepatitis A virus (HAV), HBV, post-transfusion HCV, epidemic hepatitis E virus (HEV), Epstein-Barr virus (EBV), and CMV. In contrast to adults, most children are asymptomatic and anicteric, and many episodes of hepatitis are subclinical. In symptomatic cases a prodromal illness with vomiting, abdominal pain, lethargy and jaundice are common, as in adults. The diagnosis is suggested by elevations of serum aminotransferases (ALT and AST $10-100 \times$ normal) and confirmed by specific viral serology. Liver biopsy is not required for diagnosis unless the clinical course is complicated. Centrilobular necrosis and inflammation are typical histologic changes of acute viral hepatitis.

Management
Uncomplicated acute hepatitis is managed at home. Hospital admission is required only if the child has severe vomiting leading to dehydration, abdominal pain or lethargy, if coagulation parameters are prolonged or transaminase activity remains high. Acute liver failure is a complication in less than 5% of icteric pediatric cases. The main differential diagnoses are metabolic liver disease (e.g. Wilson disease) or drug-induced liver disease.

Chronic hepatitis
HBV and HCV are the most common causes of chronic viral hepatitis in childhood, but are unlikely to lead to serious liver disease until adolescence or adult life.

Hepatitis B virus infection
Children are infected in childhood by vertical transmission from a carrier mother; horizontal transmission from parents and other family members; by infected blood products; sexual abuse; or, in adolescents, drug abuse. There is an increased risk of environmental transmission in residential institutions and hemodialysis centers. Perinatal transmission occurs mainly through placental tears, trauma during delivery, or contact of the infant mucous membrane with infected maternal fluid. Intrauterine transmission has been reported, but is not a major route of transmission. HBV carrier mothers, who are HBe antigen positive, have the highest infectivity with a 70–90% risk of transmission. Those mothers who are HBe antigen negative, but HBe antibody positive may also transmit infection, and their infants are particularly at risk of developing acute liver failure, secondary to mutant HBV. About 70% of infants infected perinatally will become chronic carriers unless immunized at birth.

The natural history of chronic HBV infection in childhood is not yet established. Children are usually asymptomatic without signs of chronic liver disease. Biochemical parameters indicate mild elevation of aminotransferases (80–150 IU/L) with normal albumin, coagulation and alkaline phosphatase. Liver histology indicates a chronic hepatitis in over 90% of the carriers, which may be mild or non-specific in 40% of children. Progression to cirrhosis is likely and has been reported in Mediterranean populations, although the exact incidence is unknown.

Children with chronic HBV are not only a continuing source of infection, but are at risk of developing cirrhosis and/or primary hepatocellular carcinoma. Chronic carriers should, therefore, remain under medical supervision so that the family may be supported and counseled, as well as to screen and immunize family members. In addition, the patient should be monitored for evidence of seroconversion or progressive liver disease and/or hepatocellular carcinoma.

Annual review should include HBV serology and viral markers of HBV DNA, standard liver tests, α-fetoprotein and abdominal ultrasound.

Management
The indications for treatment in childhood are persistently raised serum aminotransferases, presence of HBe antigen with detectable HBV DNA in serum, and features of chronic hepatitis on liver biopsy. Interferon-α ($5-10$ MU/m^2 thrice weekly) by subcutaneous injection for 6 months has a sustained clearance rate of 40–50% of those treated. Children who have active histology, low HBV DNA levels (<1000 pg/mL), high serum aminotransferase enzymes, and horizontal transmission are more likely to respond to interferon. Pretreatment with corticosteroids remains unproven in the short term, but may have a long-term effect on seroconversion over 3–4 years. Lamivudine has similar results in children as in adults with 26% seroconversion after 12 months treatment. The incidence of YMDD mutants is approximately 18% increasing with duration of therapy. Adefovir dipoxivil is currently under evaluation.

The most important strategy to prevent HBV transmission in childhood includes routine antenatal screening of all women during pregnancy, with immunization of at-risk infants, or universal immunization of all infants. The implementation of universal immunization continues to be controversial, although a number of countries in Europe and North America have adopted this policy.

Hepatitis C virus infection

The importance of hepatitis C virus infection in children lies in its propensity to develop chronic liver disease. Children infected with HCV form three main groups: those who were parenterally infected prior to blood product and donor organ screening in 1990; children who have been vertically infected; and a group of children who have been sporadically infected but the route of acquisition remains obscure. In contrast to HBV infection, vertical transmission of HCV is unusual, ranging from 2 to 10% of offspring born to HCV-RNA-positive mothers. The risk of transmission is increased up to 48% by coexisting maternal HIV infection and in those who have high HCV RNA titers. Breast feeding is not contraindicated.

Diagnosis

The diagnosis is made by screening children at risk. Serum aminotransferases are typically normal or very slightly elevated, HCV serology will indicate anti-HCV antibodies and the presence of HCV RNA by reverse transcriptase polymerase chain reaction (RTPCR). Histology reveals classic features of chronic hepatitis C, which include mild portal tract inflammation, lymphoid aggregates, and mild periportal piecemeal necrosis with steatosis and apoptosis. Giant cell hepatitis in association with HCV infection has been described in neonates.

Management

The first step is to establish the diagnosis by measuring not only anti-HCV antibody, but confirming that active infection is present by detecting HCV RNA by RTPCR (**Fig. 26.10**).

The range of genotypes identified in childhood resembles that in adult populations and does not help in diagnosis, but may provide long-term data on epidemiology and prognosis. The natural history of chronic HCV in childhood is not known, but the spontaneous seroconversion rate is 20% in children who have received blood products, and slightly less in perinatally infected children.

Children who have persistent positivity of HCV RNA and evidence of liver disease should be selected for therapy. Meta-analysis of interferon-α therapy in adults has indicated that monotherapy with interferon is unlikely to produce sustained clearance of HCV RNA or biochemical remission in more than 25% of patients. A number of studies have confirmed similar results in children. The combination of interferon and ribavirin given for 12 months has an overall sustained viral response rate of 45%, with higher response rates (70%) in children with genotypes 2 and 3. Clinical trials with pegylated (PEG) interferon and ribavirin are in progress.

Autoimmune hepatitis

Autoimmune hepatitis is a chronic inflammatory disorder affecting the liver, which is usually responsive to immunosuppressive drugs. It may affect children of any age from 6 months onwards,

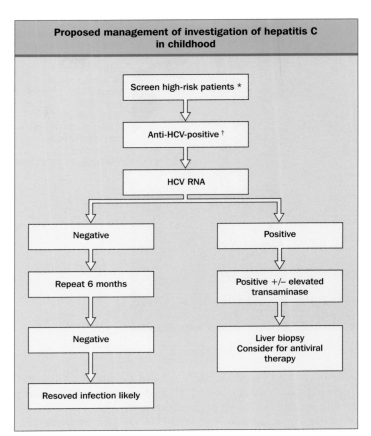

Proposed management of investigation of hepatitis C in childhood

Screen high-risk patients *

Anti-HCV-positive †

HCV RNA

Negative → Repeat 6 months → Negative → Resoved infection likely

Positive → Positive +/– elevated transaminase → Liver biopsy Consider for antiviral therapy

Figure 26.10 Prolonged management of investigation of hepatitis C in childhood. *High risk patients include recipients of multiple transfusions/pooled blood products, and infants of hepatitis C virus (HCV) positive mothers. †Anti-HCV by third generation assay. May be positive in infants of HCV positive mothers up to 9 months by passive transfer.

and there is a 3:1 female preponderance. Both forms of autoimmune hepatitis type I [antinuclear antibodies (ANA), and smooth muscle antibodies (SMA)] and type II [liver, kidney microsomal antibodies (LKM)] present in childhood.

Clinical features

In type I autoimmune hepatitis, the median age of onset is 10 years and the clinical presentation varies from acute hepatitis with autoimmune features to the insidious development of cirrhosis, portal hypertension and malnutrition. The association of multiorgan disease is higher in type I hepatitis with autoimmune thyroiditis, celiac disease, inflammatory bowel disease, hemolytic anemia and glomerulonephritis being the most common (**Fig. 26.11**).

In type II autoimmune hepatitis, the age of onset is younger (median age 7.4 years); the clinical presentation is more likely to be severe with acute liver failure in 11%; and multiorgan disease is less common. The form LKM II may develop in association with hepatitis C or secondary to drugs such as antiepileptic drugs.

The diagnosis is made in the same way as in adults by the identification of:

• elevated serum aminotransferases;
• increased total globulin or IgG concentrations greater than 1.5 times above the normal limit;

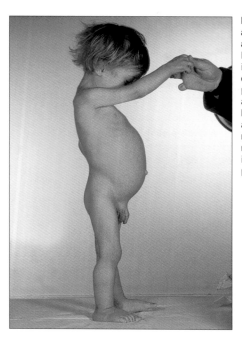

Figure 26.11 Boy with autoimmune hemolytic anemia. Autoimmune liver disease has an insidious onset in childhood and may present with cirrhosis and portal hypertension. Type I autoimmune hepatitis may also present with multisystem involvement, as in this patient.

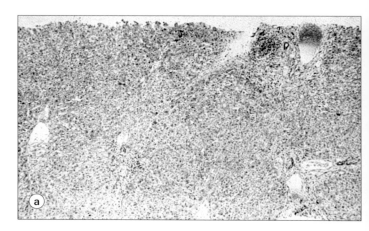

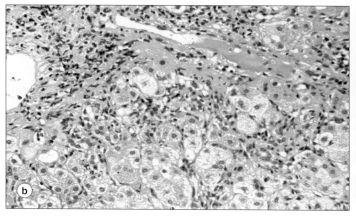

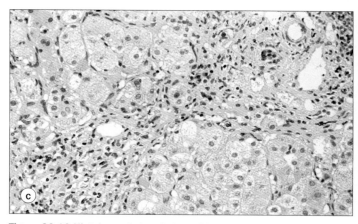

Figure 26.12 Histology of chronic hepatitis. The features of chronic hepatitis in childhood are very similar to those in adults, with an increase in inflammatory infiltrate in the portal tracts **(a)**. This may extend beyond the limiting plate [piecemeal necrosis **(b)**] leading to bridging fibrosis **(c)**. Differential diagnosis is between an autoimmune hepatitis, chronic viral hepatitis, or Wilson disease.

- seropositivity for ANA, SMA or LKM I antibodies with titers greater than 1:40 (up to 25% of children may not have detectable autoantibodies on presentation);
- characteristic histologic features of chronic hepatitis (**Fig. 26.12**); and
- exclusion of hepatitis C and Wilson disease.

Management

Both forms of autoimmune hepatitis respond to immunosuppression with prednisolone 2 mg/kg/day (maximum 60 mg) in association with azathioprine 0.5–2 mg/kg/day. About 90% of children will respond to the above regimen, but cyclosporine (2–4 mg/kg/day), tacrolimus (1–2 mg/day) or mycophenolate mofetil (20 mg/kg/day) may be helpful in inducing or maintaining remission. There has been no established optimal duration of treatment. Discontinuation of corticosteroids and/or azathioprine may be considered if liver tests have been normal for at least 1 year, but up to 80% of children will relapse following discontinuation of treatment.

Despite a biochemical response to immunosuppression, histologic progression may develop over many years. Failure of medical treatment is more likely in patients presenting at an early age, those who have type II autoimmune hepatitis, coagulopathy, high bilirubin, and established cirrhosis at presentation. Indications for liver transplantation include a presentation with acute liver failure, progression to end-stage chronic liver disease, or intolerable side-effects or failure of medical treatment. Transplantation may not provide a complete cure as the recurrence rate is approximately 25%, although this is relatively easy to control with corticosteroids.

Sclerosing cholangitis

The spectrum of sclerosing cholangitis in childhood includes neonatal sclerosing cholangitis and autoimmune sclerosing cholangitis in association with type I autoimmune hepatitis or immunodeficiency (**Table 26.8**).

Clinical features include abdominal pain, weight loss, intermittent jaundice resembling autoimmune hepatitis; and cholestasis with cholangitis and pruritus or cirrhosis with portal hypertension. Laboratory investigation will indicate elevated alkaline phosphatase (>16 × normal) and γ-GT (50–100 × normal). Bilirubin levels may be normal or intermittently elevated in at least 50% of patients; serum aminotransferases are moderately elevated (3–5 × normal); and prothrombin times and albumin levels are usually normal early in the disease.

Diseases associated with sclerosing cholangitis in childhood	
Disease	*(%)*
Autoimmune hepatitis 1	? 50
Inflammatory bowel disease	33
Histocytosis X	19
Immunodeficiency	12
Other	3
Neonatal onset	18
No associated disease	22

Table 26.8 Diseases associated with sclerosing cholangitis in childhood.

Elevated prothrombin time may be due to fat-soluble vitamin deficiency and is responsive to vitamin K. The diagnosis is confirmed by cholangiography [either operative, percutaneous, transhepatic, endoscopic or magnetic resonance imaging (MRI)], which reveals typical lesions of irregular intrahepatic ducts, focal saccular dilatations, short annular strictures, an abnormally large gallbladder, or extrahepatic ductular irregularities. Histology may demonstrate pathognomonic fibrous obliterative cholangitis with periductular fibrosis, but more often indicates features of chronic hepatitis with cholestasis.

Management

Immunosuppression is only of benefit in sclerosing cholangitis associated with autoimmune hepatitis. Treatment of inflammatory bowel disease does not prevent progression of sclerosing cholangitis. Medical therapy is directed towards treatment of cholestasis with fat-soluble vitamin supplementation, nutritional support, and management of pruritus. Treatment with ursodeoxycholic acid (20 mg/kg/day) may be of benefit, although there are no control data available in children. Isolated biliary strictures may require radiologic or surgical intervention but surgical drainage procedures are not generally indicated and may increase the risk of ascending cholangitis and progression of liver disease.

The majority of children will progress to liver failure and develop the complications of portal hypertension. Median survival or time to transplantation is 10 years from the onset of disease. Indications for liver transplantation include progressive cholestasis and intractable pruritus or the development of cirrhosis and portal hypertension. Extrahepatic disease, such as colitis may become more severe following liver transplantation.

Non-alcoholic steatohepatitis (NASH)

The increase in childhood obesity and the recognition of insulin resistance in a number of inherited disorders has led to the diagnosis of this disorder in childhood. As in adults, children may have simple steatosis or steatohepatitis which may progress to cirrhosis in childhood. The main difference is the frequent association with inherited syndromes associated with insulin resistance. NASH has also been reported after hypothalamic surgery, perhaps as a result of hyperphagia. The long-term outcome is not determined, but there may be a response to weight reduction and exercise. Therapeutic trials with metformin and other drugs have not been evaluated in childhood.

Drug-induced liver disease

The mechanisms leading to drug-induced liver damage are similar in adults and children, although there is less risk of adverse drug reactions in younger children compared with adults, which may reflect polypharmacy or concurrent disease. However, there is a specific increased risk of valproate hepatotoxicity in children less than 3 years of age (see page 416).

Acetaminophen (paracetamol) poisoning

Acetaminophen toxicity is the most common cause of drug-induced acute liver failure. It leads to a direct dose-dependent hepatotoxic effect. Children have a lower incidence of liver failure with acetaminophen overdose than adults (unless taken with alcohol), perhaps because the rate of glutathione resynthesis is higher.

Aspirin

Aspirin gives rise to dose-dependent hepatotoxicity that is mild, asymptomatic and reversible. Adverse effects are associated with levels exceeding 15 mg/dL in 90%, which may occur in children treated for juvenile chronic arthritis. Hepatic features include an asymptomatic elevation in aminotransferases with a normal bilirubin level, which usually occurs 6 days after initiation of treatment. In less than 5% of children, severe hepatocellular injury may ensue with prompt recovery on withdrawal of treatment.

Reye syndrome may be defined as an acute, non-inflammatory encephalopathy with hepatic injury occurring without a recognized cause. It has been associated in children with ingestion of aspirin in 90% of cases, especially in children who have intercurrent illnesses such as chickenpox or influenza. The pathogenesis is multifactorial and may reflect a genetic predisposition with a mitochondrial enzyme abnormality in which the viral infection or aspirin ingestion may have induced the hepatocellular insult. There is no relationship between salicylate level and severity of hepatic dysfunction. Reye syndrome in association with aspirin ingestion is now almost unknown due to the recommendation that aspirin should not be prescribed in children under the age of 12 years.

Metabolic disease in older children

Metabolic disease in older children presents with hepatomegaly often in the absence of jaundice and with or without splenomegaly or neurologic involvement. The main causes of metabolic liver disease in older children include α_1-antitrypsin deficiency, cystic fibrosis, Gaucher disease, tyrosinemia type I, glycogen storage diseases, hereditary fructose intolerance and Wilson disease.

Glycogen storage disease

The hepatic glycogen storage disorders (GSD) are a group of inherited disorders affecting the metabolism of glycogen to glucose. Characteristic findings include hepatomegaly, growth failure and hypoglycemia. The diagnosis is based on demonstrating the respective enzyme deficiency. All are autosomal recessive, except for phosphorylase kinase deficiency which is X-linked.

Glycogen storage disease type Ia

Glucose-6-phosphatase is a microsomal enzyme found in hepatocytes, renal tubular epithelium, pancreatic and intestinal mucosa, and is essential for hepatic glucose export. Deficiency of the enzyme results in complete dependency on exogenous carbohydrate. The clinical and biochemical effects of the disease result from hypoglycemia and the body's response to hypoglycemia.

Infants usually present with hypoglycemic seizures, hepatomegaly and failure to thrive. Biochemical investigations reveal fasting hypoglycemia (<1.5 g/L) with lactic acidosis (>5 mmol/L), hyperlipidemia (cholesterol >6 mmol/L and triglycerides >3 mmol/L), and hyperuricemia. Hepatic aminotransferases are usually normal or mildly elevated. Liver histology reveals steatosis and glycogen storage with no fibrosis. Histochemical stains for glucose-6-phosphatase are negative and the enzyme will not be detected in the liver.

The initial aim of dietary treatment is to provide a continuous supply of exogenous glucose in order to maintain normal blood sugars and suppress counter-regulatory responses. This is best achieved in infants by frequent day-time feeding, use of oral uncooked corn starch which is hydrolyzed in the gut to release glucose slowly over hours, and continuous nocturnal enteral glucose feeds. If dietary control is strict in infancy, normal growth and development will take place, although hepatomegaly and hyperlipidemia persist. Long-term complications include osteoporosis, renal dysfunction and calculi, and hepatic adenomata which have the potential for malignant transformation. Liver transplantation will correct the hepatic metabolic defect, but is not indicated for metabolic control. The gene for glucose-6-phosphatase has been isolated and many mutations described. Antenatal diagnosis by chorionic villus sampling is possible if a known mutation has already been identified within the family.

Glycogen storage disease type I non-a (previously known as Ib, Ic, Id)

In this disorder glucose-6-phophatase is present but dysfunctional due to a defect in glucose-6-phosphate transport into the microsome. The clinical and biochemical features are similar to GSD type Ia. In GSD type Ib, neutropenia with recurrent infections from oral ulcers and inflammatory bowel disease has been reported. The gene defect in GSD 1 non-a has been characterized and antenatal diagnosis is possible.

Glycogen storage disease type 3

In this disorder there is deficiency in the debrancher enzyme or amylo-1-6-glucosidase deficiency. The metabolic defect is mild as other routes of gluconeogenesis are intact and there is no renal involvement. The defect is expressed in muscle in 85% of cases (type 3a). The clinical presentation is similar to GSD type 1, without renal involvement. In time a peripheral myopathy and cardiomyopathy may develop. As the abnormally structured residual glycogen is fibrogenic, hepatic fibrosis and cirrhosis are complicating features. Diagnosis is by identifying the deficient enzyme in leukocytes or liver tissue.

Dietary treatment is similar to that of GSD type I, but a higher protein intake is recommended due to the demand of gluconeogenic amino acids. Most metabolic abnormalities diminish at puberty and long-term outcome is determined by the development of myopathy, cardiomyopathy or cirrhosis. Antenatal diagnosis is possible by enzyme measurement or mutation analysis on chorionic villi samples.

Glycogen storage disease type 4

This rare disease is due to a deficiency of the branching enzyme. It usually presents with evidence of severe liver disease in late infancy but there may be cardiac, muscle and neurologic involvement. Hepatic histology demonstrates cirrhosis and accumulation of abnormally shaped glycogen that is diastase resistant. Dietary treatment is as for other forms of GSD. There is rapid development of cirrhosis necessitating liver transplantation in the first 5 years of life. Progression of extrahepatic disease has been reported post-transplantation.

Glycogen storage disease types 6 and 9

These variants are due to defects in hepatic phosphorylase and phosphorylase kinase, respectively. The phenotype of both GSD types 6 and 9 is milder than in other forms of GSD. Children present with hepatomegaly and growth failure, but hypoglycemia is rare. Hyperlipidemia and ketosis may occur. Hepatic aminotransferases are often slightly raised, but progression to cirrhosis is unusual. Dietary treatment other than nocturnal corn starch is rarely necessary and spontaneous catch-up growth occurs before puberty. Neither cardiomyopathy nor myopathy has been recognized, and the long-term outlook is excellent.

Hereditary fructose intolerance

This autosomal recessive disorder is due to the absence or reduction of fructose-1-phosphate aldolase B in liver, kidneys and small intestine. The incidence has been estimated at 1:20 000 live births. The genetic mutation has been identified and is on chromosome 9. Clinical presentation is related to the introduction of fructose or sucrose in the diet. Vomiting is a prominent feature with failure to thrive, hepatomegaly and coagulopathy. Occasionally infants may present with acute liver failure with jaundice, encephalopathy and renal failure. Renal tubular acidosis and hypophosphatemic rickets occur (**Fig. 26.13**). Older children demonstrate aversion to fructose-containing food.

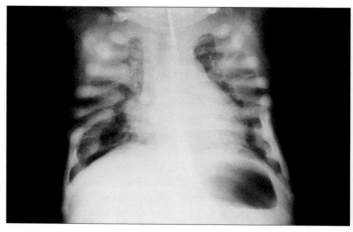

Figure 26.13 Chest radiograph demonstrates an enlarged heart secondary to fluid overload, and severe rickets secondary to renal tubular acidosis. The most likely diagnosis is between tyrosinemia type I and hereditary fructosemia.

Biochemical liver tests indicate raised hepatic aminotransferases, hypoalbuminemia, and hyperbilirubinemia. Plasma amino acids may be elevated secondary to liver dysfunction and there may be hyperuricacidemia and hypoglycemia. Hematologicabnormalities such as anemia, acanthocytosis and thrombocytosis are associated. Urinary investigations will indicate fructosuria, proteinuria, amino aciduria, and organic aciduria in association with a reduction in the tubular re-absorption of phosphate.

Diagnosis is suggested by reducing substances in the urine and confirmed by a reduction or absence of enzymatic activity in liver or intestinal mucosal biopsy or by mutation analysis. Hepatic pathology varies from complete hepatic necrosis to diffuse steatosis and periportal intralobular fibrosis which may progress to cirrhosis if fructose is continued. Fructose elimination reverses hepatic and renal dysfunction. Antenatal diagnosis is possible by chorionic villi sampling.

Gaucher disease

This autosomal recessive disorder is secondary to a deficiency of glucosylceramide-β-glucosidase which is deficient in leukocytes, hepatocytes and amniocytes. It may present in infancy with acute liver failure, but is more usual in late childhood with hepatosplenomegaly, and respiratory, neurologic and bone disease. The diagnosis is suggested by the identification of large multinucleated Gaucher cells in bone marrow aspirate and liver and confirmed by enzyme assay. Hepatic fibrosis may be severe leading to cirrhosis. Recent therapy for Gaucher disease includes enzyme replacement, substrate deprivation for the non-neuronopathic form, bone marrow or liver transplantation.

Wilson disease

Wilson disease is an autosomal recessive disorder with an incidence of 1:30 000 live births. The Wilson disease gene is on chromosome 13 and encodes a copper-binding ATPase.

Clinical features

Clinical features in childhood include hepatic dysfunction (40%) and psychiatric symptoms (35%). Children under the age of 10 years usually present with hepatic symptoms. The hepatic presentation of Wilson disease resembles that of adults who have hepatomegaly, vague gastrointestinal symptoms, acute or subacute liver failure and chronic hepatitis or cirrhosis. Children may present with deteriorating school performance, abnormal behavior, lack of coordination and dysarthria. Renal tubular abnormalities, renal calculi, and acute hemolytic anemia are associated features. The characteristic Kayser-Fleischer rings are not usually detected before the age of 7 years and may be absent in up to 80% of older children.

Diagnosis

Biochemical liver tests indicate chronic liver disease with low albumin [<3.5 g/dL (<35 g/L)], minimally elevated aminotransferases, and a low alkaline phosphatase (<200 IU/L). There may be evidence of hemolysis on blood film. The diagnosis is established by detecting a low serum copper [<1 mmol/dL (<10 mmol/L)], a low serum ceruloplasmin [<20 mg/dL (<200 mg/L)], excess urine copper (>1 mmol/24 h), particularly after penicillamine treatment (20 mg/kg/day), and an elevated hepatic copper (>250 mg/g dry weight of liver). Approximately 25% of children may have a normal or borderline ceruloplasmin as it is an acute phase protein. Radioactive copper studies are only indicated in children who have equivocal copper and/or ceruloplasmin values in whom liver biopsy is contraindicated.

Histologic features of Wilson disease depend on the clinical presentation. There may be microvesicular fatty infiltration of hepatocytes, chronic hepatitis (see Fig. 26.12), hepatocellular necrosis, multinucleated hepatocytes and Mallory hyaline, hepatic fibrosis and cirrhosis. In children who have acute liver failure the histologic features are those of severe hepatocellular necrosis with underlying cirrhosis.

Management

Current management includes a low copper diet and penicallimine (20 mg/kg/day), which is effective if started before the development of significant hepatic fibrosis. If penicillamine toxicity is unacceptable, alternative therapy includes trientine (triethylene tetramine) 25 mg/kg/day, in addition to oral zinc. In asymptomatic children or in those who have minimal hepatic dysfunction, the outlook is excellent, although acute liver failure with hemolysis may occur if treatment is discontinued. Liver transplantation is essential for children who present with acute liver failure and in children with advanced cirrhosis and portal hypertension.

It is essential for the family to be screened in order to treat asymptomatic patients and to detect heterozygotes. Mutation analysis is now more reliable than measurement of serum copper and ceruloplasmin, although the basal 24-h urinary copper is still a sensitive test.

Cystic fibrosis liver disease

The incidence of liver disease in children who have cystic fibrosis varies from 4.5 to 20%, depending on age and the definition of significant liver disease.

Pathophysiology

The etiology of cystic fibrosis liver disease has only been partially explained. Despite major advances in the understanding of the genetic defects in cystic fibrosis, no definite genetic mutation has been associated with the development of liver disease. A low familial concordance of the development of liver disease within siblings suggests that environmental factors may be important. There is an increased frequency of the HLA antigens A2, C7, DR2 (DRW15) and DQW6, suggesting that genetic factors controlling the lymphocyte-mediated immune response might be implicated. The discovery of the cystic fibrosis transmembrane receptor in the apical membrane of biliary epithelial cells has been a major step in the understanding of the etiology.

Bile acid malabsorption is a constant finding in untreated children who have cystic fibrosis. In the duodenum the total concentration of bile salts is decreased, but increases in the glycine/taurine ratio, and the percentage of potentially toxic dihydroxy bile salts have been noted. The abnormally low duodenal pH secondary to pancreatic insufficiency further exacerbates bile acid malabsorption and impairs micellar formation. Supplementation with taurine improves the glycine/taurine ratio of bile salts in the serum but not in the duodenum. It is possible that the abnormalities in bile salt concentration and the increase in hydrophobic and toxic bile acids may play an important role in the production of viscous bile and/or biliary sludge, which may lead to partial biliary obstruction and focal biliary fibrosis.

Clinical features

Most children who have cystic fibrosis and liver disease are asymptomatic in the early stages. In infants, cholestatic neonatal hepatitis may be a presenting feature (see above), but more commonly the presentation is associated with asymptomatic hepatosplenomegaly or the complications of portal hypertension.

Diagnosis

Early detection of liver disease using standard liver tests is unsatisfactory. In general, there will be transient abnormalities of alkaline phosphatase in up to 50% of patients and increases in γ-GT in 30% of males and 60% of females. Serum bilirubin levels and coagulation times remain normal until late in the disease. Ultrasonography detects increased echogenicity (41%) (but does not differentiate fatty infiltration from fibrosis) microgallbladder (10–40%) and gallstones (20–25%). Hepatobiliary scanning demonstrates pooling in intrahepatic bile ducts, which may be a normal finding, or the presence of biliary strictures.

Liver histology may indicate fatty infiltration, focal biliary cirrhosis and multilobular cirrhosis. Steatosis is the commonest finding at biopsy and includes a mixture of micro- and macro-vesicular fatty infiltration. Non-specific mild inflammation around the portal tracts is commonly found in association with chemical cholangitis (granular eosinophilic secretions in bile ducts in association with ductal proliferation of bile ducts). Fibrosis develops initially around the portal tracts and gradually extends between portal tracts until cirrhosis has developed. Cholestasis and bile plugs are rarely identified. Liver biopsy should be performed to establish the extent and severity of liver disease and is indicated when there is persistent transaminitis, hepatic echogenicity on ultrasound, hepatomegaly and/or spleno-megaly, or evidence of hepatic dysfunction.

Management

Treatment consists of nutritional support and the prevention and management of hepatic complications. Nutritional support is critically important in children who have cystic fibrosis, regardless of whether they have liver disease. If cystic fibrosis is complicated by clinically significant liver disease, then the following is recommended:

- increasing energy intake to 150% of average requirements by carbohydrate supplements, such as glucose polymer, or by increasing the percentage of fat;
- increasing the proportion of medium chain triglyercides to 50% of the fat content; and
- supplementation with fat soluble vitamins, including vitamin A (5–15 000 IU/day), vitamin E (100–500 mg/day), vitamin D (50 ng/kg), and vitamin K (1–10 mg/day).

The use of ursodeoxycholic acid in the management of cystic fibrosis liver disease is now accepted despite the absence of good clinical trials. There is clear evidence that treatment with ursodeoxycholic acid improves the biochemical indices of liver function, and is effective when prescribed before the development of significant liver disease.

The main hepatic complication of cystic fibrosis liver disease is the development of portal hypertension and the development of esophageal varices, which should be diagnosed by endoscopy. Prophylactic sclerotherapy is not recommended, but injection sclerotherapy or banding is usually effective once variceal hemorrhage develops. In order to avoid repeated anesthetics for sclerotherapy or banding, inserting a transjugular intrahepatic portal systemic shunt (TIPSS), which can be performed in quite young children, may be preferable.

Current data indicate that cystic fibrosis liver disease is a progressive disease leading eventually to cirrhosis and portal hypertension in all cases. Indications for liver transplantation include the development of end-stage liver failure with jaundice, ascites and coagulopathy, which are late features in this disease. Liver transplantation is indicated in children who have cystic fibrosis liver disease before the development of significant pulmonary complication (<50% of normal function) in order to prevent the necessity for heart, lung and liver transplantation. The use of pulmonary DNAse preoperatively is recommended. Perioperative antibiotics should be based on the sensitivity of colonized pulmonary bacteria. The outcome following liver transplantation is similar to that in children transplanted for other causes of liver disease and lung function may improve after transplantation.

Hepatic tumors

Liver tumors are relatively rare in childhood and occur in the region of 0.5–2.5 per million population. Hepatocellular carcinoma in childhood occurs at an older age than hepatoblastoma in association with underlying cirrhosis secondary to hepatitis B, hepatitis C, or α_1-antitrypsin deficiency. A rare fibrolamellar hepatocellular tumor is occasionally seen in childhood and occurs in non-cirrhotic livers. Hepatoblastoma is most commonly seen in children under the age of 18 months and is rare after the age of 5 years. There is a male predominance of 3 to 2. The commonest presenting feature is of an abdominal mass and distention, and rarely anorexia, weight loss, pain, vomiting and jaundice. Hepatoblastoma is sometimes associated with sexual precocity due to the release of human chorionic gonadotropic hormones (β-HCG). Osteoporosis may occur in up to 20% of cases leading to bone fractures and vertebral compression. Hepatoblastoma occurs with certain well-recognized associations, in particular familial adenomatous polyposis coli.

Diagnosis

Laboratory investigations will demonstrate:

- a normocytic normochromic anemia in 50% of children;
- thrombocytosis (greater than 1000×10^9/L) in 30% of children;
- normal liver tests in hepatoblastoma, but these may be abnormal in hepatocellular carcinoma due to underlying cirrhosis;
- α-fetoprotein may be a useful diagnostic and prognostic marker and is elevated in 90% of hepatoblastoma patients and 60% of hepatocellular carcinoma patients; and
- transcobalamin-1 may be a useful marker in fibrolamellar hepatocellular carcinoma.

Abdominal ultrasound, computed tomography (CT) scanning or MRI imaging will determine the site and extent of the lesion, and establish the presence of any metastases while providing information as regards suitability for surgical resection. Vascular structures are best identified on angiography or MRI imaging and are an essential investigation before surgery. Chest radiograph and CT scanning are important baseline investigations to define the presence of pulmonary metastases. Liver biopsy is necessary for histologic confirmation and selection of chemotherapy, despite the risk of disseminating tumor.

Hepatoblastoma may be classified into four groups: fetal, embryonal, macrotrabecular and small-cell undifferentiated tumors. Microscopic features distinguishing hepatocellular carcinoma from hepatoblastoma are the presence of tumor cells that are larger than normal hepatocytes with frequent tumor giant cells, broad cellular trabeculi, nuclear pleomorphism, and the absence of hematopoiesis. The fibrolamellar variant of hepatocellular carcinoma consists of plump tumor cells with deeply eosinophilic cytoplasm and a marked fibrous stroma separating epithelial cells into trabeculi.

It is important to differentiate hepatoblastoma and hepatocellular carcinoma from other undifferentiated embryonal sarcoma and this is only possible on histologic criteria. Benign vascular tumors such as hemangioma or hemangioendotheliomas are usually differentiated by the radiologic appearance on CT scanning and histology. Focal nodular hyperplasia is a rare benign tumor of childhood which may be single or multiple.

The malignant tumors must also be differentiated from hepatic adenomas which present with a pattern similar to that seen in adults. They may occur at any age, including in neonates and have even been reported in the fetus in utero. There is no link between maternal contraceptive use and childhood adenoma. Adenomas have been reported in patients receiving anabolic steroids, GSD type I, familial diabetes mellitus, hemosiderosis, and galactosemia. Histologically, the tumors may be partially encapsulated, and consist of thick cords of benign hepatocytes lacking portal structures and bile duct. It may be particularly difficult to distinguish between adenoma and well-differentiated hepatocellular carcinoma.

Management

About 90% of hepatoblastomas will respond to chemotherapy and surgery. A minority will require liver transplantation for unresectable tumors. Current chemotherapy includes a combination of cisplatinum and doxorubicin (PLADO), which will reduce the tumor in the majority of patients. Of the total, 71% will be amenable to surgical resection with an 82% 5-year survival rate. Tumors which are multifocal, central in situation or involving the portal vein are not amenable to resection and these children should be considered for liver replacement. An increasing number of patients have been successfully transplanted with a 5-year survival rate of 80%.

Hepatocellular carcinomas are less responsive to treatment and only 50% will respond to PLADO chemotherapy. Surgical resection is also less successful. The recent addition of carboplatin to PLADO may improve the response rate in these tumors. Response to therapy may be monitored by serial measurement of α-fetoprotein levels. Patients who have good responses to chemotherapy will have a rapid fall of serum α-fetoprotein, but persistent elevation suggests residual disease or metastases.

ACUTE LIVER FAILURE IN INFANCY AND CHILDHOOD

The standard definition of acute liver failure used in adults is hard to apply in pediatric practice for a number of reasons.

Acute liver failure in children	
Etiology	*Diagnostic investigations*
Infection	
Viral hepatitis A, B, C, undefined, EBV, CMV	Viral serology
Poison/drugs	
Acetaminophen (paracetamol)	Acetaminophen levels
Isoniazid, halothane	Halothane antibodies
Amanita phalloides	
Autoimmune hepatitis	Autoimmune screen
Metabolic	
Wilson disease	Serum copper, ceruloplasmin
Tyrosinemia	Urinary succinylacetone
Reye syndrome	Microvesicular fat in liver Urinary dicarboxylic acids

Table 26.9 Acute liver failure in children.

Firstly, many infants present with acute liver failure from an inborn error of metabolism implying pre-existing disease. Secondly, encephalopathy may be difficult to detect in infants and small children and be less severe than coagulopathy in the early stages. Thus, caution is required when defining acute liver failure in infancy. The etiology of acute liver failure includes many causes common in adult practice, in addition to the high incidence of acute liver failure associated with metabolic liver disease (**Table 26.9**).

Acute liver failure in infancy

Acute liver failure in infancy usually presents with multisystem involvement. The diagnosis may initially be difficult as jaundice may be a late feature. Infants are usually small for gestational dates, with hypotonia, severe coagulopathy and encephalopathy. Neurologic problems such as nystagmus and convulsions may be secondary to cerebral disease or encephalopathy. Renal tubular acidosis is common. Investigations include a search for multi-organ disease.

Galactosemia

This rare autosomal disorder is secondary to a deficiency of galactose-1-phosphase uridyltransferase. Acute illness results from the accumulation of the substrate galactose-1-phosphate (gal-1-P) following the introduction of milk feeds. Infants present with collapse with sepsis, hypoglycemia and encephalopathy in the first few days of life or with progressive jaundice and liver failure. Cataracts are present. The disease may be complicated by Gram-negative sepsis, which stimulates a life-threatening severe bleeding diathesis.

The diagnosis is established by the detection of urinary reducing substances in the absence of glycosuria, and confirmed by reduced enzyme activity in erythrocytes. Hepatic pathology demonstrates fatty change, periportal bile duct proliferation, and iron deposition with extra medullary hematopoiesis. If galactose ingestion persists, hepatic fibrosis and cirrhosis may develop or may even be present at birth.

Liver function improves following exclusion of galactose from the diet unless liver failure or cirrhosis has developed. Galactose elimination is life long, but efficacy may be limited by endogenous synthesis of gal-1-P. The long-term outcome is disappointing. Learning difficulties and growth disturbance are described and are more common in girls, 75% of whom also develop ovarian failure. Detection of galactosemia in a neonatal screening program will lead to early detection, except for infants who present with acute liver failure. Antenatal diagnosis is possible by chorionic villi sampling.

Neonatal hemochromatosis

This presumed autosomal recessive disorder is the most common cause of acute liver failure in the neonate. It is characterized by the prenatal accumulation of intrahepatic iron, due either to a primary disorder of fetoplacental iron handling, or a secondary manifestation of fetal liver disease. Intrauterine growth retardation and premature delivery is common. Clinical features include hypoglycemia, jaundice and coagulopathy within the first 2 weeks, with a fatal outcome without treatment.

Biochemical liver tests demonstrate elevated bilirubin, and reduced aminotransferases and albumin. Serum iron binding capacity is low and hypersaturated (90–100%), with a grossly elevated ferritin level (>1000 ng/L). Diagnostic liver biopsy is not feasible because of the coagulopathy, but extrahepatic siderosis is found in minor salivary glands obtained by lip biopsy. MRI may confirm excess hepatic or extrahepatic iron. Liver histology at autopsy demonstrates pericellular fibrosis, giant cell transformation, ductular proliferation and regenerative nodules. The distribution of siderosis is similar to adult hereditary hemochromatosis, with hepatocellular and extrahepatic parenchymal deposition, and sparing of the reticuloendothelial systems.

Medical management includes supportive therapy for acute liver failure and an 'antioxidant cocktail', which combines N-acetylcysteine (150 mg/kg/day), vitamin E (25 mg/kg/day), selenium (2–3 mg/kg/day), prostaglandin E$_1$ (0.4–0.6 mg/kg/h), and desferrioxamine (30 mg/kg/day). Some children have responded to this regimen, but the majority require liver transplantation. Extrahepatic iron is mobilized following successful liver transplantation.

Currently early antenatal diagnosis is not possible, but the diagnosis may be suspected by the detection of non-specific abnormalities such as hydrops fetalis or intrauterine growth retardation. Prenatal iron accumulation may be detectable by MRI, but the sensitivity is unknown. A recent report of maternal autoimmune disease preceding this syndrome (presence of anti-Ro and anti-La antibodies) may be relevant to etiology. Administration of immunoglobulin to the mother from 20 weeks' gestation may reduce the severity of this disease in an affected infant.

Disorders of mitochondrial energy metabolism

This group of disorders includes a wide range of clinical phenotypes with any mode of inheritance: autosomal recessive; autosomal dominant; or transmission through maternal DNA. A number of different defects involving the electron transport chain have been described. The clinical features develop secondary to electron transport chain dysfunction, which results in cellular ATP deficiency and the generation of toxic free radicals. Clinical symptoms vary, depending on the nature of the primary defect, the tissue or organ distribution and abundance, and the importance of aerobic metabolism in the affected tissue. The constituent proteins of the electron transport chain are encoded in two genomes, either nuclear DNA or mitochondrial DNA (mDNA) which is maternally inherited. In the context of liver failure, two entities are relevant: isolated deficiencies of the electron chain enzymes and mDNA depletion syndromes.

Deficiencies of the electron transport chain enzyme

The most common isolated defects are complexes 4 and 1, although multiple deficiencies have been reported. Infants present with multisystem involvement manifesting hypotonia, cardiomyopathy and proximal renal tubulopathy and a severe metabolic acidosis. Relevant diagnostic investigations include elevated blood lactate, lactate:pyruvate ratio >20, increased 3-OH-butyrate:acetoacetate ratio >2, or an increase in lactate, possible ketone bodies and, following a glucose load (2 g/kg × 50 g), the detection of specific organic acids such as urinary 3-methyl-glutaconic acid or other Krebs cycle intermediates. Coagulopathy is usually extreme, and may prevent liver or muscle biopsy, or cerebrospinal fluid (CSF) examination. The definitive diagnosis is based on demonstrating biochemical dysfunction of electron chain function in liver or muscle by histochemistry or enzyme analysis in fresh tissue. Demonstration of an elevated CSF lactate compared with plasma lactate indicates neurologic involvement.

Supportive management is usually the only option. Liver transplantation is only successful if the defect is confined to the liver, but is contraindicated if multisystem involvement is obvious as neurologic deterioration persists or may develop post-transplant. Antenatal diagnosis is rarely possible as the underlying gene defects are unknown.

Mitochondrial DNA depletion syndromes

Mitochondria normally contain more than one copy of mDNA and replication is regulated by a number of factors encoded by nuclear genes. Mutations in these nuclear genes lead to a reduction in copy numbers of mDNA resulting in mitochondrial depletion. The clinical presentation and biochemical findings are similar to those of infants presenting with isolated electron transport chain deficiencies. In most patients tissue measurement of electron chain activities show deficiencies in complexes 1, 3 and 4, although activity may be within the normal range. The diagnosis is confirmed by demonstrating an abnormally low ratio for mDNA:nuclear DNA in affected tissue. Treatment is supportive as liver transplantation is contraindicated. Antenatal diagnosis is not currently possible.

Tyrosinemia type I

Tyrosinemia type I is an autosomal recessive disorder due to a defect of fumarylacetoacetase (FAA), which is the terminal enzyme in tyrosine degradation. The gene for FAA is on the short arm of chromosome 15 and many mutations have been described. Intermediate metabolites such as maleyl- and fumarylacetoacetate are highly reactive compounds that are locally toxic within the liver. The secondary metabolite succinylacetone has local and systemic effects, including inhibition of porphobilinogen synthase, and is thought to be responsible for cardiac, renal and neurologic disease.

Clinical features

This is heterogeneous, even within the same family. Acute liver failure is a common presentation in infants between 1 and 6 months of age who present with mild jaundice, coagulopathy, encephalopathy and ascites. Hypoglycemia is common, either due to liver dysfunction or hyperinsulinism from pancreatic islet cell hyperplasia. In older infants, failure to thrive, coagulopathy, hepatosplenomegaly, hypotonia and rickets are common (Fig. 26.13). Older children may present with chronic liver disease, a hypertrophic cardiomyopathy, renal failure or a porphyria-like syndrome with self-mutilation. Renal tubular dysfunction and hypophosphatemic rickets may occur at any age. There is a high risk of hepatocellular carcinoma.

Diagnosis

Biochemical liver tests reveal an elevated bilirubin, amino-transferases, alkaline phosphatase and a reduced albumin. Plasma amino acids indicate a three-fold increase in plasma tyrosine, phenylalanine and methionine with grossly elevated α-fetoprotein levels. Urinary succinyl acetone is a pathognomonic but not an invariable finding. The diagnosis is confirmed by measuring FAA activity in fibroblasts or lymphocytes. Proximal tubular dysfunction may be suspected if there is phosphaturia and aminoaciduria, and confirmed by a reduction in renal tubular absorption of phosphate (<80%).

Echocardiography may reveal a hypertrophic cardiomyopathy, while radiologic examination may indicate severe hypophosphatemic rickets. Hepatic histology is non-specific with steatosis, siderosis and cirrhosis, which may be present in infancy (**Fig. 26.14**). Hepatocyte dysplasia is common and is associated with a risk of hepatocellular carcinoma.

Management

Initial management is with a phenylalanine and tyrosine-restricted diet which may improve overall nutritional status and renal tubular function, but does not affect progression of liver disease. The recent discovery of 2(2-nitro-trifluoromethylbenzoyl)-1, 3-cyclohexenedione (NTBC), which prevents the formation of toxic metabolites, has altered the natural history of this disease in childhood. Worldwide more than 100 children have been treated with NTBC. There is rapid reduction of toxic metabolites, normalization of tubular function, prevention of porphyria-like crises, and improvement in both nutritional status and liver function, particularly in those who have acute liver failure.

The long-term outcome of children who have tyrosinemia type I treated with NTBC is unknown. These children require long-term monitoring and follow-up with 6-monthly abdominal ultrasounds and CT scans, or MRI and α-fetoprotein estimation for early detection of hepatocellular carcinoma (**Fig. 26.15**). The current indications for liver transplantation for this condition include the development of acute or chronic liver failure unresponsive to NTBC, or suspicion of development of hepatocellular carcinoma. Antenatal diagnosis is possible either by chorionic villi sampling which measures FAA directly, or from mutation analysis, or by measurement of succinyl acetone

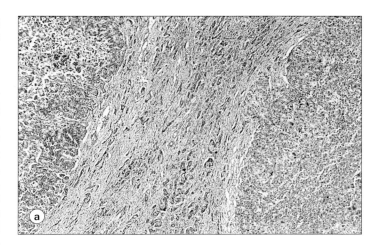

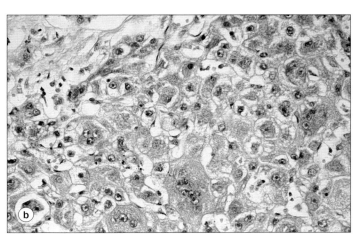

Figure 26.14 Histology of a liver biopsy. (a) Indicating non-specific steatosis and fibrosis. **(b)** There is early hepatic dysplasia, which is a frequent finding in tyrosinemia type I. A focus of hepatocellular carcinoma was found elsewhere in the liver at transplantation.

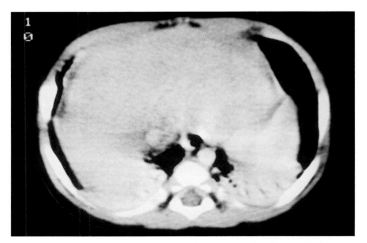

Figure 26.15 Computed tomography (CT) scan indicating multiple nodules in a patient who has tyrosinemia type I. These nodules may represent regenerative nodules or foci of hepatocellular carcinoma.

in the amniotic fluid. Prospective affected siblings may benefit from early NTBC therapy.

Familial hemophagocytic lymphohistocytosis

This rare disorder may be inherited as an autosomal recessive condition, or be secondary to a viral illness. There is progressive visceral, neurologic and bone marrow infiltration with lymphocytes and large erythrophagocytic histioctyes. Children present with fever, hepatosplenomegaly, jaundice, skin rash, edema and encephalopathy in the first year of life. There is a pancytopenia, coagulopathy, and biochemical features of acute liver failure, hypofibroginemia, and hypotriglyceridemia. Diagnosis is established by identifying the characteristic erythrophagocytic histiocytes in bone marrow, liver and CSF. The disease is usually fatal, although treatment with antimetabolites and corticosteroids, or bone marrow transplantation may be helpful. Liver transplantation is contraindicated if there is extensive bone marrow or neurologic involvement.

Acute liver failure in older children

Acute liver failure

All forms of acute viral hepatitis may present in childhood and the presentation will be similar to that of acute liver failure in adults, except where specified below. In infants, infection with herpes simplex virus (HSV-1, HSV-2, HSV-6, varicella-zoster virus, or CMV) may cause particularly severe forms of hepatic failure, often in immunocompromised hosts. In older children, hepatitis A is the most common defined viral cause of acute liver failure. However, the commonest cause of acute liver failure, as in adults, is sporadic non-A–E or seronegative hepatitis, which accounts for almost two thirds of children with acute liver failure. As in adults, this carries a particularly poor prognosis.

Drugs and toxins

Liver injury due to drugs and toxins is the second most common cause of acute liver failure in older children. Sodium valproate has been associated with more than 150 cases of fatal hepatotoxicity worldwide, although the mechanism is unclear. Valproate has a complex metabolic fate undergoing partial mitochondrial β-oxidation, forming acyl compounds with coenzyme A and carnitine and inhibiting cellular carnitine uptake. Hepatotoxicity has occurred in patients who have abnormalities of fatty acid oxidation, mitochondrial energy metabolism, the urea cycle, and those who have presumed metabolic disorders such as Alpers syndrome, suggesting that the normal response to valproate may precipitate hepatotoxicity in those who have abnormal intermediary metabolism.

Hepatotoxicity may occur at any age, but is more likely in children aged <2 years, those on multiple epileptic therapy, and those who have previous neurologic abnormalities or developmental delay. Clinical features usually develop within 6 months of starting therapy and include nausea, vomiting, increasing seizure frequency, jaundice, edema, and hypoglycemia leading to drowsiness and coma. Biochemical investigations reveal moderate increases in hepatic aminotransferases and bilirubin, and severe coagulopathy. Hepatic histology demonstrates severe microvesicular fatty change with hepatocellular necrosis and occasionally cirrhosis.

Once liver disease is established, the outlook is poor unless valproate has been promptly discontinued. Carnitine is not effective in preventing or treating hepatotoxicity, but *N*-acetylcysteine may have a hepatoprotective role. Liver transplantation may be contraindicated as neurologic disease may progress.

Progressive neuronal degeneration of childhood (Alpers disease)

The etiology of this familial disorder is unknown. It is thought to be autosomal recessive, and in some cases an electron chain transport defect has been identified. Despite a normal neonatal period, there may be both physical and developmental delay followed by the sudden onset of intractable seizures between the ages of 1 and 3 years. Although biochemical evidence of liver dysfunction is often present at this stage, clinical liver involvement is a preterminal event. Hepatic disease presents as jaundice, hepatomegaly, and coagulopathy with rapidly progressive liver failure.

There are no specific biochemical features. Electroencephalogram demonstrates high amplitude polyspikes and CT or MRI scans show areas of low density in the occipital and posterior temporal areas. There is a gradual extinction of visual evoked responses. Liver histology characteristically shows microvesicular fatty change, bile duct proliferation, focal necrosis leading to bridging fibrosis and cirrhosis (**Fig. 26.16**). Neuropathology reveals cortical involvement with neuronal cell loss and astrocyte replacement.

The condition is uniformly fatal, with most children dying before the age of 3 years and within a few months of developing overt liver disease. It is important to avoid the use of valproate as it is likely to accelerate the development of liver disease. Liver transplantation is contraindicated, as neurologic progression continues after transplant. Antenatal diagnosis is currently impossible.

Immune and metabolic mechanisms

Autoimmune hepatitis type II [associated with liver, kidney and microsomal antibodies (LKM)] is a relatively common cause of acute liver failure in childhood. The diagnosis is established by identifying elevated serum immunoglobulins and LKM antibodies (see Table 26.7). A minority of patients will respond to immunosuppressant therapy in this situation but most will require liver transplantation. Acute liver failure has also been

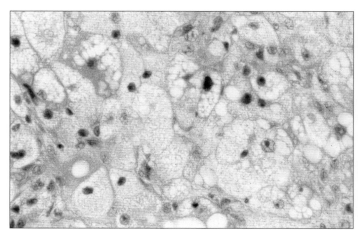

Figure 26.16 Histology of liver biopsy taken at autopsy. It indicates microvesicular fatty infiltration in hepatocytes, which is characteristic of Reye syndrome, Alpers disease or mitochondrial disorders.

recorded in association with juvenile rheumatoid arthritis, despite immunosuppressive agents being more effective in this setting. Although most inborn errors of metabolism present early in infancy, Wilson disease, tyrosinemia type I or Alpers disease present in older children.

Clinical manifestations of acute liver failure

The onset of liver disease varies according to etiology. There may be a prodromal illness with lethargy, fatigue, malaise, vomiting, diarrhea and jaundice with the subsequent development of coagulopathy and encephalopathy. Encephalopathy is difficult to detect in infants and may present with drowsiness, irritability or day/night reversal of sleep rhythm. Older children become aggressive, which is misinterpreted as antisocial behavior. The later stages of encephalopathy and hepatic coma are similar in older children and adults. A poor prognosis is indicated if any of the following features are present:

- rise in bilirubin [>18 mg/dl (>300 μmol/L)];
- a fall in aminotransferases without clinical improvement and increasing coagulopathy;
- prothrombin time >60 s;
- metabolic acidosis (pH <7.3);
- hypoglycemia (glucose less than 4 mmol/L);
- a decrease in liver size (not usual in metabolic liver disease); and
- increasing hepatic coma grade to II or III.

Supportive management for acute liver failure in childhood includes:

- maintaining blood glucose levels greater than 4 mmol/L with 10–50% dextrose;
- fluid restriction (50–75% of standard maintenance) using colloid to maintain circulating volume;
- prevention of gastrointestinal hemorrhage from stress erosions using H_2 receptor antagonists;
- prevention of sepsis with broad-spectrum antibiotics;
- prophylactic antifungal therapy; and
- treatment of coagulopathy if required with fresh frozen plasma and intravenous vitamin K (2–10 mg).

Hepatic encephalopathy is managed in the early stages with reduction of protein intake to 1–2 g/kg and provision of high calorie feeds using glucose polymer (8–10 g/kg) and oral lactulose. Increasing encephalopathy unresponsive to conservative management requires elective ventilation. The development of cerebral edema, detected by clinical signs or on CT scan, is an ominous sign. Conservative management includes fluid restriction (<50% of maintenance), mannitol, and elective hyperventilation. The role of intracranial pressure monitoring is controversial. Electrodes may be difficult to insert in children who have severe coagulopathy, particularly as the blood product replacement may exacerbate cerebral edema. Intracranial pressure monitoring may improve selection for transplantation but does not affect overall survival.

Liver transplantation should be carefully considered in all children who have acute liver failure, but difficulties arise in the selection of infants who have inborn errors of metabolism, because of the difficulty in excluding multisystem disease. Liver transplantation is indicated in those children who have poor prognostic factors, namely seronegative hepatitis, rapid onset of coma grade III or IV, or severe coagulopathy (may be more severe than coagulopathy in metabolic disease). There should be

no evidence of irreversible brain damage on CT scans or evidence of multisystem disease (normal muscle biopsy, normal electrocardiogram, etc).

The mortality rate is greater than 70% for children who are in grade III or IV coma, or who have persistently abnormal coagulation (prothrombin time >60 s). Prognosis may be better in children who have hepatitis A or who have taken an acetaminophen overdose. The causes of death in children not transplanted were sepsis (15%), hemorrhage (50%), renal failure (30%), and cerebral edema (56%). There is a 50–70% 1-year survival rate following liver transplantation, which is less than transplantation for children who have other indications. Survivors with liver transplantation face the psychologic sequelae of such a procedure and the long-term complications of this operation.

Of the hepatic support systems under evaluation, only exchange blood transfusion, plasmapheresis and possibly MARS, have had any value in pediatric practice in reducing coagulopathy and prolonging life until a donor liver was obtained.

LIVER TRANSPLANTATION

The success of pediatric liver transplantation has revolutionized the prognosis for many infants and children who would otherwise die of liver failure. The main factors in improving survival in this age group include advances in preoperative management such as the treatment of hepatic complications, nutritional support and selection for transplantation. The rapid developments in innovative surgical techniques to expand the donor pool have extended liver transplantation to the neonatal age group, while improvements in postoperative management including immunosuppression have led not only to increased survival, but also improved quality of life. The range of indications for liver transplantation in children now includes semi-elective liver replacement and transplantation for inborn errors of metabolism with extrahepatic disease and unresectable hepatic tumors.

Indications

As in adults, most children are transplanted for chronic liver failure. Biliary atresia is the most common indication for children transplanted under the age of 2 years (**Fig. 26.17**).

As many children who have cirrhosis and portal hypertension have well-compensated hepatic function, the timing of liver

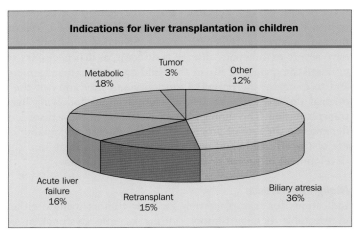

Figure 26.17 Indications for liver transplantation in children. Birmingham Program, 1988–1998.

transplantation may be difficult to decide. In general, the most useful guide is a serial estimation of hepatic function, such as:

- persistent rise in total bilirubin [6 mg/dL (>100 mmol/L)];
- prolongation of prothrombin time [international normalized ratio (INR) >1.4];
- progressive fall in serum albumin [<3.5 g/dL (<35 g/L)];
- the development of malnutrition resistant to nutritional management (deterioration in measurements of triceps skinfolds, midarm muscle area, negative growth velocity); and
- hepatic complications such as chronic hepatic encephalopathy, refractory ascites, intractable pruritus, or recurrent variceal bleeding unresponsive to optimal medical management.

Children who have chronic liver disease have a significant reduction in developmental motor skills which may be reversed following liver transplantation. Thus, these children should be transplanted before the complications of their liver disease impair the quality of their lives and before growth and development are irreversibly delayed.

Acute liver failure

The indications for liver transplantation for children who have acute liver failure depend on the etiology and the extent of the multisystem disease. In general children who have acute liver failure should be referred early to a specialist unit in the field of transplantation in order to provide time for stabilization and consideration for liver transplantation.

Children who have a poor prognosis and, therefore should have early listing for liver transplantation, include those who have:

- seronegative hepatitis;
- rapid onset of coma with progression to grade III or IV hepatic coma;
- diminishing liver size; and
- a fall in serum aminotransferases associated with increasing bilirubin [>18 mg/dL (>300 μmol/L)] and persistent coagulopathy (>50 s).

Liver transplantation is contraindicated for children who have evidence of multisystem involvement (e.g. mitochondrial disease) or irreversible brain damage from cerebral edema or hypoglycemia.

Inborn errors of metabolism

Liver transplantation is indicated for inborn errors of metabolism if the hepatic enzyme deficiency leads to irreversible liver disease or liver failure and/or hepatoma (e.g. tyrosinemia type I, Wilson disease) or severe extrahepatic disease. Selection of patients who have severe extrahepatic disease is difficult, as it is necessary to evaluate the quality of life of the child on medical management and to compare the potential mortality and morbidity of their original disease with the risk of complications following liver transplantation. The timing of transplantation in these disorders depends on the rate of progression of the disease, the quality of life of the affected child on conservative management, and the development of severe reversible extrahepatic disease.

Malignant disease

Indications for transplantation for liver tumors include either unresectable benign tumors causing hepatic dysfunction or unresectable malignant tumors refractory to chemotherapy without evidence of extrahepatic metastases.

Evaluation

The aim of the evaluation process is to:

- assess the severity of liver disease and the extent of hepatic complications;
- consider the technical aspects of the operation with regard to vascular anatomy and size;
- exclude any significant contraindications to successful transplantation; and
- prepare the child and family psychologically.

The histologic diagnosis of the original disease should be reviewed and the severity and extent of hepatic function determined by evaluating:

- albumin [3.5 g/dL (<35 g/L)];
- coagulation time (INR>1.4);
- bilirubin – rise in bilirubin [9 mg/dL (>150 μmol/L)] is usual is cholestatic patients, but may be a late feature in other diseases such as cystic fibrosis; and
- the extent of portal hypertension - this should be estimated by visualizing esophageal and gastric varices by gastrointestinal endoscopy.

It is normal to establish baseline renal function, hematologic parameters, and background serology, which includes CMV status. The most important technical information required is the vascular anatomy and patency of the hepatic vessels. Most of this information may be obtained by color-fluid Doppler ultrasound, and examination of the liver and spleen. Occasionally MRI or angiography may be required to clarify abnormal anatomy in the hypovascular syndrome or to determine the extent of portal vein thrombosis. Liver transplantation causes important hemodynamic changes during the operative and anhepatic phases, and thus baseline information on cardiac and respiratory function is essential and may be obtained from an electrocardiogram, echocardiogram or oxygen saturation study.

One of the main aims of liver transplantation is to improve quality of life post-transplant, and thus it is essential to exclude any neurologic or psychologic defects that may be irreversible after transplantation. The psychologic and developmental assessment of children may be performed using the standard tests, such as the Griffith developmental scale (children under the age of 5 years), the Bailey developmental scales, or Stanford B and A intelligence scales for children of all ages.

Chronic liver disease has an adverse effect on the dentition of young children, which includes hypoplasia, staining of the teeth and gingival hyperplasia. As gingival hyperplasia may be a significant problem post-transplant, good methods of dental hygiene should be established before transplantation.

Contraindications to transplantation

As medical and surgical expertise is improved, there are fewer contraindications to pediatric liver transplantation based on technical restrictions of age and size. Increased experience has indicated that certain medical conditions are not curable by transplantation and these include:

- the presence of severe systemic sepsis, particularly fungal sepsis;
- malignant hepatic tumors with extrahepatic spread;
- severe extrahepatic disease which is not reversible post-transplant, including severe cardiopulmonary disease (not amenable to corrective surgery),or severe structural brain damage; and
- mitochondrial disease with multisystem involvement.

Preparation for transplantation

Most live vaccines are contraindicated post-transplant, and thus it is essential to ensure that routine immunizations are complete, namely diphtheria, pertussis, tetanus and polio, pneumovax as protection from streptococcal pneumonia, and *Hemophilus influenzae* type b vaccine. In children older than 6–9 months, measles, mumps, rubella and varicella vaccination should be offered. Hepatitis A and B vaccinations may also be prescribed pretransplant.

The treatment of specific hepatic complications is an important part of preoperative management. Acute variceal bleeding should be managed in a standard way with resuscitation, endoscopic sclerotherapy or esophageal banding, vasopressin or octreotide infusions. Esophageal banding is preferable to injection of sclerotherapy, if technically possible, as the inevitable development of postsclerotherapy variceal ulcers may be further adversely affected by post-transplant immunosuppression. In children who have uncontrolled variceal bleeding, the insertion of a transjugular intrahepatic portal systemic (TIPS) shunt has proved an effective management strategy, even in quite small children. Sepsis, particularly cholangitis and spontaneous bacterial peritonitis, should be appropriately treated with broad-spectrum antibiotics. In children who have acute liver failure, antifungal therapy should be started while awaiting liver transplantation.

Fluid retention leading to ascites and cardiac failure is inevitable in most children who have liver failure. It is managed with a combination of salt and fluid restriction (to two-thirds of maintenance fluids), diuretics and albumin infusions. Hemodialysis or hemofiltration are rarely required for children who have chronic liver failure, but may be essential in managing fluid retention and cerebral edema in children who have acute liver failure.

The development of effective nutritional strategies has been an important advance in the preoperative management of children who have chronic liver failure and may have improved morbidity and mortality post-transplant. A high calorie protein feed should provide between 150 and 200% of average energy requirements. Problems arise providing these high energy feeds in fluid-restricted patients and therefore modular feeds provided by a nocturnal nasogastric enteral feeding or continuous feeding may be useful. Parenteral nutrition may be required if enteral feeding is not tolerated due to ascites and variceal bleeding.

Psychologic preparation

One of the most important aspects of the transplant assessment is the psychologic counseling and preparation of both child and family. A skilled multidisciplinary team, which includes a play therapist and psychologist, is essential to the success of this preparation and may be successfully achieved through innovative play therapy and toys and books suitable for children. Particularly careful counseling is required for parents of children referred for liver transplantation because of an inborn error of metabolism, which has not led to liver failure. These parents may find it more difficult to accept the risks and complications of the operation, the potential mortality, and the necessity for long-term immunosuppression. Parents of children who require transplantation for acute liver failure may be too distressed to appreciate fully the significance and implications of liver transplantation and may require ongoing counseling and education postoperatively.

Innovative surgical techniques

The traditional form of operation, whole-graft orthotopic liver transplantation, is now a rare occurrence in pediatric liver transplantation due to the shortage of size-matched organs for young children. This scarcity of size-matched donors led to a high waiting list mortality but the development of reduction hepatectomy, in which left lateral segments of a larger liver are cut down to fit a child, have reduced the waiting list deaths from 15% to less than 5%, and extended the range of liver transplantation to young infants under the age of 1 year. Although morbidity may be higher in children receiving reduction hepatectomy, there is no long-term difference in outcome or survival compared with orthotopic liver transplantation. Another innovation has been the development of split-liver transplantation in which a single donor liver is offered to two recipients. Recent results, which involve in situ liver splitting has improved both graft and patient survival. Of particular relevance for pediatric liver transplantation is the development of living related transplantation. There are a number of ethical problems associated with this procedure that are related to the donor morbidity and potential mortality. The main advantages are related to the greater flexibility in timing the transplant, the use of 'good quality grafts', and the reduction in pressure on the organ donor pool.

Recent results demonstrate that there is 91% survival in children receiving living related grafts transplanted electively, but survival in children who have acute liver failure is only 57%, which is comparable with the results using cadaver donors. The choice of living related transplantation in the management of children who have acute liver failure remains controversial, as not only is graft survival less likely, but it is difficult for parents to make clear decisions in this emotional situation.

Auxiliary liver transplantation is a particularly attractive technique in which part of the donor liver is inserted beside or in continuity with the native liver, and it has been used in metabolic disease and in acute liver failure. In the former, it is retained in case of graft failure or for future gene therapy, and it is particularly appropriate for children who have a functionally normal liver but severe extrahepatic disease. Auxiliary liver transplantation is now the operation of choice for children who have Crigler-Najjar type I and has proved successful in reducing the levels of unconjugated bilirubin and improving quality of life. Its role in other metabolic diseases, such as organic acidemias, has yet to be established. In the context of acute liver failure, auxiliary transplantation is targeted at patients who have the capacity for recovery in the native liver (see Ch. 33).

Hepatocyte transplantation with hepatocyte transfusion through the portal vein may be of value in metabolic disease or acute liver failure, but is still at an early stage of development.

Postoperative management

The immediate postoperative period is concerned with monitoring graft function, initiating immunosuppression and preventing or managing complications. The majority of children remain in the intensive therapy unit for 24–48 h, unless there are complications of graft function or cardiac difficulties. Graft function is evaluated in the standard way by measuring acid–base status, blood glucose levels, coagulation times, serum bilirubin, aminotransferases and alkaline phosphatase. There is considerable variation in the details of the immunosuppression regimens in use, but, as in adults, calcineurin inhibitor and corticosteroid-based regimens dominate with anti-interleukin-2 antibodies, mycophenolate and sirolimus being used in selected cases.

Prophylactic antibiotics may be prescribed for 48 h unless there is continuing infection. The incidence of stress ulcers and excess gastric acid secretion is particularly high in children recovering from liver transplantation and warrants appropriate prophylaxis. Antiplatelet drugs, such as aspirin and dipyridamole, are often prescribed to prevent vascular thrombosis that is particularly high in children, but these are typically discontinued at 3 months.

Early complications after liver transplantation

- Early graft failure is a fairly rare occurrence but may be secondary to primary non-function (within 48 h), hyperacute rejection (up to 4 days), or hepatic artery thrombosis (0–10 days). The only successful treatment is retransplantation, but the mortality of retransplantation is up to 50%.
- Hepatic artery thrombosis is more common in children than in adults because of the small size of the vessels and occurs in 10% of children. The incidence has fallen following the introduction of reduction hepatectomy with the use of larger donor blood vessels.
- Oliguria may develop in association with poor graft function, hypovolemia, or immunosuppressive therapy. Most children improve with conservative management and less than 10% require dialysis for renal failure unless transplanted for acute liver failure.
- Hypertension from cyclosporine, tacrolimus or prednisolone therapy is common and responds to fluid restriction and standard antihypertensive therapy.
- Acute cellular rejection responsive to increased immuno-suppression occurs in 50–80% of children at 7–10 days. It is less common in infants (20%), possibly as a result of immune tolerance. Most acute rejection episodes respond to corticosteroids. Tacrolimus is more effective in preventing steroid resistant rejection without an increase in toxicity as compared to cyclosporine in children.
- Chronic rejection is less common, but may occur at any time post-transplant. There may be a response to an increase in immunosuppression, addition of other drugs (such as mycophenolate mofetil or sirolimus) but many children require retransplantation.
- Biliary complications occur in 18–20% of children and are more common in those receiving reduction hepatectomies than in those receiving full liver grafts. Biliary strictures may be secondary to anastomotic stricture, edema of the bile ducts or hepatic artery ischemia, whereas biliary leaks may be secondary to leakage from the cut surface of the liver in reduction hepatectomy or more commonly from hepatic artery ischemia. Most biliary leaks will settle with conservative management, but large leaks leading to biliary peritonitis, biliary abscess or sepsis will require surgical drainage and reconstruction. Many biliary strictures are amenable to endoscopic or percutaneous dilatation and placement of a biliary stent. Long-term ursodeoxycholic acid may be useful in these patients.
- Bacterial sepsis remains the commonest complication following liver transplantation and may be related to central line insertion.

- Fungal infections (*Candida albicans* or aspergillosis) have been documented in up to 20% of patients, particularly those receiving liver transplantation for acute liver failure.

Late complications after liver transplant
Cytomegalovirus and Epstein-Barr virus infections
CMV and EBV infections are common as the majority of children undergoing liver transplantation are negative for both CMV and EBV, while the majority of donor livers (particularly reduction hepatectomies from adults) are likely to be CMV and/or EBV positive. The risk of CMV disease is directly related to receiving a CMV-positive donor, but may be treated effectively with ganciclovir, valganciclovir or hyperimmune CMV globulin.

The development of primary EBV infections is a significant long-term problem. As many as 65% of children undergoing liver transplantation will be EBV-negative, and 75% of this group will have a primary infection within 6 months of transplantation. It is important to diagnose primary EBV infection as early as possible [EBV early capsid antigen and polymerase chain reaction (PCR)], so that immunosuppression may be reduced to prevent further progression to lymphoproliferative disease.

Lymphoproliferative disease
There is a close relationship between primary EBV infection and the development of lymphoproliferative disease, ranging from benign hyperplasia to malignant lymphoma. In the majority of children the clinical features mimic infectious mononucleosis, but a minority develops isolated lymphoid involvement or malignant lymphoma. The diagnosis is based on histology from the affected tissue, which may also demonstrate polymorphic B-cell proliferation or lymphomatous features. It may be necessary to differentiate monoclonal from polyclonal infiltrates using immunofluorescence staining for heavy and light chain immunoglobulins. Although almost every organ in the body may be affected, the liver and gut are most usually involved. It is clear that lymphoproliferative disease is more likely in the presence of intense immunosuppression, particularly with OKT3 or multiple agents. Treatment includes reduction of immunosuppression, ganciclovir or the infusion of cytotoxic T cells programmed against EBV. Chemotherapy with standard lymphoma regimens is used when the lymphoproliferative disease becomes overtly malignant.

Side-effects of immunosuppression
These are numerous and in the main are similar to those seen in adults. The major difference in pediatric practice is the effect of corticosteroids on growth and ultimate height. Hirsuitism and gingival hyperplasia, which are well-known side-effects of cyclosporine, have an important effect on quality of life, particularly in adolescents. The prevention of nephrotoxicity, which is common to both cyclosporine and tacrolimus, needs careful monitoring of immunosuppressive levels to minimize this long-term effect.

Late technical problems
These include biliary strictures and hepatic artery or portal vein thrombosis; management is the same as in adult patients.

Growth failure

Growth failure affects approximately 20% of children after liver transplantation. The most important factors related to growth failure are:

- excessive corticosteroid dosage;
- recurrent hepatic complications and cholestasis;
- intercurrent illnesses, such as EBV and CMV; and
- behavioral problems which interfere with calorie intake.

Successful management of growth failure involves a skilled multidisciplinary team, including a dietitian and psychologist, ensuring adequate calorie intake (by nasogastric tube, if necessary) and early reduction or discontinuation of corticosteroid therapy.

Recurrence of disease

This is an increasingly important problem. As with adults, hepatitis B and C can recur, but the scale of the problem is much less. Recent data indicates that up to 25% of children transplanted for autoimmune hepatitis will have a recurrence, both immunologically and histologically. Giant cell hepatitis with autoimmune hemolytic anemia is a rare disorder that has been shown to recur post-transplant and is now considered a contra-indication to transplantation. The outcome for children transplanted for malignant hepatic tumors is related to the rate of recurrence, which is low if there are no extrahepatic metastases present at the time of surgery.

De novo autoimmune hepatitis

A number of recent studies have documented the development of autoantibodies (ANA, SMA, LKM) after transplantation in both children and adults in recipients who did not have auto-immune hepatitis pretransplant. The incidence is in the order of 2–3%. The histology is typical of autoimmune hepatitis and it can progress to fibrosis. The etiology is unknown, but there is usually a good response to steroid therapy, with or without azathioprine.

Long-term renal function

The development of nephrotoxicity with both cyclosporine and tacrolimus is common although only 4–5% of patients develop severe chronic renal failure requiring renal support or trans-plantation. The use of low dose calcineurin inhibitors or renal sparing drugs such as mycophenolate mofetil or sirolimus for maintenance immunosuppression reduces renal dysfunction. Acute postoperative hypertension is seen in 65% of children, but only persists in 28%.

Hyperlipidemia

Cyclosporine and sirolimus both increase serum lipids, particularly cholesterol, which resolves on transfer to tacrolimus or mycophenolate.

Non-compliance with therapy

Non-compliance with immunosuppressive therapy is probably underestimated in liver transplant recipients. Although it is possible that children who were grafted at a young age are more likely to accept medication through their adolescence than those transplanted later in life, this has yet to be proven.

Survival

Current results indicate that 1-year survival after pediatric liver transplantation may be as high as 90%, while long-term survival rates (5–8 years) range from 60 to 80%. Patients receiving elective living related transplantation initially had a higher 1-year survival (94%) compared with those receiving cadaveric grafts (78%), but recent figures are now in excess of 95% irrespective of graft origin. Nutritional status pretransplant is a significant risk factor for morbidity and mortality, as data indicating that children who had malnutrition had a 60% chance of surviving the first year compared with 95% in better-nourished children, highlighting the necessity for intensive preoperative nutritional support. It is clear that short-term survival is better in children transplanted electively compared with those transplanted for acute liver failure who continue to have 1-year survival rates of 60–70%, which is related not only to the severity of the liver disease, but is also due to multiorgan failure.

Outcome after metabolic liver transplantation

In α_1-antitrypsin deficiency, Byler disease and Wilson disease, there are both phenotypic and functional cures of the original disease. In tyrosinemia type I, liver transplantation corrects hepatic enzyme deficiency and prevents the development of liver cancer, although the kidney continues to produce toxic metabolites. Long-term nephrotoxicity from immunosuppressive agents is, therefore, a problem in this group of children. In Crigler-Najjar type I, urea cycle defects and primary oxalosis, the metabolic defect is completely corrected, and rehabilitation depends on the extent of extrahepatic disease pretransplant.

In organic acidemia, such as proprionic acidemia and methylmalonic acidemia, the metabolic defect is widespread throughout body tissue, but liver replacement provides sufficient hepatic enzyme to prevent metabolic acidosis, under normal conditions. The majority of these children is able to take a normal protein intake, but will be at risk of mild metabolic acidosis during intercurrent infections.

Quality of life after transplantation

Children who survive the initial 3-month post-transplant period without major complications should achieve a normal lifestyle, despite the necessity for continuous immunosuppressive monitoring. Prospective studies have indicated a rapid return to normal nutritional status in over 80% of children within 1-year post-transplant. Linear growth may be delayed between 6 and 24 months post-transplant, which is directly related to corticosteroid dosage and to malnutrition and preoperative stunting.

Early studies of neuropsychologic development pre- and post-transplant demonstrated that the rate of improvement post-transplant is related to the extent of motor or psychologic developmental delay pretransplant, thus highlighting the necessity for early transplantation, particularly for infants who have chronic liver disease. Prospective studies have shown that there is an initial deterioration in psychosocial development post-transplant, which may be related to the prolonged hospital-ization, and to stress of the transplant operation. Following the resumption of normal life there is a return to pretransplant psychosocial scores within 1–2 years. Most children return to nursery or normal school within 3 months of transplantation.

Long-term studies have shown that children surviving liver transplantation enter puberty normally, girls will develop menarche, and both boys and girls will have pubertal growth spurts. Successful pregnancies have been reported.

FURTHER READING

Acute liver failure

Beath SV, Boxall EH, Watson RM, et al. Fulminant hepatitis B in infants born to anti-HBe hepatitis B carrier mothers. Br Med J 1992; 304:1169–1170.

Durand P, Debray D, Mandel R, et al. Acute liver failure in infancy: a 14-year experience of a pediatric liver transplantation center. J Pediatr 2001; 139:871–876.

Rivera-Penera T, Gugig R, et al. Outcome of acetaminophen overdose in pediatric patients and factors contributing to hepatotoxicity. J Pediatr 1997; 130:300–304.

Autoimmune disease

Gregorio GV, Portmann B, Reid F, et al. Autoimmune hepatitis in childhood: a 20-year experience. Hepatology 1997; 25:541–547. *A good paper on outcome of rare disease.*

Cholestatic disease

Balistreri WF. Bile acid therapy in pediatric hepatobiliary disease: the role of ursodeoxycholic acid. Pediatr Gastroenterol Nutr 1997; 24:573–589.

Bull LN, Carlton VE, Stricker NL, et al. Genetic and morphological findings in progressive familial intrahepatic cholestasis (Byler disease [PFIC-1] and Byler syndrome): evidence for heterogeneity. Hepatology 1997; 26:155–164. *Outstanding description of genetic disorders.*

Crosnier C, Attie-Bitach T, Encha-Razavi F, et al. Jagged-1 gene expression during human embryogenesis elucidates the wide phenotype spectrum of Alagille syndrome. Hepatology 2000; 32(3):574–581.

Lindblad A, Glaumann H, Srandvik B. A 2 year prospective study of the effect of ursodeoxycholic acid on urinary bile acid excretion and liver morphology in cystic fibrosis associated liver disease. Hepatology 1998; 27:166–174.

McKiernan PJ, Baker AJ, Kelly DA. The frequency and outcome of biliary atresia in the UK and Ireland. Lancet 2000; 355:25–29.

Mieli-Vergani G, Howard ER, Portman B, et al. Late referral for biliary atresia – Missed opportunities for effective surgery. Lancet 1989; 1:421–423. *Highlights the difficulty in educating medical professionals.*

Metabolic disease

Holme E, Lindstedt S. Tyrosinaemia type I and NTBC (2-2 nitro-4-trifluormethylbenzoyl)-1, 3-cyclohexanedione). J Inherit Metab Dis 1998; 21:507–517.

Rashid M, Roberts E. Non alcoholic steatohepatitis in children. J Ped Gastroenterol Nutr 2000; 30:48–53.

Thomson R, Strautnieks S. Inherited disorders of transport in the liver. Curr Opin Genet Dev 2000; 10(3):310–313. *Summarizes recent genetic advances and highlights link with bile salt transport.*

Whitington PF, Hibbard JU. High-dose immunoglobulin during pregnancy for recurrent neonatal hemochromatosis. Lancet 2004; 364 (9446): 1690–8.

Transplantation

De Ville de Goyet J, Hausleithner V, Reding R, et al. Impact of innovative techniques on the waiting list and results in paediatric liver transplantation. Transplantation 1993; 56:1130–1136.

Haque T, Wilkie GM, Taylor C, et al. Treatment of Epstein-Barr-virus-positive post-transplantation lymphoproliferative disease with partly HLA-matched allogeneic cytotoxic T cells. Lancet 2002; 360(9331): 436–442.

Kelly D, Jara P, Rodeck B. Tacrolimus dual therapy versus cyclosporin-microemulsion triple therapy in paediatric liver transplantation: Results from a multi-centre randomised trial. Am J Trans 2002; 2:351.

Moukarzel AA, Najm I, Vargas J, et al. Effect of nutritional status on outcome of orthotopic liver transplantation in paediatric patients. Transplant Proc 1990; 22:1560–1563.

Thomson M, McKiernan P, Buckels J, et al. Generalised mitochondrial cytopathy is an absolute contraindication to orthotopic liver transplantation in childhood. Liver Transplant Surg 1995; 1:428.

Van Mourik IDM. Long term nutrition and neurodevelopmental outcome of liver transplantation in infants aged less than 12 months. J Ped Gastroenterol Nutr 2000; 30:269–276.

Yandza T, Gauthier F, Valayer J. Lessons from the first 1000 liver transplantation in children at Bicetre Hospital. J Pediatr Surg 1994; 29:905–911.

Viral disease

Bortolotti F, Jara P, Diaz C, et al. Post-transfusion and community-acquired hepatitis C in childhood. J Pediatr Gastroenterol Nutr 1994; 18(3): 279–283.

Bortolotti F, Iorio R, Resti M, et al. An epidemiological survey of hepatitis C virus infection in Italian children in the decade 1990–1999. J Paediatr Gastroenterol Nutr 2001; 32(5):562–566.

Gibb DM, Neave PE, Tookey PA. Active surveillance of hepatitis C infection in the UK and Ireland. Arch Dis Child 2000; 82:286–291.

Jonas MM, Kelly DA, Mizerski J, et al. Clinical trial of lamivudine in children with chronic hepatitis B. N Engl J Med 2002; 346(22):1706–1713. *Controlled trial of therapy for hepatitis B.*

Kelly DA, Bunn S, Apelian D, et al. Safety, efficacy and pharmacokinetics of interferon α 2B plus ribavirin in children with chronic hepatitis C. Hepatology 2001; 34:342A. *Preliminary study of combination therapy in children.*

Sira JK, Boxall E, Sleight, et al. Long-term treatment of chronic hepatitis B carrier children in the UK. Hepatology 1997; 26:427A.

CHAPTER
27

Benign Tumors of the Liver

John Karani

INTRODUCTION

There are very few issues in clinical hepatology that evoke as much debate as the pathogenesis, diagnosis and management of benign liver tumors. The advances in radiologic techniques have led to an improvement in lesion conspicuity that allows the demonstration of small liver tumors that would not have been detected a decade ago. The number of pathologic entities that are now diagnosed, both independently and in association with chronic liver diseases or multisystem disorders, continues to increase. Although didactic algorithms defining lines of investigation and management are of value, there will always be a variance in observation and expertise in radiologic and pathologic interpretation that may adversely affect or advance the diagnostic pathway. In addition, the natural history of many of these tumors, particularly the rarer types, is not yet clearly established and therefore predicting prognosis may be erroneous. However, any individual clinical practice should establish the basic principles of management recognizing the key radiologic and pathologic characteristics and the spectrum of their clinical presentations.

PRINCIPLES OF INVESTIGATION AND MANAGEMENT

A common clinical scenario is that a focal lesion has been detected on imaging. Often this will be an incidental finding unrelated to the patient's symptoms. There is a differential diagnosis that will include tumors of a wide pathologic spectrum. Each of these tumors will require different treatment and carry a different prognosis. The role of clinical and radiologic investigations is to predict the pathology of these tumors and reserve surgical or image guided biopsy for lesions that demonstrate indeterminate characteristics. It is important in the clinical assessment to ascertain whether the tumor has arisen within normal hepatic parenchyma or if there is clinical and biochemical evidence of diffuse parenchymal liver disease. There is an association of certain benign lesions with multisystem disorders and therefore this possibility should be evaluated in the clinical examination and serologic investigations. Liver function tests will be normal in the majority of patients with benign tumors. As a general rule any asymptomatic lesion in a patient with normal liver function that exhibits the pathognomonic radiologic characteristics of an individual benign tumor should be managed conservatively. Surveillance imaging can be used to confirm that the size and morphology of the lesion does not change.

The indications for surgery are difficult to define and are often not dependent upon the type of tumor. Hepatic resection and embolization carry a significant morbidity but are indicated and may be life-saving in those patients presenting with severe spontaneous hemorrhage. If pain is the presenting feature and is attributable to the tumor and also cannot be controlled by medical management, then surgery is indicated. This has to be preceded by a thorough risk versus benefit analysis for each individual patient for any surgical resection will carry short-and long-term morbidity, irrespective of whether the tumor is benign or malignant.

HISTOLOGIC CLASSIFICATION

Benign tumors can arise from all of the cellular components of the liver. Hepatocytes can give rise to hepatocellular adenomas; cystadenomas can arise from biliary epithelium and hemangiomas from mesenchymal tissue and a combination of cells may be found in the tumor-like lesions such as focal nodular hyperplasia. **Table 27.1** represents an abbreviated version of the pathologic classification that is now accepted worldwide. The specific pathologic characteristics of the more important of these lesions are described in the following text.

RADIOLOGY

There are now a number of techniques to detect and characterize benign liver lesions, including ultrasound (US), computed tomography (CT), magnetic resonance imaging (MRI), nuclear

Histological classification	
Benign epithelial tumors	Liver cell adenoma Bile duct adenoma Bile duct cystadenoma Biliary papillomatosis
Benign non-epithelial tumors	Hemangioma Infantile hemangioendothelioma Lymphangioma Angiomyolipoma Pseudolipoma Fibroma (fibrous mesothelioma) Leiomyoma
Tumor-like lesions	Cysts Fibropolycystic disease Focal nodular hyperplasia Nodular regenerative hyperplasia Mesenchymal hamartoma Biliary hamartoma (von Meyenburg complex) Inflammatory pseudotumor

Table 27.1 Histological classification.

scintigraphy and arteriography. Each of these has their own merit but in practice none is pre-eminent. The correct diagnosis is usually made by a correlative imaging strategy interpreted by an experienced radiologist who has knowledge of the clinical spectrum and associations of these lesions.

The following text outlines the simple questions that these techniques have to answer either singularly or in combination.

- Is the lesion cystic or solid or a combination of both these features? This question is reliably answered by US, supplemented by CT or MRI to determine the relative proportion of the cystic and solid elements.
- Is this a single lesion or are other tumors present and do they have similar characteristics indicating the same pathology? It is important to remember that lesions of >5 mm can be detected by all these techniques.
- Is the lesion vascular or avascular? This can be determined by contrast enhanced CT, US or MRI and the pattern of enhancement through the arterial, portal venous and delayed phases of these studies will be a differentiating characteristic between lesions. For example if there is centripetal enhancement with delayed 'filling in' then this is characteristic, but not pathognomonic, of a cavernous hemangioma. Arteriography can confirm the pattern of vascularity but in addition the arterial pattern may be characteristic of an individual tumor. Focal nodular hyperplasia and cavernous hemangioma are such examples.
- Are Kupffer cells present in the lesion? ^{99m}Tc sulfur colloid scintigraphy or MRI with intravenous supermagnetic iron oxide particles (SPIO) will define the distribution of Kupffer cells in the lesion.
- Are hepatocytes present in the lesion? ^{99m}Tc-iminodiacetic acid (IDA) derivative scintigraphy or MRI with the paramagnetic chelate manganese dipyridoxyl diphosphonate (Mn-DPDP) will define the distribution of hepatocytes in the lesion.
- Is there another specific tissue characteristic present by which the tumor can be reliably diagnosed? The presence of a capsule, calcification or hemorrhage is a recognized diagnostic feature of certain types of tumors.
- Is there evidence of chronic parenchymal liver disease or portal hypertension?
- Is the lesion resectable? The segmental anatomy and vascular relationships of the lesion have to be accurately assessed by CT or MRI.
- At what stage can the investigations stop? It may be possible to stop the radiologic pathway after a single investigation. For example, cavernous hemangiomas of <3 cm generally have pathognomonic features on US. They are echogenic with posterior acoustic enhancement and lie peripherally but close to a major hepatic vein. If these features are observed in an asymptomatic patient then the investigative sequence should stop.
- Is a biopsy required and can this be safely performed? As a general rule, all lesions that have indeterminate radiologic characteristics should be biopsied. If the lesion is large and symptomatic and will be resected independent of its pathologic characteristics then preoperative image guided biopsy is not necessary.

The following text outlines pathogenesis, pathology, radiology and basic principles of management of the more common benign lesions.

BENIGN EPITHELIAL TUMORS

Liver cell (hepatocellular) adenoma

This is the most studied benign tumor of the liver with a spectrum of lesions now defined. The majority of liver cell adenomas are related to the use of the oral contraceptive pill. The estimated annual incidence has been put at 3.4/100 000 contraceptive users equivalent to approximately 300 cases per year in the USA. Case control studies and epidemiologic evidence have shown that the development of liver cell adenoma in a woman relates to the dose, duration of usage and increasing age. Low dose oral contraceptives in current use carry little or no risk of tumor development.

Although 'spontaneous' liver cell adenoma occurs in both men, women and children, it is more commonly a sequela of therapy with androgenic anabolic steroid therapy for impotence, or to enhance muscle development in body builders and athletes. Children of either sex treated with the same drugs for Fanconi syndrome, refractory anemias and bone marrow aplasia carry an equivalent risk of liver cell adenoma development. All the compounds incriminated have been 17-alkyl (α-ethinyl) substituted derivatives of the basic steroid structure with methyltesterone, oxymethalone and norethandrolone the most commonly implicated drugs.

Rarer etiologic factors are glycogen storage disease type 1a, familial diabetes mellitus and Kleinfelter syndrome and therapy with clomifene, danazol and norethisterone.

The simultaneous occurrence of liver cell adenoma and focal nodular hyperplasia has been observed but this is uncommon. Peliosis hepatis is often present and may be extensive if the tumor is due to anabolic androgenic steroids. Reports of spontaneous regression after drug withdrawal and progression or malignant change are rare. Most gonadal steroid related liver tumors do not produce α-fetoprotein and do not metastasize despite a frequently equivocal histologic appearance which makes it difficult to distinguish from hepatocellular carcinoma.

Pathology

Macroscopically the tumors arise in an otherwise normal liver and are typically large, often measuring up to 10 cm at presentation. Pedunculation is present in approximately 10% of cases. The majority of these lesions are solitary and well demarcated but are seldom encapsulated on sectioning. The color varies from yellow to tan and they are highly vascular with areas of hemorrhage, with infarction being a characteristic feature. Rarer instances of multiple tumors occur. This disorder is termed liver cell adenomatosis and probably represents a distinct pathologic entity of differing etiology.

Microscopically the tumor is composed of liver cells arranged in plates that are two or three cells thick, separated by compressed sinusoidal spaces lined by endothelium. Enzymatically active Kupffer cells may be demonstrated by periodic acid-Schiff (PAS) diastase or Perle stains. Mitoses are absent or few with uniform cell nuclei. Excess glycogen or fat may present in larger than normal hepatocytes producing pale and eosinophilic cytoplasm. Bile ducts are absent but bile may be present as droplets within the cytoplasm or as plugs in distended canaliculi.

Radiology

With all the imaging techniques the characteristics of a liver cell adenoma depend upon its size, the degree of hemorrhage or

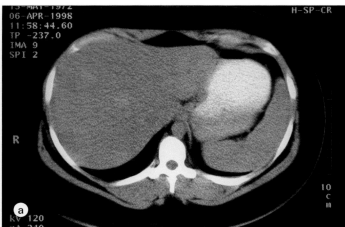

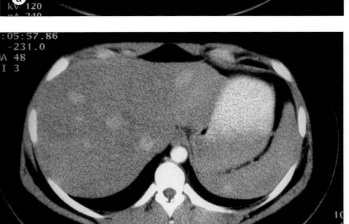

Figure 27.1 Liver cell adenoma. Computed tomography demonstrates multiple liver cell adenoma appearing as hyperdense nodules within a fatty liver on the unenhanced scan (a). Following intravenous contrast the lesions become more conspicuous due to their enhancement in the arterial phase of the scan (b).

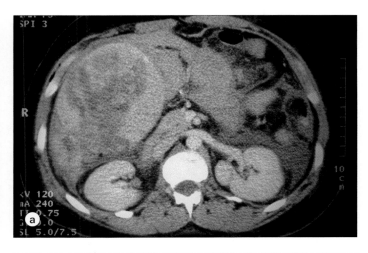

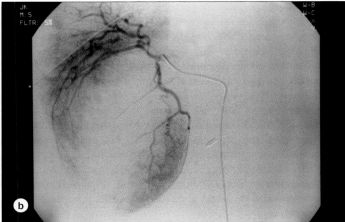

Figure 27.2 Ruptured liver cell adenoma. Computed tomography demonstrates a hypervascular adenoma that has undergone spontaneous rupture with development of a hemoperitoneum (a). Selective hepatic arteriography demonstrates the abnormal vessels on the periphery of the lesion with the central avascular area representing the line of rupture with contained hemorrhage (b).

infarction complicating the tumor or the amount of fat or glycogen present. Supportive diagnostic features may be present such as diffuse fatty replacement of the liver supporting a pre-existing storage disorder or the presence of free intraperitoneal hemorrhage.

Sonography typically demonstrates a large hyperechoic mass with central anechoic areas corresponding to zones of internal hemorrhage. Severe necrosis may develop following infarction resulting in a complex cystic sonographic appearance. Color flow and spectral scanning demonstrate the enhanced peripheral vascularity of the tumor.

Unenhanced CT usually demonstrates a hypodense or isodense lesion that, in the presence of severe fatty replacement, the tumor may appear of higher density than the surrounding abnormal hypodense parenchyma. Hyperdense areas of fresh hemorrhage may be present. Typically, the non-necrotic and non-hemorrhagic regions of the lesion will show transient enhancement during the arterial phase with a centripetal pattern of enhancement developing through the portal and late venous phases (**Fig. 27.1**) Unlike hemangiomas, this pattern of peripheral enhancement does not persist with the lesion becoming

isodense or hypodense by the portal venous phase because of arteriovenous shunting.

On MRI studies, variable characteristics are present but adenomas may show increased signal intensity on T_1-weighted images resulting from the presence of fat or glycogen. The presence of an increased signal on T_2-weighted images and enhancement following gadolinium are supportive as diagnostic features. No adenomas have been reported with uptake by ferrite reflecting a lack of Kupffer cells.

Characteristic angiographic features are of a hypervascular mass with centripetal flow and abnormal peripheral arteries. A more generalized abnormality of the liver may be present with an abnormal hepatogram phase characteristic of peliosis.

Clinical features

Symptomatic patients present with episodic or acute abdominal pain. The latter is invariably secondary to hemorrhage within the tumor. This may be further complicated by rupture into the peritoneum (**Fig. 27.2**). If not recognized and appropriately treated this sequela carries a mortality of approximately 10%. The factors that adversely influence the risk of spontaneous rupture are the size of the tumor, pregnancy and menstruation.

Management

Current opinion is that adenomas >10 cm carry sufficient risk of hemorrhage to warrant surgical excision. In a patient presenting with acute abdominal pain, severe active hemorrhage and shock, emergency radiologic intervention with arterial embolization is indicated as a prelude to resection. At the other end of the clinical spectrum is the patient on oral contraceptives where the tumor has been detected as an incidental finding on imaging. In this clinical scenario a conservative approach can be followed, as the natural history is not so well defined that the prognosis can be predicted. Complete resolution and progression on withdrawal of estrogen are both documented. A policy of close observation by imaging can be adopted. Should the tumor enlarge or the patient develops symptoms attributable to the lesion, then these are clear indications for surgery. With successful surgical resection, the long-term prognosis is good.

An elective radiologic approach using selective arterial embolization with coils and particulate material to ablate the vascularity of the tumor can provide a therapeutic alternative particularly if the lesions are multiple and their anatomy mitigates against low risk hepatic resection. As with many uncommon liver tumors of variable presentation, management and biological activity, establishing patients and then recruiting them onto a long-term case controlled study to investigate the role of radiologic intervention as alternatives to surgery and conservative management is difficult. However, individual experience and reports indicate that this approach merits consideration.

Bile duct cystadenoma

This is a rare tumor that is not unique to the liver as tumors with similar characteristics are reported in the pancreas and ovary. They constitute less than 5% of cysts of biliary origin with 85% arising from the intrahepatic biliary tree with the remainder arising from the extrahepatic bile ducts or gallbladder. With regard to pancreatic neoplasms, this similarity is explainable on the similar development of the pancreas and the biliary system from the endodermal diverticula of the gut. The primordial germ cells normally migrate from the posterior wall of the yolk sac along the wall of the hindgut through the yolk stalk, a structure that is intimately related with the gut from which the primordia of the hepatobiliary system and pancreas arise. This embryologic association may explain the ovarian-like stroma visible in these tumors, which is reported as a feature carrying a better prognosis.

Pathology

The cystadenomas are usually large multiloculate cystic tumors lined by columnar, mucin-producing epithelium. Categorization of the tumor into benign or a malignant cystadenocarcinoma is largely dependent upon the histologic assessment of the epithelium which may show internal papillary structures or cystic invaginations. Foci of cellular atypia, particularly nuclear enlargement and hyperchromasia, multilayering or solid epithelial masses indicate 'borderline' change with capsular invasion an indicator of malignant change.

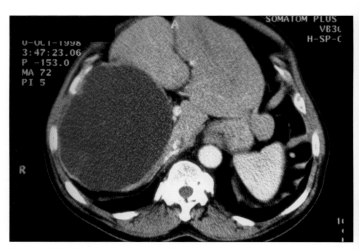

Figure 27.3 Biliary cystadenoma. This appears on computed tomography as a large hypodense lesion with mural nodularity. There is atrophy of the posterior segments of the right lobe of the liver.

Radiology

The tumors are slow growing and by the time of presentation usually measure over 10 cm. They are therefore easily detected by imaging (**Fig. 27.3**). Specific radiologic features are the complex cystic appearance of the tumor with multiple loculi containing mucinous fluid that may be detected by all techniques. The tumors are characteristically avascular on angiography. There are no specific radiologic criteria to differentiate cystadenocarcinoma and cystadenoma but an increased mural nodularity favors malignant change. Therefore the role of imaging is threefold: firstly to give an indication as to the potential diagnosis, secondly to define the segmental anatomy and vascular relationships prior to liver resection, and finally to exclude a pancreatic or ovarian primary cystadenocarcinoma metastatic to the liver.

Clinical features

The majority of these tumors occur in women with a peak incidence in the fifth decade. Patients present with pain or discomfort and a palpable mass. Biliary cystadenomas do not communicate with the biliary tree although compression or projection into major bile ducts may occur and result in obstructive jaundice or recurrent cholangitis.

Management

If anatomically possible, surgical resection is the treatment of choice and carries a good prognosis even if there is histologic evidence of malignant transformation.

Bile duct adenomas and microhamartomas

Bile duct adenomas are rare tumors, with hamartomatous features formed by numerous small non-malignant ducts separated by mature connective tissue. They are usually an incidental finding at laparotomy or autopsy appearing as single, pale well-circumscribed nodules. Over 90% are subcapsular in position and therefore are easily resected.

Microhamartomas or von Meyenburg complexes represent as not uncommon finding in wedge biopsies or at autopsy. They are tiny, usually multiple lesions composed of small dilated, angulated bile ducts in a stroma of fibrous tissue. They lie within or adjacent to portal tracts. They are usually asymptomatic but have been reported in association with portal hypertension akin to congenital hepatic fibrosis and, rarely, the development of cholangiocarcinoma within the complexes.

BENIGN NON-EPITHELIAL TUMORS

Hemangioma

This is the most common benign tumor of the liver with a reported incidence from 1 to 20%. This latter figure is a result of a prospective autopsy study in which a dedicated search for this lesion was performed. Most reports suggest a predominant prevalence in women. Although this tumor may occur in any age group, it is most commonly found in the third, fourth and fifth decades. Serial longitudinal growth studies have shown that most hemangiomas remain stable, although they may occasionally increase or decrease in size. Hormonal influences in growth have also been documented with enlargement of some tumors during pregnancy and regression of others after steroid therapy.

Pathology

Hemangiomas may be single or multiple, intraparenchymal or pedunculated, with a size varying from a few millimeters to greater than 20 cm. However, most hemangiomas are solitary, of less than 5 cm, and are found in a subcapsular site in the right lobe adjacent to peripheral divisions of the hepatic vein. Histologically, they are derived from mesodermal elements and are composed of cavernous vascular spaces lined by a single layer of flat epithelium and filled with blood. Thin fibrous septae separate the vascular channels. They have a predisposition to thrombosis with subsequent development of fibrosis, dystrophic calcification or ossification. Larger hemangiomas have a propensity to involute, developing a central fibrocollagenous scar as vascular occlusion and organization of central thrombi occurs, with central necrosis a potential sequela. Rarely, vascular occlusion may lead to total sclerosis of the hemangioma and formation of a fibrous nodule.

Radiology

Each radiologic technique has characteristic features by which hemangiomas may be reliably diagnosed but there is a significant minority that will be atypical. These require a combination of radiologic techniques to establish the diagnosis. The appearances will reflect the varying representation of the histologic elements within the tumor. Larger tumors often have mixed or atypical features and the differentiation from other benign or malignant tumors, of differing prognosis and management, may be difficult.

Characteristic appearances on US are of a well-circumscribed hyperechoic lesion of <3 cm, exhibiting posterior acoustic enhancement. They lie in a subcapsular position adjacent to a hepatic vein. If fatty infiltration of the liver is present then the tumors may be hypoechoic. Demonstration of blood flow on color Doppler flow imaging is a variable feature occurring in between 10 and 50% of hemangiomas in published series. Larger (>3 cm) or giant (>10 cm) will have varying degrees of hemorrhage, calcification or fibrosis modifying their US appearance.

On CT hemangiomas are characteristically of low density although in the presence of fatty infiltration they may appear hyperdense relative to the surrounding hepatic parenchyma. After administration of intravenous contrast agent, there is nodular peripheral enhancement of the tumor by the large

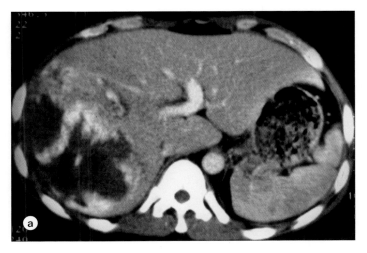

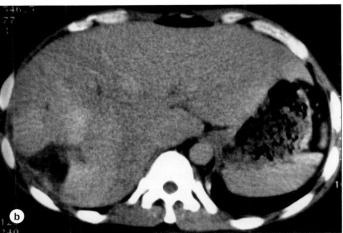

Figure 27.4 Hemangioma. Computed tomography demonstrates a giant cavernous hemangioma with centripetal enhancement in the early vascular phase (a) and 'filling in' in the delayed phase (b).

feeding vascular nidus of the tumor. Centripetal enhancement then occurs with 'filling in' of the tumor (**Fig. 27.4**). Although small lesions 'fill in' completely, large hemangiomas may show central avascular zones corresponding to the central fibrotic scar (**Fig. 27.5**). The rate of 'filling in' of the tumor is variable and is dependent on the flow dynamics of the hemangioma and on the timing of the acquisition of the scan relative to the bolus of contrast, and may be delayed for up to 20 min after the injection. It is important to emphasize that only approximately 54% of large hemangiomas have this characteristic perfusion pattern. However, only 2% of other primary and malignant tumors exhibit these features so their presence typically should allow a confident diagnosis of a hemangioma to be made. The converse argument is that up to 46% of hemangiomas exhibit atypical features of either absent, mixed or central enhancement or incomplete 'filling in' on delayed scans so clear differentiation from malignant tumors may not be possible in these cases. Therefore, it is an important rule that in the CT evaluation of a patient with a documented extrahepatic malignancy, strict adherence to these criteria must be made to ensure a metastasis is not misinterpreted as an atypical hemangioma.

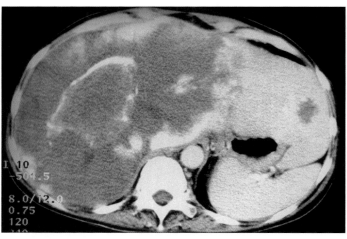

Figure 27.5 Hemangioma. Computed tomography demonstrates a central scar within a cavernous hemangioma of the right lobe of the liver. There is a small hemangioma in the left lobe that also exhibits centripetal enhancement.

With MRI hemangiomas characteristically demonstrate marked hyperintensity on T_2-weighted images that may contain low intensity areas correlating with the pathologic zones of fibrosis. After administration of the vascular phase contrast agent gadolinium diethylenetriaminepentaacetic acid (Gd-DTPA) there is early peripheral nodular enhancement with 'filling in' on delayed scans paralleling the characteristics of CT. Smaller hemangiomas more often demonstrate uniform enhancement, potentially indistinguishable from the appearances of hyper-vascular metastases or hepatocellular carcinomas (**Fig. 27.6**). Increasing the T_2-weighting of the acquisition may improve the discrimination, with hemangiomas usually being of higher signal intensity than malignant nodules. As hemangiomas do not contain Kupffer cells or normal hepatocytes they do not enhance with either superparamagnetic iron oxide particles or Mn-DPDP.

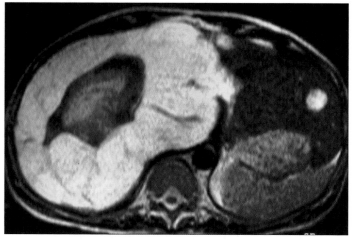

Figure 27.6 Hemangioma. T_2-weighted magnetic resonance imaging scans of same case as Figure 27.3 demonstrate the characteristic hyperintensity of the hemangioma with the central hypointense scar. The smaller lesion in the left lobe appears uniformly hyperintense.

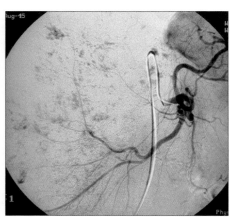

Figure 27.7 Hemangioma. Selective hepatic arteriography demonstrates the characteristic features of a hemangioma with pools of contrast and absent venous shunting.

Hemangiomas cause a focal defect on both hepatobiliary excretion and sulfur colloid scintigraphy that is accompanied by normal uptake in the surrounding liver. Tagged red blood pool scans may be diagnostic with again the features of centripetal uptake with 'filling in' on delayed scans.

Angiography is usually reserved for the atypical tumors where assessment by non-invasive techniques singularly or in combination has not resulted in a definitive diagnosis. The appearances are pathognomonic with small pools of contrast, which persist beyond the late venous phase without evidence of tumor neovascularity or arteriovenous shunting (**Fig. 27.7**).

None of these techniques is pre-eminent and it is often a correlative imaging analysis by an experienced hepatobiliary radiologist that allows the diagnosis to be made.

Clinical presentation and management

The vast majority of hemangiomas will remain asymptomatic and are discovered as an incidental finding on imaging investigations for an unrelated condition. In most instances knowledge of the characteristic features should allow a definitive diagnosis to be made and obviate the need for any further investigations. Abdominal pain may occur with larger lesions with hemorrhage, infarction or compression of adjacent viscera complicating the tumor. Thrombocytopenia from platelet sequestration, hypofibrinogenemia from deposition of an intravascular fibrin clot, and spontaneous rupture are all rare complications. It is the severity of the clinical presentation rather than any specific morphologic characteristic of the hemangioma that directs management. Rupture and hemorrhage are at the extreme of the clinical spectrum, and the requirement for surgical intervention is without question. In the patients with abdominal pain, the clinical analysis is frequently more difficult. If it is clear that the patient's symptoms are attributable to a large hemangioma and if radiologic assessment confirms that the lesion is resectable then surgery is indicated. Radiologic intervention with particulate embolization of the arterial supply is a therapeutic alternative but as yet there is no controlled trial to confirm its efficacy. Neither of these interventions, with their inherent morbidity, should be undertaken unless an objective risk benefit analysis of the patient's symptoms has been undertaken.

Infantile hemangioendothelioma

This is the commonest mesenchymal tumor of the liver and may represent part of a generalized mesenchymal disorder with cutaneous hemangiomata present in over 50% of cases. Less commonly accompanying lesions in the gastrointestinal tract, trachea, pulmonary parenchyma or central nervous system may also occur. More than 80% are diagnosed in the first 6 months of life with an approximately equal sex incidence. Complications include congestive cardiac failure secondary to arteriovenous shunting, rupture, and consumptive coagulopathy with anemia, thrombocytopenia and hemolytic jaundice as presenting features. Occasionally these lesions present as an asymptomatic mass that resolves spontaneously without complication, although there is an increased risk of hepatic hemorrhage from trauma.

Pathology

The tumors can be solitary or multicentric, varying in size from a few millimeters to >15 cm. They are well demarcated but non-encapsulated with the cut surface exhibiting a reddish-brown appearance with a spongy consistency which may show central areas of focal hemorrhage, scarring or calcification. Histologically the tumor is composed of anastomosing vascular channels lined by a solitary (type 1) or multiple layers (type 2) of plump endothelial cells. The infiltrative growth pattern between the liver cell plates is the feature that distinguishes the tumors from cavernous hemangiomas. The tumor cells are benign and mitoses are rare. Extra medullary hemopoiesis is a frequent finding. Low grade angiosarcomas, which may also present in infancy, and which carry differing management and prognostic implications, are the most important histologic diagnostic differential of the type 2 lesions.

Radiology

The radiologic features reflect the degree of arterialization and arteriovenous shunting within the tumor. High volume shunts are associated with a hyperdynamic arterial flow, dilatation of the draining hepatic veins and features of cardiac failure with cardiomegaly and pulmonary plethora. The infants who present within the first few days of life with these features are often misdiagnosed as having congenital heart disease with an intra-cardiac shunt. The role of radiology is to examine the extent of replacement of the normal liver parenchyma by the hemangio-endothelioma, assess the degree of vascularity and pathologic shunting and to determine whether any other organs are involved.

The US features of these tumors vary. Many of the tumors are well circumscribed, but their internal structure may differ in characteristics. Diffuse alteration in the parenchymal pattern with complete replacement of the normal liver pattern may be present, even in the presence of normal synthetic liver function. Doppler US characteristics are diagnostic in the majority of infants with a high volume systolic and end diastolic arterial flow and dilatation of anatomically normal main hepatic veins.

CT demonstrates the focal vascular spaces as enhancing masses on both the arterial and portal venous phases of contrast enhancement. The degree of persistence of tumor enhancement on the delayed phase will be dependent on the degree of arteriovenous shunting. The tumors with high volume shunts will be characterized by a rapid clearance of contrast and dilated hepatic veins (**Fig. 27.8**). Those without a major arteriovenous shunt will show persistent and increasing enhancement with 'filling in' resembling adult cavernous hemangiomata (**Fig. 27.9**).

MRI will demonstrate the tumors as hyperintense vascular spaces on T$_2$-weighted images. The enlarged hepatic arteries and

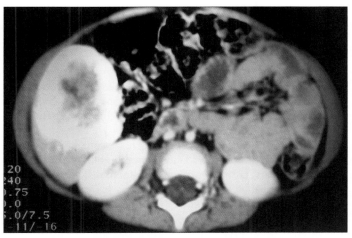

Figure 27.8 Hemangioendothelioma. Segmental hemangioendothelioma presenting in an infant appearing as a hypervascular mass on computed tomography.

decompressing hepatic veins are demonstrable on conventional multiplanar imaging or dedicated vascular image acquisition techniques (magnetic resonance angiography). Areas of focal calcification, hemorrhage and necrosis, which have variable representation within the tumors, will all have their characteristic appearances with the individual techniques.

Angiography provides a conclusive diagnosis, detailed anatomy of the tumor and its feeding arteries. Hypervascular tumor vessels are present with varying degrees of arteriovenous shunting and enlargement of the hepatic veins and hepatic artery. There is often diminution in the size of the abdominal aorta distal to the origin of the enlarged hepatic artery, as a consequence of the steal of blood through the liver.

Management

The management of these tumors is dependent on the severity of the clinical presentation. This is a rare benign tumor and yet there are many treatments advocated in published series and

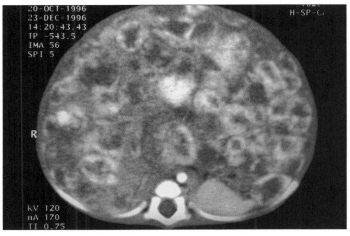

Figure 27.9 Hemangioendothelioma. Diffuse hepatic hemangioendothelioma of infancy with multiple enhancing nodules within an enlarged liver.

individual case reports. Mild degrees of cardiac failure may be treated with digitalis and diuretics, but the response to steroids and interferon seems to vary from center to center. Radiotherapy has been used but all these non-surgical management lines have to be judged by the natural history of these tumors that may undergo spontaneous regression and involution in the first few months of life without any intervention. Surgery is mandatory for intraperitoneal hemorrhage, but treatment in the presence of severe cardiac failure, unresponsive to medical treatment, is more contentious. Hepatic resection, hepatic artery ligation or embolization and transplantation all have a potential role. Hepatic artery ligation is a well-established technique with numerous published reports of its efficacy. It remains to be seen whether it is totally replaced by embolization as a method of occluding the arterial inflow to the hemangioendothelioma. Occluding the arterial supply with a metallic spring embolus delivered following percutaneous catheterization of the hepatic artery should result in the same alteration in hemodynamics as with surgical ligation but without the operative morbidity.

Resection is a surgical option when the tumor is confined to a lobe or segment but this occurs in the minority of cases. The greatest risk from resection lies in intraoperative hemorrhage. Liver transplantation may be the only option if arterial ligation fails with development of early arterial collateralization of the tumor and recurrence of severe cardiac failure.

Lymphangioma

Hepatic lymphangiomas commonly occur as multiple masses of dilated lymphatic channels containing proteinaceous fluid or blood. Multiple organ involvement, including the spleen, peritoneum, kidneys, lungs, gastrointestinal tract and skeleton may be present, especially in children.

Lipomatous tumors

Hepatic lipomas are uncommon benign tumors that are generally asymptomatic incidental findings on imaging. They may be composed solely of fat cells, or may contain varying proportions of adenomatous, angiomatous and myomatous tissue resulting in adenolipomas, myelolipomas and angiomyolipomas. Approximately 10% of patients with tuberous sclerosis and renal angiolipomas will have hepatic fatty tumors, either lipoma or angiomyolipoma. There is no sex predilection and they have been reported in a broad adult age range (24–70 years).

Pathology

The tumors are composed of vessels, smooth muscle, fat and hemopoietic tissues in various combinations. The unusual histologic appearances may cause diagnostic difficulty especially in the leiomyomatous element which may be either spindle or epithelioid. Electron microscopy and immunocytochemistry readily identify the various components of the tumor.

Radiology

The radiologic appearance of these fatty lesions is dependent on their internal composition. Fat has specific tissue characteristics. On US it is of increased echogenicity with acoustic enhancement posterior to the lesion. It has a specific density on CT of −20 to −115 Hounsfield units (HU) and on magnetic resonance it is hyperintense on both T_1- and T_2-weighted acquisitions. The presence of angiomatous or myomatous tissue will necessarily alter the homogeneity of these characteristic features. Although pure lipomas do not enhance after vascular phase contrast agents, fatty hepatic tumors with angiomatous or adenomatous elements may show variable enhancement and make diagnosis by imaging more difficult and a tissue diagnosis by image guided biopsy may be necessary.

Management

If a definitive histologic or radiologic diagnosis is made in an asymptomatic patient then no treatment is indicated. The tumors that are characterized by the presence of angiomatous features may present with hemorrhage and abdominal pain. In these rare instances surgical resection or embolization will have to be considered.

TUMOR-LIKE LESIONS

Focal nodular hyperplasia

Although rare focal nodular hyperplasia (FNH) is the second most common tumor, constituting approximately 8% of primary hepatic tumors found at autopsy. It is found most commonly in females during their reproductive years. Fewer than 20% are found in children and these account for 2% of childhood tumors. The etiology of the lesion is unknown. The preponderance in women, as with adenomas, suggests an association with estrogens, but the prevalence of oral contraceptive use in these cases is similar to that of a matched control population. Patients with FNH frequently have other vascular and neuroendocrine anomalies including cavernous hemangiomas, glioblastomas, astrocytomas, pheochromocytomas and multiple endocrine neoplasias. Lesions in children have been described in association with glycogen storage disease type 1, sickle cell disease and cyanotic congenital heart disease.

The pathogenesis of FNH has been related to neoplastic change, hamartomatous malformation or focal liver injury. The current view is that it represents a hyperplastic response to an abnormal blood flow caused by a pre-existing vascular malformation within the liver or abnormal or absent portal venous flow. It has been suggested that increased and turbulent blood flow results in platelet disruption with arterial thrombosis and release of platelet derived growth factors that may then stimulate liver cell hyperplasia.

Pathology

This lesion is typically solitary and forms a well-circumscribed fibrous lobular mass. The majority of tumors are smaller than 5 cm, with a mean diameter of 3 cm at the time of diagnosis. They are rarely encapsulated and 20% are pedunculated. The lesion tends to bulge on its cut surface and displays multiple yellow–brown nodules of liver parenchyma separated by fibrous septa. Histologically it resembles cirrhosis but is focal and surrounded by normal liver parenchyma. A central stellate scar is often seen and it may contain thick-walled vessels. The frequent finding of bile duct proliferation around the liver cell nodules may be in response to cholestasis. The nodules consist of normal liver cells arranged in plates two or three cells thick and contain increased amounts of glycogen or fat. FNH is distinguished from liver cell adenoma by its multinodularity, and the presence of septa and proliferating bile ductules.

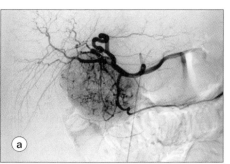

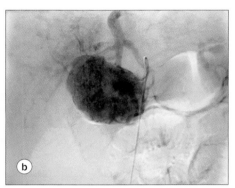

Figure 27.11 Focal nodular hyperplasia. Arteriography demonstrates the characteristic signs of focal nodular hyperplasia with a centrifugal 'spoke-wheel' arterial pattern (a) and an intense blush with draining veins (b).

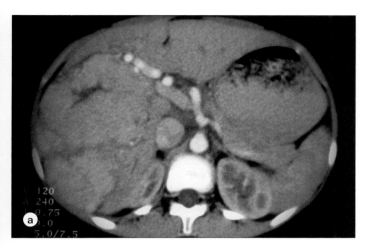

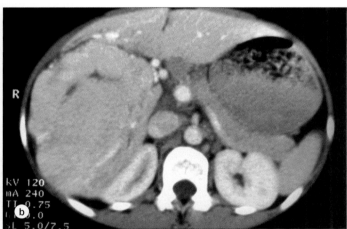

Figure 27.10 Focal nodular hyperplasia. Characteristic features of increased density, with enlarged peripheral arteries and stellate scars exhibited in the arterial phase computed tomography (a). The lesion becomes isodense in the portal venous phase (b).

Radiology

Up to 60% of FNH lesions contain Kupffer cells with reticulo-endothelial cellular function and these lesions may therefore demonstrate normal or increased uptake on sulfur colloid scintigraphy. The remainder may be seen as a photon defect. If uptake is present this may provide a differentiating feature from an adenoma. Hepatobiliary excretion scans show tracer uptake in the majority of cases, and isotope excretion can be observed in 50% of delayed scans. In practice, nuclear scintigraphy has a very limited role both in the detection and tissue characterization of focal liver lesions such as FNH with greater reliance placed upon other imaging techniques.

Sonographically, FNH may have a variable appearance, but the majority of these lesions are well-demarcated lesions that are hyperechoic or isoechoic relative to the surrounding liver. Although a central scar is a common feature, it is not specific to FNH and also it may not be visible on US. The color flow Doppler characteristics mimic the angiographic and macroscopic feature of increased blood flow with a pattern of blood vessels radiating peripherally from a central feeding artery.

On unenhanced CT studies, FNH is typically hypodense or isodense to the liver parenchyma. Its presence can often be inferred by an alteration in the surface contour of the liver and a hypodense central scar. The degree of enhancement following iodinated contrast medium is variable, but they generally rapidly enhance in the arterial and early portal venous phase becoming isodense in the late portal phase (**Fig. 27.10**). Apart from a possible central scar, which will maintain its hypodensity, enhancement of the tumor is uniform throughout these phases. It is this feature and the rapidity at which they occur which may distinguish FNH from cavernous hemangioma where the centripetal pattern of enhancement and 'filling in' is considerably slower to develop. Spontaneous intratumoral hemorrhage and a capsule are not features and if present favor the diagnosis of an adenoma.

On MRI most lesions are isointense or hypointense on T_1-weighted images and show increased signal on T_2. However, some lesions are isointense on both sequences and, as with the isodense tumors on CT, may only be detected by the expansion of the liver surface they create by their mass effect and a central scar if present. Following intravenous gadolinium a rapid intense blush may occur that rapidly fades leaving the tumor close to isointensity in the equilibrium delayed phase of the examination. Delayed and increasing enhancement of the central scar on delayed scans is a characteristic of FNH. It is proposed that this feature is due to the presence of vascularized myxoid tissue in the scar. Fibrolamellar hepatocellular carcinomas and malignant cholangiocellular tumors contain scars but these do not demonstrate this radiologic sign.

Angiographically, FNH is a hypervascular tumor with a centrifugal arterial supply creating a 'spoke-wheel' pattern in the majority of lesions. During the capillary hepatogram phase an intense blush develops with large draining veins visible (**Fig. 27.11**).

Clinical presentation and management

The majority of lesions are discovered incidentally and only approximately 15% result in symptoms. These are often of non-specific abdominal discomfort. Rupture and hemoperitoneum are rare. In the asymptomatic patient it is important to establish the diagnosis by confirming the presence of characteristic imaging features. Image guided biopsy for a histologic diagnosis is reserved for lesions that demonstrate atypical or indeterminate radiologic features. In those rare patients presenting with spontaneous hemorrhage, surgical resection or embolization is indicated. In those patients with non-specific abdominal pain this decision is far more difficult. It must be clear that the patient's symptoms are attributable to this lesion by excluding any other cause and conducting a careful analysis of the risks of morbidity from surgery versus the potential symptomatic benefit to every individual patient.

Nodular regenerative hyperplasia

This is a rare entity that is known by numerous synonyms, including nodular transformation of the liver, non-cirrhotic nodulation, miliary hepatocellular adenomatosis and adenomatous among others, but the current term of nodular regenerative hyperplasia (NRH) is now universally accepted. Autopsy series have shown prevalence as high as 0.6% but only one-third of these cases had clinical features in life potentially attributable to this diagnosis. It has been reported in all age groups with equal sex incidence. NRH is the major cause of non-cirrhotic portal hypertension in the Western world.

Various systemic diseases are associated with NRH including rheumatoid arthritis, Felty syndrome, polyarteritis nodosa, CREST syndrome (calcinosis cutis, Raynaud phenomenon, esophageal hypomobility, sclerodactyly, telangiectasia), subacute bacterial endocarditis, tuberculosis, diabetes, myeloproliferative disorders, lymphomas and after steroid or cytotoxic therapy and in recipients of bone marrow, renal and liver transplants where therapy with azathioprine has been implicated.

Common to all these disorders is a circulatory or vascular disorder and it has been postulated that NRH is a secondary and non-specific adaptation of the liver parenchyma to an alteration in total liver blood flow. This condition may not involve the whole liver and may be accentuated near the porta hepatis and therefore termed partial nodular transformation.

Pathology

Confirming the diagnosis by liver biopsy is difficult and many cases are only diagnosed at surgery or autopsy. The liver is divided into nodules that vary in size between 0.1 and 1 cm, although rarely nodules measuring up to 10 cm have been reported. Histologically the nodules are composed of cytologically normal hepatocytes arranged in abnormal cell plates that are two or more cells thick. The features are of pure liver cell nodularity, enlarging and distorting acini or lobules but not replacing them. Histologically, this disorder can be distinguished from micro-nodular cirrhosis by the absence of fibrous septa between the nodules. Obliterative vascular changes may also be present.

Radiology

The radiologic features are those of portal hypertension with splenomegaly, varices, ascites and variable alteration in the hepatic parenchyma. Nodules may be present on all imaging techniques but the liver parenchyma may remain uniform. Differentiation from cirrhotic portal hypertension may be difficult on imaging appearances alone but venous pressure studies in confirming the hemodynamic profile of presinusoidal portal hypertension with a patent portal vein are important diagnostic criteria.

Clinical presentation and management

Clinical manifestations may be non-specific, including malaise, fatigue and abdominal pain, particularly if it has developed in association with a multisystem disorder. Alternatively it may be related to complications of portal hypertension with ascites and variceal hemorrhage. Synthetic liver function is usually preserved with minimal elevation of the serum aminotransferases, bilirubin and prothrombin time.

Management is dependent on the degree of portal hypertension commencing with medical therapy and local management of the varices, proceeding to shunting and portal decompression in those patients with recurrent variceal hemorrhage if these first-line therapeutic measures fail.

Mesenchymal hamartoma

This lesion probably represents a failure of normal development in utero of the ductal plate. Histologically, there is a mixture of mesodermal and endodermal structures in a loose connective tissue stroma and fluid filled spaces without an endothelial lining. Bile duct, liver cell and angiomatous elements are present and the appearance is of well-differentiated ductal structures surrounded by loose mesenchyme containing fibroblasts. The characteristic natural history of progressive enlargement of the lesion is secondary to degeneration and fluid accumulation within the cystic component. The prominent mesenchymal and cystic components that are visible on histology and radiologic investigations will allow differentiation from FNH and liver cell adenoma.

These lesions are benign and account for approximately 6% of primary tumors presenting in childhood. The majority will present in childhood with two-thirds of patients presenting in the first year of life. Almost all patients will present before the age of 5 years but rarely this may be delayed until adolescence or early adult life. There is a slight male preponderance.

The commonest presentation is with symptoms of progressive abdominal enlargement. Less commonly, infants may present with respiratory depression or peripheral edema from the mass effect of the lesion.

US and CT assessment will demonstrate a well-circumscribed complex cystic lesion with internal septation (**Fig. 27.12**). With contrast enhancement or angiography, the lesion is predominantly avascular but neovascularity is seen in the more solid elements. The MRI appearances depend on whether an individual lesion is predominantly stromal or cystic. The lesions with a fibrotic stroma predominating will appear hypointense relative to the surrounding liver on T_1-weighted images. Alternatively, if the lesion is mainly cystic its major feature will be its hyperintensity on the T_2-weighted images. The fibrous stroma and internal septation are the features that will distinguish this tumor from a simple cyst.

As the natural history of these lesions is of progressive enlargement, treatment is removal by a combination of resection and enucleation. Marsupialization into the peritoneal cavity or transplantation are alternative treatments for unresectable lesions.

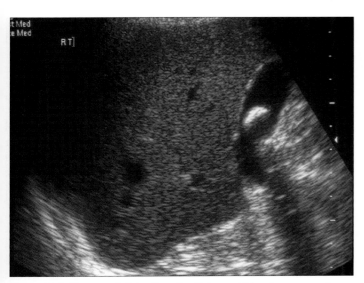

Figure 28.3 Ultrasound detection of gallstones. This ultrasonograph demonstrates a gallstone within the gallbladder lumen. Criteria for diagnosis include: echogenic concretions in the lumen, shadowing of the ultrasonographic beam, and mobility of the concretions with positioning of the patient. (Courtesy of Dr H. Irving.)

secondary bile acid is more lithogenic than its respective primary bile acid, cholate, promoting formation of gallstones and further inhibiting the motility of the gallbladder.

Clinical manifestations of gallstones

Asymptomatic gallstones

Most patients with gallstones are asymptomatic and will remain asymptomatic for several years. Such patients are regularly detected on routine ultrasonography (**Fig. 28.3**). One study of the natural history of truly asymptomatic gallstones indicated that only 20% of these patients will develop symptoms when followed up to 25 years. It has been suggested that the asymptomatic gallstone population is really comprised of two populations: those that will ultimately become symptomatic (usually within the first 5 years of follow-up) and those that never will develop symptoms. The risk of developing symptoms is 1–3%/year for the first 5–10 years, but then drops to 0.1–0.3% with prolonged observation. The risk of developing serious complications from gallstones (acute cholecystitis, cholangitis, pancreatitis, sepsis, gangrenous gallbladder) is low, only about 0.1%/year. In the most comprehensive long-term study of natural history, biliary colic always preceded any serious complication by several months. Given the costs associated with cholecystectomy, the relatively benign natural history, and the fact that biliary colic nearly always precedes more serious complications, prophylactic cholecystectomy is not recommended for asymptomatic patients. However, prophylactic cholecystectomy may be considered in the following circumstances: patients with large ileal resections, patients with known gallstones who will be traveling or working in remote regions of the world, and certain populations or medical conditions that are associated with high rates of complications or cancer (Pima Indians, calcified gallbladder, porcelain gallbladder and gallstones associated with sickle cell disease). One

decision analysis suggested that patients with diabetes mellitus do not benefit from prophylactic cholecystectomy.

In general, most gallstones do not spontaneously dissolve or exit the gallbladder asymptomatically. In the National Cooperative Gallstone Study, 1% of patients experienced spontaneous clearance of gallbladder stones over a period of 2 years while taking placebo. Even this low rate of clearance was questioned as the technique used to detect gallstones was oral cholecystography, which is much less sensitive than the currently recommended method of real-time ultrasonography (98% sensitivity and specificity). In contrast, two recent ultrasonographic studies suggested that one-third of cholesterol gallstones that develop during pregnancy dissolve. The type of stone that is more likely to dissolve is small (<0.5 cm diameter) and composed predominantly of cholesterol. In general, calcified stones, pigment stones and stones that have persisted over several years are not likely to dissolve spontaneously. Gallstones that are symptomatic are not likely to disappear spontaneously.

Symptomatic gallstones

Biliary colic is the most specific symptom of cholelithiasis and is defined as pain that is localized to either the right upper quadrant of the abdomen or epigastrium. It is characterized by a short crescendo period of increasing pain (5–15 min), a plateau of steady pain (15 min to several hours), and a decrescendo period of decreasing pain and resolution of pain (15 min to 2 h). Patients are asymptomatic between attacks of colic. Non-specific symptoms that do not correlate well with gallstones include the following: nausea, vomiting, dyspepsia, diarrhea, weight loss or gain and heartburn. Elderly, diabetic and immunocompromised patients may develop serious complications of gallbladder disease (gangrenous gallbladder, empyema of the gallbladder, perforation of the gallbladder, suppurative cholangitis) and exhibit few or no localizing abdominal complaints or findings on physical examination. In these patients gallbladder disease may present as fever, altered mental status, loss of appetite and weight loss, or sepsis.

The best data that address the natural history after an episode of biliary colic are from the National Cooperative Gallstone Study. Patients entering the trial had a preceding history of biliary colic and were then randomized to receive one of two doses of chenodeoxycholate or placebo. A total of 305 patients were enrolled in the placebo arm and were followed clinically. Patients with frequent attacks of biliary-type pain 12 months before entry into the trial continued to experience frequent attacks of pain. Some developed complicated biliary disease, and many required cholecystectomy. In contrast, those who had infrequent attacks of pain continued to have few attacks, experienced a lower complication rate and had lower rates of cholecystectomy. In general, patients with biliary colic can be expected to continue to experience biliary colic during follow-up. The severity of the attacks is highly variable but may be relatively consistent within a given individual. Patients with frequent, severe episodes may be at greatest risk for complicated gallbladder disease.

Rarely, a large gallstone in the gallbladder will erode through the gallbladder wall into an adjacent viscus (usually duodenum), traverse the bowel, impact at a point of narrowing (usually terminal ileum), and cause bowel obstruction or gastric outlet obstruction (Bouveret syndrome).

Therapeutic options

Medical treatment

Medical treatment for gallstones include oral bile acid therapy with either chenodeoxycholic acid or ursodeoxycholic acid, contact dissolution with methyl-tert-butyl ether (MTBE) or extracorporeal shock-wave lithotripsy. Generally, these forms of treatment are of historical interest only and are seldom, if ever, used today. Small cholesterol gallstones that are newly formed after rapid weight reduction or pregnancy may be particularly amenable to dissolution with oral bile acids. However, high recurrence rates (10%/year for first 5 years) limit long-term effectiveness. The great success and high patient acceptance of laparoscopic cholecystectomy have virtually eliminated the clinical application of oral bile acid dissolution therapy, shock-wave lithotripsy and percutaneous puncture of the gallbladder for MTBE treatment.

Endoscopic sphincterotomy

Endoscopic sphincterotomy is recommended for the treatment of choledocholithiasis and its complications of obstructive jaundice, cholangitis or pancreatitis. Numerous studies of endoscopic sphincterotomy for choledocholithiasis have verified its efficacy at nearly eliminating the risk of subsequent complications of passage of additional bile duct stones. Patients who are reasonable surgical candidates should undergo cholecystectomy, because the risk of acute cholecystitis in patients who have had endoscopic sphincterotomy but whose gallbladder has been left in place is 5–20% during a 3–5 year follow-up. Preoperative endoscopic retrograde cholangiopancreatography (ERCP) and sphincterotomy should be restricted to patients with a high probability of choledocholithiasis such as those with jaundice, abnormal liver tests and ductal dilatation on abdominal ultrasonography. The common duct of patients suspected of having choledocholithiasis can be adequately evaluated by intraoperative cholangiogram at the time of laparoscopic cholecystectomy. Either postoperative ERCP with sphincterotomy or laparoscopic common bile duct (CBD) exploration (when surgical proficiency in this technique is available) is equally safe and efficacious in achieving stone clearance.

Surgery for symptomatic gallstones

A conservative non-interventional approach is only warranted for patients with asymptomatic gallstones. Once gallstones become symptomatic the gallbladder should be removed. Chronic use of analgesics in the treatment of biliary pain is discouraged as it merely masks symptoms and may increase the likelihood that the patient will only present later with more serious complications of the disease. Most clinicians recommend cholecystectomy for symptomatic disease based upon the high likelihood of recurrent symptoms and the risk of developing serious complications once biliary colic has occurred. Diabetic patients may be at particularly high risk for complications as compared with non-diabetics. Complications include severe cholecystitis, gangrenous gallbladder, empyema of the gallbladder and perforated gallbladder. The operative mortality of emergency surgery for complicated gallstone disease in diabetic patients has been reported to be as high as 15–20%, or four to five times higher than that for matched groups of non-diabetic patients.

Elective cholecystectomy is the preferred treatment for symptomatic cholelithiasis. The indications for cholecystectomy include biliary colic, cholecystitis, symptomatic gallbladder polyps, gallstone pancreatitis, symptomatic biliary dyskinesis, calcified gallbladder wall, large gallstones (>2 cm), non-functioning gallbladder and being a chronic typhoid carrier. There are two basic techniques: open laparotomy or laparoscopy. Until the late 1980s, open laparotomy and cholecystectomy were the standard surgical methods against which all other therapies were judged. In 1988, it was shown that the gallbladder could be safely and effectively removed by laparoscopic technique. Since then most surgeons performing cholecystectomy have switched from the open to the laparoscopic technique and several studies have compared results of the two methods. Advantages of laparoscopic cholecystectomy include: short duration of hospital stay, lower hospital cost, early return to home and job, high patient acceptance, and low rate of complications, particularly in certain populations such as morbidly obese patients (**Table 28.1**). Disadvantages include: higher risk of major morbidity when the surgery is done by technically inexperienced surgeons, higher rate of serious bile duct injuries, and potential need to convert an elective cholecystectomy to an urgent cholecystectomy if complications occur. The risk of conversion to open cholecystectomy is increased in patients with acute disease, pancreatitis, bleeding disorders, unusual anatomy and prior abdominal surgeries. Open cholecystectomy may still be the preferred approach for patients with complex gallbladder disease [empyema, infarction, perforation causing generalized peritonitis or subphrenic abscess, biliary-enteric fistula leading to bowel obstruction (gallstone ileus) and bacterial cholangitis]; although at the present time no specific contraindications exist for laparoscopic cholecystectomy other than poor surgical risk factors.

The reported operative mortality rates for diabetics and non-diabetics are shown in **Table 28.2**. Stable diabetics who undergo elective cholecystectomy have no major increase in expected operative mortality. In contrast, diabetics who are poorly controlled and who undergo cholecystectomy for complicated biliary tract disease do experience increased morbidity and mortality. For these reasons, the development of biliary colic in a diabetic patient with gallstones is an indication for early elective cholecystectomy.

Postcholecystectomy syndrome

Approximately 5% of patients will experience persistent or recurrent non-specific symptoms after cholecystectomy. Most commonly patients complain of dyspepsia or upper abdominal pain. The differential diagnosis is extensive and includes recurrent or retained calculi in the cystic or CBD, pancreatitis, cholangitis, papillary stenosis or operative injury to the biliary tree. Once anatomic or mechanical factors have been eliminated it is necessary to consider the possibility of disordered biliary motility (biliary dyskinesis) as the basis for pain. Biliary dyskinesis implies a disorder of the normal contraction of the gallbladder or altered function of the sphincter of Oddi. After removal of the gallbladder, the source of biliary dyskinesis is limited to the sphincter of Oddi. The latter may be responsible for postcholecystectomy syndrome in 5–15% of patients. The diagnosis of sphincter of Oddi dysfunction is dependent upon accurate measurement of the basal pressure of the sphincter via biliary manometry at ERCP. Patients with basal sphincter pressures greater than 40 mmHg can experience relief of their pain after endoscopic sphincterotomy (**Table 28.3**). Additional

Surgical series of laparoscopic cholecystectomy						
Author	Year of study	Patients	Percentage to open	Mortality	Major complications	Bile duct injury
Larson	1992	1963	4.5	0.1	2.1	0.3
Southern Surg Club	1991	1518	4.7	0.07	1.5	0.5
Cuschieri	1991	1236	3.6	0	1.6	0.3
Soper	1992	618	2.9	0	1.6	0.2
Spaw	1991	500	1.8	0	1.0	0
Lillemoe	1992	400	4.0	0	5.0	0.5
Wolfe	1991	381	3.0	0.9	3.4	0
Deziel	1993	77 604	1.2	0.04	0.19	0.59
Wherry	1994	5607	8.08	0.04	0.5	0.57
Russell	1996	15 221				0.25
MacFadyen	1998	114 005	2.16	0.06		0.5
Hannan	1999	24 385		0.23	1.17	
Modified from Soper et al (94) by permission of N Engl J Med.						

Table 28.1 Surgical series of laparoscopic cholecystectomy. Large series confirm low complication rates after laparoscopic cholecystectomy with conversion rates to open cholecystectomy under 5%.

Mortality rates from acute complications of biliary tract disease: effect of diabetes mellitus						
		Mortality rates (%)				
		Diabetes mellitus			No diabetes	
Period	Surgery	No surgery	Total	Surgery	No surgery	Total
1953–1958	31	13	20	10	3	4
1960–1981	7	0	7	2	8	3

Table 28.2 Mortality rates from acute complications of biliary tract disease: effect of diabetes mellitus. Mortality rates from biliary tract disease are consistently higher in patients with diabetes mellitus.

features that support the diagnosis and a response to sphincterotomy are: dilated CBD, abnormal liver tests and prolonged retention of contrast in the biliary system at the time of ERCP. Some patients have postcholecystectomy pain but lack any objective evidence for biliary disease ('type III' sphincter of Oddi dysfunction). In most cases, these patients do not respond to sphincterotomy, suggesting that sphincter function is not related to their symptoms. One group examined these patients for underlying visceral hyperalgesia in response to balloon distention of rectum and duodenum and selectively reproduced symptoms with duodenal distention. They also found that these patients were characterized by somatization, depression, obsessive-compulsive behavior and anxiety.

Acute cholecystitis

Cholecystitis may or may not be associated with the presence of gallstones. Calculous cholecystitis occurs in over 90% of cases

Effectiveness of endoscopic sphincterotomy for sphincter of Oddi dysfunction								
	SO pressure <40 mmHg					SO pressure >40 mmHg		
Patient group				Outcome (%)				
	n	Good	Fair	Poor	n	Good	Fair	Poor
Sham	12	31	18	67	12	15	10	75
ES								
ES	12	7	12	58	11	80	11	9
	(P = NS)				(P <0.05)*			

Table 28.3 Effectiveness of endoscopic sphincterotomy for sphincter of Oddi dysfunction. Sphincter of Oddi (SO) pressures >40 mmHg identify the patients most likely to benefit from endoscopic (ES) sphincterotomy.

and implies gallbladder inflammation in the presence of gall-stones. The presence of gallstones may cause persistent obstruction of the gallbladder outlet because of impaction in the neck of the gallbladder, Hartmann's pouch, or cystic duct. These events lead to the release of a number of potential inflammatory mediators such as prostaglandins, cholesterol-supersaturated bile, lysolecithin and phospholipase A. The increase in intra-luminal pressure also causes gallbladder distention that leads to wall edema and may compromise venous and lymphatic drainage resulting in ischemia and necrosis of the gallbladder. Although bile is sterile, acute cholecystitis may lead to secondary infection with positive bile cultures in 20–75% of patients. The most common organisms isolated from cultures of gallbladder bile are *Escherichia coli*, *Klebsiella* and *Enterococccus*. Clinical features of calculous cholecystitis include fever, right upper quadrant abdominal pain with tenderness to palpation that may radiate to the back, right scapula or right clavicular area, leukocytosis and ultrasonographic images that demonstrate cholelithiasis. Additional ultrasonographic features of cholecystitis may include thickening of the wall of the gallbladder and pericholecystic fluid.

Gallbladder sludge refers to gallbladder mucin with entrapment of particulate matter nucleated from bile (**Fig. 28.4**). Sludge formation occurs within the gallbladder when gallbladder emptying is slow and incomplete. It is often associated with prolonged fasting or lack of stimulation of intestinal release of cholecystokinin. Although sludge is a reversible stage in gallstone pathogenesis, gallstones may develop, leading to symptomatic biliary tract disease. Sludge is a risk factor for gallstones, but it may be evacuated from the gallbladder and gallstone formation may be prevented.

Acalculous cholecystitis is inflammation of the gallbladder in the absence of gallstones and represents 2–12% of cases of proven acute cholecystitis. Although the pathogenesis is unknown, multiple factors such as gallbladder stasis, paresis and ischemia may play a role. Acalculous cholecystitis is more likely to occur in critically ill patients and these patients tend to have higher morbidity and mortality rates. Risk factors for acute acalculous cholecystitis include: prior surgical procedure (non-biliary), male gender, severe trauma, burns, TPN, multiorgan failure, diabetes mellitus, acute renal failure, immunocompromised host (AIDS, cancer chemotherapy, leukemia/lymphoma, uremia) and old age.

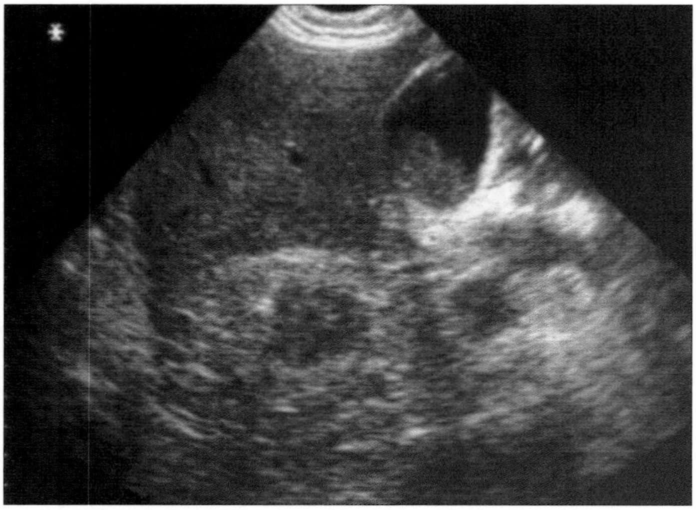

Diagnosis

Murphy's sign, which is also known as 'inspiratory arrest', is a valuable sign of acute cholecystitis. The patient is asked to take a deep inspiration while the examining fingers are held under the liver border, usually around the tip of ninth rib where the gallbladder may descend upon them. Inspiration is arrested in midcycle by painful contact with the fingers. Carcinoma of the gallbladder may produce a similar sign when it has invaded through the gallbladder wall involving the serosa or visceral peritoneum overlying the gallbladder.

One may be nearly certain of the diagnosis in the appropriate clinical situation when the following are present: leukocytosis, fever and right upper quadrant tenderness to palpation. In the absence of the latter findings, one must rely upon imperfect confirmatory radiologic studies [ultrasonography, dimethyl iminodiacetic acid (HIDA)-scintigraphy]. Findings on ultrasono-graphy that support the diagnosis of cholecystitis are: a thickened edematous gallbladder wall and a pericholecystic fluid col-lection. Although patients with acalculous cholecystitis may have sludge within the gallbladder lumen, sludge alone may not be pathologic. Sludge may be present in the absence of cholecystitis and absent in the presence of cholecystitis. A positive scan by HIDA-scintigraphy for acute cholecystitis is characterized by normal uptake and clearance of HIDA by the liver, rapid excretion into the biliary system, visualization of the extrahepatic bile ducts, and appearance of HIDA in the intestine, but no visualization of the gallbladder. This finding implies cystic duct obstruction from either inflammation or an impacted stone. False-positive scans may occur in patients on TPN, alcoholics, or those who have had a prolonged fast or who have just eaten. In addition, in acalculous cholecystitis, the cystic duct may be patent and allow entry of radionuclide into the gallbladder lumen, resulting in a false-negative scan. Positive findings on ultrasonography or HIDA-scintigraphy need to be assessed carefully before proceeding to cholecystectomy.

Clinical management

The immediate management of acute cholecystitis consists of fasting, fluid and electrolyte correction and pain management. Definitive therapy is cholecystectomy although certain peri-operative medical complications increase morbidity and mortality (**Table 28.4**). Empiric antibiotic coverage is prescribed for patients presenting with systemic signs such as high fever, leukocytosis, tachycardia or hypotension; or if there is no clinical improve-ment after 12 h of conservative management. About 20% of patients will require emergent surgery for complications such as peritonitis or perforation. For the remaining patients, early laparoscopic surgery (within 48–72 h of presentation) has been shown to be superior to delayed surgery (6–12 weeks after the attack) due to an easier dissection, reduced hospital stay and reduced rates of complications of recurrent gallstone disease. However, there may be a slightly increased risk of gallstone and bile spillage, with the subsequent risk of abscess formation with early laparoscopic surgery.

Mirizzi syndrome is a clinical syndrome of cholecystitis and jaundice that develops when a stone impacts in Hartmann's

Figure 28.4 Biliary sludge. This ultrasonograph demonstrates 'sludge' within the gallbladder lumen. In contrast to the features of cholelithiasis, sludge is echogenic and mobile but fails to cast an ultrasonographic shadow. (Courtesy of Dr H Irving.)

Factors independently associated with operative mortality after cholecystectomy			
Characteristic	Number of patients (Total = 29 271)	Number of deaths (Total = 180)	Adjusted odds ratio (95% Conf. interval)
Emergent surgery	9023	141	3.2 (2.0–5.1)
Acute myocardial infarction	63	15	14.1 (7.0–28.0)
Cardiac arrhythmia	1636	59	7.4 (1.5–3.7)
Pneumonia	252	15	5.2 (3.2–8.3)
Renal failure	190	24	8.8 (5.2–15.0)
Cancer	420	29	5.2 (3.2–8.3)
Laparoscopic surgery (versus open surgery)	14 131	21	0.22 (0.13–0.37)

Table 28.4 Factors independently associated with operative mortality after cholecystectomy.

pouch. The resulting inflammation compresses and obstructs the common hepatic duct or CBD. Obstruction of the bile duct further promotes the development of cholangitis. The stenosis of the bile duct can mimic a malignant stricture. Acute cholecystitis is often associated with mildly abnormal liver tests, but a serum bilirubin greater than 85 μmol/L (5 mg/dL) strongly suggests CBD obstruction. If untreated, the stone may erode into the CBD and create a biliobiliary fistula. Management involves drainage of the biliary system, antibiotic therapy, intravenous fluids and cholecystectomy.

Acute cholangitis

Acute cholangitis results from impaction of a gallstone in the bile duct and ascending infection behind the obstruction. Right upper quadrant pain, jaundice and fever (with chills and rigors) occurring together constitute the Charcot triad, which indicates acute cholangitis. The triad occurs in 70% of cases of acute cholangitis and is the most common complication of choledo-cholithiasis. Hypotension and mental confusion secondary to sepsis in a patient with Charcot triad constitutes the Raynold pentad. Only 10% of patients with acute suppurative cholangitis present with all five of these features. The most common cause of cholangitis in the USA is choledocholithiasis secondary to cholelithiasis. Primary bile duct stones are more common in oriental countries where oriental cholangiohepatitis is endemic. Other causes of cholangitis include: obstructing primary tumors of the ampulla, bile ducts or pancreas; primary sclerosing cholangitis, and post procedural effects (e.g. after ERCP). Relatively rare causes include: hemobilia, parasites and hereditary abnormalities of the biliary tree.

Diagnosis

The incidence of bile duct stones increases with increasing age and is more likely to occur in patients with multiple gallstones. The diagnosis of CBD stones is suggested by biliary colic, abnormal liver tests, pale stools, dark urine and dilatation of the bile duct on ultrasonography or CT scanning. However, CBD stones may be present without dilatation of the CBD or abnormal liver tests. The diagnosis is established by cholangiography. Magnetic resonance cholangiopancreatography (MRCP) is accurate for detecting choledocholithiasis and delineating biliary anatomy, but the use of this test is probably of limited value in acute cholangitis. The preferred diagnostic test is ERCP, because the retained stone may also be easily treated with a sphincterotomy.

Clinical management

Therapy for cholangitis should be individualized because of the wide spectrum of severity of illness. Antibiotic therapy and intravenous hydration should be initiated promptly on an empiric basis. Antibiotics are tailored to the types of organisms associated with acute cholangitis: *Escherichia coli*, *Klebsiella pneumoniae*, *Streptococcus faecalis*, *Pseudomonas aeruginosa* and *Bacteroides fragilis*. In the elderly or immunocompromised patient, anaerobic coverage is necessary since these patients are at increased risk for developing suppurative cholangitis. Effective antibiotic regimens include: ampicillin (or amoxicillin) plus an aminoglycoside, piperacillin alone, third generation cephalosporin or fluoroquinolones. In cases where bacteroides is suspected, the addition of metronidazole is recommended. Sulfonamides are not recommended for acute cholangitis. It is important to remember that antibiotics are viewed as adjuncts to the primary therapy, CBD drainage.

About 70% of patients will respond with a stabilization of their clinical course. Patients failing to respond to empiric therapy within 24 h should be considered for immediate biliary decompression since mortality rates approach 100% in this subgroup of patients without biliary drainage. The latter may be accomplished by endoscopic sphincterotomy with removal of the impacted stone, endoscopic placement of a biliary stent or nasobiliary drainage tube, percutaneous transhepatic drainage (radiology), or cholecystectomy plus CBD exploration or placement of T-tube. The choice of each of these modalities depends upon the expertise of the available specialists, the condition of the patient and estimated operative risk. In general, either endoscopic or surgical treatment is recommended. Radiologic placement of drainage catheters is usually restricted to the circumstance where endoscopy is unsuccessful. Several trials have examined the role of urgent endoscopy versus early surgery and have demonstrated that ERCP done early in the course of acute cholangitis is safe and effective in controlling biliary tract sepsis (**Tables 28.5** and **28.6**). It has not yet been determined whether the outcome is superior with the combination of early ERCP combined with sphincterotomy, CBD stone extraction

Severe acute cholangitis: mortality			
Cause	Surgery group (n = 41)	Endoscopic drainage group (n = 41)	
Heart failure (n)	2	0	
Bronchopneumonia (n)	2	2	
Renal failure (n)	1	0	
Multiorgan failure (n)	4	2	
Sepsis (n)	3	0	
Cerebellar hemorrhage (n)	1	0	
Total	13	4	P <0.03

Table 28.5 Severe acute cholangitis: mortality. Mortality in patients with severe acute cholangitis: a randomized trial comparing urgent biliary tract surgery to endoscopic cholangiography and drainage. This randomized study confirmed lower mortality rates with endoscopic therapy.

Severe acute cholangitis: morbidity			
Complication	Surgery group (n = 41)	Endoscopic drainage group (n = 41)	
Heart failure (n)	1	3	
Bronchopneumonia (n)	15	7	
Wound dehiscence (n)	1	0	
Wound infection (n)	7	1	
Gastrointestinal bleeding (n)	2	0	
Renal dysfunction (n)	11	7	
Bleeding after papillotomy (n)	0	1	
Disseminated intravascular coagulopathy (n)	2	0	
Total	39	19	P <0.05

Table 28.6 Severe acute cholangitis: morbidity. Morbid complications in patients with severe acute cholangitis: a randomized trial comparing urgent biliary tract surgery to endoscopic cholangiography and drainage. This randomized study confirmed lower complication rates with endoscopic therapy.

and drainage of the biliary system followed by elective laparoscopic cholecystectomy as compared with urgent cholecystectomy, CBD exploration and T-tube placement. There also have been no critical evaluations of costs associated with each of these two approaches.

Pancreatitis and gallbladder carcinoma
Additional complications of CBD stones include obstructive jaundice and gallstone pancreatitis. Endoscopic retrograde cholangiopancreatography with sphincterotomy is recommended for removal of CBD stones, even in the setting of active gallstone pancreatitis. If complete stone extraction is not possible due to medical, technical or anatomic reasons, then palliative placement of biliary and/or pancreatic stents is indicated to relieve the intraductal pressure and prevent recurrent obstruction. Elective cholecystectomy, either open or laparoscopic, is indicated after the first episode of gallstone pancreatitis to prevent future recurrence of pancreatitis.

Carcinoma of the gallbladder is the most common malignant lesion of the biliary tract and the fifth most common among malignant neoplasms of the digestive tract. Approximately 0.1–3% of gallbladders removed for symptomatic cholelithiasis or cholecystitis, especially in the elderly, contain adenocarcinoma. Pima Indians, who have an extremely high prevalence of gallstones, also have the highest rate of gallbladder cancer and mortality in the USA. Calcified (porcelain) gallbladders pose an extreme risk for development of carcinoma, as high as 25%. Gallbladder polyps are another predisposing factor for gallbladder neoplasm. In a retrospective series of 100 patients, 88% of polyps larger than 10 mm were malignant polyps. Therefore patients with polyps >10 mm should undergo elective cholecystectomy even in the absence of symptoms.

CYSTIC DISEASES OF THE LIVER

The fibrocystic diseases of the liver are autosomal-dominant polycystic disease, solitary hepatic cysts, congenital hepatic fibrosis, choledochal cysts and Caroli disease. Histopathologically they are characterized by ectasia of intrahepatic bile ducts, cysts of biliary epithelial cell origin, portal fibrosis and persistence or lack of remodeling of the embryonic ductal plate (ductal plate malformation). The clinical spectrum ranges from an asymptomatic state to cholangitis or manifestations of liver failure. Polycystic liver disease is highlighted since there have been many recent advances in its natural history, genetics and treatment.

Polycystic liver disease
Classification
Human polycystic liver disease is due to mutations in four distinct genes and is one of the most common inherited disorders involving the liver (**Table 28.7**). Mutations in two of these genes, *PKD1* and *PKD2*, are associated with autosomal dominant polycystic kidney disease (AD-PKD). In AD-PKD, renal cystic disease tends to dominate the clinical picture. Hepatic cysts are the most common extrarenal manifestation. *PKD1* mutations account for 85–90% of cases of AD-PKD; nearly all of the remaining 10–15% are due to mutations in *PKD2*. The possibility of a 'PKD3' gene has been proposed since families with AD-PKD, unlinked to *PKD1* or *PKD2*, have been occasionally reported in the literature. Patients with mutations in *PKD2* tend to have later-onset disease and greater life expectancy compared to patients with mutations in *PKD1*. Mutations in a third gene, *PRKCSH*, and a recently identified fourth gene, *SEC63*, cause the comparatively rare, isolated form of autosomal dominant polycystic liver disease (PCLD). The latter patients with PCLD are distinguished from AD-PKD patients by lack of renal cystic disease.

Natural history
The natural history of polycystic liver disease, regardless of etiologic mutation, is strikingly similar. The prevalence and number of hepatic cysts in patients with AD-PKD increase with

Genetic and phenotypic classification of polycystic disease

Inheritance	Gene	Protein	Disease expression
Autosomal dominant (adults)[1]			
AD-PKD 1	PKD1	polycystin-1	Liver and kidney
AD-PKD 2	PKD2	polycystin-2	Liver and kidney
PCLD 1[2]	PRKCSH	hepatocystin	Liver
PCLD 2[2]	SEC63	sec63	Liver
Autosomal recessive (pediatrics)			
AR-PKD	PKHD1	fibrocystin	Kidney[3]

AD-PKD, autosomal dominant polycystic kidney disease; PCLD, isolated polycystic liver disease; AR-PKD, autosomal recessive polycystic disease.
[1]Autosomal dominant forms of polycystic disease tend to present clinically in late adolescence or adult life. In contrast, autosomal recessive polycystic kidney disease is a serious renal disease in pediatric populations.
[2]The SEC63 gene mutations for PCLD have only recently been described and the designations of PCLD 1 and PCLD 2 not yet established.
[3]The most common hepatic association of AR-PKD is congenital hepatic fibrosis.

Table 28.7 Genetic and phenotypic classification of polycystic disease.

increasing age, female gender, severity of renal cystic disease and severity of renal dysfunction (**Fig. 28.5**). By age 60 nearly 80% of AD-PKD patients have hepatic cysts. While men and women have equal lifetime risk to develop hepatic cysts, women experience greater numbers and larger cysts. Severe hepatic cystic disease correlates with both the numbers of pregnancies and the use of exogenous female steroid hormones. One longitudinal study of anovulatory women with AD-PKD treated with hormone replacement suggested that estrogens selectively increase the severity of hepatic cystic disease (**Fig. 28.6**). Female tendency toward more extensive hepatic cystic disease has also been noted in PCLD.

Genetics (Table 28.7)

The 14.1 kb *PKD1* gene has been cloned and sequenced and the resultant protein of 4304 amino acids, polycystin-1 (PC-1), has been characterized. There are over 230 mutations of the *PKD1* gene associated with disease which are evenly dispersed without evidence for clustering. However, some studies have suggested that the type or position of mutation may predict intracranial aneurysms. Furthermore, a study of 80 families with AD-PKD due to mutations in *PKD1* indicated that the location of the mutation in the 5′ end of the gene predicted more rapid progression to, and greater severity of, end-stage renal disease, but more severe disease has also been attributed to mutations within the N-terminus. Any correlation between the type or position of the mutation and variation in hepatic cystic disease has not been demonstrated.

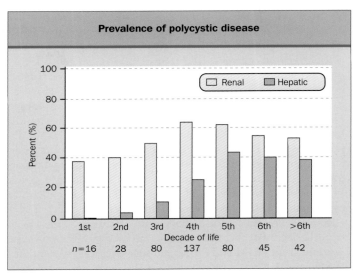

Figure 28.5 Prevalence of polycystic disease. The frequency of renal and hepatic cysts is displayed by age in a population at risk for autosomal dominant polycystic kidney disease (AD-PKD). Cysts were detected by real-time ultrasonography. The population at risk included 239 patients with AD-PKD and 189 unaffected family members. The number of subjects in each decade is indicated at the bottom.

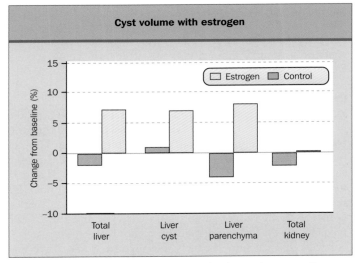

Figure 28.6 Cyst volume: postmenopausal estrogen increases liver volume. Percentage of volume change in liver and kidney at the end of 1 year of follow-up is shown. Estrogen-treated patients are depicted by the green bar and non-treated controls as an orange bar.

The *PKD2* gene is smaller than *PKD1* (only 5.3 kb) and codes for a 968 amino acid protein, polycystin-2 (PC-2). There are over 60 identified mutations of *PKD2* and, like the mutations of *PKD1*, they are evenly dispersed throughout the gene without clustering at any one position. The severity of disease may vary with site of mutation in *PKD2* and the functional consequence on the resultant PC-2 protein. The relationship of the site of mutation of *PKD2* to phenotypic expression of polycystic disease is under study but no clear relationships have yet been reproducibly defined.

The first demonstration that PCLD was genetically distinct from *PDK1* and *PKD2* was from phenotypic and genetic studies of three generations of a family affected by polycystic liver disease without renal cysts. It was later determined that PCLD was due to mutations in protein kinase C substrate 80K-H gene (*PRKCSH*) on chromosome 19p13. *PRKCSH* encodes for hepatocystin. Mutations that affect mRNA splicing or truncate hepatocystin have been reported in PCLD families. However, the distribution of mutations within the gene and the genotype–phenotype relationships remain speculative. Further studies indicated that the *PRKCSH* locus was probably not responsible for all cases of PCLD, and suggested the presence of a second PCLD gene. Davila studied 10 families by linkage analysis and identified a locus on chromosome 6q as containing a second PCLD gene. An analysis of genes in that region identified mutations in *SEC63* as causing PCLD in eight families. *SEC63* encodes a protein in the endoplasmic reticulum. The authors hypothesized that the protein could interact with the polycystin proteins from *PKD1* and *PKD2* and suggested that disruption of this interaction could be relevant for the development of cystic disease.

Characteristics of liver cyst epithelium
Liver cysts arise from intrahepatic bile duct epithelial cells. The bile duct epithelium normally comprises 2–4% of the liver cell mass and serves to dilute and alkalinize bile in a hormone-dependent fashion. Secretin stimulates cyclic adenosine monophosphate (cAMP)-dependent Cl^- and HCO_3^- secretion by biliary epithelia. Liver cyst epithelial cells retain differentiated secretory function as AD-PKD liver cysts secrete fluid and generate a positive luminal pressure after intravenous secretin administration.

Characteristics of polycystin-1 and polycystin-2
PC-1 is a large (around 460 kDa) integral membrane protein with a prominent extracellular NH2-terminal domain, 11 putative transmembrane domains, and a small intracellular COOH-terminal domain. PC-1 might regulate Ca^{2+} or G-protein signaling and may interact with PC-2. PC-2 is a 110 kDa integral membrane protein with intracellular NH2- and COOH-terminal tails. The transmembrane domains share marked homology with voltage-gated cation channels and the COOH terminus has an EF-hand domain, a motif often expressed in voltage-gated calcium channels. Biophysical studies have confirmed that PC-2 functions as a cation channel. Together, the PC-1 and PC-2 complex is predicted to form a signal transduction unit that translates extracellular cues into intracellular information. Additional studies demonstrated that PC-1 and PC-2 form a mechanotransduction complex co-localized to the primary cilium of epithelial cells. Interestingly, two other proteins that give rise to epithelial cysts, polaris and cystin, also localize to the primary cilium of epithelial cells. Furthermore, fibrocystin, the protein linked to autosomal recessive PKD (ARPKD), is localized to the primary cilium of biliary epithelia and reduction of fibrocystin expression leads to loss of ciliary structure.

Contributory events in cyst expansion
Proliferating epithelial cells form nascent cysts that detach from the original duct to form autonomous structures that no longer communicate directly with the duct. Expansion of these autonomous cysts can be promoted by luminal fluid secretion, remodeling of the underlying matrix and neovascularization.

Normal intrahepatic bile duct cells function as both absorptive and secretory epithelium where net absorption is favored under basal conditions. Secretion is triggered by hormonal signaling, primarily via secretin. Retaining characteristics of intrahepatic bile duct epithelial cells, human hepatic cysts generate a positive intraluminal pressure under basal conditions and have increased rates of fluid secretion following intravenous administration of secretin. For cyst epithelium to invade the surrounding tissues, the extracellular matrix must be remodeled. Matrix remodeling occurs through the secretion of metalloproteases into the surrounding matrix, vascularization for metabolic support, and production and secretion of a rich cocktail of cytokines and growth factors.

Molecular diagnostics
The molecular diagnostic approaches to AD-PKD have advanced considerably with the availability of direct gene sequencing (**Table 28.8**). Using commercially-available methods, pathologic mutations are detected in 44–76% of families with mutations of *PKD1* and 75% of families with mutations of *PKD2*.

Molecular genetic testing is relatively new and consensus guidelines are lacking. Ultrasonography is a reasonable screening tool in adults (**Fig. 28.7**). In young (age < 30 years), presymptomatic individuals at risk of AD-PKD, molecular genetic testing may offer a number of advantages over other approaches. In this group, ultrasonography may lack sensitivity and linkage analysis is impractical. The identification of a *PKD1* or *PKD2* mutations could affect family planning or choice of future diagnostic studies. Discovery of AD-PKD mutations may also encourage regular blood pressure monitoring and screening for associated conditions such as cerebral aneurysms or mitral valve prolapse. Genetic testing may also have a role in the evaluation of young family members being considered as living donors for renal transplantation to another family member with renal failure from AD-PKD. Clarifying the mutation status as negative in such potential donors would reduce future risks to both the donor and the recipient.

Clinical genetic testing for PCLD is also available in Europe and includes genetic sequencing of *PRKCSH*. Clinical testing for *SEC63* mutations will likely be available soon. Because the sensitivity of ultrasonography in PCLD is undefined, use of *PRKCSH* testing (and ultimately *SEC63* testing also) to identify presymptomatic patients at risk of the disease, may have even more relevance than in AD-PKD. While genetic testing results may not immediately alter the management of a PCLD-affected patient, the ability to screen other asymptomatic, at-risk family members (and potential transplant donors) for mutations is important for patient care. As patients are frequently concerned about the risks to their offspring, formal genetic counseling is recommended even when the mutation status is unknown.

Clinical features
Patients with small (<2 cm) or few hepatic cysts tend to be clinically asymptomatic. In contrast, patients who develop massive hepatic cystic disease, based upon a definition for massive as a total liver cyst:parenchymal volume ratio >1, become symptomatic with abdominal pain or discomfort, early postprandial fullness, or shortness of breath. Rarely, patients can experience complications of advanced liver disease such as portal hypertension with variceal hemorrhage. The consequences of

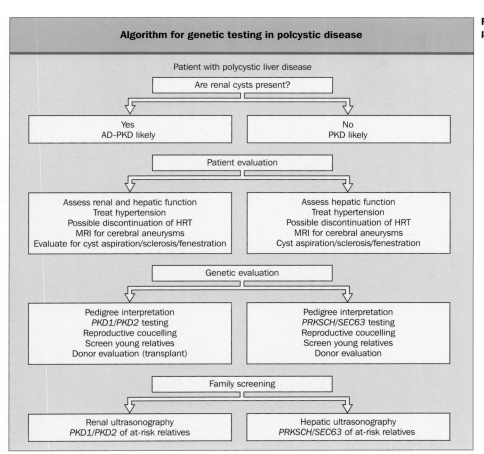

Figure 28.7 Algorithm for genetic testing in polycystic disease.

Algorithm for genetic testing in polcystic disease

Patient with polycystic liver disease

Are renal cysts present?

Yes
AD-PKD likely

No
PKD likely

Patient evaluation

Assess renal and hepatic function
Treat hypertension
Possible discontinuation of HRT
MRI for cerebral aneurysms
Evaluate for cyst aspiration/sclerosis/fenestration

Assess hepatic function
Treat hypertension
Possible discontinuation of HRT
MRI for cerebral aneurysms
Cyst aspiration/sclerosis/fenestration

Genetic evaluation

Pedigree interpretation
PKD1/PKD2 testing
Reproductive coucelling
Screen young relatives
Donor evaluation (transplant)

Pedigree interpretation
PRKSCH/SEC63 testing
Reproductive coucelling
Screen young relatives
Donor evaluation

Family screening

Renal ultrasonography
PKD1/PKD2 of at-risk relatives

Hepatic ultrasonography
PRKSCH/SEC63 of at-risk relatives

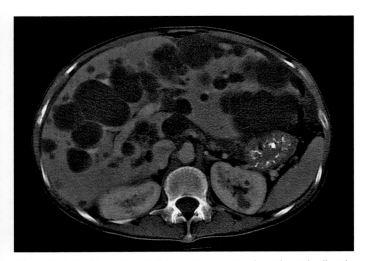

Figure 28.8 Cysts on CT. Multiple cysts are seen throughout the liver in a patient with polycystic liver disease. (Courtesy of Dr H. Irving.)

progressive AD-PKD include renal failure, requirement for hemodialysis and renal transplantation. Dialysis, in particular, is thought to increase the risk for hepatic complications. A single center reported that 21% of polycystic patients on dialysis experienced hepatic complications, mainly hepatic cyst infection, hemorrhage or cyst adenocarcinoma, a finding that was not confirmed in a subsequent report by a different center.

Typically, liver parenchymal volume is preserved despite extensive hepatic cystic disease and extraordinary distortion of the hepatic architecture. The only blood test abnormality is a modest elevation of γ-glutamyltransferase, which correlates with hepatic cyst burden. Rarely, a patient with polycystic liver disease will experience hepatic decompensation and variceal hemorrhage, ascites or encephalopathy.

The most common, clinically-relevant complications arising in hepatic cysts are intracystic hemorrhage, infection or post-traumatic rupture (**Table 28.9**). Cyst adenocarcinoma, biliary obstruction, Budd-Chiari syndrome or hepatic failure is rarely reported. Associated conditions include mitral valve prolapse, diverticulosis, inguinal hernia and cerebral aneurysm.

Therapy
Medical treatment
There are no effective medical therapies for polycystic liver disease. Somatostatin analogs, which block the effects of secretin, failed to demonstrate any significant effect on hepatic cyst growth or size. As noted above, hepatic cystic disease, but not renal cystic disease, worsens under the influence of female gender, pregnancy or use of exogenous female steroid hormones. These observations suggest that women with polycystic livers should avoid estrogen replacement therapy. However, proof that avoidance of estrogen effectively alters the course of hepatic cystic disease is lacking. The clinician must individualize hormonal replacement therapy in polycystic patients by weighing the

Complications of polycystic liver disease			
Classification	*Specific type*	*Diagnostic tests*	*Treatment*
Arising within cyst			
	Infection	MRI, In[111] WBC scan	Fluoroquinolones Drainage
	Hemorrhage	CT or MRI	Pain control Drainage (rare)
	Carcinoma	CT or MRI Aspiration cytology	Surgery
Compression by cyst			
	Biliary obstruction	ERCP	Stent placement Cyst decompression
	Venous obstruction		
	– Hepatic	Hepatic venography	Cyst decompression Resection Transplantation
	– Portal	MRI/MRA Mesenteric angiography	Cyst decompression Resection Transplantation
Hepatic dysfunction	Portal hypertension	Endoscopy (varices) US/CT/MRI	Band ligation Cyst decompression Resection Transplantation
	Hepatic failure	Exceedingly rare Look for other cause	Transplantation
CT, computed tomography; ERCP, endoscopic retrograde cholangiopancreatography; In-WBC scan, Indium-labeled white blood cell scan; MRI, magnetic resonance imaging; US, ultrasonography.			

Table 28.8 Complications of polycystic liver disease.

potentially deleterious effect on hepatic cystic disease against other potential benefits and risks.

Radiologic cyst aspiration and sclerosis

Symptomatic patients with one or a few dominant cysts may be considered for cyst aspiration and sclerosis. Most patients with polycystic disease have too many cysts or the cysts are of insufficient size to warrant this approach. Cyst sclerotherapy requires ultrasonographic or computed tomography (CT) guided percutaneous puncture of the targeted cyst and placement of an intracystic drainage catheter. Success in obliterating individual cysts in polycystic patients is approximately 70–90%.

Cyst fenestration

Cyst fenestration is a common surgical approach to symptomatic, massive hepatic cystic disease. Two approaches have been used: open laparotomy and, more recently, laparoscopy. Several series of open laparotomy, encompassing large numbers of patients, indicate that this approach results in general amelioration of symptoms. However, open laparotomy is associated with prolonged hospitalizations, morbidity i.e. bleeding, infection, bile leak, ascites (0–50%), and even mortality (<1%). Because it is less invasive, laparoscopic cyst fenestration is gaining increasing acceptance as an alternative surgical technique (**Fig. 28.8**). The advantages of laparoscopic surgery include: less morbidity,

reduced hospital stay and the potential for outpatient surgical management. One recent review, totaling 40 cases, indicated that symptoms recurred in about half necessitating repeat laparoscopic cyst fenestration. Although there were no deaths, surgical conversion to open surgical cyst fenestration occurred in 10% of cases and 35% of patients experienced complications.

Liver resection

One center reported their experience with partial liver resection in the management of 31 patients with highly symptomatic, massive hepatic polycystic disease. Patients ages ranged from 34 to 69, the gender ratio (M:F) was 3:28, and renal function varied from normal to dialysis-dependent. Nearly all patients experienced significant relief from symptoms and sustained reduction in symptoms was common (>95%). However, over 50% of the patients experienced significant perioperative morbidity and there was one perioperative death (due to rupture of an intracranial aneurysm). Therefore, most surgeons reserve hepatic resection for those cases that are refractory to cyst decompression.

Liver transplantation

Polycystic liver patients with symptoms (e.g. severe abdominal pain or severe weight loss due to early satiety) refractory to other treatments or symptomatic hepatic cystic disease associated with end-stage renal cystic disease may be considered for

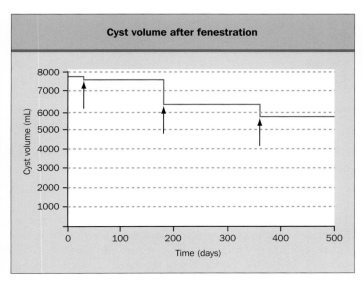

Figure 28.9 Cyst volume after fenestration. The reduction in liver volume achieved by sequential laparoscopic cyst fenestration in a single patient is shown. Initial liver volume was 7710 mL, and the final volume after three procedures (arrows indicates the days of laparoscopic cyst decompression) was 5677 mL.

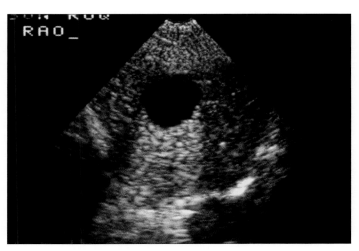

Figure 28.10 Solitary hepatic cyst. Ultrasonography of a solitary cyst in the right lobe of the liver. (Courtesy of Dr H. Irving.)

liver or combined liver-kidney transplantation. Rare indications for hepatic transplantation include variceal hemorrhage, ascites, obstruction of hepatic venous outflow (Budd-Chiari equivalent), or biliary tract obstruction by extensive cystic disease not amenable to other interventions. Survival at 1, 3 and 5 years for patients undergoing isolated hepatic transplantation (n = 128) are 78.1, 71.7 and 68.7%, respectively. Survival at 1, 3 and 5 years for patients undergoing combined liver-kidney transplantation (n = 78) are 79.5, 75.5 and 75.5%, respectively. The genetic basis of polycystic liver disease warrants caution with respect to living donor liver transplantation.

Solitary hepatic cyst
Characteristics
Solitary hepatic cysts are relatively common, usually asymptomatic, and most often are discovered incidentally during the evaluation of a wide variety of abdominal symptoms or disorders. The exact prevalence of solitary hepatic cysts for the US population is unknown, but the female:male ratio is approximately 4:1. A recent Taiwanese study used ultrasonography in a large-scale community-based screening program for simple hepatic cysts to explore the age- and sex-specific prevalence, and in a hospital-based study to record the size of simple hepatic cysts. A total of 3600 subjects in eight communities underwent screening ultrasonography, and 156 simple hepatic cysts were detected in 132 study subjects. The overall prevalence was, therefore, 3.6%. The prevalence increased with age, ranging from 0.8% below age 40 to 7.8% in subjects over 60 years of age. The size of 219 hepatic cysts in 167 hospitalized patients were as follows: 53% had diameters between 1 and 3 cm, and only 7% were larger than 5 cm. Cysts occurred more commonly in the right lobe and were twice as common in women. All of these cysts were asymptomatic and none of the patients suffered clinical consequences (**Fig. 28.9**).

Treatment
Asymptomatic solitary hepatic cysts are best managed conservatively. The preferred treatment of symptomatic cysts is ultrasound- or CT-guided percutaneous cyst aspiration followed by alcohol (or doxycycline) sclerotherapy. This approach is more than 90% effective in controlling symptoms and ablating the cyst cavity. The recurrence rate after successful ablation is only 5–15%. If the radiologically guided, percutaneous approach is ineffective or unavailable, treatment may include either laparoscopic or open surgical cyst fenestration. The laparoscopic approach is increasingly utilized for anatomically accessible cysts and greater than 90% efficacy is reported.

Congenital hepatic fibrosis
Characteristics
Congenital hepatic fibrosis is an uncommon, autosomal-recessive, inherited disorder that is most often associated with autosomal recessive polycystic kidney disease (ARPKD). Mutations responsible for ARPKD, and presumably congenital hepatic fibrosis, arise in the *PKDH 1* gene which encodes the protein fibrocystin (Table 28.7). Other clinical associations of congenital hepatic fibrosis include renal dysplasia, nephronophthisis, Meckel-Gruber syndrome, Ivemark syndrome, Jeune syndrome, vaginal atresia and tuberous sclerosis. Congenital hepatic fibrosis can also coexist with other fibrocystic liver diseases such as Caroli disease and choledochal cyst. The histopathologic features may vary, but in nearly all cases there is fibrous enlargement of the portal tracts, which contain abnormally shaped bile ducts. Congenital hepatic fibrosis typically involves all lobes of the liver equally, but on occasion one lobe of the liver may be preferentially affected. Von Meyenburg complexes (VMCs), also referred to as bile duct microhamartomas, are dilated, ectatic, intra- and interlobular bile ducts embedded in a fibrous stroma, and occur in nearly all patients with congenital hepatic fibrosis (VMCs are also commonly found in both ADPKD and Caroli disease).

Clinical features
Congenital hepatic fibrosis presents in three clinical forms: portal hypertension, recurrent cholangitis and asymptomatic or

latent disease. The first two forms are usually diagnosed in early childhood in patients who present with variceal hemorrhage or unexplained biliary sepsis, respectively. In contrast, some patients will be detected later, during their adult years, when they are evaluated for unexplained hepatomegaly or portal hypertension. Rarely, patients present with evidence of both portal hypertension and cholestasis, the latter due to either associated biliary anomalies (Caroli disease) or to intrinsic destructive cholangiopathy. In general, hepatic function is well preserved, despite portal hypertension or bouts of cholangitis, although some patients experience progressive hepatic failure in long-term follow-up.

Treatment

The first-line treatment of variceal hemorrhage is endoscopic variceal eradication (either sclerotherapy or ligation treatment), followed by institution of β-adrenergic blockade. In most cases, varices may be successfully obliterated by the endoscopic approach, thereby controlling this potentially life-threatening complication. Surgical shunts or transjugular intrahepatic portosystemic shunt (TIPS) are reserved for patients who fail endoscopic therapy, bleed from gastric varices or who have portal hypertensive gastropathy. Occasionally patients will experience progressive hepatic fibrosis and hepatic dysfunction after long-standing portosystemic shunt surgery, and development of this complication may necessitate consideration for liver transplantation.

In patients with cholangitis, radiologic imaging [ultrasonography, biliary radioscintigraphy, CT or magnetic resonance imaging (MRI)] may be required to determine whether the patient with congenital hepatic fibrosis has concomitant biliary cystic disease. If the latter is present, the treatment of cholangitis is centered on provision of adequate biliary drainage, relief of obstruction (papillotomy with stone extraction or stricture dilatation), and control of infection with antibiotics. In the absence of biliary cystic disease or cholangiocarcinoma (said to occur in as many as 6% of cases of congenital hepatic fibrosis), cholestasis may be related to idiopathic inflammatory destructive cholangiopathy and respond to ursodeoxycholic acid therapy. Indications for hepatic transplantation include variceal hemorrhage or hemorrhage from portal hypertensive gastropathy that is not responsive to endoscopic treatment or amenable to portosystemic shunt surgery or TIPS, recurrent cholangitis that is not amenable to medical, endoscopic, radiologic or surgical therapy; and hepatic failure (development of coagulopathy, biochemical deterioration, ascites or portosystemic encephalopathy).

Choledochal cyst
Characteristics

Choledochal cysts are usually present since childhood but do not cause sufficient symptoms to lead to their detection until adulthood in at least 20% of patients. Choledochal cysts are cystic dilatations that may occur throughout the macroscopic intra- and extrahepatic biliary tree. Although the term choledochal cyst has been used for any cystic dilatation of the biliary tree, isolated choledochal cysts are usually restricted to only the common hepatic or bile duct. Despite the uncommon occurrence of choledochal cysts, there are hundreds of reports in the literature encompassing over 3000 cases. Choledochal cyst is a rare condition in the Western hemisphere, but it is relatively more common among Japanese and other Asian populations. Several classifications of choledochal cysts have been proposed but the most commonly cited in the medical literature by Todani (77) is outlined in **Figure 28.10**. In this system, the most common cyst is a type I cyst, representing more than 80% of cases. The pattern of inheritance is unclear and there have been no definitive studies of either the genetic markers or molecular biology of choledochal cysts.

The pathogenesis of choledochal cysts is unknown. Histologically, the cyst walls are made up of fibrous tissue representing a chronic inflammatory process and the epithelial lining is either partially or completely absent.

Clinical features

The most common clinical presentation of choledochal cyst is a relatively young patient (child or adolescent) with pain, a mass in the right upper quadrant or epigastrium and jaundice. In one series of 740 cases, jaundice was the most common and consistent presenting feature. In infants, jaundice is often the only sign and the disorder may be difficult to distinguish from biliary atresia. The majority of the patients are diagnosed before 30 years of age and the male:female ratio in most series is about 1:4.

Reported complications include spontaneous or traumatic rupture, rupture during pregnancy, liver abscess, cirrhosis and complications related to portal hypertension including gastroesophageal varices and development of cholangiocarcinoma. The incidence of cholangiocarcinoma ranges from 2.5 to 17.5%, which is 5–35 times greater than the population at large. The incidence of carcinoma increases throughout life and approaches 50% by age 50 years. Internal drainage procedures without cyst excision appear to accelerate the development of cholangiocarcinoma. Bacterial overgrowth and increased levels of secondary bile acids may contribute to cyst metaplasia and carcinoma. The tumors may originate in different parts of the pancreatobiliary system, including the liver, gallbladder, intrahepatic ducts, pancreatic ducts or pancreas.

Diagnosis

The diagnosis of a choledochal cyst should always be suspected in a child presenting with recurrent abdominal pain, jaundice and raised serum amylase. Initial imaging of the biliary tree by ultrasonography or radioscintigraphy (HIDA scans) is usually diagnostic. Confirmation and anatomic definition may require CT, ERCP or a percutaneous transhepatic cholangiogram (PTC). Patients with extrahepatic choledochal cysts have an increased incidence of anomalous pancreaticobiliary junction, which requires ERCP when planning for excision of the cyst. In recent years, MRCP has shown to be equivalent to ERCP in detecting and defining not only choledochal cysts but also the presence of an anomalous union of the pancreatic and bile ducts. MRCP can also define the length of extrahepatic bile duct involved with the cyst which is important when planning a surgical approach. Particularly in the pediatric population, MRCP offers an attractive non-invasive diagnostic alternative with the lack of ionizing radiation. Endoscopic ultrasonography has also been a useful imaging method for patients with suspected anomalous pancreaticobiliary junction. Prenatal ultrasonography can detect choledochal cysts in utero, which may help antenatal counseling since early neonatal cyst excision and duct revision may be required.

CHAPTER
29

Malignant Tumors of the Liver

Philip J. Johnson

Tumors of the liver enter into the differential diagnosis of many patients presenting to the hepatologist and tend to be managed by hepatologists and hepatobiliary surgeons rather than by oncologists. A sound knowledge of these tumors is therefore required by all involved in the practice of clinical hepatology. In many parts of the world primary liver cell cancer (PLCC) or 'hepatocellular carcinoma' (HCC) is a common malignant tumor and represents a major public health problem. The liver is also the most frequent, and often the clinically predominant, organ site of metastatic malignant disease. This chapter deals firstly with the most common primary malignant tumor of the liver, HCC, then some other primary liver tumors, and finally secondary liver tumors.

HEPATOCELLULAR CARCINOMA

Hepatocellular carcinoma, which accounts for 70–80% of all primary liver tumors, is the sixth most common cancer in the world (fifth in men, ninth in women), and the 500 000 to 1 million cases that occur each year account for at least 5% of all new cancers. It tends to present late in its natural history because small tumors cause few or no symptoms and the large size of the liver precludes easy palpation of the tumor until it has gained considerable dimensions. The large functional reserve of the liver also delays symptomatic presentation with disturbances such as jaundice or ascites. Patients who are carriers of the hepatitis B virus (HBV), hepatitis C virus (HCV), or those who have cirrhosis of any other etiology, are at a very high risk of HCC development. Physicians managing such patients need to maintain a high index of suspicion (**Table 29.1**).

Epidemiology and pathogenesis
Elucidation of the epidemiology of HCC has led to one of the great medical success stories of the 20th century. Not only have many of the most important risk factors been identified and their impact quantified, but also preventive measures based on these results are now being implemented.

Age-adjusted incidence rates for HCC vary from around 2–3/100 000 in Northern Europe, the USA and Australia, up to more than 100/100 000 in parts of sub-Saharan Africa and the Far East (**Table 29.2**). These figures may hide important information. For example, within the USA, where the overall incidence rate is low, there is marked variation in relation to ethnicity with rates per 100 000 of 18, 4 and 2 for Chinese, black Americans and white Americans respectively. Furthermore, within individual countries there may be very striking geographic differences in incidence, even among ethnically homogenous peoples. Thus, in some parts of China incidence rates are below 10/100 000 whereas in others, rates exceed 100/100 000

Key features of hepatocellular carcinoma (HCC) and secondary liver tumors	
HCC	*Secondary liver tumors*
HCC usually presents late, when the tumor is already large	Liver metastases are present in 40% of patients who have extrahepatic malignancy who come to autopsy
The non-tumorous liver is usually cirrhotic	Survival is directly related to the size of the tumor
Resection offers the only hope of long-term survival, but is only an option for a minority of patients because: the tumor has already metastasized, or liver function is too poor, or the tumor is too large	All solitary lesions should be investigated for the possibility of surgical resection
Recurrence after resection or transplantation is common particularly when the tumor is large or there is histologic evidence of vascular invasion	In patients who have good performance status cytotoxic chemotherapy should be considered, either given as a standard intravenous regimen or as a chronic infusion
HBV vaccination should ultimately decrease the incidence of HCC in many high incidence areas	Postoperative adjuvant treatment improves survival and decreases the risk of hepatic metastases in patients who have Duke stage C colorectal cancer
HBV, hepatitis B virus	

Table 29.1 Key features of hepatocellular carcinoma (HCC) and secondary liver tumors.

(**Fig. 29.1**). Rates are consistently higher for men than for women. The incidence of HCC rises with age in all areas of the world, and peaks between 35 and 75 years, the peak being earlier in higher incidence areas (**Fig. 29.2**). Around 70–90% of cases of HCC are associated with cirrhosis and among patients with cirrhosis the annual rate of HCC development is in the order of 1–5% per annum.

All factors linked to the development of HCC, including chronic HBV, HCV infection and excessive alcohol consumption, also cause cirrhosis. Once cirrhosis is established, even if the causative factor is withdrawn (for example, alcohol in alcoholic cirrhosis, or iron in the case of hemochromatosis), the increased risk of HCC remains. The incidence in the West appears to be rising, perhaps in relation to the increased

453

Age adjusted incidence rates of hepatocellular carcinoma (HCC) (per 100 000 of population) in various countries			
	Country	*Male*	*Female*
Low incidence areas	UK	1.6	0.8
	USA (white)	2	1
	Australia	1.1	0.5
	Germany	4	1.2
	Denmark	3.6	2.3
Intermediate incidence areas	Italy	7.5	3.5
	Spain	7.5	4
	Romania	11.8	7.9
	Argentina	8	5
High incidence areas	Japan	20	5
	Hong Kong	32	7
	Mozambique	113	31
	Zimbabwe	65	25
	Senegal	25	9
	Taiwan	85	–
Where figures for different areas of the same country are available, typical values have been given. Most registries do not distinguish between HCC and other primary tumors, so the figures should, at best, be considered as a rough guide.			

Table 29.2 Age adjusted incidence rates of hepatocellular carcinoma (HCC) (per 100 000 of population) in various countries.

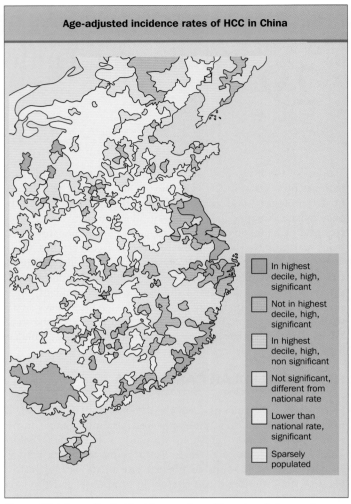

Age-adjusted incidence rates of HCC in China

In highest decile, high, significant

Not in highest decile, high, significant

In highest decile, high, non significant

Not significant, different from national rate

Lower than national rate, significant

Sparsely populated

Figure 29.1 Age-adjusted incidence rates of hepatocellular carcinoma (HCC) in China in relation to the national average. Note that, although the prevalence of hepatitis B carriage is fairly constant throughout China, there is a great deal of geographic variation, with cases tending to cluster (red and purple areas) strongly around the coastal strip.

prevalence of chronic HCV infection (see Ch. 16), but caution should be exercised. Over the last 30 years diagnostic tools have become much more sensitive, and lesions which would not have been detected in the 1970s are now routinely picked up by new imaging techniques.

Hepatitis B virus infection

From a worldwide perspective, HBV infection is the major etiology of HCC accounting for perhaps 75% of all cases. Areas of the world with the highest HCC incidence have carriage rates for hepatitis B surface antigen (HBsAg) of greater than 10% (**Fig. 29.3**). A landmark prospective study of 22 707 male Chinese civil servants, about 15% of whom were HBsAg seropositive, showed conclusively that chronic HBV infection precedes HCC development and the relative risk for a male HBsAg carrier for HCC was about 100. In other areas of the world the relative risk for HBV carriers is much lower and this probably reflects variable impact of additional risk factors such as aflatoxin exposure and the age at which the infection was contracted. Other cancers do not develop with undue frequency among HBV carriers. The association of HBV and HCC is confined to *chronic* HBV infection, particularly when acquired at birth or during childhood. The period from acquisition of the virus to tumor development can be as short as 4 years and as long as 80 years.

Although the weight of epidemiologic evidence linking chronic HBV infection to the subsequent development of HCC is now overwhelming, elucidation of the mechanism has proved elusive. Hepatitis B virus DNA, integrated into the host genome, can be detected in most cases, even in the absence of serologic evidence of HBV infection. However, there does not appear to be a consistent integration site and HBV does not contain recognized oncogenes. Preliminary evidence from Taiwan where mass vaccination against HBV was introduced in 1984 for children of mothers who were HBsAg carriers, and universally in 1986, shows that a steady decrease in the number of children who develop HCC, aged 6–14 years, is already evident. The incidence rate has fallen from 0.7/100 000 (1981–1986) to 0.57 (1986–1990) and to 0.36 (1990–1994).

Hepatitis C virus infection

With the development of tests for antibodies to HCV in 1989 it became apparent, at least in Japan and the West, that HCV was as important as HBV in the pathogenesis of HCC. In Europe, HCV positivity in patients who have HCC ranges from 20 to 76%, with a tendency to increase from north to south (**Table 29.3**) and in the USA it accounts for about 50% of cases. There appears to be a very long incubation period as assessed by following up patients who have hemophilia and in whom the time of acquisition could be accurately documented. Since HCV has no reverse transcriptase activity and is not a retrovirus, it should, in theory, have no direct oncogenic potential. Most

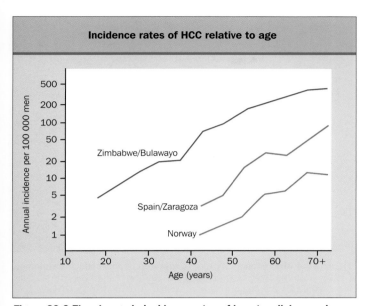

Figure 29.2 The change in incidence rates of hepatocellular carcinoma (HCC) according to age in three different geographic areas. Reproduced from Munoz & Bosch in Okuda & Ishak (87) by permission of Springer Science and Business Media.

Country	Anti-HCV positivity	
	Percentage of HCC patients	Percentage of control population
Italy	76	<1
France	58	<1
Spain	75	7.5
Greece	40	6
UK	10	<1
USA	20	1
Japan	68	7

Rate of positivity for anti-hepatitis C virus (anti-HCV) among patients who have hepatocellular carcinoma (HCC) in various countries compared with a control population from the same country

There is considerable variation within country and figures may even depend on the particular assay used. Figures should therefore only be taken as rough estimates.

Table 29.3 Rate of positivity for anti-hepatitis C virus (anti-HCV) among patients who have hepatocellular carcinoma (HCC) in various countries compared with a control population from the same country.

authors have attributed the association with HCC to the chronic liver disease that HCV may cause.

There is now good evidence that effective antiviral treatment for both hepatitis C and hepatitis B is decreasing the risk of HCC development particularly if disease control is established before the onset of cirrhosis. Co-infection with HBV and HCV is associated with a very high risk of HCC development. Chronic carriers of HCV, particularly in areas of the world where the infection is common, are at a significantly increased risk of B-cell non-Hodgkin lymphoma and this should be borne in mind when investigating focal hepatic lesions in such patients.

Aflatoxin exposure and other possible etiologic factors

Aflatoxins are mycotoxins generated by the fungi *Aspergillus flavus* and *Aspergillus parasiticus*. These mycotoxins are among the most potent naturally occurring carcinogens known. Humans are exposed following ingestion of nuts and meal that are stored under hot humid conditions where these molds grow. The relative risk of HCC for individuals exposed to aflatoxin is very high, similar to that for HBV carriage, but for individuals who have both risk factors the relative risk is increased in a multiplicative manner. These are likely to be major etiologic factors in humid

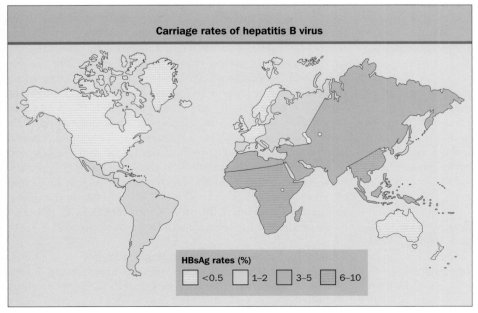

Figure 29.3 Worldwide carriage rates of the hepatitis B virus. Note that the areas with the highest carriage rates coincide with the areas that have the highest incidence of hepatocellular carcinoma (HCC).

parts of China and Africa, and may account for the wide variation of incidence in these continents.

There is a strong association between the use of contraceptive preparations and benign hepatic adenomas (see Ch. 27). Although there may be an increased risk of HCC development after prolonged usage, the absolute risk remains extremely small.

Clinical features and disease associations

The most common mode of presentation of HCC is with the triad of abdominal pain in the right upper quadrant, weight loss and hepatomegaly. Patients who present in this manner usually have a tumor larger than 6 cm in diameter and diameters of over 15 cm are not uncommon. The pain is usually a dull ache, sometimes referred to the shoulder. Sudden attacks of more severe pain may be caused by spontaneous bleeding into the tumor. Hepatomegaly, often massive, is an invariable feature of symptomatic malignant liver tumors. The liver feels firm or stony hard. Usually, the symptoms will have been present for only a few weeks in high incidence areas or for a few months in lower incidence areas. Delay in seeking medical advice is seldom a reason for late diagnosis or a factor that can be held responsible for delayed intervention. Less common presentations are listed below.

Hepatic decompensation

In a male who has previously well-controlled cirrhosis and who develops ascites, recurrent variceal hemorrhage or encephalopathy, HCC must always enter the differential diagnosis. The ascites becomes difficult to control with standard diuretic therapy and may be bloodstained. Jaundice of the hepatocellular type becomes steadily progressive.

Gastrointestinal hemorrhage

About 10% of cases will present with gastrointestinal bleeding. In 40% of the cases the bleed will have been from esophageal varices; this is much more frequent if the patient has portal vein invasion by the tumor. Bleeding from duodenal ulceration and other benign causes accounts for the remaining 60% of cases. The patient may have cutaneous stigmata of chronic liver disease, but this is by no means always the case. The majority of patients who present with HCC, as well as having no history of chronic liver disease, have no clinical signs thereof. The failure to detect clinical signs of chronic liver disease does not imply its absence.

Tumor rupture – 'hemoperitoneum'

Spontaneous rupture is a particularly dramatic presentation of the tumor (**Fig. 29.4**). There is a sudden onset of abdominal pain and swelling. Although hemoperitoneum is a frequent event late in the course of the disease, it may occasionally be a presenting feature. The patient presents with shock and a rigid, silent abdomen. The diagnosis is established by paracentesis, which reveals bloodstained fluid or frank blood.

Asymptomatic presentation

Increasingly, because of surveillance programs, tumors are being detected before any symptoms develop (see below). With current imaging procedures, tumors as small as 0.5–1 cm can be detected. The frequency of asymptomatic diagnosis is entirely dependent on the intensity of the screening program. In most countries those cases detected at this stage remain a small

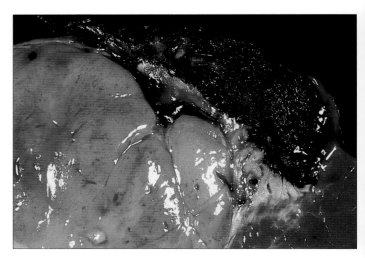

Figure 29.4 Macroscopic picture of ruptured hepatocellular carcinoma (HCC). Note the large blood clot on the surface of the liver. The vessels responsible for the hemorrhage are visible. (Courtesy of Dr CT Liew.)

fortunate minority. Not surprisingly, the natural history of these very early lesions is different from symptomatic tumors and apparent survival is much better. Surgical resection or liver transplantation may be curative in this group.

Endocrine, paraneoplastic syndromes, other rare modes of presentation

HCC has a reputation for paraneoplastic presentations, but this is largely due to highly selective reporting. Overall less than 1% of all cases will present with any of these syndromes, although asymptomatic cases will be detected more frequently if sought assiduously. Among the paraneoplastic syndromes, a high red cell count (erythrocytosis) is well recognized, and is presumed to be related to ectopic production of erythropoietin or an erythropoietin-like substance. Two types of hypoglycemia are recognized. The first ('type A') occurs during the terminal stage of a rapidly growing tumor and is seldom symptomatic. A much greater clinical problem is type B disease, in which severe symptomatic hypoglycemia occurs relatively early in the disease course. The hypoglycemia does not respond consistently to any therapeutic approach and the physician usually resorts to long-term enteral glucose administration. Other even rarer presentations include gynecomastia, hypercalcemia and hyperthyroidism. Spread to involve the hepatic vein is a cause of the Budd-Chiari syndrome with massive tense ascites. Obstructive jaundice may be due to compression of the bile ducts by tumor rather than hepatocellular failure. In approximately half the cases the site of obstruction is extrahepatic. Other rare causes of jaundice include direct growth of the tumor into the bile duct or bleeding from the tumor into the biliary system (hematobilia). HCC has occasionally been reported as a cause of 'pyrexia of unknown origin' (PUO). The PUO occurs late in the disease and leads to diagnostic difficulties during management. Diarrhea of uncertain pathogenesis is also a frequent symptom.

Clinical features of specific histologic subtypes

Two rare, histologically defined, primary liver cancers deserve special consideration since they have specific clinical correlates. The fibrolamellar variant of HCC has several distinctive clinical

New UICC/AJCC staging system for hepatocellular carcinoma (HCC)	
Primary tumor (T)	
TX	Primary tumor cannot be assessed
T0	No evidence of primary tumor
T1	Solitary tumor without vascular invasion
T2	Solitary tumor with vascular invasion or multiple tumors ≤5 cm
T3	Multiple tumors more than 5 cm or tumor involving a major branch of the portal or hepatic vein
T4	Tumor(s) with direct invasion of adjacent organs other than the gallbladder or with perforation of visceral peritoneum.
Regional lymph nodes (N)	
NX	Regional lymph nodes cannot be assessed
N0	No regional lymph node metastases
N1	Regional lymph node metastases
Distant metastases (M)	
MX	Distant metastases cannot be assessed
M0	No distant metastases
M1	Distant metastases

Stage grouping			
Stage I	T1	N0	M0
Stage II	T2	N0	M0
Stage IIIA	T3	N0	M0
Stage IIIB	T4	N0	M0
Stage IIIC	Any T	N1	M0
Stage IV	Any T	Any N	M1

Histologic grade (G)	
Gx	Grade cannot be assessed
G1	Well differentiated
G2	Moderately differentiated
G3	Poorly differentiated
G4	Undifferentiated
Fibrosis score (F)	
F0	Fibrosis score (no fibrosis to moderate fibrosis)
F1	Fibrosis score (severe fibrosis to cirrhosis)

Table 29.5 New UICC/AJCC staging system for hepatocellular carcinoma (HCC).

(AHPBA) recently endorsed the use of the CLIP (Cancer of the Liver Italian Program) score for staging of HCC. This score takes into account liver function (Child-Pugh class), tumor morphology, serum AFP and portal vein invasion and appears to accurately predict patient survival.

Management

Physicians searching the literature for effective treatment of HCC should be aware that clinical trials are often undertaken on patients who have characteristics that suggest a better prognosis within the above mentioned spectrum of prognoses. The results are then compared (usually favorably) with figures for the overall group, leading to an overstatement of the therapeutic potential in an unselected population of patients who have HCC. At the time of writing the only potentially curative treatment is surgical resection including transplantation. Unfortunately, however, most cases will fall within the category of being unresectable. The major reasons why patients cannot undergo conventional resectional surgery with a view to cure are the extent of the tumor (including metastases), the implications of the associated cirrhosis, extrahepatic metastases, or unrelated co-morbidity. The presence of cirrhosis does not preclude resection, but the results are best in patients who have Child class A cirrhosis. Liver transplantation is feasible in patients who have small tumors, irrespective of the Child category. Extensive, bilobar disease and/or invasion of the major vessels including the inferior vena cava, main portal vein, and common hepatic artery generally preclude surgical resection.

Surgical approaches

Liver resection is a major operation that carries an operative mortality of up to 5% in non-cirrhotic, and up to 10% in cirrhotic patients. No single liver function test can predict the survival of an individual patient undergoing liver resection, but once the liver disease decompensates, patients almost always develop liver failure after resection. Child grade C cirrhosis is therefore usually considered to be a contraindication to surgery, but liver failure can still occur after resection in those who have Child grades A or B. It has been proposed that the presence of portal hypertension, as judged by a hepatic venous pressure gradient of >10 mmHg, is the best single test predicting postoperative liver failure. However, the amount of intraoperative blood loss, the duration and degree of hypotension and size of the remaining liver remnant also influence survival.

Although cirrhosis is no longer considered an absolute contraindication, the operative mortality is significant for several reasons. Many cirrhotic patients have a coagulopathy and a low platelet count because of hypersplenism. Portal hypertension increases the risks of bleeding because of the opening up of portosystemic collaterals in the retroperitoneum. The cirrhotic liver is firm, difficult to manipulate, and does not readily take suture material. Most of these problems are now surmountable with technical advances, but surgical successes are often negated by postoperative complications. Estimates of the functional capacity of the residual tissue are difficult to determine preoperatively and this may prove to be inadequate after surgery. Initial adequate function may deteriorate secondary to infection and cirrhotic patients are intrinsically immunocompromised and at high risk of sepsis. A patient who has a normal liver can tolerate resection of about 75% of the liver, but in a cirrhotic liver a right lobectomy (55% resection) is the upper limit of surgical resectability.

Surgical resection

CT is the usual preoperative investigation. This shows the site and extent of the disease, but may miss up to one-third of nodules detected at surgery. Angiography has the potential to delineate the vascular anatomy, confirm patency of the portal vein, and may detect tumor not seen on CT (**Fig. 29.9**). The most reliable way of detecting macroscopic abdominal spread and assessing the extent of liver involvement is during laparotomy. Intraoperative ultrasound locates otherwise undetected small primary and secondary lesions and tumor thrombus in portal and hepatic veins. It also helps to determine the resection margins and the plane of liver transection in relation to the hepatic vasculature, thereby helping to preserve as much functioning liver tissue as possible.

The liver can be divided into eight segments, each receiving its hepatic arterial, portal venous and biliary duct branches. The hepatic venous branches are distributed between, rather than within, the individual segments. Accurate delineation of the segments to be excised has been facilitated by intraoperative ultrasound, and by the injection of dyes into the portal or arterial blood supply. The five commonly used lobar and/or segmental resections are shown in **Figure 29.10**. In a right trisegmentectomy, the right lobe of the liver and medial segment of the left lobe are removed. In a left trisegmentectomy, the left lobe of the liver and the anterior segment of the right lobe are removed. An extended right hepatectomy usually refers to a right trisegmentectomy, but may also refer to a slight modification of a right lobectomy in which the hepatic parenchyma is transected well to the right of the falciform ligament rather than at this ligament, thus sparing most of the medial segment. An extended left lobectomy should not be confused with the left trisegmentectomy, since it does not result in removal of the full anterior segment of the right lobe. Non-anatomic resection refers to resection of the liver along non-anatomic planes. In

general, this results in more bleeding and can leave behind parts of the liver remnants deprived of their blood supply and subject to necrosis.

Improvements in perioperative support have radically decreased the morbidity associated with surgical resection. Nonetheless after major resection cholestasis and fluid retention and impaired synthetic function may combine to increase hospital stay. A major risk factor for postoperative complications is the 'future liver volume'. Percutaneous portal vein remobilization has recently been advocated as a method for increasing liver cell mass – by inducing selective hypertrophy of the non-diseased liver (usually of the left lobe). A key aspect to the planning for this procedure is calculation, on the basis of CT scan, of the future liver volume.

About 10–15% of patients who have HCC will come to resection and about one-third to one-half of these will survive for 5 years. Postoperative disease recurrence, usually intrahepatic, is the main cause of death.

Orthotopic liver transplantation

Orthotopic liver transplantation potentially overcomes the problems of intrahepatic tumor distribution, clears micrometastatic liver tumors and relieves hepatic insufficiency all of which limit the application of conventional resection. Many of the first patients to achieve long-term survival in the 1970s after transplantation had malignant liver disease. Many tolerated the operation well and recovered rapidly but, despite careful preoperative assessment that attempted to exclude those who had extrahepatic spread, tumor recurrence was common. By the early 1990s a multicenter registry showed only an 18% survival at 5 years with only 9% disease free at 2 years. Presumably this stemmed from undetectable extrahepatic micrometastases, perhaps promoted by the requisite immunosuppression. This experience led many groups to abandon transplantation for malignant disease other than when the tumor was found incidentally in a patient undergoing transplantation for advanced cirrhosis.

More recently it has become apparent that the number of nodules, maximum tumor size and/or the degree of vascular invasion (either microvascular invasion or portal vein invasion) are the major adverse factors influencing recurrence rates (**Fig. 29.11**). Guidelines proposed by Mazzaferro et al (1996) limit transplantation to those with a single tumor less than 4 cm in diameter or up to three nodules with the largest being less than 3 cm in diameter. With these criteria, 5-year survival of around 75% can be expected. Small tumors not numbering more than two have a prognosis similar to those cirrhotic patients without HCC who undergo liver transplantation.

Despite these excellent results, there is a growing discrepancy between the number of patients awaiting liver transplantation and the number of donor livers that become available (see Ch. 37). This means that units tend to be strict in confining transplants to those who meet the above criteria. Live donor transplantation may increase the supply but this approach is not widely used at present. Several groups are investigating the possibility of 'bridging' the gap between diagnosis and going on the transplant list, and the time at which a donor liver becomes available. TACE, percutaneous ethanol injection (PEI) and radiofrequency ablation (RFA) have all been used but there is no consensus about their benefit.

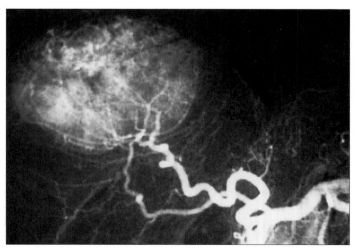

Figure 29.9 Hepatic angiography of a large hypervascular hepatocellular carcinoma (HCC) in the dome of the liver. (Courtesy of Dr Wei Tse Yang.)

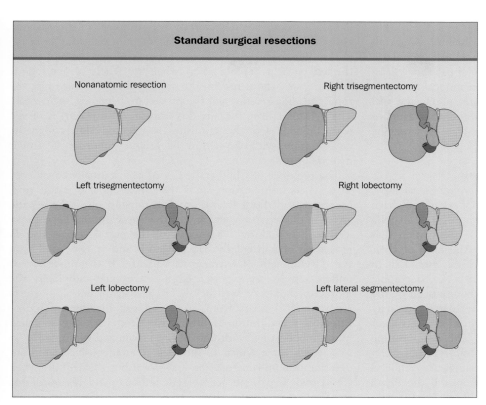

Figure 29.10 Standard surgical resections.

The question whether, in a particular patient, resection or transplantation is to be preferred is controversial. When the patient has decompensated liver disease the answer is clearly transplantation, but in other circumstances, and while the results with liver transplantation are still improving, referral for an opinion to a center where both options can be considered should be undertaken. In addition to the surgical considerations, the potential for further de novo malignant change in the cirrhotic tissue left in situ can influence the decision. Trials assessing the extent to which ablative therapies such as RFA may be as effective as surgical resection is currently underway. Pre- and postoperative adjuvant treatments are often given but are not, as yet, of proven benefit.

Management of the patient who has inoperable disease

The physician must clearly define the aims and limitations of any proposed treatment. These aims should be set out before the patient in a manner that, while realistic, avoids destroying all hope. There are now so many options for the management of patients who have inoperable disease that it is easy to lose sight of certain basic principles. For the vast majority of cases the aim is good palliation; no treatment has yet been convincingly and consistently proven to increase survival, other than perhaps in a subset of patients treated with TACE.

Non-surgical treatment can be classified as locoregional, including intra-arterial or percutaneous local ablative approaches, a combination of the two, or systemic. When regional lymph nodes are involved or there are extrahepatic metastases, locoregional treatment is seldom indicated. Intra-arterial treatment is also contraindicated when there is involvement of the main portal venous system. It is among the patients who are unsuitable for any of the above treatments, that systemic chemotherapy is usually considered.

'Liver failure' as indicated by overt jaundice, recurrent or diuretic resistant ascites, recurrent gastrointestinal hemorrhage or encephalopathy unexplained by other factors will, in the view of most authorities, preclude any form of active treatment other than liver transplantation. In such patients prognosis is primarily

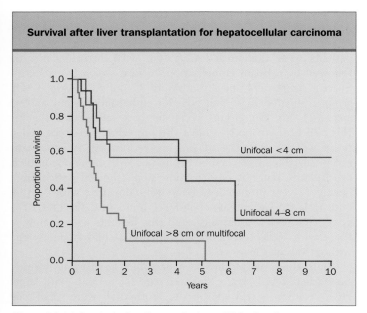

Figure 29.11 Survival of patients who have HCC after liver transplantation in relation to tumor size and number. Reproduced from McPeake et al (95) by permission of Elsevier.

defined by the underlying liver function rather than the tumor; effective antitumor therapy may not necessarily improve overall survival. Figures will vary from center to center, and around the world, but as a very broad generalization 15% of patients will be considered for surgical resection, 50% for non-surgical therapies and 35% will be unsuitable for any active treatment, and will receive best supportive care. These figures will change as more patients are detected in the asymptomatic stage by screening programs.

Intra-arterial therapy – the theoretical basis

With the disappointing results seen with systemic therapy, several approaches that aim to target the tumor specifically have been developed. There are two ways in which targeting may be achieved. The first approach is based on the observation that primary and secondary liver tumors derive the bulk of their blood supply from the hepatic artery. This approach to selectivity may be further enhanced by new arteriographic procedures that permit 'super selective' catheterization of the tumor feeding artery. Direct infusion of cytotoxic agents may increase the drug exposure (the time/concentration interval) of the tumor to the drug by up to 400-fold. The dose-limiting toxicity then becomes regional (i.e. hepatic), rather than systemic. The extent to which regional advantage is obtained depends on both the rate of drug elimination and the blood perfusion rate. Thus, drugs with a short half-life are particularly appropriate for this route of administration and measures to decrease liver blood flow may be expected to enhance their activity. Nonetheless, if the tumor is maximally sensitive at drug levels achieved by systemic administration there will be no advantage with this approach.

On pharmacologic grounds, the most appropriate drugs are 5-fluorouracil (5-FU) and 5-fluorodeoxyuridine (FUDR), both of which have half-lives of only a few minutes. Unfortunately, 5-FU, at least as a single agent, falls into the category of ineffective therapy for patients who have HCC.

A second source of selectivity is the use of lipiodol as a vehicle for cytotoxic chemotherapy. This oily based contrast medium, when injected into the hepatic artery at the time of arteriography, is cleared from normal hepatic tissues but accumulates in malignant tumors, probably because of the leaky character of neovascular tissue, combined with the lack of lymphatic clearance from tumor tissue. The lipiodol forms an emulsion with the cytotoxic agent and then acts as a reservoir for the prolonged delivery of the agent to the tumor, and perhaps enhances uptake by the tumor cells. The extent to which the lipiodol acts as an embolizing agent in itself remains controversial.

Regional drug delivery and transcatheter oily chemoembolization (TACE)

There seems no doubt that, compared with systemic administration, drugs given intra-arterially are more effective, although it must not be forgotten that patients treated in this manner invariably have a better performance status than those treated with systemic therapy. For this reason, better results would be expected regardless of any inherent increased efficacy of the treatment.

Following hepatic angiography to identify the arterial anatomy and the blood supply of the tumor a catheter is placed in the appropriate vessel. Not infrequently angiography

identifies tumor not detected by CT scanning. In the past the entire liver has been covered by placement of the catheter in the proper hepatic artery but nowadays it is more common to use the left or right hepatic artery when the whole of one lobe is involved, or, where feasible, to selectively catheterize just the tumor feeding arteries and the procedure becomes 'segmental'. The cytotoxic drug (usually doxorubicin or cisplatin) is mixed with lipiodol and the emulsion is injected slowly. Finally, embolization with 0.5–1 mm of gelatin cubes or a similar material is undertaken.

The presence of Child grade C cirrhosis is usually considered to be a contraindication, as is thrombosis of the portal vein, because the cirrhotic liver is crucially dependent on the hepatic artery in this situation, and any further interruption thereof may lead to liver failure. Thrombosis of the portal vein is also an indication of particularly bad prognosis and is associated with the development of extrahepatic disease. If the procedure is undertaken by an experienced interventional radiologist the mortality should be well below 5% and significant side-effects are rare (1%) apart from occasional gall bladder infarction. Effective embolization is often associated with the so-called 'post embolization syndrome' of fever, pain and vomiting for up to a week after which it subsides spontaneously. Significant deterioration in liver function may occur but usually only when Child grade C patients are treated. Although widely regarded as standard treatment for almost 15 years, and clear evidence that tumor necrosis was indeed caused, early controlled trials did not show an increase in survival and the consensus was that although the 'primary effect' (i.e. causing tumor volume reduction) is good, there is little effect on long-term survival for which other factors such as the tumor type, degree of spread and serum AFP level are more significant than the treatment.

However, more recently, two trials and a systematic review have, for the first time, provided evidence that TACE may indeed, in selected cases, improve survival. In the first of these, randomized 80 subjects, to either TACE (with cisplatin in lipiodol followed by gelatin sponge embolization) or best supportive therapy (Fig. 29.13b). The survival figures at 1, 2 and 3 years were 57, 31 and 26% compared to 32, 11 and 3%, respectively ($p=0.006$). In the second study, from Spain, 112 patients were randomized to TACE with doxorubicin again followed by gelfoam embolization, or best supportive therapy. Survival figures at 1 and 2 years were 82 and 63% in the TACE group compared to 75 and 50% for embolization alone and 63 and 27% for the groups receiving best supportive therapy (**Fig. 29.12**a). In both studies the procedure was repeated if there was no evidence of progressive disease. A systematic review suggested that chemoembolization with either doxorubicin or cisplatin, but not embolization alone showed a significant benefit (2-year probability of survival, compared with control, odds ratio 0.53 with 95% confidence limits of 0.32–0.89). The systematic review again suggested that benefits were mainly in those with well-preserved liver function (Child grade A) and without vascular invasion.

Whilst these two studies have, according to many authorities, established TACE as the standard care for patients with larger HCC, caution is still appropriate. Both trials were small, and some criticisms about how well the treatment and control groups were balanced have been raised. Furthermore, and of particular importance in designing further comparative studies,

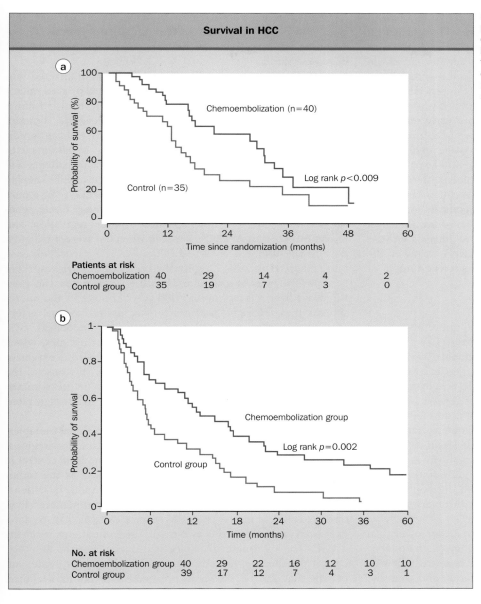

Figure 29.12 Survival curves from two prospective randomized trials of arterial chemoembolization for the treatment of hepatocellular carcinoma (HCC). Survival curves from two prospective randomized trials of arterial chemoembolization for the treatment of HCC. (For references see Llovet and Bruix 2003) (a) From Spain. (b) From Hong Kong.

there remains considerable controversy as to what is actually meant by the term 'chemoembolization' and the relative importance of the 'embolization' and the 'chemotherapy' aspects of the treatment. It is notable that different cytotoxic agents were used in the two trials. Some in the field aim to develop extensive tumor necrosis by the embolization whilst others use the embolic material to slow down the blood flow to the tumor and not to permanently occlude the vessels and thereby permit repeat procedures.

Percutaneous ethanol (alcohol) injection

Ultrasound or CT-guided percutaneous injection of sterile absolute alcohol into liver tumors, via a 19–22 gauge needle, under local anesthetic consistently induces vascular thrombosis and coagulative necrosis. A total of between 2 and 100 ml of alcohol is injected during the course of several sessions (depending on the tumor size) and distributed as uniformly as possible throughout the lesion. The most suitable patients are those with small tumors (<3 cm), with good underlying liver function (Child grade A). In such patients, 'complete response' is obtained in around 80% with survival figures at 3 and 5 years in the order of 75 and 50% respectively. In such patients it seems likely that results may be as good as surgical resection.

The benefits of PEI decrease markedly in larger lesions; the procedure becomes more tedious and it is more difficult to generate complete necrosis, in part because of the presence of septa within the lesion but also because of 'run off' of the alcohol into the vasculature; most centers will not consider PEI for lesions larger than 5 cm.

The procedure is cheap, simple to perform, does not require a general anesthetic and is virtually free of any associated mortality. The only complications are intense pain if the alcohol is allowed to leak out into the peritoneal cavity, transient pyrexia, occasional episodes of hemoperitoneum (<5% of cases) and, rarely, tumor seeding along the needle tract. Nonetheless, as with surgical resection, in 50–70% of cases there will be intrahepatic recurrence. This is particularly so in larger lesions and those that are multifocal to begin with. Most will occur within 2 years of the initial procedure.

How should one decide between surgical resection and PEI in a patient with a solitary small liver tumor before prospective randomized clinical trials directly comparing the procedures are available? There are no hard and fast rules and it is probably fair to say that there is a trade-off between more early morbidity and mortality with surgical resection and more late deaths with PEI. If the patient is young, there are no coexisting medical conditions and liver function is good, most would still favor surgical resection. This has the added theoretical benefit of removing surrounding tissue that may be the site of micrometastatic disease. If there is any factor indicating significant operative risk, co-morbidity, or the patient is elderly and frail, then PEI is probably preferable. In the future it is likely that the current position of PEI will be challenged by RFA largely on the grounds that the lesions can be dealt with in a fewer number of sessions.

Thermal and laser ablation

Both heating and cooling locally administered under ultrasound control, have been used to induce tumor necrosis. 'Cryotherapy', which relies on a 'freeze–thaw' process is undoubtedly effective in delivering local tumor control even in larger lesions (up to 8 cm) but the probe needs to be large (up to 10 mm in diameter) and the treatment needs to be delivered under general anesthetic at the time of laparotomy. RFA, in which heat is developed from an alternating electric current in the radiofrequency range, can result in complete necrosis of a 3 cm tumor in less than 1 h and in one session. RFA is considered to be 'minimally invasive', the needle electrodes being only 15-gauge. Depending on tumor size and site it may be administered percutaneously, intraoperatively or laparoscopically. Some lesions, particularly those near to large vessels, may be technically difficult to access.

Overall the complication rate is under 10%, rather lower than that reported for cryotherapy as is the mortality. Such opinions should be taken cautiously as the size of tumor treated with RFA tends to be smaller than with cryoablation and thus the inherent risks of the procedure are also smaller. Nonetheless there is a general trend toward RFA and away from cryotherapy. Moreover, the more rapid achievement of complete tumor necrosis and easier access to tumor margins has also led to a general trend towards RFA over PEI. Indeed such is the enthusiasm for RFA that prospective randomized trials comparing RFA with surgical resection are currently underway.

Other technologies are being developed to achieve similar ends to RFA and PEI and these include photodynamic therapy and laser thermal ablation. The latter has yielded encouraging results, and has the advantage that it can be carried out under magnetic resonance guidance, the whole procedure being monitored with near real time thermal imaging to assess the efficacy of tissue necrosis.

Radiotherapy and internal irradiation with intra-arterial radioisotopes

The application of external beam irradiation for the treatment of liver tumors has been severely limited by the radiosensitivity of normal hepatocytes. Maximum tolerance of normal liver to radiation is generally accepted to be between 2500 and 3000 cGy; above this level the risk of radiation hepatitis (veno-occlusive disease with perivenular congestion and fibrosis) increases rapidly.

Therapeutic doses of radioisotopes can be administered into the hepatic artery using ^{90}Y tagged to resin-based or glass microspheres or ^{131}I in conjunction with lipiodol. Lipiodol-^{131}I emits mainly γ-radiation. The volume of radioactive lipiodol administered is limited by the size and vascularity of the tumor; thus in practice, radioactive lipiodol is used only in patients with tumors less than 5 cm in diameter. About 40% of patients will gain objective remissions with minimal toxicities while keeping the radiation dose to a normal liver below 2000 cGy. ^{90}Y, a pure β-emitter, is more powerful than ^{131}I with a mean tissue penetration of about 2.5 mm. Optimal tumor regression and reduction of serum AFP level are seen when the average radiation dose to the tumor is above 12 000 cGy. The partial response rate is more than 50%. Despite the presence of cirrhosis, there is little evidence of radiation hepatitis, even when the non-tumorous liver receives up to 7000 cGy. Leakage of the microspheres into the right gastric artery or gastroduodenal artery may occasionally cause radiation gastritis or duodenitis. Systemic leakage of the microspheres to involve the lungs, which are also sensitive to irradiation, may occur if there is extensive arteriovenous shunting within the tumor. For this reason, the degree of lung shunting must be determined before administration of the radioisotope by using a ^{99m}Tc macroaggregated albumin (^{99m}Tc-MAA) scan (**Fig. 29.13**).

From the above it is clear that all these locoregional therapies, and indeed surgical resection, the definitive locoregional treatment, are all capable of delivering complete local control in a percentage of cases, the percentage decreasing as the tumor size increases. It seems likely that all these would, in patients without underlying liver disease or with well compensated liver disease, result in improvement in survival but this has, to date, only been demonstrated in two small series of patients receiving TACE. The treatment of choice will depend on the ease and cost of the therapy, its complication and acceptability rate, and benefit that can be shown in prospective randomized clinical trials. The problem for all these remains that recurrence is the rule. What is needed therefore is effective chemotherapy to supplement local control. To date this has not been demonstrated but remains the long-term goal.

Systemic therapy

Almost all the cytotoxic agents used in oncologic practice have been evaluated, and none has been shown (as a single agent or in combination with other agents) consistently to improve survival or to achieve a response rate of greater than 20%. The most widely used agent has been Adriamycin (doxorubicin). In a review of several published trials involving more than 600 patients, the objective response rate was 19% with a median survival of 4 months. A reasonable approach is to administer three courses and to reassess at 2 months. If there is evidence of a response, in terms of a greater than 50% fall in serum AFP or a decrease in liver or tumor size as determined by ultrasound or CT scanning, then treatment should be continued to a maximum dose of 550 mg/m². Above this cumulative dose, cardiotoxicity becomes increasingly frequent. In the absence of response, active treatment should be abandoned or changed. Recently a

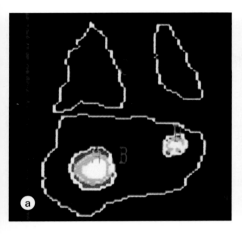 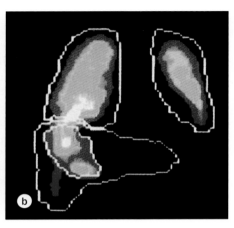

Figure 29.13 γ scan of the liver after injection of technetium-labeled macroaggregated albumin. This serves as a simulation to examine the distribution of yttrium-labeled microspheres that will occur when these are given as treatment for hepatocellular carcinoma (HCC). In (a) the activity is concentrated in the two liver tumors, indicating a high tumor to normal ratio and no shunting to the lungs. In (b) there is massive lung shunting. If this latter patient were given yttrium treatment, radiation pneumonitis would be very likely to occur. (Courtesy of Dr Stephen Ho.)

regimen known as PIAF (platinum, interferon, Adriamycin, and 5-FU) has been shown to convert about 10–20% of unresectable tumors to resectable ones, but this regimen should remain experimental until controlled trials have been completed. It is noteworthy that the most common primary liver tumor in childhood, hepatoblastoma, is significantly more chemosensitive, and it is now common practice to administer chemotherapy before surgical resection. The most usual regimen is PLADO (cisplatin 80 mg/m^2 over 24 h by continuous infusion) and doxorubicin (60 mg/m^2 as an intravenous infusion over 48 h). Using this regimen, more than 80% of cases of hepatoblastoma will achieve remission, and initially unresectable tumors can often be resected after four courses.

The last decade has seen interest in altering the hormonal environment of the tumors and small studies suggested survival benefit from antiandrogenic, antiestrogenic agents and octreotide. However, recent large-scale prospective randomized controlled studies have generally failed to find any support for these contentions. It should be recognized that these systemic treatments tend to be studied in patients with advanced disease and the possibility that they would be more effective if instituted earlier can not be excluded.

Screening programs for hepatocellular carcinoma

Whole population screening is not an option, but there are well-defined high risk groups – patients who have chronic liver disease and those who carry the HBV and/or HCV – who may benefit from HCC surveillance programs (although in a proportion of patients who develop HCC, the underlying liver disease is 'silent' and would thus never present for surveillance). The lifetime risk of HCC development for a male who has cirrhosis in any of these groups is in the range of 10–40%. In such an individual, who has access to the necessary resources, it seems likely that a 3–6 monthly AFP estimation and ultrasound examination will lead to the detection of tumor development before it becomes clinically apparent. If liver transplantation is available, a case can be made for screening all those at risk. If not then screening is only appropriate in those with good liver function, who would be candidates for resection with curative intent if a tumor is detected.

Surveillance programs are commonly promoted in the West, but it should be stressed that, at the time of writing, this practice is not supported by evidence showing that it is either cost effective or leads to improved survival and the practical problems associated with surveillance should not be underestimated. Other, non-HCC lesions may be picked up, including macroregenerative nodules, dysplastic nodules and hemangiomas, and these are not easy to confirm histologically particularly when small. Furthermore the patient undergoing resection or transplantation faces a 5–10% chance of perioperative mortality, whereas without operation the survival with an asymptomatically detected tumor may be up to 3 years.

OTHER PRIMARY LIVER TUMORS

The ratio of HCC:cholangiocarcinoma:other primary malignant liver tumors is in the order of 100:10:1. It follows that in most units physicians and pathologists will have only a very limited experience of 'other' primary liver tumors. It is, however, important that such diagnoses are established accurately since some of the tumors described below have a significantly better prognosis than HCC and are more often cured by surgery. Histologic review by a pathologist who has a special interest in liver tumors is always recommended if there is any doubt whatsoever about the diagnosis. Fibrolamellar carcinoma is considered a 'variant' of HCC and has been described above.

Sarcomas

Angiosarcomas present in a manner similar to those of other malignant tumors of the liver, usually with hepatomegaly, pain and weight loss, or hemoperitoneum. In about 25% of cases a history of occupational exposure to vinyl chloride (VC), thorotrast or arsenic can be obtained. Precursor features are well recognized and include periportal and subcapsular fibrosis and evidence of activation of hepatocytes in the sinusoid lining cells. Exposure to VC is now strictly controlled during the production of polyvinyl chloride so that the number of cases is likely to decrease significantly. A similar situation exists with thorotrast, a radiologic contrast medium containing a colloidal suspension of thorium dioxide (a powerful emitter of α particles), which was first used in the 1920s but has been withdrawn since 1950. The minimum period between exposure and tumor development is 15 years, but cases are still being encountered more than 40 years after the agent was withdrawn from use. The radioactive emission of the thorotrast can be readily detected by autoradiography and the particles of thorotrast can be seen by electron microscopy. The tumors are usually multifocal and, apart from the occasional patient with localized disease where the tumor is amenable to resection, the prognosis is less than 1 year with no therapy having been shown to alter the natural history.

Epithelioid hemangioendotheliomas

Epithelioid hemangioendotheliomas represent the malignant end of a spectrum starting with the typical hemangioma. There are no specific presenting features and they are most often seen in young and middle-aged females. The tumors are usually multiple at presentation and metastases are detectable in about half of all cases. Although the tumor may appear epithelioid on routine histologic examination, its endothelial origins can be confirmed by staining for factor-VIII-related antigen, and the malignant cells have characteristic ultrastructural features. The prognosis is very variable. Most patients will die from the tumor, but prolonged survival periods of up to 10 years, even without treatment, have been reported. The standard surgical approaches of resection where this is possible, or liver transplantation, are still recommended.

Primary hepatic lymphomas

Such tumors are even rarer than those mentioned above. Their diagnosis remains controversial since it is often difficult to establish that they are truly primary. Occasionally cases can be cured by resection or palliated with chemotherapy, but the prognosis is very poor in the majority of cases.

Malignant liver tumors in childhood – hepatoblastoma

Malignant liver tumors are rare in children, but when present are usually hepatoblastomas. Of hepatoblastomas, 90% occur within the first 5 years of life and they outnumber HCC in this age group by a ratio of 2:1. The usual presentation is with an enlarging upper abdominal mass together with pain, weight loss and anorexia. Association with congenital abnormalities is well described as are cases of precocious puberty related to β-human chorionic gonadotropin (HCG) production by the tumor cells. Serum AFP is consistently elevated, often to very high levels. It accurately reflects tumor mass and is useful in monitoring treatment. On imaging the tumor is hypervascular, usually solitary and often exhibits calcification.

Primary liver tumors in childhood are uniformly fatal without resection. As with adult HCC, the main hope of cure is complete surgical resection. About 50% will be suitable for resection and half of these will survive long term. However, the tumor is highly sensitive to chemotherapy (usually Adriamycin and cisplatinum) and postoperative adjuvant therapy, even in the presence of incomplete resection, has been found to improve survival rates. Currently, in several centers, preoperative chemotherapy is given to all patients irrespective of the perceived degree of operability. Long-term survival rates in the order of 80% are being achieved. All children who have hepatoblastoma should be managed in centers conversant with a multimodality approach to treatment.

SECONDARY LIVER TUMORS

Until recently the approach to the patient who has hepatic metastases has been largely nihilistic and the detection of metastases immediately heralded withdrawal of all active therapy. However, it is now recognized that, with careful selection, a small percentage of patients may be cured by surgery, a proportion may have their survival prolonged, and others can be offered a useful improvement in quality of life by cytotoxic chemotherapy. Equally, however, administration of cytotoxic therapy to patients who have poor performance status and widely disseminated disease may significantly decrease their quality of life during their few remaining months. A carefully balanced approach is therefore needed. Hepatic metastases are often only one site of metastatic disease and the overall management of such cases is the purview of the oncologist. The following section briefly summarizes the situation for those in which the liver is the sole or predominant site of disease.

Liver metastases are found at 1% of all autopsies. After lymph nodes, the liver is the most common site of metastatic disease, being involved in 40% of adult patients who have primary extrahepatic malignancy and up to 75% of those with primary tumors drained by the portal venous system (pancreas, large bowel and stomach). About 20% present with synchronous metastases (the figure is higher if metastases are sought by intraoperative US) and a further 20% of hepatic metastases develop during the course of the disease. The tumors may be solitary or multiple, but unlike HCC they tend to be umbilicated and infiltrate the normal liver tissue (**Fig. 29.14**). Around 25% of cases will have solitary liver metastases and thus be candidates for some form of surgical resection; this figure is much lower for other primary tumors such as those of breast and lung.

Clinical features and disease associations

Patients who have hepatic metastases present with pain, weight loss, anorexia and hard hepatomegaly in which discrete masses can often be palpated. The abdomen may be distended with ascites and there may be other, extrahepatic, signs of malignancy. These are all signs of advanced disease. Patients who have hepatic metastases who may be candidates for surgical resection often have their tumors detected before symptoms develop. Certain metastatic tumors, particularly carcinoid and other 'neuroendocrine' tumors including islet cell carcinomas, appear to involve the liver with relatively little disruption of hepatic function (see below).

Diagnosis

Routine liver tests are not very helpful in diagnosing liver metastases, although metastases are unlikely if all routine liver tests are entirely within their reference ranges. Any abnormality of standard liver function, particularly a raised activity of hepatic alkaline phosphatase, is an indication for further imaging of the liver.

Contrast-enhanced CT of the abdomen is now widely considered as a routine investigation in patients presenting with colorectal cancer and has sensitivity in the order of 85%. With intraoperative US scanning the sensitivity reaches 100% (by definition, as this is the gold standard by which other techniques are judged). If isolated hepatic metastases are detected, CT of the chest and pelvis should be undertaken, if not part of the initial investigation. It should be stressed that the figures quoted above refer to the detection of metastases when the reporting radiologist has been specifically requested to examine the liver with a view to detecting tumors. Metastases show lower

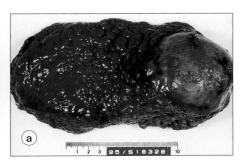
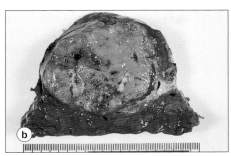
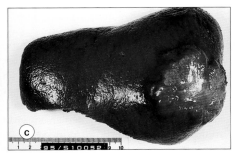
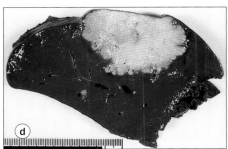

Figure 29.14 Comparison of the macroscopic appearances of primary and secondary liver tumors. Note that the primary tumor (hepatocellular carcinoma (HCC)) arises as a well-circumscribed, solitary nodule in an extensively macrocirrhotic liver and bulges from the surface of the liver (a & b). In marked contrast the secondary tumor arises in a non-cirrhotic liver, is infiltrating in nature, and umbilicated (c & d). (Courtesy of Dr CT Liew.)

attenuation than the surrounding liver, both before and after contrast, and often show peripheral ring enhancement on ultrasound examination (**Fig. 29.15**). In contrast to primary liver tumors, metastases tend to be umbilicated and do not expand and distort the liver surface to the same extent (Fig. 29.15). About 20% of patients who have hepatic metastases from colorectal cancer will show calcification on CT or US and as such seem to have a significantly better prognosis. Estimation of the serum concentration of CEA is used mainly to detect recurrence after resection of the primary colorectal tumor and, as such should be a part of routine initial investigation. A rising CEA level in this situation usually heralds metastases, most often in the liver.

All too frequently patients present with malignant liver disease (usually reported as adenocarcinoma on biopsy), but no obvious primary extrahepatic site can be detected after full physical examination. Extensive radiologic investigations such as barium meal, barium enema and intravenous pyelography are not indicated as the occult tumor is seldom situated in the gut or kidney and both false-positive and false-negative results are frequent. CT scanning is the most rewarding investigation, but in a proportion of these patients the primary is never identified.

Histology

Histologic confirmation of suspected hepatic metastases is not always indicated, particularly when active treatment is not contemplated. However, if the source of the primary tumor is not known, biopsies are usually done to exclude some of the more treatable forms of metastatic disease such as lymphoma or breast cancer. In addition, when the lesion is solitary, biopsy is indicated unless resection is to be undertaken. The presence of metastases obviously has major implications for the patient, but this diagnosis should not be presumed if a solitary lesion is detected as this may be an unrelated benign lesion. When the primary tumor from which a hepatic metastasis has originated is not apparent, histologic examination may provide a clue to the site of the primary (**Fig. 29.16**). Adenocarcinomas are usually of colorectal or pancreatic origin, but intrahepatic cholangio-carcinomas also have a similar appearance. Anaplastic tumors are usually of bronchial origin. Recently developed histological methods involving special stains, immunocytochemistry, and electron microscopy often permit determination of the origin of these highly anaplastic tumors. Thus, the CK7/CK20 profile often gives clues as to the primary site of the lesion, and positive nuclear staining for TTFI is suggestive of a primary lung tumor.

Natural history and prognosis

In the absence of treatment there is an inverse linear relation between percentage of liver involved and log survival time (from diagnosis) with secondary liver tumors. About 50% of patients are alive at 3 months and less than 10% at 1 year, although individual cases may show wide variations. Patients who have multiple metastases have a significantly worse prognosis than

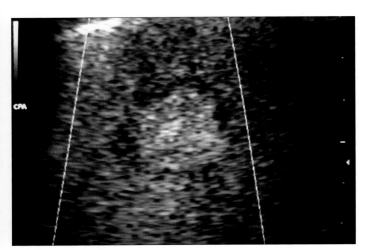

Figure 29.15 Characteristic liver secondary seen on ultrasound examination as a 'target' lesion with a hypoechoic rim and a hyperechoic center. (Courtesy of Dr Wei Tse Yang.)

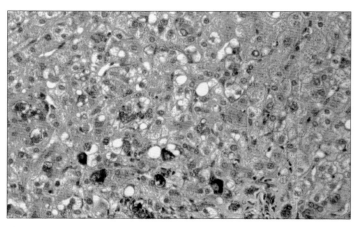

Figure 29.16 Hepatic metastasis for a primary melanoma. The site of a secondary tumor can seldom be confidently made on routine histologic examination. Here the presence of melanin confirms metastasis from a primary melanoma. (Courtesy of Dr Bernard Portmann.)

those who have solitary metastases, as do those who have any evidence of other, extrahepatic, metastases. Among those who have solitary lesions receiving no active treatment, a 20% 3-year survival rate has been quoted. This observation should not be forgotten when assessing the efficacy of surgical resection of solitary metastases in uncontrolled studies. Metastases from primary carcinoid tumors are the only secondary tumors to exhibit a significantly better prognosis, survival periods of up to 10 years not being uncommon. With the wide use of more sophisticated radiologic techniques the diagnosis is being established earlier, often while the patient is asymptomatic, and this makes for an apparent increase in survival.

Management

As with primary tumors, the first aim of investigation is to identify that small subgroup that might benefit from surgical resection, the only hope of cure. In about 25% of cases of metastatic colorectal cancer disease is confined to the liver and overall, about 20% of all patients who have hepatic metastases will be candidates for surgical resection with curative intent. A review of the literature shows that survival at 1, 3, 5 and 10 years is of the order of 85, 50, 35 and 20% respectively. Although the complication rate can be high, the perioperative mortality should now be well below 5%. The precise indications vary from unit to unit. Some consider that any cases in which all macroscopic disease can be removed should be candidates. Others confine surgical resection to those who have solitary lesions, or at most, three small lesions confined to one lobe. Such decisions remain a matter of philosophy and resource. Resection appears less likely to be curative as the tumor size increases, the number of nodules decreases, and as the time between resection of the primary tumor and the detection of liver metastases decreases. An involved margin after resection is usually a harbinger of subsequent recurrences. The optimal follow-up strategy remains unclear and although there is now evidence from randomized controlled trials that post operative adjuvant therapy with intravenous and/or intra-arterial administration of 5-FU based therapy decreases the recurrence rate and improves survival, this approach has not yet entered routine practice.

Surgical resection of hepatic metastases is an area of intense research at present and much of the current dogma is being actively challenged. The wider application of 2-[fluorine-18] fluoro-2-deoxy-D-glucose-positron emission tomography (FDG-PET) and intraoperative ultrasound scanning prior to resection is frequently demonstrating lesions not detected on the original imaging. Several groups are examining the possibility, in carefully selected cases, of resecting both the liver and lung lesions, and combining surgical resection with RFA when the complete surgical resection cannot be attained. Preoperative cytotoxic chemotherapy, to render an initially unresectable lesion resectable, is also an area of intense investigation.

Management of inoperable hepatic metastases

Steady incremental advances are improving the outlook for patients with unresectable metastatic colorectal cancer. 5-FU in combination with folinic acid (FA) remains the foundation of treatment and the standard infusional regimens lead to response rates of around 20% and an improvement in median survival from 6 months to 12 months. Two recently introduced drugs (oxaliplatin and irenotecan), in combination with 5-FU-FA, can each increase the response rate to 30–50% with a median overall survival of 15–20 months. With the addition of bevacizumab [an anti-vascular endothelial growth factor (anti-VEGF) monoclonal antibody] the figure for median survival appears now to exceed 20 months. Similar results can be obtained with hepatic arterial infusion of 5-FU-FA although the toxicity is quite distinct from that seen with systemic administration of 5-FU. Nausea, vomiting, diarrhea and myelosuppression are all uncommon. The toxicity relates to ulcer disease and hepatic toxicity. The most common lesion is a sclerosing cholangitis, probably due to primary damage of the blood vessels feeding the bile ducts, which also derive their blood supply from the hepatic artery. The overall cost, inconvenience, and side-effects of chronic intra-arterial chemotherapy still limit this approach. However, in highly motivated patients, with good performance status and modest disease burden, controlled studies have shown that significant improvement in quality of life can be obtained (**Fig. 29.17**).

Hepatic metastases from the neuroendocrine tumors

Hepatic metastases often dominate the clinical picture in patients with neuroendocrine tumors particularly carcinoid tumors, even in the absence of the 'carcinoid syndrome'. The syndrome, which affects about 20% of patients with carcinoid tumors, comprises facial flushing, abdominal cramps and diarrhea and, less often, wheezing, and right-sided cardiac complications attributable to the episodic release of vasoactive peptides such as serotonin, kallikrein, 5-hydroxytryptophan and neurotensin. Since the liver can readily metabolize serotonin, the primary peptide produced, the carcinoid syndrome only develops when the liver is bypassed or there are metastases within the liver; the development of the carcinoid syndrome thus invariably implies metastatic spread from a primary lesion in the small bowel to the liver. Abdominal pain or discomfort is often due to hepatic involvement although the pain may be due to obstruction by the primary small bowel tumor. Diagnosis is based on an elevated level of urinary 5-hydroxyindoleacetic acid (5-HIAA), the characteristic histological pattern of a neuro-endocrine tumor involving the liver (staining for synaptophysin

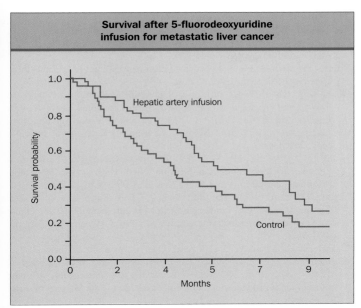

Figure 29.17 Improvement in survival, with a normal quality of life after chronic infusion with 5-fluorodeoxyuridine (FUDR). Reproduced from Allen-Marsh TG et al (94) by permission of Elsevier.

and CD 56 are very characteristic as is chromogranin, although the latter marker can be negative in poorly differentiated tumors), and disease distribution can be assessed by an octreotide scan. Because the synthetic analogs of somatostatin bind with high affinity to somatostatin receptors present on the great majority of carcinoid tumors, radiolabeled octreotide can be used for localization tumors, being more sensitive than conventional imaging procedures such as CT scanning, and being positive in over 80% of cases. It is highly characteristic that the patient's general clinical state and standard liver function tests can be remarkably good, even in the presence of massive liver involvement.

In the absence of symptoms, there is probably no indication for active treatment of hepatic carcinoid metastases unless complete surgical resection is feasible. Symptoms of the carcinoid syndrome may be controlled by reduction of tumor mass (by surgery, arterial embolization, or cytotoxic chemotherapy) or pharmacologic interference with production or action of the tumor products. Some of these approaches may have unpleasant side-effects and should be employed only when symptoms become severe.

By the time the carcinoid syndrome has developed, the tumor is usually too widespread for curative resection to be attempted, but it may be feasible in 5–10% of cases. 'Debulking' surgery or 'shelling out' metastases may relieve symptoms, but as better approaches to pharmacologic control of symptoms become available and with the advent of hepatic artery embolization, it is being used much less widely. Embolization, with or without cytotoxic chemotherapy (doxorubicin, streptozocin and 5-FU) in various combinations control symptoms in most patients when disease is predominant in, or confined to, the liver. About 80% of patients achieve complete resolution of symptoms, which may last for 1 month to several years (median, 1 year). The procedure can be repeated and some patients have had multiple embolizations over several years. Liver transplantation has been employed in carefully selected cases.

Pharmacological control

α-Methyl-dopa and parachlorophenylalanine, which inhibit key enzymes in the biosynthesis of serotonin from tryptophan, have now been largely superseded by the long-acting somatostatin analog octreotide. Octreotide is usually dramatically effective against diarrhea and frequently against flushing too, with associated decrease in the 5-HIAA levels. The disadvantage has been that it has needed to be administered subcutaneously two or three times per day (50–100 μg). Most patients, however, learn to administer the drug themselves, and effective slow release formulations that only require monthly injections are now available. The aim of therapy is symptom control; significant tumor shrinkage occurs in less than 10% of cases. Some authorities believe that somatostatin analogs have a role in carcinoid tumors even in the absence of the syndrome, where they may 'stabilize the disease'. When octreotide becomes ineffective, the addition of interferon-α may further control symptoms.

Control of diarrhea with codeine phosphate or loperamide and careful avoidance of precipitating factors such as alcohol, stress and certain foods may also be effective. Streptozocin is the most active cytotoxic agent to have been used but it leads to a reduction in tumor mass in only 30% of cases. The addition of other agents, such as adriamycin and 5-FU, may give rather higher response rates but at the cost of considerably greater toxicity. Cytotoxic chemotherapy should be the treatment of last resort and only used after embolization and pharmacologic approaches have failed. All these approaches to decreasing tumor bulk may be associated with the massive release of vasoactive peptides from the tumor tissue. To prevent the resultant complications, patients are treated with octreotide.

FURTHER READING

Epidemiology
Beasley RP. Hepatitis B virus the major etiology of hepatocellular carcinoma. Cancer 1988; 61:1942–1956. *The definitive summation of the data implicating, and in the case of Taiwan, quantifying the risk of HCC in chronic carriers of the hepatitis B virus.*
Editorial Committee. Atlas of cancer mortality in the People's Republic of China. China Map Press.
Melia WM, Wilkinson ML, Portmann BC et al. Hepatocellular carcinoma in the non-cirrhotic liver: a comparison with that complicating cirrhosis. Quarterly Journal of Medicine, New Series 1. 1984 III; 211:391–400.
Munoz and Bosch in Okuda and Ishak, eds. Neoplasms of the liver. Tokyo: Springer Verlag, 1987, pp. 3–9.

Ross RK, Yuan JM, Yu MC, et al. Urinary aflatoxin biomarkers and risk of hepatocellular carcinoma. Lancet 1992; 339:943–946.

Diagnosis and staging
Di Bisceglie AM. Liver tumors. Clin Liver Dis 2001; 5(1).
Llovet JM, Beaugrand M. Hepatocellular carcinoma: present status and future prospects. J Hepatol 2003; 38:S136–S149.
Vauthey J-N. Primary and metastatic liver cancer. Surg Oncol Clin N Am 2003; 12(1).

Miscellaneous liver tumors

Kemeny MM, Adak S, Gray B, et al. Combined-modality treatment for resectable metastatic colorectal carcinoma to the liver: surgical resection of hepatic metastases in combination with continuous infusion of chemotherapy – an intergroup study. J Clin Oncol 2002; 20(6): 1499–1505.

McPeake JR, Portmann B. Hepatic malignancy, Budd-Chiari syndrome and space-occupying conditions. In: Williams R, Portmann B, Tan KC, eds. The practice of liver transplantation. London: Churchill Livingstone; 1995:57–71.

Metz DC, Jensen RT. Endocrine tumors of the gastrointestinal tract and pancreas. In: Rustgi AK, Crawford JM, eds. Gastrointestinal cancers. Edinburgh: Saunders; 2003:681–717.

Perilongo G, Shafford E, Maibach R, et al. Risk-adapted treatment for childhood hepatoblastoma. Final report of the second study of the International Society of Paediatric Oncology—SIOPEL 2. Eur J Cancer 2004; 40(3):411–421. *Documents the remarkable success of treatment of the childhood cancer hepatoblastoma and shows the power of integrated international trials that the pediatric community has pioneered.*

Van Kaick G, Muth H, Kaul A, et al. Results of the German thorotrast study. In: Boice JD Jr, Fraumeni JF Jr, eds. Radiation carcinogenesis epidemiology and biological significance. New York: Raven Press; 1984: 253–262.

Treatment and prevention

Allen-Marsh TG, Earlam S, Fordy C, et al. Quality of life and survival with continuous hepatic-artery floxuridine infusion for colorectal liver metastases. Lancet 1994; 344:1255–1260.

Bruix J, Sherman M, Llovet JM et al. Clinical management of hepatocellular carcinoma. J Hepatol 2001; 35: 421–430.

Chang MH, Chen CJ, Lai MS, et al. Universal hepatitis B vaccination in Taiwan and the incidence of hepatocellular carcinoma in children. N Engl J Med 1997; 336:1855–1859. *The first evidence that universal vaccination against the HBV may decrease the incidence of HCC. A landmark paper.*

Leung TWT, Patt YZ, Lau WY, et al. Complete pathological remission is possible with systemic combination chemotherapy for inoperable hepatocellular carcinoma. Clin Cancer Res 1999; 5:1676–1681.

Llovet JM, Bruix J for the Barcelona – Clinic Liver Cancer Group. Systematic review of randomised trials for unresectable hepatocellular carcinoma: chemoembolisation improves survival. Hepatology 2003; 37: 429–442.

Mazzaferro V, Regalia E, Doci R et al. Liver transplantation for the treatment of small hepatocellular carcinoma in patients with cirrhosis. N Engl J Med 1996; 334: 693–699. *Defines the most widely accepted criteria for transplantation in patients with HCC (the Milan criteria).*

CHAPTER
30
Vascular Diseases of the Liver

Dominique-Charles Valla

INTRODUCTION

The vasculature of the liver is unusual in that it has both a venous and an arterial blood supply. Poorly oxygenated blood from the low pressure portal venous system supplies the hepatic parenchyma. Richly oxygenated blood from the high pressure arterial side is mainly directed to the bile ducts. Arterial blood is eventually collected into small veins that drain into the intrahepatic portal venous system. Thus, the hepatic sinusoids are exclusively supplied with venous blood, 65% of which comes directly from the portal vein, and 35% indirectly from the hepatic arteries. There is a poorly understood mechanism whereby the hepatic artery and portal vein work together to maintain a constant blood flow to the liver. Sinusoids drain into central veins which in turn drain into hepatic veins entering the inferior vena cava close to the right atrium.

In this chapter, diseases that affect the vascular structures of the liver will be considered with the exception of parenchymal or biliary diseases that secondarily affect the hepatic vasculature. Likewise, vascular disorders that occur secondary to systemic circulatory disturbances such as cardiac failure or cardiogenic shock will not be discussed further.

HEPATIC ARTERIAL DISEASES

Hepatic artery occlusion

Over 50% of hepatic arterial blood flow is distributed to the intrahepatic bile ducts (through the peribiliary plexus), with the rest going to the large blood vessels (through the vasa vasora), to the portal tracts, and to the liver capsule (**Fig. 30.1**). In addition to the main hepatic arteries that enter the liver at the hepatic hilum, there are numerous accessory arteries that directly penetrate the liver through the capsule. The branches of the hepatic arteries are interconnected. The peribiliary plexus drains into small veins that ultimately reach the intrahepatic portal venous system.

Hepatic arterial occlusion is relatively uncommon. The above characteristics explain why hepatic arterial obstruction gives rise to clinical sequelae only in particular circumstances. In essence, ischemic bile duct damage occurs when the peribiliary plexus is involved or when all main and accessory arteries are simultaneously blocked. Concurrent impairment of portal venous and hepatic arterial inflow results in liver infarction.

Etiology and pathogenesis
Occlusion of the main arteries may result from arterial constriction within a malignant tumor (most frequently a carcinoma of the bile duct or pancreas). Iatrogenic occlusion may be intentional or unintentional, and occur in the context of surgery (liga-

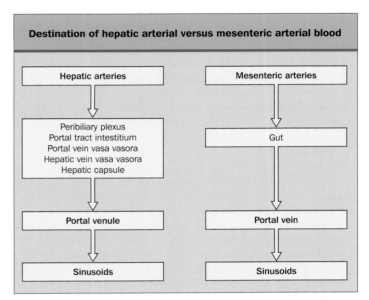

Figure 30.1 Destination of hepatic arterial and mesenteric arterial blood. There are striking similarities. Because over 50% of hepatic arterial blood is destined for the bile ducts, occlusion of the hepatic arteries can impact not only on the hepatic parenchyma but also on the bile ducts.

tion, suture, anastomosis, injury), or percutaneous catheterization (therapeutic embolization, inadvertent dissection). Stenosis or occlusion can be related to blunt or penetrating trauma; to systemic arteritis (e.g. polyarteritis nodosa, giant cell arteritis, Wegener granulomatosis, Behçet disease and systemic lupus erythematosus); or to systemic infection (e.g. bacterial endocarditis, tuberculosis, syphilis). Atheroma of the hepatic artery is rare compared with other arteries.

Outside the liver transplant setting, occlusion limited to the main hepatic arteries or their large branches is without consequences. The opening of pre-existing intrahepatic or extrahepatic anastomoses is seen at imaging within a few hours of the occlusion. In the context of decreased portal blood inflow, such as circulatory failure or portal vein occlusion, sudden obstruction of a main artery results in parenchymal infarction. When hepatic arterial occlusion gives rise to infarction, this is usually segmental with the central pale area surrounded by a hemorrhagic region.

Selective injury to the peribiliary plexus can be observed after transcatheter embolization of small-sized particles (less than 120 μm in diameter); after intrahepatic arterial infusion of toxic substances (fluoruridine or alcohol); and in patients with systemic disorders characterized by microcirculatory impairment (e.g. sickle-cell disease, systemic lupus erythematosus,

473

antiphospholipid syndrome, paroxysmal nocturnal hemoglobinuria, polyarteritis nodosa). Injury to the peribiliary plexus induces ischemic bile duct injury, with destruction of the biliary epithelium. The cellular debris can mix with bile components to form biliary casts. There may be complete necrosis of the bile duct wall with extravasated bile forming around bile infarcts within the liver. Bile infarcts can become cystic (bilomas), or superinfected. Healing of the areas of necrosis can give rise to fibrous stenoses or, conversely, to cystic dilatation of the bile ducts. When areas of stenosis or dilatation are multiple, this aspect of the biliary tree mimics the findings that are seen in primary sclerosing cholangitis.

In the setting of liver transplantation, the bile ducts and the liver are particularly vulnerable to arterial occlusion. This can be explained by the devascularization of the liver capsule (preventing collaterals from developing from accessory arteries) and to preservation injury to the endothelium of the peribiliary plexus. Arterial thrombosis may contribute to the formation of a stricture at the site of bile duct reconstruction.

Clinical features

The classic features of hepatic infarction are severe right upper quadrant abdominal pain accompanied by tachycardia, hypotension, fever and leukocytosis. Serum aminotransferase levels are markedly increased.

Ischemic bile duct injury can develop in the absence of clinical features and be revealed by increased serum alkaline phosphatase levels, several weeks or months after arterial occlusion has occurred. High fever, jaundice and right upper quadrant pain may be present when there is acute severe necrosis of the bile ducts, particularly with biliary cast formation. Bilomas may be silent, and only detected at imaging; or they may become infected giving rise to the features of single or multiple liver abscesses. Unpredictable episodes of recurrent cholangitis occur when there are stenoses or dilatation, particularly when there are secondary stones. In some patients, chronic cholestasis leads to secondary biliary fibrosis and portal hypertension.

Diagnosis

The diagnosis of hepatic infarction is established by computed tomography (CT) or magnetic resonance (MR) imaging showing a triangular zone with a peripheral base without any enhancement at the arterial and portal phase of contrast injection. An associated portal vein thrombosis or an episode of shock may be present.

Bile duct injury is suggested by ultrasonography (US) or CT, and confirmed by MR cholangiography. In selected cases, endoscopic retrograde cholangiography is needed to show diffuse beading, or single or multiple narrowing that usually predominates at the confluence of the left and right hepatic ducts and in the upper part of the main bile duct. The main differential diagnosis is primary sclerosing cholangitis. Bilomas are demonstrated using US, CT or MR imaging. A superinfected biloma is difficult to differentiate from an abscess of other origin.

The diagnosis of arterial thrombosis should be suspected whenever the above features are found in a patient with a history of hepatic surgery, radiologic intervention involving the hepatic artery, abdominal trauma, systemic vasculitis or infection. Diagnosis will usually be suggested by Doppler ultrasonography and confirmed using CT or MR angiography. Arteriography is considered in selected cases or as a first step when being performed as part of a therapeutic procedure.

Natural history and prognosis

The outcome for patients who have hepatic artery occlusion depends to a great extent on the anatomic position of the occlusion, the rate of the occlusion, and the status of the portal circulation. The underlying condition is a major determinant of prognosis.

Focal infarction at the periphery of the liver has little clinical sequelae. The infarcted area undergoes atrophy while there is hypertrophy of the rest of the parenchyma. However, when several segments of the liver are involved, either contiguously or as multiple lesions, liver failure may develop.

Similarly, focal bile duct lesions have limited clinical consequences if they are located at the periphery of the biliary tree. The parenchymal area corresponding to the bile duct lesion may undergo atrophy or abscess formation. When the bile duct lesions are centrally located, they will impact on the whole liver and transplantation may be required.

If hepatic artery occlusion follows soon after liver transplantation, the outcome is poor without urgent recanalization of the hepatic artery or retransplantation.

Management

The management of patients who have hepatic artery occlusion depends upon the clinical sequelae. If acute liver failure develops, then management should be instituted as described in Chapter 33. Bile duct damage may require percutaneous drainage of bilomas or abscesses, biliary drainage and insertion of stents for stenoses as described in Chapters 20, 28 and 33. In patients who have less severe complications, management may be expectant. Anticoagulation should be started in patients with portal venous thrombosis. Antibiotics should be used to prevent secondary infection in infarcted liver tissue and whenever there is acute cholangitis.

In the transplant patient with hepatic artery occlusion, reconstruction or recanalization of the hepatic artery must be considered urgently, using interventional radiology or surgery, as discussed later in this chapter. Outside the transplant setting, a decision to attempt recanalization must take into consideration the severity of the clinical sequelae, the location and the mechanism of the occlusion, and the association with portal vein thrombosis.

Hepatic artery aneurysms

Aneurysm of the hepatic artery is a rare condition, the cause of which may be: atheroma, fibromuscular dysplasia, polyarteritis nodosa, systemic infections (e.g. endocarditis, tuberculosis, and syphilis), or intra-abdominal sepsis; due to trauma [for example following liver biopsy or transjugular intrahepatic portosystemic shunt (TIPS) insertion] or congenital. The aneurysms can be either intra- or extrahepatic. They may show considerable variation in size. A distinction is made between a true aneurysm where the dilatation involves all three layers of the arterial wall, and a false aneurysm where the dilatation results from a rupture of the intima and of the media with preservation of the adventitia. Most aneurysms due to trauma or infection are of the false type. Dissections and aneurysms may thrombose or may

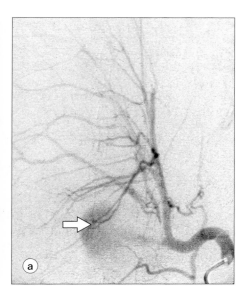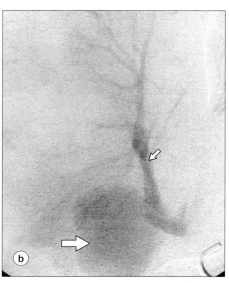

Figure 30.2 Hepatic arterial aneurysm.
(a) Traumatic hepatic arterial aneurysm filling with radiographic contrast (arrow). (b) The same aneurysm now filled (arrow). Early filling of a portal vein branch has occurred via an arteriovenous fistula (small arrow).

rupture into the peritoneal cavity, the liver, the bile ducts (causing hemobilia), or the intra or extrahepatic portal vein (causing arterioportal fistula).

Hepatic artery aneurysms are most common in middle-aged men and are often asymptomatic for long periods. The most common symptom is abdominal pain which can be severe particularly if there is arterial dissection. The risk of rupture increases with the size and the number of aneurysms. A diameter below 2 cm indicates a low risk of rupture. When compared with atheroma, fibromuscular dysplasia and polyarteritis nodosa have a greater risk of rupture. Pregnancy can precipitate the rupture of pre-existing aneurysms. Large extrahepatic aneurysms may cause obstructive jaundice or portal vein thrombosis.

Doppler-US, and CT or MR angiography are the key diagnostic investigations as described in Chapter 8. The use of arteriography should be limited to therapeutic evaluation.

The prognosis for a ruptured hepatic artery aneurysm is poor; mortality as high as 40% has been reported. Expectant management with imaging follow-up at regular intervals is appropriate in patients with silent intrahepatic aneurysms less than 2 cm in diameter. Percutaneous transarterial embolization or stenting has become the preferred therapy for large or symptomatic lesions. A ruptured aneurysm is best managed using emergency embolization therapy after appropriate resuscitation. Surgery can be used where interventional radiology fails or is unsuitable. (**Fig. 30.2**).

Solitary arterioportal fistula

In most cases, an arterioportal fistula is produced by the rupture of a false aneurysm of the hepatic artery into the neighboring portal vein branch (see above for causes of false aneurysm). Previous needle liver biopsy is probably the most common cause of the small arterioportal fistulas detected with current imaging techniques. Abdominal trauma is the most common cause of large arterioportal fistulas. Small peripheral arterioportal fistulae are common findings at CT or MR imaging in patients with cirrhosis or hepatocellular carcinoma.

Even with large arterioportal fistulae, the increase in portal pressure is usually moderate and does not reach a clinically significant level. In patients where an arterioportal fistula is associated with clinically significant portal hypertension, underlying chronic liver disease should be considered. Such an association may not be totally fortuitous since traumatic injury is more common in alcoholics or drug addicts. Large fistulae can induce mesenteric to hepatic arterial stealing resulting in intestinal ischemia. A hepatic bruit is usually present. The diagnosis is usually made by either Doppler-US or by CT or MR imaging.

Treatment of arterioportal fistulae depends on their size and position. Small intrahepatic fistulae may require no treatment. Extrahepatic fistulae can be managed with embolization using a transarterial or a transhepatic portal approach. However, spreading or dislodgment of the embolized material can lead to portal or mesenteric vein thrombosis.

Hereditary hemorrhagic telangiectasia (HHT)

Hereditary hemorrhagic telangiectasia is characterized by malformations of the small vessels resulting in arteriovenous fistulae. The condition is inherited as an autosomal dominant trait with one of two possible genes involved: endoglin on chromosome 9, and an activin receptor-like kinase on chromosome 12. Both genes code for a receptor of the transforming growth factor (TGF)-β superfamily and are mainly expressed on endothelial cells. Involvement of the skin and of nasal and gastrointestinal mucosae is common. Hepatic involvement is rare. Fistulae may be predominantly arteriovenous or arterioportal. Under the microscope, randomly distributed telangiectasias are surrounded by various degrees of fibrous tissue. Nodular hyperplasia and sinusoidal fibrosis are common. Among HHT patients liver involvement without obvious extrahepatic involvement is rare.

Massive arteriovenous shunting within the liver may cause high output cardiac failure in the absence of liver dysfunction or portal hypertension. Ischemic bile duct injury may occur due to blood-stealing away from the peribiliary plexus. When present, portal hypertension is related to either the association of nodular regenerative hyperplasia and perisinusoidal fibrosis, or to arterio-portal shunting, or to post-transfusion chronic viral hepatitis. Ascites is rare.

The diagnosis of HHT is based on the cardinal features of the disease (recurrent epistaxis, cutaneous telangiectasias, familial history). Hepatic involvement is demonstrated by Doppler-US on the basis of a marked enlargement of the hepatic arteries with increased blood flow velocity. CT or MR imaging usually confirm the enlargement of the hepatic arteries and allow better characterization of gross architectural changes including large regenerative nodules.

Embolization of the hepatic artery has been associated with both encouraging short-term results, and severe – sometimes lethal – ischemic damage to the liver or bile ducts. Therefore, embolization should be considered only in patients with severe biliary involvement or progressive cardiac dysfunction when liver transplantation is contraindicated. Although liver transplantation will not cure the other complications of HHT, its results are good provided it is performed before severe cardiac dysfunction has occurred.

PORTAL VEIN DISEASE

Disorders of the portal vein include aneurysm, fistulae and obstruction. The so-called portal vein cavernoma corresponds to the network of hepatopetal collaterals that develop following permanent obstruction of the portal vein, of its main radicles, or of its main branches.

Portal aneurysm

Aneurysm is usually defined as an increase in portal vein diameter taking a fusiform or a saccular aspect. This is an extremely uncommon condition the cause of which is unknown; it may be congenital. Aneurysms may rupture or thrombose. Most cases of portal aneurysm are recognized fortuitously at abdominal imaging. Expectant management is reasonable. Acute thrombosis of a previously normal portal vein can be associated with a marked but transient enlargement of the thrombosed portion which may lead to an erroneous diagnosis of pre-existing portal aneurysm.

Spontaneous portacaval fistula

These fistulae are characterized by a large-sized communication between the portal vein and the inferior vena cava in the absence of chronic liver disease. Two entities have been described. In the first entity, 'congenital absence of the portal vein', the extrahepatic portal vein is not seen at mesenteric or celiac angiography because of a total fistula between a mesenteric vein and the inferior vena cava. In the second entity, one or several intrahepatic fistulae are demonstrated. For both entities, evidence for a congenital anomaly stems from their recognition in neonates screened for congenital galactosemia (portosystemic shunting induces hypergalactosemia), and from their association with other developmental anomalies. However, similar intrahepatic shunts can develop in patients with acquired chronic liver disease suggesting that a block in the intrahepatic circulation may actually cause intrauterine development of a portacaval fistula. In most cases, there is no evidence for familial transmission.

Enlargement of the hepatic arteries suggests compensatory arterialization. Morphometry may show a paucity of intrahepatic portal veins. Macroregenerative nodules (resembling focal nodular hyperplasia) or nodular regenerative hyperplasia may develop which may be explained by an imbalance between increased arterial perfusion and abolished portal inflow. There are anecdotal reports of adenoma, hepatoblastoma or hepatocarcinoma.

Although liver function is well maintained, patients may develop portal-systemic encephalopathy, usually after the age of 50.

Diagnosis is established by Doppler-US and CT or MR angiography. Most patients will not require any treatment. In patients with debilitating portal-systemic encephalopathy, percutaneous transhepatic embolization of the shunt should probably be attempted first, keeping liver transplantation as an ultimate option. Proper characterization of the macronodules may require limited surgical resection. Large hepatic resections should be avoided because there is concern that regeneration can be impaired by the lack of portal inflow.

Extrahepatic portal vein obstruction
Etiology and pathogenesis
Primary adenocarcinomas of the liver, pancreas or bile ducts may invade or constrict the portal vein. When not related to a tumor, portal venous obstruction is due to thrombosis. Causes of portal vein thrombosis (PVT) can be systemic or local. Causes are usually not apparent at the time of presentation. Therefore, investigations have to be systematic. As showed in **Table 30.1**, all the known hereditary or acquired thrombogenic factors have been incriminated, with primary myeloproliferative disorders and protein S deficiency as the leading causes. Chronic portal

Thrombogenic conditions that cause portal vein thrombosis or primary Budd-Chiari syndrome		
	Approximate prevalence in patients with	
	Portal vein thrombosis (%)	Budd-Chiari syndrome (%)
Myeloproliferative disorder	25	50
Antiphospholipid syndrome	13	20
Paroxysmal nocturnal hemoglobinuria	1	5
Behçet disease	0	5
Factor V Leiden	5	25
Factor II gene mutation	13	5
Primary protein C deficiency	3	25
Primary protein S deficiency	25	3
Primary antithrombin deficiency	1	1
Homozygous *C677T MTHFR* mutation	13	13
Combination of two or more of the above factors	15	25

Table 30.1 Thrombogenic conditions that cause portal vein thrombosis or primary Budd-Chiari syndrome.

hypertension per se induces a decrease in the levels of protein C, protein S or antithrombin, which makes recognition of a primary defect difficult. Likewise, iron deficiency, hypersplenism and hemodilution may mask the peripheral blood features of myeloproliferative disorders. It is unclear whether pregnancy or administration of estrogen/progesterone precipitates PVT. Local factors are identified in 30% of patients at the time when they present with acute thrombosis, and in a lesser proportion when they present at the late stage of portal cavernoma. Common local factors include portal venous injury (e.g. cannulation, section, ligation, anastomosis, splenectomy); portal venous stasis (due to cirrhosis, obliterative portal venopathy or hepatic venous outflow block); and inflammatory conditions in the splanchnic area (e.g. appendicitis, diverticulitis, inflammatory bowel disease, pancreatitis, cholangitis, liver abscesses). Surgery for portal hypertension has been a major provider of PVT in the past. Several systemic causes, or systemic and local causes are frequently combined. Currently, about 25% of PVT cases remain unexplained despite extensive investigation.

In patients with cirrhosis but no hepatocellular carcinoma, the risk of extrahepatic PVT is related to the severity of liver disease, being less than 1% in Child-Pugh class A patients, and up to 15% in candidates for liver transplantation or portosystemic shunting. In the native livers from patients coming to transplant, about 50% of intrahepatic portal veins are found to be thrombosed. Decreased portal blood velocity, which occurs with progressive worsening of cirrhosis, probably explains PVT in patients with advanced liver disease. However, there is evidence that extrahepatic PVT in a Child-Pugh class A patient is precipitated by an underlying or incidental thrombogenic state.

Upstream from the portal vein thrombus, preserved mesenteric venous arches prevent ischemic damage to the gut, whereas involvement of these arches produces intestinal ischemia. Downstream, the liver is protected from clinically significant ischemia by an increased arterial blood flow (the buffer response), and by a rapid development of hepatopetal collaterals (the cavernoma) (**Fig. 30.3**). These collaterals, however, do not relieve the extrahepatic block, so portal hypertension ensues.

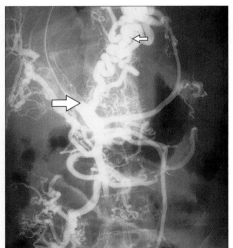

**Figure 30.3
Transhepatic venogram showing thrombosis in the portal vein (arrow).** There is widespread collateral circulation (small arrow).

There are particular consequences to the obstruction of one major branch of the portal vein, with the other branches remaining patent. In the obstructed territory, the hepatic parenchyma undergoes atrophy due to apoptosis and necrosis. Sinusoids are dilated. In the unobstructed territory, however, the hepatic parenchyma undergoes hypertrophy related to hepatocellular proliferation. The mechanisms signaling this adaptation are not yet understood.

Clinical features
Acute thrombosis
Many cases of extrahepatic PVT are now recognized at the acute stage of recent thrombosis (acute pylephlebitis) in patients with abdominal pain, often associated with fever. When thrombosis is precipitated by an abscess in the splanchnic area, spiking fever with chills and positive blood cultures indicate septic pylephlebitis. Patients in whom portal vein thrombosis complicates intra-abdominal inflammation or malignancy may present with obvious features of the underlying disorder such as a perforated viscus or necrotizing pancreatitis.

Chronic portal vein thrombosis
When the initial episode goes unnoticed, the condition is recognized at the stage of portal cavernoma, usually as a fortuitous discovery of portal hypertension in the investigation of thrombocytopenia, splenic enlargement, or esophageal varices. Gastrointestinal bleeding has become an uncommon presentation of PVT. Presentation with ascites or encephalopathy is rare, although these features may transiently accompany gastrointestinal bleeding. Biliary complications may be the presenting features of a portal cavernoma.

Investigations and diagnosis
Liver specific tests are generally normal in patients who have portal vein thrombosis not secondary to parenchymal liver disease, although mild abnormalities may be present in adults who have portal vein thrombosis. In such patients liver biopsy typically shows normal hepatic parenchyma. However, some patients with superimposed or pre-existing intrahepatic portal vein thrombosis may show some histological alterations (see below). Complete blood counts may show thrombocytopenia and leukopenia with or without anemia related to hypersplenism. However, blood cell counts may be increased or high normal which, in a patient with massive splenic enlargement, suggests that a primary myeloproliferative disorder is present. Wedged hepatic venous pressure in portal hypertension due to portal vein thrombosis is normal, but where the thrombosis is secondary to hepatic disease, wedged hepatic venous pressure may be elevated.

CT scan and Doppler-US are the key diagnostic procedures, as described in Chapter 8. At the acute stage, diagnosis is based on the absence of flow in the portal vein lumen which is occupied by solid material. Differential diagnosis includes a tumor invading the vein. At CT scanning, spontaneous hyperdensity of the portal vein prior to contrast injection indicates recent thrombosis (**Fig. 30.4**). Arterial phase enhancement of the endoluminal material indicates invasion by a malignant tumor. At the late stage, diagnosis of portal cavernoma is made by showing that the normal portal vein is replaced by winding venous structures. There may be calcifications of the portal vein wall indicating previous mural thrombi.

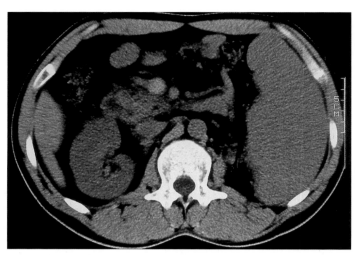

Figure 30.4 Uninjected computed tomography (CT) scan showing spontaneous hyperdensity in the mesenteric vein. This is diagnostic of recent venous thrombosis. Note that the spleen is enlarged due to a myeloproliferative disorder.

Identification of a possible cause is difficult. Local factors are investigated with abdominal imaging. Due to acute portal hypertension, intestinal and gallbladder walls are thickened and the head of the pancreas is enlarged in the absence of ischemic damage or primary inflammatory lesions.

Underlying prothrombotic disorders require systematic hematological investigations. Even without direct proof from laboratory investigation, a family or personal history of deep vein thrombosis represents circumstantial but significant evidence for an underlying prothrombotic condition. A myeloproliferative disorder may be readily identified by traditional hematologic investigations, but in some patients the culture of bone marrow cells is necessary to identify increased spontaneous formation of erythroid colonies. Primary deficiency in antithrombin, protein C or protein S is firmly established when screening discloses an affected first degree relative.

Natural history and prognosis

When there is extension, or recurrence, of thrombosis into the small mesenteric veins, there is a risk of intestinal necrosis, peritonitis and multiorgan failure. At this stage, even after resection of the infarcted gut, mortality rates may reach 50%.

Recurrent gastrointestinal bleeding from portal hypertension is the major complication of long-standing PVT. The prognostic factors for bleeding include the size of the esophageal varices and a past history of bleeding. The second major complication is recurrent thrombosis, usually in the portal venous territory and less commonly in other venous beds. The main prognostic factor for recurrent thrombosis is the presence of an underlying prothrombotic condition. Compression of the bile ducts by portal collaterals is emerging as an important source of morbidity including bacterial cholangitis, cholecystitis, and chronic cholestasis. The likelihood of these biliary complications increases with time elapsed from initial obstruction.

The prognosis of patients who have chronic portal vein thrombosis is to a large degree dependent upon any associated underlying disorder, such as cirrhosis. In those patients in whom no associated condition is identified, the outlook is good.

Tolerance, for example, to gastrointestinal bleeding is better than in patients who have cirrhosis because of the preserved liver function. In children who present with variceal bleeding secondary to portal vein thrombosis, the risk of hemorrhage decreases after adolescence and hepatic dysfunction may occur years later associated with atrophy and portal tract fibrosis.

Management

PVT treatment is discussed differently at the stage of recent thrombosis versus at the stage of cavernoma. Recanalization of a recently thrombosed portal vein can be expected in over 75% of the cases promptly treated with anticoagulation alone. Spontaneous recanalization appears to be rare. Anticoagulation should be maintained for at least 6 months before concluding lack of success. When reperfusion has been achieved, current data support continued anticoagulation in patients with permanent underlying prothrombotic disorders and no contra-indication. Successful thrombolysis for acute portal vein thrombosis has been reported. However, the high rate of reperfusion on anticoagulation alone and the risk of dreadful complications from thrombolysis question the value of the latter treatment.

In patients with portal cavernoma, pharmacological or endoscopic treatments for prevention of first or recurrent gastrointestinal bleeding appear useful. There is some evidence that anticoagulation can be given for decreasing the risk of recurrent thrombosis without increasing the risk or the severity of gastrointestinal bleeding. Therefore, anticoagulation can be proposed for patients with portal cavernoma, particularly when there is an underlying thrombogenic condition and when no treatable local factor has been documented. The outcome is excellent in patients treated according to the above considerations. In elderly patients mortality is largely related to unlinked diseases.

In occasional cases, portal venous angioplasty may be successfully undertaken. A TIPS is not normally indicated in this situation and would usually be impossible to establish.

Obstruction of intrahepatic portal veins
Schistosomiasis

Worldwide, the major cause for the obstruction of intrahepatic portal veins is schistosomiasis, which is beyond the scope of this chapter. In brief, adult worms residing in the small mesenteric veins lay their eggs in the intestinal wall for fecal elimination. When infestation is massive, eggs are transported downstream along the portal venous system to the liver where they block the small intrahepatic portal veins. The granulomatous reaction leads to fibrosis of the portal tracts and neighboring sinusoids. Portal hypertension ensues. In many patients, concurrent hepatitis C or hepatitis B add their own lesion to the formation of the intrahepatic block.

Obstructive portal venopathy

Obstructive portal venopathy is similarly characterized by the obstruction of small intrahepatic portal veins. It has been reported under numerous other names, including non-cirrhotic intrahepatic portal hypertension in clinically-based reports, and hepatoportal sclerosis or non-cirrhotic portal fibrosis in pathologic studies. In Western countries, exposure to arsenicals, vinyl chloride monomer, and thorium sulfate has been recognized to cause obliterative portal venopathy in the past. Recent

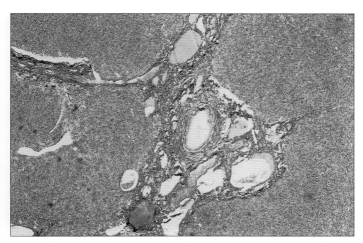

Figure 30.5 Histologic features of obliterative portal venopathy. The normal portal vein is no longer visible. It should be much larger than the interlobular bile duct that is visible at the center of the portal tract. The normal portal vein is replaced by several thin walled channels that constitute a microscopic cavernoma. There are slender fibrous expansions of the portal tract.

studies indicate that an underlying thrombogenic condition similar to those discussed above for extrahepatic portal vein thrombosis is found in over half the patients. Still, a proportion of cases remain cryptogenic. It is generally admitted that the obstruction is related to phlebitis or thrombosis.

The portal tracts are devoid of normal veins. The small intrahepatic portal veins are absent, thrombosed or replaced by a fibrous scar. Characteristically, multiple small vascular channels (a microscopic equivalent to the cavernoma) are found within the portal tracts, at their periphery, or at random within the lobule (**Fig. 30.5**). Fibrous enlargement of the portal tracts, nodulation of the parenchyma, patchy sinusoidal dilatation and sinusoidal fibrosis are common. The atrophy of the parenchyma is reflected by the approximation of the portal tracts and of the central veins.

Clinical features and prognosis

The clinical presentation almost always includes portal hypertension. Liver failure is rare or occurs after a course of several decades. The prognosis is better than for cirrhotic portal hypertension, and is mostly related to accompanying diseases. Superimposed extrahepatic PVT is seen in half the patients. There is no specific therapy. Anticoagulation can be proposed when an underlying thrombogenic condition is present. Portal hypertension can be managed as recommended for cirrhotic patients.

Diagnosis

Diagnosis is suspected when portal hypertension is found in the absence of extrahepatic portal vein thrombosis and in the absence of the common causes of cirrhosis. Liver biopsy is the clue to the diagnosis by showing the abnormal portal veins or, in the case of schistosomiasis, the ova. The hepatic venous pressure gradient can be normal or raised. A gradient below 12 mmHg in a patient with previous bleeding from portal hypertension and a patent main portal vein suggests that small intrahepatic portal veins are obstructed.

Splenic vein thrombosis

The most common causes of splenic vein thrombosis are pancreatitis with or without pancreatic pseudocysts and pancreatic tumors. Retroperitoneal infections or fibrosis, cirrhosis, and upper abdominal surgery are unusual causes. When no obvious local cause is found, an underlying prothrombotic disorder should be suspected as for PVT.

Thrombosis of the splenic vein gives rise to the development of collateral vessels between the spleen and the portal vein, namely portoportal shunts, or between the spleen and the vena cava or azygos vein, namely portosystemic shunts. In particular, a collateral circulation develops via the short gastric veins into the gastric fundus, and then to the left gastric vein and portal vein. The result is prominent gastric varices, with few or no varices in the lower esophagus. The classic clinical feature is splenomegaly.

In many patients splenic vein thrombosis is identified following gastrointestinal bleeding usually from gastric varices since esophageal varices are less common. Other patients may present with features related to the associated underlying disorder such as pancreatic neoplasia or chronic pancreatitis. In some patients, diagnosis is made fortuitously in the investigation of splenomegaly, gastric varices or collateral veins at abdominal imaging.

The diagnosis would generally be confirmed by Doppler-US, but CT or MR angiography may be required. Hematologic investigations may reveal evidence of hypersplenism.

Prognosis depends to a large extent on the underlying predisposing cause. In those without serious underlying pathology the prognosis is good.

In patients in whom thrombosis is confined to the splenic vein, splenectomy is the definitive treatment and is curative. However, in patients with underlying thrombogenic factors, splenectomy may initiate portal or mesenteric vein thrombosis. Endoscopic treatment using a cyanoacrylate glue injection may be superior to band ligation or sclerosis. Prophylactic splenectomy has been proposed for patients in whom splenic vein thrombosis was identified before variceal bleeding. The benefit:risk ratio of this approach is unclear, and generally, splenectomy is reserved for those patients who have bled.

HEPATIC VENOUS OUTLET OBSTRUCTION

Budd-Chiari syndrome (BCS) is characterized by an obstruction of the hepatic venous outflow tract at the level of small hepatic veins, large hepatic veins, or suprahepatic segment of the inferior vena cava (IVC). Secondary BCS is related to invasion or compression of the veins by an extravenous lesion, whereas primary BCS is related to primary phlebitis or thrombosis. Veno-occlusive disease is now considered not to be a primary disorder of the hepatic veins and will be discussed below as sinusoidal obstruction syndrome.

Etiology and pathogenesis

BCS is a rare condition. Causes of secondary BCS include malignancies prone to invade their venous outflow tract (adenocarcinoma of the liver, kidney or adrenals), or developing in the vicinity of the terminal portion of the IVC (leiomyosarcoma and myxoma). Alveolar hydatid disease behaves like a malignant tumor of the liver. Focal nodular hyperplasia or liver

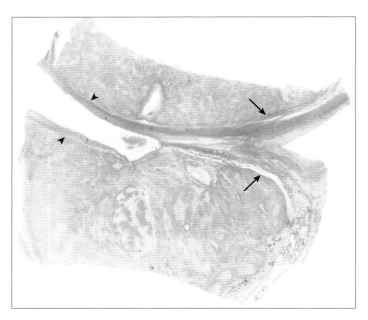

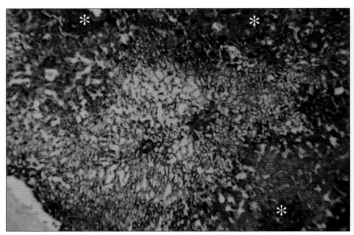

Figure 30.7 Histologic features of hepatic venous outflow block. Centrilobular necrosis is visible as a loss of hepatocytes in the center of the photograph while hepatocytes are preserved in the periportal areas (indicated by asterisks). There is also marked dilatation of the centrilobular sinusoidal remnants (Masson trichrome).

Figure 30.6 Membranous stenosis of the left hepatic vein ostium. Low magnification view of the termination of the left hepatic vein (small arrows) into the inferior vena cava (arrowheads) in a patient with a myeloproliferative disorder. There is a 'web' occluding the ostium.

cysts can block the termination of the hepatic veins in the IVC but rarely produce clinically significant obstruction, probably because of their slow development.

As shown in Table 30.1, half the cases of primary BCS are related to a myeloproliferative disease, 25% to factor V Leiden mutation and 25% to protein C deficiency. All other thrombogenic disorders have also been implicated. BCS is particularly common in patients with paroxysmal nocturnal hemoglobinuria. There is good evidence for an association with some inflammatory disorders (e.g. granulomatous venulitis, Behçet disease, inflammatory bowel disease, amebic abscess), with oral contraceptive use and with pregnancy. The local factors that cause thrombosis at this uncommon site usually remain unidentified. A combination of causes is common (25% of cases).

Hepatic vein or IVC involvement by thrombosis can take three different aspects depending on the stage at which it is discovered: a fresh thrombus, a localized fibrous or membranous stenosis, or complete obliteration of the vein. In the Far East, a membranous obstruction of the terminal IVC is the predominant form of BCS whereas in the West, a thrombus or a localized stenosis of the hepatic veins appears to be more frequent (**Fig. 30.6**). In rare cases, thrombosis is limited to the small hepatic veins.

Obstruction of the hepatic venous outflow tract has dual consequences. First, sinusoidal pressure rises, explaining congestion (**Fig. 30.7**), portal hypertension, increased lymph production (resulting in the formation of protein-rich ascitic fluid), and the development of collaterals that bypass the obstructed portion of the hepatic veins or inferior vena cava. Second, there may be a sudden interruption in hepatic venous blood outflow, explaining ischemic necrosis (Fig. 30.7) and the resulting liver insufficiency. Hepatic perfusion is restored through the following mechanisms: increased arterial blood flow; increased portal pressure; the redistribution of intrahepatic portal flow from

obstructed areas toward unobstructed areas and the development of intrahepatic and extrahepatic venous collaterals (which should be distinguished from portosystemic collaterals). Fibrosis develops is the areas of ischemic necrosis.

At the advanced stage of the disease, thrombosed intrahepatic portal veins are found in an irregular distribution. The areas where both portal veins and hepatic veins are thrombosed undergo infarction or parenchymal extinction (i.e. transformation into a fibrous area devoid of parenchymal cells). By contrast, the areas with thrombosed portal veins, but patent hepatic veins, undergo hypertrophy (nodular regenerative hyperplasia), sometimes in an exuberant form (regenerative macronodules). Extrahepatic PVT occurs in about 20% of cases.

Clinical features
Hepatic vein or IVC thrombosis can run a long asymptomatic course and be discovered incidentally in up to 20% of cases. There is little clinicopathologic correlation, an acute presentation being frequently associated with histopathologic features of chronic damage with superimposed features of recent injury. The acute presentation includes upper abdominal pain, hepatomegaly, ascites of recent onset, increased serum aminotransferases, decreased coagulation factors, and impaired renal function. A chronic presentation as decompensated liver disease is most common (60% of cases).

Diagnosis
Diagnosis should be considered whenever patients with a known prothrombotic disorder develop liver disease; whenever patients with acute and severe liver disease have an enlarged painful liver and massive ascites; in patients with ascitic fluid protein content more than 3.0 g/dL; and in all patients presenting with chronic liver disease that remains unexplained once all common viral, autoimmune and metabolic causes have been ruled out.

Diagnosis is made on the basis of the findings at Doppler-US and MR imaging. The most specific and sensitive signs are an altered flow pattern within the hepatic veins, a hepatic venous

Gut 2002; 51:275–280. Non-cirrhotic intrahepatic portal hypertension revisited.

Perkocha LA, Geaghan SM, Yen TS, et al. Clinical and pathological features of bacillary peliosis hepatis in association with human immunodeficiency virus infection. N Engl J Med 1990; 323:1581–1586. *A landmark study showing that peliosis in immune deficient patients can be related to the infection with agents later identified as* Bartonella *sp.*

Vauthey JN, Tomczak RJ, Helmberger T, et al. The arterioportal fistula syndrome: clinicopathologic features, diagnosis, and therapy. Gastroenterology 1997; 113:1390–1401.

CHAPTER 31

Liver Diseases in Pregnancy

Rebecca W. Van Dyke

Liver diseases that occur during pregnancy can be divided into three categories: liver diseases that are unique to pregnancy; liver diseases that occur more commonly with or because of pregnancy; and acute or chronic liver diseases that exist coincidentally with pregnancy (**Table 31.1**). The first category contains diseases such as intrahepatic cholestasis of pregnancy (ICP), pre-eclampsia/eclampsia/HELLP syndrome (named for the laboratory features of *h*emolysis, *e*levated *l*iver enzymes and *l*ow *p*latelet count), and acute fatty liver of pregnancy (AFLP). The latter two categories include many types of liver diseases; however, this chapter will focus on liver diseases that are affected by the pregnant state or liver diseases that have special therapeutic implications in the setting of pregnancy. For example, the pregnant state is a risk factor for common problems such as the development of gallstones and biliary colic as well as rare diseases, such as Herpes simplex hepatitis and Budd-Chiari syndrome. Other liver diseases can be more devastating for the pregnant woman (e.g. hepatitis E) or may have, like hepatitis B, implications for the newborn infant. Finally, in any patient with chronic liver disease, the consequences of pregnancy must be considered carefully, both for the mother and the child.

EPIDEMIOLOGY

Liver disease is uncommon during pregnancy; however, jaundice, which is often a sign of significant liver disease, is reported in approximately 1 in 1500 to 1 in 5000 pregnancies. The most common reason for jaundice during pregnancy in the USA is viral hepatitis, a reflection of the prevalence of viral hepatitis in the general population. Other than hepatitis E, which is rarely encountered in the USA, the incidence and course of hepatitis A, B and C are not different in the pregnant patient as opposed to the non-pregnant patient. The second most common cause of jaundice is a disease unique to pregnancy, intrahepatic cholestasis of pregnancy, which accounts for up to 20% of jaundice in pregnancy. The most common cause of new abnormal liver tests in pregnancy is pre-eclampsia-related liver disease.

NORMAL CHANGES IN LIVER TESTS AND PHYSICIAL EXAMINATION DURING PREGNANCY

Although most liver functions are not affected by normal pregnancy, some laboratory and physical findings occur during normal pregnancy that may be mistaken for evidence of liver disease. On physical examination, normal pregnant women may have peripheral edema as a result of an expanded intravascular volume, decreased serum albumin and/or pressure exerted by a gravid uterus. Spider nevi and palmar erythema are common findings in normal pregnancy, occurring in up to 67% of women, particularly in the second and third trimester. These vascular phenomena are related to increases in serum estrogen levels and generally disappear after delivery. Transient small esophageal varices have been observed in some pregnant women without liver disease due to compression of the inferior vena cava and increased flow in the azygous system.

During pregnancy a number of biochemical tests may also be affected (**Table 31.2**). Plasma albumin levels are decreased as a result of increasing plasma volume. Serum alkaline phosphatase and leucine aminopeptidase values increase throughout pregnancy to as much as two times the upper limits of normal as a result of placental production. By contrast, serum alanine aminotransferase (ALT) and aspartate aminotransferase (AST) values do not normally exceed the upper limits of normal, thus consistent increases are a reliable clue to liver disease. Other liver tests such as the prothrombin time, 5′ nucleotidase, γ-glutamyl-transpeptidase and bilirubin either remain unchanged or may actually decrease with normal pregnancy. A variety of other serum proteins and lipids either increase or decrease during normal pregnancy (Table 31.2). Finally, pregnancy is associated with a mild subclinical cholestasis as indicated by decreases in bile formation and in hepatic transport of bile salts; however these changes are not detected with routine laboratory studies.

Liver biopsies from normal pregnant women may show modest changes, including reactive Kupffer cells, variation in nuclear size

Liver disease in pregnancy		
Liver diseases unique to pregnancy	Liver diseases occurring more commonly in pregnancy	Pre-existing liver diseases coincident with pregnancy
Hyperemesis gravidarum	Gallstones (symptomatic)	Hepatitis B and C
Intrahepatic cholestasis of pregnancy	Fulminant hepatitis E	Autoimmune hepatitis
Pre-eclampsia/HELLP	Budd-Chiari syndrome	Wilson disease
Acute fatty liver of pregnancy	Herpes simplex hepatitis	Cirrhosis Liver transplantation Liver adenoma

Table 31.1 Liver disease in pregnancy.

Expected changes in laboratory tests in normal pregnancy		
Values increase	*Values not changed*	*Values decrease*
Alkaline phosphatase (to 2 ×)	Alanine and aspartate aminotransferases	Albumin
Leucine aminopeptidase (to 2 ×)	Prothrombin time	Antithrombin III
Bile acids (to 2 ×)		Protein S
Globulins		γ-glutamyltranspeptidase
Fibrinogen		
Triglycerides		

Table 31.2 Expected changes in laboratory tests in normal pregnancy.

Clinical findings in intrahepatic cholestasis of pregnancy		
Incidence	0.2–1.5% of pregnant women	
Onset	3rd trimester (median onset, 29 weeks)	
Symptoms and signs	Pruritus	100%
	Jaundice	10–25%
Laboratory findings		
Alkaline phosphatase	3–5-fold increase	
Bilirubin	1–4 mg/dL	
Aminotransferases	2–4-fold increase	
Serum bile salts	3–10-fold increase	
Prothrombin time	Modest increase in 20% of patients	

Table 31.3 Clinical findings in intrahepatic cholestasis of pregnancy.

and shape, proliferation of smooth endoplasmic reticulum and giant mitochondria, which are of no known clinical significance.

PATHOPHYSIOLOGY AND CLINICAL FEATURES

Liver diseases unique to pregnancy
Hyperemesis gravidarum
Hyperemesis gravidarum is an idiopathic syndrome of severe nausea and vomiting that generally occurs in the first trimester of pregnancy, typically before 10 weeks of gestation. Risk factors for hyperemesis gravidarum include young age, obesity, nulliparity, tobacco use and twin gestation. In many patients with severe vomiting and dehydration, abnormal biochemical liver tests may be observed, usually elevations of serum bilirubin and/or aminotransferases. The elevations are usually mild with bilirubin levels up to 4 mg/dL and aminotransferases levels up to 200 U/L. Liver biopsy shows mild fatty change, mild cholestasis or no abnormality. Liver test abnormalities resolve with resolution of vomiting and dehydration.

Cessation of oral feeding may be necessary to reduce nausea and vomiting and total parenteral nutrition may be necessary in severe cases.

Intrahepatic cholestasis of pregnancy
ICP, also called benign cholestasis of pregnancy, cholestasis of pregnancy or obstetric cholestasis, occurs in 0.2–1.5% of pregnant women and usually presents in the third trimester at a mean gestation time of 29 weeks (**Table 31.3**). Patients may have a family or personal history of pruritus during pregnancy or prior oral contraceptive use and the disease is more common in Scandinavia and Chile. Patients typically present with generalized pruritus. As with other pruritic syndromes, the itching is usually worse at night and can become very intense, leading to skin excoriations, infections, insomnia, fatigue and depression.

Frank jaundice occurs in about 10–25% of patients, usually after the onset of pruritus. The jaundice is generally not severe, and bilirubin levels rarely rise above 6 mg/dL. Alkaline phosphatase levels usually rise above what is expected from normal pregnancy to three to five times the upper limits of normal and this alkaline phosphatase is of hepatic, not placental, origin. Serum aminotransferases can also increase from 2- to 10-fold. Serum bile acids are increased to 10- to 100-fold. In severe cases, with clinically obvious jaundice, steatorrhea and vitamin K deficiency may occur owing to intestinal bile salt deficiency. Liver biopsy, which is rarely necessary, shows a 'bland' cholestasis with minimal or no inflammation (**Fig. 31.1**). Imaging studies such as ultrasound or computed tomography (CT) scans are normal but usually are not necessary.

In both humans and animals, exogenous estrogen impairs hepatic uptake and biliary secretion of bilirubin and bile salts. ICP is thought to be due to an increased sensitivity to these cholestatic effects of estrogen, likely in conjunction with minor mutations in genes coding for hepatic canalicular transporters or other proteins involved in bile formation. For example, in one family, ICP occurred in six women, all of whom had a mutation in the gene for the MDR3 canalicular phospholipid pump. ICP appears to be decreasing in prevalence, however, suggesting environmental factors may play a role as well.

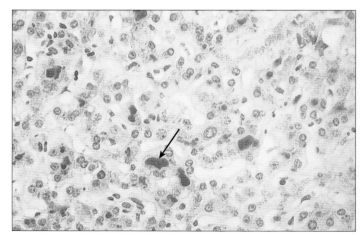

Figure 31.1 Liver biopsy from a patient with intrahepatic cholestasis. Cholestatic changes are shown including bile accumulation in canalicular spaces (arrow).

Medical treatments for pruritus include divided doses of ursodeoxycholic acid (10–15 mg/kg/day) or cholestyramine (8–16 g/day). These drugs should be started early in symptomatic cases as they may take time to be fully effective. No maternal or fetal toxicities related to these agents have been observed, other than an increase in maternal steatorrhea with cholestyramine. Indeed, data suggests that fetal outcomes also may be improved by treatment of mothers with ursodeoxycholic acid. Other suggested treatments for which efficacy is less well established include S-adenosyl-L-methionine (800 mg/day i.v.), dexamethasone (12 mg/day for 7 days and then tapered over 3 days) and phenobarbital (90 mg at bedtime). The treatment of choice for severe ICP is delivery of the infant, which is followed by resolution of pruritus. However the risks to an immature fetus of early delivery should be balanced against maternal symptoms. Finally, vitamin K should be administered to jaundiced women near the time of delivery to decrease postpartum bleeding, especially for women who received cholestyramine.

Infants of mothers with ICP appear to be at increased risk of fetal distress, low birth weight, sudden intrauterine death and perinatal mortality. Thus, pregnancies should be monitored closely from at least 34 weeks on, although fetal stress tests may not prevent all sudden fetal deaths. Prompt delivery should take place as soon as fetal distress is identified. In the absence of evidence of fetal distress, delivery is recommended by 36 weeks for severe cases (such as women with jaundice) and by 37 weeks for women with mild disease.

While ICP resolves quickly after delivery, it will likely recur in future pregnancies or if women use oral contraceptives, although its severity may vary. Women who have experienced ICP have a greater lifetime risk of developing gallstones.

Pre-eclampsia

Pre-eclampsia, a common disease in pregnancy, is characterized by the triad of hypertension, proteinuria and edema. It begins in the late second trimester, third trimester or in the first few days postpartum, occurs in 7–10% of all pregnancies and is the major cause of maternal morbidity and mortality. Eclampsia is a more severe stage of the disease with extreme hypertension (≥160/100), proteinuria (≥5 g/24 h) and seizures. Pre-eclampsia has been associated with a spectrum of liver injury, including the HELLP syndrome and hepatic infarcts, hematomas or rupture. The liver complications of pre-eclampsia account for up to 70% of new abnormal liver tests during pregnancy and up to 20% of maternal mortality is due to pre-eclampsia. Risk factors for the development of pre-eclampsia/eclampsia include procoagulant disorders (such as antiphospholipid antibody syndrome), pre-existing hypertension, extremes of childbearing age, first pregnancy and the presence of multiple gestations.

Although the pathogenesis is unclear, pre-eclampsia/eclampsia is a systemic disease of abnormal endothelial reactivity that can affect multiple organs. The initial event may be abnormal trophoblastic implantation leading to reduced placental perfusion. Mothers exhibit endothelial dysfunction, decreased plasma volume, increased systemic vascular resistance, decreased perfusion of various organs, abnormal endothelial reactivity with vasospasm, deposition of fibrin in vascular spaces and activation of the coagulation cascade. These lead to ischemic damage of multiple organs, including the liver in about 10% of cases. On liver biopsy, fibrin thrombi are present in the periportal sinusoids

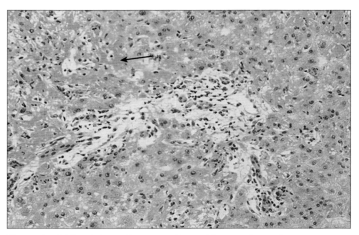

Figure 31.2 Liver biopsy from a patient with pre-eclampsia. Characteristic fibrin thrombi (arrow) are seen in the periportal sinusoidal space.

with ischemic hepatocyte necrosis and periportal hemorrhage with little inflammation (**Fig. 31.2**). Occasional patients also exhibit microvesicular fatty change.

The frequency and severity of liver function test abnormalities, such as aminotransferase elevations, reflects the degree of hepatocellular necrosis that correlates somewhat with the severity of the underlying pre-eclampsia/eclampsia. HELLP syndrome, the most common clinical manifestation of pre-eclampsia-related liver disease, denotes a subset of women who exhibit evidence of microangiopathic hemolytic anemia, thrombocytopenia (platelet count less than 100 000), and elevated liver tests. HELLP syndrome occurs in about 10% of women with pre-eclampsia with an overall incidence of 0.5–1.0% of pregnancies (**Table 31.4**). Patients with HELLP syndrome may present with asymptomatic laboratory abnormalities or with liver-related symptoms including nausea and vomiting or right upper quadrant pain and tenderness. Characteristic laboratory abnormalities include increases in serum aminotransferases from 5 to 100 times normal. Because of the associated hemolysis, serum lactic dehydrogenase (LDH) and bilirubin are also elevated and red blood cell morphology is often abnormal. The prothrombin time may be normal despite these abnormal liver enzymes or it may be elevated. Antithrombin III levels are characteristically low and evidence of intravascular coagulopathy may develop, especially in severe disease. Renal involvement is indicated by elevated blood urea nitrogen (BUN) and creatinine levels. Liver biopsy is diagnostic but usually not indicated as the diagnosis is often made clinically.

Pre-eclampsia also affects the fetus, which is at high risk of growth retardation and sudden fetal death due to poor placental perfusion or infarction. Since maternal pre-eclampsia and liver involvement resolve quickly after delivery, the principal treatment for both mother and child involves rapid assessment of fetal lung maturity, administration of corticosteroids to improve fetal lung function and to speed improvement of HELLP (if time permits) and prompt delivery. Mothers should be observed closely after delivery as the disease may transiently worsen for 1–2 days. Although maternal morbidity can be considerable, maternal mortality is usually 2.5% or less. Fetal outcome is less

Clinical findings in HELLP* syndrome	
Incidence	~ 1% of all pregnancies, especially first pregnancies ~ 10% of women with pre-eclampsia
Onset	3rd trimester (median onset, 33 weeks)
Symptoms and signs	
Hypertension, proteinuria and edema	~100%
Headache	up to 60%
Nausea and vomiting	35%
Abdominal pain	80%
Laboratory findings	
Thrombocytopenia	100%, early onset
Abnormal red blood cells	Frequent (fragments, schistocytes)
Prothrombin time	Modest increase (late)
Fibrin degradation products	Increased (early)
Aminotransferases	5- to 100-fold increase
Alkaline phosphatase	Up to ~2-fold increase
Bilirubin	Low, unless extensive hemolysis and/or hepatic necrosis occur
Serum creatinine	Mild increase

*HELLP, laboratory features of hemolysis, elevated liver enzymes and low platelet count.

Table 31.4 Clinical findings in HELLP syndrome.

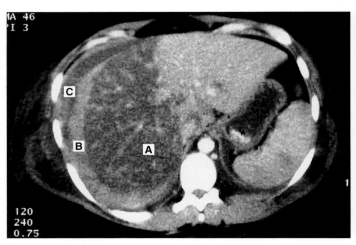

Figure 31.3 Contrast enhanced computed tomography scan of a patient with pre-eclampsia. The patient developed hepatic infarction with segmental hypoperfusion of the right lobe (A) and subcapsular hematoma (B) that ruptured, creating extrahepatic hemorrhage (C).

good with fetal losses of 6–25% depending on disease severity. HELLP syndrome recurs in about 3–5% of subsequent pregnancies. It is recommended that women who had HELLP syndrome be screened for procoagulant disorders.

Hepatic infarction, subcapsular hematoma, and hepatic rupture are estimated to occur in 1:15 000–45 000 pregnancies and in 1–2% of women with pre-eclampsia. Patients usually present in the third trimester or the immediate postpartum period with abdominal pain, hypotension, fever, leukocytosis, nausea, vomiting, shock and abnormal liver tests similar to those in severe HELLP syndrome. These likely represent a progression from the milder HELLP syndrome to confluent hepatic infarction, to subcapsular hematoma, and subsequently, to hepatic rupture. Because it may be difficult to differentiate a contained subcapsular hematoma from free hepatic rupture, on clinical grounds, CT is very helpful in the evaluation of these patients (**Fig. 31.3**). Patients with hepatic infarction or contained liver hematoma should undergo volume resuscitation, if necessary, and urgent delivery. Contained hematomas do not need specific treatment and resolve slowly after delivery. For hepatic rupture, a cesarean section should be performed emergently with volume resuscitation and surgical drainage and packing of the liver. Selected cases may be treated by hepatic artery embolization. Emergent liver transplantation has been performed in a few cases. Due to the severity of maternal disease, fetal loss is as high as 60–70% and maternal mortality from hepatic rupture is up to 50%.

Acute fatty liver of pregnancy

AFLP occurs in approximately 1 in 900–6000 pregnancies primarily in the third trimester or the first few days postpartum.

AFLP is one of a group of diseases known as the hepatic microvesicular steatoses that includes Reye syndrome, Jamaican vomiting sickness and toxicity of several drugs (tetracycline, sodium valproate and fialuridine). They are characterized by infiltration of hepatocytes with microvesicular droplets of fat and profound liver dysfunction (manifested by changes in PT, glucose, bilirubin) with modest increases in AST/ALT levels.

The pathogenesis of AFLP is thought to involve abnormalities in β-oxidation of fatty acids, in mitochondrial function and in ATP syntheses. Hepatic metabolism of triglycerides and fatty acids increases greatly during pregnancy. AFLP may occur when this increased load of fatty acids is delivered to a liver that also exhibits impaired mitochondrial β-oxidation of fatty acids due to elevated estrogens and one or more other factors including genetic abnormalities in acyl-CoA dehydrogenases, inflammatory cytokines and/or drugs such as salicylates or non-steroidal anti-inflammatory drugs. Under these conditions, fatty acids and reactive oxygen species may cause damage to mitochondria and reduce ATP synthesis leading to energy deprivation in hepatocytes, reduction in many hepatocyte functions, lactic acidosis and liver cell dysfunction. Most cases of AFLP are sporadic and non-recurring. However genetic abnormalities in fatty acid oxidation, especially long chain 3-hydroxyacyl-CoA dehydrogenase (LCHAD) deficiency, account for up to 20% of cases. For example, when a mother heterozygous for LCHAD deficiency is pregnant with a homozygously affected fetus, AFLP occurs in most pregnancies. Therefore it is recommended that all infants and mothers who experience AFLP be tested for LCHAD deficiency. A list of clinical laboratories that perform this test can be found at www.genetests.org.

The early clinical signs of AFLP are non-specific but include fatigue, malaise, nausea and vomiting accompanied by abdominal pain, particularly in the right upper quadrant or epigastrium (**Table 31.5**). Signs of liver failure such as hepatic encephalopathy may ensue within days. Physical findings include right upper quadrant tenderness, jaundice and a normal or small liver. Signs and symptoms of pre-eclampsia are seen in 30–40% of cases. The development of coma portends a poor outcome.

Laboratory studies show relatively modest increases in AST and ALT, rarely greater than 10 times normal, increased

Clinical findings in acute fatty liver of pregnancy	
Incidence	1 in 900–6000 pregnancies
Onset	3rd trimester (median onset, 35 weeks)
Symptoms and signs	
Nausea and vomiting	Up to 80%
Abdominal pain	60%
Hypertension, proteinuria, edema	20–30%
Jaundice	90% (if disease severe)
Encephalopathy	70% (if disease severe)
Hypoglycemia	25% (if disease severe)
Laboratory findings	
Alkaline phosphatase	2- to 5-fold increase
Bilirubin	2–30 mg/dL
Aminotransferases	5- to 10-fold increase
Prothrombin time	Marked increase in severe disease to >20 s
Platelet count	Decrease late in severe disease with evidence of DIC*
Serum uric acid	Modest elevation
*DIC, Disseminated intravascular coagulation.	

Table 31.5 Clinical findings in acute fatty liver of pregnancy.

PT and international normalized ratio (INR), bilirubin levels and hypoglycemia. Elevated uric acid levels and renal insufficiency are common, possibly owing to microvesicular steatosis in renal tubular cells. Disseminated intravascular coagulation (DIC) may occur in severe cases.

On liver biopsy, the pathognomonic finding is that of centrilobular microvesicular fatty infiltration with little or no inflammation (**Fig. 31.4**a, b). The periportal hepatocytes are relatively spared. A frozen section of the liver biopsy stained for fat with an oil red O stain can be very helpful, especially if fatty infiltration is not obvious on a hematoxylin and eosin stain (Fig. 31.4c).

Ultrasound examination may show a hyperechoic liver and CT may identify a fatty liver with a liver density less than that of the spleen, but these imaging studies have poor sensitivity for AFLP and are often normal or non-specific.

Since AFLP resolves after delivery, the principal management involves fetal assessment and prompt delivery. In mild cases involving an immature fetus, gestation could be allowed to continue for some days but only with close monitoring by an experienced team of obstetricians and physicians expert in the care of liver failure. Like pre-eclampsia, AFLP can worsen transiently in the immediate postpartum period but then resolves rapidly. Maternal morbidity may be considerable and a few patients have required liver transplants. However, most women recover and maternal and fetal mortality are in the 5–20% range. Postpartum hemorrhage is common in women with coagulopathy. AFLP can recur in subsequent pregnancies, although this is very rare unless genetic abnormalities in fatty acid oxidation are present.

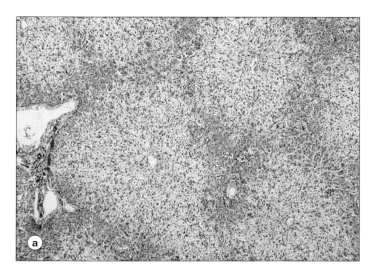

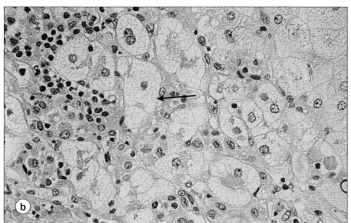

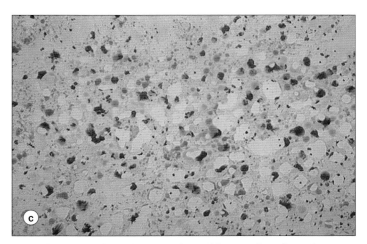

Figure 31.4 Liver biopsy from a patient with acute fatty liver of pregnancy. Microvesicular fatty change in pericentral hepatocytes (arrow); (a) low power, (b) high power, (c) Oil red O stain.

Liver diseases occurring more commonly with pregnancy
Cholesterol gallstones
Pregnancy is a risk factor for the development of biliary sludge and cholesterol gallstones. This may be related to pregnancy-induced decreases in gallbladder motility due to elevated progesterone levels as well as increases in biliary cholesterol

secretion and possibly impaired bile salt excretion related to high estrogen levels. Indeed, ultrasound studies have documented transient formation of sludge and stones in 33% and 10% of normal pregnancies, respectively. Women with a history of ICP are at even higher risk of gallstone formation. Moreover, gallstones are more likely to cause symptoms during pregnancy. Clinically, pregnant women with gallstone disease present in a manner similar to that of the non-pregnant patient, and the management is the same, although elective cholecystectomy is usually deferred until after delivery. Endoscopic retrograde cholangiopancreatography (ERCP) and laparoscopic cholecystectomy can be performed during pregnancy with excellent maternal outcome and low fetal loss rates (<5–10%).

Budd-Chiari syndrome

Budd-Chiari syndrome, or hepatic vein thrombosis, may occur during pregnancy. Pregnancy, like the use of oral contraceptives, is thought to contribute to a hypercoagulable state that increases the risk of thrombotic diseases. In addition to pregnancy, patients with Budd-Chiari syndrome may also have other underlying hypercoagulable states (e.g. mutations in coagulation factors, myeloproliferative disorders) that are uncovered during pregnancy. The syndrome typically occurs postpartum with the sudden onset of abdominal pain and ascites. The diagnosis is confirmed by venography. Liver biopsy shows centrilobular congestion. Treatment options are discussed elsewhere in this book (Ch. 37).

Herpes simplex virus

Herpes simplex virus (HSV) hepatitis is a rare acute hepatitis that occurs predominantly in pregnant women and immunocompromised patients. It represents a form of disseminated primary herpes infection, and most cases are caused by HSV type 2. All of the reported cases have occurred in the second or third trimester. Systemic symptoms are common, including fever, chills, malaise and nausea. Mucocutaneous lesions characteristic of HSV, if present, are helpful in making the diagnosis. Anicteric liver failure is the hallmark of this disease, often associated with considerable right upper quadrant pain. The serum aminotransferases are usually extremely elevated, rising to levels of 25- to 40-fold normal. In contrast, serum bilirubin usually is only mildly elevated to a level about 2- to 3-fold that of normal. Marked hepatocellular dysfunction is as indicated by an increased INR. Although CT may show multiple non-enhancing low-density lesions, these are not specific findings. A liver biopsy is usually diagnostic, and both immunoperoxidase staining for HSV and viral culture should be performed. Histologically, the liver shows patchy and confluent hepatic necrosis with hemorrhage but little inflammation. At the periphery of the necrosis, there may be intranuclear eosinophilic Cowdry type A inclusions (**Fig. 31.5**). Early recognition is essential as treatment with aciclovir is effective if begun early. After delivery, the infant should also receive of treatment. Maternal and fetal mortality can be as high as 50%.

Other liver diseases that occur coincidentally with pregnancy

Acute viral hepatitis

Any liver disease can exist concurrently with pregnancy. Acute viral hepatitis in well-nourished patients is not different in pregnant patients except that the rate of fetal loss is higher in severely affected women. The exception is hepatitis E in which

pregnant woman experience a very high rate (20% or greater) of fulminant liver failure.

Pre-existing liver disease

Patients with pre-existing liver disease, such as Wilson disease, autoimmune hepatitis, hepatitis C, chronic hepatitis B and alcoholic liver disease, have lower rates of fertility; however, pregnancies do occur. In general, pregnancy does not change the course of the underlying liver disease. However during pregnancy women with hepatitis C usually exhibit normalization of elevated AST and ALT values with return to prepregnant values after delivery.

The outcome of pregnancy may depend on the clinical condition of the patient. In Wilson disease and autoimmune hepatitis, it is important to not stop therapy as these diseases can flare during pregnancy with potentially serious adverse effects on both mother and fetus. Drugs such as azathioprine or penicillamine may have rare teratogenic effects on the fetus, but the risk of this possibility is far outweighed by the benefit of continued therapy. In general, a higher incidence of fetal wastage and premature births occurs in these pregnancies, probably related to the poorer clinical condition of the mothers. Further, up to 43% of women with autoimmune hepatitis experience a flare of their disease within 6 months of delivery.

Pregnant women with cirrhosis have approximately a 25% chance of experiencing variceal bleeding during the pregnancy, especially in the latter half of gestation. This increased risk probably reflects the increased circulatory volume of late pregnancy. In addition, as the gravid uterus enlarges, there may be an obstruction of the inferior vena cava with peripheral venous return forced through collateral systems. Patients should be aware of the risk; screening for varices could be performed prior to pregnancy and the option of a therapeutic abortion may be considered. In patients with documented varices, multiple different therapies have been used with variable results. β-blocker therapy, shunt surgery (for women with non-cirrhotic portal hypertension), and elective sclerotherapy have all been used successfully to treat variceal bleeding in pregnancy, but no prospective trials are available to assess the true efficacy of these

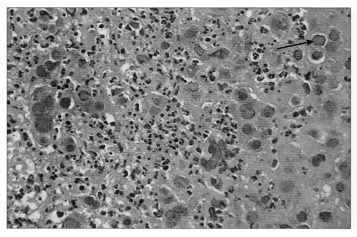

Figure 31.5 Liver biopsy from a patient with Herpes simplex hepatitis. Widespread hepatocyte necrosis is shown with many characteristic eosinophilic intranuclear viral inclusions (arrow).

treatments. There have been no reports, as yet, of using transjugular intrahepatic portosystemic shunts (TIPS) or variceal band ligation in pregnancy, but these therapeutic modalities may also be considered. In patients who are actively bleeding from esophageal varices, standard therapy should be undertaken including volume resuscitation, intravenous octreotide, variceal banding or sclerotherapy and, if necessary, a Sengstaken-Blakemore tube and placement of a TIPS. The use of vasopressin should be avoided, given the risk of inducing labor with this medication. Maternal mortality can be 10% or higher and these women experience higher rates of fetal loss and premature birth.

Vertical transmission of virus

In cases of acute or chronic viral hepatitis, vertical transmission of virus from mother to child is an important issue. Transplacental transfer of hepatitis A is extremely rare. The infant is at risk of infection during delivery if the acute infection occurs within 2 weeks before or after delivery. If that is the case, a single intramuscular injection of immune serum globulin shortly after birth is recommended.

Transplacental transmission of hepatitis B has not been reported, but vertical transmission at the time of delivery is common with the risk estimated to be approximately 25% if the mother is hepatitis B surface antigen (HBsAg)-positive and 80–90% if she is also hepatitis B e antigen (HBeAg)-positive. Many infants infected at birth develop chronic infections and perpetuate infection to the next generation. All pregnant women should be screened for HBsAg and infants born to HBsAg-positive mothers, regardless of HBeAg status, should be given both active and passive immunization with hepatitis B vaccine (0.5 ml i.m. at the time of birth and at 1 and 6 months of age) and hepatitis B immune globulin (0.5 ml i.m. at the time of birth). Although this regimen is highly effective, babies born to highly viremic mothers, who exhibit HBV DNA of 1.2×10^9 viral particles (or gene equivalents)/mL, may experience better protection if mothers also are treated with lamivudine during the last 1–2 months of pregnancy. Other family members should be tested and vaccinated if negative for HBsAg and HBsAB.

Since hepatitis B is a common infection worldwide, and because of lifelong risks of infections, universal vaccination has been recommended in the USA for all infants. All other infants born in the USA (to mothers without hepatitis B infection) should receive three doses of hepatitis B vaccine, one dose at about 0–2 months of age, one at 1–4 months of age (at least 1 month after the first dose) and the last dose at 6–18 months of age.

Vertical transmission of hepatitis C is uncommon, occurring in about 8% of births, but is greatly increased in infants born to women with HIV infection. No treatment is available to prevent this vertical transmission, however some infants appear able to control and eliminate this virus even if they are infected at birth. Babies born to women with hepatitis C receive maternal antibody against hepatitis C and may only express true infection at 6 months of age or greater. Therefore it is recommended that infants born to infected mothers be checked for hepatitis C, using a polymerase chain reaction (PCR)-based test for hepatitis C RNA, at 3, 6 and 18 months of age and only those positive at 6 or 18 months be considered chronically infected. Treatment for those infants that do become chronically infected is being evaluated.

Liver transplantation

Liver transplantation often allows return of normal menstrual function in women of child-bearing age and pregnancies have been reported as early as several months after successful transplant. Pregnancies after liver transplantation are considered high risk with rates of maternal pregnancy-related hypertension and pre-eclampsia of at least 25%. Although immunosuppressive drugs are potentially teratogenic, few congenital anomalies have been described. Pregnancy after transplant does result in increased fetal growth retardation, fetal loss and premature birth. However if the liver graft is functioning well and mother and fetus are followed closely by an experienced team, most mothers and babies have done well. Reports from small series indicate a risk of rejection of about 20% during or immediately after pregnancy, although most episodes were mild and treatable.

Liver adenomas

Liver adenomas may enlarge under the influence of estrogen during pregnancy and potentially might become symptomatic and/or rupture. The actual risk of rupture during pregnancy is unknown but is likely related to size and/or rapid growth. Large adenomas identified prior to pregnancy could be considered for surgical resection. Treatment of a ruptured adenoma during pregnancy includes volume resuscitation, rapid delivery and use of angiographic and/or surgical means to stop bleeding and remove the adenoma.

DIFFERENTIAL DIAGNOSIS

The differential diagnosis of liver disease in pregnancy includes all types of liver diseases, but in this section we focus on diseases that are either unique to pregnancy or more common in pregnancy. Diagnosis can be divided based on the stage of pregnancy (**Table 31.6**). In the first trimester of pregnancy, the only disease

Differential diagnosis of liver disease according to stage of pregnancy		
First trimester	*Second trimester*	*Third trimester*
Acute viral hepatitis	Acute viral hepatitis	Acute viral hepatitis
Hyperemesis gravidarum	Gallstone disease	Intrahepatic cholestasis of pregnancy*
Gallstone disease	Herpes simplex hepatitis	Acute fatty liver of pregnancy*
		Pre-eclampsia related liver disease (HELLP, hepatic infarction, hematoma, rupture)*
		Gallstone disease
		Herpes simplex hepatitis
*These can rarely occur in the second trimester or immediately postpartum. HELLP, laboratory features of hemolysis, elevated liver enzymes and low platelet count.		

Table 31.6 Differential diagnosis of liver disease according to stage of pregnancy.

Diagnostic features distinguishing causes of liver disease in pregnancy					
Tools	Intrahepatic cholestasis of pregnancy	Pre-eclampsia/eclampsia related liver disease	Acute fatty liver of pregnancy	Viral hepatitis	Biliary tract disease
Onset (trimester)	3	3 or postpartum	3 or postpartum	Any	Any
Family history	Often	No	Rare	No	No
Recurrence in subsequent pregnancy	Likely	Possible	Rare	No	Possible if stones not removed
Symptoms	Pruritus	Malaise, nausea, vomiting, abdominal discomfort, fever, headache	Malaise, anorexia, nausea, vomiting, abdominal discomfort, somnolence	Malaise, nausea, vomiting	Nausea, abdominal pain, fever
Signs	Skin excoriations Jaundice	Pre-eclampsia (hypertension, proteinuria, edema) Evidence of shock may indicate hepatic rupture	Up to 40% with concurrent pre-eclampsia Hepatic encephalopathy Bleeding due to coagulopathy Signs of liver failure	Liver tenderness Jaundice Signs of liver failure (uncommon)	RUQ pain/ tenderness Jaundice
Serum liver tests	Bilirubin rarely >6 mg/dL Alkaline phosphatase 3–5 normal Serum transaminase level variable, 2–10 × normal Increased PT (rare)	Variable elevations of AST/ALT (5–100 × normal) Extreme elevations of transaminase suggests hepatic infarction Bilirubin variable	Variable bilirubin of up to 10 × normal Variable serum aminotransferase levels, rarely greater than 10 × normal Increased PT	Significant elevations of aminotransferases from 5 to 25 times normal Variable degree of liver dysfunction	Elevated bilirubin Elevated alkaline phosphatase
Serum tests: Other	Serum bile acid 10–100 × normal	Hemolysis, thrombocytopenia Renal insufficiency Increased uric acid DIC	Renal insufficiency Hypoglycemia Increased uric acid DIC Leukocytosis	Hepatitis serology: anti-HAV IgM, anti-HBc IgM, HBsAg, HBeAg, anti-HCV, and HCV RNA	None
Hepatic imaging	Normal	Useful for diagnosing hepatic infarcts, hematomas, and rupture	Can show fatty liver but not sensitive	Not useful	Useful to show gallstones, sludge and/or dilated bile ducts if present
Liver biopsy	Cholestasis with little or no inflammation	Periportal hemorrhage with sinusoidal fibrin deposition	Microvesicular fatty infiltration of centrilobular hepatocytes	Intense portal and periportal inflammation with lobular necrosis	Normal or periportal edema, PMN infiltration, cholestasis

ALT, alanine aminotransferase; AST, aspartate aminotransferase; DIC, disseminated intravascular coagulation; HAV, hepatitis A virus; HBc, hepatitis B core; HBeAg, hepatitis B e antigen; HBs Ag, hepatitis B surface antigen; HCV, hepatitis C virus; IgM, immunoglobulin M; PMN, polymorphonuclear neutrophil; PT, prothrombin time; RUQ, right upper quadrant.

Table 31.7 Diagnostic features distinguishing causes of liver disease in pregnancy.

unique to pregnancy is hyperemesis gravidarum, which should be easily differentiated from acute viral hepatitis by more severe nausea and vomiting in the former and much more elevated AST/ALT values in the latter and by serologic testing for hepatitis viruses. Gallstone disease, like hyperemesis gravidarum, may present with nausea and vomiting and mild liver test abnormalities, but significant abdominal pain should only be present in the former.

In the second trimester of pregnancy, the possibility of herpes simplex hepatitis should be considered in patients with fever, abdominal pain and marked elevations in serum aminotransferases and mild elevations of bilirubin. This disease may present similar to other causes of viral hepatitis (e.g. hepatitis A and B) but can be differentiated by serology, liver biopsy and, if present, skin lesions.

In the third trimester of pregnancy, various diseases can occur, which may be differentiated based on clinical presentation (**Tables 31.6 and 31.7**). A cholestatic pattern of liver tests in the setting of pruritus will differentiate ICP from other liver diseases (e.g. HELLP, acute fatty liver of pregnancy and viral hepatitis).

Treatment of diseases unique to pregnancy	
Disease	*Treatment*
Hyperemesis gravidarum	Supportive care with rehydration, correction of underlying metabolic and electrolyte imbalance Nutritional support with total parenteral nutrition in severe cases
Intrahepatic cholestasis of pregnancy	Ursodeoxycholic acid (10–15 mg/kg/day or 1 g/day) Cholestyramine (8–16 g/day) Parenteral vitamin K, especially near the time of delivery Monitor beginning at 34 weeks with prompt delivery for fetal distress or by 36 weeks (severe disease) or 37 weeks (mild disease)
Pre-eclampsia related liver disease/HELLP*	Treatment of pre-eclampsia Corticosteroids (in selected cases) Prompt delivery
Hepatic hematoma/ rupture	Close observation and prompt delivery for contained hematoma Prompt delivery with cesarean section for patients with suspected rupture Laparotomy with drainage and packing of rupture Hepatic artery embolization for rupture in selected cases
Acute fatty liver of pregnancy	Prompt delivery Supportive care of liver failure
*HELLP, laboratory features of hemolysis, elevated liver enzymes and low platelet count.	

Table 31.8 Treatment of diseases unique to pregnancy.

Fulminant hepatic failure can result from acute fatty liver of pregnancy, viral hepatitis or severe HELLP syndrome, and these can be differentiated with serology and/or liver biopsy. Differentiation of acute viral hepatitis from ICP, HELLP syndrome, and acute fatty liver of pregnancy is particularly important, because the treatment for the latter three is early delivery. A summary of the treatments for liver disease unique to pregnancy is shown in **Table 31.8**.

PROGNOSIS

For patients with chronic liver disease who become pregnant, the maternal outcome and prognosis depend greatly on the underlying liver disease. Pregnancy does not alter the outcome of most liver diseases, but the presence of cirrhosis and portal hypertension greatly increases the risk of gastrointestinal bleeding, which then portends a poor prognosis. For the fetus, the perinatal mortality is increased, with a higher incidence of prematurity, stillbirth and intrauterine growth retardation, but there is no increased risk of birth defects.

For patients with hyperemesis gravidarum, maternal survival is excellent if dehydration, metabolic disorders and malnutrition are treated (**Table 31.9**). Mean infant birth weight is decreased if the hyperemesis is severe, for example, with a greater than 3% decrease in maternal body weight. In ICP, maternal survival is not affected, but there is up to a 70% chance of a recurrence with subsequent pregnancies. Furthermore, there is some perinatal morbidity and mortality, owing to prematurity, stillbirth and fetal death. The prognosis for HELLP and AFLP is somewhat worse, with maternal mortality rates of 2–20%. This is an improvement on historical reports, likely caused by advances in intensive care, early diagnosis, early delivery and recognition of milder cases. Recurrence has been variable with rates of 3–27% for HELLP and is rare, but not absent, for AFLP.

Prognosis of liver diseases unique to pregnancy		
Disease	*Maternal outcome*	*Fetal outcome*
Hyperemesis gravidarum	Excellent maternal outcome with good supportive care	Decreased mean birth weight in severe cases
Intrahepatic cholestasis of pregnancy	Resolves with delivery Increased risk of postpartum hemorrhage Recurrence is common with subsequent pregnancies and/or use of oral contraceptives Increased lifetime risk of gallstone formation	Increased risk of intrauterine growth retardation (10%), meconium staining, spontaneous preterm labor, and intrapartum fetal distress resulting in increased perinatal mortality (2% or more)
Pre-eclampsia related liver disease/HELLP*	Adverse effect on maternal outcome with mortality of 2–3% No long-term sequelae	Intrauterine growth retardation. Increased perinatal mortality of 6–25%, related to severity of maternal disease
Acute fatty liver of pregnancy	Maternal mortality of 2–20%. No long-term sequelae Recurrence is rare in absence of genetic mutation in fatty acid metabolism	5–20% or higher fetal mortality, related to severity of maternal disease
*HELLP, laboratory features of hemolysis, elevated liver enzymes and low platelet count.		

Table 31.9 Prognosis of liver diseases unique to pregnancy.

FURTHER READING

Changes in liver during pregnancy

Bacq Y, Zarka O, Brechot J, et al. Liver function tests in normal pregnancy: A prospective study of 103 pregnant women and 103 matched controls. Hepatology 1996; 23:1030–1034.

Liver diseases unique to pregnancy

Abell TL, Riely CA. Hyperemesis gravidarum. Gastroenterol Clin North Am 1992; 21:835–849.

Intrahepatic cholestasis of pregnancy

Germain AM, Carvajal JA, Glasinovic JC, et al. Intrahepatic cholestasis of pregnancy: an intriguing pregnancy-specific disorder. J Soc Gynecol Investigation 2002; 9:10–14.

Bacq Y, Sapey T, Brechot M-C, et al. Intrahepatic cholestasis of pregnancy: a French prospective study. Hepatology 1997; 26:358–364.

Roncaglia N, Arreghini A, Locatelli A, et al. Obstetric cholestasis: outcome with active management. Eur J Obstet Gynecol Reprod Biol 2002; 100:167–170. *This recent review discusses the pros and cons of active management of ICP including close monitoring and early delivery of the fetus and evidence for improved fetal outcomes.*

Diaferia A, Nicastri PL, Tartagni M, et al: Ursodeoxycholic acid therapy in pregnant women with cholestasis. Int J Gynecol Obstet 1996; 52:133–140.

Ertan AK, Wagner S, Hendrik HJ, et al. Clinical and biophysical aspects of HELLP-syndrome. J Perinat Med 2002; 30:483–489. *This is an excellent recent review of the HELLP syndrome.*

Martin JN, Thigpen BD, Rose CH, et al. Maternal benefit of high-dose intravenous corticosteroid therapy for HELLP syndrome. Am J Obstet Gynecol 2003; 189:830–834.

Marsh FA, Kaufmann SJ, Bhabra K. Surviving hepatic rupture in pregnancy – a literature review with an illustrative case report. J Obstet Gynaecol 2003; 23:109–113.

Acute fatty liver of pregnancy

Treem WF. Mitochondrial fatty acid oxidation and acute fatty liver of pregnancy. Seminars in Gastrointestinal Disease 2002; 13:55–66.

Yang Z, Zhao Y, Bennett MJ, et al. Fetal genotypes and pregnancy outcomes in 35 families with mitochondrial trifunctional protein mutations. Am J Obstet Gynecol 2002; 187:715–720.

Tyni T, Ekholm E, Pihko H. Pregnancy complications are frequent in long-chain 3-hydroxyacyl-coenzyme A dehydrogenase deficiency. Am J Obstet Gynecol 1998; 178:603–608.

Liver diseases occurring more commonly with pregnancy

Davis A, Katz VL, Cox R. Gallbladder disease in pregnancy. J Reprod Med 1995; 40:759–762.

Tham TCK, Vandervoort J, Wong RCK, et al. Safety of ERCP during pregnancy. Am J Gastroenterol 2003; 98:308–311.

Walker ID. Thrombophilia in pregnancy. J Clin Pathol 2000; 53:573–580.

Valla D-C. The diagnosis and management of the Budd-Chiari Syndrome: Consensus and controversies. Hepatology 2003; 38:793–803.

Kang AH, Graves CR. Herpes simplex hepatitis in pregnancy: a case report and review of the literature. Obstet Gynecol Surv 1999; 54:463–468.

Liver diseases occurring coincidentally with pregnancy

Heneghan MA, Norris SM, O'Grady JG, et al. Management and outcome of pregnancy in autoimmune hepatitis. Gut 2001; 48:97–102.

Cirrhosis and pregnancy

Russell MA, Craigo SD. Cirrhosis and portal hypertension in pregnancy. Semin Perinatol 1998; 22:156–165. *This and the following article are the best recent reviews of a topic in which there is little published experience outside of case reports.*

Aggarwal N, Sawnhey H, Suri V, et al. Pregnancy and cirrhosis of the liver. Aust NZ J Obstet Gynaecol 1999; 39:503–506.

Viral hepatitis and pregnancy

Euler GL, Copeland JR, Rangel MC, et al. Antibody response to post exposure prophylaxis in infants born to hepatitis B surface antigen-positive women. Pediatr Infect Dis J 2003; 22:123–129.

Advisory Committee on Immunization Practices, CDC. Hepatitis B virus: a comprehensive strategy for eliminating transmission in the United States through universal childhood vaccination: recommendations of the Immunization Practices Advisory Committee (ACIP). Morbidity and Mortality Weekly Report 1991; 40(RR-13):1–19. *This classic paper, available through the CDC website, is an excellent review of the problem of vertical transmission of hepatitis B and the scientific evidence for current recommendations for vaccination of infants, both children born to infected mothers and children born to uninfected mothers.*

Van Zonneveld M, van Nunen AB, Niesters HGM, et al. Lamivudine treatment during pregnancy to prevent perinatal transmission of hepatitis B virus infection. J Viral Hepat 2003; 10:294–297.

Resti M, Bortolotti F, Vajro P, et al. Guidelines for the screening and follow-up of infants born to anti-HCV positive mothers. Dig Liver Dis 2003; 35:453–457. *An Italian study group reviewed clinical data and compiled recommendations for evaluating infants born to hepatitis C infected mothers.*

Resti M, Jara P, Hierro L, et al. Clinical features and progression of perinatally acquired hepatitis C virus infection. J Med Virol 2003; 70:373–377.

Pregnancy after liver transplantation

Armenti VT, Herrine SK, Radomski JS, et al. Pregnancy after liver transplantation. Liver Transpl 2000; 6:671–685.

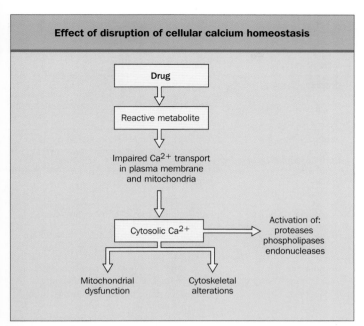

Figure 32.4 Effect of disruption of cellular calcium homeostasis.

Drug-induced liver disease and autoantibody expression	
Drug	*Autoantibody*
Nitrofurantoin	ANA, SMA
Methyldopa	ANA, SMA
Chlorpromazine	ANA (AMA negative)
Tienilic acid	LKM$_2$
Diclofenac	ANA
Sulfonamides	ANA
Iproniazid	AMA (E6 moiety)
Halothane	PDH (E2 moiety)
Nimesulide	ANA
Alverine	ANA
ANA, antinuclear antibody; SMA, smooth muscle antibody; AMA, antimitochondrial antibody; LKM$_2$, liver kidney microsomal type 2; PDG, pyruvate dehydrogenase.	

Table 32.5 Drug-induced liver disease and autoantibody expression.

Immunologic mechanisms may also be involved in idiosyncratic drug-induced hepatotoxicity (type B reactions). The term immunologic idiosyncrasy assumes an allergic basis for drug-induced liver injury. However, the mechanism of the immune response is still not fully understood. The basis of the injury is thought to be hypersensitivity which develops after a period of 1–5 weeks, recurs quickly on readministration of the drug, and is accompanied by fever, rash, eosinophilia, lymphocytosis and an inflammatory infiltration of the liver. In some cases, the liver is involved as part of a systemic hypersensitivity reaction. For drugs to induce an immune response, it is generally assumed that they covalently alter an endogenous macromolecule forming a carrier hapten-conjugate, which then acts as an immunogen and elicits a humoral and/or a cellular immune response directed against the liver. The immune response may be directed against three types of antigenic determinants (epitopes) of the altered macromolecule: epitopes that include the bound drug metabolite (haptenic epitopes); novel epitopes of the carrier molecule, namely neoantigens that result from the covalent modification; and native or autoantigen epitopes normally seen as self molecules but rendered immunogenic by covalent modifications (Fig. 32.3).

Autoantibodies have been documented in the sera of patients taking the antihypertensive diuretic, tienilic acid (**Table 32.5**). These patients developed a high incidence of anti-liver-kidney microsomal type 2 (anti-LKM$_2$) autoantibodies that recognize epitopes specific to CYP2C9, the major cytochrome P450 involved in the biotransformation of tienilic acid. Anti-LKM$_2$ autoantibodies are highly specific for drug-induced autoimmune-like chronic hepatitis and have a different pattern of immunofluorescence staining from the anti-LKM$_1$ autoantibodies found in type 2 autoimmune hepatitis. Another example of autoantibodies associated with drug-induced liver injury is the recognition of the E2 subunit of pyruvate dehydrogenase complex (PDC) by sera of patients with a history of halothane hepatitis. E2, the major autoantigen recognized by antimitochondrial antibodies in primary biliary cirrhosis, mimics the epitope common to several trifluoroacetylated proteins produced as a result of halothane exposure, representing an example of molecular mimicry. Non-tissue-specific autoantibodies, such as antinuclear and antismooth muscle antibodies, may occur in drug hepatitis caused by nitrofurantoin, methyldopa, and minocycline. Major histocompatibility antigens (MHC) class I and class II molecules present antigenic peptides to T lymphocytes, and as human leukocyte antigen (HLA) molecule expression is genetically polymorphic it is possible that certain haplotypes may modulate the immune response. Weak associations have been reported with the MHC complex HLA-A11 for halothane-induced and diclofenac-induced hepatotoxicity, and HLA-DR6 for nitrofurantoin-induced liver injury. Other drugs that are thought to mediate immunologic-mediated liver damage include phenytoin, dapsone and sulfonamides. Idiosyncratic hepatotoxicity not associated with hypersensitivity is thought to depend on metabolic idiosyncrasy and examples include isoniazid and valproic acid. **Table 32.6** compares the features that suggest immunoallergy or metabolic idiosyncrasy.

Hepatotoxicity is normally prevented or limited by a number of protective mechanisms. Cytochrome P450 can be inactivated by the reactive metabolites themselves when they covalently bind to the apoprotein of cytochrome P450. Reactive epoxides undergo transformation by epoxide hydrolases to stable compounds. Other enzymes such as glutathione peroxidase and catalase protect against lipid peroxidation. Failure of these protective mechanisms therefore contributes to drug-induced liver injury.

PATTERNS OF DRUG-INDUCED HEPATOTOXICITY

Two broad categories of liver injury are commonly recognized i.e. cholestasis and hepatocellular (or cytolytic) damage. The former is characterized by a predominantly elevated alkaline phosphatase and γ-glutamyltransferase (γ-GT), while in the latter the

Comparison of drug-induced immunologic and metabolic idiosyncrasy		
Feature	Immunologic type	Metabolic type
Frequency	0.01% exposed	0.1–2% exposed
Gender	More common in women	Slightly more common in women
Latent period	Relatively constant	Highly variable
Response to rechallenge	Invariably fever in 12–72 h	Abnormal liver function tests after 3–30 days
Fever	Common	Less striking
Rash, arthralgia	Common	Rare
Eosinophilia	20–70% cases	Less than 10% cases
Granulomas	Common	Rare
Autoantigens	Common	Rare
Examples	Diclofenac Methyldopa	Isoniazid Ketoconazole

Table 32.6 Comparison of drug-induced immunologic and metabolic idiosyncrasy. Modified from Farrell (94).

Morphologic classification of drug-induced acute liver injury	
Type of injury	Examples
Hepatocellular (cytolytic)	
Zonal necrosis	Acetaminophen, CCl$_4$, halothane
Steatosis: macrovesicular microvesicular	Ethanol, methotrexate Tetracycline, valproic acid, methotrexate
Hepatitis	Methyldopa, isoniazid
Cholestatic	
Hepatocanalicular (pericholangitis)	Amoxicillin–clavulanic acid, chlorpromazine
Canalicular (non-inflammatory)	Estrogens, 17 α-substituted steroids (anabolic)
Vascular	
Hepatic vein occlusion	Estrogens
Veno-occlusive disease	Antineoplastic agents, pyrrolizidine alkaloids
Peliosis hepatitis	Anabolic steroids

Table 32.7 Morphologic classification of drug-induced acute liver injury.

Morphologic classification of drug-related chronic liver injury	
Type of injury	Examples
Chronic hepatitis	
Autoimmune-like	Methyldopa, dantrolene, sulfonamides, diclofenac
Viral hepatitis-like	Amiodarone, isoniazid, halothane, aspirin
Chronic cholestasis	
Ductal (sclerosing cholangitis)	Floxuridine (FUDR)
Ductopenia	Flucloxacillin, tricyclic antidepressants
Hepatocanalicular	Chlorpromazine, barbituates, cimetidine, phenytoin, tolbutamide, amitriptyline
Granulomas (more than 50 drugs implicated)	Sulfa drugs, allopurinol, carbamazepine, chlorpromazine, diazepam, diltiazem, gold, phenytoin, penicillin, nitrofurantoin, tolbutamide, quinidine, isoniazid
Chronic steatosis	Ethanol, methotrexate, antineoplastic agents
Phospholipidosis	Amiodarone, perhexiline maleate, thioridazine
Vascular	
Nodular regenerative hyperplasia	Azathioprine, 6-thioguanine
Non-cirrhotic portal hypertension	Vinyl chloride, azathioprine, 6-thioguanine
Hepatic vein occlusion	Estrogens
Veno-occlusive disease	Antineoplastic agents, pyrrolizidine alkaloids
Peliosis hepatitis	Anabolic steroids
Neoplasms	
Adenoma	Estrogens
Hepatocellular carcinoma	Estrogens, anabolic steroids, vinyl chloride
Angiosarcoma	Vinyl chloride, thorotrast
Fibrosis	Methotrexate, vitamin A, vinyl chloride

Table 32.8 Morphologic classification of drug-induced chronic liver injury.

aminotransferases, alanine (ALT) and aspartate (AST), are significantly elevated, although mixed patterns of abnormalities are common. Hepatocellular injury can be acute or chronic and includes necrosis, steatosis and hepatitis in various combinations. A variety of chronic lesions related to vascular damage, neoplastic change or fibrosis has also been described. These patterns of hepatotoxicity are summarized in **Tables 32.7** and **32.8**.

Necrosis

Necrosis induced by intrinsic hepatotoxins is often zonal (centrilobular or zone 3, midzonal or zone 2, and periportal or zone 1), whereas that produced by idiosyncratic reactions is more diffuse and similar to that observed with viral hepatitis. Some drugs such as halothane are associated with diffuse as well as zonal necrosis. The predominance of necrosis in selected areas is not fully understood, but zone 3 necrosis is thought to relate to the abundance of the cytochrome P450 metabolizing systems in centrilobular hepatocytes and a vulnerability of this area to hypoxia. This distribution is likely to be influenced by other factors such as rate of drug uptake, drug concentration and

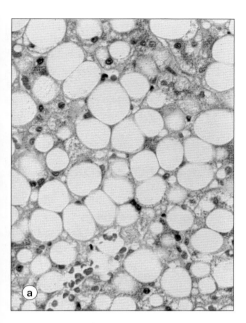 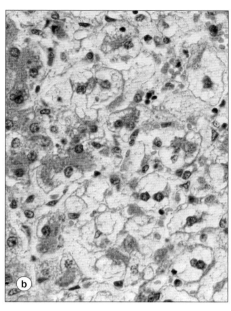

Figure 32.5 Steatosis. (a) Macrovesicular steatosis; **(b)** microvesicular steatosis.

concentrations of cellular protective components such as GSH. Examples of drugs or toxins causing zone 3 necrosis include acetaminophen, CCl₄, chloroform, *Amanita phalloides* toxin, and pyrrolizidine alkaloids. Periportal or zone 1 necrosis is characteristic of ferrous sulfate overdoses, yellow phosphorus and toxins such as allylalcohol. Agents causing midzonal necrosis include beryllium and furosemide (frusemide).

Steatosis

Steatotic liver injury frequently precedes liver necrosis and two types are described according to their pathologic patterns. Steatosis may predominate in either the centrilobular or periportal region. Occasionally, the fat cells may coalesce to form fatty cysts or become surrounded by histiocytes to form lipogranulomas. Triglyceride is the predominant lipid that accumulates and this occurs when the rate of formation exceeds that of disposal into lipoproteins or hydrolysis to fatty acids. In macrovesicular steatosis, the hepatocyte contains a single large droplet of fat, which displaces the nucleus to the periphery of the cell giving it the appearance of an adipocyte (**Fig. 32.5**a). This pattern of fat is also seen with obesity, diabetes, ethanol, malnutrition and jejunoileal bypass.

In microvesicular steatosis, the hepatocyte contains numerous small droplets of fat that leave the nucleus centrally placed so that the cell retains its hepatocyte-like appearance (Fig. 32.5b). The pathogenesis appears related to inhibition of the mitochondrial oxidation of fatty acids. Candidate drugs include valproic acid and tetracycline. Another form of lipid accumulation is phospholipidosis, which occurs when amphiphilic drugs accumulate within lysosomes forming a stable complex with phospholipids. Phospholipidosis can histologically resemble alcoholic hepatitis. The liver injury induced is usually mild but can be associated with Mallory hyaline, and can progress to overt disease. Cirrhosis has been observed in patients taking amiodarone and perhexiline maleate. Alcohol-like liver injury without phospholipidosis has also been reported in patients taking nifedipine and diltiazem.

Hepatitis

Non-specific hepatitis is typical of many types of drug-induced hepatotoxicity. It lacks the typical appearance of autoimmune hepatitis and is associated with scattered foci of necrosis and a variable inflammatory infiltrate. It is usually not associated with progressive liver disease. Chronic hepatitis that resembles autoimmune hepatitis in its histologic and clinical features has been described for a number of drugs (see Table 32.8). Pathologic changes include portal and periportal inflammatory infiltration by lymphocytes and plasma cells, often associated with degeneration of surrounding cells (piecemeal necrosis). Autoantibodies are frequently present in the sera. Granulomatous hepatitis is characterized by aggregates of epithelioid histiocytes and accompanying inflammatory cells. Drug-induced granulomas are usually non-caseating and their presence suggests an immunologic idiosyncrasy (see Table 32.6).

CHOLESTASIS

Intrahepatic cholestasis is a common manifestation of hepatotoxicity. It is predominantly noted as centrilobular bile staining of hepatocytes and as bile casts in the canaliculi. If the cholestasis is severe, the periportal area is also involved and bile plugs occur. Several forms of cholestatic liver disease have been described (see Table 32.7 and Table 32.8).

Bland, pure or canalicular cholestasis

This is characterized by a bland accumulation of bile in canaliculi and cells with little or no necrosis or inflammatory features (**Fig. 32.6**). Anabolic and contraceptive steroids are candidate drugs.

Hepatocanalicular cholestasis

This form of cholestasis is accompanied by a portal and lobular inflammatory infiltrate. Necrosis may also occur. This type of liver injury is observed with chlorpromazine and erythromycin.

503

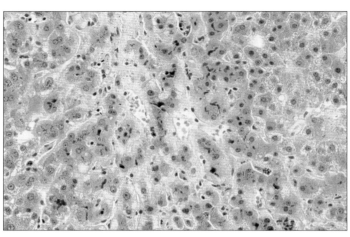

Figure 32.6 Bland or pure cholestasis following anabolic steroid use.

Ductopenic cholestasis

An inflammatory cholestasis may also be accompanied by destruction of the small bile ducts resulting in ductopenic cholestasis or 'vanishing bile duct syndrome'. Drugs implicated in this form of liver injury include: chlorpromazine, tricyclic antidepressants, flucloxacillin, haloperidol, thiabendazole, tolbutamide and carbamazepine. In some cases, the bile duct destruction occurs without an inflammatory infiltration, but frank cholangitis with neutrophilic infiltration of bile ducts is more common. This form of liver injury can persist for months and even years before resolving, but may progress to secondary biliary cirrhosis.

Ductular or cholangiolar cholestasis

Another form of cholestasis associated with bile casts in the cholangiocytes is known as ductular or cholangiolar cholestasis and is exemplified by benoxaprofen.

Ductal cholestasis

Ductal cholestasis associated with intra- and extrahepatic sclerosing cholangitis has been described following intra-arterial administration of floxuridine and fluorouracil for treatment of metastatic liver carcinoma.

OTHER CHRONIC LESIONS

Chronic forms of liver disease almost always depend on continued exposure to the drug rather than a self-perpetuating process instigated by the initial insult. However, in a few cases cirrhosis may develop despite discontinuation of the drug; this may occur with amiodarone and perhexiline maleate treatment as they can persist for many months in the liver. Portal hypertension has also been described following drug-induced liver injury due to the development of portal fibrosis. This non-cirrhotic portal hypertension, or hepatoportal sclerosis, has been described with vitamin A intoxication, chronic exposure to arsenicals, vinyl chloride and copper sulfate. Periportal fibrosis has also been reported following methotrexate administration. Portal hypertension due to vascular lesions may also result from drug administration such as oral contraceptive-induced hepatic vein occlusion and antimetabolite-induced veno-occlusive disease (see Table 32.8).

Drug administration has been linked to tumor development, both benign and malignant disease. Oral contraceptives and anabolic steroids have been implicated in the pathogenesis of hepatic adenomas and hepatocellular carcinoma. Angiosarcomas have been reported in those exposed to vinyl chloride and arsenic. Cholangiocarcinoma has been reported in those using anabolic and contraceptive steroids but a causal relationship has not been definitively established.

DRUG-INDUCED LIVER INJURY ACCORDING TO DRUG CLASS

Steroids: anabolic and contraceptive drugs

Natural and synthetic steroids have a number of effects on the liver:

- pure cholestasis;
- development of tumors, hepatic adenoma, and hepatocellular carcinoma;
- architectural disturbance with the development of focal nodular hyperplasia (FNH);
- increased incidence of gallstones;
- hepatic vein occlusion; and
- peliosis hepatis.

Many of these effects have been reported for both oral contraceptive steroids (OCS) and anabolic steroids. Both groups of drugs are intrinsic hepatotoxins and the presence of an alkyl or ethinyl group on carbon 17 appears to be essential for the development of cholestatic liver disease. However, there are some differences in the type of resultant liver injury. Anabolic and androgenic steroids have been more frequently associated with malignant tumors, while contraceptive steroids are more commonly associated with benign liver tumors. Hepatic vein occlusion may relate to thrombogenic effects of the estrogen component of contraceptive steroids. Anabolic steroids more commonly produce peliosis hepatis.

Oral contraceptive steroids are associated with pure cholestasis in approximately 10/100 000 women exposed in Western Europe and 25/100 000 in Chile and Scandinavia, and it occurs within 2–3 months of commencing therapy. The estrogen component is probably responsible for the cholestasis. The injury is dose-dependent and is less common with low-dose preparations. Oral contraceptive steroid-induced cholestasis occurs in women with a history of cholestasis of pregnancy, and has also been observed in sisters, suggesting a genetic component. The mechanism by which estrogens and related steroids produce cholestasis is uncertain, but it appears to result from interference with bile excretion. Decreased bile flow, biliary secretion of bile acids, plasma membrane fluidity, and Na^+- and K^+-ATPase activity have all been reported in experimental animals. Biliary excretion of sulfobromophthalein (BSP) is also impaired. Estrogens may also alter the membrane lipid composition. Following cessation of OCS, the cholestasis resolves and the prognosis is excellent. Pure cholestasis may also complicate the use of stanozolol, a C-17 substituted testosterone, and danazol, a C-17 substituted androgen used in endometriosis.

The risk of developing hepatic adenomas and hepatocellular carcinoma appears to be increased by OCS and anabolic/androgenic use (**Fig. 32.7**), and most cases are associated with 17-α-alkylated steroids.

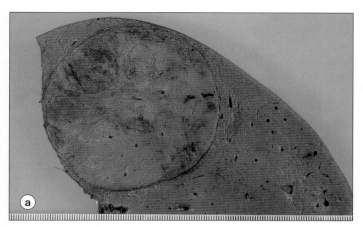 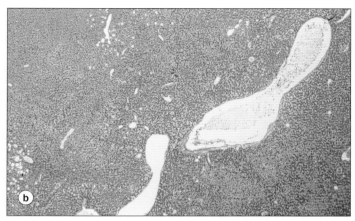

Figure 32.7 Hepatic adenoma secondary to long-term oral contraceptive steroid (OCS) usage. (a) Macropathology; **(b)** micropathology.

Adenomas have also been reported with norethisterone, a progestin, and clomifene. The true incidence of OCS-related adenomas is unknown but the risk seems to be time-dependent and the relative risk is increased 116-fold at 5 years. Adenomas may regress after cessation of the drug, but can recur with readministration of OCS or with pregnancy. Estrogen-associated adenomas are highly vascular and have a tendency to hemorrhage into the tumor or into the peritoneal cavity. Whether adenomas progress to hepatocellular carcinoma (HCC) is controversial. Foci of dysplasia or malignancy have been described in resected adenomas, and the incidence of HCC is increased when OCS have been used for periods in excess of 5 years. However, other cofactors may be important in the pathogenesis of HCC in OCS users and anabolic steroid users, such as hepatitis B and alcohol excess. Like adenomas, steroid-induced HCC may regress after cessation of the drugs. Oral contraceptive steroid use has also been linked to the development of epithelioid hemangioendothelioma, and the enlargement of existing hemangiomas. Angiosarcomas have been reported with anabolic steroid use.

The risk of hepatic vein occlusion, or Budd-Chiari syndrome, is increased 2.5-fold in OCS users, consistent with their perceived thromboembolic potential. This thrombogenic trait is ascribed to the estrogenic component of the drug which may exacerbate an underlying thromogenic disorder. Peliosis hepatis is characterized by blood-filled cavities within the hepatic parenchyma which may be lined by sinusoidal endothelium, and numerous cases have been reported in association with anabolic/androgenic steroids.

Anticonvulsant and psychoactive drugs
Anticonvulsant drugs
Phenytoin
Phenytoin causes both acute and chronic hepatotoxicity. While most patients are adults, hepatotoxic effects have been reported in patients as young as 8 months. Clinical symptoms and signs occur within 6 weeks of administration and include rash, fever, lymphoadenopathy, and eosinophilia, suggesting a hypersensitivity or immunologic basis to the injury. This is supported by the occasional occurrence of a pseudomononucleosis syndrome of lymphoadenopathy, lymphocytosis, and serum sickness-like features. Some patients exhibit manifestations of Stevens-Johnson syndrome. Histologically, the lesion resembles

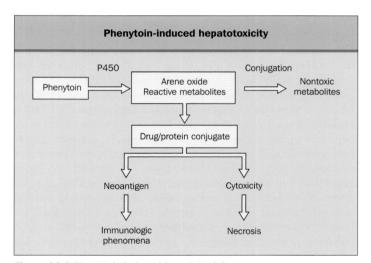

Figure 32.8 Phenytoin-induced hepatotoxicity.

acute viral hepatitis with diffuse hepatocellular degeneration, foci of necrosis, and an inflammatory infiltrate. Granulomas have also been described. However, phenytoin-induced liver injury may also result from the adverse effects of toxic intermediates, as it is metabolized by the cytochrome P450 system with the production of reactive arene oxide metabolites, which may subsequently bind covalently to tissue macromolecules, producing liver injury (**Fig. 32.8**).

Differences in individual susceptibilities to phenytoin-induced liver damage may be due to genetic differences in rates of biotransformation, as deficiencies in epoxide hydrolase activity (required for detoxification) have been reported in those affected and their family members.

Carbamazepine
Carbamazepine is similar to phenytoin in its structure and it also utilizes epoxide hydrolase in its biotransformation. Minor liver dysfunction is seen in approximately 5–10% of asymptomatic subjects using the drug. Liver damage begins within 1 month of commencing therapy and hepatocellular, cholestatic and granulomatous reactions (**Fig. 32.9**) have been described.

Carbamazepine may also cause cholangiolitis and has been reported as a cause of ductopenia.

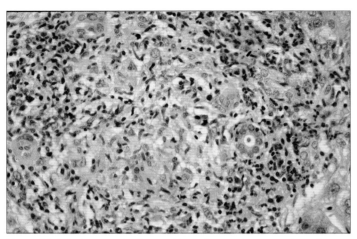

Figure 32.9 Carbamazepine-induced hepatic granulomatous liver disease.

Valproic acid

Valproic acid-induced liver injury has a particular predilection for children, especially for those less than 2 years of age. Symptoms occur between 10 and 12 weeks of therapy and seem to be dose-related in some cases. Between 1978 and 1984, the fatality rate from acute liver failure was approximately 1:500 in children up to 2 years of age and 1:12 000 in older children and adults receiving antiepileptic polytherapy. In patients treated with valproic acid as a monotherapy, the fatality rate was lower, reaching 1:7000 in children up to 2 years of age and 1:45 000 in older children and adults. Since 1984, the fatality rate has dropped, probably as a consequence of improved knowledge about the adverse effects of valproic acid. Risk factors for acute liver failure include concomitant treatment with enzyme inducers [e.g. carbamazepine, phenytoin, phenobarbital and rifampin (rifampicin)], concomitant treatment with drugs that inhibit hepatic β-oxidation (e.g. aspirin), and pre-existing metabolic diseases associated with impaired hepatic fatty acid oxidation. Thus, polypharmacy may also be a factor in valproate-induced liver injury. The pathologic lesions include submassive necrosis with microvesicular steatosis and bile duct injury. The mechanism of injury is uncertain. A branched medium-chain fatty acid itself, valproic acid inhibits mitochondrial oxidation of long-chain fatty acids, with reduction in hepatocellular acetyl coenzyme A and impairment of urea cycle enzymes. Patients with inborn errors in the urea cycle are susceptible to valproate hepatotoxicity. There is no specific antidote for valproate-associated hepatotoxicity. Because most patients with valproate-induced acute liver failure have secondary carnitine deficiency, treatment with carnitine has been studied but its effectiveness remains unproven.

Psychoactive drugs

Chlorpromazine

Chlorpromazine causes cholestatic jaundice in 1% of those taking the drug, but subclinical liver dysfunction may occur in as many as 40–50% of chronic users. It occurs within 5 weeks of therapy and is heralded by a prodrome of flu-like symptoms, followed by a rash and fever in up to 60% of cases. The histologic pattern includes cholestasis in zone 3 and portal inflammation with eosinophils in 20–50% of cases. Granulomas have been described. The prognosis is generally good, but a small

number of patients develop a prolonged cholestatic syndrome with hypercholesterolemia and xanthelasmata. In these patients, the histology can resemble primary biliary cirrhosis, but anti-mitochondrial antibodies are negative, although some patients have antinuclear antibodies in their sera. The clinical features suggest a hypersensitivity reaction, but chlorpromazine and its metabolites do directly interfere with bile secretion. Altered membrane fluidity, impaired membrane Na^+- and K^+-ATPase activity and impaired solute transport are changes that contribute to the development of chlorpromazine-induced cholestasis. Furthermore, chlorpromazine affects the cytoskeleton, causing dilatation and diverticuli in the canaliculi.

Antidepressants: tricyclic antidepressants

Many members of this class of psychotropic drugs (imipramine, amineptine, amitriptyline, and desipramine) are hepatotoxic and asymptomatic liver dysfunction may occur in approximately 10% of users. The injury can be either cholestatic or hepatocellular, although amitriptyline has caused a prolonged cholestatic lesion with portal fibrosis and inflammation. The mechanism of hepatotoxicity is thought to be due to reactive arylating intermediates.

Antidepressants: monoamine oxidase inhibitors

Hepatotoxicity is commonly seen in this group with jaundice reported in 1–2% of patients. Iproniazid, an amine oxidase inhibitor, was originally used to treat tuberculosis, but occasionally resulted in fatal liver necrosis with a mortality of 20% in those who developed jaundice. Clinical features occur within 4–5 weeks of treatment. Histology reveals diffuse hepatocellular necrosis that can progress to massive necrosis in some patients, resembling that associated with acute viral hepatitis. Iproniazid hepatitis is usually associated with anti-M6 antimitochondrial antibody. Angiosarcomas have been reported in experimental animals following administration of phenylhydrazine.

Cocaine

Cocaine use may result in severe liver damage with associated systemic failure, rhabdomyolysis and renal failure. Pathologic examination reveals zone 3 centrilobular necrosis but also microvesicular steatosis, suggesting impaired fatty acid oxidation. It is metabolized by the cytochrome P450 enzyme system to the active hepatotoxic metabolite norcocaine nitroxide which causes oxidative stress. Hepatotoxicity may also be due to hepatic ischemia as cocaine increases the systemic levels of norepinephrine and epinephrine (noradrenaline and adrenaline), which reduce hepatic artery blood flow.

Ecstasy (3,4-methylenedioxymethamphetamine)

Several case reports have described an acute hepatotoxic syndrome similar to that seen with cocaine, that is, hyperthermia, rhabdomyolysis, and hepatic necrosis (see Ch. 33). Chronic ecstasy ingestion has been associated with recurrent episodes of acute hepatitis.

Antibiotics

Antibacterial agents

Tetracyclines

Tetracyclines can cause severe acute liver injury. The majority of cases have been in pregnant women where tetracycline was used to treat urinary tract infections. However, males and non-pregnant women are also susceptible to tetracycline-induced liver damage, especially at higher doses of more than 1.5 g/day. Within 2–3 days of intravenous administration of tetracycline, jaundice occurs with non-specific symptoms such as malaise, anorexia and vomiting.

Histologically, the main lesion is microvesicular fat (see Fig. 32.5b) resembling that seen in fatty liver of pregnancy, Reye syndrome and valproic acid hepatotoxicity. Also, tetracycline in high doses impairs hepatic mitochondrial oxidation. The mechanism of injury appears to be a toxic effect of the drug or its metabolites rather than an immunologic effect, and suggested methods of injury include failure of ATP synthesis and inhibition of protein synthesis. Similar toxic effects can be seen with oxytetracycline and chlortetracycline. Minocycline has been reported to cause liver injury with predominantly allergic features.

Erythromycin
Administration of erythromycin estolate causes hepatocellular liver injury in up to 15% of patients and results in cholestatic jaundice in approximately 1–3% of recipients. The risk of cholestatic jaundice is lower with erythromycin stearate and propionate, and is calculated at 3.6/100 000 users for all erythromycin preparations. Symptoms occur between 1 and 3 weeks after commencing treatment and rash, fever, and eosinophilia in tissue and blood have suggested an allergic mechanism of injury. However, erythromycin estolate can impair bile flow and interfere with canalicular membrane Na$^+$- and K$^+$-ATPases, which indicates a direct hepatotoxic effect. Erythromycin toxicity may also present as an acute cholangitis or cholecystitis. Liver biopsy reveals centrilobular cholestasis and a portal infiltration rich with eosinophils.

Flucloxacillin
Hepatotoxicity due to penicillins is rare, and very few cases of penicillin-G-induced liver injury have been reported. However, several semisynthetic penicillin derivatives have been associated with cholestatic or hepatocellular injury which rapidly improves on withdrawal of the drug. Flucloxacillin produces cholestatic liver disease. The risk of liver injury is estimated at 7.6/100 000 users. Symptoms usually occur within 3 weeks of treatment, and there is often a lag period between the cessation of drug administration and onset of symptoms. While most patients fully recover, some develop a syndrome of prolonged cholestasis with ductopenia, and portal and bridging fibrosis that can progress to cirrhosis.

Ampicillin and amoxicillin
These semisynthetic penicillins have little hepatotoxicity when used alone. However, when amoxicillin is used in combination with clavulanic acid, the risk of cholestasis is 1/100 000 users. Symptoms occur within 1–2 weeks of treatment but can be delayed for up to 6 weeks following withdrawal of the drug. Histology reveals cholestasis with minimal inflammation or necrosis. Granulomas may be present. The mechanism of injury probably relates to immunologic idiosyncrasy.

Sulfonamides
Sulfa drugs are associated with a wide spectrum of pathologic changes in the liver. The precise risk of injury following administration of these drugs is unknown, but the incidence of hepatic injury appears to be less than 5%. Patients infected with human immunodeficiency virus (HIV) carry a higher risk for immunologic toxic reactions, including liver injury. The risk for sulfonamide-induced liver injury appears to be increased in slow acetylators. The clinical pattern of sulfonamide hepatotoxicity is usually cholestatic or mixed hepatocellular-cholestatic and the clinical course can resemble viral hepatitis. Hypersensitivity phenomenon such as a rash, fever, arthralgia, and eosinophilia are not uncommon. Sulfonamides in combination with other drugs also cause liver injury. Sulfasalazine induces allergic-type hepatitis with low levels of serum complement and circulating immune complexes, mimicking serum sickness. Although the sulfpyridine is believed to be responsible for the liver injury, the 5-aminosalicylate moiety may also play a part (see below). Pyrimethamine-sulfadoxine, used as an antimalaria prophylaxis, causes hepatic necrosis and fatalities has been described from massive necrosis. Granulomatous hepatitis has also been described. Trimethoprim-sulfamethoxazole can lead to cholestatic hepatotoxicity, and fatalities due to acute liver failure have been recorded. However, the majority of patients fully recover when the drug is withdrawn.

Fluoroquinolones
Asymptomatic elevations of aminotransferases have been observed quite frequently with flouroquinolones. Hepatocellular liver injury with spontaneous resolution has been reported for norfloxacin. Acute liver failure has been described in patients taking ciprofloxacin and enoxacin. Cholestatic liver injury was occurs with ofloxacin, enoxacin and ciprofloxacin, but recovery within 1–2 months is the norm. Patients with liver cirrhosis appear to have an increased risk for developing seizures during treatment with pefloxacin.

Nitrofurantoin
This antibiotic is associated with a wide variety of adverse effects such as peripheral neuropathy, pulmonary infiltration, and skin reactions and it can also lead to cholestatic hepatitis with hypersensitivity features suggesting an underlying immunoallergic mechanism as the basis for the injury. It has also been associated with chronic hepatitis and cirrhosis, particularly in women over the age of 40 years who have taken the drug for longer than 4–6 months. The chronic hepatitis is associated with a number of autoimmune features such as hyperglobulinemia and positive antinuclear and antismooth muscle autoantibodies. Associations with HLA-DR6, HLA-DR2 and HLA-B8 have been reported.

Antifungal agents
Ketoconazole
Ketoconazole has been well-documented as a hepatotoxic drug, with an estimated risk of injury of 1/15 000 cases. Asymptomatic liver dysfunction occurs in 5–10% of users. Symptoms occur within 1–6 months of treatment and are commoner in women. Liver biopsy reveals a diffuse hepatocellular necrosis, occasionally with bridging necrosis, but fatalities are rare.

Griseofulvin
This antifungal agent produces hepatocellular carcinoma and a porphyria-like syndrome in experimental animal models.

Humans taking this drug may develop porphyrinuria and those with acute intermittent porphyria may relapse. Cholestatic injury has also been documented in humans, and alcohol-like lesions in mice.

Antituberculous agents

Most of the antituberculous drugs can cause hepatic damage in susceptible individuals, but as these drugs are administered in combination to prevent resistant bacterial strains emerging, it may be difficult to attribute liver dysfunction to a particular agent. Furthermore, drug interactions can potentiate hepatotoxicity.

Isoniazid

Isoniazid is one of the most important causes of drug-induced liver injury, and two types of injury are observed. Mild hepatotoxicity is seen in approximately 10–20% of users and occurs in the first few months of treatment. It produces a mild non-specific focal hepatitis (**Fig. 32.10**) that is clinically unapparent and that resolves despite continuation of the drug.

Isoniazid-induced hepatitis occurs in approximately 1% of all users, but in 2% of those over 50 years of age. It appears to be more common in women and alcoholics. For two-thirds of patients, symptoms begin within the first 3 months of treatment, but this can be delayed for up to 12 months. Clinically, the symptoms and signs are those of an acute viral illness. There is a rising serum transaminase level and histologic findings include acute hepatitis, bridging necrosis, submassive necrosis and chronic hepatitis. The drug must be stopped once hepatitis is diagnosed. The mortality for clinically jaundiced patients is 10%. The mechanism of injury involves the production of toxic metabolites. Isoniazid first undergoes biotransformation in the liver by acetylation, producing the harmless acetylisoniazid which then undergoes hydrolysis to monoacetylhydrazine. This product is oxidized by the cytochrome P450 system to form reactive metabolites that covalently bind to tissue macromolecules. It has been suggested that the rate of acetylation of isoniazid to subsequent toxic metabolites may be important for individual susceptibility to hepatotoxicity and rapid acetylators appear to be at greatest risk of injury. However, it has also been suggested that slow acetylation status may be as important a risk factor for hepatic injury.

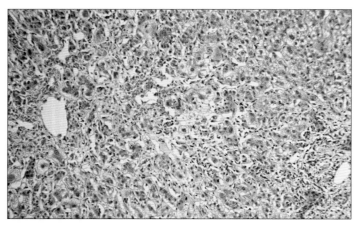

Figure 32.10 Mild hepatitis secondary to isoniazid administration.

Rifampin (rifampicin)

Rifampin (rifampicin)-induced liver injury occurs in approximately 1–4% of users and occurs within 3 weeks of therapy. It is usually given in combination with isoniazid. Clinically, it produces an acute hepatitis similar to that seen with isoniazid. The histology reveals hepatocellular injury and necrosis is common. Rifampin (rifampicin) impairs the hepatic uptake of bile acids and bilirubin in a dose-dependent manner, and impaired BSP excretion is observed in experimental animals. It induces drug-metabolizing systems in the endoplasmic reticulum and this may explain the higher incidence of hepatotoxicity in recipients of combination therapy compared with those using monotherapy.

Analgesic and anti-inflammatory drugs
Acetaminophen

Acetaminophen (paracetamol) is a widely used analgesic and antipyretic drug that has a good safety profile when used at the recommended dose (0.5–4 g daily). Higher doses, however, can lead to liver damage in one of two ways. The commonest is intentional overdosing and this is commonly encountered in the USA and UK. Hepatotoxicity is also seen with therapeutic use involving doses above the recommended range (4–8 g daily), when other factors are present that influence the susceptible individual. These include chronic alcohol ingestion, co-ingestion of drugs that induce the cytochrome P450 metabolizing system, pre-existing liver disease, and conditions that are associated with low GSH stores such as malnutrition. Individuals with Gilbert syndrome may also have an increased susceptibility to acetaminophen-related liver injury due to their deficiency of hepatic UDP-glucuronyltransferase. Acetaminophen is an intrinsic hepatotoxin; the effect on the liver is predictable and dose-dependent.

Clinically, there are three phases:
- phase 1 (1–24 h) when the patient complains of nausea vomiting and diaphoresis;
- phase 2 (24–48 h) during which time there may be no symptoms or clinical evidence of liver disease, and
- phase 3 (3–10 days) with the onset of overt acute liver dysfunction or failure (see Ch. 33).

The characteristic histologic lesion is centrilobular or zone 3 necrosis that may develop into submassive or massive hepatic necrosis (**Fig. 32.11**).

The zone 3 location of the initial histologic change is a consequence of the location in this area of the cytochrome P450 enzyme that is involved in metabolizing the drug (CYP2E1). At low doses, acetaminophen is largely conjugated with sulfate or glucuronic acid (**Fig. 32.12**) and these conjugates are then excreted in the urine.

A small proportion of the drug (approximately 5%) is metabolized by the CYP2E1 isoenzyme resulting in the formation of the highly toxic and reactive electrophile N-acetyl-p-benzoquinone imine (NAPQI). This is rendered harmless by conjugation with GSH and, after further conversion to acetylcysteine derivatives, is excreted in the urine as a mercapturic acid (Fig. 32.12). GSH, therefore, normally provides protection against the toxic intermediate at low levels of acetaminophen ingestion. However, with larger doses of acetaminophen, the sulfate and glucuronide pathways are saturated and therefore a larger amount of drug is available for

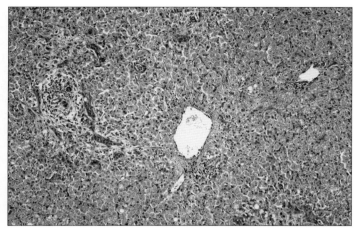

Figure 32.11 Acetaminophen-induced submassive hepatic necrosis.

biotransformation via the P450 enzyme system. Subsequent detoxification depends on conjugation with GSH and therefore tissue levels of GSH are critical to the development of hepatic necrosis. When doses of acetaminophen are large enough to deplete GSH stores by more than 70%, detoxification of NAPQI cannot be sustained; it can then covalently bind to tissue macromolecules which are essential for cellular homeostasis, resulting in structural and functional disruption of key cellular components by oxidation of protein and non-protein thiols. Lipid peroxidation is a late event and may be the result rather than the cause of tissue necrosis. Through the covalent modification of plasma membrane and mitochondrial proteins, intracellular calcium homeostasis is destroyed, resulting in a cascade of endonuclease-, phospholipase-, and protease-induced cellular damage that ends in cell death. N-acetylcysteine and methionine increase hepatic GSH stores by promoting GSH synthesis. Other agents that inhibit the CYP2E1 isoenzyme, such as cimetidine, offer protection against liver injury in experimental animals, but do not appear to be of benefit in humans.

Salicylates

Aspirin is another intrinsic hepatotoxin with a dose-dependent and reversible form of liver injury. Hepatic injury may occur with high therapeutic doses in children and adults with chronic rheumatologic or collagen vascular diseases, or following a deliberate overdose. The injury is usually associated with serum salicylate levels of greater than 2.5 mmol/L (25 mg/dL) but can occur at lower serum drug levels. Hypoalbuminemia may predispose to aspirin-induced hepatotoxicity by increasing the unbound fraction of the drug. The hepatotoxic effects of aspirin may be involved in the development of Reye syndrome. In most cases, it presents as an asymptomatic dysfunction in liver function and jaundice occurs in less than 5% of cases. Liver biopsy is compatible with a non-specific focal hepatitis with minimal inflammatory changes in the portal areas. Recovery is complete on cessation of drug ingestion.

Non-steroidal anti-inflammatory drugs

The hepatotoxicity induced by this group of drugs is not uniform. Most cause hepatocellular damage but several lead to cholestasis. Likewise, the frequency of liver damage that they produce is variable; for example, mefenamic acid rarely causes liver injury unlike ibufenac, which caused fatal liver damage and was ultimately withdrawn from the market. Although the mechanism of injury appears to be idiosyncrasy, for some drugs it is immunologically mediated with accompanying hypersensitivity phenomena. Others appear to have a metabolic basis for their injury. The risk of hepatotoxicity for the group as a whole is estimated to be approximately 3.7–9.0/100 000 users. The incidence was highest for sulindac (148/100 000 users), lowest for ibuprofen (1.6/100 000 users), and intermediate for mefenamic acid (2.5/100 000 users), diclofenac (3.6/100 000 users), and naproxen (3.8/100 000 users). Associated risk factors for liver injury include old age, renal disease and alcohol excess.

Diclofenac

Women and patients with osteoarthritis appear to be more susceptible than others to diclofenac-induced hepatotoxicity which causes asymptomatic liver dysfunction in 15% of users. Duration of administration before the onset of liver dysfunction is widely variable, ranging from 1 to 14 months. Allergic features are rare. Liver biopsy demonstrates a non-specific acute hepatitis with zonal necrosis. Recovery is usual but fatalities have been recorded. Diclofenac has also been associated with an autoimmune-like chronic hepatitis. Monitoring of serum

Figure 32.12 Schematic representation of acetaminophen biotransformation.

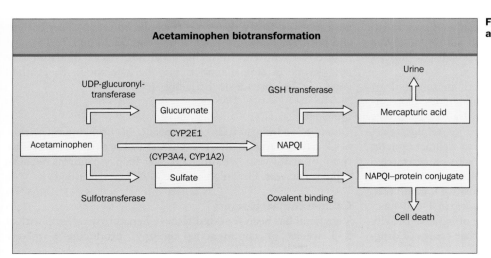

aminotransferases every 3 months is recommended in patients with prolonged ingestion of diclofenac.

Phenylbutazone

This drug has been associated with clinically apparent liver injury in 0.25% of users. Symptoms usually begin within 6 weeks of treatment and are similar to a viral hepatitis. Rash, fever and arthralgia are common. The histology may vary from hepatocellular necrosis to bridging necrosis to granulomatous hepatitis. Less commonly, cholestasis with minimal hepatocellular features can be seen.

Sulindac

As with diclofenac, the mechanism of injury with sulindac appears to be hypersensitivity-based. The illness begins within 6 weeks of drug administration. The liver biopsy reveals a cholestatic injury in most patients, although hepatocellular features have been recorded in some patients. Approximately 5% of jaundiced cases are fatal. Recovery may take months.

Ibuprofen

This drug appears to be one of the least commonly implicated NSAIDs in the generation of liver injury despite its frequent use. It is associated with hepatocellular injury that has many of the clinical hallmarks of the hypersensitivity syndrome.

Nimesulide

This agent is a new NSAID of the sulfonanilide class and is a more selective cyclo-oxygenase type 2 (cox-2) inhibitor than cox-1 inhibitor. Nimesulide-induced hepatotoxicity may occur as hepatocellular necrosis or pure cholestasis. Autoantibodies may be detected in serum and some patients demonstrate hypersensitivity features.

Cardiovascular drugs
Antihypertensive agents
Methyldopa

Both acute and chronic liver disease has been described in patients taking methyldopa, although the incidence has fallen as it has been replaced by newer antihypertensive agents. Asymptomatic liver dysfunction occurs in 5–30% of users within 1–6 weeks, and may resolve despite continued use of the drug. Overt hepatic disease occurs in 1% of users. The commonest histologic lesion resembles acute viral hepatitis with hepatocellular necrosis. Portal and periportal inflammation is prominent. More importantly, methyldopa can cause an autoimmune-like chronic hepatitis that has been reported to progress to fibrosis and macronodular cirrhosis in some patients.

The mechanism of injury appears to be both an immunologic and metabolic idiosyncrasy. Methyldopa undergoes biotransformation via the cytochrome P450 system by oxidation to a reactive metabolite thought to be a quinone or semiquinone. These intermediates may covalently bind to cellular macromolecules, resulting in a conjugate that can act as a neoantigen becoming a target for immune recognition. Evidence for immunologic disturbance is suggested by a positive Coomb test, positive autoantibodies and inhibition of cytotoxic T-cell function. Despite these findings, clinical evidence of hypersensitivity is rare. The mortality is similar to that for other causes of drug-induced hepatocellular injury, with a rate of 10% in those who develop clinically apparent jaundice.

Angiotensin-converting enzyme inhibitors

This class of drugs occasionally produces liver damage. Acute hepatocellular injury occurs over a widely variable period of time. The mechanism of injury is unknown although hypersensitivity phenomena have been described with captopril. Cross-reactivity of hepatotoxicity can occur between captopril and enalapril.

Thiazide diuretics

Despite widespread use, thiazide diuretics rarely cause liver injury, but cholestatic hepatitis has been reported with chlorthiazide. In mice, furosemide causes zone 3 necrosis.

Hydralazine

This vasodilator can cause a variety of liver injuries including hepatocellular hepatitis and granulomatous hepatitis, particularly on a background of a lupus-like syndrome. The drug can also produce an effect mimicking acute cholangitis. Non-specific organ antibodies are found in the serum and anti-liver microsomal antibodies directed against CYP1A2 have been reported.

Antiarrhythmic agents
Amiodarone

Amiodarone is an amphophilic drug with a lipophilic ring complex and a hydrophilic side chain, a structure that results in its accumulation in lysosomes. Within the lysosomes, it binds to phospholipids and prevents their degradation by phospholipases, thereby producing secondary phospholipid storage. This results in increased density on computed tomography (CT) scanning due to the iodine content of the stored drug. Toxicity is not confined to the liver and lysosomal inclusions are also found in other tissues. The range of liver injury sustained with amiodarone is diverse, and both acute and chronic liver disease has been reported. Approximately 15–50% of users develop an asymptomatic rise in liver tests, while clinically apparent disease occurs in less than 3% of patients. Jaundice is rare. Acute hepatitis in those taking the drug for a few weeks usually resolves upon cessation of therapy. Chronic injury can be insidious and patients may present with complications of cirrhosis. Histologic appearances include granulomas, cholangitis and micronodular cirrhosis, but the typical appearance is that of alcoholic hepatitis with steatosis, focal necrosis, centrilobular fibrosis, Mallory hyaline and polymorphonuclear infiltration (**Figs 32.13** and **32.14**).

Interference with mitochondrial fatty acid oxidation by amiodarone in animal models may be a factor in the pathogenesis of this pseudoalcoholic liver injury.

Quinidine

Quinidine administration may result in liver injury within 6–12 days of treatment. The clinical symptoms are similar to those of acute viral hepatitis and liver biopsy confirms hepatocellular necrosis. Granulomas have also been described.

Calcium channel blockers

Verapamil has been reported to have hepatotoxic effects within 2–3 weeks of commencing therapy, producing a mixed

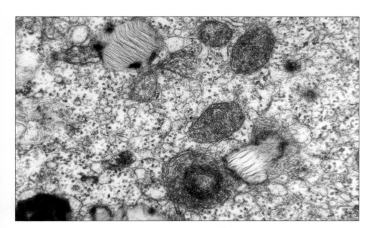

Figure 32.13 Amiodarone-induced phospholipidosis. Electron microscopy reveals phospholipidic inclusions.

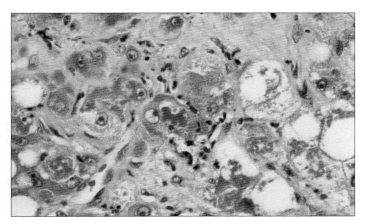

Figure 32.14 Amiodarone-induced liver disease demonstrating Mallory bodies and hepatic fibrosis.

cholestatic and hepatocellular pattern. Nifedipine can cause steatosis and zone 3 necrosis. It has also been implicated in pseudoalcoholic liver disease. Diltiazem may rarely cause fatal hepatotoxicity.

Anti-anginal agents
β-Adrenergic blocking drugs
Most of the drugs in this group rarely induce liver disease. However, labetalol can cause hepatocellular necrosis within 2 months of treatment, and fatalities have been recorded. Metoprolol is metabolized by the CYP2D6 isoenyzme, which is also responsible for debrisoquin (debrisoquine) metabolism. It induces an acute hepatitis.

Perhexiline maleate
A lipophilic drug that accumulates in lysosomes, this agent produces pseudoalcoholic liver disease similar to that described for amiodarone, which can also progress to cirrhosis despite cessation of drug ingestion. Deficiency of the CYP2D6 metabolizing isoenzyme, which is responsible for perhexiline hydroxylation, may be a predisposing factor for perhexiline-induced liver damage. Susceptibility to perhexiline hepatotoxicity has been associated with HLA-B8 phenotype.

Antihyperlipidemic agents
3-Hydroxy-3-methylglutaryl coenzyme A reductase inhibitors (statins)
Asymptomatic elevation in aminotransferases occurs in 1–5% of users in the first few weeks of treatment and this abnormality is usually dose-related. The mechanism of liver function abnormality may be the accumulation of metabolites whose conversion to cholesterol has been blocked by inhibiting the 3-hydroxy-3-methylglutaryl coenzyme A reductase enzyme.

Clofibrate
Clofibrate may also produce asymptomatic elevation in aminotransferases. Cholestasis, granulomatous inflammation and an increased incidence of gallstones have been reported following clofibrate administration. In animal models they cause an increase in hepatocyte peroxisomes that may be related to the development of hepatic neoplasms in these animals.

Immunomodulatory drugs
Immunomodulatory drugs, a group of drugs that includes antineoplastic drugs, antimetabolites, immunosuppressant agents and antiviral drugs, produce a wide spectrum of hepatotoxicity ranging from mild hepatocellular hepatitis to cirrhosis. However, it can be difficult to identify the cause of the injury due to the multiple potential causes of liver dysfunction in patients receiving these drugs. The differential diagnosis may include the underlying disease itself, metastatic disease, opportunistic infection, sepsis and polypharmacy with multiple drug interactions.

Antimetabolites
Methotrexate
The potential for hepatotoxicity with long-term use of methotrexate includes fatty liver, liver fibrosis and cirrhosis. The risk of liver injury seems to be related to the duration of therapy but other contributing factors may include obesity, diabetes, alcohol excess, underlying liver disease and renal impairment. Several studies show that the risk for development of fibrosis or cirrhosis is dose-dependent. For every gram of methotrexate ingested, the risk for progression of one histologic grade is approximately 6%. The progression of methotrexate-induced liver injury is usually subclinical, and it has been argued that a liver biopsy should be performed after cumulative doses in excess of 1.5 g. Patients with rheumatoid arthritis appear to have lower susceptibility to methotrexate-induced hepatotoxicity. Although fibrosis can progress despite the liver tests being normal, monitoring of liver function is advisable as methotrexate has been associated with hepatocellular toxicity and acute liver failure. Histologic abnormalities include steatosis, necrosis, a mixed portal inflammatory infiltrate and ultimately cirrhosis. The mechanism of liver injury is unclear.

Antipurines
Azathioprine, frequently used to treat chronic liver disease, is metabolized in the liver to produce 6-mercaptopurine. Liver injury induced by this drug ranges from portal inflammation with cholestasis to peliosis hepatis, nodular regenerative hyperplasia, veno-occlusive disease and hepatoportal sclerosis (or idiopathic portal hypertension), suggesting a susceptibility of the vascular endothelium to injury by azathioprine. There is a

strong association between male renal transplant recipients and azathioprine-induced veno-occlusive disease. After kidney transplantation, liver injury appeared 4–143 months after surgery at an average dose of 2.5 mg/kg/day in approximately 2% of the patients. 6-Mercaptopurine, used to treat leukemia, is also hepatotoxic. It can produce jaundice in 5–40% of users, although hepatocellular injury is more common than cholestatic injury. 6-Thioguanine produces histologic hepatotoxicity similar to that described for azathioprine, in particular veno-occlusive disease, nodular regenerative hyperplasia and hepatoportal sclerosis. Cytosine arabinoside produces a mild cholestatic injury.

Antipyrimidines

One of the most important drugs that causes hepatotoxicity in this group is 5-fluorouracil, which produces little liver damage when administered orally as a single agent. However, the co-administration of a pyrimidine synthesis inhibitor (phosphono-acetyl-l-asparate), used to enhance the efficacy of 5-fluorouracil, results in cholestatic injury. A derivative of 5-fluorouracil, floxuridine, has been reported to cause irreversible sclerosing cholangitis and cholecystitis when infused into the hepatic artery as treatment for metastatic liver disease.

Alkylating agents

Many drugs in this group are capable of hepatic injury. Cyclophosphamide, used in high dosage or in combination with other agents for bone marrow pre-conditioning, can lead to veno-occlusive disease (**Fig. 32.15**).

Busulfan, at high doses used in bone marrow preconditioning, produces a similar lesion but may also induce a cholestatic hepatitis. The nitrogen mustards are rarely hepatotoxic. Chlorambucil can produce hepatocellular injury that has been reported to progress to cirrhosis.

Antiviral agents
Nucleoside analogs

Zidovudine (AZT) hepatotoxicity has been documented in patients with HIV. The typical histologic abnormality is a severe macrovesicular steatosis with minimal necrosis or inflammation. However, acute liver failure has been reported following its use. The mechanism of injury is uncertain, but seems to relate to a toxic effect on mitochondrial function with subsequent fat accumulation, lactic acidosis and multiorgan failure.

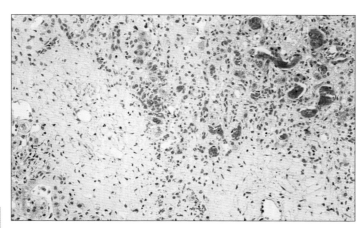

Figure 32.15 Cyclophosphamide-induced veno-occlusive disease.

Naturally occurring immunomodulatory agents
L-asparaginase

This agent usually induces a mild steatosis that resolves with cessation of the drug. Large doses can cause hepatic necrosis. Toxicity may result from impaired hepatic protein synthesis as deamination of asparagine is facilitated by asparaginase, resulting in depletion of asparagine stores.

Alkaloids

These agents rarely cause liver injury, but when used in combination with irradiation, vincristine and vinblastine can lead to a severe hepatitis. Pyrrolizidine alkaloids induce veno-occlusive disease. Etoposide and other podophylline alkaloids in high doses can cause hepatic necrosis.

Adriamycin (doxorubicin hydrochloride)

This agent and the related minomycin have been implicated in the development of veno-occlusive disease. Bleomycin can induce steatosis.

Cyclosporin

Hepatotoxicity is a fairly trivial component of the side-effect profile of cyclosporin but both hepatocellular and cholestatic liver disease have been described in patients after organ transplantation or with autoimmune disease. Most patients have increased serum bile acids and some also have increased conjugated serum bilirubin concentrations, which may be caused by inhibition of canalicular excretion of anions. Cyclosporin-associated liver injury is dose-dependent and usually disappears upon reduction of the dose; only a few patients have developed chronic liver disease. Both cholestatic and hepatocellular liver injury was more pronounced in patients with parenteral nutrition, which may be a risk factor for cyclosporin-associated liver injury.

Tacrolimus

The context of tacrolimus hepatotoxicity is very similar to that for cyclosporin. Liver toxicity is predominantly cholestatic and considered to be dose-dependent. Decreased hepatic activity of CYP3A has been identified as a risk factor for renal toxicity with tacrolimus. The dose-dependent nature of the hepatotoxicity raises the possibility that decreased activity of CYP3A could also be a risk factor for liver injury.

Anesthetic agents
Halothane

Halothane is the prototype for anesthetic-induced hepatotoxicity. The risk of liver injury ranges from 1/35 000 to 1/10 000 anesthetics administered. Risk factors for developing halothane-induced hepatotoxicity include obesity, female sex, advancing age and repeated exposure to the agent (implying a sensitization process). The risk of injury has been reported to be 7/10 000 in those who had previously experienced this anesthetic agent. Asymptomatic liver dysfunction occurs in approximately 20–25% of those exposed. Non-specific symptoms appear within 2 weeks of exposure (but may occur as quickly as 2–3 days in those previously exposed) and resemble those of acute viral hepatitis. Histologic features include zone 3 necrosis that can progress to massive necrosis. Other less severe lesions include spotty necrosis, diffuse hepatitis and bridging necrosis. Increased incidence after repeated exposure, shortened period between exposure and the onset of symptoms, and clinical and histologic findings suggest an immunologic mechanism. However, the centrilobular location of hepatocyte necrosis suggests a toxic mechanism produced by biotransformation. In humans, 20% of halothane is metabolized, producing bromide ion and trifluoroacetic acid (TFA), which are not hepatotoxic. In animal studies, reactive metabolites of halothane covalently bound to tissue macromolecules and induced liver injury only in the presence of tissue hypoxemia. TFA-protein conjugates have been demonstrated in the sera of patients who have been exposed to halothane anesthesia and seem to act as neoantigens, producing antibodies in patients with severe liver injury. These antibodies may cross-react with endogenous proteins; antibodies to the E2 component of PDH have been reported. This may explain the hypersensitivity phenomena such as fever, rash, eosinophilia and increased frequency of toxicity with repeated exposure.

Other anesthetic agents
Enflurane-induced liver injury is less common than that due to halothane but produces a similar clinical and histologic picture. Isoflurane is metabolized less extensively than halothane and therefore is less commonly implicated as a cause of anesthesia-related liver dysfunction.

Industrial and naturally occurring toxins
Carbon tetrachloride
Occupational exposure to CCl_4 may occur in those in contact with dry-cleaning, grain fumigants or working with fire-fighting equipment. Inhalation and ingestion are the commonest modes of exposure. Starvation and alcohol excess appear to enhance the toxicity of CCl_4, possibly by inducing the microsomal metabolizing enzyme system, in particular the CYP2E1 isoenzyme. Hypoxia enhances the conversion of CCl_4 to the reactive metabolite CCl_3. Symptoms occur within 24 h of exposure, and jaundice appears after 2–4 days. Renal impairment often coexists. Histology shows zone 3 necrosis and fatty change is not uncommon.

Yellow phosphorus
Yellow phosphorus-induced hepatic injury occurs by inhalation or ingestion of rat poison, and produces a clinical syndrome similar to that described for CCl_4. It is characterized by rapidly deteriorating liver and renal function, and can lead to acute liver failure within 3–4 days of exposure. The breath, vomitus and feces typically have a garlic odor and are phosphorescent. The pathologic findings are zone 1 necrosis with macrosteatosis.

Selenium
At low concentrations this essential trace element protects against lipid peroxidation. However, in higher concentrations selenium is hepatotoxic and inhibits protein synthesis with subsequent deficiency of methionine and cysteine. Acute toxicity results in microvascular steatosis. Like phosphorus toxicity, the breath and excreta have a garlic odor.

Vinyl chloride
Vinyl chloride has been associated with a range of liver pathologies, including angiosarcoma, fibrosis and hepatoportal sclerosis. Liver injury appears to be related to duration of exposure, but other factors may include smoking and alcohol.

The most characteristic histologic lesion is capsular and subcapsular fibrosis. Angiosarcomas are often peripherally placed and associated with terminal retroperitoneal hemorrhage. Vinyl chloride at a low concentration can be metabolized by alcohol dehydrogenase, but at higher levels, metabolism is performed by the microsomal enzyme systems. Extrahepatic manifestations of vinyl chloride toxicity include Raynaud phenomenon and scleroderma-like skin changes.

Pesticides (insecticides, herbicides, fungicides)
Pesticides have rarely produced significant liver injury in humans despite experimental evidence of perivenular necrosis in rodents. However, their potential for hepatotoxicity and hepatocarcinogenesis is a concern as they are stored for a long time in body fat and in the liver. The pesticide dichlorodiphenyltrichloroethane (DDT) is listed by the World Health Organization as a carcinogen. Cholestasis with bile duct degeneration and necrosis has been reported following paraquat ingestion, but the clinical relevance of this is superseded by the pulmonary and gastrointestinal manifestations.

Arsenic
Acute ingestion of this poison produces acute and chronic liver injury. Features of hypersensitivity are prominent and the histologic abnormalities include hepatocellular necrosis and severe steatosis. Alternatively, patients may present with a cholestatic syndrome, reflected histologically by cholestasis and portal infiltration, which may progress to a primary biliary cirrhosis-like entity. Chronic arsenic exposure is associated with hepatosclerosis, cirrhosis, hepatocellular carcinoma and angiosarcoma.

Mushroom poisoning
Ingestion of *Amanita phalloides* (death cap) and *Amanita verna* (destroying angel) is associated with severe liver injury, especially in children. *Amanita phalloides* is recognized by its green–brown cap, white gills and stem. Toxicity is due to the amatoxins, which bind to RNA polymerase and inhibit the formation of messenger RNA, and phallotoxins, which impair cell membrane function by interfering with the polymerization–depolymerization cycle. As little as three mushrooms can be fatal as they contain approximately 7 mg of amatoxins. Symptoms occur within 8–12 h of ingestion followed by a period of apparent improvement before clinically overt liver dysfunction occurs (see Ch. 33). Histology reveals zone 3 hemorrhagic necrosis with severe steatosis. In those that survive, a minority can progress to have a histologic picture of chronic autoimmune-like hepatitis with autoantibodies, hyperglobulinemia and circulating immune complexes in the serum.

Aflatoxins
Aflatoxins are derived from the *Aspergillus* species and have been identified as a contaminant of nuts, corn, wheat, barley, soy beans and rice. There are 12 naturally occurring parent forms, and they have been classified into two major groups: aflatoxin B and aflatoxin G. The former toxin is the most common aflatoxin contaminant found in food. Hepatotoxicity is due to impairment of RNA synthesis, possibly due to inhibition of RNA polymerase or interaction with nuclear chromatin. Ingestion of aflatoxin-contaminated food results in acute hepatotoxicity heralded by nausea, vomiting and jaundice with subsequent development of portal hypertension. Liver biopsy demonstrates cholestasis with

periductal fibrosis. Chronic ingestion in animals results in veno-occlusive disease and hepatocellular carcinoma; aflatoxins are also carcinogenic in humans. They have been postulated as cocarcinogens with hepatitis B virus.

Herbal medicines

The increasing use of alternative medicines has led to an increased awareness of their potential toxicity. The association with hepatotoxicity may be difficult to establish as many patients fail to disclose the use of herbal remedies on routine enquiry. Germander, which is used to treat obesity, has been associated with acute hepatitis and acute liver failure. Symptoms of abdominal pain and jaundice develop within 3–18 weeks of germander administration in capsular form or as tea. Histology reveals a non-specific hepatocellular necrosis. Symptoms resolve quickly on withdrawal of the agent, but rapidly reappear upon re-exposure. Animal studies have reported depletion of GSH and protein thiols due to germander-derived reactive metabolites, activated by the cytochrome P450 enzyme system. Chinese herbal remedies have also been associated with acute hepatitis, in particular xiao-chai-hu-tang, used as an antidote to the common cold, but also used to treat liver diseases in Japan. Acute hepatitis may also follow administration of mistletoe (*Viscus album*) used to treat asthma, skullcap (*Scutellaria*) and valerian (*Valeriana officinalis*) used to treat stress, and chaparral leaf. Pyrrolizidine, ingested as Bush Tea in the Caribbean, causes veno-occlusive disease.

Miscellaneous drugs

Retinoids

Both etretinate and its pro-drug acitretin can cause asymptomatic hepatocellular liver injury in up to 20% of patients at the beginning of therapy. In most patients, elevated aminotransferases normalize despite continued administration of the drug; liver histology is not available in such patients. However, some patients develop chronic hepatitis that can progress to cirrhosis and chronic liver failure, necessitating transplantation.

Tetrahydroaminoacridine (tacrine)

This drug is a centrally active non-competitive inhibitor of acetyl cholinesterase, which is used for the treatment of patients with Alzheimer disease. It is associated with hepatocellular liver injury in approximately 50% of patients but does not normally cause cholestatic liver injury. Liver injury manifests typically 6–8 weeks after exposure, and most patients stay free of symptoms. In patients with aminotransferases more than three times the upper limit of normal or jaundice, treatment should be withdrawn. The mechanism of toxicity is uncoupling of oxidative phosphorylation of hepatic mitochondria.

CLINICAL FEATURES OF DRUG-INDUCED LIVER INJURY

There are few, if any, clinical features associated with drug-induced hepatotoxicity that are pathognomonic for drug-induced injury to the liver. Many drugs cause a non-specific viral hepatitis-type picture with an initial prodrome of nausea, anorexia and vomiting followed by abdominal pain and jaundice (**Fig. 32.16**).

Fever, rash, and arthralgia are hallmarks of hypersensitivity which may indicate an immunologic idiosyncrasy to drugs, but

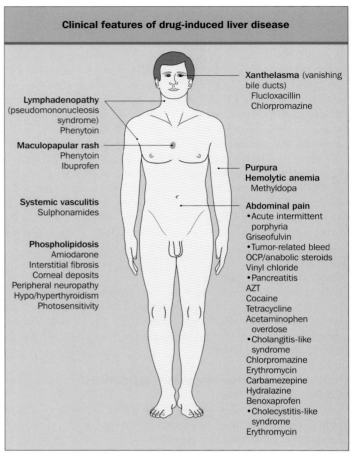

Figure 32.16 Clinical associations of drug-induced liver disease.

these signs also occur with viral hepatitis. Classical indicators of toxin-induced liver injury, such as the garlic odor of breath, vomitus and feces of yellow phosphorus hepatotoxicity, are rare. Syndromes of acute liver disease occur in three phases as characterized by injury due to acetaminophen, hepatotoxic mushrooms and CCl_4: early severe gastrointestinal and neurologic symptoms; a period of apparent improvement; and finally overt liver injury with subsequent multiorgan involvement. Some drugs mimic clinical entities such as cholecystitis (erythromycin) and cholangitis (chlorpromazine), pseudomononucleosis, lymphadenopathy and serum sickness-like syndromes (phenytoin, sulfonamides, sulindac, dapsone), bone marrow suppression (immunomodulatory drugs), and systemic vasculitis (allopurinol, sulfonamides). Hepatic adenomas may present as a painless abdominal mass or hemoperitoneum following rupture of the tumor.

DIAGNOSIS OF DRUG-INDUCED LIVER INJURY

Because the majority of clinical manifestations of drug-induced liver injury are non-specific, making the correct diagnosis at an early stage is extremely difficult. Furthermore, liver deterioration may represent progression of the underlying disease, a complication of the underlying disease, or an unrelated clinical episode such as sepsis. In addition, the administration of multiple drugs in seriously ill patients further complicates the process of drug-induced liver damage. A low threshold of suspicion is therefore necessary to make the correct diagnosis at an early stage in the illness when withdrawal of the offending agent should result in complete recovery. Central to the diagnosis is a thorough history including recent and past drug exposure (including herbal remedies, vitamins and homeopathic medicines), and occupational hazards with exposure to potential toxins. Ideally, the diagnosis should be based on a history of illness subsequent to drug ingestion and improvement on cessation of therapy. Confirmation of the diagnosis by a drug rechallenge is rarely justifiable. In recent years, a clinical scale for the diagnosis of drug-induced hepatitis has been developed and validated (**Table 32.9**).

Investigations
Liver tests
It has been suggested that drug-induced liver injury is diagnosed as hepatocellular when the ALT and AST are greater than twice the upper limit of normal or when the ALT/alkaline phosphatase ratio is equal to or greater than 5. The injury is cholestatic where the alkaline phosphatase is twice the upper limit of normal or where the ALT/alkaline phosphatase ratio is less than or equal to 2. However, many drug reactions frequently cause a mixed pattern of liver function abnormality. Hypo-albuminemia is particularly associated with salicylate toxicity, but this may just reflect the severity of the underlying liver disease, if present.

Full blood count
Lymphocytosis and eosinophilia are associated with immuno-logic phenomena. Leukopenia and thrombocytopenia may reflect bone marrow suppression as a result of drug toxicity or as a secondary toxic event following liver failure. A low platelet count may also indicate disseminated intravascular coagulation (DIC) which may follow acute toxic injury to the liver.

Coagulation screen
A prolonged international normalized ratio (INR) or activated partial thromboplastin time (APTT) reflects deteriorating liver function. These indices are the most useful prognostic markers of acute liver failure following acetaminophen overdose. A DIC screen (fibrinogen, fibrin degradation products or D-dimers) is also useful.

C-reactive protein
This is an acute phase protein which can be elevated as a non-specific response to a hypersensitivity reaction.

Autoimmune screen
Autoantibodies found in association with drug-related liver impairment are listed in Table 32.5. Elevated immunoglobulin-G (IgG) levels are observed with autoimmune-like syndromes. Increased IgE levels have been described following gold and carbamazepine administration.

Electrolytes and renal function
A markedly elevated K^+ may indicate rhabdomyolysis associated with acute liver failure, in particular, cocaine-induced liver injury.

Toxicology screen
This can be useful to aid the diagnosis of a suspected drug overdose.

Drug-induced liver injury diagnostic scale	
	Score
Temporal relationship between drug intake and the onset of clinical picture	
Time from drug intake until the onset of first clinical or laboratory manifestations:	
4 days to 8 weeks (or less than 4 days in cases of re-exposure)	3
Less than 4 days or more than 8 weeks	1
Time from withdrawal of the drug until the onset of manifestations:	
0–7 days	3
8–15 days	0
More than 15 days*	–3
Time from withdrawal of the drug until normalization of laboratory values**:	
Less than 6 months (cholestatic or mixed patterns) or 2 months (hepatocellular)	3
More than 6 months (cholestatic or mixed) or 2 months hepatocellular)	0
Exclusion of alternative causes***	
Viral hepatitis	
Alcoholic liver disease	
Biliary tree obstruction	
Other (pregnancy, acute hypotension):	
Complete exclusion	3
Partial exclusion	0
Possible alternative cause detected	–1
Probable alternative detected	–3
Extrahepatic manifestations	
Rash, fever, arthralgia, eosinophilia (>6%), cytopenia:	
4 or more	3
2 or 3	2
1	1
None	0
Intentional or accidental re-exposure to the drug	
Positive rechallenge test	3
Negative or absent rechallenge test	0
Previous report in the literature of cases of DILI associated with the drug:	
Yes	2
No (drugs marketed for up to 5 years)	0
No (drugs marketed for more than 5 years)	–3
Total score	

*Except cases of prolonged persistence of the drug in the body after drug withdrawal (e.g. amiodarone). **Normalization: decrease to values below 2× the upper limit of normal values. ***Use the exclusion criteria considered appropriate in each case. Definite drug associated injury >17, probable 14–17, possible 10–13, unlikely 6–9, excluded <6.

Table 32.9 Drug-induced liver injury (DILI) diagnostic scale. Description of the component elements and scores attributed. Modified from Maria (97).

Others

Amylase, creatine phosphokinase (CPK) and lactate may indicate muscle necrosis secondary to rhabdomyolysis. A rapidly rising lactate accompanies impaired mitochondrial fatty acid oxidation.

Radiology

Ultrasound and CT examination can be useful to rule out non-drug-related causes of liver dysfunction. Hepatic adenomas and carcinomas can be diagnosed and subsequently confirmed by angiography. Fatty infiltration of the liver may be first suggested by ultrasound screening. Amiodarone produces a classical CT appearance with increased liver density due to the iodine content of the retained drug stored within the lysosomes. Examination of hepatic vein patency by CT and Doppler studies may aid the diagnosis of drug-related Budd-Chiari and veno-occlusive disease.

Liver biopsy

Histologic features suggestive of drug-related liver disease are listed in **Table 32.10**.

MANAGEMENT

The main treatment for drug-induced hepatotoxicity is withdrawal of the offending agent. While the majority of patients will recover completely, for some the adverse effects continue to deteriorate, despite cessation of therapy. The basic principles of management involve supportive care and alleviation of symptoms such as pruritus. Colestyramine, antihistamines, opiate antagonists, and odansatron may alleviate pruritus, but

Histologic features that implicate a drug-induced etiology
Zonal necrosis
Microvesicular steatosis
Granulomas
Eosinophilic inflammatory infiltration
Pure cholestasis
Peliosis hepatis
Veno-occlusive disease

Table 32.10 Histologic features that implicate a drug-induced etiology.

some patients may require plasmapheresis. Rifampin (rifampicin) has also been used to treat pruritus. Corticosteroids have no established role in the treatment of drug-related liver injury, but may be used in the setting of immunologic idiosyncrasy to suppress features of hypersensitivity or in autoimmune-like syndromes. Specific antidotes exist for overdose of some drugs such as acetaminophen, where N-acetylcysteine can replenish hepatic GSH stores. Carnitine has been suggested in cases where defects in mitochondrial fatty acid defects are prominent, but there is little evidence to indicate that this is of major benefit. Hyperbaric oxygen has been suggested as an adjunct to therapy in cases of CCl_4 toxicity as hypoxemia potentiates the hepatotoxic effects. Liver transplantation may ultimately be necessary if clinical and biochemical parameters continue to deteriorate (see Ch. 37).

FURTHER READING

General reviews

Farrell GC. Drug-induced liver disease. Edinburgh: Churchill Livingstone; 1994:1–673.

Lee WM. Drug-induced hepatotoxicity. N Engl J Med 1995; 333:1118–1127.

Pathogenesis

Beaune PH, Lecoeur S. Immunotoxicology of the liver: adverse reactions to drugs. J Hepatol 1997; 26(suppl 2):37–42. *An excellent review of the mechanisms of liver injury following drug administration.*

Berson A, Freneaux D, Larrey D, et al. Possible role of HLA in hepatotoxicity. An exploratory study in 71 patients with drug-induced idiosyncratic hepatitis. J Hepatol 1994; 20:336–342.

Fromenty B, Pessayre D. Impaired mitochondrial function in microvesicular steatosis. Effects of drugs, ethanol, hormones and cytokines. J Hepatol 1997; 26 (suppl 2):43–53. *This is a superb review of drug-induced steatosis, covering normal mitochondrial function, inborn errors of metabolism and acquired impairment of β-oxidation.*

Larrey D, Pageaux GP. Genetic predisposition to drug-induced hepatotoxicity. J Hepatol 1997; 26(suppl 2):12–21. *This is a fascinating and in-depth review of the detoxification mechanisms of the liver and the genetic predisposition to variation in these systems.*

Pohl LR. Drug-induced allergic hepatitis. Semin Liver Dis 1990; 10:305–315.

Watkins PB. Role of cytochrome P450 in drug metabolism and hepatotoxicity. Semin Liver Dis 1990; 10:235–250.

Specific drugs

Ellis AJ, Wendon JA, Portmann B, et al. Acute liver damage and ecstasy ingestion. Gut 1996; 38:454–458.

Gitlin N. Clinical aspects of liver disease caused by industrial and environmental toxins. In: Schiff L, Schiff ER, eds. Diseases of the liver. Philadelphia: Lippincott; 1993:1018–1050.

Gut J, Christen U, Huwyler J, et al. Molecular mimicry of trifluoroacetylated human liver protein adducts by constitutive proteins and immunochemical evidence for its impairment in halothane hepatitis. Eur J Biochem 1992; 210:569–576.

Larrey D. Hepatotoxicity of herbal remedies. In: Arroyo V, Bosch J, Bruguera M, et al, eds. Therapy in liver diseases. Barcelona: Masson; 1997:233–238.

Larrey D, Vial T, Pauwels A, et al. Hepatitis after germander (*Teucrium chamaedrys*) administration: another instance of herbal medicine hepatotoxicity. Ann Intern Med 1992; 117:129–132.

Makin AJ, Wendon J, Williams R. A 7-year experience of severe acetaminophen-induced hepatotoxicity (1987–1993). Gastroenterology 1995; 109:1907–1916. *A comprehensive study of the clinical and biochemical parameters of acetaminophen-induced liver failure from a single center.*

Steenbergen WV, Peeters P, De Bondt J, et al. Nimesulide-induced acute hepatitis: evidence from six cases. J Hepatol 1998; 29:135–141.

Diagnosis

Maria VAJ, Victorino RMM. Development and validation of a clinical scale for the diagnosis of drug-induced hepatitis. Hepatology 1997; 26:664–669. *A useful guide for determining the likelihood of drug-induced liver injury when the diagnosis is uncertain.*

CHAPTER
33

Acute Liver Failure

John G. O'Grady

Acute liver failure is a complex medical emergency that evolves after a catastrophic insult to the liver. The liver damage is sufficiently severe to trigger the development of encephalopathy within a matter of days or weeks of the liver injury. Acute liver failure is a heterogeneous condition incorporating a range of clinical syndromes. The dominant factors that give rise to this heterogeneity include the underlying etiology, the age of the patient and the duration of time over which the disease evolves. The natural history of the condition is very variable within this spectrum and survival rates without recourse to transplantation range from 10 to 90% for different cohorts. The treatment involves an integrated, multidisciplinary strategy with the hepatologist, intensivist and transplant surgeon playing pivotal roles. The key components of the management are the assessment of the severity of the disease and the associated prognosis, prevention or treatment of the complications that may arise and the use of transplantation when spontaneous survival is considered unlikely. Consequently, this condition should ideally be managed in specialist centers where these integrated care protocols are achieving survival rates in the range of 40 to in excess of 90% depending on the underlying etiology.

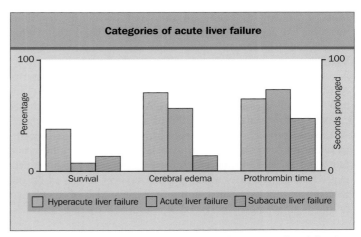

Figure 33.1 Categories of acute liver failure. Hyperacute liver failure has the best prognosis despite the high incidence of cerebral edema and marked prolongation of prothrombin time. Acute liver failure shares the same characteristics but has a much poorer prognosis. The outcome in subacute liver failure is poor despite the low incidence of cerebral edema and less marked prolongation of prothrombin time. The survival figures relate to the period 1973–1985 before liver transplantation confused natural history studies, and the survival rate for the hyperacute group is now considerably higher.

DEFINITIONS

The terms fulminant hepatic failure and acute liver failure are used interchangeably. Fulminant hepatic failure was first used in the late 1960s and was defined as the development of encephalopathy within 8 weeks of the onset of symptoms in patients with no previous history of liver disease. Late-onset hepatic failure was later described for a complementary group of patients in whom the first symptom to encephalopathy interval ranged between 9 and 26 weeks. A French nomenclature from the 1980s defined fulminant hepatic failure as the onset of encephalopathy within 2 weeks of the onset of jaundice (rather than the less precise first symptom), and subfulminant hepatic failure as the development of encephalopathy 3–12 weeks after becoming jaundiced.

In the 1990s another classification was proposed in an attempt to achieve a closer alignment between the patient subgroups and the associated natural history and pattern of clinical features observed (**Fig. 33.1**). This used the core term acute liver failure to describe the development of encephalopathy within 12 weeks of the onset of jaundice, and prefixed the terms hyper- and sub- to describe subgroups with distinct clinical characteristics in which this interval is up to 7 days and 5–12 weeks, respectively. This definition excluded patients with previous symptomatic liver disease but allowed the inclusion of subclinical chronic liver disease characteristic of Wilson disease and some patients with hepatitis B related liver failure.

Hyperacute liver failure is defined as the development of encephalopathy within 7 days of the onset of jaundice. This group has the highest likelihood of recovery with medical management despite the characteristic rapid deterioration, high incidence of cerebral edema and severe prolongation of prothrombin time that are observed. In acute liver failure the encephalopathy develops between 8 and 28 days after the onset of jaundice. This group has a high mortality, a high incidence of cerebral edema and prolongation of prothrombin time that is as severe as in hyperacute liver failure. The interval between the onset of jaundice and the development of encephalopathy in subacute liver failure ranges from 4 to 12 weeks. This group also has a high mortality rate despite a very low incidence of cerebral edema and much less severe prolongation of prothrombin time.

Young children with acute liver failure may not develop classical encephalopathy until late in the disease process. Increasingly in this group the diagnosis of acute liver failure is made on the basis of a coagulopathy. It has also been argued that in adults with severe liver damage, drugs like benzodiazepines may mimic encephalopathy and that coagulopathy is a more reliable parameter to differentiate severe hepatitis or liver injury from acute liver failure.

517

ETIOLOGY AND PATHOGENESIS

There is considerable geographic variation in the etiology of acute liver failure (**Fig. 33.2**). Viruses and drugs account for the majority of cases. However, a significant number of patients have no definable viral cause and have no history of exposure to drugs or toxins. This condition is referred to as seronegative hepatitis in this chapter but is also known as non-A-E hepatitis and acute liver failure of indeterminate etiology. The overall incidence of acute liver failure complicating acute hepatitis in the USA is 0.9% and this equates to about 2000 deaths annually. Most of the drug-induced cases are rare idiosyncratic reactions, but some like acetaminophen are in part dose related toxic events.

Viral

Acute liver failure is a very uncommon complication of hepatitis A infection, occurring in 0.14–0.35% of hospitalized cases, and in 0.4% of all cases seen in the USA. As hospitalized and notified cases represent only a proportion of all cases of acute hepatitis A, the real prevalence is probably considerably lower. Exposure to hepatitis A in childhood is associated with a very low mortality and induces immunity. However, in Western countries the overwhelming majority of the population now enters adulthood with no immunity against hepatitis A. The risk of acute liver failure is significantly increased in adults and there is a positive

correlation with age. This trend may be reversed by vaccination of populations at risk. The diagnosis of acute hepatitis A is made by the detection of the immunoglobulin M (IgM) antibody in serum and this is present in 95% of cases at the time of presentation. The remaining 5% become positive on repeat testing.

The incidence of acute liver failure following acute hepatitis B is 1–4% of hospitalized patients. Women appear to have a higher risk and a number of interesting cases have been described where sequential female sexual partners of hepatitis B carriers have developed acute liver failure. In early studies, hepatitis D co-infection or superinfection was thought to increase the risk of acute liver failure as hepatitis D virus (HDV) was found in 34–43% of patients with acute liver failure due to hepatitis B, as compared to 4–19% of less severe cases. However, the prevalence of hepatitis D appears to have decreased dramatically in recent years. The presence of the IgM antibody to hepatitis B virus (HBV) core-antigen in serum is the most accurate way of diagnosing acute liver failure due to de novo hepatitis B infection. Hepatitis B surface antigen (HBsAg) may be undetectable in serum at the time of presentation in a minority of patients, and HBV DNA levels tend to be low in most instances. These observations reflect the role of an aggressive immune response to the HBV in the pathogenesis of the acute liver failure. It is now recognized that acute liver failure-like syndromes occur in chronic hepatitis B in association with spontaneous surges in

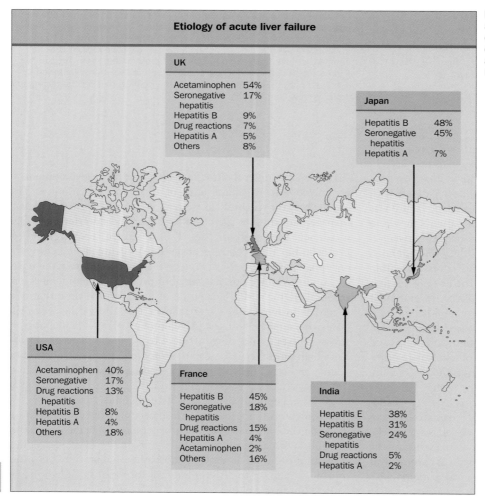

Etiology of acute liver failure

UK

Acetaminophen	54%
Seronegative hepatitis	17%
Hepatitis B	9%
Drug reactions	7%
Hepatitis A	5%
Others	8%

Japan

Hepatitis B	48%
Seronegative hepatitis	45%
Hepatitis A	7%

USA

Acetaminophen	40%
Seronegative	17%
Drug reactions hepatitis	13%
Hepatitis B	8%
Hepatitis A	4%
Others	18%

France

Hepatitis B	45%
Seronegative hepatitis	18%
Drug reactions	15%
Hepatitis A	4%
Acetaminophen	2%
Others	16%

India

Hepatitis E	38%
Hepatitis B	31%
Seronegative hepatitis	24%
Drug reactions	5%
Hepatitis A	2%

Figure 33.2 Etiology of acute liver failure. There are considerable geographic variations in the etiology of acute liver failure. Acetaminophen is especially common in the UK, while hepatitis B and hepatitis E are particularly prominent in France and India, respectively.

viral replication (HBV DNA levels typically markedly elevated), seroconversion from hepatitis B 'e' antigen (HBeAg) to hepatitis B 'e' antibody (HBeAb) and with exposure to immunosuppressive or cytotoxic drugs. Studies of the role of mutants, especially the pre-core mutants that are unable to secrete HBeAg, have failed to conclusively link them to the pathogenesis of hepatitis B related acute liver failure. Vaccination and antiviral therapy with drugs such as lamivudine and adefovir should alter the observed pattern of hepatitis B related acute liver failure.

The risk of developing acute liver failure after exposure to hepatitis C appears to be very low and in a number of studies of patients with acute liver failure the overall hepatitis C positivity rate was only 2%. Contrary reports have emerged from series of Japanese and Hispanic Californian patients, but these populations have relatively high carrier rates for hepatitis C and the association is probably not causal. Post-transfusion hepatitis, which is usually due to hepatitis C, rarely leads to acute liver failure. It has been suggested that chronic hepatitis C infection may be a cofactor with acute hepatitis B infection increasing the risk of developing acute liver failure.

Seronegative hepatitis is a common cause of acute liver failure in some parts of the Western world. The diagnosis remains one of exclusion. There is now considerable doubt whether this is a viral infection as most cases are sporadic and unidentified toxins or autoimmune processes may be the underlying mechanisms. Middle-aged females are most frequently affected and the risk of developing acute liver failure has been calculated at 2.3–4.7% of hospitalized cases.

Hepatitis E is common in parts of Asia and Africa and the risk of developing acute liver failure ranges from 0.6–2.8 to over 20% in pregnant women, being particularly high during the third trimester. Hepatitis E is also encountered in Europe and the USA and may account for up to 8% of cases that would previously have been described as seronegative hepatitis. A history of travel to a high endemic area was not always present in these cases. Unusual causes of viral acute liver failure include herpes simplex 1 and 2, herpesvirus-6, varicella zoster, Epstein-Barr virus and cytomegalovirus. The cases due to herpes simplex may have external manifestations of herpetic infection and there is often a positive therapeutic response to aciclovir. Herpes simplex was implicated in 3% of cases of adult cases of acute liver failure in France.

Drugs

Acetaminophen (paracetamol) overdose is the commonest cause of acute liver failure in the UK and the USA. It appears to be increasing in other English speaking countries but remains rare in continental Europe and the rest of the world. It is usually taken with suicidal or parasuicidal intent, but up to 8% cases in the UK resulted from the therapeutic use of acetaminophen. This is either because of unintentional overdosing or accelerated metabolism in people with liver enzyme induction as a consequence of anti-epileptic therapy or regular alcohol usage. The pattern in the USA may be somewhat different as one small urban study suggested that 70% of cases were suicidal and 30% were unintentional in undernourished or alcoholic subjects. The patients developing acute liver failure represent only about 2–5% of those presenting at hospital with acetaminophen overdoses. The median dose of acetaminophen causing acute liver failure in the UK was 40 g (range 5–210 g), and the mortality

Drug causes of acute liver failure	
Category 1	*Category 2*
Acetaminophen	Benoxyprofen
Halothane	Phenytoin
Isoniazid/rifampin (rifampicin)	Isoflurane
Non-steroidal anti-inflammatory drugs (NSAIDs)	Enflurane
	Tetracycline
Sulfonamides	Allopurinol
Flutamide	Ketoconazole
Sodium valproate	Monoamine oxidase inhibitors (MAOIs)
Carbamazepine	Disulfiram
Ecstacy	Methyldopa
	Amiodarone
	Tricyclic antidepressants
	Propylthiouracil
	Gold
	2, 3-Dideoxyinosine (ddI)

Table 33.1 Drug causes of acute liver failure. The drugs that cause acute liver failure are divided into two categories; category 1 includes frequent causes and category 2 includes occasional causes.

was highest at doses exceeding 48 g. Unintentional overdosing in the USA averaged 12 g of acetaminophen, as compared with 20 g in the suicidal group, but resulted in higher rates of coma (33 versus 6%) and death (19 versus 2%).

Estimates of the risk of developing acute liver failure as a result of an idiosyncratic reaction range from 0.001% for non-steroidal anti-inflammatory drugs to 1% for the isoniazid/rifampin (rifampicin) combination. The diagnosis is made on the basis of a temporal relationship between exposure to the drug and the development of acute liver failure. The more common offending drugs are listed in **Table 33.1**. Most cases develop during the first exposure to the drug but some, like halothane, occur in sensitized individuals on the second or subsequent exposure. Non-therapeutic drugs also cause acute liver failure. Ecstacy (methylenedioxymethamphetamine) has been associated with a number of clinical syndromes ranging from rapidly progressive acute liver failure associated with malignant hyperthermia to subacute liver failure.

Other etiologies

Acute liver failure associated with pregnancy tends to occur during the third trimester. Although three discrete entities have been described, in reality considerable overlap is frequently observed. Acute fatty liver of pregnancy usually occurs in primigravids carrying a male fetus, and is characterized by severe microvesicular steatosis, which may be detectable by ultrasound. Serum uric acid levels are markedly elevated in these patients. The HELLP syndrome is defined as the combination of hemolysis, elevated liver enzymes and low platelets. Acute liver failure complicating pre-eclampsia or eclampsia typically exhibits

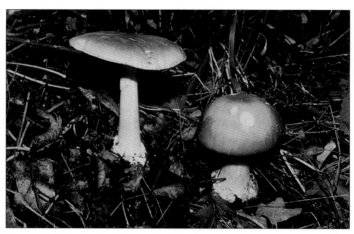

Figure 33.3 A classical view of the poisonous *Amanita phalloides*.

very high serum transaminase levels and abnormal tissue perfusion patterns on computed tomography (CT) scanning that reflect the microvascular infarction characteristic of this condition.

Wilson disease may present as acute liver failure, usually during the second decade of life. It is characterized clinically by a Coomb negative hemolytic anemia and demonstrable Kayser-Fleischer rings in the majority of cases. The serum ceruloplasmin levels are usually, but not invariably, low and the serum and urinary copper levels are increased. Although the latter is the most specific feature of Wilson disease, increases of lesser magnitude can occur in other causes of acute liver failure. A serum alkaline phosphatase/total bilirubin ratio of <2.0 had been suggested as an accurate discriminator of Wilson disease from other causes of acute liver failure.

Poisoning with *Amanita phalloides* (mushrooms) is most commonly seen in central Europe, South Africa and the west coast of the USA (**Figure 33.3**). Severe diarrhea, often with vomiting, is a typical feature and commences 5 h or more after ingestion of the mushrooms. Liver failure develops 4–5 days later. Autoimmune chronic hepatitis may present as acute liver failure but it is usually beyond rescue with corticosteroid or other immunosuppressive therapy. Anti-liver-kidney-microsomal antibodies may be the only detectable autoantibody in these cases. The diagnosis may be difficult to establish as autoantibodies in low titers are found in a proportion of patients with seronegative hepatitis. The Budd-Chiari syndrome may present with acute liver failure and the diagnosis is suggested by hepatomegaly and confirmed by the demonstration of hepatic vein thrombosis. Malignancy infiltration, especially with lymphoma, is another rare cause of acute liver failure that is typically associated with hepatomegaly. Ischemic hepatitis is being increasingly recognized as a cause of acute liver failure, especially in older patients. Other unusual causes of acute liver failure include heatstroke and sepsis.

Pediatric causes

Children are at risk of developing most of the causes of acute liver failure discussed above but also have some unique underlying causes especially in the category of metabolic disease. Neonatal hemochromatosis presents within the first few weeks of life and has been treated by liver transplantation as early as

5 days of age. Acute liver failure due to mitochondrial disorders may be triggered by bacterial infections and are characterized by high lactate levels in blood. Other metabolic causes include tyrosinemia, galactosemia and fructose intolerance. Young infants can develop acute liver failure with viral infections such as adenovirus, coxsackie and cytomegalovirus.

CLINICAL SYNDROME

Acute liver failure causes a syndrome of multisystem failure potentially involving all of the major body systems. Jaundice is present in most patients but some cases of hyperacute liver failure develop encephalopathy before jaundice becomes clinically apparent. Most of the other classical signs of liver failure are notable by their absence. Fetor and asterixis are not prominent features of the encephalopathy of acute liver failure, although are more likely to be seen with subacute liver failure. Portal hypertension can occur but clinical manifestations are unusual. Ascites is characteristic of Wilson disease and can occur in subacute liver failure, whilst bleeding from esophageal varices has been documented occasionally.

Encephalopathy

All patients with acute liver failure have some degree of encephalopathy. Patients with grades 1 and 2 encephalopathy exhibit degrees of drowsiness or disorientation, but they can be roused and they respond appropriately to verbal stimuli. Progression to grade 3 encephalopathy is often heralded by a short period of extreme agitation before the patient becomes very confused and at best obeys simple commands. Grade 4 encephalopathy signifies deep coma with the patients being responsive at best to painful stimuli. In acetaminophen-induced acute liver failure, the encephalopathy develops on the third or fourth day after drug ingestion, but in other etiologies the onset and rate of progression of the encephalopathy is variable.

The pathogenesis of the encephalopathy is incompletely understood but is likely to be multifactorial (Ch. 11). Ammonia levels are classically elevated in serum but in amounts inadequate to independently cause encephalopathy. Furthermore, there is an absence of a close correlation between the ammonia levels and grade of encephalopathy. Phenols, fatty acids, middle-molecular weight substances and mercaptans have also been proposed as possible causative agents. These toxins interfere with neuronal energy metabolism, and may also contribute to alterations in blood–brain barrier permeability by direct toxicity. The inhibitory neurotransmitter γ-aminobutyric acid (GABA) is increased in acute liver failure and this may act independently or in synergy with the benzodiazepine receptor, which forms a supramolecular complex with the GABA receptor on neuronal plasma membranes. Other possible mechanisms include the development of false neurotransmitters e.g. octopamine, and imbalances in the ratios of plasma and intracerebral amino acids.

Intracranial hypertension

Early clinical studies suggested intracranial hypertension occurred in 70% of patients with hyperacute liver failure, 55% of patients with acute liver failure and 15% of patients with subacute liver failure who developed grade 3–4 encephalopathy.

Main changes seen with intracranial hypertension			
	Early	*Intermediate*	*Late*
Baseline intracranial pressure	Normal	Increased	Increased
Surges in intracranial pressure	Yes	Possible	May occur
Mean arterial pressure	Normal or increased	Normal or low	Low
Cerebral perfusion pressure	Normal	Normal or low	Low
Cerebral oxygen metabolism	Normal or increased	Normal or reduced	Reduced
Cerebral autoregulation	Maintained	Lost	Lost
Potential cause of death	Brainstem herniation	Brainstem herniation	Hypoxic brain

Table 33.2 Intracranial hypertension. This is a breakdown of the main changes in the key parameters as intracranial hypertension progresses through a spectrum of increasing severity from early to late stages.

However, there is some evidence that the incidence of cerebral edema is decreasing with modern management protocols. Nevertheless, it remains a major cause of death and frequently disqualifies patients from transplantation.

The term intracranial hypertension covers a range of events including increased blood flow, astrocyte swelling, brainstem herniation and hypoxic injury through sustained impairment of cerebral perfusion (**Table 33.2**). In the early phase, the baseline intracranial pressure is normal but sudden surges in pressure occur either spontaneously or in response to tactile or auditory stimuli. There is an associated increase in mean arterial pressure so that cerebral perfusion pressure is maintained and neuronal oxygenation is satisfactory. The risk to life at this stage is by means of classical brainstem herniation. With time, the baseline intracranial pressure gradually increases but sudden surges may continue to increase the pressure to dangerous levels. Auto-regulation is lost and the systemic arterial pressure response becomes less predictable so that cerebral perfusion is variably reduced with an associated reduction in oxygen delivery to the brain. In the later stages, either the intracranial pressure is so high or the mean arterial pressure is so low that adequate cerebral perfusion no longer occurs and death results from hypoxic brain damage.

The clinical features of cerebral edema include systemic hypertension, 'decerebrate' posturing, hyperventilation, abnormal pupillary reflexes and ultimately impairment of brainstem reflexes and functions. Papilledema however is rarely seen. The outcome with medical management is either full recovery or death, although a few survivors with residual neurologic deficits have been described. Failure of neurological recovery has been observed following otherwise successful liver transplantation.

Renal failure

This occurs in 75% of patients developing grade 4 encephalopathy following an acetaminophen overdose and 30% of other etiologies of acute liver failure. Renal failure after an acetaminophen over-dose is a consequence of direct renal toxicity and develops early in the course of the illness. Early renal dysfunction is also seen in Wilson disease and pregnancy related syndromes. In the other etiologies, renal impairment develops relatively late and pro-gresses from a stage of 'functional' or prerenal failure (urinary sodium <10 mmol/L, urine/plasma osmolarity ratio >1.1) to

acute tubular necrosis. Urea synthesis is impaired in acute liver failure and serum creatinine levels are preferred for the purposes of monitoring renal function.

Metabolic disorders

Hypoglycemia is common and can induce reversible impairment of consciousness prior to the onset of classical encephalopathy. The signs and symptoms of hypoglycemia are often masked and regular blood glucose monitoring is required. Metabolic acidosis is present in 30% of patients developing acute liver failure after an acetaminophen overdose and is associated with a particularly high mortality – >90% if the pH of arterial blood is <7.30 on the second or subsequent days after the overdose. This acidosis precedes the onset of encephalopathy and is independent of renal function. In contrast, a metabolic acidosis is found in 5% of patients with other etiologies of acute liver failure, occurring later in the disease process and also associated with a poor out-come. Increased serum lactate levels have been documented in patients with metabolic acidosis, and these correlate inversely with mean arterial pressure, systemic vascular resistance and oxygen extraction ratios. The hyperlactatemia possibly reflects tissue hypoxia resulting from impaired oxygen extraction as a result of microvascular shunting of blood away from actively respiring tissues. In most etiologies of acute liver failure, alkalosis is the dominant acid–base abnormality and it may be associated with hypokalemia. Hyponatremia may reflect sodium depletion in patients with vomiting or it may be dilutional due to excessive antidiuretic hormone secretion or intracellular sodium shifts. Hypophosphatemia is most frequently encountered in acetaminophen-induced acute liver failure when renal function is preserved.

Hemodynamics

The hemodynamic changes in acute liver failure are very similar to those observed in the systemic inflammatory response syn-drome (SIRS). The early hemodynamic profile reflects a hyper-dynamic circulation with increased cardiac output and reduced systemic peripheral vascular resistance. Profound vasodilatation may cause relative hypovolemia and invasive monitoring is used to determine appropriate fluid regimens and adequate intra-vascular volumes. Progressive disease leads to circulatory failure either as a result of a falling cardiac output or an inability to maintain an adequate mean arterial pressure. This is a common cause of death in acute liver failure. Cardiac dysrhythmias occur and may be due to a definable precipitating event e.g. hypo- or hyperkalemia, acidosis, hypoxia, or cardiac irritation by a catheter, especially Swan-Ganz catheters.

Pulmonary complications

Patients with grade 3–4 encephalopathy are usually intubated and mechanically ventilated to provide airway protection and to facilitate monitoring and treatment. Prior to intubation, hyperventilation may be observed due to early intracranial hypertension or as a response to a coexisting metabolic acidosis. Impaired oxygen exchange is common, usually as a result of acute lung injury with or without infection. Sputum plugs and intrapulmonary hemorrhage can also contribute to the challenge of maintaining adequate oxygenation.

Hematology

The liver is responsible for the synthesis of most of the coagulation factors (except factor VIII which is produced by endothelial cells) and some of the inhibitors of coagulation and fibrinolysis. In acute liver failure circulating levels of fibrinogen, prothrombin and factors V, VII, IX and X are reduced, and the prothrombin time is widely used as an indicator of the severity of liver damage. In addition to decreased synthesis of coagulation factors by the liver, there is evidence of increased peripheral consumption. Overt disseminated intravascular coagulation (DIC) is occasionally observed, especially in the pregnancy related syndromes, but sensitive investigative techniques point to the presence of a low-grade process in most patients. Both quantitative and qualitative defects in platelet function are well described in acute liver failure and platelet counts of $<100 \times 10^9/L$ are seen in up to 70% of patients. Platelet aggregation is impaired, but there is an increase in platelet adhesiveness, a pattern that may be due to increased levels of circulating von Willebrand factor.

There is a fairly poor correlation between the laboratory and clinical manifestations of the coagulopathy. The highest risk of bleeding is seen in those with an associated thrombocytopenia or a frank DIC syndrome. Gastrointestinal hemorrhage was common and was attributed to gastric erosions, but the incidence and severity have been decreased by gastric mucosal protection regimens. The other main sites include nasopharynx, lungs, kidneys, retroperitoneum and skin puncture sites.

Anemia not related to bleeding may be due to hemolysis or bone marrow disease. A Coomb negative hemolytic anemia is a characteristic of Wilson disease and a Coomb positive hemolytic anemia may be seen in acute liver failure secondary to autoimmune hepatitis. Aplastic anemia is associated with seronegative hepatitis especially in younger patients, and has been seen in up to one-third of cases in pediatric series. This may be related to parvovirus B19 infection, although this is not necessarily the cause of the associated acute liver failure. Erythrohemophagocytosis is an increasingly recognized occurrence in acute liver failure.

Infection

Patients with acute liver failure are at increased risk of infections and this has been calculated as twice the expected rate for similarly ill patients without liver disease. It is another of the common causes of death playing an integral role in the evolving cycle of hemodynamic instability and multisystem failure. It also frequently disqualifies potential candidates from emergency liver transplantation. Infection may be difficult to detect with confidence as there is a poor correlation between the presence of infection and body temperature or white cell counts. Clinical studies found that patients with at least grade 2 encephalopathy had proven bacterial infection in up to 80% and fungal infection in 32% of cases. The source of positive cultures included blood, urine, sputum and vascular cannulae. The predominant bacteria were *Staphylococcus aureus*, streptococci and coliform bacteria, while *Candida* species accounted for most of the fungal infections. The fungal infections were particularly difficult to diagnose and were detected antemortem in only 50% of cases. The risk factors for both bacterial and fungal sepsis include coexisting renal failure, cholestasis, treatment with thiopentone and liver transplantation. Surveillance cultures are required on a daily basis.

Diagnosis

The diagnosis of acute liver failure is a clinical one based on the detection of evidence of encephalopathy in patients with acute liver disease. Formal psychometric testing may be useful in patients with subacute liver failure to detect subtle changes to mental state, but in most patients the diagnosis of encephalopathy is made on overt clinical criteria. Commonly hypoglycemia and unusually uremia may mimic hepatic encephalopathy in patients with acute liver failure, and these need to be excluded before the diagnosis is confirmed.

The etiology of acute liver failure must be accurately identified and the appropriate investigations are outlined in **Table 33.4**. The laboratory investigation of acute liver failure is dealt with in **Table 33.5**. Histologic assessment of liver tissue may aid the diagnosis of the cause of acute liver failure but this is often only available after death or transplantation. Confluent necrosis is the commonest histological finding and this may be zonal or involve all of the parenchyma. Necrosis that is zonal within the acinus and coagulative or eosinophilic is more likely to be secondary to a toxic insult or ischemia (**Fig. 33.3**). The features of necrosis and parenchymal collapse may he interspersed with evidence of regeneration (**Fig. 33.4**). The regeneration may either occur in a diffuse pattern of small areas throughout the liver or in randomly occurring larger nodules that give the 'map-like pattern' that has been described in this condition (**Figs 33.5** and **33.6**). The latter pattern is most commonly seen in patients with subacute liver failure. The defined viral causes of acute liver failure have similar histologic appearances and in true acute hepatitis B infection there are usually no tissue markers detectable to implicate hepatitis B as the cause. The detection of hepatitis B markers suggests seroconversion to HBeAb positivity, a surge in hepatitis B replication or superinfection with δ viruses or viruses unrelated to hepatitis B as the cause of the acute liver failure.

Histologic features may suggest specific diagnoses including sodium valproate toxicity, malignant infiltration, Wilson disease, pregnancy related syndromes and the Budd-Chiari syndrome. Sodium valproate toxicity is characterized by microvesicular steatosis. Screening for malignant infiltration as the cause of acute liver failure is one of the stronger indications for performing

Underlying etiology of acute liver failure		
Etiology	Investigation	Comment
Hepatitis A virus (HAV)	IgM anti-HAV	95% positive initially – 100% on repeat testing
Hepatitis B virus (HBV) acute infection	IgM anti-core	Always positive but HBsAg often undetectable
seroconversion	Full HBV profile	HbsAg positive, HBeAg negative, HBeAb initially negative, HBV DNA negative
increased replication	Full HBV screen	HBsAg positive, HBeAg positive, HBV DNA markedly elevated
Hepatitis D virus (HDV)	IgM anti-HDV	IgM anti-core may be positive (co-infection) or negative (superinfection)
Hepatitis E virus (HEV)	Anti-HEV	IgM antibody test not routinely available
Seronegative hepatitis	All tests	Diagnosis of exclusion
Acetaminophen	Drug levels in blood	May be negative on third or subsequent days after overdose
Halothane	Antibody test	Diagnosis usually made on clinical grounds
Idiosyncratic drug reactions	Eosinophil count	Most diagnoses based on temporal relationship
Ecstacy	Blood, urine, hair analysis	Medium-term exposure can be mapped from analysis of hair
Autoimmune	Autoantibodies, IgGs	High titers or anti-KLM suggest diagnosis
Pregnancy-related syndromes: fatty liver	Ultrasound, uric acid, histology	First pregnancy
HELLP syndrome toxemia	Platelet count	Disseminated intravascular coagulation a prominent feature
	Serum aminotransferases	Very high transaminase, appropriate obstetric history
Wilson disease	Urinary copper, ceruloplasmin	Deeply jaundiced, anemic, second interruption in drug compliance
Amanita phalloides		History of ingestion of mushrooms, diarrhea
Budd-Chiari syndrome	Ultrasound or venography	Ascites, prominent caudate lobe on imaging
Malignancy	Imaging and histology	Imaging may be interpreted as normal
Ischemic hepatitis	Aminotransferases	Aminotransferases very high
Heatstroke	Myoglobinuria	Rhabdomyolysis a prominent feature

Table 33.3 Underlying etiology of acute liver failure. The investigations required to establish the underlying cause of acute liver failure.

a liver biopsy in this condition. The benefit from a histologic diagnosis is strongest when lymphoma is the underlying diagnosis, as this may be responsive to chemotherapy. Patients with Wilson disease presenting as acute liver failure usually have established cirrhosis, commonly associated with interface hepatitis resembling autoimmune disease, hepatocyte ballooning and steatosis. Liver histology may be very useful in making a precise diagnosis within the spectrum of pregnancy related liver diseases, ranging from the fatty infiltration characteristic of acute fatty liver of pregnancy (**Fig. 33.7**), to the fibrin microthrombi and associated necrosis that is a feature of liver dysfunction secondary to pre-eclampsia or eclampsia. The histologic features of the Budd-Chiari syndrome are extreme sinusoidal dilatation, congestion and coagulative necrosis.

PROGNOSIS

The range of parameters that correlates with prognosis in acute liver failure is extensive. The grade of encephalopathy, not unsurprisingly, correlates strongly with outcome and this is true for both the grade of encephalopathy at the time of presentation to a specialist unit and the maximum grade attained. The prognosis deteriorates further when grade 4 encephalopathy is complicated by cerebral edema and even further when the latter coexists with renal failure (**Fig. 33.8**). Reliance on the development of these clinical complications to determine prognosis is not helpful when defining the scope and application of liver transplantation in this condition. Furthermore, subsets of patients have very poor prognoses without the development of cerebral or renal

Interpretation of laboratory parameters in acute liver failure

Investigation	Interpretation
Hemoglobin	Hemorrhage, hemolytic or non-hemolytic anemia, aids fluid replacement
White cell count	Partial indicator of presence of sepsis
Platelet count	Important risk factor for bleeding, DIC syndrome, erythrohemophagocytosis, may be very low in acetaminophen cases
Serum bilirubin	Very variable, levels > 700 µmol/L (41 g/dL) indicate hemolysis
Aminotransferases	Very variable and of no prognostic value
Serum albumin	Normal early but falls with disease progression, very low in hyperthermia
Prothrombin time	Very variable but of strong prognostic value
Serum sodium	Often low and may reflect sodium deficiency or dilution
Serum potassium	Low initially but rising with onset of renal failure
Serum phosphate	Low in acetaminophen cases with preserved renal function
Blood glucose	Regular estimations the only reliable screen for hypoglycemia
Acid–base status	Alkalosis common but acidosis associated with a poor prognosis
Arterial oxygen	Best screen for pulmonary disease even when chest X-ray is normal
Serum creatinine	Best indicator of renal dysfunction
Serum amylase	Essential to screen for co-existing pancreatitis

Table 33.4 Interpretation of laboratory parameters. Abnormalities in investigations are interpreted in the context of acute liver failure. DIC, disseminated intravascular coagulation.

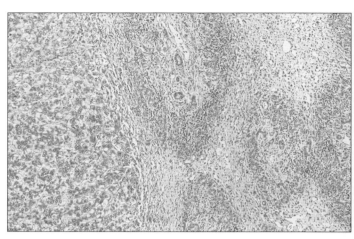

Figure 33.5 Liver histology. Adjacent regeneration (right) and severe collapse (left) occurring in a patient who has subacute liver failure. This appearance can overestimate the likelihood of spontaneous recovery. (Courtesy of Professor B. Portmann.)

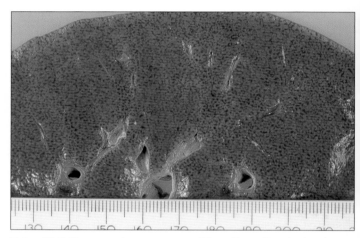

Figure 33.6 Macroscopic appearance of liver. The uniformly shrunken liver is characteristic of hyperacute liver failure. (Courtesy of Professor B. Portmann.)

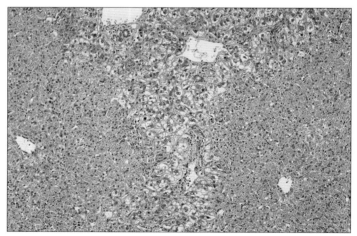

Figure 33.4 Liver histology. Submassive eosinophilic necrosis following an acetaminophen overdose showing few viable hepatocytes. This appearance can underestimate the capacity for regeneration to occur and the likelihood of spontaneous recovery. (Courtesy of Professor B. Portmann.)

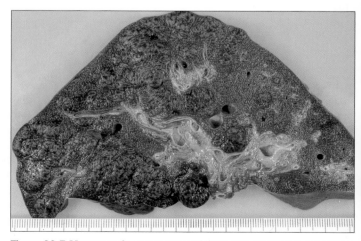

Figure 33.7 Macroscopic appearance of liver. The areas of regeneration randomly interspersed with collapse gives the 'map-like' pattern. The areas of regeneration may achieve significant volumes without improving the clinical condition. (Courtesy of Professor B. Portmann.)

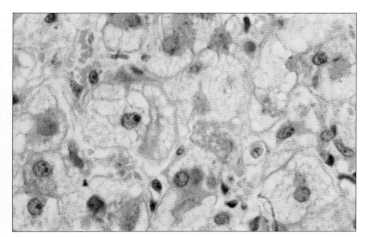

Figure 33.8 Diagnostic biopsy. This biopsy from a pregnant woman who has acute liver failure shows extensive fatty infiltration and is an example of the minority of biopsies that establish a specific diagnosis. (Courtesy of Professor B. Portmann.)

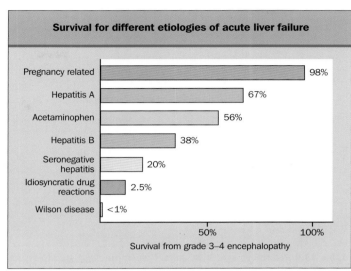

Figure 33.10 Impact of etiology on prognosis. The survival rates attained at King's College Hospital with medical management of patients progressing to acute liver failure is given for the underlying etiology. Similar results have been reported from Japan.

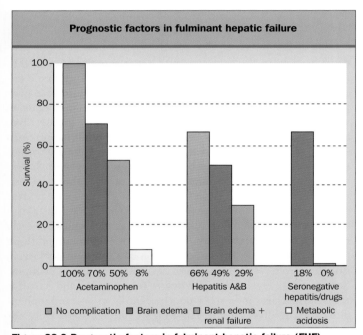

Figure 33.9 Prognostic factors in fulminant hepatic failure (FHF). Survival is related to etiology of the syndrome as well as to the development of complications. Data from O'Grady et al (89).

Referral to specialist units following acetaminophen ingestion

Any of these criteria should prompt referral		
Day 2	*Day 3*	*Day 4*
Arterial pH <7.30	Arterial pH <7.30	INR >6 or PT >100 s
INR >3.0 or PT >50 s	INR >4.5 or PT > 75 s	Progressive rise in PT to any level
Oliguria	Oliguria	Oliguria
Creatinine >200 µmol/L (1.5 mg/dL)	Creatinine >200 µmol/L (1.5 mg/dL)	Creatinine >300 µmol/L (2.3 mg/dL)
Hypoglycemia	Encephalopathy	Encephalopathy
	Severe thrombocytopenia	Severe thrombocytopenia

Table 33.5 Referral to specialist units. Criteria are suggested to select patients with acetaminophen-induced liver damage for referral to a specialist center. INR, international normalized ratio; PT, prothrombin time.

failure. The use of transplantation intensified the need for early indicators of prognosis so that those in need of this intervention could be identified as quickly as possible.

The prognosis of acute liver failure varies greatly with the underlying etiology (**Fig. 33.9**), as well as a number of other factors. Determination of prognosis drives two key management issues when assessing patients with acute liver failure i.e. the need for referral to specialist centers and the indications for transplantation. Indications for referral to specialist units have been suggested for acetaminophen and other etiologies of acute liver failure (**Tables 33.6 and 33.7**). Separate criteria have been identified for use within specialist centers to identify the cohort

most in need of liver transplantation; these King's College criteria, which are widely used, are given in **Tables 33.8 and 33.9**. One of the problems with the criteria is the difficulty applying the coagulation parameters outside the UK. The scale on which prothrombin times are reported in the USA is dramatically shorter than in the UK reflecting differences in technique and the reagents used. The use of the INR (international normalized ratio) did not entirely resolve this problem because of loss of accuracy at higher readings. In France, the factor V levels are used in preference to either the prothrombin time or INR. Factor V levels <20% in patients under the age of 30 years and <30% in older patients are indicative of a poor prognosis once

Referral to specialist units in non-acetaminophen etiologies		
The presence of any of the following criteria should prompt referral		
Hyperacute	*Acute*	*Subacute*
Encephalopathy	Encephalopathy	Encephalopathy
Hypoglycemia	Hypoglycemia	Hypoglycemia (less common)
PT >30 s	PT >30 s	PT >20 s
INR >2.0	INR >2.0	INR >1.5
Renal failure	Renal failure	Renal failure
Hyperpyrexia		Serum sodium <130 mmol/L (130 mEq/L)
		Shrinking liver volume

Table 33.6 Referral to specialist units. Criteria are suggested to select patients with non-acetaminophen-induced liver damage for referral to a specialist center. INR, international normalized ratio; PT, prothrombin time.

Indicators of a poor prognosis in acetaminophen-induced acute liver failure			
Parameter	*Sensitivity*	*Specificity*	*Positive predictive*
Arterial pH <7.30	49%	99%	81%
All 3 of the following concomitantly:			
Prothrombin time >100 s or INR >6.5, Creatinine >300 µmol/L (2.3 mg/dL) and Grade 3–4 encephalopathy	45%	94%	67%

Table 33.7 Indicators of a poor prognosis. The King's College criteria indicating a poor prognosis in acetaminophen-induced acute liver failure. INR, international normalized ratio.

Indicators of a poor prognosis in nonacetaminophen etiologies of acute liver failure			
Parameter	*Sensitivity*	*Specificity*	*Positive predictive*
Prothrombin time >100 s or INR >6.7	34%	100%	46%
Any 3 of the following:			
Unfavorable etiology (seronegative hepatitis or drug reaction), age <10 or >40 years, acute or subacute categories, serum bilirubin > 300 µmol/L (2.3 mg/dL), PT >50 s or INR >3.5	93%	90%	92%

Table 33.8 Indicators of a poor prognosis. The King's College criteria indicating a poor prognosis in causes of acute liver failure other than acetaminophen. INR, international normalized ratio; PT, prothrombin time.

encephalopathy develops. Factor V levels have not been used extensively in clinical practice outside France. A study from the UK assessed the prognostic value of factor V levels and validated their use in non-acetaminophen causes of acute liver failure, but found that they were not discriminatory in cases secondary to acetaminophen.

The King's College criteria, which are early indicators of prognosis, pre-empt advanced encephalopathy and have a major advantage in that largely they can be applied quickly and before the patient progresses to the advanced stages of encephalopathy. In non-acetaminophen cases, etiology, the age of the patient and the interval between the onset of jaundice and the development of encephalopathy are the static variables used to assess prognosis (Table 33.9). These are combined with two commonly used dynamic parameters, serum bilirubin and prothrombin time, to complete the model. In acetaminophen cases, the pH of arterial blood has the strongest predictive value, and a pH <7.30 suggests a very poor prognosis. In patients who did not

develop acidosis, the coexistence of a prothrombin time >100 s (INR 6.7), serum creatinine >300 µmol/L and grade 3 encephalopathy was necessary to be reasonably certain of a poor prognosis. However, despite the prompt identification of patients with a poor prognosis after an acetaminophen overdose, liver transplantation could only be achieved in a minority of cases because of very rapid progression of the disease. The criteria are still used as originally described with a few exceptions. In the original analysis, the discriminatory power of a metabolic acidosis with an arterial pH <7.30 on the second or subsequent day after an acetaminophen overdose was very strong (95% mortality), but the more liberal use of N-acetylcysteine and aggressive early rehydration appear to have improved the outcome in these patients. As a result, the interpretation of a transient acidosis in isolation from other prognostic indicators is more cautious. Serum lactate levels above 3.5 before resuscitation and 3.0 after resuscitation also indicate a poor prognosis in acetaminophen-induced acute liver failure. The King's College criteria were not validated in a number of rarer etiologies particularly pregnancy-related syndromes, Wilson disease and *Amanita phalloides* poisoning.

Assessment of the volume of viable hepatocytes by histologic examination is considered by some to be of prognostic value. The critical mass that suggests a good prognosis has been calculated at between 25 and 40%. This parameter has been used in isolation and in combination with other criteria to select patients for liver transplantation, but the potential for sampling error is considerable. A biopsy taken from an area of total collapse will show few viable hepatocytes even though the adjacent tissue may be regenerating. In addition, the poor prognosis in patients with subacute liver failure may not be apparent from the relative healthy appearance of a biopsy taken from a regenerative nodule (Fig. 33.4).

A small liver on clinical or radiologic assessment, or more particularly a liver that is found to be shrinking rapidly, is a poor prognostic indicator. This feature is especially useful in subacute liver failure when the degree of encephalopathy and the severity of the derangement of coagulation may not be particularly marked. In Japan, CT scanning has been used to assess both the size of the liver and the functional reserve and this was useful in determining prognosis. Serial ultrasonic assessments are commonly used to detect changes in liver size, but the ease with which this can be done has to be weighted against the relatively subjective assessment of liver volume with this technique.

A number of parameters have been shown to have prognostic value in certain circumstances. Patients with acute hepatitis B who have cleared HBsAg from serum are more likely to survive than those with persistent HBsAg in blood. Serum α-fetoprotein levels are higher in patients surviving acute liver failure due to hepatitis B. Serial arterial ketone body ratios have also been shown to identify likely survivors in a number of studies. Although these parameters are of academic interest they are not routinely used to guide decision making in clinical practice.

MANAGEMENT

Overall strategy

The management starts with identification of etiology and an initial assessment of prognosis. Appropriate patients should then be referred to specialist centers where appropriate monitoring is instituted and a decision on the need for immediate liver transplantation is made. Patients are then monitored for the complications that may develop and these are treated as they emerge to the point of recovery, death or transplantation. Patients not initially considered for transplantation may change status on the basis of prognostic indicators or the pattern of clinical complications that emerges. Likewise, patients listed for transplantation may develop complications that preclude this intervention or occasionally may show unexpected signs of recovery before a donor organ becomes available. The final decision on transplantation is made when an organ is available. The potential to develop 'bridges to transplantation' using hepatectomy and/or extracorporeal liver support devices is likely to be increasingly tested in the forthcoming decade.

General measures

There has been scant reward from decades of research activity seeking the panacea for acute liver failure. Efforts have focused on reducing tissue injury, removing accumulated toxins and promoting hepatocyte regeneration (**Table 33.10**). Initial promising reports of efficacy followed by disappointing negative trials have been a recurring theme. There is no role for corticosteroid therapy and controlled studies suggest that in general they are contraindicated. Occasional patients with late-onset hepatic failure are steroid responsive but they are not yet readily identifiable on the basis of serologic markers. Insulin and glucagon infusions have been used to promote hepatic regeneration without convincing evidence of efficacy. Circulating interferon levels were markedly reduced in one study of patients with acute liver failure of viral etiology, and improved survival rates were reported for patients treated with interferon for 3 or more days. However, this observation has also been refuted in a larger study. Similarly an initial enthusiastic report of the benefits of prostaglandins could not be reproduced within the construct of a controlled trial.

There are a few drugs with well-defined roles in specific etiologies of acute liver failure. N-acetylcysteine is established in the management of acetaminophen-induced acute liver failure. It was initially used to prevent liver damage when administered orally within 8 h and intravenously within 15 h of acetaminophen ingestion. The drug is given on the basis of the level of acetaminophen in blood by time after the ingestion of the drug. Standard curves have been developed in the UK and the USA to indicate when N-acetylcysteine is indicated, and a third line has recently been proposed for high-risk patients (**Fig. 33.10**). The latter include patients taking enzyme inducing drugs e.g. antiepileptic therapy, regular alcohol consumers and malnourished patients. An extended role for this drug in acetaminophen-induced acute liver failure was first suggested by a retrospective study of 100 patients showing that N-acetylcysteine given 10–36 h after drug ingestion was associated with a significant decrease in mortality (37 versus 58%), despite the development of comparable prolongations in prothrombin time. These observations were confirmed in a prospective

General management measures in acute liver failure		
Measure	*Controlled trials*	*Comment*
Corticosteroids	Yes	Old study but no benefit seen
Interferon	No	Initial positive report but no benefit seen in larger study
Insulin and glucagon	Yes	Early anecdotal suggestion of benefit but not confirmed in controlled study
Prostaglandin E$_1$	Yes	No survival benefit when controlled trial was performed
N-acetylcysteine	Yes	Beneficial in acetaminophen cases, broader use not yet confirm in clinical studies
Bowel decontamination	Yes	Inconclusive results
Charcoal hemoperfusion	Yes	No survival benefit, re-emerging as component of some extracorporeal circuits incorporating hepatocytes
Resin hemoperfusion	No	Preliminary studies only, inconclusive
Extracorporeal circuits	Yes	One large negative trial

Table 33.9 General management measures. Almost all specific treatments applied to acute liver failure have been found to be ineffective.

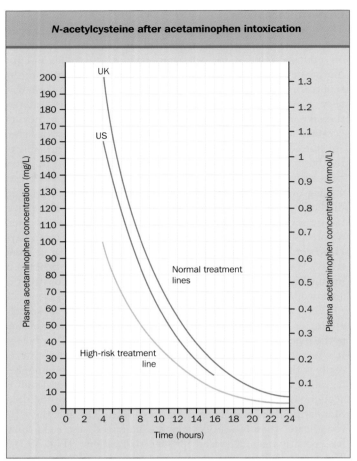

N-acetylcysteine after acetaminophen intoxication

Figure 33.11 *N*-acetylcysteine after acetaminophen intoxication. The nomogram shows the blood levels that indicate a high risk of hepatotoxicity after acetaminophen ingestion in the UK and the USA. The lowest line is used in high-risk patients including the malnourished, chronic alcohol consumers and patients taking enzyme inducing drugs (e.g. antiepileptics).

controlled trial of 50 patients, in which patients in the active treatment limb were commenced on *N*-acetylcysteine 36–80 h after drug ingestion. Although adequate studies of the overall effect of *N*-acetylcysteine on survival have not been reported for other etiologies of acute liver failure, it is increasingly used empirically in ischemic and toxic insults, as well as a modulator of cellular oxygen metabolism. Penicillin, and possibly silymarin, should be added at the earliest opportunity to the standard supportive measures in patients with *Amanita phalloides* toxicity.

Charcoal hemoperfusion was extensively assessed as a system to reduce circulating toxins. A study of 76 patients suggested a significant increase in survival with hemoperfusion when it was commenced while the patient was in grade 3 rather than grade 4 encephalopathy. Subsequently, controlled trials to assess the efficacy and optimal duration of hemoperfusion were carried out in 137 patients. Seventy-five patients with grade 3 encephalopathy were randomized to receive 5 or 10 h of hemoperfusion daily, and there was no difference in survival between the two groups (51.3 versus 50.0%). Sixty-two patients with grade 4 encephalopathy were randomized to receive either no hemoperfusion or 10 h of hemoperfusion daily, and survival rates

were also similar in the two groups (39.3 versus 34.5%). Even though these studies included 137 patients, it has been argued that the numbers may have been inadequate to detect a significant clinical effect, and this illustrates the difficulty in designing controlled studies in acute liver failure. Other non-biological systems that have been inconclusively evaluated include plasmapheresis and albumin dialysis (MARS).

A number of biological extracorporeal bioartificial liver support systems have been developed for clinical assessment in recent years. The hybrid bioartificial liver (BAL) intermittently exposed separated plasma to a cartridge containing porcine liver cells attached to collagen-coated microcarriers after the plasma has been passed through a charcoal column designed to remove substances toxic to the hepatocytes. A controlled trial failed to establish survival benefit in the overall population, although there were indications that subgroups of patients including acetaminophen-induced hepatotoxicity and hyperacute/acute liver failure benefited from therapy with BAL. Another extracorporeal liver assist device (ELAD) continuously exposed whole blood to cartridges containing approximately 200 g of well-differentiated human hepatoblastoma cells. The pilot studies performed suggested a benefit in successfully bridging patients to transplantation but definitive trials have not been performed. Ex-vivo perfusion using pig or human livers that are unsuitable for transplantation has also been described as a bridge to transplantation in a small number of patients. Hepatocyte transfusions are also attracting some interest as a method of augmenting liver function, but as yet no significant clinical outcomes have been reported with this approach.

Liver transplantation

Liver transplantation has revolutionized the management of acute liver failure by offering a lifeline to those cases that have a poor prognosis despite all the advances that have occurred in supportive care. It is now an integral part of the management of acute liver failure.

Grafts and graft allocation

Acute liver failure now accounts for 5% of all liver transplant activity in the USA and 11% in Europe. Most donor organ allocation systems prioritize acute liver failure; in the United Network for Organ Sharing (UNOS) system it is classified as status 1 with regional sharing of organs for patients in this status and in the UK it is the only primary diagnosis on the 'super-urgent' registration list. Living-related donation is well established in Asia, where cadaveric donation is limited, and is being increasingly used in Western countries. Series from specialized centers in the US, continental Europe and the UK are remarkably consistent in showing that 45–51% of patients admitted with acute liver failure underwent liver transplantation (**Fig. 33.11**). In 13–27% of cases, liver transplantation was considered to be contraindicated at the time of admission, and between 6 and 18% of patients were removed from the waiting list or died before an organ became available. The UK figures exclude cases due to acetaminophen and only 7–9% of these underwent transplantation.

The waiting times for donor organs are pivotal in determining the policy on liver transplantation in the management of acute liver failure. The USA and UK allocation systems now result in the majority of patients being transplanted within 48 h of

Management of specific complications
Neurologic

The specific management options for encephalopathy are limited. Patients with subacute liver failure may benefit from dietary protein restriction, lactulose or bowel decontamination. However, these approaches are ineffective in the treatment of the more rapidly progressive encephalopathy characteristic of the hyperacute and acute syndromes. No convincing data have emerged to support the use of branched chain amino acids. Clinical and electroencephalogram (EEG) assessed responses to flumazenil have been transient and unpredictable and have not indicated a role for this drug in the management of the encephalopathy of acute liver failure. A transient improvement in encephalopathy has also been noted during many of the studies of extracorporeal liver support devices, but ultimately without survival benefits.

Mannitol is the mainstay of treatment of surges in intracranial pressure that may compromise brainstem function (**Fig. 33.22**). The overall beneficial effect of mannitol was established in a controlled trial and the mechanism of action was considered to be its property as an osmotic diuretic. It has also been suggested that the rapidity of action of mannitol is more consistent with its function of increasing cerebral blood being the basis for the therapeutic response. A rapid bolus of 0.3–1.0 g/kg is recommended to achieve the maximal diuretic effect, and in anuric patients a diuresis is simulated by ultrafiltrating three times the administered volume over the subsequent 30 min. This process is repeated as determined by the pattern of clinical relapses until the serum osmolarity exceeds 320 mOsm. More recent studies showed that the administration of mannitol was followed by an increase in cerebral blood flow associated with an increase in cerebral metabolic rate for oxygen and reduced brain lactate formation.

Sodium thiopentone (phenobarbital) was shown to control cerebral edema that had become unresponsive to mannitol in an uncontrolled study. A priming dose of between 185 and 250 mg (median 250 mg) given over 15 min was followed by a 4-h infusion of between 50 and 250 mg/h. Another study documented a 73% response rate to barbiturates, but this was followed by an 80% relapse rate after thiopentone was withdrawn. Thiopentone has neither been subjected to a controlled trial nor shown to improve the survival rate. Its role is limited by loss of efficacy and hemodynamic instability following its administration. There is an additional concern that the use of thiopentone results in an increase in infective complications in those surviving this phase of the illness. Acute, but not chronic, hyperventilation was reported to be of benefit. Nevertheless, hyperventilation to partial pressure of CO_2 levels below 25 mmHg is routinely incorporated as a first line treatment in protocols in the USA. Acute hyperventilation using low-tidal volumes (to prevent increases in intrathoracic pressure reducing venous return from the head) combined with 80–100% inspired oxygen may control surges in intracranial pressure that are unresponsive to mannitol and thiopentone. Hypothermia and hypertenonic saline infusions have also been shown in small studies to be useful adjuncts in the management of intracranial hypertension.

In the later stages of the neurologic complications, the emphasis of management changes to the preservation of cerebral perfusion pressure, increased oxygen delivery to the brain and manipulation of the neuronal microcirculation to promote cerebral oxygen extraction. The patient is now nursed with the trunk at 0–10 degrees to the horizontal. The options for increasing the mean arterial pressure and consequently improving cerebral perfusion pressure are outlined in the section dealing with hemodynamics. These adjustments are made to maintain a cerebral perfusion pressure greater than 50 mmHg where possible. If it becomes difficult to maintain adequate cerebral perfusion pressure, spontaneous recovery is unlikely without liver transplantation, and hepatectomy is useful to secure transient improvement.

N-acetylcysteine and prostaglandin I_2 infusions have been shown to increase cerebral blood flow and cerebral metabolic

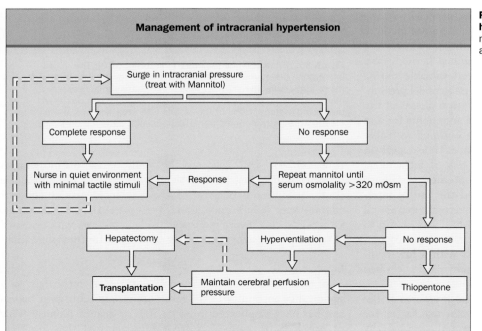

Management of intracranial hypertension

Figure 33.23 Management of intracranial hypertension. The therapeutic alternatives in the management of this serious complication of acute liver failure.

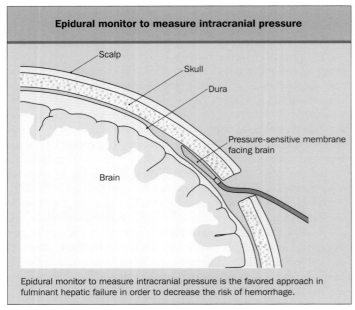

Epidural monitor to measure intracranial pressure

Scalp
Skull
Dura
Pressure-sensitive membrane facing brain
Brain

Epidural monitor to measure intracranial pressure is the favored approach in fulminant hepatic failure in order to decrease the risk of hemorrhage.

Figure 33.24 Epidural monitor to measure intracranial pressure. This is the favored approach in acute liver failure in order to decrease the risk of hemorrhage.

Arguments for and against intracranial pressure monitoring in acute liver failure

For	Against
Only way of getting effective insight into condition	Complication rate too high
Allows early diagnosis	Clinical features allow diagnosis
Drives intelligent treatment	Never proven to improve survival
Monitors effect of potentially hazardous interventions	Good management protocols prevent potentially hazardous interventions
Modern devices are easy to place	Requires neurosurgical input
Aggressive correction of coagulopathy not necessary	Aggressive correction of coagulopathy necessary
	False readings may arise and confuse management

Table 33.10 Intracranial pressure monitoring. The arguments for and against the use of pressure monitoring in acute liver failure are presented.

rate for oxygen and are considered to improve microcirculatory stability. Occult seizure activity may contribute to neurologic instability in patients with grade 4 encephalopathy. Phenytoin and diazepam are effective therapies, despite the theoretic consideration that the latter may aggravate the underlying encephalopathy. There is no established role for other diuretics or antihypertensive agents in the management of cerebral edema in acute liver failure.

The use of intracranial pressure monitoring (**Fig. 33.23**) is controversial and has not been subjected to clinical trials. Early detection of cerebral edema and the facility to constantly monitor this complication help to optimize therapeutic interventions. Intracranial pressure monitoring allows earlier and more accurate detection of pressure changes, especially in the ventilated patient in whom most of the clinical signs are masked. It also facilitates careful monitoring of the intracranial pressure during high-risk therapeutic interventions, such as hemodialysis and tracheal suctioning. It is also considered valuable during orthotopic liver transplantation as increases in intracranial pressure often occur during the dissection and reperfusion phases of the transplant operation. The main points of the arguments for and against intracranial pressure monitoring are outlined in **Table 33.11**. The most commonly used system places transducers on or through a small nick in the dura. The risk of intracranial hemorrhage is a deterrent, although the studies that have systematically addressed safety have favored the use of intracranial pressure monitoring, especially using fiberoptic extradural or subdural devices. Proponents argue that it has been shown to be effective and relatively safe, despite the attendant coagulopathy. Epidural transducers were associated with a low complication rate at 3.8%, but subdural and parenchymal devices had higher complication rates at 20 and 22% respectively.

One study has shown that high intracranial pressures at the time of insertion of the device were the main risk factor for intracranial hemorrhage, rather than the expected coagulopathy

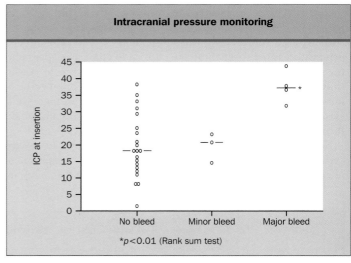

Intracranial pressure monitoring

ICP at insertion

No bleed   Minor bleed   Major bleed

*$p < 0.01$ (Rank sum test)

Figure 33.25 Intracranial pressure monitoring (ICP). The initial intracranial pressures are shown for patients developing major and minor intracranial bleeds after insertion of intracranial pressure monitors. High pressures correlated more strongly with risk than prothrombin times. None of the bleeds was fatal and two of the major bleeds were asymptomatic frontal lobe bleeds detected on scanning.

(**Fig. 33.24**). This suggests the routine use of intracranial pressure monitoring in all patients with hyperacute and acute (but not subacute because of the low incidence of cerebral edema) liver failure once grade 3–4 encephalopathy develops. Others advocate its use more selectively in patients with evidence of cerebral edema, or those being considered for transplantation.

Infection
The high incidence of bacterial and fungal infections is a significant contributor to the mortality rate in acute liver failure and has been implicated in up to 50% of deaths. Clinical trials of prophylactic antibiotics have demonstrated that systemic

antibiotics reduce the incidence of culture-positive bacterial infection by half but this strategy is associated with the emergence of highly resistant organisms in up to 10% of cases. However, this reduction in infection rates was not accompanied by a significant impact on major clinical outcomes (mortality, progression to transplantation) or economic considerations (duration of intensive care unit and hospital stay, overall cost of antimicrobials). Small bowel decontamination was not effective in altering the pattern of infection. Systemic antibiotics are recommended when infection is suspected and the precise regimens used are determined by local antibiotic policy.

The use of prophylactic systemic antifungal therapy has not been subjected to controlled trials. It may be appropriate in patients with risk factors for systemic fungal infection like renal failure, severe cholestasis, previous or concomitant thiopentone therapy or liver transplantation. Systemic fungal infection is notoriously difficult to diagnose in the setting of acute liver failure, and a high index of suspicion is required especially in the high-risk group outlined above and in those cases where there is an arrest in the recovery of coagulation activity. The latter is a valuable sentinel marker of infection that often predates clinical manifestations by some days. *Candida* spp. account for the vast majority of fungal infections, and there are no data to show superiority of any of the available therapies.

Hemodynamic instability and oxygen debt

Circulatory failure is considered to be a significant contraindication to transplantation and a common mode of death in acute liver failure, often occurring against the background of sepsis and multiorgan failure. Invasive hemodynamic monitoring is routinely initiated in patients with grade 3 encephalopathy and filling pressures are normalized with appropriate combinations of colloid, crystalline fluids and blood products. Hypotension occurring despite adequate intravascular volumes (pulmonary capillary wedge pressure 10–14 mmHg) is treated with vasopressor agents, using norepinephrine if the cardiac index exceeds 4.5 L/min/m^2 or epinephrine if the cardiac output needs to be boosted above this threshold. The initial stabilizing dose to achieve a mean arterial pressure above 60 mmHg ranged between 0.2 and 1.8 mg/kg/min of epinephrine and 0.2 and 2.0 mg/kg/min of norepinephrine. Vasopressor agents may cause or aggravate an oxygen debt and prostacyclin infused at a rate of 5 ng/kg/min has been shown to improve parameters of oxygen metabolism (delivery, consumption and extraction ratio) when used in conjunction with both epinephrine and norepinephrine. N-acetylcysteine infusion (10 mg/kg/min for 15 min followed by 0.2 mg/kg/min for 4 h) caused less vasodilatation than prostacyclin, independently increased mean arterial pressure and was as effective as prostacyclin in improving oxygen metabolism. The combination of prostacyclin and N-acetylcysteine was more beneficial to oxygen metabolism than either drug alone (**Fig. 33.25**). Patients developing resistance to inotropes have been shown to have a hypoadrenal profile that responds to hydrocortisone.

Renal failure

The prophylactic use of dopamine has been common practice but its benefits have been challenged, especially in the setting of profound vasodilatation that is typical of acute liver failure. The appropriate clinical studies have not been performed in this

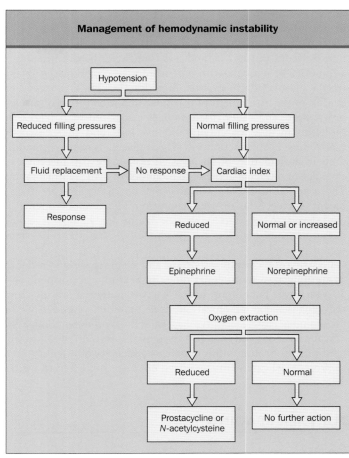

Figure 33.26 Management of hemodynamic instability. A care pathway for the management of hemodynamic instability.

setting. Extracorporeal renal support was required in 75% of cases of acetaminophen-induced acute liver failure and 30% of other etiologies that progressed to grade 3–4 encephalopathy. The metabolic complexity of combined liver and renal failure suggests early intervention with hemodialysis, pre-empting standard indications, is prudent. Continuous filtration or dialysis systems are associated with less hemodynamic instability and run a lower risk of aggravating latent or established cerebral edema than intermittent hemodialysis. The coagulopathy of acute liver failure does not negate the need for anticoagulation and paradoxically heparin requirements have been shown to be increased during hemodialysis The heparin doses required to prevent platelet depletion showed considerable variation and are best determined by functional assays such as the activated clotting time. Antithrombin III supplementation in a dose of 3000 units prior to hemodialysis reduced heparin requirements. Prostacyclin infusions in doses between 2 and 5 ng/kg/min proved superior to heparin anticoagulation in continuous systems with respect to the functional duration of the filters and the hemorrhagic complications experienced.

Coagulopathy

Prophylactic repletion of coagulation factors with fresh frozen plasma has been practiced and requirements of up to a mean of 40 mL/kg/day to maintain the prothrombin time within 5–10 s of normal have been reported. The possible potential advantages of reduced bleeding and infection (as a consequence of repletion of opsonins) have not been established by clinical studies. A controlled trial of fresh frozen plasma failed to demonstrate an improvement in survival, and was thought to be detrimental in a minority of patients with a consumptive coagulopathy. Fresh frozen plasma administration impedes the use of coagulation studies in the assessment of prognosis and monitoring of disease progression, and other disadvantages associated with aggressive repletion include potential fluid overload and hyperviscosity syndromes. Prophylactic fresh frozen plasma is more commonly used in anticipation of an invasive procedure e.g. insertion of cannulae or intracranial pressure monitors, or liver transplantation. There are limited data available yet on the utility of recombinant factor VIa in this condition. Thrombocytopenia is considered to an important risk factor for hemorrhage and maintenance of platelets counts above 50–70 $\times$ 10^9/L has been recommended.

Gastric protection is important and hemorrhage was reduced by prophylaxis with cimetidine in a study performed over 20 years ago. Sucralfate, which has the potential advantage of reducing gastric colonization and pulmonary infection by maintaining gastric acidity, has gained favor even though its efficacy has not been formally assessed. Likewise, the efficacy of ranitidine or proton pump inhibitors which are also widely used to protect the gastric mucosa have not been subjected to formal assessment.

Nutrition

Although the standard patient with acute liver failure is well nourished at the onset of the illness, it is important to institute nutrition as soon as possible. The catabolic rate increases in patients with acute liver failure and this is most apparent in those with complicating sepsis and those undergoing liver transplantation. The theoretical problems that limit nutritional options are legion – gastrointestinal ileus, desire to minimize gastrointestinal protein, difficulty maintaining isoglycemia, fluid restrictions secondary to renal failure, theoretical role of amino-acid ratios in mediating encephalopathy, difficulty handling lipids, aggravation of sepsis by intravenous feeding, etc. Despite all of these considerations, adequate nutrition can be obtained in the majority of patients. An element of enteral nutrition is desirable to help maintain the integrity of the small intestinal mucosa, and this is titrated against the volume of gastric aspirates and the development of diarrhea. Pilot studies showed that parenteral feeding is tolerated considerably better than would be expected from theoretical considerations. Lipid solutions (10%) are cleared from serum and standard amino-acid preparations do not appear to have a clinically relevant impact on the encephalopathy profile. Continuous renal support systems give good flexibility with regard to the management of fluid loads and assiduous attention to the maintenance of feeding lines keeps the septic complications within the expected pattern of frequency.

FURTHER READING

Etiology

O'Grady JG, Schalm SW, Williams R. Acute liver failure: redefining the syndromes. Lancet 1993; 342:273–275. *This article discusses the very important role that definitions play in defining prognosis and the clinical course of acute liver failure.*

Rolando N, Wade J, Davalos M, et al. The systemic inflammatory response syndrome in acute liver failure. Hepatology 2000; 32:734–739.

Prognosis

Bernal W, Donaldson N, Wyncoll D, et al. Blood lactate as an early indicator of outcome in paracetamol-induced acute liver failure. Lancet 2002; 359:558–563.

O'Grady JG, Alexander GJ, Hallyar KM, et al. Early indicators of prognosis in fulminant hepatic failure. Gastroenterology 1989; 97:439–445. *This seminal article details a scheme to accurately determine prognosis using commonly available variables to rapidly identify which patients will likely need transplantation or not. The scheme has been repeatedly tested by other systems, and has still stood the test of time.*

Complications

Blei AT, Olafsson S, Webster S, et al. Complications of intracranial pressure monitoring in fulminant hepatic failure. Lancet 1993; 16; 341:157–158. *An excellent review from most of liver transplant programs in the United States detailing the use of and complications from intracranial pressure monitoring in patients with fulminant hepatic failure, demonstrating primarily its relative safety.*

Harry R, Auzinger G, Wendon J. The clinical importance of adrenal insufficiency in acute hepatic dysfunction. Hepatology 2002; 36:395–402.

Murphy N, Auzinger G, Bernel W, et al. The effect of hypertonic sodium chloride on intracranial pressure in patients with acute liver failure. Hepatology 2004; 39:464–470.

Strauss GI, Knudsen GM, Kondrup J, et al. Cerebral metabolism of ammonia and amino acids in patients with fulminant hepatic failure. Gastroenterology 2001; 121(5):1109–1119.

Treatment

Demetriou AA, Brown RS, Busuttil RW, et al. Prospective, randomised, multicenter, controlled trial of a bioartificial liver in treating acute liver failure. Ann Surg 2002; 239:660–670. *A report of the largest clinical trial of cell-based, liver support therapy in the treatment of patients with acute liver failure. It shows that such devices may play a role in the management of patients with acetaminophen-induced acute liver failure, and acute liver failure caused by hepatitis A and B. It also highlights the problems with performing studies with liver support devices.*

Ellis AJ, Hughes RD, Wendon JA, et al. Pilot-controlled trial of the extra-corporeal liver assist device in acute liver failure. Hepatology 1996; 24:1446–1451.

Jalan R, Damink SW, Deutz NE, et al. Moderate hypothermia for uncontrolled intracranial hypertension in acute liver failure. Lancet 1992; 354:1164–1168.

O'Grady JG, Gimson AE, O'Brien CJ, et al. Controlled trials of charcoal hemoperfusion and prognostic factors in fulminant hepatic failure. Gastroenterology 1988; 94:1186–1192.

Transplantation

Bernal B. Changing patterns of causation and the use of transplantation in the United Kingdom. Semin Liver Dis 2003; 23:227–237.

CHAPTER
34

The Liver in Systemic Disease

Andrew Ross and Lawrence S. Friedman

The liver is the second largest and most biochemically complex organ in the body. Multiple interactions exist between the liver and other organ systems and, as a result, the liver is often affected by systemic disease processes. This chapter reviews liver involvement in some of these systemic diseases and is limited to those processes not covered in more detail in other chapters.

ENDOCRINE DISORDERS

Diabetes mellitus

Patients with obesity and diabetes mellitus, especially type II diabetes mellitus, may present with elevated serum aminotransferase levels or massive hepatomegaly (Table 34.1). The most common histologic abnormality observed in affected persons is fatty change, or steatosis, reflected by deposition of large, macronodular fat droplets in liver parenchymal cells. These histologic findings may be found in asymptomatic obese or diabetic patients without liver enzyme elevations and fall within the pathologic spectrum of non-alcoholic fatty liver disease (NAFLD) (Fig. 34.1) (see Ch. 22).

A peculiar type of subcapsular focal fatty change is found in diabetic patients on continuous ambulatory peritoneal dialysis (CAPD). It is thought that glucose and insulin from the dialysis solutions diffuse through the hepatic capsule and accumulate in the thin rim of subcapsular hepatocytes. The high insulin con-

centrations in the subcapsular hepatocytes result in localized steatosis by inhibiting the oxidation of free fatty acids and stimulating the synthesis of triglycerides (Table 34.2).

Thyroid disease

The liver plays an integral role in thyroid hormone metabolism through the production of thyroxine-binding globulin (TBG),

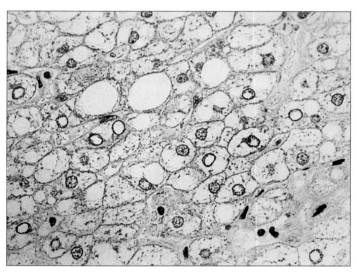

Figure 34.1 Glycogenated nuclei. Microvesicular and macrovesicular fat are present.

Diabetes and associated liver diseases
Hepatic disease caused by diabetes
Glycogen deposition (Mauriac syndrome)
Fatty liver
Cirrhosis
Biliary tract disease
Liver diseases associated with therapy of diabetes
Viral hepatitis (needle stick)
Injury due to oral hypoglycemic drugs
Liver disease associated with diabetes
Hemochromatosis
Chronic active autoimmune hepatitis
Hepatogenic diabetes

Table 34.1 Diabetes and associated liver diseases

Causes of liver steatosis
Increased fatty acid mobilization 　Obesity 　Insulin deficiency 　Corticosteroid excess 　Starvation 　Alcohol 　Inflammatory bowel disease
Increased fatty acid synthesis 　Alcohol 　Hyperalimentation
Decreased synthesis of apoproteins 　Tetracycline 　Yellow phosphorus
Decreased transport and release of lipoproteins 　Colchicine 　Ethanol 　Orotic acid

Table 34.2 Causes of liver steatosis

prealbumin and albumin, to which over 88% of circulating thyroid hormone is bound. In addition, the liver is the major site of peripheral thyroid hormone metabolism and is involved in the conjugation, biliary excretion, oxidative deamination and extra-thyroidal deiodination of thyroxine (T_4) and triiodothyronine (T_3) and the conversion of T_4 to reverse T_3 (rT_3). Thyroid hormones are also important for normal hepatic function and bilirubin metabolism. The expression of low-density lipoprotein (LDL) receptors and the activity of hepatic enzymes that are important in lipid metabolism are regulated, in part, by thyroid hormone. In addition, thyroid hormone appears to play an important role in regulating the activity of uridine 5′-diphosphate (UDP) glucuronosyltransferase, the hepatic enzyme that is primarily responsible for the conjugation of bilirubin prior to excretion.

Hyperthyroidism

Liver injury is common in patients with thyrotoxicosis and can be hepatocellular or cholestatic (**Table 34.3**). Increased serum aspartate aminotransferase (AST) and alanine aminotransferase (ALT) levels have been reported in up to 37% of patients with thyrotoxicosis who have no overt signs of hepatic impairment. The liver enzyme elevations are thought to result from an increase in hepatocyte oxygen requirements without a compensatory increase in hepatic blood flow. Liver biopsy specimens in patients with mild hyperthyroidism-related hepatic injury may reveal lobular inflammation with an infiltrate

consisting of polymorphonuclear leukocytes, eosinophils and lymphocytes, hepatocyte nuclear changes, and Kupffer cell hyperplasia. A small percentage of patients may exhibit more progressive injury with centrilobular necrosis and perivenular fibrosis. Clinically, these patients typically present with self-limited hepatitis, but fulminant hepatic failure has been described in patients with severe thyrotoxicosis.

Elevated serum levels of alkaline phosphatase have been described in up to 64% of patients with thyrotoxicosis, but only 17% have an elevated γ-glutamyltranspeptidase level and 5% an elevated total bilirubin level. Liver biopsy specimens from patients with cholestatic thyrotoxicosis-induced liver injury reveal non-specific lobular inflammation with intrahepatocytic cholestasis. Jaundice is rare in patients with thyrotoxicosis, and its presence should prompt a search for other complications of hyperthyroidism, such as cardiac failure, or sepsis.

It is unclear whether hepatic injury in patients with thyrotoxicosis is an effect of thyroid hormone on hepatocytes alone or the result of associated conditions such as congestive heart failure, infection and malnutrition. In all likelihood, the cause is a combination of these factors. In the majority of cases, the hepatic abnormalities reverse following restoration of a euthyroid state.

Hypothyroidism

The clinical picture of hypothyroidism can be confused with advanced chronic liver disease because of similarities in presenting

Hepatic abnormalities associated with various thyroid conditions and therapies			
Condition	Clinical and laboratory findings	Liver biopsy findings	Outcome
Thyrotoxicosis	Elevated aminotransferase levels (in up to 37% of patients); Elevated serum alkaline phosphatase levels (in up to 64% of patients)	Lobular inflammation; hepatocytes nuclear changes; Kupffer cell hyperplasia	Laboratory abnormalities and liver biopsy findings are reversible in the majority of patients with the restoration of the euthyroid state
		Centrilobular necrosis and perivenular fibrosis in rare cases	Fulminant hepatic failure has been reported
		Non-specific lobular inflammation; intrahepatocytic cholestasis	
Hypothyroidism	Elevated serum AST levels, myalgias, fatigue; elevated serum bilirubin levels; ascites	Centrilobular fibrosis in patients with ascites	Clinical findings and laboratory abnormalities are usually reversible within weeks of the initiation of thyroid replacement therapy
Propylthiouracil therapy	Elevated serum AST and ALT levels (up to 30% of patients)	Non-specific hepatocellular injury	Hepatotoxicity is typically dose-related; full recovery occurs in the majority of patients
		Hepatocellular necrosis in less than 1% of patients	Persistent hepatitis occurs in less than 1% of patients
			Fulminant hepatic failure has been reported
Methimazole and carbimazole therapy	Rare elevations in serum bilirubin and alkaline phosphatase levels	Intrahepatic cholestasis	Liver test abnormalities and biopsy findings may persist after therapy is discontinued

Table 34.3 Hepatic abnormalities associated with various thyroid conditions and therapies. ALT, alanine aminotransferase; AST, aspartate aminotransferase

symptoms and laboratory findings (Table 34.3). Myalgias, fatigue, muscle cramps and an elevated AST level (resulting from myopathy in patients with hypothyroidism) are findings that are common to both liver disease and hypothyroidism. In addition, myxedema coma and ascites with a high serum-ascites albumin gradient (SAAG) can be seen in hypothyroidism. The cause of ascites in patients with hypothyroidism remains in dispute. Although it has long been thought that ascites in patients with hypothyroidism results from right-sided heart failure, right heart pressures are often normal in these patients. However, histologic demonstration of central congestive fibrosis of the liver in patients with myxedema ascites supports a role for right-sided heart failure as an etiology. An alternative explanation for ascites in patients with severe hypothyroidism is enhanced vascular endothelial permeability. Regardless of the underlying patho-physiology, ascites in patients with hypothyroidism typically resolves with thyroid replacement therapy.

Cholestatic jaundice has been described in several case reports of patients with hypothyroidism. Gallstones in patients with hypothyroidism may result from reduced bile flow, hyper-cholesterolemia, and gallbladder hypotonia. Hepatic dysfunction associated with hypothyroidism typically resolves within weeks of initiation of thyroid replacement therapy.

Liver injury associated with antithyroid therapy

Propylthiouracil (PTU) can cause hepatocellular injury, which occasionally may be severe, sometimes resulting in hepatic failure or death. Elevated serum AST and ALT levels occur in up to 30% of patients taking PTU, and the effect appears to be dose-related, with peak aminotransferase levels occurring soon after the initiation of therapy (Table 34.3). The elevated amino-transferase levels typically fall following a reduction in the dose of PTU, and the majority of patients experience a full recovery after discontinuation of the drug. In less than 1% of patients, hepatitis persists, with evidence of hepatocellular necrosis on liver biopsy. The hepatitis is an idiosyncratic reaction to PTU that typically occurs in women younger than 30 years of age during the first few months of therapy. Patients usually recover completely after therapy is discontinued, but fulminant hepatic failure requiring liver transplantation has been reported. Patients who experience asymptomatic, mild (= 2 × normal) elevations in serum aminotransferase levels while taking PTU can continue the drug with close monitoring, but the medication should be stopped immediately if aminotransferase levels rise further.

Methimazole and carbimazole cause liver test elevations less frequently than does PTU (Table 34.3). Hepatotoxicity from these agents is typically cholestatic, with elevations in serum bilirubin, alkaline phosphatase, and γ-glutamyltranspeptidase levels.

Thyroid abnormalities resulting from liver disease

Thyroid test abnormalities are common in patients with liver disease. Patients with cirrhosis often have a reduced level of total and free T_3 with an elevated level of rT_3, reflecting the 'sick euthyroid' state. The changes result from a decrease in the activity of deiodinase type 1, thereby leading to reduced con-version of T_4 to T_3. In turn, T_4 is converted to rT_3. This sequence is regarded as an adaptive hypothyroid state that reduces the basal metabolic rate within hepatocytes and preserves body protein stores.

Patients with acute hepatitis and fulminant hepatic failure initially have increased serum levels of total T_4; this is attributed to an increased synthesis of TBG as an acute-phase reactant. Levels of free T_4 remain normal. With increasing severity and duration of liver disease, total T_4 levels may decrease because of reduced hepatic TBG synthesis. Levels of T_3 may vary, but the ratio of free T_3 to free T_4 correlates inversely with the severity of liver disease.

Other forms of chronic liver disease may be associated with thyroid disease. Up to 25% of patients with primary biliary cirrhosis (PBC) have associated autoimmune hypothyroidism. Thyroid dysfunction is also common in patients with auto-immune hepatitis: Grave disease occurs in up to 6% of patients with autoimmune hepatitis, and autoimmune thyroiditis occurs in up to 12%. Patients with primary sclerosing cholangitis also have an increased incidence of Hashimoto thyroiditis, Grave disease and Riedel thyroiditis. Antiviral therapy of chronic hepatitis B and C with α-interferon and pegylated interferon has been associated with both hypothryroidism and hyper-thyroidism. Up to 10% of patients with hepatitis C treated with α-interferon develop thyroid dysfunction, presumably as a result of the induction of antithyroid and antithyrotropin anti-bodies by interferon.

RHEUMATIC DISEASES

The incidence and clinical significance of hepatic abnormalities in rheumatic (collagen vascular) disorders are poorly defined, in part because liver biopsy is usually not performed in patients with mild liver biochemical test abnormalities. In addition, the medications used to treat collagen vascular disorders may cause hepatotoxicity, and distinguishing between drug-induced liver disease and liver disease associated with the underlying systemic rheumatic disease may be difficult.

Systemic lupus erythematosus

Hepatic involvement in systemic lupus erythematosus (SLE) has been difficult to characterize. Initially, hepatic manifestations of SLE were thought to be rare. However, a retrospective obser-vational study performed by Runyon et al (1980) described hepatomegaly in up to 39% of 238 patients with SLE, with associated jaundice in 24%. Overall, 21% of these patients had abnormal liver chemistries and liver biopsy results that could not be explained by other causes.

Hepatic involvement in SLE may be caused by the underlying disease, a coexisting disorder, or medications. Differentiating autoimmune hepatitis (formerly called lupoid hepatitis) from SLE-related hepatic manifestations is based in part on the detection in serum of smooth muscle antibodies and anti-mitochondrial antibodies in patients with autoimmune hepatitis; both antibodies are rare in SLE. This distinction is important because patients with autoimmune hepatitis typically have more serious, progressive liver disease as compared to patients with hepatic involvement in SLE. Coexisting liver disease such as viral hepatitis and primary biliary cirrhosis can often be seen in patients with SLE. Findings in two retrospective studies and a prospective study describing the association between SLE and liver disease are summarized in **Table 34.4**.

Hepatomegaly is the most consistent reported clinical finding in patients with hepatic manifestations of SLE. Jaundice and

Liver findings in systemic lupus erythematosus (SLE)	
Number of patients	551
Number with evidence of liver disease	146 (26.5%)
Etiology	
Drug-related	50 (9%)
Liver disease not related to SLE	17 (3%)
Venous congestion	8 (1.5%)
Unknown	72 (13%)
Clinically significant liver disease	22 (4%)
Death due to liver disease	3 (<1%)

Table 34.4 Liver findings in systemic lupus erythematosus (SLE)

splenomegaly have also been described. Non-specific liver chemistry abnormalities with mild elevations of serum AST, ALT, bilirubin and alkaline phosphatase levels have been described.

The most common hepatic histologic finding in patients with SLE is steatosis, often not attributable to corticosteroid use or other risk factors for steatosis. Additional histologic findings include granulomatous hepatitis, centrilobular necrosis, chronic hepatitis and cirrhosis.

Patients with SLE are especially susceptible to salicylate toxicity from prolonged high-dose salicylate therapy. Salicylate hepatotoxicity in SLE is characterized by diffuse hepatocyte injury, disruption of the limiting plate, and stellate cell activation with a plasma cell-predominant chronic portal infiltrate, occasional lymphoid follicles and fibrosis. A more acute pattern of injury is characterized by centrilobular ballooning of hepatocytes, scattered acidophilic bodies and moderate portal inflammation. Other reported findings include microabscesses from bacterial infection, hemosiderosis from blood transfusion, PBC and drug toxicity. Successful treatment of SLE or discontinuation of offending medications typically leads to improvement in associated hepatic biochemical and histologic abnormalities.

Criteria for treating SLE-related liver disease are not well defined. Liver biochemical abnormalities improve in the majority of patients treated with corticosteroids. In patients who have persistent liver test abnormalities despite treatment, a thorough evaluation, including liver biopsy, should be considered. Attention should be paid to the patient's medication history, particularly salicylate therapy.

Rheumatoid arthritis

Abnormalities in liver chemistries, primarily elevated serum alkaline phosphatase and γ-glutamyltranspeptidase levels have been reported in up to 6% of patients with rheumatoid arthritis (RA). Elevated alkaline phosphatase levels may also be of bone origin. Liver biopsy findings from patients with abnormal liver chemistries and RA are non-specific and include Kupffer cell hyperplasia, steatosis and a periportal mononuclear cell infiltrate. As in patients with SLE, medications used in the treatment of RA, such as methotrexate, gold salts, non-steroidal anti-inflammatory drugs (NSAIDs), and corticosteroids, may result in hepatotoxicity that is difficult to distinguish from hepatic disease caused by RA.

Sjögren syndrome

Among 300 patients with primary Sjögren syndrome (kerato-conjunctivitis sicca) investigated by Skopouli et al (1994) for liver involvement, 7% had abnormal liver chemistries. Of these patients, 6.6% had antimitochondrial antibodies, 92% of whom had features of PBC. Although the exact frequency of PBC in patients with primary Sjögren syndrome is unknown, an overlap between the two conditions has been well described, related perhaps to the similar underlying pathogenic mechanisms of the two diseases. Patients with primary Sjögren syndrome and abnormal liver chemistries should be tested for antimitochondrial antibodies for possible PBC.

Primary antiphospholipid antibody syndrome

Primary antiphospholipid antibody syndrome (APS) is defined by the clinical features of recurrent arterial or venous thrombosis, recurrent pregnancy loss and thrombocytopenia in the presence of antiphospholipid antibodies (anticardiolipin antibody and the lupus anticoagulant). Diagnosis of APS requires detection of antibodies on two separate occasions 6 months apart. The hepatic manifestations of APS are usually related to vascular abnormalities. Several cases of hepatic vein thrombosis (Budd-Chiari syndrome) have been reported in patients with APS. In addition, a recent report suggests a role for antiphospholipid antibodies in the pathogenesis of nodular regenerative hyperplasia of the liver (see Ch. 35). This rare disorder is characterized by diffuse micronodular transformation of hepatic parenchyma resulting in elevated liver chemistries and portal hypertension.

Scleroderma

While hepatic involvement in scleroderma is rare, limited cutaneous scleroderma, or the CREST (calcinosis cutis, Raynaud phenomenon, esophageal dysmotility, sclerodactyly, and telangiectasia) syndrome has been described in 3–17% of patients with PBC. The prevalence of PBC in patients with scleroderma is unknown. Scleroderma typically precedes PBC by a mean of 12 years (age 36 years versus 48 years). Raynaud phenomenon is the most common presenting symptom. Anti-centromere antibodies are relatively specific for the CREST syndrome and have been found in the serum of 10–29% of patients with PBC but in up to 100% of patients with PBC and CREST syndrome. Up to 90% of patients with scleroderma and PBC also have evidence of Sjögren syndrome; the acronym 'PACK' (PBC, anticentromere antibodies, CREST and kerato-conjunctivitis sicca) has been used to describe this constellation.

Systemic vasculitis

Many of the systemic vasculitides may involve the liver. Poly-arteritis nodosa (PAN) primarily affects small- and medium-sized arteries and is associated with chronic hepatitis B virus infection in over 50% of cases. Although lymphocytic infiltration in the intima and media of the hepatic arteries is rarely detected in percutaneous liver biopsy specimens, this finding can be observed on larger specimens obtained at autopsy in up to 50% of patients with PAN. Hepatic pathology in patients with PAN is generally related to chronic hepatitis B.

Polymyalgia rheumatica (PMR) and giant cell arteritis (GCA) typically involve large arteries, and abnormal liver chemistries, usually an elevation of the serum alkaline phosphatase level, are seen in up to one-third of patients. Liver biopsy specimens from patients with PMR and GCA typically show arterial wall invasion by giant cells.

SICKLE CELL DISEASE

Homozygous sickle cell anemia, or sickle cell disease (SCD), affects 1 in 600 African-American children. Liver chemistry abnormalities are universal in patients with SCD; most patients with the disease have elevated serum unconjugated bilirubin and AST levels secondary to ongoing hemolysis. Serum alkaline phosphatase elevations are typically of bone origin.

Acute syndromes secondary to SCD are common. Acute sickle hepatic crisis (ASHC) presents with tender hepatomegaly, jaundice, nausea and low-grade fever. Serum AST and ALT levels are usually less than 300 U/L, and serum bilirubin levels are typically less than 15 mg/dL. The syndrome is self-limited and usually resolves following therapy with intravenous fluids and analgesics.

In contrast to ASHC, sickle cell intrahepatic cholestasis (SCIC) is a rare complication of SCD that carries a more ominous prognosis. The presenting clinical symptoms and signs are similar to those of ASHC. In addition, acute renal failure is usually found in patients with SCIC, and progressive encephalopathy, coagulopathy and death are common. SCIC may present as fulminant hepatic failure. Differentiating ASHC from SCIC is based on clinical and laboratory findings. Serum AST and ALT levels are usually greater than 1000 U/L in SCIC, and serum bilirubin levels are strikingly high because of a combination of hemolysis, renal failure and intrahepatic cholestasis. The underlying pathophysiology of SCIC is related to sickling of red blood cells within the hepatic sinusoids and resulting anoxic hepatocyte damage. Liver biopsy typically shows ballooning of hepatocytes, sinusoidal 'sickling', and intracanalicular cholestasis. Treatment is largely supportive with the use of exchange transfusion. Successful liver transplantation for SCIC has been reported.

Chronic liver disease associated with SCD is also common. Autopsy series reveal cirrhosis in up to 29% of patients who die of complications of SCD. Most cases of chronic liver disease associated with SCD are thought to be secondary to hepatic iron overload following numerous blood transfusions or from infection by hepatitis B or C virus acquired by transfusion of contaminated blood products before the implementation of universal screening of the blood supply. Following the implementation of universal screening of donated blood in the USA the incidence of viral hepatitis in patients with SCD has decreased substantially.

Patients with SCD are particularly prone to the development of pigmented gallstones. Up to 58% of patients with SCD develop cholelithiasis, and approximately 17% are found to have choledocholithiasis at the time of cholecystectomy.

AMYLOIDOSIS

The three major categories of amyloidosis are primary amyloidosis, or light-chain amyloidosis (AL); secondary amyloidosis associated with amyloid protein A (AA); and familial amyloidosis. In primary amyloidosis, which includes amyloidosis related to multiple myeloma, amyloid fibrils are derived from the variable portion of the immunoglobulin light chain (kappa or lambda). In secondary amyloidosis, the amyloid fibrils form as a result of proteolytic cleavage of serum amyloid protein A, an acute-phase reactant. The causes of secondary amyloid include rheumatoid arthritis, osteomyelitis, tuberculosis, Hodgkin disease and other lymphomas, familial Mediterranean fever, long-term heroin abuse, subclinical ankylosing spondylitis and lepromatous leprosy. Familial amyloidosis is rare and includes type I familial amyloid polyneuropathy (FAP), an autosomal dominant disorder caused by a mutation on chromosome 18 that leads to hepatic production of a variant prealbumin, transthyretin (TTR). The disease is manifested by a progressive mixed chronic polyneuropathy (sensory, motor and autonomic) that presents after the age 20 years and is universally fatal. Early recognition is important because liver transplantation has been demonstrated to halt progression and even improve the neurologic symptoms. In all types of amyloidosis, amyloid deposition occurs most commonly in the heart, kidneys and peripheral nervous system; hepatic dysfunction may result from passive congestion caused by cardiac dysfunction.

Regardless of the type of amyloidosis (AL, AA, FAP), the hepatic manifestations of amyloidosis are similar. Although hepatic amyloidosis is common and rarely causes clinical manifestations, it carries an ominous prognosis. The median survival in patients with biopsy-proven hepatic amyloidosis is 9 months, with 5- and 10-year survival rates of 13 and 1%, respectively. Clinical symptoms of hepatic amyloidosis are non-specific and may include weight loss, fatigue, abdominal pain, anorexia, early satiety and nausea. Hepatomegaly is the most common physical finding in hepatic amyloidosis and occurs in up to 81% of patients; purpura and ascites can also be seen. Other stigmata of chronic liver disease, including spider angiomata, palmar erythema and Dupuytren contractures, are rarely observed.

Abnormalities in liver chemistries are common in patients with hepatic amyloidosis. A series from the Mayo Clinic described an elevated serum alkaline phosphatase level in 86% of patients with hepatic amyloidosis, with the level greater than 500 U/L in the majority of cases. Elevated serum AST and bilirubin levels were found in 37 and 21% of cases, respectively. Hepatomegaly on physical examination was associated with a higher likelihood of abnormal liver chemistries. The prothrombin time may be prolonged in patients with primary hepatic amyloidosis; however, the risk of bleeding is not increased. In up to 89% of patients, proteinuria is present on urinalysis. Thrombocytosis and Howell-Jolly bodies can be seen in the peripheral blood smear as a result of amyloid-induced hyposplenism.

The diagnosis of hepatic amyloidosis can be made by transcutaneous liver biopsy, but transcutaneous liver biopsy is associated with an increased bleeding risk in patients with hepatic amyloidosis. Amyloid appears as a pale pink homogenous amorphous protein on liver biopsy when stained with hematoxylin and eosin (**Fig. 34.2**). Up to 95% of patients suspected of having hepatic amyloidosis have evidence of amyloid deposition on fat pad aspirate or bone marrow biopsy. Because demonstration of hepatic involvement rarely changes management, biopsy of lower-risk sites is usually warranted when the diagnosis of hepatic amyloidosis is in question.

Management of hepatic amyloidosis is limited primarily to supportive care or treatment of the underlying predisposing condition. A recent trial comparing regimens containing

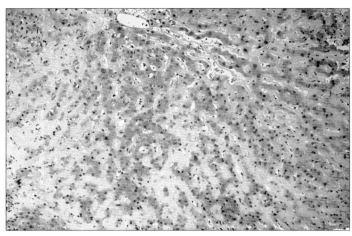

Figure 34.2 Deposition of amyloid. Liver biopsy specimen demonstrating marked deposition of amyloid within the space of Disse with resulting compression of the hepatic trabeculae (hematoxylin and eosin).

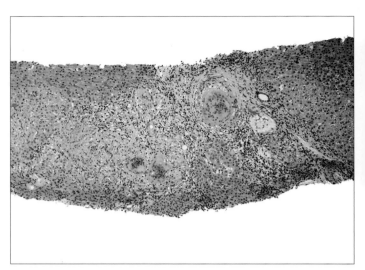

Figure 34.3 Portal tract with non-caseating granulomas. Liver biopsy specimen demonstrating a portal tract with non-caseating granulomas in a patient with sarcoidosis (hematoxylin and eosin).

melphalan, prednisone and colchicine in patients with primary amyloidosis found that median survival was significantly longer in patients treated with a combination of melphalan and prednisone than in those treated with colchicine alone or a regimen containing all three drugs. Liver transplantation may be of benefit in rare patients with FAP.

SARCOIDOSIS

Sarcoidosis is a chronic systemic disorder of unknown etiology that is characterized by an accumulation of T lymphocytes and macrophages leading to granuloma formation in affected organs. Organ dysfunction occurs from distortion of the normal architecture by the inflammatory infiltrate or by development of fibrosis associated with chronic inflammation.

Hepatic involvement is seen in 60–90% of patients with sarcoidosis when liver biopsy is performed. Sarcoidosis accounts for up to 30% of all cases in which hepatic granulomas are present on a liver biopsy specimen. Granulomas typically predominate around portal tracts and show no evidence of caseation necrosis (**Fig. 34.3**). In the vast majority of patients with hepatic sarcoidosis, liver disease is asymptomatic; however, progressive liver disease characterized by hepatomegaly, cholestasis and the development of portal hypertension has been described. Biochemically, serum immunoglobulin G levels are usually raised, the serum bilirubin is normal, and the alkaline phosphatase is mildly elevated. Serum aminotransferase levels may or may not be elevated. Evidence of mild hepatomegaly can be demonstrated by ultrasound or computed tomography in up to 50% of patients with hepatic sarcoidosis.

In patients with sarcoidosis, the presence of splenomegaly and ascites does not always imply portal hypertension or hepatic involvement. Splenomegaly is most commonly caused by granulomatous infiltration rather than portal hypertension. Ascites formation in sarcoidosis can be related to cor pulmonale resulting from progressive pulmonary disease, hypoalbuminemia resulting from hepatic dysfunction, or, rarely, peritoneal sarcoid granulomas. Hepatic sarcoidosis usually follows a benign clinical course, and there are no data to suggest that corticosteroid administration reduces the risk of progression of the disease.

Therefore, uncomplicated hepatic involvement by sarcoidosis is not an indication for corticosteroid therapy.

In a minority of cases, progressive destruction of the intra-hepatic bile ducts may lead to chronic intrahepatic cholestasis. Although an association may exist between sarcoidosis and PBC, antimitochondrial antibodies are not present in patients with sarcoidosis-related chronic intrahepatic cholestasis, and testing for antimitochondrial antibodies is recommended because of the similar clinical presentations of the two conditions. Other causes of cholestasis in patients with sarcoidosis include sarcoid involvement of the extrahepatic bile ducts, common bile duct compression by hilar lymphadenopathy and pancreatic sarcoidosis.

Biliary cirrhosis may develop in the later stages of hepatic sarcoidosis and patients with end-stage liver disease should be considered for liver transplantation. Portal hypertension is rare in patients with sarcoidosis. In patients with portal hypertension related to hepatic sarcoidosis, complications such as bleeding esophageal varices may be the initial clinical presentation. Affected patients are typically young and black; among Caucasians, women over age 40 are affected most commonly. Liver biopsy specimens in patients presenting with portal hypertension may show fibrosis, cirrhosis or nodular regenerative hyperplasia. Portal hypertension in patients without advanced fibrosis on a liver biopsy specimen has been proposed to result from granulomatous phlebitis or granulomatous infiltration of small portal vein branches with resulting presinusoidal portal hypertension. In some patients, there may be superimposed sinusoidal obstruction from extensive fibrosis. In approximately 25% of patients, portal hypertension is related to secondary biliary cirrhosis. Rarely, associated PBC or primary sclerosing cholangitis account for hepatic fibrosis and portal hypertension in patients with sarcoidosis. The cornerstones of management of the portal hypertension associated with sarcoidosis have been non-selective β blockade and endoscopic management of variceal bleeding. A surgical portosystemic shunt or transjugular intrahepatic portosystemic shunt may be considered in appropriate candidates. Corticosteroids do not appear to affect disease outcome, and in patients with severe hepatic sarcoidosis and limited extrahepatic disease, liver transplantation should be considered.

CONGESTIVE HEART FAILURE

The hepatic manifestations of congestive heart failure result from a decrease in hepatic blood flow due to poor left ventricular function; passive hepatic congestion due to impaired right ventricular function; and decreased arterial oxygen saturation. Clinically, congestive heart failure typically manifests as jaundice secondary to hepatic congestion and hepatocellular necrosis secondary to impaired perfusion. 'Cardiac cirrhosis' refers to a characteristic hepatic fibrosis related to prolonged, severe congestive heart failure. A summary of the clinical and biochemical manifestations of hepatic involvement in congestive heart failure is shown in **Table 34.5** and **Table 34.6**.

Whereas decreases in both hepatic blood flow and arterial oxygen saturation can occur in a variety of conditions that result in circulatory collapse, elevated hepatic venous pressure with passive hepatic congestion is usually the result of congestive heart failure. Chronic passive hepatic congestion, or 'congestive hepatopathy', typically presents with hepatomegaly with or without ascites and splenomegaly; other clinical manifestations of chronic liver disease such as spider angiomata and esophageal varices are rare in such patients. Physical examination may reveal a pulsatile liver and hepatojugular reflux. Encephalopathy,

resulting from reduced cerebral perfusion, has been reported to occur in a minority of patients.

Jaundice may be seen and may occasionally be profound (although it is characteristically mild in patients with constrictive pericarditis). The mechanism of hyperbilirubinemia in congestive heart failure is thought to be related to multiple insults including hepatocellular dysfunction, hemolysis, pulmonary infarction and elevated hepatic vein pressures leading to bile canalicular obstruction and bile thrombi. In addition, patients with severe congestive heart failure may be treated with medications that can contribute to the development of jaundice.

Liver chemistry abnormalities are typically mild in patients with congestive hepatopathy. An elevated serum bilirubin level, usually no higher than 3 mg/dL, is seen in up to 70% of patients. The alkaline phosphatase level is elevated in only 10% of patients; absence of a significant elevation of the alkaline phosphatase is helpful in excluding obstructive jaundice in patients who present with marked elevations in the serum bilirubin. Elevations in serum aminotransferase levels, typically two to three times the normal value, may be seen in up to one-third of patients. Patients with severe heart failure may present with marked elevations of the aminotransferases and bilirubin that mimic the findings in acute hepatitis. Levels of serum albumin are decreased in up to 50% of patients with congestive heart failure but are rarely less than 2.5 g/dL. Ascites associated with congestive hepatopathy is usually protein-rich, with an ascitic total protein level greater

Clinical features of congestive hepatopathy and hepatic failure		
Clinical features common to both conditions	Features suggestive of congestive hepatopathy	Features suggestive of hepatic failure
Fatigue	Dyspnea	–
Altered mental status	Orthopnea	–
Hepatomegaly	Neck venous distention	Spider angiomata
Ascites	Hepatojugular reflux	Palmar erythema
Edema	Cardiac gallop	Caput medusae
Jaundice	Cardiomegaly on radiograph	–

Table 34.5 A comparison of the clinical features showing the similarities and differences between congestive hepatopathy and hepatic failure due to chronic liver disease

Liver test abnormalities in congestive hepatopathy					
Liver test	Abnormal	Right-sided CHF; acute versus chronic	Correlation with clinical or pathologic findings	Improvement with CHF resolution	Normalization with CHF resolution
AST	Common	Acute > chronic	Centrilobular necrosis	1–3 days	3–7 days
ALT	Less common	Acute > chronic	Centrilobular necrosis	1–3 days	3–7 days
Alk phos	Uncommon	Acute = chronic	Hepatomegaly	No	No
Bilirubin	Common	Acute > chronic	Centrilobular necrosis	1–3 days	3–7 days
PT	Common	Acute = chronic	No	Yes	2–3 weeks
Alb	Less common	Acute = chronic	No	1–2 days	Less common

Table 34.6 Liver test abnormalities in congestive hepatopathy. CHF, congestive heart failure; AST, aspartate aminotransferase; ALT, alanine aminotransferase; PT, prothrombin time; Alb, albumin

than 2.5 g/dL and a serum-ascites albumin gradient greater than 1.1.

Liver biopsy specimens from patients with congestive hepatopathy reveal sinusoidal engorgement, variable degrees of zone 3 hemorrhagic necrosis, steatosis and cholestasis, with occasional bile thrombi in the canaliculi. With chronic or recurrent episodes of congestive heart failure, the reticulin network surrounding the central vein may collapse, and a stromal reaction of fibrotic bands radiating outward from the central vein can be observed. A pattern of 'reverse lobulation' is characteristic of cardiac cirrhosis and occurs when these radiating fibrotic bands reach adjacent central veins (**Fig. 34.4**).

The management of congestive hepatopathy relies on the treatment of the underlying congestive heart failure. Improvements in jaundice, hepatic congestion and ascites are typically seen following institution of diuretic therapy. Optimization of cardiac output may prevent further hepatocellular injury related to poor left ventricular performance. Caution should be utilized in the administration of medications that are metabolized by the liver. Morbidity and mortality related to the hepatic manifestations of congestive heart failure are rare and are more often related to the underlying cardiac diseases. Early treatment of congestive heart failure may result in reversal of the histologic liver abnormalities and avoid progression to cardiac cirrhosis. The presence of cardiac cirrhosis does not portend an unfavorable prognosis; synthetic function appears to be similar to that in patients with passive congestion alone, and portosystemic shunting and variceal bleeding typically do not occur.

Diffuse hepatic injury resulting from acute hypoperfusion of the liver is commonly referred to as ischemic hepatitis. In the majority of cases, ischemic hepatitis occurs in the clinical setting of congestive heart failure, and many of the clinical, laboratory and pathologic features are similar to those seen in patients with congestive hepatopathy. Patients with ischemic hepatitis typically have experienced a period of systemic hypotension prior to the finding of abnormal liver chemistries. Most patients are asymptomatic at presentation, and the diagnosis is only entertained after routine measurement of liver chemistries. In rare patients, nausea, vomiting, anorexia, malaise, right upper quadrant pain and jaundice may be the presenting symptoms.

Liver biopsy specimens from patients with ischemic hepatitis reveal zone 3 necrosis. Centrilobular architectural collapse varies depending on the duration of ischemia, and necrosis can extend to midzonal hepatocytes. Changes consistent with passive congestion often coexist with those of ischemic hepatitis, especially in patients with severe, decompensated congestive heart failure. A dramatic rise in the levels of serum aminotransferases to 25 to 250 times the upper limit of normal is typical in patients with ischemic hepatitis. Peak serum aminotransferase levels are reached within 1 to 3 days of the hypotensive episode and are usually accompanied by an early rise in serum lactate dehydrogenase (LDH) levels, a finding that may help discriminate ischemic hepatitis from acute viral hepatitis. The serum bilirubin level usually rises to no more than 4 times the upper limit of normal after the serum aminotransferase levels begin to decline. Serum alkaline phosphatase levels usually do not rise above two times the upper limit of normal. Liver biopsy is rarely warranted in these patients, as the diagnosis can usually be made on the basis of clinical and liver chemistry findings.

The course of ischemic hepatitis is usually self-limited, with only mild impairment in hepatic synthetic function, if the patient survives the cardiac insult. Mental status changes in patients with ischemic hepatitis are related to cerebral hypoperfusion rather than hepatic encephalopathy. Hepatic regeneration and recovery of normal function occur in the majority of cases; fulminant hepatic failure leading to death is rare. The prognosis of ischemic hepatitis is related to that of the underlying cardiac disease.

CONSTRICTIVE PERICARDITIS

Constrictive pericarditis results from diffuse thickening of the pericardium with a consequent restriction in ventricular filling and a rise in right atrial and vena caval pressures. The clinical features and hepatic changes are similar to those in the Budd-Chiari syndrome and cardiac cirrhosis resulting from other causes of congestive heart failure. All three conditions lead to hepatomegaly and frequently splenomegaly, ascites and jaundice in the latter stages. A list of causes of constrictive pericarditis is shown in **Table 34.7**. The diagnosis of hepatopathy caused by constrictive pericarditis is made clinically on the basis of an increased jugular venous pressure with a paradoxical rise in inspiration and characteristic wave form (prominent 'x' and 'y' descents) and a loud third heart sound. A chest radiograph may show pericardial calcification, but computed tomographic scanning or magnetic resonance imaging, together with cardiac catheterization, are usually required to confirm the diagnosis. Cardiac Doppler studies may demonstrate abnormalities in ventricular filling. Treatment is directed toward the pericarditis. If pericardiectomy is possible, the prognosis of the liver disease is good, although recovery is slow. Even the fibrosis of cardiac cirrhosis can partially reverse.

LYMPHOMA

The liver is part of the reticuloendothelial system and may be involved by lymphomas. Life-threatening complications of

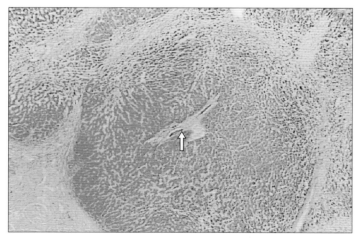

Figure 34.4 Histologic appearances of cardiac cirrhosis. Regenerative nodules form within the liver, due to fibrous linking of perivenular areas that come to surround the unaffected portal tract (arrow). This is associated with atrophy of the zone 3 hepatocytes, and sinusoidal dilatation, in contrast to regenerative activity in periportal hepatocytes. (Courtesy of Dr J. Wyatt.)

CHAPTER
35 Non-cirrhotic Portal Hypertension

Shiv Kumar Sarin

INTRODUCTION

Non-cirrhotic portal hypertension (NCPH) represents a group of disorders in which portal vein pressure is elevated (>10 mmHg) in the absence of cirrhosis of the liver. In these conditions, hepatic parenchymal function is normal but portal hypertension (PHT) exists. Conventionally, the definition not only includes the absence of cirrhosis but also the absence of hepatic venous outflow obstruction, such as exists in veno-occlusive disease and Budd-Chiari syndrome. Hence, NCPH comprises a heterogeneous group of diseases, which are characterized by an increase in portal pressure due to intrahepatic or prehepatic lesions, in the absence of cirrhosis, i.e. regeneration and bridging fibrosis. A second component of the definition is that the hepatic venous pressure gradient (HVPG), i.e. the difference between the wedged hepatic vein pressure (WHVP) and the free hepatic vein pressure (FHVP) is normal (<5 mmHg) or only mildly elevated and significantly lower than the actual portal vein pressure. The pathology in NCPH is generally vascular, present in the portal vein, its branches or in the perisinusoidal area of the liver.

The majority of these diseases, which are grouped under the term NCPH (**Table 35.1**), have PHT as a late manifestation of the primary disease. These diseases will not be covered individually as several are covered elsewhere in this textbook. However, two diseases, which are particularly common in the developing countries, present only with features of PHT. These two con-ditions, non-cirrhotic portal fibrosis (NCPF), and extrahepatic portal vein obstruction (EHPVO), are the prototype diseases, which fall under the heading NCPH (**Fig. 35.1**). For this reason, the pathophysiology, etiology, clinical features, management and natural history of these two diseases are described in detail in this chapter.

Historical perspective

Banti et al from Northern Italy at the end of the nineteenth century first drew attention to the clinical manifestations of cirrhosis including congestive splenomegaly, anemia, with or without gastrointestinal bleeding and ascites. Awareness of a similar clinical condition, yet histologically distinct from cirrhotic causes of PHT emerged in the Indian subcontinent in the late 1950s with the identification of patients having 'tropical splenomegaly syndrome' or 'Bengal splenomegaly'. In 1962, Indian scientists drew attention to an entity of splenomegaly in the absence of cirrhosis in North Indian patients. Almost at the same time, a similar group of patients were described from Japan. Subsequently, Boyer et al (67), while working at Calcutta, reported a series of similar patients and termed the condition as idiopathic portal hypertension (IPH). Mikkelsen et al (65) described 36 patients in USA with PHT but without cirrhosis who had phlebosclerosis of intra- and extrahepatic portal veins and coined the term hepatoportal sclerosis. However, in a majority of these patients, the portal vein was partly or completely occluded. In 1969, a workshop organized by the Indian Council of Medical Research (ICMR) reviewed all

Common causes of non-cirrhotic portal hypertension[†]
Extrahepatic portal venous obstruction*
Non-cirrhotic portal fibrosis or idiopathic portal hypertension
Schistosomiasis
Primary or secondary biliary cirrhosis (precirrhotic stage)
Congenital hepatic fibrosis
Veno-occlusive disease*
Nodular regenerative hyperplasia
Partial nodular transformation
Hepatoportal sclerosis
Peliosis hepatitis

*May present acutely.
[†]Most causes are chronic conditions.

Table 35.1 Common causes of non-cirrhotic portal hypertension[†].

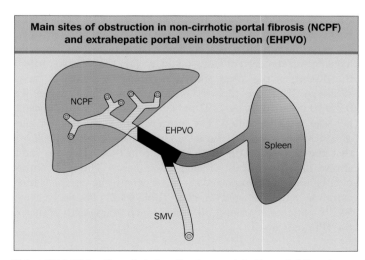

Main sites of obstruction in non-cirrhotic portal fibrosis (NCPF) and extrahepatic portal vein obstruction (EHPVO)

NCPF

EHPVO

Spleen

SMV

Figure 35.1 Main sites of obstruction in non-cirrhotic portal fibrosis (NCPF) and extrahepatic portal vein obstruction (EHPVO). SMV, superior mesenteric vein.

Comparison between non-cirrhotic portal fibrosis and idiopathic portal hypertension		
	NCPF	*IPH*
Age (years)	25–35	43–56
Male:female ratio	2:1	1:3
Hematemesis/melena (%)	94	40
Mass in LUQ (%)	6	40
Ascites (%)	2	10
Autoimmune features	Rare	Common
Pathology		
Irregular parenchymal nodules (%)	53	29
Bile duct proliferation (%)	38	4
Wedged hepatic venous pressure	Normal/mildly raised	Moderately raised
IPH, idiopathic portal hypertension; LUQ, left upper quadrant; NCPF, non-cirrhotic portal fibrosis.		

Table 35.2 Comparison between non-cirrhotic portal fibrosis and idiopathic portal hypertension.

available information on this condition, carefully excluding patients with cirrhosis and extrahepatic portal vein thrombosis and termed this distinct clinicopathologic entity 'non-cirrhotic portal fibrosis' (NCPF). While there are some differences, the patients with NCPF and IPH (the term commonly used in Japan) represent the same disease entity (**Table 35.2**). This condition has since then been reported in varying frequencies from all over the world. However, it clearly is more common in developing counties.

NON-CIRRHOTIC PORTAL FIBROSIS

Epidemiology

NCPF accounts for nearly 10–20% of all cases of variceal bleeding in the developing world. The disease is common in those of the lower or lower–middle socioeconomic strata of society. Improved hygiene and standard of living could explain the relative rarity of the disease in the West and its declining incidence in Japan. While in 1985 the reported incidence of IPH in Japan was 0.75/10 population, by 1992 only an average of 11 new patients per year were identified. The incidence of NCPF has not been prospectively studied in the Indian subcontinent but it is believed that the disease is still quite common in this region. In India, almost all series indicate a male predominance. This is in contrast to IPH in Japan, Europe and the USA, where the disease is more common in middle-aged females (**Table 35.2**). The mean age of NCPF patients is around 30 years, much younger than that of the IPH patients.

Etiology

The pathogenesis of NCPF is not clear and a number of hypotheses have been proposed.

Occult portal vein bacteremia

Non-cirrhotic portal fibrosis has been commonly seen in patients from a low socioeconomic background. Thus, intra-abdominal infections at birth and in early childhood are common in these patients and have been alleged to play an important role. Umbilical sepsis, bacterial infections and diarrheal episodes in infancy and in early childhood are proposed to lead to portal pyemia and pylephlebitis, resulting in thrombosis, sclerosis and obstruction of small- and medium-sized portal vein radicals.

The histologic changes seen in the liver in patients with IPH, together with the development of PHT, have been seen after injecting killed non-pathogenic colon bacilli into the portal vein of rabbits and dogs. In a rabbit model of indwelling cannulation of the gastrosplenic vein, repeated injections of *Escherichia coli* lipopolysaccharide also resulted in the development of spleno-megaly and a significant increase in the portal pressure. No parenchymal hepatic injury was discernible. The rabbit model also clearly showed a hyporesponsiveness of the vascular bed suggestive of peripheral vasodilatation, and a hyperdynamic circulatory state. The precise mechanism as to how the endotoxemia causes the rise in portal pressure is not clear, but it is quite possible that activation of hepatic stellate and Kupffer cells could play a role.

Exposure to trace metals and chemicals

Prolonged ingestion of arsenic has been incriminated in the causation of NCPF. Liver histology in patients with chronic arsenic ingestion reveals periportal fibrosis, incomplete septal fibrosis, with or without development of neovascularization within the expanded portal zones suggestive of NCPF or IPH. Previous exposure to arsenic as Fowler's solution for the treatment of psoriasis was reported in one study. These patients had florid skin stigmata of arsenicosis, something not commonly experienced in the Indian population. Furthermore, patients diagnosed with NCPF did not have elevated arsenic content in the liver, as assayed by electron probe microanalysis. In animal studies, arsenic was found to induce a 4–14-fold increase in hepatic hydroxyproline and hepatic collagen content compared with control mice, but features of NCPF or PHT did not develop in any animal. These observations suggest that although arsenic ingestion might induce hepatic fibrogenesis, it cannot be directly incriminated in the causation of most cases of NCPF.

In patients from Iran, a history of pica was obtained in nearly half the patients. A histologic picture resembling NCPF has also been observed following chronic exposure to vinyl chloride monomers, copper sulfate (vineyard sprayers), protracted treatment with methotrexate, hypervitaminosis A and in renal allograft recipients receiving treatment with 6-mercaptopurine or azathioprine, and corticosteroids.

Immunological alterations

Evidence supporting immunological derangements as an etiology includes:

- a reduction in the suppressor/cytotoxic T lymphocytes (T8) in NCPF patients and a decreased T4/T8 lymphocyte ratio;
- a reduction in the cell-mediated immune status in NCPF patients; and,
- a poor autologous mixed lymphocyte reaction (MLR).

In Japan, IPH is frequently associated with autoimmune disorders including systemic lupus erythematosus (SLE), progressive systemic sclerosis (PSS), thyroiditis and mixed connective tissue disease (MCTD). Nearly two-thirds of Japanese female patients with IPH test positive for anti-double-stranded DNA and one-quarter test positive for antinuclear antibody. Such a high prevalence of associated autoimmune conditions has not been the experience in the Indian subcontinent. However, familial aggregation and a high frequency of HLA-DR3 have been found in these patients.

Experimental studies
Repeated injections of splenic extract, Freund's adjuvant and egg albumin have been shown to produce splenomegaly and histologic lesions similar to IPH in rabbits. Injection of splenic extract in sensitized rabbits resulted in the development of an NCPF-like picture, with splenomegaly and an increase in portal pressure with negligible parenchymal injury.

Procoagulant factors
There is limited and controversial data on the role of procoagulant factors in the causation of thrombosis of the portal vein branches. Deficiency of protein C and S has been proposed along with mutations in the factor V Leiden in small series of patients. However, a cause and effect remains to be confirmed.

Proposed hypothesis for the pathogenesis of NCPF
Based on the available information, a hypothesis for the development of NCPF and even possibly extrahepatic portal vein obstruction has been proposed. Both of these venous inflow tract diseases could develop if portal pyemia or endotoxemia develops in a subject born with an underlying procoagulant state. This could precipitate thrombosis in the portal vein or its radicals. If it is a major thrombotic event, occurring at an early age in life, the main portal vein becomes occluded, leading to the development of EHPVO (**Fig. 35.2**). However, if the event is minor but repeated, only small or medium size branches of the portal vein could develop microthrombi. Since this process may have many repeated episodes, the syndrome of NCPF would develop at a later age e.g. in a young adult.

Pathology
When NCPF was first recognized, the salient histologic features characteristic of this condition were described. In fact, NCPF was considered a distinct clinicopathologic entity. The initial histologic descriptions were based on the systematic study of wedge hepatic specimens, obtained from patients in surgery. In patients with NCPF, the liver is usually normal grossly, but may be irregular (**Fig. 35.3**). This irregularity, only seen in 10–15% of all cases of NCPF, is confined to the liver surface. The portal vein and its branches are prominent and have sclerotic walls. Autopsy series commonly show thrombosis in the medium and small (diameter $<300\,\mu m$) portal vein branches. In the early stages of disease, the sclerosis may be less marked and thrombi may not be evident.

Histologic changes in NCPF were aptly coined as 'obliterative portovenopathy of liver'. Portal fibrosis is common in NCPF (**Fig. 35.4**). There is a marked, but patchy, segmental subendothelial thickening of the large and medium-sized branches of the portal vein. These changes are summarized in an excellent

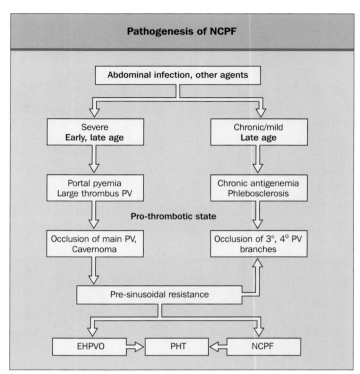

Figure 35.2 A proposed hypothesis for the pathogenesis of non-cirrhotic portal fibrosis (NCPF) and extrahepatic portal vein obstruction (EHPVO). MPV, main portal vein.

review (**Table 35.3**). The intimal thickening of intrahepatic portal venous channels, associated with obliteration of small portal venules and emergence of new aberrant portal channels, is characteristic of NCPF. Evidence of previous phlebothrombosis is suggested by the presence of old mural thrombi incorporated into the wall, and mural thickening of the extrahepatic portal vein. Coexistence of lesions characteristic of NCPF and EHPVO may occur in the same patient. While many investigators believe that thrombosis is an initial event leading to sclerosis, the Japanese investigators consider thrombosis to be secondary to a primary sclerosis of the portal vein branches. In wedge biopsy specimens from Japan, thrombi in the peripheral portal vein branches have not been found.

A widening of the space of Disse with haphazardly arranged collagen bands in the perisinusoidal space leading to capillarization of sinusoids may also be seen. Whether these electron microscopic changes correlate with the severity of PHT or occurrence of ascites, which is seen in a small proportion of NCPF patients, has not been determined.

Hemodynamics
In patients with NCPF, the WHVP is generally normal but may be slightly elevated in up to half the patients. However, the intrasplenic and portal vein pressures are markedly elevated. Two sites of increased resistance to flow (**Fig. 35.5a**) have been identified: a distinct pressure gradient between the spleen (intrasplenic pressure; ISP) and the liver (intrahepatic pressure; IHP) and another between the liver (IHP) and the WHVP (**Fig. 35.5b**). Variceal pressure measurements in these patients are comparable to that in cirrhotic PHT (**Fig. 35.6**). Splenic and portal vein

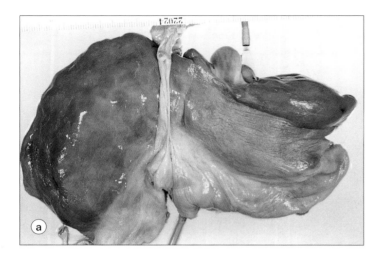

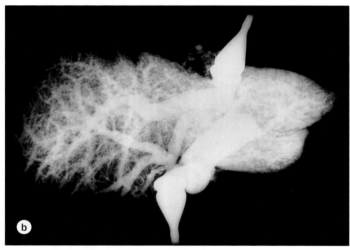

Figure 35.3 Idiopathic portal hypertension. (a) The liver in idiopathic portal hypertension. The surface is smoothly irregular but has no diffuse nodules. (b) Postmortem portography and venography of a liver with idiopathic portal hypertension. The portal branches are seen all the way toward the periphery with no sign of thrombosis. [(a) and (b), Courtesy of Prof. M. Okudaira.]

Histologic findings in idiopathic portal hypertension		
	Frequency (%)	
	Mild	*Moderate to severe*
Dense portal fibrosis and portal venous obliteration	48	52
Portal inflammation		47
Irregular intimal thickening of portal veins	75–100*	
Organizing thrombotic and/or recanalization of portal veins	20–100*	
Nodular hyperplasia of the parenchyma	40	
Abnormal blood vessels in the lobules	75	
Intralobular fibrous septa		95
Subcapsular atrophy		70
Periductal fibrosis of interlobular bile ducts	50	
Modified from Nakanuma et al (89) by permission of Acta Pathol Jpn based on a study of 66 patients with idopathic portal hypertension. *100% abnormalities were observed only in autopsy specimens.		

Table 35.3 Histologic findings in idiopathic portal hypertension.

blood flow are both markedly increased in IPH patients from Japan, even more than that seen in patients with cirrhosis and portal hypertension suggestive of a hyperdynamic circulatory state. Pulmonary hemodynamics in patients with NCPF has also been reported and pulmonary hypertension has been observed. Doppler ultrasound studies have shown that the hepatic and splenic blood flow is increased in the IPH patients.

Clinical profile

Over a 12-year period (1983–1995), our institutional experience of PHT was 2137 patients, 1133 of whom had gastrointestinal bleeding. NCPH was the cause of PHT in 35.4% of all bleeders but only 4.1% of non-bleeders. NCPF was diagnosed in 207 patients, while EHPVO was diagnosed in 236 patients. The clinical and laboratory profiles of these patients are shown in **Table 35.4**.

NCPF occurs predominantly in young patients with slight male preponderance. Patients may present with one or more well-tolerated episodes of gastrointestinal hemorrhage, splenomegaly

or consequences of hypersplenism. Development of ascites, jaundice and hepatic encephalopathy are uncommon and are only seen after an episode of gastrointestinal hemorrhage. The patients have normal growth and physical development. As compared to other causes of PHT, the spleen is disproportionately large, particularly so in patients with NCPF. It is not uncommon to see patients presenting with repeated attacks of left upper quadrant pain due to perisplenitis and splenic infarction. The clinical presentation of NCPF is distinct from IPH in several regards (Table 35.2). Like cirrhosis, NCPF may present occasionally with unusual disease associations such as glomerulonephritis or hypoxemia secondary to hepatopulmonary syndrome. Cardiac dysfunction has been described in both patients with NCPF and EHPVO.

Laboratory features

Conventional tests of liver function are, by and large, normal in NCPF patients. In addition, semi-quantitative tests of liver function, such as monoethylglycinexylidide (MEGX) extraction are also comparable to healthy individuals. The frequency of hepatitis B and C in non-transfused NCPF patients is comparable to that found in the general population excluding a role for these viruses in the causation of NCPF.

Anemia is found in the majority of NCPF patients. This may be microcytic, hypochromic (due to gastrointestinal blood loss), normocytic or normochromic (hypersplenism). Leukopenia (<4000/mm³ leukocytes) and thrombocytopenia (platelets <50 000 /mm³) may also be present. The bone marrow is hypercellular. Coagulation and platelet function anomalies have been

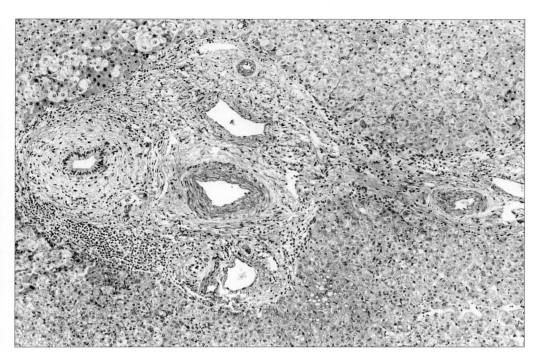

Figure 35.4 Portal fibrosis in idiopathic portal hypertension. The portal tract is markedly fibrosed with no evidence of cirrhosis. The size of the portal vein is about the same as an artery within the same portal area; normally, it should be five times the artery in diameter. The venous wall is also thickened.

observed in NCPH patients (**Table 35.5**). A state of mild compensated disseminated intravascular coagulation secondary to endotoxemia or portosystemic collaterals has been reported in a fair proportion of these patients.

Gastroesophageal varices are present in 85–95% of patients with NCPF (**Fig. 35.7**). In a series from North India, large varices were far more common in NCPH (90%) than in patients with cirrhosis (70%). Similarly, anorectal varices were also more commonly reported in NCPH than in cirrhosis (90 versus 56%), and were likely to be larger in those with NCPH. Variceal pressures (using pressure gauge) are similar in NCPH and cirrhosis, but patients with cirrhosis are more likely to bleed for any given variceal pressure. They found the prevalence of red signs and the Northern Italian Endoscopy Club (NIEC) index to be similar in these two groups of patients. Portal hypertensive gastropathy is relatively uncommon in NCPF patients and is a usual cause of upper gastrointestinal bleeding at presentation.

Imaging

Splenoportovenography, often used in the past, shows a dilated and thickened vein with venous collaterals. There are areas of poor opacification of peripheral portal vein branches suggesting narrowing or occlusion of the second and third order branches. By ultrasonography (**Fig. 35.8**), the portosplenic axis is seen to be dilated and patent. Occasionally, thrombus is seen in an intrahepatic branch of the portal vein. The wall thickness (echogenic boundary of portal vein) of the main portal vein and its branches has been found to be significantly greater in NCPF than for other etiologies of PHT. Spontaneous splenorenal shunts are also seen more frequently in NCPF patients than in patients with cirrhosis.

Hepatic venography and radionuclide scintigraphy (using ^{99m}Tc phytate or sulfur colloid) have been used to distinguish between NCPF and cirrhosis. High marrow uptake on scintigraphy is almost pathognomonic of cirrhosis. Computed tomography (CT) portography and CT hepatic angiography have been used to show aberrant vessels in the periphery of hepatic parenchyma in these patients (**Figs 35.9** and **35.10**). Magnetic resonance (MR) angiography is also a very useful technique to assess the patency of the portal and hepatic veins and the presence of spontaneous shunts (**Fig. 35.11**).

Portal cholangiopathy, defined as anomalies of the biliary system and gallbladder in patients with PHT, is commonly seen in patients with EHPVO. It is mild and less common in NCPF patients and in general is of little clinical consequence.

Differential diagnosis

Non-cirrhotic portal fibrosis can easily be differentiated from acute or chronic portal vein thrombosis (**Table 35.6**). NCPF generally develops insidiously, while acute portal vein thrombosis often has an acute presentation (upper gastrointestinal bleeding, abdominal pain and ascites). In chronic portal vein thrombosis, there is cavernous transformation of the portal vein. NCPF, however, can not be excluded if there is only thrombosis in one branch of the portal vein.

Child Class A cirrhosis may clinically mimic NCPF, but liver histology (lobular disarray, pseudolobule formation) will distinguish between the two. Moreover, a disproportionately large spleen with a dilated and thickened portal vein favors the diagnosis of NCPF. Tropical splenomegaly syndrome (TSS) is another condition, sometimes seen in the tropics, which presents with massive splenomegaly. However, PHT is uncommon in patients with TSS and the WHVP is within normal limits. Elevated serum immunoglobulin M (IgM) levels and high malarial antibody titers are also common in TSS patients. Histologically, NCPF needs to be distinguished from conditions like nodular regenerative hyperplasia (**Fig. 35.12**), partial nodular transformation and incomplete septal cirrhosis.

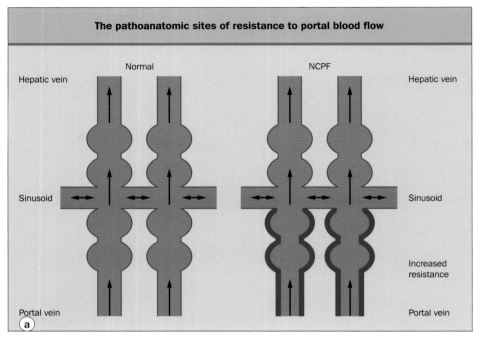

Figure 35.5a The pathoanatomic sites of resistance to portal blood flow. Sites of resistance in patients with non-cirrhotic portal fibrosis (NCPF), namely presinusoidal and perisinusoidal, caused by thickening and obstruction to the medium-sized and small branches of portal veins and the collagenization of the space of Disse, respectively.

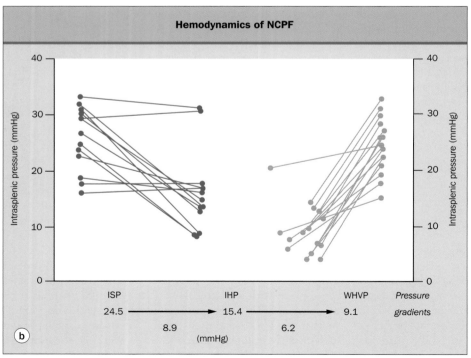

Figure 35.5b Pressure gradients in patients with non-cirrhotic portal fibrosis (NCPF). Two pressure gradients, between the spleen and liver [intrasplenic pressure (ISP) – intrahepatic pressure (IHP)] and between the liver and the wedged hepatic venous pressure (IHP–WHVP) are observed in patients with NCPF. In effect, they represent presinusoidal and perisinusoidal resistance to portal blood flow.

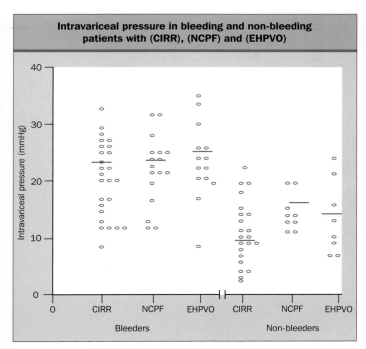

Figure 35.6 Intravariceal pressure. Intravariceal pressure measured by direct needle puncture in bleeding and non-bleeding patients with cirrhosis (CIRR), non-cirrhotic portal fibrosis (NCPF) and extrahepatic portal vein obstruction (EHPVO).

Coagulation and platelet function in non-cirrhotic portal hypertension

Parameter (normal range)	NCPF (n = 18)	EHPVO (n = 18)
INR	1.8 ± 0.68*	1.7 ± 0.4*
PTT (28–31 s)	29 ± 4.2	30 ± 4.2*
Fibrinogen (250–350 mg%)	196 ± 57**	199 ± 61**
Fibrinogen degradation products (<8 μg/mL)	<8	>8**
Platelet aggregation (40–60%)	33 ± 16.5	22 ± 11.3**
Platelet MDA (6–12 nmol/mL)	9.0 ± 3.6	9.6 ± 3.8

*$P < 0.05$, **$P < 0.001$ compared with controls.
EHPVO, extrahepatic portal vein obstruction; INR, international normalized ratio; MDA, malondialdehyde; NCPF, non-cirrhotic portal fibrosis; PTT, partial thromboplastin time.

Table 35.5 Coagulation and platelet function in non-cirrhotic portal hypertension.

Profile of non-cirrhotic portal fibrosis and extrahepatic portal vein obstruction patients

	NCPF (n = 207)	EHPVO (n = 236)
Mean age (years)	30.7	13.9
Sex (males : females)	117 : 90	168 : 68
Hemetemesis/melena (%)	84.5	94.5
Mass in LUQ (%)	13.5	3.5
Ascites (transient) (%)	10	12.7
Jaundice (%)	–	12.7
Liver function tests	Near normal	Near normal
Esophageal varices (%)	92	94
Gastric varices (%)	22.3	40.7
Portal gastropathy		
Presclerotherapy (%)	1.6	0.5
Postsclerotherapy (%)	17	15
Portal biliopathy (%)	40	90
Portal colopathy (%)	40	44

Data are based on the experience at the GB Pant Hospital, New Delhi, India (unpublished data). NCPF, non-cirrhotic portal fibrosis; EHPVO, extrahepatic portal vein obstruction.

Table 35.4 Profile of non-cirrhotic portal fibrosis and extrahepatic portal vein obstruction patients.

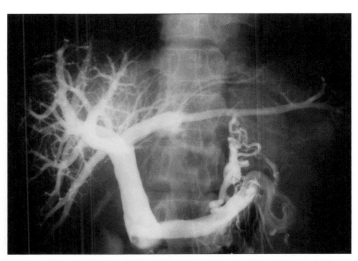

Figure 35.7 Idiopathic portal hypertension. An early case of idiopathic portal hypertension. Percutaneous transhepatic portogram shows a dilated splenic vein and portal trunk and unobturated portal vein branches. A large spleen is indirectly recognized from the size of the splenic vein in its hilum.

Management

Gastrointestinal hemorrhage is the major concern in the management of NCPF. For acutely bleeding patients, endoscopic variceal ligation (EVL) and endoscopic sclerotherapy (EST) are equally efficacious (95% success in the control of an acute bleed). Emergency shunt surgery is required in less than 5% of cases. If required, selective shunting (e.g. distal splenorenal shunt), is preferred because of a lower incidence of post-shunt encephalopathy. The number of sessions of banding or sclerotherapy required for obliteration of varices is similar in patients with cirrhosis and NCPH. Variceal recurrence has been reported in approximately 20% of cases, but recurrent bleeding is quite

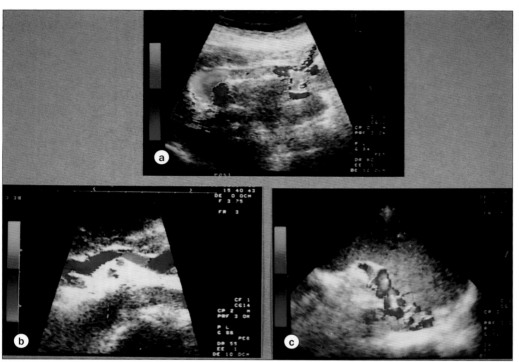

Figure 35.8 Color Doppler ultrasonography for the diagnosis of portal hypertension. (a) Markedly enlarged paraumbilical vein with flow within it. (b) An enlarged left gastric vein flowing into the esophageal varices. (c) Splenorenal shunt at the splenic hilum. Doppler signal (colors) indicates winding blood channels.

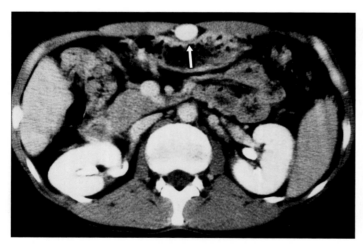

Figure 35.9 Computed tomography of a large paraumbilical vein. Paraumbilical vein (arrow) in the midline of the abdomen is obvious in this contrast-enhanced computed tomography scan.

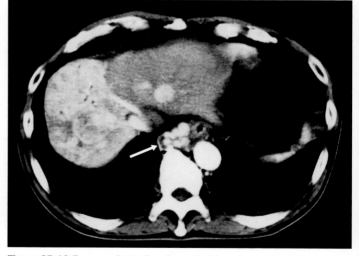

Figure 35.10 Paraesophageal varices. A widened paraesophageal structure was identified as paraesophageal varices (arrow) upon injection of contrast medium. The lobar attenuation difference is due to portal invasion of hepatocellular carcinoma.

uncommon (approximately 3%) once obliteration is achieved. Primary prophylaxis using β blockers and EVL were found to be comparable and efficacious, even in non-cirrhotic patients. There have been no large randomized controlled trials of pharmacologic versus endoscopic therapies in the primary prophylaxis of NCPF. Gastric varices are seen in nearly one-quarter of NCPF patients, more often than that seen in cirrhotic patients. These varices can be managed with cyanoacrylate glue injection and rarely require surgical intervention.

A number of interventional radiologic procedures have been reported to be effective in IPH patients. These include splenic embolization, percutaneous transhepatic obliteration and trans-

jugular intraheptic portosystemic shunts (TIPS). Whether patency rates of TIPS in patients with NCPF are similar to those with cirrhosis is unclear. Shunt surgery has been reported to be an effective back-up in patients who fail to respond to endoscopic therapy. Surgery may also be indicated for patients with symptomatic hypersplenism, spontaneous bleeding episodes or severe anemia requiring transfusion or repeated splenic infarcts. Elective shunt surgery is also a reasonable option for patients who live remote from good medical facilities or who prefer a single therapeutic intervention. The most important cause of

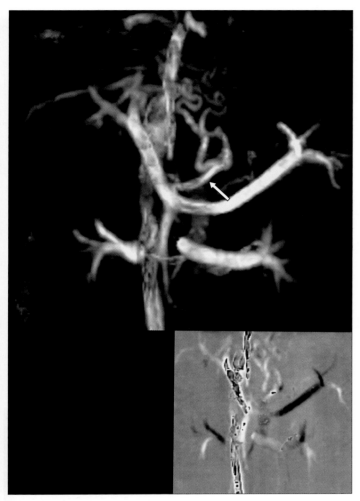

Figure 35.11 Magnetic resonance angiography of the hepatofugal left gastric vein. Magnetic resonance angiography by the phase-contrast technique (without contrast medium) clearly demonstrates the hepatofugal left gastric vein (arrow). The black and white colors in the inset indicate the flow direction. The left gastric vein is flowing cephalad, away from the liver. (Courtesy of H. Abe.)

death in NCPF or IPH patients is exsanguination. Certain Japanese workers have advocated prophylactic devascularization.

Surgical mortality after emergency shunts is approximately 10%. Shunt occlusion, chronic portosystemic encephalopathy and rebleeding after elective shunt surgery are seen in approximately 10% of patients. The morbidity and mortality after shunt surgery and the limited expertise available to perform these procedures have restricted the use of surgery in the management of patients with NCPF. Recently, the development of membranoproliferative glomerulonephritis and other renal anomalies have been reported following shunt surgery in NCPF patients.

EXTRAHEPATIC PORTAL VEIN OBSTRUCTION

Definition
Extrahepatic portal vein obstruction (EHPVO) is a common cause of portal hypertension in the developing countries but less so in the West. It is characterized by obstruction in the pre-hepatic portion of the portal vein. This may be accompanied by thrombosis of the splenic or superior mesenteric veins. Portal vein thrombosis is also a known complication of liver cirrhosis. However, the term EHPVO should be restricted to a group of patients with portal hypertension, who have obstruction of the main portal vein in the absence of cirrhosis of the liver (**Fig. 35.13**).

EHPVO is the most common cause of major upper gastro-intestinal bleeding in children. In children, EHPVO is usually an isolated condition and is only recognized when the child develops symptoms. In adults, the diagnosis is made earlier because the patients are already under observation for another disease. After cirrhosis, this is the second commonest cause of PHT, even in the West. The most common site of blockage is at the site of portal vein formation (90%) and total blockage of splenoportal axis is seen in only 10%.

Differentiating features between extrahepatic portal vein obstruction, non-cirrhotic portal fibrosis and cirrhosis of liver			
Parameter	EHPVO	NCPF	Cirrhosis
Mean age (years)	10	28	40
Ascites after bleed	Absent/transient	Absent/transient	+ to +++
Encephalopathy	–	–	+
Jaundice/signs of liver failure	–	–	+
Liver function tests	Normal*	Normal	Deranged
Liver			
Gross	Normal/small	Normal, rarely irregular	Shrunken, nodular
Microscopic	Normal	Normal/portal fibrosis	Necrosis, regeneration
Splenoporto-venography/US	Portal/splenic vein block	Normal splenoportal axis, 'withered tree' appearance, periportal fibrosis	Dilated, patent portal and splenic vein

* Occasional impairment may be observed.
EHPVO, extrahepatic portal vein obstruction; NCPF, non-cirrhotic portal fibrosis; US, ultrasound.

Table 35.6 Differentiating features between extrahepatic portal vein obstruction, non-cirrhotic portal fibrosis and cirrhosis of liver.

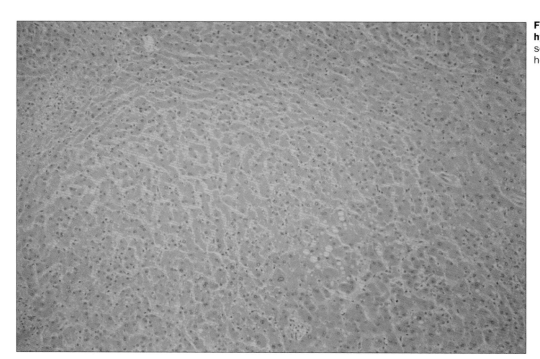

Figure 35.12 Nodular regenerative hyperplasia. A regenerative nodule is seen compressing the surrounding hepatocytes.

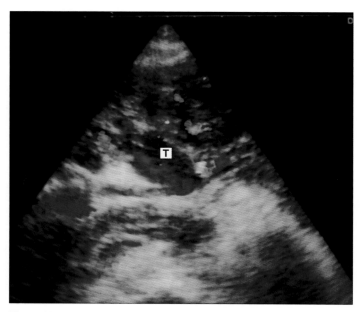

Figure 35.13 Color Doppler scan of a portal thrombus (T). A hepatopetal blood flow along the thrombus is recognized.

Etiology

The etiology of EHPVO in children is unknown, although various hypotheses have been proposed. The proposed mechanisms could be categorized as: direct causes, which lead to portal vein injury and subsequent obstruction, such as neonatal peritonitis, abdominal trauma, iatrogenic operative trauma to the portal vein, and cysts and tumors encroaching upon the portal vein within the porta hepatis. Next are congenital abnormalities such as

portal vein stenosis, and portal vein atresia or agenesis. Third are factors that are indirectly associated with portal vein thrombosis such as neonatal systemic sepsis from non-intra-abdominal sources, dehydration, multiple exchange transfusions and hypercoagulable states. The latter includes myeloproliferative disorders such as polycythemia vera, inherited deficiencies of natural anticoagulants such as antithrombin III, deficient protein C and protein S deficiency, and factor V Leiden mutation.

The most common predisposing condition is neonatal umbilical sepsis. In this condition, the inflammatory process begins in the umbilical stump before normal obliteration of vein and proceeds proximally to involve the portal venous system. Several investigators believe that umbilical vein cannulation and umbilical sepsis are responsible for portal vein thrombosis in a significant proportion of patients. Others, however, disagree with these observations (**Table 35.7**). The discrepancies between these observations are probably because the earlier studies have been retrospective and clinical. In a review of 11 major studies, a positive history of umbilical vein catheterization was found in 9% and umbilical sepsis in another 9% of patients with EHPVO. These findings suggest some role for these two factors, but the association is possibly weak. Umbilical vein catheterization was complicated by portal vein thrombosis in 40% after 25–48 h and 100% after 3 days, but was not associated with long-term occlusion. It is possible that the untreated and presumably more severe umbilical sepsis, which may result after deliveries conducted at home or in unhygienic conditions, could still result in portal thrombosis.

Some studies suggest that EHPVO is a developmental abnormality of the portal venous system. Obstruction can occur anywhere along the line of left and right vitelline veins from which the portal vein develops. Other congenital defects, usually of the cardiovascular system, have also been reported in associ-

Etiology of extrahepatic portal vein obstruction										
Etiology	Children Shalaons Sherlock (1962)	Maddrey et al (1968)	Lindsay et al (1979)	Houshham et al (1983)	Carlim et al (1992)	Orazoo et al (1994)	Stringer et al (1994)	Children Boles et al (1986)	Adults Vlegger (1997)	Crloff (1994)
Number of patients	160	37	97	32	132	38	53	43	21	162
Umbilical sepsis	9	5	12	0	23	1	1	8	2	12%
Intra-abdominal sepsis	1	–	26	7	24	0	10	1	1	6%
Umbilical catheterization	1	–	6	2	0	0	8	3	0	8%
Prothrombotic disorders	–	–	3	0	7	7	5	0	6	2%
Pancreatitis	–	2	0		3	2	0	–	0	–
Trauma	–	1	2		12	2	4	–	1	4%
Idiopathic	5	29	48 (51%)	17 (59%)	54 (41%)	17 (45%)	26 (49%)	31	11	68%

Table 35.7 Etiology of extrahepatic portal vein obstruction.

ation with EHPVO. Congenital defects are common in patients with extrahepatic portal obstruction of unknown cause.

As the occurrence of venous thrombosis of the splenoportal axis is the predominant pathology, the presence of a prothrombotic state has been proposed. An animal model for EHPVO has not yet been produced to support the contention that a prothrombotic state is the initiating event. Myeloproliferative disorders, overt or occult, are an important cause of EHPVO in adults. It has been suggested that the progression of the underlying hematologic disease with 'ongoing thrombosis' might influence the course of bleeding in these patients, particularly in the long term, and, therefore, must be looked for in every patient. In one series, a latent myeloproliferative disorder in 58% was detected in patients with EHPVO of unknown etiology and 57% of these developed an overt myeloproliferative disorder during follow-up. One or more prothrombotic disorder could be detected in 72% adult patients with portal vein thrombosis in another study. Primary myeloproliferative disorders were the leading causal factor (30% cases); primary deficiencies in natural coagulation inhibitors (protein C, protein S, antithrombin III), prothrombin gene mutation (G-20210A), methylene tetrahydrofolate reductase gene mutation (C677T) and factor V gene (Leiden) mutation accounting for the rest. The etiology of blocked portal vein is obscure in ~ 50% of patients.

Pathology

The macroscopic appearance of the liver varies from smooth to finely granular. The architectural pattern of liver is preserved. Mild or sometimes moderate hepatic fibrosis is seen in up to 40% of the adult patients, partly as a result of parenchymal extinction. Such periportal fibrosis could arise from non-specific or specific inflammation or from chemical irritation as a result of hepatocellular breakdown products. Vascular lesions have been demonstrated in approximately 48% of cases in the form of multiple portal vein channels in small portal tracts in addition to portal fibrosis of a mild degree in the majority. Phlebo-thrombosis of intrahepatic portal vein branches was seen in a

few patients though much less commonly than in NCPF cases and it was suggested that phlebothrombosis is a common pathogenic denominator in NCPF and EHPVO.

While the pathology of the liver is not very characteristic in EHPVO, the pathology of the portal vein is typical and is termed cavernous malformation of the portal vein. It is made up of a cluster of variable-sized vessels arranged haphazardly within a connective tissue support and the original portal vein cannot be identified. It is usually located at the hilum of the liver and can extend for a variable length inside and outside the liver. Although, hamartomatous and neoplastic theories have been proposed, most authors feel that these features are an end result of thrombosis of the portal vein.

Pathophysiology of EHPVO

The prehepatic block of EHPVO with normal hepatic sinusoidal pressure and a high pressure in the obstructed splanchnic bed, results in the formation of multiple hepatopetal thin winding collaterals. These collaterals are seen on angiography as 'cavernous transformation' and have been shown by ultrasound Doppler studies to provide a significant contribution to the total hepatic blood flow in these patients. These collaterals join the intrahepatic portal vein branches at various levels. This is a kind of neovascularization to compensate for the portal vein block.

Functional status of liver

Impairment of the hepatic storage capacity and transport maximum for bromsulfathaline has been documented. It has been suggested that periportal fibrosis prevents normal portal venous blood flow, thus making the liver in EHPVO more dependent upon hepatic arterial blood and these pathologic changes may lead to a decreased functional status of the liver.

Clinical presentation (Table 35.8)

EHPVO can present as early as 6 weeks after birth or may not become manifest until adulthood. The typical presenting symptoms in infancy are variceal bleeding, ascites and growth failure. Later in childhood and early adult life, variceal bleeding

Clinical presentations of extrahepatic portal venous obstruction								
	Maddrey (1968)	Lindsay (1979)	Househam (1983)	Cardin (1992) Adults	Orozco (1994) Adults	Mikkelsem (1965)	Stringer	Boles
Age at presentation (years)	19.8	20.9				38		
Bleed	32/37	53/97	13/32					
Splenomegaly	5/37	23/97	11/32					
Ascites		7/97	5/32	23/32	–	5/13		
Ascites (post bleed)	(5/37)	6/97	7/32	23/32	–	5/13		
Etiology								
Umbilical sepsis	5/37	12	–	23/32	1/38		1/53	8/43
Pancreatitis	2	–	–	3	2		0	–
Trauma abdomen	1	2	–	12	2		4	–
Splenomegaly	100%	–	100%					
Hepatomegaly	8/37	–						
Site of block		–						
Hilar PV	17	–						
PV formation	13							
Splenic vein	7	–						
Cavernomatous transformation	21	–						
Intra-abdominal infection	–	26	7	24	–		10/53	1
Exchange transfusion	–	6	2	–	–		8	3
Idiopathic	29/37	51%	176(59%)	54 (41%)	17 (45%)		26 (49%)	31
PV, portal vein								

Table 35.8 Clinical presentations of extrahepatic portal venous obstruction.

and hypersplenism are the main presenting clinical problems. Abdominal pain and thrombocytopenia due to splenomegaly may occur as well. Rarer problems seen in adults with portal venous thrombosis (PVT) include venous infarction of the bowel, hemobilia and pulmonary emboli.

The most usual presentation for patients with portal venous obstruction is sudden, unexpected, and often massive hematemesis. The patients withstand the hemorrhages remarkably well and hepatocellular failure is not a problem. Ascites develops during the course of the disease in up to 20% of patients, but it is generally transient following hemorrhage or surgery. Ascites is more frequent in adult patients than in children suggesting that the duration of portal hypertension could determine whether ascites develops. It also has been suggested that ascites may be related to the deterioration of liver function and fall in serum albumin with increasing age.

Jaundice may also be a presenting feature of portal vein occlusion. Jaundice may result from venous collaterals running in the vicinity of common bile duct and compressing the bile duct. A rise in serum bilirubin has also been attributed to acceleration in the normal aging process of the liver as a result of impaired blood supply. Hypoxemia has also been documented in case reports in patients with EHPVO, as a result of intrapulmonary vascular dilatation.

The clinical course is usually one of recurrent episodes of gastrointestinal hemorrhage from esophageal or gastric varices, but it is not possible to predict which patients will bleed repeatedly. The splenic size and portal pressure do not correlate with the incidence or severity of hematemesis. Except for occasional reports, there is no definitive data to suggest that the frequency of variceal bleeding decreases after puberty.

Growth

The hepatotrophic effect of portal blood has been well established in several experimental studies. It has been shown that young rats undergoing portal vein ligation or portosystemic shunt surgery gain significantly less body weight compared with sham-operated control animals. Growth patterns in patients with EHPVO indicate that nearly one-third of patients are short in stature and have significantly diminished growth velocity (**Fig. 35.14**). Growth spurts have been observed after shunt surgery in patients with EHPVO.

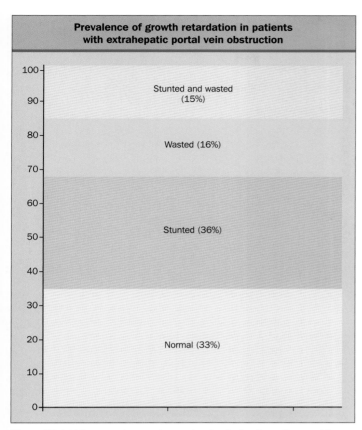

Figure 35.14 The prevalence of growth retardation in patients with extrahepatic portal vein obstruction (EHPVO).

Portal biliopathy

The term 'portal biliopathy' refers to abnormalities of the extrahepatic and intrahepatic bile ducts with or without anomalies of the gallbladder wall in patients with portal hypertension. Biliary tract abnormalities have been reported in 80–100% of patients with EHPVO by endoscopic retrograde cholangiopancreatography (ERCP). The changes include indentations of paracholedochal collaterals on bile duct, localized strictures, angulation of ducts, displacement of ducts and stones in the common bile duct and focal narrowing, dilatations, irregular walls and clustering of intrahepatic branches in the hepatic ducts (**Fig. 35.15**). Gall bladder varices are quite common and carry significant amount of blood around the gall bladder. These do not affect gall bladder contractility. The frequency of gallstones has been reported to be higher in EHPVO patients.

The biliary abnormalities may be explained either by compression of bile ducts by prominent paracholedochal and epicholedochal collaterals (indentations and wall irregularities) or ischemic injury of the bile ducts as a result of thrombosis of veins draining the bile duct (stricture formation). These two mechanisms may not be mutually exclusive as some changes like indentations; smooth strictures and caliber irregularity disappear after shunt surgery due to disappearance of paracholedochal collaterals while others like angulation and ectasia persist suggesting fixed obstruction due to ischemia.

Although biliary abnormalities have been reported in 80–100% of cases, few are symptomatic. There are case reports

of jaundice caused by the presence of cavernous transformation of the portal vein. Symptomatic patients are usually adult, indicating that portal biliopathy is a progressive disease.

Hemodynamic studies

WHVP within normal limits and significantly elevated intrasplenic pressure indicates the presinusoidal nature of the block. Total hepatic blood flow is normal or decreased. However hepatic arterial flow is increased after portal venous obstruction. Systemic vascular resistance is significantly lower and cardiac output is significantly higher in patients with EHPVO, indicating a hyperdynamic circulatory state, similar to that found in patients with cirrhosis.

Autonomic dysfunction

Impaired cardiovascular autonomic reflexes occur in subjects with portal hypertension due to EHPVO. The role of autonomic nervous dysfunction in the pathogenesis of characteristic hemodynamic disturbances of portal hypertension is controversial. It has been suggested that disturbances in autonomic cardiovascular reflexes may contribute to the hemodynamic abnormalities in cirrhosis but only to a small extent in EHPVO patients.

Coagulation abnormalities

Coagulation abnormalities have been variably reported in patients with EHPVO. While one study found normal coagulation studies, others have reported abnormal prothrombin time, partial thromboplastin time and platelet function. It has been suggested that abnormal coagulation in patients with EHPVO results from mild compensated disseminated intravascular coagulation secondary to portosystemic shunting.

Immune status

The humoral immunity is normal in patients with EHPVO when compared to patients with cirrhosis in whom it is grossly abnormal. The cell-mediated immunity shows qualitatively similar defects in patients with EHPVO and chronic liver disease. The defects in cell-mediated immunity result, in part, from sequestration of T cells by the spleen and partly from the presence in serum of factors that influence the kinetics of lymphocyte response.

Diagnosis

The presence of esophageal varices in a child with normal or near-normal liver function tests should alert the clinician to the possibility of EHPVO. In an adult, compensated cirrhosis may produce a similar picture. A number of radiologic techniques have been successfully used to study the portal venous system including splenoportography, celiac angiography, percutaneous transhepatic portography, duplex sonography, color Doppler flow imaging (CDFI), arterial portography, CT arterial portography, CT percutaneous transplenic portography and MR angiography.

Splenoportography or arterial portography (selective celiac or superior mesenteric angiography) provide images of the portal venous system of sufficiently high quality to permit identification of the site of obstruction (**Fig. 35.16**). However, large collateral flow rate can often divert the contrast and prevent adequate visualization of patent intrahepatic radicles.

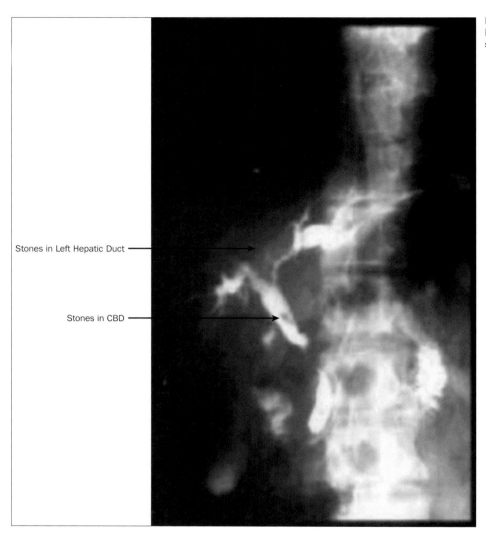

Stones in Left Hepatic Duct

Stones in CBD

Figure 35.15 ERCP picture showing intrahepatic and extrahepatic bile duct strictures and stones.

Ultrasound is a reliable non-invasive alternative with high accuracy (sensitivity 94–100% and specificity 96%), particularly if cavernous transformation of the portal vein has occurred. Cavernous transformation produces a distinctive tangle of tortuous vessels in the porta hepatis and represents collateral flow around the portal vein (Fig. 35.16). Two potential errors are noteworthy: first, a new thrombus that is virtually anechoic may not be detected if color Doppler is not used; and second in patients with portal hypertension, low velocity or 'to-and-fro' portal flow may be very difficult to detect, causing a false impression of occlusion.

Management

The management of EHPVO depends very much upon the age of the patient, the site of obstruction and the clinical manifestations. Variceal hemorrhage is the major complication requiring therapy. Patients with portal hypertension who have not bled from varices can be observed as bleeding may not occur for many years. In general, hypersplenism is not an indication for surgical intervention, but in an occasional patient, profound thrombocytopenia with bleeding, repeated infections or physical discomfort caused by massive splenomegaly may be sufficiently severe to merit splenectomy.

Treatment of variceal bleeding

Since the EHPVO patients have essentially normal livers and tolerate bleeding well, therapy should be individualized. If the obstruction is confined to splenic vein, splenectomy alone is curative. The problem is not so straightforward when the portal vein is involved.

Endoscopic variceal eradication

Both endoscopic sclerotherapy and band ligation have been found to be effective. With sclerotherapy, the risk of spread of the thrombus is not real. Long-term follow-up studies have found that sclerotherapy prevented bleeding in 88% patients after variceal eradication. In general, EVL has yielded even better results with fewer complications than sclerotherapy, particularly in smaller children. However, variceal eradication alone without alleviation of portal hypertension cannot lead to normal growth of these patients and also does not prevent the development of portal biliopathy and formation of gastric and ectopic varices.

Shunt surgery

A variety of shunt procedures are available for those who fail endoscopy therapy. These include non-selective shunts including a central splenorenal shunt with splenectomy, mesocaval,

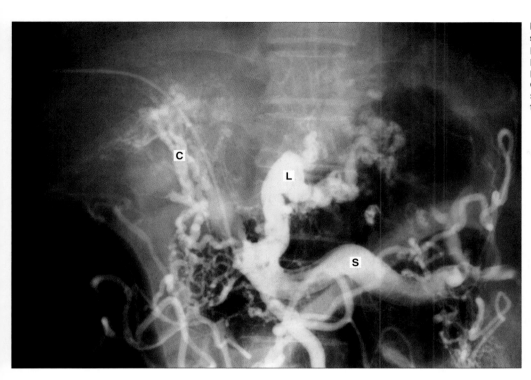

Figure 35.16 Catheter penetration of a soft thrombus. The catheter passed percutaneously through the liver penetrated a soft thrombus in the portal vein. Injected contrast medium opacified an enlarged left gastric (L), splenic vein (S), and cavernous transformation (C).

portacaval and 'makeshift' shunts. Initial rebleeding rates, although better than with ablative procedures, are still high. More recent series have shown improved patency rates even in small children. A 10% rebleeding rate was noted in children less than 6 years old who had undergone non-selective shunting with an average vein size of 6.5 mm. Others have since reported rebleeding rates with central splenorenal shunts and mesocaval shunts ranging from 4 to 33%.

The selective shunts, designed to decompress gastroesophageal varices without compromising portal blood flow, include distal splenorenal shunts (DSRS), distal splenocaval shunts, gastro-epiploic to left renal vein shunts and left gastric vein to left renal vein shunts. An overall patency rate of 92% at 5 years was reported with selective shunts and resulted in low rebleeding rates. However, selective shunts cannot be performed in patients who have thrombosis of the splenic vein, which is common in EHPVO, or who have had a previous splenectomy and only around a third of patients prove to be suitable candidates for this intervention. In addition, hypercoagulable disorders are frequently associated with EHPVO, with an increased consequent risk of thrombosis in any kind of shunt.

Other approaches that directly treat the gastroesophageal varices include transesophageal ligation of varices, esophago-gastrectomy and gastric devascularization with splenic artery ligation and splenopneumopexy. In general, these procedures have extremely high rates of rebleeding, approaching 70–80%. Therefore, they are not recommended as primary procedures especially when surgical shunting is an option. In patients with failed shunts or in patients where shunting is not possible, these ablative procedures may be considered.

Hypersplenism

Since splenomegaly, thrombocytopenia and leukopenia are common in EHPVO patients, the question often arises whether splenectomy should be performed, even prior to variceal bleeding. In general, splenectomy should not be performed, as it has no permanent effect on portal hypertension. Moreover, removal of the spleen can lead to thrombosis of the splenic vein making future shunt operations more difficult.

Thrombocytopenia, often below 50 000/mm^3, is more alarming to the physician than to the patient. Although reduced in number, these platelets function normally. Symptomatic hypersplenism is seen in only around 5% of patients with EHPVO. Distal splenorenal shunt will relieve splenic congestion, resulting in a reduction in the spleen volume and a modest increase in the platelet count in some patients.

Portal biliopathy

Symptomatic portal biliopathy is predominantly due to compression of the bile ducts (**Fig. 35.17**) and is indication for intervention. Although choledocholithiasis can be managed by endoscopic sphincterotomy, the biliary obstruction persists and the risk of recurrent stone disease remains high. For those with biliary obstruction, portosystemic shunting usually leads to amelioration of biliary obstruction and prevents further stone formation. In patients with persistent obstruction, hepatico-jejunostomy may be needed to treat the biliary obstruction, with access to the region being made possible by an initial portosystemic shunt. Symptomatic portal biliopathy is one of the few indications for portosystemic shunting in the absence of variceal bleeding. An algorithmic approach to such patients is helpful (**Fig. 35.18**).

Anticoagulant therapy

It was suggested that long-term anticoagulation might prevent both extension of thrombosis to the splanchnic veins and thrombosis in other deep veins once the role of prothrombotic disorders was recognized in the pathogenesis of PVT. The avail-

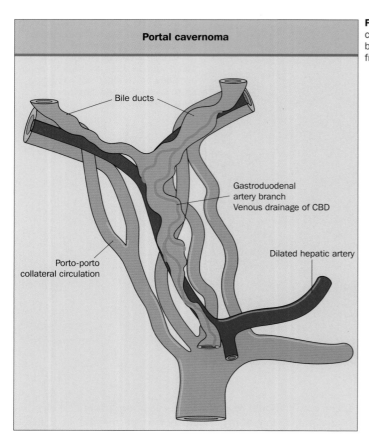

Portal cavernoma

Bile ducts

Gastroduodenal artery branch
Venous drainage of CBD

Dilated hepatic artery

Porto-porto collateral circulation

Figure 35.17 Portal cavernoma. A schematic diagram showing the portal cavernoma, the collaterals joining the extrahepatic to the small intrahepatic branches of portal vein and the pressure on the bile duct radicals (Modified from Lebrec D.).

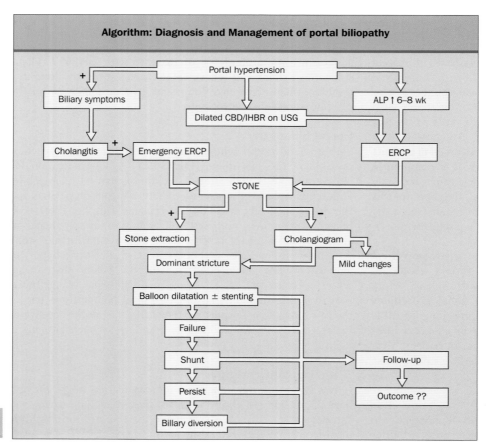

Algorithm: Diagnosis and Management of portal biliopathy

Portal hypertension

+ Biliary symptoms

Dilated CBD/IHBR on USG

ALP ↑ 6–8 wk

Cholangitis + → Emergency ERCP

ERCP

STONE

+ Stone extraction − Cholangiogram

Dominant stricture ← Mild changes

Balloon dilatation ± stenting

Failure

Shunt → Follow-up

Persist → Outcome ??

Biliary diversion

Figure 35.18 Algorithm to manage patients with portal cholangiopathy. ALP, alkaline phosphatase; CBD, common bile duct; ERCP, endoscopic retrograde cholangiopancreatography; IHBR, intrahepatic biliary radicles; USG, ultrasound.

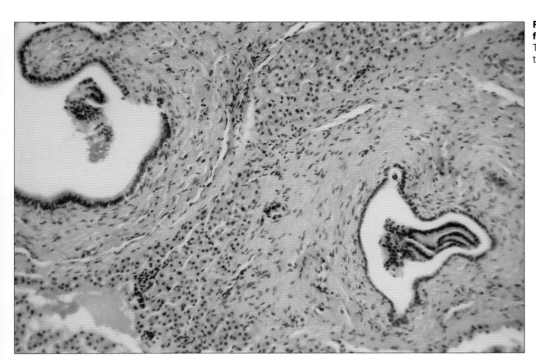

Figure 35.19 Congenital hepatic fibrosis containing dilated bile ducts. The liver parenchyma is sandwiched by thick fibrous bands in the portal tracts.

able preliminary data suggest a possible benefit with no evidence of an increase in either the incidence or severity of gastro-intestinal bleeding. Recanalization of fresh portal vein thrombosis has been reported following anticoagulation. Acute PVT can occasionally be treated by thrombolysis, or by removal of the thrombus through the transjugular route.

NODULAR REGENERATIVE HYPERPLASIA AND PARTIAL NODULAR TRANSFORMATION

Nodular regenerative hyperplasia (NRH) of the liver is a local hyperplastic response of hepatocytes probably due to vascular anomalies. In NRH, 1–2 mm nodules of regenerating hepato-cytes occur diffusely, compressing the intervening liver parenchyma (Fig. 35.12). There is no fibrosis associated with the nodules. About 75% of these patients have antiphospholipid antibodies, especially anticardiolipin antibodies. NRH has been associated with collagen vascular disease, lympho- and myeloproliferative disorders, and other blood dyscrasias.

Partial nodular transformation on the other hand relates to the presence of a large regenerative nodule near the hepatic hilum leading to the development of portal hypertension. Such nodules are a result of portal circulation disturbances and have also been seen in IPH. Nodules form in the areas of the liver where there is adequate portal perfusion in compensation for the parenchymal atrophy caused by decreased portal perfusion in other areas as a result of vascular changes.

CONGENITAL HEPATIC FIBROSIS

Congenital hepatic fibrosis (CHF) (**Fig. 35.19**), presents in child-hood with liver enlargement and portal hypertension. The most common clinical presentation is bleeding from gastroesophageal varices. This condition is generally inherited in an autosomal recessive fashion and is often associated with polycystic kidney disease in children (Ch. 28). In this condition, the liver cells are normal ultrastructurally, and these patients have normal liver function. While there are bands of fibrous tissue that diffusely percolate through the liver, this condition is differentiated from cirrhosis by the absence of regenerative nodules. Within the bands of fibrous tissue is often striking numbers of dilated and cystic bile ductules. This condition is thought to be related to a failure of normal ductal development. Because these patients have normal liver function, the variceal bleeding tends to be well tolerated. Treatment of patients with CHF is primarily geared towards control of variceal hemorrhage. In general, the first level of treatment is endoscopic variceal band ligation or endoscopic sclerotherapy. Patients who fail endoscopic therapy are also excellent candidates for a selective shunt, because this disease is not progressive and they do not have impaired liver function. In general, these patients also do not develop ascites and rarely require liver transplantation. However, in the patients with CHF associated with polycystic kidney disease, renal failure ultimately becomes the predominant clinical problem.

FURTHER READING

Non-cirrhotic portal fibrosis

Banti G. Splenomegalic mit Leberzirrhose. Beitrage sur pathologischen. Anat Allgemeinen Pathol 1889; 24:21–33.

Boyer JL, Sengupta KP, Biswas SK, et al. Idiopathic portal hypertension: comparison with the portal hypertension of cirrhosis and extrahepatic portal vein obstruction. Am Intern Med 1967; 66:41–68.

Dhiman RK, Chawla Y, Vasishta RK, et al. Non-cirrhotic portal fibrosis (idiopathic portal hypertension): experience with 151 patients and a review of the literature. J Gastroenterol Hepatol 2002; 17:6–16.

Mikkelsen WP, Edmondson HA, Peters RL, et al. Extra- and intrahepatic portal hypertension without cirrhosis (hepatoportal sclerosis). Ann Surg 1965; 162:602–620.

Nakanuma Y, Nonomura A, Hayashi M, et al. Pathology of the liver in idiopathic portal hypertension associated with autoimmune disease. Acta Pathol Jpn 1989; 39:586–592. *Excellent review of the histopathology of the liver in non-cirrhotic portal hypertension.*

Okudaria M, Ohbu M, Okuda K. Idiopathic portal hypertension and its pathology. Semin Liver Dis 2002; 22:59–71.

Proceedings of the workshop on non-cirrhotic portal fibrosis. Indian Council of Medical Research, New Delhi 1969.

Sarin SK. Non-cirrhotic portal fibrosis. Gut 1989; 5:336–351.

Sarin SK, Agarwal SR. Idiopathic portal hypertension. Digestion 1998; 59:420–423. *Good overall review.*

Sarin SK, Sethi KK. Tropical splenomegaly syndrome versus non-cirrhotic portal fibrosis: is there a hemodynamic correlation. Hepatology 1988; 8:1459.

Sarin SK, Sethi KK, Nanda R. Measurement and correlation of wedged hepatic, intrahepatic, intrasplenic and intravariceal pressure in patients with cirrhosis of liver and non-cirrhotic portal fibrosis. Gut 1987; 28:260–266.

Sarin SK, Kapoor D. Non-cirrhotic portal fibrosis: current concepts and management. J Gastroenterol Heptol 2002;17:526–534.

Extrahepatic portal vein thrombosis

Ando H, Kaneko K, Ito F, et al. Anatomy and etiology of extraheptic portal vein obstruction in children leading to bleeding esophageal varices. J Am Coll Surg 1996; 183:543–547.

Shah SR, Mathur SK. Presentation and natural history of variceal bleeding in patients with portal hypertension due to extraheptic portal venous obstruction. Indian J Gastroenterol 2003; 22:217–220.

Stringer MD, Heaton ND, Karani J, et al. Patterns of portal vein occlusion and their aetiological significance. Br J Surg 1994; 81:1328–1331. *Thoughtful description of pattern of thrombosis.*

Webb LJ, Sherlock S. The aetiology, presentation and natural history of extrahepatic portal venous obstruction. Q J Med 1979; 192:627–639. *Good clinical review of 97 cases.*

Zargar SA, Yattoo GN, Javid G, et al. Fifteen-year follow up of endoscopic injection sclerotherapy in children with extrahepatic portal venous obstruction. J Gastroenterol Hepatol 2004; 19:139–145.

Sarin SK, Bansal A, Sessan S, Nigam A. Portal vein obstruction in children leads to growth retardation. Hepatology 1992;15:229.

Sarin SK, Agarwal SR. Extrhepatic portal vein obstruction. Semin Liver Dis. 2002;22:43–58.

Complications of non-cirrhotic portal hypertension

Chandra R, Kapoor D, Tharakan A, et al. Portal biliopathy. J Gastroenterol Hepatol 2001; 16:1144–1148. *Description of important complication of EHPVO.*

Khuroo MS, Yattoo GN, Zargar SA, et al. Biliary abnormalities associated with extrahepatic portal venous obstruction. Hepatology 1993; 17:807–813.

Mehta S, Gondal R, Saxena S, et al. Profile of hypersplenism in cirrhotic and non-cirrhotic portal hypertension. Hepatology 1994.

Sarin SK, Bhatha V, Makwane U. 'Portal biliopathy' in extrahepatic portal vein obstruction. Indian J Gastroenterol 1992; 11:A82.

Treatment of non-cirrhotic portal hypertension

Condat B, Pessione F, Hillaire S, et al. Current outcome of portal vein thrombosis in adults: risk and benefit of anticoagulant therapy. Gastroenterology 2001; 120:490–497. *Interesting data on controversial topic.*

Hirota S, Ichikawa S, Matsumoto S, et al. Interventional radiologic treatment of idiopathic portal hypertension. Cardiovasc Intervent Radiol 1999; 22:311–314.

Kochar R, Goenka MK, Mehta SK. Outcome of injection sclerotherapy using absolute alcohol in patients with cirrhosis, non-cirrhotic portal fibrosis, and extrahepatic portal venous obstruction. Gastrointest Endosc 1991; 37:460–464.

Malkan GH, Bhatia SJ, Bashir K, et al. Cholangiopathy associated with portal hypertension: diagnostic evaluation and clinical implications. Gastrointest Endosc 1999; 49:344–348.

Mitra SK, Rao KL, Narasimhan KL, et al. Side-to-side lienorenal shunt without splenectomy in non-cirrhotic portal hypertension in children. J Pediatr Surg 1993; 28:398–401.

Sarin SK, Govil A, Jain AK, et al. Prospective randomized trial of endoscopic sclerotherapy versus variceal band ligation for esophageal varices; influence on gastric varices and variceal recurrence. J Hepatol 1994; 26:826–832.

Sarin SK, Lamba GS, Kumar M, et al. Comparison of endoscopic ligation and propranolol for the primary prevention of variceal bleeding. N Engl J Med 1999; 340:988–993.

Warren WD, Henderson JM, Millikan WJ, et al. Management of variceal bleeding in patients with noncirrhotic portal vein thrombosis. Ann Surg 1988; 207:623–634. *Classic series describing 70 cases.*

Other causes of non-cirrhotic portal hypertension

Al-Mukhaizeem KA, Rosenberg A, Sherker AH. Nodular regenerative hyperplasia of the liver: an under-recognized cause of portal hypertension in hematological disorders. Am J Hematol 2004; 75:225–230.

Klein R, Goller S, Bianchi L. Nodular regenerative hyperplasia (NRH) of the liver – a manifestation of 'organ-specific antiphospholipid syndrome'? Immunobiology 2003; 207:51–57.

CHAPTER
36
Hepatobiliary Surgery

Andrew M. Smith and J. Michael Henderson

INTRODUCTION

As early as 2000–3000 BC, the Assyrian and Babylonian cultures used the livers of sacrificed animals to divine the future. Over the ensuing centuries, battle surgeons debrided small bits of liver protruding from abdominal wall stab and gunshot wounds. However, formal entry into the peritoneal cavity to control hemorrhage due to trauma or to remove tumors and drain cysts had to await the development of general anesthesia and antisepsis.

The first successful liver resection was performed in Berlin by Dr Carl von Langenbuch in 1887. He removed a pedicled tumor from the left lobe of a 30-year-old woman. Later that evening, however, the patient required re-exploration to control hemorrhage. Liver surgery entered the modern era in the 1950s, and remarkable progress has occurred over the past 50 years. The factors responsible for the progress include an understanding of the segmental anatomy of the liver as described by Couinaud in 1954, advances in the techniques of liver resection, a better understanding of liver diseases, the dramatic improvements in techniques to image the liver, and the ability to support patients metabolically both intraoperatively and postoperatively.

HEPATIC ANATOMY AND DEFINITION OF RESECTIONS

The liver is divided into a left and right half based on the incoming vascular structures. Externally, a plane between the gallbladder fossa and the inferior vena cava (IVC) divide the right and left lobes; the falciform ligament further divides the left lobe into medial and lateral segments. The liver has segmental anatomy as defined by Couinaud (**Fig. 36.1**). Each liver segment has independent biliary drainage and vascular inflow and outflow. Consequently it is possible to remove an individual segment without disrupting the blood flow or biliary drainage of the remaining segments. Based on the Brisbane 2000 Terminology of Hepatic Anatomy and Resection, the liver can be divided into four sections: the right anterior section (segments V and VIII), right posterior section (segments VI and VII), left medial section (segment IV) and left lateral section (segments II and III). A right lobectomy or hepatectomy removes segments V–VIII; a left lobectomy excises segments II–IV. Removal of segments IV–VIII comprises an extended right lobectomy; the medial segment of the left lobe is resected in addition to the entire right lobe. Segments II–VI are excised in an extended left lobectomy; the anterior portion of the right lobe in addition to the entire left lobe. A wedge resection removes the tumor along with a 1–2 cm margin of normal parenchyma in a non-anatomic manner.

HEPATIC SURGERY

Intraoperative monitoring and resuscitation

Precise intraoperative monitoring and resuscitation are crucial for the success of liver resection. Mean arterial pressure and central venous pressure are added to the routine monitoring of the heart rate, blood pressure, electrocardiogram and oxygen saturation. A Swan-Ganz catheter is reserved for patients with cardiac problems who require even more precise monitoring. A Foley catheter and nasogastric tube are placed after the induction of general anesthesia. Excessive intraoperative blood loss has been demonstrated to be the major determinant of adverse perioperative outcome. Minimizing blood loss during hepatectomy is therefore essential. Low central venous pressure anesthesia (below 5 mmHg) is fundamental, and is maintained by restricting fluid infusion and limiting intraoperative blood transfusion unless more than 25% of the blood volume is lost. Other techniques to reduce blood loss include vascular inflow and outflow control and placing the patient in the Trendelenburg position.

Surgical techniques

Preliminary laparoscopy may be used in some patients with primary hepatocellular carcinoma (HCC) or metastatic colorectal cancer to the liver who have not had previous upper abdominal surgery. If laparoscopy reveals metastatic disease, bilobar disease, cirrhosis or significant fatty change in the non-tumor-bearing portion of the liver, the procedure is terminated. The patient is spared a laparotomy and can be discharged within 24 h. Laparoscopy is less useful in patients who have had prior upper abdominal surgery since they have adhesions from prior surgery which will limit the visibility of laparoscopy and increase the risk of iatrogenic injury to the bowel. In patients with prior upper abdominal surgery a limited right subcostal incision is made and if extrahepatic and bilobar disease are not found, the incision is extended into a chevron with a midline extension. Once the laparotomy has been performed, the abdomen is again inspected for any extrahepatic disease.

The liver is mobilized by dividing the right and left triangular ligaments and the falciform ligament. The mobilization facilitates intraoperative ultrasound and parenchymal transactions later. There are three basic techniques for anatomic hepatectomies:

- Hepatectomy with preliminary vascular ligation was described by Lortat-Jacob in 1952. The initial maneuver is the ligation and division of the left or right side of the portal pedicle at the hilum, followed by ligation and division of the appropriate hepatic veins and finally the sectioning of the liver parenchyma. The dissection of the hepatic veins can be hazardous and control of the suprahepatic and infrahepatic inferior vena cava is

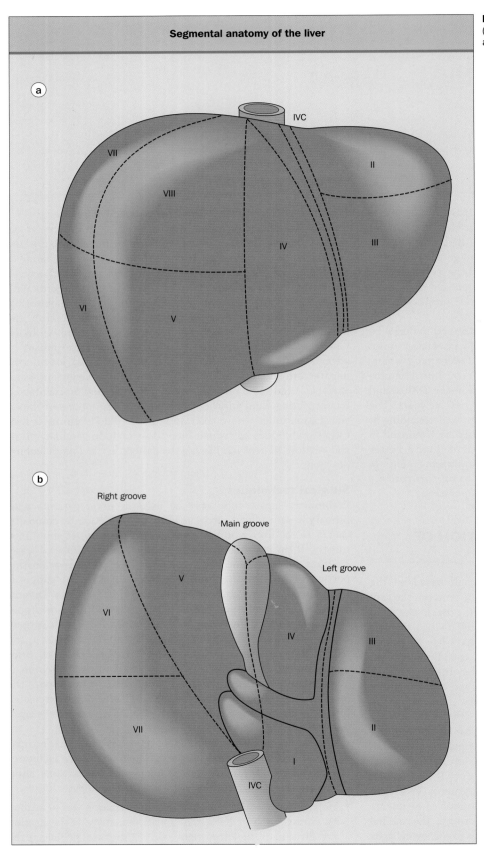

Segmental anatomy of the liver

Figure 36.1 Segmental anatomy of the liver.
(a) Anterior view of segments II–VIII. (b) Inferior aspect of the segmental anatomy.

recommended. This technique has two advantages: it reduces intraoperative blood loss and it produces a clear line of demarcation between the ischemic and the normally vascularized liver. The disadvantage of this technique, besides the risk of injury to major veins, is the danger of erroneous ligation of an element in the porta hepatis.

- Hepatectomy by primary parenchymal transection was described by Ton That and Nguyen-Duong-Quang. The hepatic parenchyma is divided along the line of the middle hepatic vein, and glissonian elements are ligated within the liver, without prior control. Division of the hepatic vein is performed within the liver toward the end of the procedure. The main attraction of this technique is that the risk from anatomic variants is minimized as the portal elements are approached above the hilum. The disadvantage of this technique is that bleeding can be considerable if the resection is not performed quickly, and continuous or intermittent clamping of the hepatic pedicle may be necessary.

- The final method is hepatectomy with extrahepatic vascular control and intrahepatic ligation. The hilar dissection is initially performed, gaining control of the arterial and portal elements of the side to be resected and clamping them without ligation. The appropriate side of the vena cava is freed without dissecting the hepatic vein. The liver is then divided along the main scissural line and, as in the technique of Ton That, the portal elements are located as the parenchyma is transected. Ligation of the vessels is, therefore, performed distal to the clamps. At the end of the liver transection, the hepatic vein is ligated within the liver and the clamps are removed. This technique has the advantages of minimizing blood loss by prior vascular control and of safe, accurate division and ligation of the vessels and biliary branches within the liver.

Controlling the bleeding from the parenchyma at the time of its transection remains the most challenging portion of a liver resection. Over the years, several techniques have evolved to reduce the bleeding. The 'Pringle' maneuver is performed by occluding all the vascular inflow into the liver. This is carried out by applying a non-crushing vascular clamp to the hepatoduodenal ligament. However, this maneuver does not control bleeding from the hepatic veins. Intermittent inflow occlusion – 15 min occluded, 5 min reperfusion – has gained popularity recently because of its additional benefit in reducing ischemia/reperfusion injury. The technique of total vascular exclusion (TVE) has some proponents. The dissection is identical to that performed for a total hepatectomy for a liver transplant. In addition to occluding the portal inflow, the IVC both above and below the liver are controlled. Therefore, all the vascular inflow and outflow are occluded. The technique of TVE does reduce cardiac output by 25–30%, but the majority of patients remain hemodynamically stable with additional volume (approximately 500–1000 cm^3). The technique allows parenchymal transection in a virtually bloodless field. However, clamp times should be kept to less than 60 min, particularly if the remaining parenchyma has either fibrosis or fatty change.

The liver tissue may be divided by several methods, including the finger fracture technique, the Kelly clamp, and the Cavitron ultrasonic dissector (Cavitron Surgical Systems, Stamford, CT). The aim of all these methods is to divide only the parenchymal tissue, exposing the vessels and the biliary structures. The ultrasonic dissector consists of a vibrating device that oscillates at a frequency of 23 kHz. It fragments preferentially the water-filled parenchymal cells that are removed by a coaxial irrigation apparatus. The collagen and elastic tissue of the vessels are preserved so that they can be dissected cleanly before accurate coagulation or ligation (**Fig. 36.2**). In most cases, nothing more is needed than meticulous suture or ligation of the larger vessels, and coagulation of smaller vessels as the resection proceeds. The raw surface is cauterized with an argon beam coagulator or the Tissue-Link coagulator. Both result in tissue desiccation and good hemostasis. Bile channels run with the portal pedicles and are simultaneously dealt with by suture ligation during the resection. Small bile leaks on the raw surface should be actively looked for and oversewn with fine sutures. When hemostasis has been achieved, drains are left in the subphrenic and subhepatic areas, although recent data indicates a lower morbidity if no drains are placed. The abdomen is then closed.

Postoperative care

The majority of patients who undergo a liver resection enjoy a relatively uncomplicated postoperative course. This is particularly true if the intraoperative effort was problem free. Relatively few patients require more than an overnight stay in a monitored unit. The main points of emphasis are: absence of bleeding, control of pain, satisfactory liver function, minimizing the risk of infection, and return of gastrointestinal function. Intravenous fluids and blood products are given as needed; antibiotics are continued for the first 24 h. The nasogastric tube is removed on the first postoperative day and the diet is advanced as tolerated. The majority of patients have an epidural catheter inserted for pain control; this is removed on the fourth or fifth postoperative day, if the coagulation profile is normal. The Foley catheter is removed on the same day.

Laboratory studies, which include a complete blood count, liver and renal tests, and a prothrombin time, are obtained daily for at least the first 3 days. Initially, the aminotransferases are elevated, ranging from a few hundred U/L to more than a thousand; however, they should normalize rapidly over the next 5–7 days. The prothrombin time and serum bilirubin level may also be elevated; the former may require the administration of vitamin K or fresh frozen plasma. The severity of the derangement of the postoperative liver studies depends on the magnitude of the resection, the duration of the clamp time (warm ischemia), the integrity of the remaining parenchyma, and the intraoperative course. A difficult resection associated with hypotension and the administration of large volumes of fluid and blood products results in more postoperative liver dysfunction. The cholestatic enzymes, alkaline phosphatase, and γ-glutamyltranspeptidase (γ-GT) are initially normal and then tend to rise toward the end of the first week. Both of these tests are markers of regeneration and may stay elevated for a few weeks. The most worrisome biochemical profile 7–10 days following a major liver resection involves a rising serum bilirubin and prothrombin time, accompanied by a normal alkaline phosphatase level.

The mortality following a major liver resection in patients without cirrhosis should be <10% and in major centers is <2%. Mortality results from liver failure/severe dysfunction, infection, multisystem failure and cardiac events. The mortality in patients with cirrhosis is significantly higher. A recent series reported 14% mortality in a group of patients with Child class A cirrhosis. Morbidity ranges from 24 to 40% following liver resection and

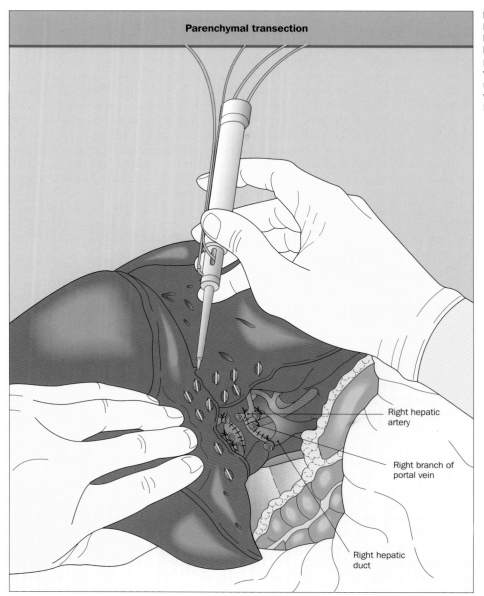

Parenchymal transection

Right hepatic artery

Right branch of portal vein

Right hepatic duct

Figure 36.2 Parenchymal transection. A right hepatic lobectomy is depicted. The right branches of the hepatic artery, portal vein, and bile duct have been ligated and divided. The liver parenchyma is being transected with the CUSA, which is an instrument that uses ultrasound to melt away the parenchyma and expose the vessels and bile ducts which are then clipped or ligated, depending on their size, and divided.

may be procedure-specific, or similar to that reported after any major abdominal operation, such as atelectasis, a urinary tract infection or a wound infection. Procedure-specific complications include liver dysfunction, renal dysfunction (usually as a result of the liver dysfunction), bile leaks, bleeding from the operative site, pleural effusions, ascites and subphrenic fluid collection.

RADIOFREQUENCY ABLATION

Although surgical resection is the gold standard in the treatment of patients with primary and secondary liver tumors, most patients are not candidates for surgery because of either large tumor burden or accompanying comorbidities. Because medical therapy has limited benefit, regional treatment methods such as percutaneous ethanol injection, cryoablation, and perhaps most promising radiofrequency (RF) ablation have emerged as alternative treatment options for a large number of these patients with liver-predominant disease.

In 1990 McGahan and Rossi independently published the first descriptions of the use of RF thermal ablation for the creation of deep thermal injuries in the liver. Rapidly alternating current is applied via an uninsulated electrode tip into the liver tissue. Heat is generated when the local ionic agitation leads to localized frictional heating of the tissue surrounding the electrode. Cell death occurs in 1 s at 55° C and is instantaneous at 60°C. Heating also causes desiccation and if temperatures are high enough, carbonization. Because electrical heating occurs only very close to the electrode, the creation of high temperatures in a large sphere around the electrode is due to heat exchange. Liver and tumor tissue has high thermal conductivity. However blood vessels act as a heat sink by convective cooling, moving heat away from the intended target. This can seriously affect the zone of ablation. However it protects the blood vessel; unfortunately bile ducts do not have such protection.

RF ablation can be performed at open laparotomy, at laparoscopy or by percutaneous means. It is clear that open RF ablation is more effective than the percutaneous method. Around 35% of patients examined by conventional imaging are found to have unsuspected disease at the time of open surgery. The electrode is passed into the center of the lesion under ultrasound control. Currently lesions up to 5 cm can be ablated. The extent and completeness of RF ablation is difficult to assess intra-operatively. 'Outgassing' is the appearance of microbubbles in the tissue and this indicates heating, but there is no reliable correlation between outgassing and tissue kill. RF ablation incurs few complications. The major risk is bile duct injury from improper placement of electrodes too close to the major bile ducts.

The clinical results of RF ablation can be divided into results of treatment of colorectal cancer metastases, HCC and other tumors. Unfortunately the literature in this area includes no randomized trials and very few long-term follow-up studies. Published studies demonstrate that the procedure is safe; only 2–8% of patients have complications. Reviewing RF ablation in patients with colorectal cancer shows there is good control of disease at the RF ablation site, with a reported recurrence of 2–21%. However as expected with advanced disease, new metastases develop in 27–66% of cases. Currently RF ablation is indicated for certain unresectable liver tumors and at the present time there is little justification for using this treatment on resectable liver tumors except for those cases deemed unfit. The results of long-term studies are awaited.

MALIGNANT NEOPLASMS

Hepatocellular carcinoma

HCC is the fifth most common cancer worldwide, being responsible for about 1 million deaths each year. The age adjusted incidence rate of HCC varies widely between 20 and 28 cases/100 000 in East Asia and in sub-Saharan Africa. In the USA a significant increase in incidence from 1.4 to 2.4 cases/100 000 has been observed during the last two decades. Risk factors associated with the development of HCC include cirrhosis (the 5-year cumulative incidence ranges between 7 and 20%), hepatitis B virus (HBV) or hepatitis C virus (HCV) infection, male gender, thorotrast, aflatoxin B1, parasites and certain metabolic liver diseases (e.g. hemochromatosis). The tumor normally develops within pathologically altered liver tissue. Because carcinoma itself and not the accompanying hepatic disorder accounts for disease-specific mortality, early tumor detection with an intent of curative treatment, either in terms of local resection or liver transplantation, presents the key issue in the management of the population at risk.

The clinical presentation of HCC varies considerably from an asymptomatic condition, in the case of an incidentally discovered small lesion, to general deterioration, upper abdominal pain, weight loss, jaundice, hepatic dysfunction and a palpable abdominal mass. The laboratory studies most likely to be abnormal involve alkaline phosphatase, γ-GT, and bilirubin. α-fetoprotein (AFP) is a glycoprotein which may help in diagnosis when serum levels are greater than 500 µg/L (normal in most laboratories is between 10 and 20 µg/L). However, not all tumors secrete AFP, and serum concentrations are normal in up to 40% of small HCCs. Ultrasound is the most common imaging study for detecting HCC because it is often used in screening. Further diagnostic imaging usually requires computed tomography (CT) or magnetic resonance imaging (MRI). The ability of CT to detect HCCs has improved with the development of helical CT technology. This technique involves the rapid administration of contrast material in combination with extremely fast imaging. The arterial phase of enhancement allows for detection of hypervascular HCCs as small as 3 mm. The sensitivity of helical CT for detecting HCC may be as high as 90%. On MRI, HCC appears as a high intensity pattern on T_2-weighted images, and a low intensity pattern on T_1-weighted images. MRI has better sensitivity and specificity compared to CT in cirrhotic patients in whom it can be difficult to distinguish an HCC from regenerative nodules. It is also more likely to reveal multicentric disease or a more extensive tumor than demonstrated by CT (**Fig. 36.3**). A needle biopsy, either a core or an aspiration for cytology, is often diagnostic. If a needle biopsy of the tumor is performed, a biopsy of the non-tumor bearing portion of the liver should also be carried out to rule out the presence of cirrhosis, particularly if splenomegaly is demonstrated in the imaging studies. Splenomegaly suggests the diagnosis of portal hypertension and cirrhosis. The key issue in the surgical management of HCC is to confirm the diagnosis quickly with the least invasive techniques. The debate at present is whether small HCC in good risk patients should be managed by liver transplantation or by resection, both of which can be performed safely and with a good chance of success. For more advanced HCC, other treatment modalities come into play.

Once the diagnosis of HCC has been made, further studies are necessary to rule out metastatic disease and to stage the tumor. A CT scan of the chest is required to eliminate the possibility of pulmonary spread. A bone scan may also be indicated. A number of staging systems have been proposed for HCC, none of which has been universally adopted. These schemas invariably incorporate four features that have been recognized as being important determinants of survival: the size of the tumor, the severity of underlying liver disease, extension of the tumor particularly with vascular invasion, and the presence of metastases. Clinical staging of HCC was first done using the Okuda system and, more recently, refined by the CLIP (Cancer of the Liver Italian Program) and Barcelona Clinic Liver Cancer

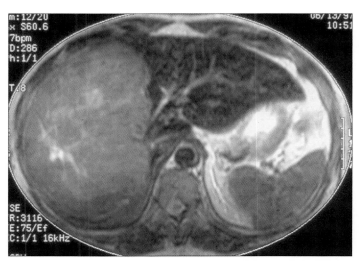

Figure 36.3 Hepatocellular carcinoma (HCC). A magnetic resonance image of a large HCC that required an extended right lobectomy.

Group (BCLC) scores. These can all be applied to patients at the time of presentation and initial evaluation is made using clinical, laboratory and basic imaging data. The tumor, node, metastasis (TNM) system is of limited relevance as it only considers tumor variables for post-resection pathologic staging.

If no metastatic disease is detected, and the patient is not a transplant candidate, the patient should be further assessed for a possible resection, by excluding other comorbid conditions, such as heart or lung disease. Early detection strategies for HCC has significantly increased the number of patients undergoing liver resection for non-cirrhotic conditions, and with Child-Pugh class A liver cirrhosis with normal or moderately elevated bilirubin values (<1.9 mg/dL) in the absence of portal hypertension. The resection rate remains low, around 15%, in high volume centers in the USA. Improvements in patient selection and surgical techniques have reduced the operative mortality to the range of 2–15%. Risk factors that increase operative morbidity and mortality include cirrhosis, significant fatty change, prolonged (greater than 1 h) vascular occlusion (warm ischemia), major blood loss, a major resection, coronary artery disease and an elevated preoperative bilirubin. Death is usually from liver failure or severe dysfunction and multiorgan failure. A major liver resection carries a morbidity rate of 25–40%. A recent review of hepatic resections for HCC reports 3-year and 5-year survival rates from 68 to 76% and 51 to 68%, respectively. The favorable determinants of survival by univariate analysis include no vascular invasion, asymptomatic status, a solitary tumor, a histologically negative margin, an encapsulated tumor and a tumor less than 5 cm in diameter. Multivariate analysis shows lack of vascular invasion to be the most reliable favorable factor. Preoperative portal vein embolization (PVE) is a valuable adjunct to major liver resection in the appropriate patient with the goal of hypertrophy of the future liver remnant to enable resection that would otherwise leave a remnant liver insufficient to support life following partial hepatectomy. There are three potential benefits to this technique:

- Post-resection morbidity is diminished, as evidenced by minimal changes in post-resection liver function and decreased length of hospitalization.
- Patients who were initially unresectable because of insufficient remaining normal hepatic parenchyma can undergo resection for potential cure.
- Subclinical disease or rapid progression may be detected prior to definitive surgery on post embolization imaging studies, thus sparing the patient an unnecessary operation.

The role of preoperative hepatic artery chemoembolization (HAC) in the treatment of HCC remains unclear. The impetus to evaluate neoadjuvant therapies arises from the belief that recurrences occur not because of inadequate surgical resection, but because of pre-existing clinically occult microscopic tumor foci. HAC has been used in the following three settings:

- treatment of large unresectable HCC;
- prior to resection; and
- prior to transplant.

When used as a primary treatment for large unresectable HCC, approximately 35% have an objective antitumor response. However its role prior to resection is not defined. One randomized controlled study has shown that HAC prior to surgical resection may be associated with increased mortality.

Fibrolamellar HCC (FLHCC) is a rare variant of hepatoma that was first described in 1956. In contrast to the more common type of HCC, FLHCC is found in young patients (mean age 23 years), and is not associated with either chronic hepatitis or cirrhosis. It usually occurs in the left lobe. The most common presenting symptoms are a palpable mass, abdominal pain, weight loss, malaise and anorexia. The variant FLHCC is thought to be biologically relatively more indolent than HCC because it usually becomes quite large before it is detected. Neurotensin may be a serum marker.

Two series reporting FLHCC have been published. In one series there were 10 patients with a mean tumors of 8 cm. The 5- and 10-year survival rates were 70%. Recurrence occurred in half of the patients and three had a repeat liver resection. Of the 20 patients in the other report, 14 were resected and six underwent liver transplantation. The 5-year survival was 36%. A review of the literature reveals a 5-year survival rate of 56%. When matched stage for stage, the survival of patients with FLHCC is no better than that for non-FLHCC patients. No patient with stage III disease survived for 5 years. Because intrahepatic recurrence is frequently observed and these tumors are slow growing, transplantation has been proposed. In two series, the results of resection and transplantation have been compared. In these studies the long-term results are comparable suggesting resection when possible is preferred to transplantation.

METASTATIC TUMORS

The most frequently encountered liver tumors are metastatic, commonly from colorectal or neuroendocrine primary sites. Other tumors that are seen include breast, melanoma, genitourinary and sarcoma, but the results of resection have been poor with these tumors. The majority of liver resections in the USA are performed for metastatic colorectal carcinoma. Approximately 150 000 new cases of colorectal carcinoma occur in the USA annually. Of these, about one-third will develop liver metastases, 20% of which will have metastatic disease confined to the liver. Approximately a quarter of this 20% (about 2000 patients) may be candidates for liver resection.

The only curative option for patients with liver-isolated colorectal metastases is surgical resection. In patients with four or fewer isolated hepatic lesions, resection may be curative, with 5-year relapse-free survival rates ranging from 24 to 38%. However, no more than 10% of patients with isolated hepatic metastases are amenable to potentially curative resection. The majority are not candidates for resection because of tumor size, location, multifocality or inadequate hepatic reserve. Nevertheless, because of its impact on survival, surgical resection is the treatment of choice when feasible. For surgical resection to be considered, there must be no evidence of involvement of the hepatic artery, major bile ducts, or main portal vein, and there must be adequate functional hepatic reserve post-resection. Furthermore, occult extrahepatic metastatic disease must be excluded.

The optimal selection of patients who appear to have isolated liver disease for resection is evolving. In the past, contraindications to liver resection were defined by retrospective series. As a result of these analyses, surgeons have been reluctant to offer resection to patients with more than three lesions, those with bilobar distribution, and those in whom it was not possible

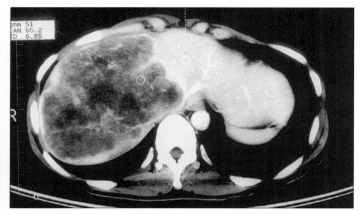

Figure 36.4 Metastatic colorectal carcinoma. Axial computed tomography image of a large metastatic lesion that was resected by an extended right lobectomy.

to achieve 1 cm margins (**Fig. 36.4**). However, these relative contraindications have been challenged. In one report of 165 patients, of whom 44 underwent complex resections (multiple tumors in both lobes), 5-year survival (37%) was similar to those with fewer or unilobar lesions. In a second report of 155 patients who underwent resection of more than four hepatic metastases, the 5-year survival was 23% overall, and 14% for those with 9–20 lesions resected. The operative mortality ranged from 3 to 8%.

Approximately 10–15% of patients are candidates for a second liver resection for recurrent disease. Almost 65–85% of patients who have a liver resection for metastatic colorectal carcinoma will develop a recurrence. About 20–30% of these patients will have a recurrence in the liver alone and 10% may be candidates for another resection. The preoperative evaluation and the operative morbidity and mortality are the same as before the first resection. The operative blood loss is higher because of adhesions from the initial surgery. The prognostic factors are also the same: obtaining a 1 cm tumor free margin and a solitary lesion. The survival is also equal to that obtained from the first resection (**Table 36.1**). Patients with a metastatic neuroendocrine tumor, such as carcinoid or an islet cell tumor of the pancreas, may also be candidates for liver resection. The patients most likely to benefit from resection are those who have symptoms from a functioning tumor that is overproducing a biologically active hormone, such as those associated with the carcinoid syndrome or a gastrinoma. A series from the Mayo Clinic included 74 patients, 50 with carcinoid and 23 with islet cell tumors. The operative morbidity and mortality were 24 and

Survival after repeat liver resection for colorectal metastases				
Resection	1 Year (%)	3 Years (%)	5 Years (%)	10 Years (%)
First	78	30	16	16
Second	85	39	25	11

Table 36.1 Metastatic tumors. A repeat liver resection for colorectal metastases has a survival comparable with that of the initial resection.

2.7%, respectively. Over 90% experienced symptomatic relief, and the 4-year survival rate exceeded 70%. In selected patients, liver resection is safe and effective palliation for patients with metastatic neuroendocrine tumors. A small percentage of these patients may also gain a survival advantage from liver resection.

BENIGN TUMORS

These lesions are reviewed in detail in Chapter 27. In this section we will describe the surgical indications for removal and techniques.

Cavernous hemangiomas

Cavernous hemangiomas are the most common benign mesenchymal hepatic tumors. Around 60–80% of cases are diagnosed in patients who are between the ages of 30 and 50 years. Hemangiomas are often solitary, but multiple lesions may be present in both the right and left lobe of the liver in up to 40% of patients. The majority are small (<5 cm). Most patients with hepatic hemangiomas are asymptomatic, have an excellent prognosis and require no intervention. The main indication for investigation is to differentiate the hemangioma from other focal liver lesions.

Only symptomatic hemangiomas need to be excised, regardless of their size. Symptoms however are more likely with larger hemangiomas, presenting with upper abdominal fullness, discomfort or early satiety. Non-specific abdominal pain and the presence of a hemangioma is not an indication for surgery. However, patients who return on more than one occasion because of upper abdominal pain for which no other cause is uncovered may be candidates for excision. Massive lesions that are clearly responsible for pain should also be excised. Size itself is not an indication for surgery; a series from the Mayo Clinic which included 36 patients with hemangiomas with an average size of 8 cm followed for a mean of 12 years reported no spontaneous bleeding. The Kasabach-Merritt syndrome, which is a low-grade local consumptive coagulopathy, is also another indication.

Enucleation is the procedure of choice for removing a cavernous hemangioma (**Fig. 36.5**). A 'friendly plane' can be developed between the hemangioma and the normal liver parenchyma. Blood loss can be minimized if the enucleation procedure is combined with control of vascular inflow (Pringle maneuver), or if the hemangioma is massive, with total vascular exclusion (TVE). Enucleation is associated with a 50% reduction of blood loss when compared with a formal resection. Resection is indicated only if the diagnosis is in doubt and there is concern that the lesion is a hemangiosarcoma. Long-term survival after removal of a cavernous hemangioma is excellent.

Hepatic cell adenoma

Hepatic adenomas are uncommon benign epithelial liver tumors that develop in a liver with an otherwise normal appearance. They are seen predominantly in young women (20–44 years-old), are frequently located in the right hepatic lobe, and are typically solitary (70–80%), although multiple adenomas have been described in patients with glycogen storage diseases (GSD) and hepatic adenomatosis. Adenomas range in size from 1 to 30 cm.

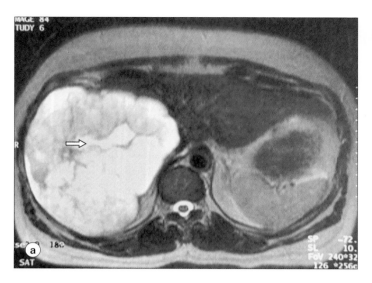

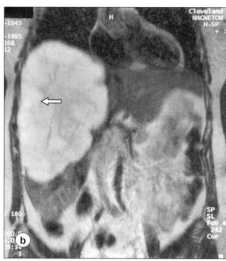

Figure 36.5 Cavernous hemangioma. (a) An axial magnetic resonance image showing a large, symptomatic hemangioma (white area; arrow). (b) A coronal view of the same lesion. The hemangioma was enucleated.

Patients with adenomas can present with abdominal pain (50%) and as many as 30% may present acutely with bleeding, either into the tumor or freely into the peritoneal cavity. Malignant degeneration has also been reported with hepatic adenomas. All symptomatic hepatic cell adenomas and those greater than 5 cm require resection because of the risk of hemorrhage and malignant degeneration. Asymptomatic lesions that are less than 5 cm may be observed by serial scans if the patient stops taking oral contraceptives. However, a low threshold to resect the adenoma must be maintained if the lesion does not significantly reduce in size within a few months. Because of the possibility of malignancy, a liver resection with a 1–2 cm margin of normal parenchyma is required for adequate treatment. The overall mortality associated with hepatic cell adenomas is 2–3%, which is virtually limited to those women who present with intraperitoneal rupture and hemorrhage; 20% of these women die.

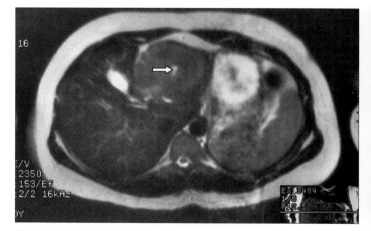

Figure 36.6 Magnetic resonance image (MRI) of focal nodular hyperplasia. An axial MRI picture of the characteristic central scar (arrow) of focal nodular hyperplasia.

Focal nodular hyperplasia

Focal nodular hyperplasia (FNH) is the most common non-malignant hepatic tumor that is not of vascular origin. FNH is seen in both sexes and throughout the age spectrum, although it is found predominantly in women (in a ratio of 8 or 9:1) between the ages of 20 and 50 years. FNH is most often solitary (80–95%), and usually less than 5 cm in diameter.

Laboratory studies are normal. CT, MRI and a technetium sulfur colloid scan are the most helpful imaging studies. Scanning by CT and MRI may reveal the typical 'central scar' – composed of abnormally large portal tracts including large feeding arteries, portal veins and bile ducts (**Fig. 36.6**). Virtually all cases (80%) of FNH should have a positive sulfur colloid scan because Kupffer cells are present as well as hepatocytes in these lesions (**Fig. 36.7**). A biopsy reveals all the elements of normal liver tissue, not just hepatocytes. Unlike adenomas, FNH rarely requires resection because there is little risk of either hemorrhage or malignant degeneration. Asymptomatic lesions, even very large ones, can be followed safely. Indications for resection include pain or increasing size as demonstrated by repeated imaging.

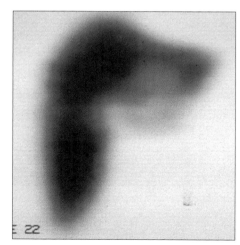

Figure 36.7 Sulfur colloid scan of focal nodular hyperplasia (FNH). A sulfur colloid scan on the same lesion as depicted in Figure 36.6. The FNH takes up the isotope because of the presence of Kupffer cells in the tumor.

CYSTIC DISEASE

Simple cysts

Simple, benign cysts of the liver occur in about 5% of the general population; however, only 5% of these patients become symptomatic. The female:male ratio is approximately 1.5:1 among those with asymptomatic simple cysts while it is 9:1 in those with symptomatic or complicated simple cysts. Although most patients have a solitary cyst, some patients may have several simple cysts. The pathogenesis of these presumed congenital, slow growing cysts is not clearly defined, but congenital lymphatic obstruction and faulty bile duct development are proposed mechanisms. The right lobe is the most frequent site of these lesions. The lesions are lined by cuboidal epithelium and most often contain clear liquid although occasionally they may contain bloody, milky or bile-stained fluid.

While most simple cysts are asymptomatic, when symptoms occur, they do so because of the very large size of the cyst or hemorrhage into the cyst. Physical examination may reveal a soft upper abdominal mass; a tender mass may be appreciated if hemorrhage has occurred. Liver specific tests are generally normal. Ultrasound and CT reveal a homogenous cystic lesion(s). The distinction between a simple cyst, cystadenoma, cystadeno-carcinoma, and echinococcal cyst can be difficult. However, the distinction is extremely important since these lesions have different clinical significance. Ultrasonography is the most useful method for the diagnosis of a simple cyst. It appears as an anechoic unilocular fluid-filled space with imperceptible walls, and with posterior acoustic enhancement. On a CT scan, a simple cyst is defined as a well-demarcated water attenuation lesion that does not enhance following the administration of intravenous contrast. Uncomplicated simple cysts are virtually never septated. However, hemorrhage into a simple cyst can lead to confusion in the sonographic differentiation from a cystadenoma or cystadenocarcinoma.

Treatment is required only if the cyst is symptomatic or if the diagnosis is uncertain. Percutaneous aspiration alone results in prompt recurrence of the cyst. Placement of a percutaneous catheter may also result in infection of the cavity. Removing as much of the cyst wall as possible is the surgical procedure of choice. Excellent results have been obtained by excising the cyst wall laparoscopically. Several centers have reported recurrence rates ranging from 0 to 14% and morbidity rates of 0 to 15% after laparoscopic unroofing of solitary simple cysts (**Fig. 36.8**).

Complete excision or liver resection is not necessary and may be hazardous because of bleeding. Any fluid that is produced by the remaining cyst wall is reabsorbed by the peritoneum. If the cyst is infected, external drainage is necessary. A cyst that contains bile must communicate with the biliary tree. Formerly, the recommendation was to sew a Roux limb to the cyst. However, the sterile cyst was then converted to an abscess. The current approach is to identify the communication with the bile duct by performing an intraoperative cholangiogram and then close the fistula by suturing. The morbidity and mortality associated with procedures to treat simple liver cysts is extremely low and the long-term prognosis is excellent.

Polycystic liver disease

Adult polycystic liver disease (APLD) is inherited as an autosomal dominant and occurs in 0.6% of the population. There is

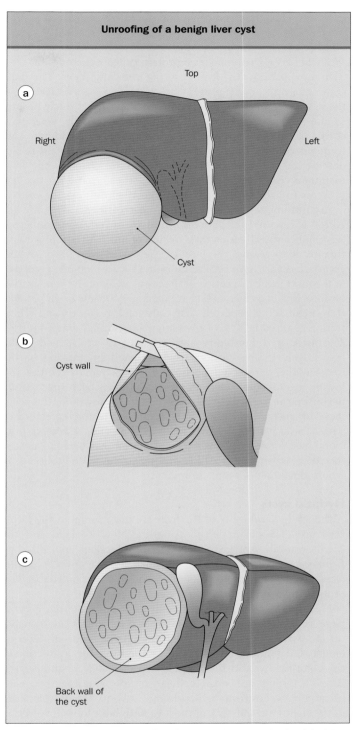

Figure 36.8 Unroofing of a benign liver cyst. (a) A cyst in the right lobe. (b) The lesion is being partially excised laparoscopically; the same procedure could be performed open. (c) Final appearance after much of the cyst wall has been excised.

an increased prevalence associated with increasing age and female sex. Of patients with APLD, 50% have polycystic kidney disease as well. The hepatic cysts are grossly and histologically similar to simple cysts of the liver. However the cysts are multiple and may extensively replace both sides of the liver. In addition to macroscopic cysts, there are usually numerous microscopic cysts and clusters of multiple bile ductules, designated as Von Meyenburg complexes. The pancreas is infrequently cystic. Hepatic cysts occurring in APLD result from a mutation in the *PRKCSH* gene that encodes a protein called hepatocystin.

In most patients the liver cysts are clinically silent. The most common symptoms, if present, are related to the massive size of the cystic liver. Abdominal distention, discomfort, early satiety, supine dyspnea, leg edema from compression of the vena cava, and hepatomegaly are the major symptoms and findings. Less frequent complications include portal hypertension and biliary obstruction. In spite of the massive cystic changes, the liver maintains its functional capability; these patients do not progress to liver failure. CT is the most helpful imaging study.

Asymptomatic patients require no treatment. Therapy for APLD is reserved for patients who have severe symptoms that are significantly affecting their quality of life. The goal of surgical therapy is to reduce the bulk of the cystic liver. Two surgical approaches that have resulted in some success include resection of the most involved portion of the liver and extensive fenestration or unroofing of as many cysts as possible. A review of 46 patients from eight series reported that combining resection and fenestration resulted in 82% of the patients becoming symptom free. The associated morbidity and mortality were 33 and 4.3%, respectively. Some authors have reported progression of the cysts in the unresected portion of parenchyma over the following several years. Liver transplantation has been successfully performed in a small number of patients. However, the technical difficulty of performing the transplant is much greater in a patient who has previously had a resection and/or fenestration. Combined kidney and liver transplantation has been advocated for patients with both APLD and polycystic kidney disease in whom renal failure seems imminent.

Hydatid cysts

Although hydatid cysts of the liver are uncommon in the USA, they are endemic in South America, New Zealand and the Mediterranean. Approximately 95% of infections are caused by *Echinococcus granulosa*; the remaining 5% are from *E. multilocularis*, which is more virulent and difficult to control because of its diffuse nature and invasive characteristics.

Hydatid cysts are most commonly unilocular and may grow as large as 20 cm. The cyst wall is about 5 mm thick and consists of an external laminated hilar membrane and an internal enucleated germinal layer which is responsible for production of the colorless hydatid fluid, brood capsules and daughter cysts. Brood capsules are small cellular masses and together with calcareous bodies form 'hydatid sand'. About 70% of lesions are in the right lobe and 15% in the left, with both lobes involved in approximately 15% of cases.

Many infections are probably contracted in childhood and remain dormant for many years. Development of symptoms is insidious. Distention of the liver capsule may produce right upper quadrant pain. Jaundice is infrequent but may be due to extrinsic biliary compression or communication with the biliary tree leading to obstruction by cystic debris. The complications associated with hydatid cysts usually result from either the cyst becoming secondarily infected with bacteria (10% of cases), or it ruptures into the peritoneal cavity, pleural space, pericardium or biliary tree. The diagnosis of hydatid disease of the liver requires a high index of suspicion, especially if the patient is

either a native of an endemic area, or has recently traveled to an endemic area. The current serum immunoelectrophoresis assay is 85–90% accurate. The most helpful study is a CT scan which demonstrates a cystic lesion in the liver that either has a calcified wall, contains daughter cysts or both.

Once the diagnosis has been established, surgery is generally required as the natural history of viable hydatid cysts is one of growth and potential complications. Medical therapy includes the anthelmintics such as albendazole and mebendazole. However, these agents have limited success. They are used preoperatively in an effort to sterilize the cyst and are reserved as definitive treatment for patients with inoperable, diffuse or recurrent disease. The principles of surgical therapy include complete evacuation of the cyst, destruction of the germinal lining, and avoiding spillage of daughter cysts. The surgical options consist of a liver resection, pericystectomy and non-resectional procedures. A liver resection is considered radical and reserved for peripheral lesions or diffuse involvement of a lobe. A pericystectomy involves removing the entire cyst; the procedure is difficult to perform and carries significant morbidity. The current preferred procedure involves complete evacuation of the cyst, instillation of 30% hypertonic saline to sterilize any remaining scolices, removing the endocyst (which contains the germinal layer), and either leaving the cavity open or packing it with omentum. With the non-resectional approach, the mortality in uncomplicated cases is 5% and the recurrence rate is 5–10%.

Neoplastic cysts

Cystadenoma and cystadenocarcinoma are rare cystic tumors of the liver. Of these tumors, 75% occur in women. Upper abdominal fullness and/or discomfort and a palpable mass are the presenting clinical manifestations. An ultrasound and/or CT scan are the most helpful imaging studies. A cystadenoma appears as a cystic mass with smooth walls and internal septa (**Fig. 36.9**); a cystadenocarcinoma has a similar appearance but with a solid component (**Fig. 36.10**). However, the distinction between a cystadenoma and cystadenocarcinoma can be difficult

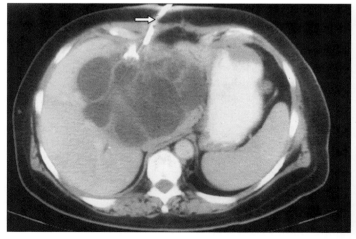

Figure 36.9 Hepatic cystadenoma. A computed tomography scan image that shows a large, multiseptated cystic mass in the central portion of the liver. Attempts to drain (arrow) the lesion were unsuccessful. The benign lesion was excised using total vascular exclusion because of its central location.

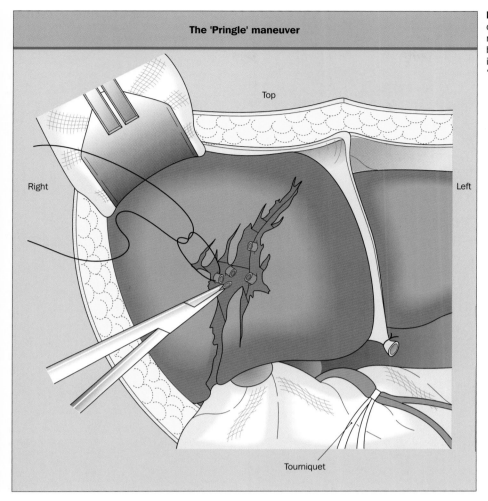

The 'Pringle' maneuver

Top

Right

Left

Tourniquet

Figure 36.16 The 'Pringle' maneuver. A large, deep laceration in the right lobe of the liver which requires control of individual vessels to arrest bleeding. The tourniquet is occluding the vascular inflow (hepatic artery and portal vein); the 'Pringle' maneuver.

arterial blood supply to the extrahepatic biliary tree, and the tension on the anastomosis.

Choledochoduodenostomy is an excellent bypass procedure for unresectable periampullary malignancies. The procedure is relatively easy to perform and requires only one anastomosis. The anastomosis is within easy reach of the endoscope therefore allowing both diagnostic and therapeutic endoscopic intervention. Benign, iatrogenic strictures are not usually amenable to a choledochoduodenostomy because of the high location of the obstruction and the associated scarring in the area of the duodenum. Ascending cholangitis was cited as a complication of choledochoduodenostomy. However, an anastomosis 2.5 cm in length will prevent this problem. Other disadvantages include the sump syndrome which results from inadequate drainage of the distal duct. This complication can also be prevented by performing a large anastomosis. An endoscopic sphincterotomy usually eliminates the sump syndrome.

Construction of a Roux limb provides an excellent conduit for biliary reconstruction. The limb may be sewn to any accessible portion of the biliary tree, particularly the common bile duct (choledochojejunostomy) or the hepatic duct (hepatico-jejunostomy). A Roux limb is the best option for either an immediately recognized bile duct injury or a subsequent benign stricture because it will easily reach the hepatic bifurcation and the anastomosis is tension free (**Fig. 36.17**). An anastomotic stricture results in cholangitis and occurs in 15–20% of patients. Many of these recurrent strictures can be successfully treated by radiographic dilatation and stenting. If stenting is not successful, the biliary-enteric anastomosis can be revised with a good long-term result in 90% of patients. Roux limb reconstruction is also the procedure of choice to restore biliary drainage following the resection of a proximal cholangiocarcinoma.

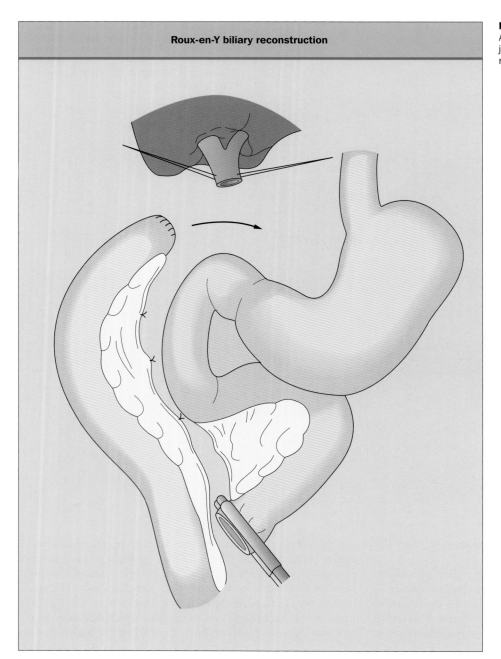

Roux-en-Y biliary reconstruction

Figure 36.17 Roux-en-Y biliary reconstruction. Anastomosis of the bile duct to a Roux limb of jejunum provides the best method for biliary reconstruction.

FURTHER READING

Surgical technique and anatomy

Skandalakis JE, Skandalakis LJ, Skandalakis PN, et al. Hepatic surgical anatomy. Surg Clin N Am 2004; 84: 413–435.

Trunkey DD. Mastery of surgery. In: Baker RJ, Fischer JE, eds. Lippincott Williams and Wilkins; 2001:1128–1147. *Reviews the current dilemmas in the management of liver trauma.*

Couinand C. Le Foie, Etudes anatomique et chirurgicales. Paris: Masson, 1957.

Lortat-Jacob JL. Hepatectomie droit reglée. Presse Med 1952; 60:549.

Hepatocellular carcinoma

Fong Y, Sun RL, Jarnigan W, et al. An analysis of 412 cases of hepatocellular carcinoma at a Western center. Ann Surg 2002; 236:397–406. *Reports the experience gained in a single centre in the management of hepatocellular carcinoma.*

Wildi S, Pestalozzi BC, McCormack L, et al. Critical evaluation of the different staging systems for hepatocellular carcinoma. Br J Surg 2004; 91(4):400–408. *A paper describing the benefits and pitfalls of current staging systems.*

Benign tumors

DeCarlis L, Pirotta V, Rondinara G, et al. Hepatic adenoma and focal nodular hyperplasia: diagnosis and criteria for treatment. Liver Transpl Surg 1997; 3:160–165.

Hugh TJ, Poston, GJ. Benign liver tumors and masses. In: Blumgart LH, Fong Y, eds. Surgery of the liver and biliary tract 2000, p. 139. Philadelphia: WB Saunders. *An excellent chapter covering the diagnosis and management of benign liver lesions.*

Trastek V, van Heerden J, Sheedy P, et al. Cavernous hemangiomas of the liver: Resect or observe? Am J Surg 1983;145:49–52.

Metastatic tumors in the liver
Adam R, Pascal G, Azoulay D, et al. Liver resection for colorectal metastases: the third hepatectomy. Ann Surg 2003; 238(6):871–883.

Choti MA, Sitzmann JV, Tiburi MF, et al. Trends in long-term survival following liver resection for hepatic colorectal metastases. Ann Surg 2002; 235(6):759–766. *A large series demonstrates that the results of hepatic surgery continue to improve.*

Siperstein AE, Garland A, Engle K. Laparoscopic radiofrequency ablation of primary and metastatic liver tumors. Technical considerations. Surg Endosc 2000; 14: 400–405.

Sutcliffe R, Maguire D, Ramage J, et al. Management of neuroendocrine liver metastases. Am J Surg 2004; 187(1):39–46.

Abscesses and cystic disease
Gigot J, Jadoul P, Que F, et al. Adult polycystic liver disease. Is fenestration the most adequate operation for long-term management? Ann Surg 1997; 225:286–294.

Huang C, Pitt H, Lipsett P, et al. Pyogenic hepatic abscess. Changing trends over 42 years. Ann Surg 1996; 223:600–609. *A large experience with liver abscesses over a long time period. The trends are clear.*

McManus DP, Zhang W, Li J, et al. Echinococcosis. Lancet. 2003; 362(9392):1295–1304.

CHAPTER
37 Indications and Patient Selection

John R. Lake

INTRODUCTION

Liver transplantation is the treatment of choice for those suffering from end-stage liver disease. The development and growth of liver transplantation has revolutionized the field of hepatology and greatly improved the outlook of patients suffering from various liver diseases. This procedure is now applied world wide as treatment for a large number of irreversible acute and chronic liver diseases for which there were previously no other treatment options (**Table 37.1**). Over the past decade there has been an enormous increase in the number of liver transplant operations performed (**Figs 37.1 and 37.2**).

The primary goals of liver transplantation are to prolong life and to improve the quality of life. Thus, it is essential to optimize patient selection and ideally time the transplant procedure so as to gain the maximum benefit. Unfortunately, because of the extreme shortage of organs for transplantation, optimal timing using deceased donor organs is not always possible. This shortage of organs has spawned great interest in new techniques for liver transplantation such as live donor transplants and splitting one liver for two recipients.

In the USA, 5330 liver transplant operations were carried out in 2002, while the equivalent figure for Europe was 4857. However, there are clear signs that the rate of expansion is slowing on both sides of the Atlantic. By contrast, the growth of liver transplantation in Asia has been explosive.

The outcomes of liver transplantation are currently excellent and much improved as compared to 20 years ago due to advances in operative technique, a better understanding of the course and prognosis of several liver diseases, and more effective post-operative care including immunosuppression. However, there are areas where we have made little progress, particularly in the management of post-transplant hepatitis C.

In recent years, there has also been a significant change in the indications for liver transplantation, so that nowadays the procedure is being offered in a wider range of more complicated conditions as well as to older patients. The most common indication is end-stage chronic liver disease in adults, which accounts for 69 and 70% of liver transplant activity in the USA and Europe, respectively (**Fig. 37.3**).

The main differences between the USA and Europe relate to the higher proportion of patients who have acute liver failure in Europe and until recently, a lower proportion of patients who have malignant disease receiving transplants in the USA (see Fig. 37.3). However, the proportion of patients receiving liver transplants for malignant disease in Europe is now decreasing and in the USA is increasing (**Fig. 37.4**).

Among patients who have cirrhosis, chronic viral hepatitis is currently the most common indication for orthotopic liver disease (OLT). In particular, chronic hepatitis C has continued to increase as an indication in both Europe and the USA over the past decade, while on both continents, the percentage of patients transplanted for chronic cholestatic liver disease is decreasing (**Fig. 37.5**).

The expansion in the indications for transplantation contrasts with the shortage of liver donors. This continues to put pressure on the field to continue to refine the selection for, and timing of, transplantation to obtain the best and most cost-effective outcomes.

TIMING OF LIVER TRANSPLANTATION

The success and increase in the number of liver transplants as a treatment option for end-stage liver disease has led to a marked shortage in donor organs and has greatly lengthened the waiting times for this procedure. As the waiting list grows, there has been an increase in the number of patients dying while awaiting the procedure. In the USA, there was an almost twofold increase in the number of patients dying while listed for liver transplantation between 1997 and 2001, with the number rising from 1198 to 2066. In the USA, this has led to a radical change in how patients are prioritized on the waiting list, making certain that organs are allocated to the seriously ill patients. This has already resulted in significantly fewer deaths in those on the waiting list, i.e. only 1814 waiting list deaths in 2003.

The timing of transplantation is necessarily influenced by access to donor organs. The current system of organ allocation in the USA, and a few other countries, is based on the prioritization of patients based on what is termed the MELD (model for end-stage liver disease) score. This prognostic score was originally developed to predict the short-term mortality risk for patients undergoing a transjugular intrahepatic portosystemic shunt (TIPS) procedure. However, it has now been well validated as an excellent predictor of 3-month mortality on the waiting list. This score utilizes three objective laboratory parameters, serum creatinine and bilirubin concentrations and international normalized ratio (INR) (**Table 37.2**). This organ allocation scheme has been in place in the USA for more than 3 years and has already led to a decrease in the waiting list mortality, while not compromising post-transplant outcomes (**Fig. 37.6**). More recently, it has also led to a reappraisal of who truly benefits from transplantation. Ideally, liver transplantation should be performed at a sufficiently late phase of the disease, where the patient's quality of life is impaired and they are at a greater risk of mortality on the waiting list than their risk of short-term mortality with transplantation. Although patients who have less advanced liver disease have excellent survival rates after the procedure, they also have been shown to survive with a

585

Indications for liver transplantation in adults	
Chronic liver disease	**Cholestatic diseases**
	Primary biliary cirrhosis
	Primary sclerosing cholangitis
	Secondary biliary cirrhosis
	Viral-related cirrhosis
	Viral B cirrhosis
	Viral B-δ cirrhosis
	Viral C cirrhosis
	Alcoholic cirrhosis
	Autoimmune cirrhosis
	Budd–Chiari syndrome
Parasitic diseases	Echinococcosis
Metabolic diseases	**With liver disease**
	Wilson disease
	Hereditary hemochromatosis
	α_1-antitrypsin deficiency
	Protoporphyria
	Gaucher's disease
	Glycogenosis type 1
	Without liver disease, but secondary to a liver metabolic defect
	Primary hyperoxaluria
	Essential hypercholesterolemia
	Familial amyloid polyneuropathy secondary to a variant transthyretin
Primary malignant tumor of the liver	Hepatocellular carcinoma
	Fibrolamellar hepatocellular carcinoma
	Epithelioid hemangioendothelioma
	Cholangiocellular carcinoma
Various	Adenomatosis of the liver
	Polycystic liver disease
	Caroli disease
Acute liver failure	Fulminant and subfulminant hepatitis
	Wilson disease (fulminant)
	Budd–Chiari syndrome (fulminant)
	Other causes of acute liver failure: post-trauma, postsurgery, postarterial embolization
	Acute alcoholic hepatitis (?)

Table 37.1 Indications for liver transplantation in adults.

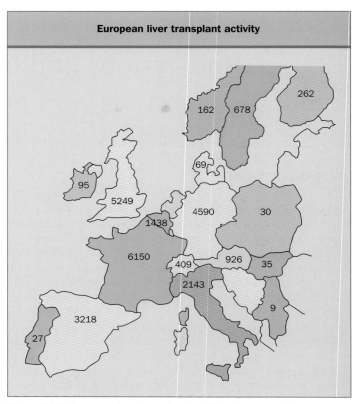

Figure 37.1 European liver transplant activity. Liver transplantation is performed in 19 European countries with 103 transplant centers, 26 538 transplants in 23 476 patients. Modified from The European Liver Registry Report.

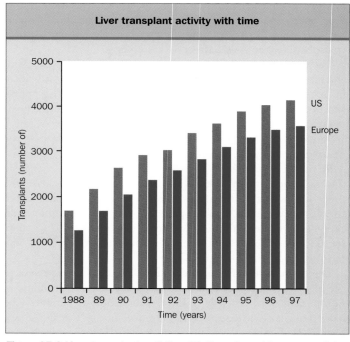

Figure 37.2 Liver transplant activity with time. Annual increases of the number of liver transplantations in Europe and the USA are decreasing as a function of the limited supply of donor organs. Modified from the United Network for Organ Sharing (UNOS) and The European Liver Registry Report.

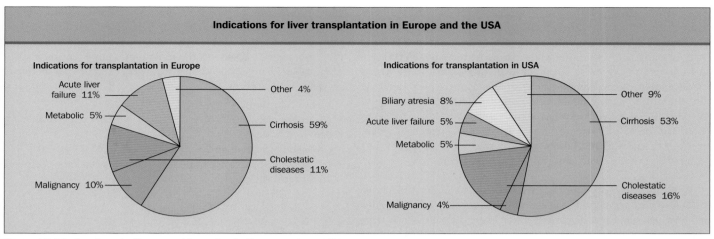

Figure 37.3 Indications for liver transplantation in Europe and the USA. The main indications for liver transplantation in Europe and the USA show subtle differences relating to acute liver failure and malignant disease. Modified from the United Network for Organ Sharing (UNOS) and The European Liver Registry Report.

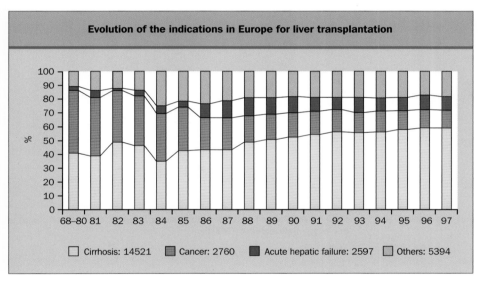

Figure 37.4 Evolution of the indications in Europe for liver transplantation. The main changes have been the progressive decrease of the patients transplanted for malignancy, the emergence of acute liver failure in the indications in 1986, and the increase of the number of patients transplanted for cirrhosis. Modified from The European Liver Registry Report.

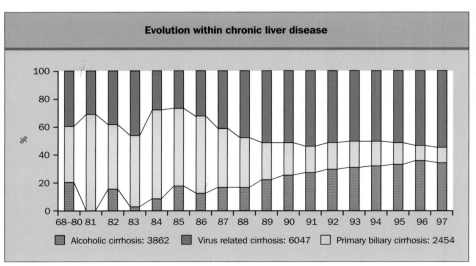

Figure 37.5 Evolution within chronic liver disease. Changes in the indications among patients transplanted for primary biliary cirrhosis (PBC), alcoholic cirrhosis and viral cirrhosis. Note the progressive decline of PBC as an indication and the increase of alcoholic and viral cirrhosis, which are now the two main indications for transplantation. Modified from The European Liver Registry Report.

reasonable quality of life for extended periods without liver transplantation. However, transplantation should also be performed at a time when the patient is in a condition that does not impair the outcome after transplantation. Certainly, patients who have more advanced liver disease are more likely to develop operative complications and have longer postoperative hospitalization and rehabilitation periods. Nonetheless, there is no MELD score that identifies when transplantation is futile as even the most ill patients have a reasonable chance of post-transplant survival, and obtain a substantial survival benefit, i.e. comparing the 1-year survival with transplantation to that without (**Fig. 37.7**).

While in the USA one might only need to understand how MELD works and the MELD scores at which your local patients achieve priority for a deceased donor liver, but this is not true throughout much of the world that does not use MELD. Likewise, it does not apply to live donor transplants. Thus, guidelines for referral or performance of the transplant in patients who have chronic liver disease likely vary as to where one practices and may vary as to whether an appropriate live donor is available. Survival models have been applied to liver transplantation for a number of diseases such as primary biliary cirrhosis (PBC) and alcoholic cirrhosis, and these have shown that a survival

benefit may not be apparent for up to 5 years after transplantation when the operation was performed relatively early in the disease. One model was developed at the Mayo Clinic for PBC, the liver disease with the most predictable natural history. This utilizes five independent prognostic variables predictive of survival:

- serum bilirubin;
- albumin levels;
- age;
- prothrombin time; and
- the presence or absence of peripheral edema (including response to diuretic therapy).

The equation for calculating the model of end-stage liver disease (MELD) score
· MELD = (0.957 × ln(creatinine) + 0.378 × ln(bilirubin) + 1.12 × ln(INR) + 0.643) × 10
· Capped at 40
INR, international normalized ratio.

Table 37.2 The equation for calculating the model of end-stage liver disease (MELD) score.

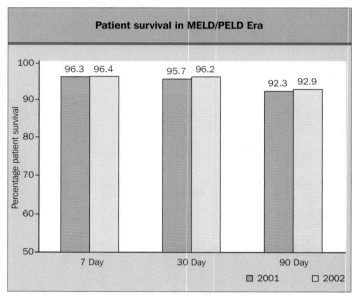

Figure 37.6 Patient survival before and after institution of the model of end-stage liver disease (MELD)

Figure 37.7 Relative risk of death with or without transplantation by model of end-stage liver disease (MELD) score.

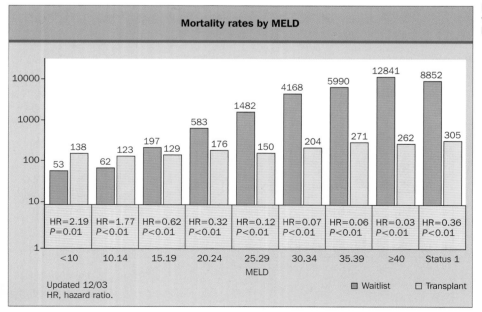

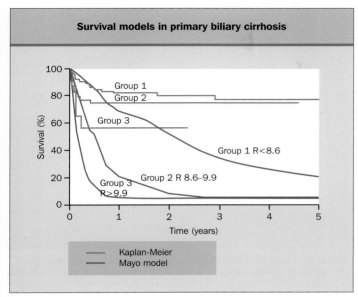

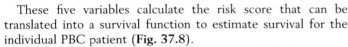

Figure 37.8 Survival models in primary biliary cirrhosis. Estimated Kaplan-Meier survival after liver transplantation in three groups of patients who had primary biliary cirrhosis versus estimated survival without liver transplantation as predicted by the Mayo model. Group 1, low risk; group 2, medium risk; group 3, high risk. Reproduced from Markus et al (89) by permission of the Massachusetts Medical Society.

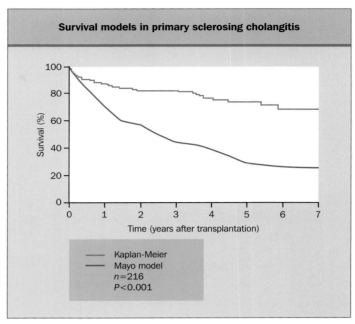

Figure 37.9 Survival models in primary sclerosing cholangitis. Actual Kaplan-Meier survival after liver transplantation in patients who have primary sclerosing cholangitis and the estimated survival without transplantation as predicted by the Mayo model simulated control. Data from Wiesner et al in Maddrey & Sorrell (95).

These five variables calculate the risk score that can be translated into a survival function to estimate survival for the individual PBC patient (**Fig. 37.8**).

The application of this model has demonstrated that liver transplantation improves survival when compared with supportive therapy in patients who have PBC. The survival benefit with liver transplantation is greater in the highest risk group, even though the survival rate is poorer in this high risk group due to the higher postoperative mortality (see Fig. 37.8). While MELD may be a better predictor of short-term mortality in PBC patients, the Mayo model will also provide prognostic information for longer term risks.

The prognostic models have also been used to evaluate objectively the efficacy of the procedure (see Fig. 37.8). The overall benefit has been clearly demonstrated for these patients. The benefit was greater in patients with the highest risk scores, but in the highest risk group, post-transplant mortality was greater. Similar data exists for MELD where a clear-cut survival benefit from transplant is not obtained in general until the patient has a MELD score >15 (Fig. 37.7). In addition, patients with a MELD score <10 have been shown to not benefit from transplantation, at least in terms of survival. A reasonable option is to consider the patient for transplantation when the expected survival is between 1 and 2 years, i.e. MELD score >15, if a live donor is available.

Effective prognostic models are present but less well-developed for other chronic liver diseases, including primary sclerosing cholangitis (PSC) and alcoholic cirrhosis (**Figs 37.9–37.11**). No model will be perfect, and they apply to a group of patients rather than an individual with that particular disease. To define the optimal timing for liver transplantation, an analysis of the natural history of the disease, together with a clinical judgment of the patient's quality of life are still the main guidelines to aid

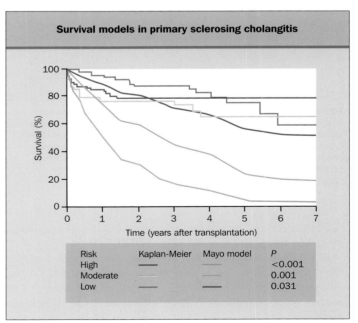

Figure 37.10 Survival models in primary sclerosing cholangitis (PSC). Actual Kaplan-Meier survival after liver transplantation in three risk groups of patients with PSC and their estimated survival without transplantation as predicted by the Mayo model. Data from Wiesner et al in Maddrey & Sorrell (95).

589

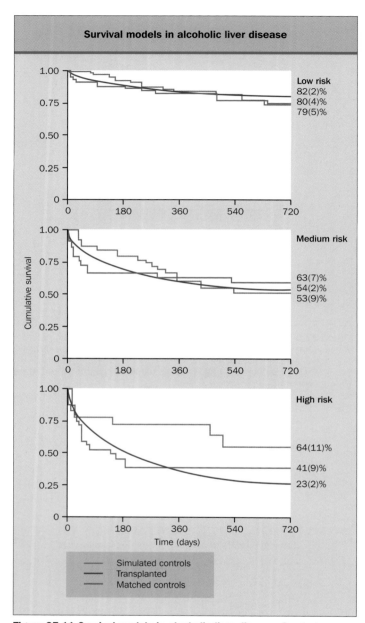

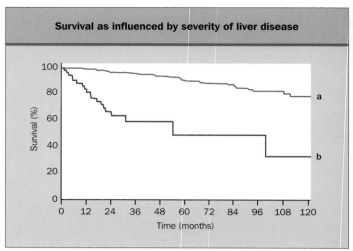

Figure 37.12 Survival as influenced by severity of liver disease. The probability of survival in patients who have compensated viral C cirrhosis (a) is greater at 91% at 5 years than after the appearance of the first major complication in patients who have decompensated viral C cirrhosis (b), which is 50% at 5 years. Reproduced from Fattovitch et al (97) by permission of the American Gastroenterological Association.

Figure 37.11 Survival models in alcoholic liver disease. Survival observed in patients transplanted for alcoholic cirrhosis, in matched and simulated controls, in a French multicenter trial. A higher survival after liver transplantation versus matched and simulated controls was observed only in the high risk group. Figures in brackets represent percentage of survival. Reproduced from Poynard et al (94) by permission of Elsevier.

the final decision. In addition, the clinical status of the disease should be taken into account (**Fig. 37.12**).

In patients who have PBC, PSC and autoimmune hepatitis, the disease process may or may not be controlled, and this will influence the decision. Likewise, in viral-related liver disease, control of viral replication is an important issue. When viral replication is controlled, e.g. using lamivudine to control hepatitis B virus (HBV) infection, the severity of the liver disease can actually improve and the clinical course either stabilizes or progresses more slowly. In contrast, if active viral replication persists and is associated already with advanced liver disease,

liver function will deteriorate more rapidly. Sometimes, either spontaneous arrest of viral replication or spontaneous viral reactivation may occur independently of any therapeutic intervention. In the latter case, the liver disease may reactivate and the prognosis in such patients may be difficult to assess. In some cases, liver function will return to baseline values after a transient period, but in others liver function will continue to deteriorate.

In patients with alcoholic cirrhosis, the discontinuation of alcohol generally and often dramatically improves prognosis. The improvement may take several months to become apparent, and this is one of the more persuasive reasons to recommend a 6-month period of abstinence from alcohol before performing transplantation in alcoholic patients.

CONTRAINDICATIONS TO LIVER TRANSPLANTATION

As more experience has been gained with liver transplantation, the number of contraindications has decreased over the years. Nowadays, there is general consensus about a number of contraindications to liver transplantation, although these are not universally agreed by all transplant centers:

- extrahepatic organ failure (heart, lungs), unless multiorgan transplantation is available;
- uncontrolled extrahepatic infection;
- extrahepatic malignant disease – the only potential exception is metastatic disease to liver from neuroendocrine tumors;
- diffuse thrombosis of the portal venous system (including the three main veins of the portal system – portal vein, superior mesenteric vein and splenic vein);
- uncontrolled immune deficiency;
- active substance abuse;
- inability to withstand the surgical procedure.

Previous contraindications no longer applicable include: an upper age limit of 55 years; previous multiple upper abdominal

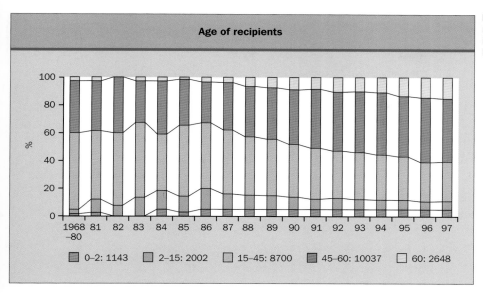

Figure 37.13 Age of recipients. Liver transplant recipients over the age of 60 years are increasing steadily. Modified from The European Liver Registry Report.

operations or previous portocaval surgical anastomosis; isolated thrombosis of the portal venous vein; and the presence of hepatitis B surface antigen (HBsAg) in patients' serum. The ultimate decision depends mainly on the criteria developed within each transplant center. There is no absolute upper limit for age as defined by the Conference Consensus held in Paris in 1993. The proportion of recipients over the age of 60 years has been increasing steadily. However, in candidates over the age of 65 years close attention to the patients' general health and, in particular, their cardiovascular health is required (**Fig. 37.13**). While in general, the outcome of older patients after liver transplantation has been similar to younger patients undergoing the same procedure, the ability of older recipients to overcome postoperative complications is clearly less than that of a 20–30 year-old patient, even with the apparent absence of specific risk factors such as coronary artery disease.

CHOLESTATIC DISEASES

Primary biliary cirrhosis
PBC is characterized by the destruction of small interlobular bile ducts, due to an inflammatory process, that mainly affects women between 40 and 60 years of age (see Ch.19). The course of the disease comprises three periods: an asymptomatic phase, lasting up to 20 years; a symptomatic phase with mild jaundice, itching and fatigue, lasting from 1 to 20 years; and a third and final stage, lasting a few months to 2–3 years, with marked jaundice, a relentless increase in serum bilirubin levels and clinical complications of portal hypertension. The course of the disease is steadily progressive, with clinical manifestations such as fatigue, pruritus, variceal bleeding, ascites and osteoporosis. It is clear that liver transplantation has dramatically improved the prognosis of PBC.

PBC was the first disease to be universally accepted as an indication for liver transplantation, and at present it is considered that the timing of intervention should be set at the onset of the third clinical stage in parts of the world where MELD is not used. This is the point where there is no prospect of spontaneous stabilization or recovery, but sufficiently early so as

not to negatively impact the outcome of transplantation. The major indication for liver transplantation is a serum bilirubin level over 10 mg/dL (>170 µmol/L). The risk of death awaiting transplantation is under 15% and the median survival when serum bilirubin level is over 6 mg/dL and 9 mg/dL is 24 and 17 months, respectively.

Other indications include variceal bleeding not controlled by endoscopic therapy or drug treatment, intractable ascites, and rarely intolerable pruritus or fatigue. With the more widespread use of ursodeoxycholic acid as a medical treatment, the indication for liver transplantation has become less frequently determined by the serum bilirubin level and more frequently by the complications of portal hypertension and by liver failure. A few patients are transplanted because their quality of life is poor despite all medical therapies. In these cases, a careful psychosocial appraisal of the quality of life and of fatigue should be performed before referral for liver transplantation.

The 10-year survival rate in these patients after transplantation is 80–90%, and the risk of recurrence seems to be ~ 10–20% at 5 years, even though the immunologic manifestations of the disease persist after transplantation. Nonetheless, the impact of recurrence on liver graft function is low, and very few recipients have been retransplanted for PBC recurrence. Interestingly, pruritus disappears immediately after transplantation in 100% of cases but fatigue improves only in ~ 70% of cases. Clearly, liver transplantation increases survival, as well as quality of life.

Primary sclerosing cholangitis
PSC is characterized by a chronic fibrosing inflammation of the bile ducts (see Ch. 20). It is commonest in men under the age of 50 years, and is associated with inflammatory bowel disease in ~ 70% of patients. It appears insidiously with pruritus, fatigue and/or jaundice initially, but later leads to biliary cirrhosis and complications of portal hypertension. There is also an increased risk of cholangiocarcinoma, with a prevalence of up to 30%. Treatment with standard doses of ursodeoxycholic acid (15 mg/kg) has not been proven to modify the course of the disease. PSC is a not uncommon indication for liver transplantation and accounts for nearly 10% of transplant activity in

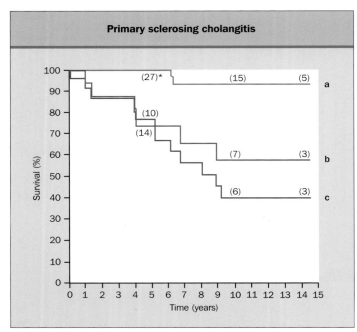

Figure 37.14 Primary sclerosing cholangitis. Survival from the time of onset of primary sclerosing cholangitis in patients not undergoing transplantation (c); in patients not undergoing transplantation after exclusion of those who had bile duct carcinoma at time of examination (b); and in patients treated by liver transplantation (a) at the Paul Brousse Center. (* actual patient numbers at that time point). Reproduced from Farges et al (95) by permission of Mosby.

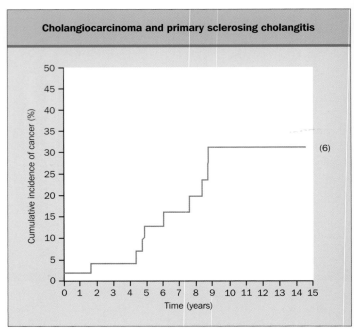

Figure 37.15 Cholangiocarcinoma and primary sclerosing cholangitis. Cumulative actuarial incidence of cholangiocarcinoma from time of onset of primary sclerosing cholangitis, emphasizing the increasing risk of developing cholangiocarcinoma. (6): number of patients at 15 years. Reproduced from Farges et al (95) by permission of Mosby.

the USA. It is the fourth most common indication in Europe in adults. Currently the main indications are:

- patients who have long-standing severe jaundice [bilirubin level over 100 μmol/L (6 mg/dL)], cholestasis and pruritus not related to an acute episode of cholangitis;
- established cirrhosis resulting in portal hypertension (ascites/ esophageal varices) and/or liver failure (prothrombin less than 50% of normal value);
- significant deterioration in the patient's quality of life; and
- recurrent episodes of cholangitis (in a few patients).

There are still some remaining questions and limitations regarding liver transplantation for PSC. The natural course of the disease and the optimal timing of liver transplantation are not totally clear. One study identified five independent clinical variables predictive of survival in PSC:

- age;
- histologic stage on liver biopsy;
- serum bilirubin level;
- hemoglobin concentration; and
- presence or absence of inflammatory bowel disease.

A recent report showed a 73% 5-year post-transplant survival rate, whereas the expected survival rate without transplantation was 28% (see Fig. 37.9). On the other hand, liver transplantation in PSC is still associated with higher morbidity and mortality due to previous surgical interventions (reported by most transplant centers), uncontrolled infection, undiagnosed cholangiocarcinoma, and, possibly, a higher risk of graft loss from chronic rejection. If the disease can be diagnosed pretransplantation, some success

has been obtained with aggressive radiotherapy and chemotherapy (see below)

Latent cholangiocarcinoma remains a problem. Cholangiocarcinoma should be in the differential diagnosis of PSC, but, in addition, the latter can be complicated by the development of cholangiocarcinoma. Progression of the tumor is often clinically silent. In addition, routine imaging studies are rarely of much benefit. Patients who otherwise would be good candidates for transplantation may have extrahepatic spread that precludes transplantation. In the explants, the incidence of cholangiocarcinoma varied from 8 to 18%, and most of these tumors were not diagnosed before transplantation. Currently, we lack the tools to recognize cholangiocarcinoma in the at-risk patient with PSC. The rapid development of persistent jaundice and pruritus, a recent clinical deterioration with weight loss, increased carcinoembryonic antigen (CEA) or CA 19-9 levels, and a long course of the disease (over 10 years) are all non-specific factors that could suggest the development of malignancy, but better methods are still needed to diagnose malignancy at an early stage (**Figs 37.14** and **37.15**). Patients who have coexisting inflammatory bowel disease should also have a colonoscopy at the time of assessment for transplantation to exclude colonic malignancy. Moreover, they need on-going frequent colonoscopy after liver transplantation as colorectal cancer is the most common cause of death beyond 1 year.

Since the results of liver transplantation are good and the procedure radically changes the prognosis of the disease, patients should be referred early after the onset of liver symptoms in order to reduce the operative risk and to prevent the development of hepatobiliary malignancy. Cases of recurrence of PSC have been described, and this can occasionally affect the outcome of the graft. In contrast, PSC-like symptoms have also been observed after liver transplantation in patients transplanted for diseases unrelated to PSC, and the real significance of recurrent disease will only become apparent with long-term follow-up.

Secondary biliary cirrhosis

The main causes of secondary biliary cirrhosis are anatomic abnormalities of the bile ducts or perioperative trauma of the extrahepatic bile ducts. Liver transplantation is indicated if surgical repair is not possible or after the development of secondary biliary cirrhosis when there is uncontrolled clinical cholestasis, jaundice, repeated episodes of cholangitis and/or portal hypertension. The timing of liver transplantation can be particularly difficult, as relief from the underlying obstruction can lead to a dramatic stabilization of the liver disease. The highest operative risk is now seen in patients who have coexisting extensive intra-abdominal adhesions and portal hypertension, and these patients are prime candidates for this unfavorable combination.

VIRAL HEPATITIS

Chronic viral hepatitis is the most common cause of end-stage liver disease world wide, and thus it is the most frequent diagnosis in patients referred for liver transplantation. However, viral reinfection and recurrence of disease after liver transplantation is a major clinical problem and may lead to allograft failure requiring retransplantation or result in death.

Hepatitis B

In spite of the success of vaccination against HBV, patients with cirrhosis due to HBV still constitute a sizable group of candidates for liver transplantation (5–10% of all recipients). However, the hope is that with the ever-expanding success of vaccination programs that this indication for liver transplantation will decrease over the next two decades. The current success of transplantation for hepatitis B-related disease represents one of the great triumphs of the past decade in the field of liver transplantation as the results of transplantation for hepatitis B are currently amongst the very best compared to other indications (**Fig. 37.16**). We are now able to prevent reinfection in >90% of recipients. Prior to this, transplantation for hepatitis B was marked by frequent HBV reinfection and in most patients, aggressive post-transplant hepatitis B that often led to death within a matter of months.

Although it is a progressive disease in the majority of cases, some patients present with an acute clinical deterioration at the time of viral reactivation or during the process of hepatitis B e antigen (HBeAg to anti-HBe) seroconversion. This can result in either irreversible liver failure and death, or a transient deterioration that is followed by a dramatic improvement of the liver disease. The main indications are similar to those for other liver diseases:
- recurrent ascites;
- spontaneous bacterial peritonitis;
- recurrent episodes of gastrointestinal bleeding not successfully controlled by medical treatment or ablative therapy;
- recurrent encephalopathy;

- liver failure with a low level of albumin, elevated serum bilirubin and low prothrombin level; and
- the development of hepatocellular carcinoma (HCC).

The risk of spontaneous HBV reinfection after transplantation is around 80%. The pretransplant HBV DNA status, traditionally detected using conventional hybridization techniques or now as $>10^5$ copies/mL using a quantitative polymerase chain reaction (PCR) technique, is the best predictor of HBV recurrence after transplantation. HBV reinfection is the consequence of either an immediate reinfection of the graft due to circulating HBV particles, or of a reinfection of the graft from HBV particles coming from extrahepatic sites. Reinfection of the graft in patients receiving anti-hepatitis B surface immunoglobulin (HBIg) is probably related to HBV in extrahepatic sites. It may be the consequence of HBV overproduction at these extrahepatic sites, a low protective titer of HBIg or emergence of escape mutants. This latter mechanism is probably important since mutations in the pre-S/S genome of HBV and in the 'a' determinant have been described.

HBV reinfection is characterized by the reappearance of HBsAg and HBV DNA in the serum. After HBsAg reappearance, HBV replication levels are usually high, and large quantities of HBV particles are present in the graft. Almost all patients reinfected with HBV will develop disease; most commonly an acute lobular hepatitis which evolves to chronic hepatitis. Some cases follow a particularly severe clinical course leading to acute liver failure, probably related to the high amount of HBsAg, HBeAg and hepatitis B core antigen (HBcAg) in the nuclei and cytoplasm of the hepatocytes. This form of post-transplant liver disease is termed fibrosing cholestatic hepatitis and is a unique histologic disease that is only seen in immunosuppressed patients. A similar disease has been shown to occur with hepatitis C (HCV).

The initial strategy developed to prevent HBV reinfection of the allograft was the administration of polyclonal HBIg (see also Ch. 42). Early studies of the use of HBIg during the anhepatic phase and short-term post-transplant period yielded disappointing results as most of the patients developed HBV reinfection (**Table 37.3**).

However, subsequent studies of the long-term administration of high doses of HBIg dramatically reduced the rate of HBV reinfection and disease recurrence. In a European multicenter study, the effect of long-term administration of HBIg produced a dramatic decrease in the rate of HBV reinfection from 75% in

HBV recurrence rate in relation to initial liver disease and HBV Ig administration			
Liver disease	No Ig (%)	Short-term Ig (%)	Long-term Ig (%)
HBV cirrhosis*	78	90	56
HBV DNA, HBeAg+	75	71	70
HBV DNA, HBeAg–	66	92	37
HDV cirrhosis*	70	56	17
FHF B	56	ND	0

Table 37.3 Hepatitis B virus recurrence rate in relation to initial liver disease and HBIg administration. *P <0.001. FHF, fulminant hepatic failure B. (From Samuel et al. N Engl J Med. 1993;329:1842–7.)

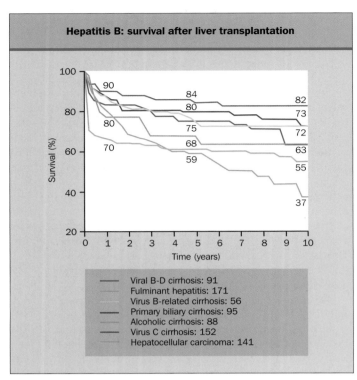

Figure 37.16 Hepatitis B: survival after liver transplantation. Actuarial 10-year survival after liver transplantation at Paul Brousse Hospital in 1106 patients transplanted from June 1984 to June 1997 in relation to the initial liver disease. Observe that using a policy of giving long-term administration of anti-hepatitis B surface immunoglobulin (HBIg), patients with B-D cirrhosis have the highest survival and those with B and C cirrhosis have the same survival. Patients who have hepatocellular carcinoma have the lowest survival and those with fulminant hepatitis have the lowest short-term survival due to higher postoperative mortality, but a relative stable survival curve in the long term. Numbers in key refer to number of patients in each group.

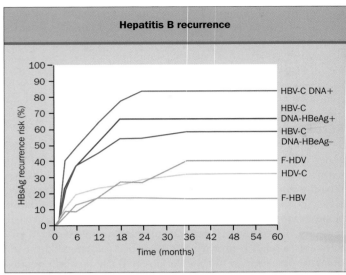

Figure 37.17 Hepatitis B recurrence. Hepatitis B virus (HBV) recurrence risk in relation with the initial liver disease in a multicenter European trial on 372 patients. Note that patients with fulminant hepatitis B (F-HBV) have a 17% risk, those with B-D cirrhosis [hepatitis D virus (HDV)-C] a 32% risk, those with fulminant B-D hepatitis (F-HDV) a 40% risk, and those with B cirrhosis (HBV-C) a 67% risk (*P*<0.01). Among the group of patients with HBV-C, the risk of recurrence was significantly higher in those who were HBV DNA-positive (80%), than in those who were HBV DNA and hepatitis B e antigen (HBeAg)-negative. Reproduced from Samuel et al (93) by permission of the Massachusetts Medical Society.

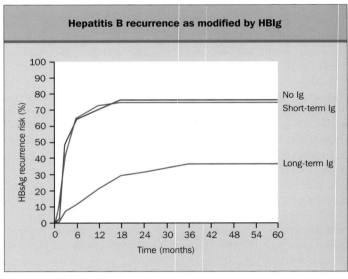

Figure 37.18 Hepatitis B recurrence as modified by HBIg. Hepatitis B virus (HBV) recurrence risk in relation to the administration of anti-hepatitis B surface immunoglobulin (HBIg) in a multicenter European trial. Note that patients receiving at least 6 months of HBIg have a significantly lower risk of HBV recurrence (32%) in contrast to those who receive either no or short-term prophylaxis (80% rate of HBV recurrence). Reproduced from Samuel et al (93) by permission of the Massachusetts Medical Society.

patients receiving no or short-term administration of HBIg, to 33% in those receiving long-term administration of HBIg. In the most aggressive protocols, up to 10 000 IU of HBIg was given during the anhepatic phase, and repeated daily during the first six postoperative days. The level of anti-HBs was determined weekly and repeated doses of HBIg were given when anti-HBs levels fell below 100 IU/L. This approach reduced the overall actuarial rates of reappearance of HBsAg in patients who had HBV cirrhosis to 17 and 29% at 1 and 2 years, respectively (**Figs 37.16–37.19**).

It is the standard to inhibit viral replication with antiviral therapy before transplantation, in order to clear HBV DNA from serum (see also Ch. 42). An ideal treatment should have a rapid and potent antiviral action without provoking a deterioration of liver function. Lamivudine, a nucleoside analog, is the most effective currently available drug to clear HBV DNA from the serum in patients who have cirrhosis awaiting liver transplantation. The drug, even when given alone, is well tolerated and is associated with a low rate of HBV reinfection. However, the major limitation to lamivudine therapy is acquired resistance, which occurs at a rate of 20–30% of patients per year. Severe disease can develop in patients developing mutations in the YMDD motif of the HBV DNA polymerase. Fortunately, new antivirals have been developed that are

effective against lamivudine-induced HBV mutants and can rescue patients who develop liver disease in this setting. Adefovir dipivoxil is one such agent. It is also well tolerated but has some risk of renal toxicity and the dose must be adjusted for

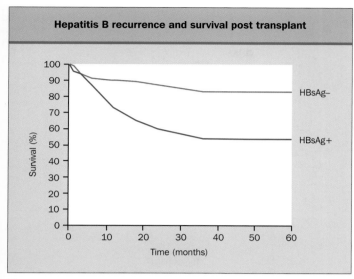

Figure 37.19 Hepatitis B recurrence and survival post-transplant. Actuarial survival in patients in relation to hepatitis B virus (HBV) recurrence in a multicenter European trial. Those HBV recurrence [hepatitis B surface antigen-positive (HBsAg+)] have a significantly lower survival rate, mostly due to HBV recurrence, than those without recurrence. This underlines the importance of prophylaxis against HBV. Reproduced from Samuel et al (93) by permission of the Massachusetts Medical Society.

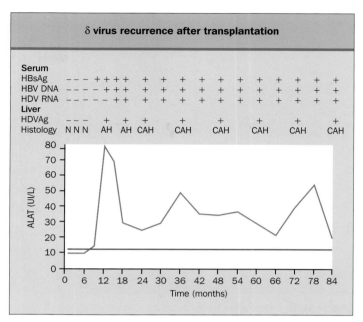

Figure 37.20 δ virus recurrence after transplantation. Classic course of a patient transplanted for B-D liver cirrhosis with hepatitis B virus (HBV) recurrence. Note the concomitant reactivation of B and D infection and the development of chronic B-D hepatitis on the graft. This outcome is present in 10–15% of cases when anti-hepatitis B surface immunoglobulin (HBIg) is administered after transplantation. (From Samuel personal communication.)

renal function. The onset of action is relatively slow compared to lamivudine but the rate of resistance is much lower (1–3% per year) and it is an excellent antiviral over the long term. Several additional antivirals (e.g. tenofovir and entecavir) with similarly low rates of resistance but with a more rapid onset of action are likely to be in clinic use in the near future. The level of anti-HBs antibody that needs to be maintained in serum with HBIg monotherapy is a subject of debate. There was a general agreement that it should be at least 100 IU/L, but this level may be insufficient in patients at high risk of recurrence such as HBV DNA-positive cirrhotic patients. In this setting, the maintenance of anti-HBs antibody over 500 IU/L may be able to prevent HBV recurrence, but this approach is very expensive. It is now clear that when HBIg is combined with an antiviral, much lower doses of HBIg are required to yield extremely low rates (<5%) of HBV reinfection. For example, a protocol developed by the Australia–New Zealand Liver Transplant Study Group has shown that doses as low as 400–800 per month can be extremely effective. Moreover, there are protocols being developed that combine active vaccination with antiviral therapy to generate endogenous anti-HBs production.

Finally, it does appear that some patients on antiviral therapy can have HBIg discontinued with a low risk of reinfection. This seems certainly true for those who are HBV DNA-negative by a PCR assay. In the future, it may be that combination antviral therapy with replace HBIg use.

Hepatitis B and D

Patients chronically infected with HBV and hepatitis D virus (HDV) are at substantially lower risk of HBsAg reappearance than patients chronically infected with HBV alone, and if re-infection does occur, the disease is less devastating than in patients who have solitary HBV infection. The rate of HBsAg

reappearance in patients who have hepatitis B and D-associated cirrhosis was around 50–60% in patients who did not receive long-term administration of HBIg, and 13–17% in those receiving HBIg. The overall lower HBV recurrence rate in these patients compared with HBV cirrhotic patients is probably due to the fact that almost all patients who have HDV cirrhosis are HBV DNA-negative at the time of liver transplantation and that HDV has an inhibitory effect on HBV replication.

In this group of patients, there is a risk of reinfection with either HBV or HDV or with both viruses. The course of HDV reinfection and its consequences on the graft are different depending on whether HBsAg reappears or not. In the first post-transplant months, HDV reinfection assessed by the presence of HDV RNA in the serum or in the liver was observed in 80% of cases. With HBV recurrence, there is viral reactivation of both viruses (**Fig. 37.20**), but HBV–HDV recurrence is in general less severe than HBV recurrence alone. In patients who remained HBsAg-negative after transplantation, HDV RNA was found transiently in serum and HDV antigen was detected in the liver. However, the amount of HDV antigen in the graft was low, the graft was histologically normal, and ultimately HDV markers progressively disappeared from the liver and serum (**Fig. 37.21**).

Hepatitis C

Liver disease due to HCV is currently the most common indication for liver transplantation in both Europe and the USA. Patient selection for liver transplantation is based on the same criteria as other causes of viral cirrhosis. The major issue after liver transplantation is disease recurrence. HCV RNA is found in more than 95% of patients transplanted for HCV cirrhosis, and HCV RNA levels increase rapidly after liver transplantation,

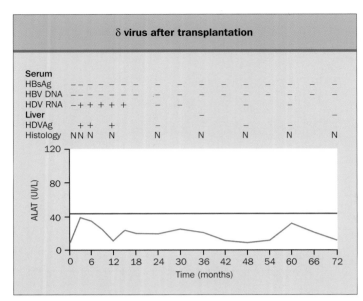

Figure 37.21 δ virus after transplantation. Classical course of a patient transplanted for B-D liver cirrhosis without hepatitis B virus (HBV) recurrence. Note the presences of D antigen in the liver and hepatitis D virus (HDV) RNA in serum in the first months, despite the absence of hepatitis B surface antigen (HBsAg) in serum; however there are no graft lesions and HDV markers disappeared after 2 years. This outcome is present in 85–90% of cases when hepatitis B immunoglobulin (HBIg) is administered after transplantation. (From Samuel personal communication.)

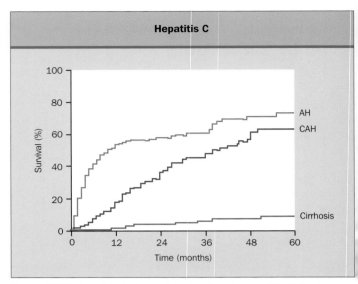

Figure 37.22 Hepatitis C. Actuarial rate of acute hepatitis (AH), chronic hepatitis (CAH), and cirrhosis in 140 patients transplanted at Paul Brousse hospital for HCV cirrhosis. Despite a 75% survival rate at 5 years, this emphasizes the need for a prevention of HCV recurrence after transplantation. Reproduced from Feray et al (94) by permission of Wiley-Liss, Inc.

reaching pretransplant levels as early as 1 week post-transplantation. The actuarial rate of occurrence of acute lobular hepatitis is 57% at 1 year and 72% at 5 years post-transplant. The actuarial rate of occurrence of chronic hepatitis was 25% at 1 year and 60% at 4 years after the occurrence of acute lobular hepatitis; 8–20% of the patients developed liver cirrhosis within 5 years of follow-up (**Fig. 37.22**). Some data suggest the recurrent disease may be increasing in severity over the past decade, although this is not generally accepted. However, it should be emphasized that the majority of the reinfected patients have a benign course and 20–40% of the patients have minimal or no lesions on histologic assessment of the graft. The actuarial 5-year patient survival rate is quite good, in the order of 75–80%.

After transplantation, HCV RNA levels increase by 10- to 100-fold, a likely consequence of immunosuppressive therapy. The severity of HCV recurrence appears to be related to both the level of HCV viremia before and consequently after trans-plantation. Other factors associated with poorer outcomes include age, more advanced liver disease, Black race, cytomegalovirus (CMV) seropositivity and more advanced pretransplant disease.

Methods to prevent HCV infection after transplantation have yet to be identified and the long-term outcome remains unclear (see also Ch. 42). Treatment of HCV pretransplantation in patients with advanced disease using interferons and ribavirin is often challenging because of side-effects. Nonetheless, one group has obtained sustained virologic responses in around 20% of patients on waiting lists using escalating doses of both inter-feron and ribavirin. The likelihood of response was around four-fold greater in those with genotype 2 and 3 as compared to those with genotype 1. In those who were subsequently transplanted, 70–80% failed to develop reinfection. Unfortunately, only a minority of patients can tolerate a full course of therapy and

thus, the search for alternative ways to prevent reinfection will continue.

ALCOHOLIC LIVER DISEASE

While alcoholic cirrhosis is a frequent cause of liver disease it accounts for a relatively small proportion of liver transplant activity. Alcohol is the second most common indication for liver transplantation in USA and Europe after HCV related liver disease. Current data indicate that with 11 000 deaths from alcoholic cirrhosis in the USA/year, only 6% of cases are receiving liver transplants. Given the limited supply of donor organs and some reluctance to transplant patients who have a 'self-inflicted' illness, several centers have developed an evaluation process (based on medical and psychiatric criteria) to identify patients who would most benefit from transplantation. The number of patients from the population who have alcohol-related cirrhosis that are candidates for liver transplantation is still limited. There are several reasons for this.

- Although alcoholic disease itself is not a contraindication, many community physicians do not refer these patients for liver transplantation, and some centers are reluctant to trans-plant these patients, due to a concern about the ethics and legitimacy of the procedure and the risk of recidivism.
- In many patients, cirrhosis develops at a later age when trans-plantation is contraindicated.
- Alcohol is also the cause of extrahepatic diseases that will not be treated by transplantation. In addition, alcoholic patients appear to be at increase risk for post-transplant malignancies.
- Most centers demand a 6-month period of abstinence from alcohol before intervention.
- Some patients may show behavior patterns that suggest the compliance with long-term immunosuppressive therapy may be erratic.

• It is still difficult to determine the prognosis of patients who have alcoholic liver disease as a dramatic clinical improvement can occur after 6 or more months of abstinence from alcohol.

In this context, guidelines for patient selection are currently directed at cirrhotic patients whose liver disease remains life-threatening despite a minimal period of 6 months of abstinence. This permits a re-evaluation of the need for, and timing of, liver transplantation and gives some insight into the patient's ability to abstain from alcohol. This interval has not achieved consensus as some programs do not adhere to such requirements while others require a longer period of abstinence. Some period of sobriety is important, but it should not be used as the sole criterion for selection and should be considered along with other psychosocial predictors of abstinence. In some cases the required duration of abstinence will allow some patients to escape transplantation because of a marked improvement of liver function. Patients participating in an alcohol-counseling program with a stable and favorable psychosocial supportive environment are most often capable of avoiding recidivism and non-compliance with immunosuppressive therapy.

Acute alcoholic hepatitis is currently regarded as a contraindication in most centers because the majority of patients is actively drinking at the time of presentation and has a higher risk of recidivism. Consequently, scarce donor organs would be allocated to patients who have a predictably inferior medical and psychiatric outcome. In selected cases, in whom the 6-month period of abstinence is impossible to achieve because of the severity of the liver disease, candidacy for liver transplantation should be addressed on an individual basis. A positive selection decision needs to be supported by a self-recognition of alcoholism with a real desire for long-term cessation of alcohol consumption, in addition to a strong psychosocial and family support network and a positive appraisal by a psychiatrist.

Several reports suggest that the short-term outcome of liver transplantation in alcoholic cirrhosis is equivalent to that in non-alcoholics, although the prognosis is unclear in patients who have acute alcoholic hepatitis. The risk of recidivism of alcoholism is estimated between 15 and 40% and it seems to be related to the duration of abstinence before transplantation and the duration of follow-up after transplantation. Most patients with recidivism have a moderate drinking pattern after transplantation without consequences to the graft, but 5–10% of patients experience severe consequences of recidivism including non-compliance with medications, steatosis, and ultimately loss of the graft. The recidivism rates indicate the importance of stringent selection criteria in this context. Psychosocial support and participation in alcohol treatment after transplantation is clearly needed. Additional studies of large numbers of patients are needed to determine the long-term relapse rate with regard to alcohol consumption. An increased rate of de novo cancer has been observed in patients transplanted for alcoholic cirrhosis, but its impact on long-term outcomes is not well defined.

AUTOIMMUNE HEPATITIS AND CIRRHOSIS

The clinical presentation of the autoimmune hepatitis is variable, classically presenting as chronic hepatitis, but it may also present with established cirrhosis and in a few cases as acute liver failure. The main characteristic of this disease is a good response to immunosuppressive treatment with steroids and azathioprine, particularly in type 1 patients.

Liver transplantation is indicated when there is clinical deterioration including the development of cirrhosis, esophageal varices and impaired coagulation despite long-term adequate immunosuppressive treatment. More urgent clinical conditions include resistant ascites, spontaneous bacterial peritonitis and encephalopathy. In this condition, it is essential to evaluate the severity as well as the activity of the disease. The level of liver enzymes and the histologic evaluation of the inflammatory infiltrate, together with intensity of hepatocyte necrosis and fibrosis, help to decide whether additional immunosuppressive treatment might improve the clinical condition and as a result postpone the need for transplantation. A short course of additional immunosuppressive treatment could be introduced under cautious supervision by transplant physicians, and in the absence of improvement, liver transplantation is indicated. Acute liver failure, in which immunosuppressive treatment is usually ineffective and potentially deleterious, is an indication for emergency liver transplantation.

The results of liver transplantation for autoimmune hepatitis are usually excellent with a 5-year survival rate over 80%. A higher risk of rejection has been reported and the role of corticosteroid treatment before transplantation in the occurrence of rejection has been debated. Well-documented cases of recurrence have been described, but they usually respond to an increase in the corticosteroid component of the immunosuppressive regimen and rarely lead to graft failure and retransplantation of the liver.

HEPATOBILIARY MALIGNANCY

From the earliest days of liver transplantation, hepatobiliary malignancy was a favored indication for liver transplantation (**Fig. 37.23**). However, that early experience yielded results that were inferior to those transplanted for other liver diseases. The key concepts in the evaluation of the role of transplantation are the different tumor types and volumes, risk of tumor recurrence, donor organ shortage, the associated liver disease and the role of immunosuppression in promoting tumor growth. Contraindications

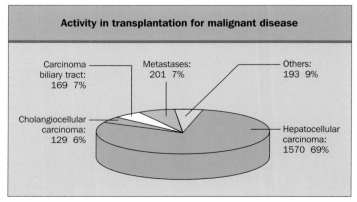

Figure 37.23 Activity in transplantation for malignant disease. The breakdown of indications shows a predominance of patients with hepatocellular carcinoma. Reproduced from The European Liver Registry Report.

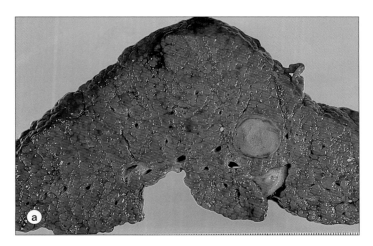

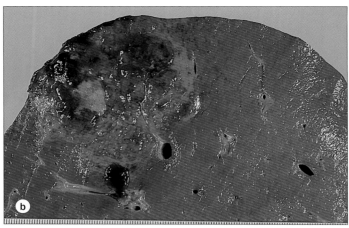

Figure 37.24 Transplantation for hepatocellular carcinoma. (a) The small, singular, circumscribed tumor in a patient with cirrhosis is an ideal candidate for transplantation, but the large tumor arising in a non-cirrhotic liver (b) is no longer considered a good risk patient. (Courtesy of Professor B. Portmann.)

to liver transplantation are advanced primary liver tumors with any extrahepatic spread, hemangiosarcoma and liver metastases from non-neuroendocrine primary tumors.

Hepatocellular carcinoma

HCC, when left untreated, has an extremely poor prognosis with only 1–24 months survival from the time of diagnosis. Early enthusiasm for this indication for transplantation was frustrated by the high incidence of tumor recurrence, in excess of 50%, over 1–2 years of follow-up. Although there is some variability, most centers currently practice a restrictive policy for transplantation for HCC (**Fig. 37.24**).

Improved patient selection criteria have led to better results. The so-called Milan Criteria are those most commonly used which include patients with a single lesion <5 cm in diameter, who have three or fewer nodules that are smaller than 3 cm in diameter, in the absence of lymph node metastases or vascular invasion (**Table 37.4**). While the Milan Criteria are most widely accepted, some groups have expanded the criteria to single lesions of up to 6.5 cm or three or less lesions each up to 5 cm in diameter. However, it is important to note that these studies are retrospective analysis based on pathologic data. The Milan Criteria, by contrast, have stood the test of time for clinical staging. Moreover, many of the programs which advocate expanding the HCC criteria used the Milan Criteria to select patients. Unfortunately this demonstrates that clinical staging can both underestimate, as well as overestimate, the amount of tumor present. Until prospective studies can show that using the expanded criteria as clinical staging still yields good results, it is hard to recommend revision of the selection criteria. From a practical standpoint, in the USA in the MELD era, patients with HCC would require more MELD points than they would receive based on liver function to achieve sufficient priority for deceased donor transplantation. The criteria for awarding additional MELD points are based on the Milan Criteria.

Overall 3-year survival rate and survival without recurrence in patients with hepatocellular carcinoma				
Liver disease	Resection (n=60)		Transplantation (n=60)	
	Survival (%)	Recurrence free survival (%)	Survival (%)	Recurrence free survival (%)
All patients	52	27	49	46
Size				
<3 cm	39	18	60	56*
>3 cm	56	32	43	39*
No. nodules				
1	53	28	46	20
>1	46	20	51	49
Combination				
< 3 cm and 1–2 nodules	41	18	83	83
> 3 cm and > 2 nodules			46	44

Table 37.4 Overall 3-year survival rate and survival without recurrence in patients with hepatocellular carcinoma treated by resection or transplantation in relation to the size and the number of nodules. Note the excellent survival in those transplanted with less than three nodules of <3 cm. *P <0.05. (From Bismuth et al. Ann Surg. 1993;218:145–51.)

Tumor invasion of the portal vein leading to intrahepatic metastasis is the most common means of HCC spread. A relationship between the risk of tumor recurrence and the presence of portal vein involvement has been established. The risk of recurrence was 100% when the tumor involved the main portal vein or the two main intrahepatic portal branches. Although the recurrence rate was lower in cases of involvement of a smaller portal branch, the risk remained significant and this should be considered as a negative prognostic factor. For this reason, the possible involvement of the portal vein or its branches with a tumor needs to be carefully evaluated in potential transplant candidates.

Preoperative evaluation must include at least a computed tomography (CT) scan of the abdomen and chest, and perhaps a bone scan. In the USA, patients are restaged at 3-month intervals after registering on the United Network for Organ Sharing (UNOS) waiting list in order to continue to receive additional MELD points. Some centers perform an exploratory laparotomy before transplantation, in order to confirm the absence of extrahepatic spread. As soon as the transplant procedure begins, it is essential to look for any sign of extrahepatic disease and to carefully inspect the hepatic pedicle for the presence of pathologic lymph nodes. A perioperative histologic analysis of suspicious tissue is mandatory, and the procedure should be abandoned before the hepatectomy in cases of confirmed extrahepatic spread. Despite the uncertain long-term benefit in some cases, and the need to compare carefully the results obtained from liver transplantation with those of other methods (e.g. early resection, alcohol injection, chemoembolization, radiofrequency ablation), it is clear that liver transplantation is the only possible curative option in many cases of HCC associated with cirrhosis. The procedure in patients who have early disease is associated with a recurrence rate of 10% and a 5-year survival rate of 75%, which is similar to that achieved for other indications for liver transplantation.

Fibrolamellar carcinoma

This is a particular histologic variant of HCC that is more common in young women who do not have underlying liver disease. The treatment of choice is liver resection, where one can be quite aggressive because of the absence of underlying liver disease. When a partial hepatectomy is not possible, liver transplantation is a good option, although there is a significant risk of recurrence since these tumors tend to be large at presentation and at transplantation. However, the slower tumor growth rates result in a significant period of survival for those requiring transplantation, even when the tumor eventually recurs. Whether the prognosis is better than in those with standard HCC is not clear.

Cholangiocarcinoma

Cholangiocarcinoma is the second most common cancer among the primary hepatic neoplasms, accounting for 5–20% of liver malignancies. The ones that arise from the epithelium of the intrahepatic bile ducts are called 'true' cholangiocarcinomas as opposed to those that arise from the extrahepatic biliary tree. A clear association between cholangiocarcinoma and PSC has been established, and the occurrence of cholangiocarcinoma seems to correlate with the duration of the latter disease. Nowadays there is considerable debate about the indications for, and results of, transplantation for this kind of tumor. Liver transplantation

does not offer either a cure or a significant duration of palliation in the majority of patients. This may be due to the fact that many of these tumors are diagnosed at an advanced stage, when the disease has metastasized to the lymph nodes. In the absence of lymph node disease, 1-year, 2-year and 3-year survival rates of 77, 64 and 51% were observed, respectively. On the other hand, with lymph node disease the 1-year survival rate dropped to 14%, and the 2-year survival rate was 0%.

Recently, the Mayo Clinic has reported very good results in a select group of patients with cholangiocarcinoma using aggressive external beam and intraductal radiation therapy, with chemotherapy in patients without evidence of extraductal disease. After this therapy, patients are explored and only those in whom no residual disease can be demonstrated are put on a waiting list and are granted additional MELD points. With this approach, they have attained medium-term survival rates of 80–85%. However, it must be emphasized that a very small minority of patients with cholangiocarcinoma will qualify for transplantation with this approach.

Epithelioid hemangioendothelioma

Epithelioid hemangioendothelioma is a rare tumor of the liver that is generally multifocal and has an endothelial origin. It is more common in younger adults and is usually quite indolent in nature. In the absence of extrahepatic dissemination, liver transplantation should be considered. In an experience of 10 patients, the 3-month survival rate was 89%, with 3-year survival rates of 76%. The recurrence rate was 30%, although little is known about the factors affecting survival and recurrence following liver transplantation. It should be noted that metastatic spread at the time of surgery does not appear to be an absolute contraindication to transplantation, and this is distinctly different from the situation in patients who have HCC or cholangiocarcinoma. Given that these tumors have a relatively benign natural history, even when untreated, the major selection issue is to identify the few individuals who will experience a survival benefit.

Metastatic liver disease

Classically, metastatic tumors of the liver have been considered a poor indication for liver transplantation, although some centers have performed this procedure in conjunction with other therapies, such as chemotherapy and radiotherapy particularly in individuals with neuroendocrine tumors. Most series have demonstrated an unacceptably high recurrence rate with non-endocrine metastases that did not justify the cost of the procedure and utilization of scarce donor organs. On the other hand, in metastases from neuroendocrine tumors, liver transplantation could be indicated for patients who have symptoms related to massive hepatomegaly or syndromes related to hormone production. Effective therapeutic alternatives are usually not available and the typical candidate for transplantation has diffuse metastases of the liver, slow-growing tumors and no extrahepatic disease. The main advantages of transplantation are a significant improvement of the quality of life in many patients and a possible cure in some of them. However, an inadequate knowledge of specific biologic and pathologic prognosis factors, the possibility of tumor growth as a consequence of immunosuppression, and the shortage of donor organs are key issues that counterbalance the argument in favor of transplantation. While the results to date have been mixed, it is believed that long-term follow-up will determine the utility of liver transplantation for neuro-endocrine liver metastases.

BUDD-CHIARI SYNDROME

The Budd-Chiari syndrome is a clinical disorder with a broad clinical spectrum resulting from the occlusion of the main hepatic veins at their junction with the inferior vena cava. It is similar clinically to veno-occlusive disease of the liver, although the latter most commonly occurs in the setting of bone marrow transplantation or occasionally due to certain hepatotoxins. The diagnosis is suggested by the absence of flow in the hepatic veins on ultrasonography and confirmed by the demonstration of thrombus on retrograde hepatic venography, together with changes in liver morphology.

A surgical portosystemic shunt, principally TIPS or a meso-caval shunt, is the most commonly used treatment in all acute and subacute forms that have not responded to other treatments. The effect of portosystemic shunting is to reduce portal pressure and induce reversal of the flow in the portal vein. The liver congestion is relieved, preserving hepatocytes and allowing liver regeneration. This ultimately leads to a reduction in ascites formation.

The first liver transplantation for Budd-Chiari syndrome was performed in 1974, and the European Liver Transplant Registry recorded 224 liver transplantations for this disease from January 1988 to June 1997. The indications for liver transplantation are the fulminant form of the disease associated with liver failure, which usually does not respond to mesocaval shunt surgery, and the chronic stage with established cirrhosis and its complications despite shunt procedures.

Although the choice of transplantation is appropriate for end-stage cirrhotic disease, it is difficult to ignore the efficacy of the long-term results of portosystemic shunting in Budd-Chiari syndrome. Conclusions on the benefits of one treatment over another might be difficult due to the rarity of the disease, the wide variety of precipitating diseases and the diversity of the clinical conditions. The final decision should be made taking into account the causative disease, a careful assessment of the degree of hepatic venous occlusion, and a precise grading of the clinical form of the disease and the hepatic dysfunction. The same is true for veno-occlusive disease. If liver transplantation is performed, it is essential to identify and treat associated pro-thrombotic disease and adhere to a rigid protocol for long-term anticoagulant therapy.

CYSTIC FIBROSIS

Cystic fibrosis is a multisystemic genetic disease with a gene carrier rate of 5% in the population. In spite of new medical therapies, life expectancy is approximately 50% at 30 years. Cirrhosis occurs in 5–15% of patients who have cystic fibrosis, with an onset in the first decade of life and later progression to portal hypertension, hypersplenism and variceal bleeding. For these patients, liver transplantation, isolated or in combination with lung or heart-lung transplantation, is the only effective treatment option to prolong survival and the quality of life. Questions have been raised regarding the suitability of such candidates for liver transplantation, because these patients are often in a poor nutritional condition as a result of severe intestinal

malabsorption and chronic infection with highly resistant bacteria. However, postoperative management does not differ significantly from that of other patients undergoing liver transplantation, except for special attention to pulmonary care, nutritional management and the risk of malabsorption of immuno-suppressive drugs.

CAROLI DISEASE

Caroli disease is an uncommon congenital disorder of the intra-hepatic biliary tree. It is characterized by multiple and segmental dilatations of the bile ducts. The clinical course is often complicated by recurrent episodes of cholangitis that seriously impair the patient's quality of life. Abdominal pain may be quite severe in some cases. Patients may also develop progressive fibrosis and portal hypertension. Treatment is difficult and depends on the location and extent of the disease. Medical treatment is worthless because bile duct dilatation and gallstone formation favor bacterial persistence after the initial colonization of the biliary tree. Antimicrobial agents provide temporary improvement, but recurrence is the rule after cessation of this therapy. Bacterial cholangitis is the most frequent and life-threatening complication of the disease. Consequently, due to poor results of both medical and surgical therapies, liver transplantation has been proposed in complicated Caroli disease that is diffuse within the liver. However, only a relatively small number of cases have been reported.

METABOLIC DISEASES

Wilson disease

In this disease, there is copper deposition in the liver, the central nervous system and the kidneys. This autosomal recessive hereditary disease is secondary to a gene mutation on chromosome 13 and results in an inability to excrete copper in bile and consequently copper accumulates in the liver. There are five main clinical presentations of liver disease:

- chronic hepatitis with a moderate increase in aminotransferases;
- decompensated liver cirrhosis with ascites and liver failure;
- acute liver failure with impaired coagulation, hemolytic anemia and encephalopathy;
- absence of clinical liver disease with a neurologic presentation or other manifestations; and
- following the diagnosis of Wilson disease in a sibling.

Most frequently, this disease is medically treatable and the drugs of choice are D-penicillamine and trientene, which act as chelators of copper and as a detoxificant of copper overload in hepatocytes. This therapy may arrest further progression of the disease and promote possible reversal of the clinical manifestations. However, liver transplantation may be indicated in the following situations:

- a fulminant course that almost invariably requires urgent transplantation;
- patients who have cirrhosis who fail to respond to 2–3 months of copper chelation therapy and supportive therapy for associated complications;
- progression of the disease despite chelation therapy; and
- severe hepatic failure and hemolysis after discontinuation of chelation therapy.

Generally, after liver transplantation, the copper balance is restored and there might be an improvement in both the neurologic and renal complications of the disease, although this is not a certainty. The prognosis is good with no evidence of reaccumulation of hepatic copper.

α_1-Antitrypsin deficiency

The diagnosis is made by the finding of a significant reduction of serum α_1-antitrypsin levels, a positive Pi ZZ phenotype, and a diagnostic liver biopsy with periodic acid-Schiff-positive diastase-resistant cytoplasmic globules. One-quarter of children who have the Pi ZZ phenotype will develop neonatal cholestasis and among this group, 50% will develop progressive liver failure at some time during childhood or adolescence. More than 50% of adults have coexistent pulmonary disease associated with α_1-antitrypsin deficiency, but the lung disease is usually mild. Clinical signs of neonatal cholestasis appear during the first days of life and are usually evident before 10 weeks of age. As there is no effective replacement therapy, liver transplantation is indicated in patients who have cirrhosis and progressive hepatic decompensation. After liver transplantation, the α_1-antitrypsin level returns to normal and the 5-year actuarial survival rate after transplantation is higher than 80%.

Hereditary tyrosinemia

This disease is characterized by progressive hepatocellular damage, renal tubular dysfunction, hypophosphatemia, and urinary excretion at concentrations of more than 100 times the normal rate of the tyrosine metabolite succinylacetone. Hepatic fibrosis develops with prominent regeneration nodules, leading to cirrhosis. Survival beyond the age of 10 years is rare. Up to 37% of children over the age of 2 years will develop HCC.

Medical treatment has not proved to be effective. Liver transplantation corrects the biochemical abnormalities and allows patients to have a normal protein intake. In patients presenting with the disease in early infancy, transplantation should be postponed for as long as possible to allow the baby to grow. In those who have a later onset of symptoms, the timing of grafting is difficult as delay may increase the risk of developing HCC. Prospective screening with ultrasound examination of the liver and serum α-fetoprotein estimates may be useful to detect tumors early enough to allow liver transplantation.

Crigler-Najjar syndrome

This is an inherited disorder that occurs in two forms (type I and II), characterized by severe, life-long, non-hemolytic, unconjugated hyperbilirubinemia. Liver transplantation is not generally indicated in the type II syndrome, which can be treated with continuous phenobarbital therapy. In type I syndrome, the serum bilirubin concentration does not decrease when phenobarbital is administered. The majority of infants will develop kernicterus and brain damage in the first 18 months of life, but the onset of kernicterus and progressive brain damage may be delayed until puberty or the early twenties. Liver transplantation may be indicated when there is failure to prevent the kernicterus despite extensive phototherapy, or in cases because of poor quality of life due to the need for prolonged phototherapy. Auxiliary partial

OLT has also been performed successfully. As irreversible brain damage has been described, the optimal timing for liver transplantation is important, in order to reduce neurologic sequelae and improve survival and quality of life after transplantation.

Hereditary hemochromatosis

Hereditary hemochromatosis is a recessive autosomal disorder leading to iron overload with a disease frequency of 5/1000 population. The disease is secondary in 95% of cases to a point mutation (C282Y) in the HFE gene located on chromosome 6. It is characterized by increased intestinal iron absorption with deposition of parenchymal iron in the liver, heart, pancreas, pituitary and joints, and a potential risk for developing cirrhosis and HCC. Liver transplantation is indicated for hemochromatosis complicated by liver failure or the presence of HCC not treatable by resection. However, the survival of patients undergoing liver transplantation for hemochromatosis is less favorable, due to cardiac involvement and the frequent coexistence of HCC. Pretransplant phlebotomy to reduce cardiac complications needs to be carefully evaluated, to determine whether it can improve survival after liver transplantation. The risk of re-appearance of iron deposits in the liver is debatable.

Protoporphyria

This is an autosomal dominant disorder characterized by photosensitivity and elevated levels of protoporphyrin in erythrocytes, plasma and feces. It is secondary to a deficiency in an enzyme responsible for heme synthesis called heme synthase or ferrochelatase. The pathogenesis of liver disease is still unclear, but is probably the consequence of accumulation of protoporphyrin pigments in the liver. Liver transplantation should be considered when jaundice, recurrent cholangitis or liver failure occurs. After transplantation a dramatic, but partial, decrease in plasma and erythrocyte levels of protoporphyrins is obtained, and this leads to a partial or complete resolution of photosensitivity. Some patients may develop recurrent disease in the graft, but long-term survival without recurrence has also been described.

Primary hyperoxaluria

Primary hyperoxaluria is a rare autosomal recessive disorder characterized by hyperoxaluria, calcium oxalate urinary lithiasis, nephrocalcinosis and consequent renal failure. There are at least two types, and type 1 is much more common and well-studied. Type 1 primary hyperoxaluria is secondary to a hepatic deficit in alanine-glyoxylate aminotransferase deficiency. Once renal failure occurs there is a dramatic acceleration in the rate of oxalate accumulation. Renal transplantation in isolation results in almost universal recurrence of oxalosis in the kidney graft and a return to hemodialysis after varying intervals. Combined liver and kidney transplantation treats both the renal failure and cures the cause of the disease, and this approach may avoid recurrence of oxalosis in the kidney graft. However, this presumes the kidney graft functions sufficiently well to clear the excess pool of calcium oxalate, but this does not necessarily happen before further damage to the graft occurs. Combined liver and kidney transplantation should be performed before the occurrence of severe complications and the ideal timing is just before or immediately after the patients are initiated on hemodialysis. Long periods of hemodialysis will significantly increase

Indications for liver transplantation in children	
Chronic liver disease	Cholestatic diseases
	Extrahepatic biliary atresia
	Byler disease
	Ductopenia (nonsyndromic)
	Alagille syndrome
	Primary sclerosing cholangitis
	Autoimmune chronic hepatitis
	Viral B cirrhosis
	Budd–Chiari syndrome
Metabolic liver disease	α_1-antitrypsin defeciency
	Hereditary tyrosinemia
	Crigler–Najjar type 1
	Protoporphyria
	Type 1 and 4 glycogenosis
	Galactosemia
Primary malignant tumor of the liver	Hepatocellular carcinoma
	Hepatoblastoma
	Cholangiocellular carcinoma
Acute liver failure	Fulminant and subfulminant hepatitis
	Wilson disease (fulminant)
	Budd–Chiari syndrome (fulminant)

Table 37.5 Indications for liver transplantation in children.

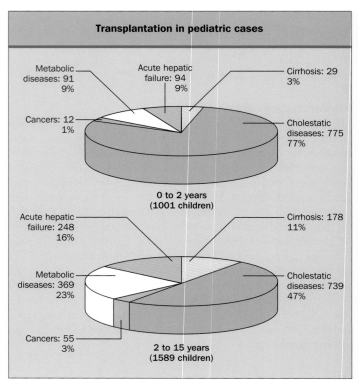

Figure 37.25 Transplantation in pediatric cases. The indications for liver transplantation up to the age of 2 years and in older children. Modified from The European Liver Registry Report.

the pool of calcium oxalate in the body. Some authors have advocated an isolated liver transplantation early in the course of the disease before the occurrence of renal failure, but this preemptive therapeutic approach remains controversial.

Familial amyloidosis with polyneuropathy

This is an autosomal dominant systemic disease usually predominantly involving the peripheral nervous system. The commonest genetic defect is a single mutation located on chromosome 18, leading to the synthesis of a variant transthyretin (also called prealbumin) that is found in plasma. It then forms amyloid plaques that are deposited in neural and visceral tissues. The disease onset is usually between 30 and 40 years of age. There is no medical treatment and patients usually die at a median of 10 years after the onset of symptoms. The principle of liver transplantation as a treatment for familial amyloid polyneuropathy is to suppress the production of the transthyretin variant, thus stopping the evolution of the disease leading to clinical improvement. The main indication is when the disease has progressed to clinically significant neuropathy but before extensive cardiac involvement has occurred. This generally happens when autonomic neuropathy leads to weight loss with changes in

bowel habit. Liver transplantation is not indicated in asymptomatic patients or advanced cases.

PEDIATRIC LIVER TRANSPLANTATION

Liver transplantation is a well-accepted treatment for children with end-stage liver disease (**Table 37.5**). Evaluation and appropriate patient selection for transplantation are becoming increasingly important issues as more and more children are submitted to the procedure (**Fig. 37.25**). The main selection criteria for liver transplantation are:

- severe jaundice;
- intractable variceal hemorrhage;
- liver failure manifested as vitamin K-resistant coagulopathy, malnutrition and hypoalbuminemia;
- hepatic encephalopathy; and
- severe malaise, weakness, and failure to grow.

The long-term results of transplantation in children are generally better than those in adults, with a 1-year survival rate of over 90% and with little further change in up to 5-years of follow-up because of the lack of recurrent disease. In addition, liver transplantation results in a dramatic improvement in quality of life, resumption of daily activities including education, psychologic transformation and a reintegration into society. In some critical clinical situations, such as age under 1 year, congenital anatomic abnormalities, multiple organ injuries and malnutrition, the outcome is not as good.

The equation for calculating the pediatric end-stage liver disease (PELD) score
· PELD = (0.436 × age*) − (0.687 × ln(albumin)) + (0.480 × ln(bilirubin)) + (1.857 × ln(INR)) + (0.667 × growth failure[†]) × 10
· No cap
Notes: * Age <1 year = 1, Age >1 year = 0; [†] growth failure = 1, no growth failure = 0; INR, international normalized ratio.

Table 37.6 The equation for calculating the pediatric end-stage liver disease (PELD) score.

The small number of pediatric donors available has necessitated the use of partial or reduced adult grafts or grafts from living related donors. There is a higher incidence of hepatic artery thrombosis after liver transplantation, and this is the main difference between pediatric and adult transplantation The exact timing of the procedure may be difficult, but if possible it should be performed in children at least 1 year old and over 10 kg in weight. On the other hand, delayed intervention can be associated with progressive complications and clinical deterioration of the patient.

With the institution of MELD, a separate, but parallel system for allocating pediatric organs was developed. A scoring system by which pediatric patients are prioritized on the waiting list goes by PELD, and includes total bilirubin concentration, INR and albumin, in the equation (**Table 37.6**). In addition, children less than 1 year of age are given some additional points as are children who experience growth failure. In contrast to MELD, which is capped at 40, there is no cap for PELD. The institution of PELD as a system for priority allocation has had a similar effect to MELD, in that it has decreased waiting list mortality for pediatric patients. It has also now been shown on retrospective analysis to be a very potent predictor of short-term mortality on the waiting list. While initially PELD was applied to all patients less than 18 years of age, it has recently been shown that MELD is a better predictor of short-term mortality on the waiting list for those pediatric patients between the ages of 12 and 17 years. Similar to MELD, the institution of PELD has had no significant impact on post-transplant mortality.

Extrahepatic biliary atresia

Biliary atresia is the most frequent cause of chronic cholestasis in infants, affecting 1:8000 to 1:12 000 live births. It is a pan-biliary disease of both the intrahepatic and extrahepatic biliary tree, probably the end result of a destructive inflammatory process leading to fibrosis and obliteration of the biliary tract. When left untreated, this condition leads to death from liver failure in early childhood, with an average survival of 12–18 months. Fewer than 10% of patients not undergoing biliary bypass surgery survive beyond 3 years.

The best primary treatment of biliary atresia remains controversial because of the limited efficacy of Kasai portoenterostomy, the success of liver transplantation, and the greater technical difficulty of transplantation in patients who have had multiple previous surgical procedures. Currently, liver transplantation for biliary atresia represents 50% of the cases of pediatric liver transplantation and between 5 and 10% of both pediatric and adult procedures. The first-line treatment should be a Kasai portoenterostomy before the age of 8–10 weeks by an experienced pediatric surgical team. Generally speaking, 25–30% of children who undergo a Kasai procedure have restoration of bile flow, with resolution of cholestasis and no progression to cirrhosis. The remaining 70–75% are potential candidates for liver transplantation because adequate restoration of bile flow was not obtained.

The current criteria for liver transplantation are an immediate failure of the Kasai procedure (30–40% of the total), leading to transplantation before 3 years of age or secondary failure (30–35% of the total) with recurrence of jaundice, leading to transplantation at a variable age. These patients develop portal hypertension and uncontrolled bleeding, uncontrolled cholangitis, ascites, intolerable pruritus and liver failure.

The timing of liver transplantation is based on the patient's clinical condition. The procedure must be performed before the onset of growth failure, irreversible complications and deteriorating nutritional status. If possible, it is preferable to postpone the procedure until the infant reaches 1 year of age or weighs 10 kg, because the survival rates increase from 50–60% to 80% if the transplant is performed after 1 year of age. Recurrence of the disease after liver transplantation has not been observed. It has become clear that the Kasai procedure and liver transplantation are complementary treatments for biliary atresia and that transplantation should be considered for cases of early or late failure of portoenterostomy. The ultimate aims of liver transplantation in these patients are the return to full quality of life and normal development.

Interlobular bile duct paucity

Two types of paucity of interlobular bile ducts are described: a syndromic type, the most common being called Alagille syndrome, with the presence of at least two major extrahepatic associated features; and a non-syndromic type that is secondary to multiple viral or metabolic insults to the liver. As liver failure is rarely responsible for death in the syndromic type, liver transplantation is rarely indicated. On the other hand, there is progressive biliary cirrhosis and liver failure in the non-syndromic type and liver transplantation is the only available therapy, being indicated at any age in which liver failure becomes clinically manifest.

Byler disease

This is a poorly understood disease for which the biochemical basis is still unknown. Clinically, it is characterized by hepatocyte failure to excrete bile, without any anatomic or histologic biliary abnormalities. Recently the use of ursodeoxycholic acid has been shown to improve cholestasis and liver function in some patients. When secondary biliary cirrhosis and liver failure develop, liver transplantation should be considered.

RETRANSPLANTATION

Due to the shortage of organ donors, the indications for retransplantation are controversial. Survival after retransplantation is lower than that after primary transplantation at around 50% at 1 year. Emergency retransplantation during the first week should be differentiated from later retransplantation. The indications for the former are in general primary graft non-function, thrombosis of the hepatic artery and, more rarely, acute rejection. The causes of later retransplantation are chronic rejection, long-term biliary consequences of arterial thrombosis, and hepatitis C or B recurrence in the graft. In these cases, survival is more dependent on the condition of the patient at the time of retransplantation, rather than on the indication for retransplantation.

In general the transplant should not be done too late, in order to offer the patient a reasonable chance of success. Retransplantation for HBV recurrence is generally considered to be contraindicated, due to a very high risk of HBV recurrence and of an accelerated and fatal course of reinfection in the second graft. However, an aggressive antiviral approach may improve the prognosis.

FURTHER READING

Alcoholic and metabolic liver disease

Belle SH, Beringer KC, Detre KM. Liver transplantation for alcoholic liver disease in the United States: 1988 to 1995. Liver Transplant Surg 1997; 3:212–219.

Holmgren G, Ericzon BG, Groth CG, et al. Clinical improvement and amyloid regression after liver transplantation in hereditary transthyretin amyloidosis. Lancet 1993; 341:1113–1116. *Early description of an interesting indication for liver transplantation.*

Poynard T, Barthelemy P, Fratte S, et al. for a multicentre group. Evaluation of efficacy of liver transplantation in alcoholic cirrhosis by a case-control study and simulated controls. Lancet 1994; 344:502–507. *Seminal paper on the role of liver transplantation in alcoholic liver disease.*

Autoimmune liver disease

Benhamou JP. Indications for liver transplantation in primary biliary cirrhosis. Hepatology 1994; 20:11S–13S.

Farges O, Malassagne B, Sebagh M, et al. Primary sclerosing cholangitis: liver transplantation or biliary surgery. Surgery 1995; 117:146–155.

Harrison J, McMaster P. The role of liver transplantation in the management of sclerosing cholangitis. Hepatology 1994; 20:14S–19S

Markus BH, Dickson ER, Grambsch PM, et al. Efficacy of liver transplantation in primary biliary cirrhosis. N Engl J Med 1989; 320:1709–1713.

Wiesner RH, Therneau TM, Porayko MK, et al. Prognastic models to assist in the timing of liver transplantation. In: Maddrey WC, Sorrell MF, eds. Transplantation of the liver. Newark: Appleton & Lange; 1995:123–144.

Malignant disease

Bismuth H, Chiche L, Adam R, et al. Liver resection versus transplantation for hepatocellular carcinoma in cirrhotic patients. Ann Surg 1993; 218:145–151.

Freeman RB. Liver allocation for HCC: a moving target. Liver Transplant 2004; 10(1):49–51.

O'Grady JG, Polson RJ, Rolles K, et al. Liver transplantation for malignant disease. Results in 93 consecutive patients. Ann Surg 1988; 207:373–379. *An early clinical experience that outlined many of the principles that still apply in malignancy.*

Pichlmayr R, Weimann A, Ringe B. Indications for liver transplantation in hepatobiliary malignancy. Hepatology 1994; 20:33S–40S.

Pediatric

Alagille D. Liver transplantation in children. Indications in cholestatic states. Transplant Proc 1987; XIX:3242–3248. *Pioneering description of role of liver transplantation in pediatric cholestatic liver disease.*

Otte JB, De Ville de Goyet J, et al. Sequential treatment of biliary atresia with Kasai portoenterostomy and liver transplantation: a review. Hepatology 1994; 20:41S–48S.

Prognosis and selection

Freeman RB Jr, Wiesner RH, Harper A, et al. UNOS/OPTN Liver Disease Severity Score, UNOS/OPTN Liver and Intestine, and UNOS/OPTN Pediatric Transplantation Committees. The new liver allocation system: moving toward evidence-based transplantation policy. Liver Transplant 2002; 8(9):851–858.

Freeman RB Jr, Wiesner RH, Roberts JP, et al. Improving liver allocation: MELD and PELD. Am J Transplant 2004; 4(suppl 9):114–131. *An excellent review of MELD and PELD, their implementation and the results of the change in US allocation policy.*

Jury of The Conference of Consensus on the Indications of Liver Transplantation. Consensus statement on indications for liver transplantation: Paris, June 22–23, 1993. Hepatology 1994; 20:63S–68S. *A summary of attempts to reach consensus in a number of controversial areas in liver transplantation.*

Kremers WK, van IJperen M, Kim WR, et al. MELD score as a predictor of pretransplant and posttransplant survival in OPTN/UNOS status 1 patients. Hepatology 2004; 39(3):764–769.

Report of the European Liver Transplantation Registry; Updating June 1997. Hopital Paul Brousse, Villejuif, France. 5/1968–6/1997. *Valuable source of data in Europe.*

Viral and infectious liver diseases

Fattovitch G, Giustina G, Degos F, et al. Morbidity and mortality in compensated cirrhosis type C. Gastroenterology 1997; 112:463–472.

Feray C, Gigou M, Samuel D, et al. The course of hepatitis C virus infection after liver transplantation. Hepatology 1994; 20:1137–1143.

Feray C, Gigou M, Samuel D, et al. Influence of the genotypes of hepatitis C virus on the severity of recurrent liver disease after liver transplantation. Gastroenterology 1995; 108:1088–1096.

Hadni SB, Franza A, Miguet JP, et al. Orthotopic liver transplantation for incurable alveolar echinococcosis of the liver: report of 17 cases. Hepatology 1991; 13:1061–1069. *A good discussion of a rare indication for liver transplantation.*

Samuel D, Muller R, Alexander G, et al and the European Concerted Action on Viral Hepatitis (EUROHEP). Liver transplantation in European patients with the hepatitis B surface antigen. N Engl J Med 1993; 329:1842–1847. *Another seminal paper.*

Samuel D, Zignego AL, Reynes M, et al. Long-term clinical and virologic outcome after liver transplantation for cirrhosis due to chronic δ hepatitis. Hepatology 1995; 21:333–339.

Wiesner RH, Sorrell M, Villamil F. International Liver Transplantation Society Expert Panel. Report of the first International Liver Transplantation Society expert panel consensus conference on liver transplantation and hepatitis C. Liver Transplant 2003; 9(11):S1–9.

CHAPTER

38

The Transplant Operation: What the Hepatologist Should Know

Michael Lewis Schilsky, Milan Kinkhabwala and Jean Crawford Emond

BACKGROUND

The liver transplant operation has evolved over the past 40 years by overcoming a spectrum of physiologic and technical problems to become the accepted treatment for end-stage liver disease and liver failure. The first description of experimental liver transplantation is attributed to CS Welch, who performed transplantation of the whole canine liver by placing the graft next to the native liver in an auxiliary position. These initial experimental efforts were based on the assumption that total removal of the native liver would be a prohibitive undertaking. The general procedure of orthotopic liver replacement in humans was defined by Starzl in 1963, but acceptance of the procedure was associated with continued technical modifications that led to more dependable outcomes.

Modifications in liver transplantation technique continue to this day. Among the most important developments was the introduction of venous bypass in 1983, in response to the significant hemodynamic instability that was common during the anhepatic phase of the transplant procedure. While some centers no longer use routine venous bypass, its widespread use in the 1980s contributed to a reduction in operative mortality. In addition to venous bypass, other key developments in liver transplantation included simplification of the multiorgan retrieval operation in the donor, and the introduction of the University of Wisconsin preservation solution. These advances collectively mitigated the logistic constraints of the transplant procedure and facilitated training of new transplant surgeons.

A major surgical triumph was the development of partial transplantation in the 1980s, driven by a scarcity of donors for small children. As a result living donor and split liver transplantation are now accepted worldwide; in many centers they account for the majority of liver transplants performed in children. More recently these techniques in partial liver transplantation have been extended to adults, similarly driven by a scarcity of donor organs. Living donation liver transplant (LDLT) introduces an enormous challenge for the transplant hepatologist. An understanding of the techniques and outcomes is necessary to properly select and counsel patients and their donors. In addition, a new array of complications is possible, increasing the complexity of postoperative management. Auxiliary liver transplantation, in which part or all of the native liver is preserved, has also been rediscovered in recent years with several potential applications. These diverse procedures are reviewed in this chapter, displaying the range of possibilities available to the transplant surgeon.

While knowledge of all of the technical aspects of the organ retrieval and performance of the transplant operation are requisite for the transplant surgeon, an understanding of the technical needs and limitations of the procedure also enhances the practice of the hepatologist, clinical coordinators and other members of the transplant team. These transplant team members can apply this knowledge to the transplant evaluation, patient selection and understanding of the potential post-transplant complications often managed by these individuals.

ORGANIZATION OF THE OPERATING ROOM FOR LIVER TRANSPLANTATION

Because of the unpredictable and often urgent nature of liver transplantation, most transplant centers utilize dedicated liver transplant operating rooms with surgical teams available around the clock. The complexity of the procedure demands a complete understanding of the operation and its potential complications by specialized nursing and anesthetic teams. While costly in terms of personnel, the expense is well justified, because even small errors in functional efficiency can lead to disastrous outcomes. The consistently high survival rates in current practice have been achieved by widespread adherence to these standards. Nowhere is this high standard in the operating room more dramatic than in the role of the liver transplant anesthetist, whose interventions must address profound alterations in homeostasis caused by the failing liver, support the circulation during periods of massive blood loss, and overcome the occasional bouts of cardiac dysfunction and dysrhythmias associated with reperfusion.

Immediate access to support services for the liver transplant operating room is essential. These services include clinical laboratory, blood bank, telephone links for in-hospital and outof-hospital calls and access to advanced monitoring devices such as transesophageal echocardiography. The operating room itself should be large enough to accommodate all of the equipment, instrumentation and personnel that are present during the transplant operation. The patient table must be electrically controlled in order to facilitate rotation of the patient during the operation. Two modern electrosurgical units and an argon beam coagulator should be available and functional at all times. A rapid infusion system permits rapid correction of volume losses, and when bypass is used the bypass pump can also serve as a reservoir for rapid infusion of blood products. To reduce blood product requirements, we also utilize a cell saver system. A sterile slush machine is required, particularly if extensive ex vivo surgery is required to prepare the allograft. A variety of cannulas and other supplies for cardiovascular procedures are required when venous bypass is used

The instrument trays should include both vascular and general surgical instruments: these trays should be open on the field for every case. Vascular trays should include instruments for fine anastomoses such as the portal vein and artery, as well as larger instruments for the vena cava. We have added a microvascular instrument set to our instrument list, which has been particularly useful for small hepatic arterial and biliary anastamoses. Several sets of mechanical retractors should be available in the inventory so that there are no delays for sterilization when multiple cases are performed. For pediatric cases, an operating microscope should be available, as it has become standard for arterial anastamoses in many centers, particularly for living donor transplants.

DECEASED DONOR HEPATECTOMY

Most organs for transplantation are now procured from multiple-organ donors. The donor operation has evolved greatly from the classical method, in which most of the dissection was performed in situ ('warm') before cooling and removal of the organs. Today most donor surgeons utilize variations of the rapid flush/en-bloc retrieval technique, in which cold perfusion of the organs with preservation solution is performed first, followed by dissection and removal of the organs under asanguinous conditions. Additionally, organs are retrieved 'en bloc', in groups of grape-like clusters that are based on common vascular pedicles. The individual organs can then be separated on the back table under controlled conditions, greatly simplifying the abdominal donor operation.

In performing donor hepatectomy, the surgeon is faced with two general tasks: first, direct assessment of the donor liver for suitability; second, removal of the liver and its hilar structures without injury. Ischemic injury due to donor hemodynamic instability, macrovesicular steatosis, cirrhosis and malignancy are potential conditions for which the surgeon may choose to discard the liver during direct assessment. When additional information is required, an intraoperative frozen section biopsy may be obtained to investigate suspected liver pathology. Donor selection is evolving as the growing crisis of the waiting list has led to re-evaluation of selection and the successful use of a scale of grafts not meeting traditional criteria; informally termed 'marginal livers', but more correctly identified as 'extended criteria donors' (ECD).

Donor hepatectomy is performed through a long midline abdominal incision and median sternotomy (**Fig. 38.1**). The pericardium and right pleural spaces are opened for later exsanguination through the vena cava. The abdomen is explored to exclude incidental malignancy. The suprahepatic vena cava is exposed by division of the falciform and triangular ligaments. The left lateral segment is mobilized, exposing the gastrohepatic ligament. An accessory left hepatic artery, if present, is carefully protected. Limited dissection of the porta hepatis is then performed in order to expose the common bile duct, which is divided distally. The extrahepatic biliary tree is flushed with saline through an incision in the gallbladder, in order to prevent bile-induced autolysis of the biliary epithelium during storage (**Fig. 38.2**).

The terminal ileum, right colon and duodenum are mobilized medially by sharp dissection along the peritoneal reflection. This maneuver affords complete exposure of the retroperitoneum. The origins of the renal veins are identified on the vena cava, and the distal aorta is encircled with a tape for later cannulation. In conventional retrieval, precooling of the liver with cold crystalloid solution is accomplished by introduction of a small catheter in the portal circulation (**Fig. 38.3**). This same catheter

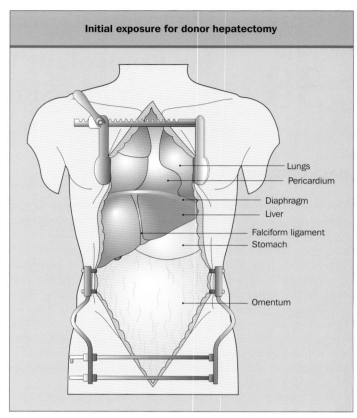

Initial exposure for donor hepatectomy

Lungs
Pericardium
Diaphragm
Liver
Falciform ligament
Stomach
Omentum

Figure 38.1 Initial exposure for donor hepatectomy.

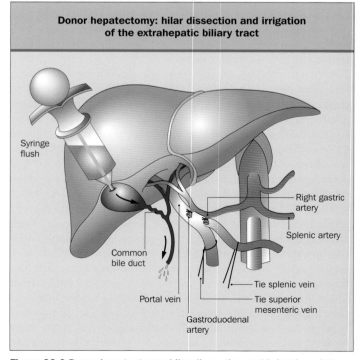

Donor hepatectomy: hilar dissection and irrigation of the extrahepatic biliary tract

Syringe flush
Right gastric artery
Splenic artery
Common bile duct
Portal vein
Tie splenic vein
Tie superior mesenteric vein
Gastroduodenal artery

Figure 38.2 Donor hepatectomy: hilar dissection and irrigation of the extrahepatic biliary tract.

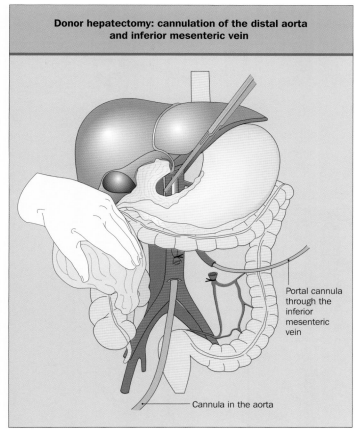

Donor hepatectomy: cannulation of the distal aorta and inferior mesenteric vein

Portal cannula through the inferior mesenteric vein

Cannula in the aorta

Figure 38.3 Donor hepatectomy: cannulation of the distal aorta and inferior mesenteric vein in preparation for in situ flush with preservation solution.

is used later in the procurement as a conduit to flush the portal vein with preservation solution. Some centers, including our own, perform neither 'precool' nor in situ portal flush routinely during en-bloc liver/pancreas procurement. In this modification the in situ flush is performed only through the arterial circulation, with the portal flush performed on the back table immediately after retrieval. In the final step before in situ flush, the supraceliac aorta is encircled with a tape at the level of diaphragmatic crus. The donor is then fully heparinized and a large-bore cannula is inserted into the distal aorta (see Fig. 38.3). The donor is exsanguinated through a large venting incision in the vena cava, while the supraceliac aorta is simultaneously clamped and cold preservation solution is flushed through the aortic and portal cannulae, allowing rapid core cooling of the abdominal organs. Concomitantly, topical cooling is accomplished by instilling ice slush into the peritoneum. Once the caval effluent has cleared, the organs can be removed sequentially: thoracic organs first, liver/pancreas second, and kidneys last. The liver is removed by first dividing the diaphragm circumferentially, encompassing the suprahepatic vena cava and the dome of the liver. The circular cuff of diaphragm is removed from the liver and cava during back-table preparation of the liver. The common hepatic artery is identified along the superior border of the pancreas and dissected proximally to the celiac trunk, sequentially ligating the principal branches: gastroduodenal, left gastric and splenic arteries. The origin of the celiac trunk on the aorta is

identified and a circular patch of aorta is fashioned around the origin ('Carrell patch'). Knowledge of variations in hepatic arterial anatomy is crucial to safe hepatectomy (**Fig. 38.4**).

The portal vein is divided at its origin behind the pancreas, ensuring adequate length for the recipient operation. The remainder of the porta hepatis is then divided, with careful attention to the identification and preservation of an accessory right hepatic artery. If an accessory right hepatic artery is identified, the entire length of the vessel together with a trunk of the superior mesenteric artery can be procured in order to facilitate back-table reconstruction.

In the final step, the infrahepatic vena cava is divided above the renal veins. The liver is then removed and placed in storage containers for transport. Before closing the abdomen, lengths of iliac artery and vein are procured for potential use as vascular conduits in the recipient.

ORTHOTOPIC LIVER TRANSPLANTATION

Like most difficult operations technical success requires mastery of anatomy, efficient surgical technique that minimizes unnecessary movement, and seamless communication between team members. Refinements in technique continue to this day, although events can be identified that have had a broad impact in shaping the liver transplant operation. For example, the technique of dissection has evolved with the introduction of improved electrocautery units and the argon beam coagulator, devices that have reduced operative time and facilitated hemostasis. It has also become standard practice to utilize mechanical retractors for exposure during liver transplantation, facilitating anatomic exposure during the liver transplant operation.

The transplant operation must also be optimized for the individual recipient. For each of the phases of the operation, knowledge of the physiologic condition of the patient, underlying comorbid disease, prior abdominal operation, presence or absence of hepatocellular carcinoma (HCC), degree of portal hypertension and coagulopathy, vascular anomalies and vascular patency, all may influence the transplant operation and perioperative patient management.

The size of the donor liver selected must take into account the recipient's size and physiologic condition. Livers that may be inadequate for sicker individuals may have predictably good success in relatively healthier recipients. Formulas that predict the normal expected liver volume still utilize height and weight as variables but do not incorporate the metabolic needs of a particular recipient based on their severity of illness. While there must be adequate hepatic mass to avoid poor function in the recipient, transplantation of an organ that is too large can lead to organ ischemia and difficulties with wound closure. Fascial closure in the presence of a large graft and significant generalized edema can result in both ventilatory and hemodynamic compromise, and rarely even abdominal compartment syndrome with failure of the graft. Post-transplant abdominal compartment syndrome is characterized by a sudden and unexpected change in hemodynamics, primary non-function of the graft, tense abdomen on examination and oliguria in an otherwise uncomplicated transplant. This is an emergency condition in which immediate re-exploration and abdominal closure with temporary mesh is indicated. At the time of re-exploration, the hepatic artery and portal vein need to be investigated for patency.

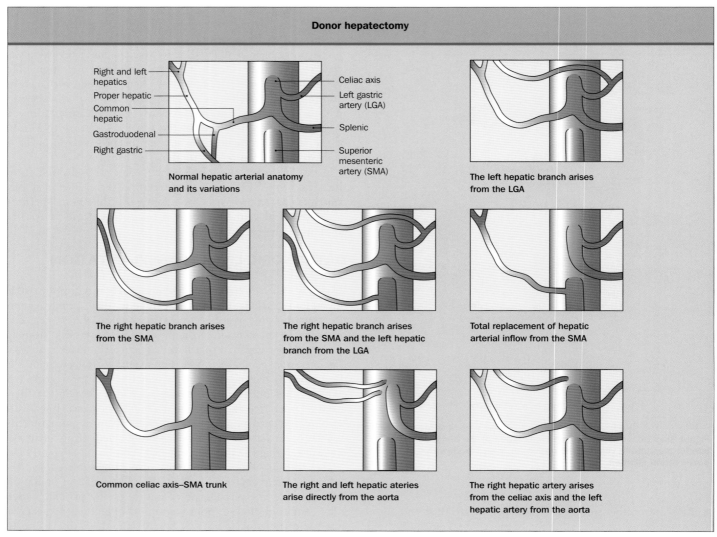

Donor hepatectomy

Right and left hepatics
Proper hepatic
Common hepatic
Gastroduodenal
Right gastric

Celiac axis
Left gastric artery (LGA)
Splenic
Superior mesenteric artery (SMA)

Normal hepatic arterial anatomy and its variations

The left hepatic branch arises from the LGA

The right hepatic branch arises from the SMA

The right hepatic branch arises from the SMA and the left hepatic branch from the LGA

Total replacement of hepatic arterial inflow from the SMA

Common celiac axis–SMA trunk

The right and left hepatic ateries arise directly from the aorta

The right hepatic artery arises from the celiac axis and the left hepatic artery from the aorta

Figure 38.4 Donor hepatectomy: variations in hepatic arterial anatomy.

Primary abdominal closure should not be reattempted until the graft function has normalized, renal and pulmonary function have been restored, and nutritional deficits addressed. Methods of addressing organ size mismatches include graft size reduction, splitting and use of prosthetic materials for closure.

There are several factors that can increase the technical difficulty of the transplant operation. The presence of prior abdominal surgery in patients often leads to adhesions and a technically more difficult hepatectomy in the recipient, particularly in recipients with severe portal hypertension. Prolonged operative time and increased blood product requirement can be anticipated. The increased use of blood products increases the possibility of life-threatening electrolyte disturbances associated with large volume transfusion, especially in recipients with underlying renal dysfunction. At our center, we make several modifications to routine practice for patients with renal dysfunction. First, arrangements are made preoperatively for intraoperative renal replacement [continuous venovenous hemofiltration (CVVH)], and lines for dialysis are placed prior to beginning the operation. Secondly, units of packed red blood cells (PRBCs) are washed to prevent life-threatening hyper-

kalemia upon reperfusion. Third, we vent 500 cc of blood through the graft upon reperfusion rather than reperfuse the initial blood directly into circulation. Finally, in patients at high risk for bleeding and without a prior history of thrombosis or hyper-coagulable state, low dose aprotinin infusion can be utilized during the hepatectomy to reduce blood loss, although randomized controlled trials have not shown a clear benefit to routine aprotinin administration in all cases. Factor VIIa has also recently become available to correct coagulopathy, although at considerable expense. The role of this novel agent in liver transplantation remains unclear and awaits further study.

Patients with sclerosing cholangitis or very small bile ducts require reconstruction using a Roux-en-Y choledochojejunostomy (biliary enteric anastamosis to a defunctionalized limb of intestine) rather than primary choledochocholedochostomy (duct to duct anastamosis), which can also lengthen the operative procedure. For patients with a history of thrombosis or those with known coagulation disorders, the use of anti-coagulation with heparin and antiplatelet aggregation agents such as aspirin should be considered after reperfusion of the new graft. This is especially important in patients with a positive lupus anticoagulant or Factor V Leiden deficiency. The known presence of HCC in the liver prior to transplant should engender a careful search for evidence for any metastatic disease prior to, but also at the time of transplant. In those with larger or multiple tumors, it is advisable to have a backup recipient candidate available in case evidence of extrahepatic tumor is discovered during the abdominal exploration. Discovery of extrahepatic malignancy is a contraindication to completion of transplantation. Patients with known portal vein thrombosis may undergo thrombectomy at the time of the transplant, or may require venous bypass. When portal venous thrombosis is known to be present prior to transplant, veins for grafting should be available in the event that thrombectomy is unsuccessful. For some patients with transjugular intrahepatic portosystemic shunts (TIPS) placed prior to their transplant surgery, careful dissection of the stent from the vena cava may be necessary. Other devices that may appear near the operative field are vena cava filters for prevention of pulmonary embolism.

There may also be other specific recipient issues that should prompt preoperative consultations. The anesthetic team should be aware of patients with known cervical disc problems or airway problems that may require special care for intubation and airway monitoring. Patients with portopulmonary syndrome and elevated pulmonary artery pressures are at increased risk for intra- and perioperative hemodynamic instability, and cardiac or pulmonary specialists should be available to work with the anesthetic team for intra- and perioperative management of these individuals, including access to intraoperative transesophageal echocardiography. Ideally, management of patients with mild to moderate cardiopulmonary disease is carefully planned prior to transplantation, as patients with severe disease are generally not candidates for transplantation. However, occasionally underlying cardiopulmonary disease may not be evident until induction of anesthesia and placement of a pulmonary artery catheter. If significant cardiopulmonary disease is discovered only at operation, a decision to proceed must be made in consultation with the surgeon, anesthesiologist and consultants from cardiology and pulmonary medicine. Transplantation in the face of severe pulmonary hypertension is generally futile. Patients with functioning neuroendocrine tumors require special management with somatostatin infusion and β blockers to prevent release of hormonal factors that could result in severe hemodynamic instability. Patients with known red-cell antibodies may require extra time for cross matching by the blood bank, which must be alerted as soon as a potential liver is available. If cross match negative blood is not available, the operation may need to be delayed or cancelled altogether.

General approaches to the operation

Three general operative strategies are available to the surgeon performing orthotopic liver transplantation: the traditional dissection without venovenous bypass, the traditional dissection with bypass and 'piggyback' placement of the liver. Each offers advantages. Traditional dissection without bypass is the most challenging, requiring both an experienced surgeon and an anesthetic team. The principal advantages are simplicity and short anhepatic times, as little as 30 min. In addition, complications associated with bypass, such as morbidity related to the cannulation sites, are avoided. Hemodynamic instability can be more severe, however, increasing demands on the anesthetic

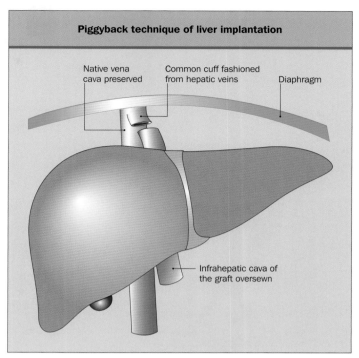

Piggyback technique of liver implantation

Native vena cava preserved
Common cuff fashioned from hepatic veins
Diaphragm
Infrahepatic cava of the graft oversewn

Figure 38.5 Piggyback technique of liver implantation. The native vena cava is preserved.

team during the anhepatic and post-reperfusion phase. Addition of bypass prolongs the operation and the anhepatic time, but mitigates the volume-associated hemodynamic changes associated with portal and vena caval clamping.

The piggyback technique is designed to circumvent the hemodynamic risks of traditional dissection without bypass by removing the native liver with preservation of the vena cava, avoiding the need to cross-clamp the vena cava during the anhepatic phase, and thereby preserving venous return to the heart (**Fig. 38.5**). This technique adds additional time and complexity during the hepatectomy and introduces an increased risk of hepatic outflow complications related to the single hepatic venous anastomosis. However, advocates of the piggyback technique have been pleased with a decrease in volume-related instability during the anhepatic phase. The piggyback technique may be most appropriate in patients with compromised cardiovascular reserve as an alternative to bypass. We have utilized the piggyback technique when recipients are unable to tolerate test clamping of the vena cava and portal vein after a period of resuscitation by the anesthesiologist. The piggyback technique is also useful when the surgeon is confronted with a large donor liver in a small recipient, because piggyback is performed without an infrahepatic caval anastamosis, which may be difficult in the presence of a significant size mismatch.

Three phases of orthotopic liver transplantation

The liver transplant operation is described in three phases: hepatectomy, anhepatic phase and reperfusion phase. The patient is prepared for operation by positioning in the supine position with the right arm tucked to facilitate placement of an assistant. Upon induction of anesthesia, vascular access lines are placed by

609

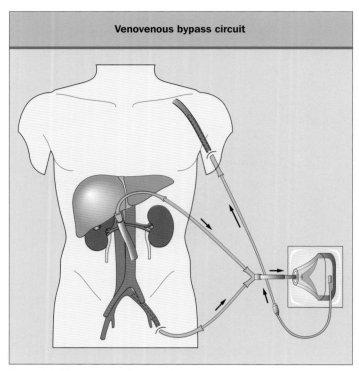

Venovenous bypass circuit

Figure 38.6 Venovenous bypass circuit.

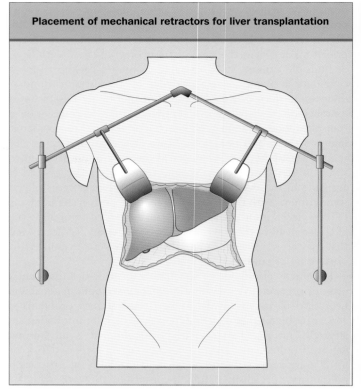

Placement of mechanical retractors for liver transplantation

Figure 38.7 Placement of mechanical retractors for liver transplantation.

the anesthetist. At least one large sheath introducer is placed in the central venous circulation, which serves as a large volume access and as a portal for a pulmonary artery catheter. An additional large volume access, usually a sheath introducer, is placed either centrally or peripherally. When venovenous bypass is used, the bypass cannulae are placed surgically after preparing and draping the entire chest, abdomen and groins. A femoral cannula is placed by cut-down on the saphenous vein. The axillary cannula, through which blood is returned to the central circulation, can be placed either percutaneously or by open cut-down on the axillary vein (**Fig. 38.6**). All of these steps are associated with postoperative morbidity, nerve injuries from positioning, vascular complications from venous or arterial lines and local wound complications.

Hepatectomy

The hepatectomy is performed through a bilateral subcostal incision with extension in the midline to the xiphoid process, which is often excised. The incision should be carried as far laterally to the right as possible in order to allow a complete and unobstructed view of the liver, especially the retrohepatic and suprahepatic vena cava. Mechanical retraction under both costal margins elevates and spreads the aperture of the rib cage in order to create a horizontal rather than convex costal margin, thereby maximizing access to the suprahepatic vena cava (**Fig. 38.7**). It should be remembered that the cirrhotic liver is often extremely small and difficult to access in its location high above the costal margin. The exposure is completed by inferior traction on the viscera, thereby clearly exposing the porta hepatis for dissection.

The technique of dissection is unique to liver transplantation and differs from traditional general surgical operations in that sharp (rather than blunt) dissection is emphasized, and the electrocautery probe is the principal dissecting tool. This unique technique was developed specifically to address the challenges of portal hypertension with engorged intra-abdominal varices, coagulopathy and thrombocytopenia, and an extensive dissection that would require several hours of work (and several hours of additional bleeding) if performed using more conventional surgical techniques. In most uncomplicated transplants, an experienced surgeon is typically able to complete the hepatectomy phase of the operation in 1–2 h using the sharp dissection/cautery technique.

The liver is mobilized completely from its ligamentous attachments (often vascularized in the presence of cirrhosis) and from the right hemidiaphragm. After the ligaments and diaphragm are completely freed, the liver can be easily elevated to expose the retrohepatic vena cava. The hilar dissection is performed after the porta hepatis is exposed by an assistant, who reflects the liver edge upward while another assistant (or mechanical retractor) holds the intestines and duodenum caudally. The goal of the hilar dissection is identification and ligation of the structures in the porta hepatis (hepatic artery, bile duct and portal vein). The general principle is that portal structures must be ligated as high in the hilum as possible in order to preserve length, which may be important during implantation of the liver allograft.

In patients previous hepatobiliary surgery (most commonly cholecystectomy), densely vascularized adhesions of the colon, stomach, duodenum and omentum present an obstacle to exposure of the hepatic hilum. In such cases, the adhesions and adherent structures must be 'shaved' off the liver surface using

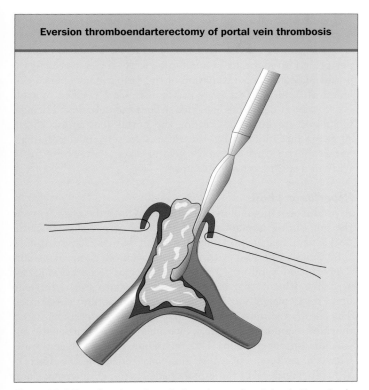

Eversion thromboendarterectomy of portal vein thrombosis

Figure 38.8 Eversion thromboendarterectomy of portal vein thrombosis.

cautery. Some surgeons delay ligation of the hepatic artery until mobilization is complete, since it is thought that the end-stage liver is predominantly dependent upon the arterial supply and the patient becomes functionally anhepatic after arterial ligation. In addition, prolonged ligation of the hepatic artery before reconstruction in the new liver may predispose to intimal injury, dissection and thrombosis. The portal vein is skeletonized in its entirety from the border of the pancreas to the bifurcation. If a TIPS is found in the extrahepatic portal vein, the first choice in strategy is to clamp proximal to the TIPS and divide the portal vein in a location that is free of stent material. Sometimes this is not possible and a clamp has to be placed across a long retropancreatic TIPS, in which case the TIPS is transected along with the portal vein in the mid portion of the porta hepatis. The wires of the transected metal stent are then individually removed, taking care not to shred the wall of the vein. If the portal vein is thrombosed, it is usually possible to re-establish flow by transecting it and removing the organized thrombus using a combination of sharp separation of the thrombus from the vein wall together with balloon thrombectomy, in a procedure that is similar to endarterectomy for atherosclerosis (**Fig. 38.8**). This dissection can be carried proximally to the junction of the mesenteric and splenic veins since this confluence is nearly always patent. If portal revascularization is not possible, a conduit of cadaveric iliac vein is placed on the superior mesenteric vein and tunneled through the root of the transverse mesocolon, to be used as an interposition graft to the portal vein of the new liver. Preoperative imaging of the portal vein using magnetic resonance angiography or high quality multiple phase computed tomography (CT) permits the surgeon to have a fairly accurate map of the portal circulation prior to transplantation.

The presence of a spontaneous or surgically constructed spleno-renal shunt, for example, can be addressed by ligation of the left renal vein. A surgical mesocaval shunt can be addressed by ligation of the mesocaval conduit, provided the native portal vein is patent and of adequate caliber. When the portal vein is unusable and a prior mesocaval shunt is present, we have, for example, even utilized the shunt for inflow to the new graft. Ultimately the surgeon must be resourceful in dealing with likely unexpected findings. After completion of the hilar dissection, the retrohepatic cava is fully dissected on the right side from the infrahepatic cava to the right hepatic vein by division of the flimsy lateral and posterior attachments with cautery. The adrenal vein is encountered in this plane and must be suture ligated. In the piggyback technique the liver is separated from the vena cava by ligation of all the small hepatic vein branches to the right lobe and the caudate until the liver is completely freed with the exception of the three main hepatic veins. This permits application of a partial occlusion clamp to preserve caval blood flow during implantation of the new liver. The left side of the retro-hepatic cava is exposed by anterior reflection of the left lateral segment and retraction of the caudate lobe with a narrow hand-held malleable retractor, allowing cautery dissection of the left side of the retrohepatic cava.

If bypass is to be used, the portal bypass cannula can be placed as the final step in the hepatectomy, after high ligation of the portal vein close to or above its bifurcation in the hilum (see Fig. 38.6). When the portal vein cannot safely be dissected because of dense scar tissue, or when portal vein thrombosis is present, it may be preferable to gain access for portal bypass using the inferior mesenteric vein. When no bypass is used, the portal vein is simply clamped proximally, near the pancreatic border. Before explanting the diseased liver, however, we perform a test clamp of the infrahepatic vena cava and portal vein to determine whether the patient will tolerate the anhepatic phase. If the blood pressure falls, typically below a mean arterial blood pressure of 60–70, then additional measures are required before repeating the test clamp, including volume loading and initiation of baseline pressor support. Finally, the infra- and suprahepatic vena cava are clamped in traditional techniques (**Fig. 38.9**). Correct placement of these clamps is important in facilitating subsequent caval anastamoses; the suprahepatic clamp should be placed as close to the diaphragm as possible in order to gain as much cuff length as possible for use in the suprahepatic caval anastomosis. We secure the suprahepatic clamp with a vascular tape in order to minimize accidental release. The infrahepatic caval clamp should be placed as distally as possible, without occlusion of the renal veins. We often transect the hepatic veins within the liver substance, in order to gain as much suprahepatic caval length as possible. Similarly, the infrahepatic cava is transected high into the liver, in order to preserve length, and the liver is removed.

Anhepatic phase

After the liver is removed, hemostasis is achieved by suture ligature and cautery of bleeding tissues in the retroperitoneum (see Fig. 38.9). The vascular anastamoses are then performed in the following order: suprahepatic cava, infrahepatic cava and portal vein. The hepatic arterial anastomosis is usually performed after portal reperfusion. The duration of the anhepatic phase, ending in portal venous reperfusion, is approximately

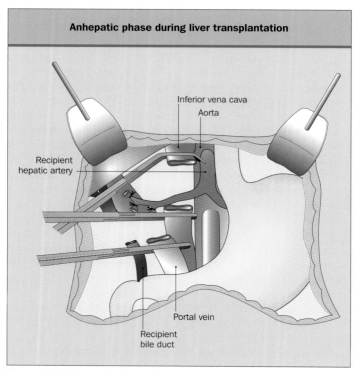

Anhepatic phase during liver transplantation

Inferior vena cava
Aorta
Recipient
hepatic artery
Portal vein
Recipient
bile duct

Figure 38.9 Anhepatic phase during liver transplantation.

30–45 min. The physiologic consequences of the anhepatic phase include progressive coagulopathy, fibrinolysis and acidosis.

When portal bypass is not used, there is also progressive bowel edema and venous engorgement. Before reperfusion, preservation solution in the liver graft must be removed to prevent arrhythmias associated with high potassium preservation solutions. We accomplish this task by flushing the portal vein of the graft on the back table with cold colloid solution (hetastarch), although this can also be performed during implantation as well. Of the three venous anastamoses performed, all have different challenges. The suprahepatic caval anastamosis has been viewed as the most difficult, because of limited exposure, the relatively short length of the cuffs available for anastamosis, and the difficulty in revising the anastamosis after completion. The surgeon therefore has to visually assess the relative diameter and lengths of the cuffs between native cava and graft, and adjust while performing the anastamosis to achieve the following goals: hemostatic suture line; intimal approximation to minimize nidus for thrombosis; and correct anterior–posterior orientation to avoid torsion and outflow obstruction. The last goal is especially important when there is substantial size mismatch between the graft and patient.

During the suprahepatic caval anastamosis, the liver graft is parachuted into the hepatic fossa and the posterior (back wall) aspect of the anastomosis is performed first, through the inside of the cava. The infrahepatic caval anastomosis is performed in a similar fashion. Assessment of the proper length of the infrahepatic cava and maintenance of the alignment of the cava on its axis are important considerations in performing the infracaval anastomosis. In the piggyback technique, the suprahepatic cava of the graft is anastomosed end to side to the confluence of the recipient hepatic veins or to a long anterior incision on the

recipient vena cava, utilizing either partial or total occlusion of the recipient vena cava. The infrahepatic vena cava of the graft is then simply oversewn. The portal vein anastomosis is performed after the caval anastamoses. A crucial aspect of the portal anastomosis is estimation of the proper donor portal vein length that allows a straight anastomosis. Care is taken to avoid constriction at the suture line. Fine sutures and delicate, meticulous technique are important during the portal anastamosis. Some surgeons intentionally tie the sutures loosely, incorporating a 'growth factor' that allows the vein to distend after reperfusion without a waist at the anastamosis.

Reperfusion phase
Byproducts of metabolism accumulate in both the graft liver and the gut during implantation of the liver, especially when the portal vein has been clamped without bypass. Reperfusion is sometimes associated with significant hemodynamic instability ('reperfusion syndrome') due to the cold, hyperkalemic and acidotic effluent that is flushed directly into the right heart upon revascularization. Transient hypocontractility is common. The anesthetist must therefore be prepared to administer hemodynamic support, including catecholamines, bicarbonate and calcium on reperfusion. The technique of reperfusion varies between centers, but most surgeons reperfuse the liver by sequential removal of the suprahepatic clamp, infrahepatic clamp and finally the portal venous clamp. After caval clamp removals any obvious suture line leaks can be oversewn and the graft can be 'prewarmed' by backbleeding caval blood and with heated irrigation before releasing the portal clamp. Upon releasing the portal vein clamp, some blood may be discarded ('vented') to eliminate some of the detrimental substances which accumulate in the mesenteric circulation during the cross-clamp. It is not clear that venting reduces the reperfusion syndrome, except in the circumstance where the patient is known to be hyperkalemic before reperfusion. We also discard initial blood perfused through the graft when there is significant graft steatosis, because of the concern of flushing lipid particles directly into the lungs. Even with preimplantation flushing of the graft with colloid solution, there is often still enough residual preservation solution and heparin within the liver graft to cause transient hyperkalemia and systemic heparin-induced anticoagulation. When T wave elevations are seen immediately after reperfusion of the portal vein, the surgeon can intermittently occlude the portal inflow manually to permit successive washes of potassium to be absorbed and dealt with pharmacologically.

The appearance of the liver upon reperfusion may often give an early indication of graft function. Severe reperfusion injury may be manifest by a bright red color and a firm, swollen appearance. The liver with good initial function and minimal reperfusion injury will rapidly and homogeneously fill with blood upon portal reperfusion and appear a dark salmon color. To palpation, the liver will remain soft and retain the sharpness of its edges. In a well-functioning liver, bile may be seen at the common duct even before arterial revascularization. Finally, the functioning liver will readily clear lactic acid and plasminogen activators, resulting in a correction of acid–base abnormalities and resolution of the complex coagulopathy that is due to a combination of fibrinolysis and dilution of platelets and coagulation factors. In livers prone to poor initial function, it is often advisable to maintain as low a central venous pressure as possible

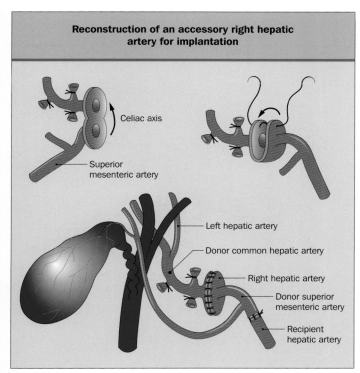

Figure 38.10 Reconstruction of an accessory right hepatic artery for implantation.

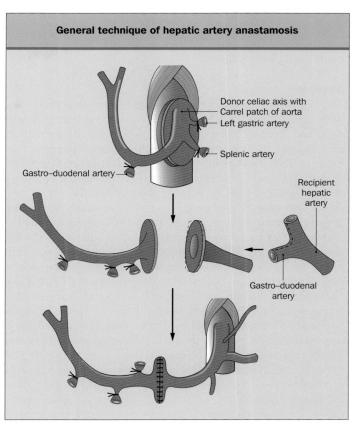

Figure 38.11 General technique of hepatic arterial anastomosis utilizing a donor aortic Carrel patch to the recipient hepatic artery branch patch.

to minimize the deleterious effects of graft engorgement in a liver with other risk factors. Volume overload is more common when no bypass is used, because of the obligatory volume loading that must occur to permit safe cross clamping. After reperfusion this excess intravascular volume can become a liability for graft function as well as oxygenation and pulmonary compliance, and constant communication between the surgeon and anesthesiologist after reperfusion is essential. Measures to reduce graft swelling can include the use of nitroglycerine and diuretics. Crystalloid volume is minimized and only blood products are administered, according to the degree of bleeding assessed by the surgeon inspecting the operative field.

Arterial anastomoses

After portal reperfusion the vascular suture lines are rapidly inspected for hemostasis before beginning the hepatic arterial anastomosis. If an accessory right hepatic artery is present in the liver graft, reconstruction of this vessel is performed ex vivo on the back table before implantation. The most common technique for hepatic arterial anastomosis is an end-to-end anastomosis of the donor aortic Carrel patch to the recipient hepatic artery (**Fig. 38.10**). The hepatic arterial anastomosis can be facilitated by preparation of the recipient hepatic artery as a 'branch patch', in which a common cuff is fashioned from a bifurcation, usually the hepatic–gastroduodenal bifurcation (**Fig. 38.11**). The recipient hepatic artery tends to be fragile and is prone to intimal dissection with even small trauma. If the recipient hepatic artery is unsatisfactory the splenic artery can be used as an alternative, or an interposition graft can be taken directly off the aorta. Before the introduction of microvascular techniques, direct

aortic implantation was in fact the most common approach in pediatric recipients.

While there has been some debate about the etiology of hepatic artery thrombosis in the past, it is now clear that precision in fashioning the arterial anastomosis is the most important factor in decreasing the risk of this complication. Fine atraumatic clamps and fine monofilament sutures (7-0) are used in the anastomosis, and growth factors are occasionally used to prevent constriction. High-power magnification has clearly been shown to decrease the thrombosis rate in pediatric liver transplantation, in which reconstruction of 2 or 3 mm arteries may be required. After releasing the arterial clamp, adequacy of flow is assessed by palpation, Doppler examination, and, in some cases, direct measurement with a flow probe. Causes of inadequate arterial flow include technical flaws in the anastomosis, clamp injury to the intima of the artery proximal to the anastomosis, or inadequate inflow due to alterations in the recipient, such as celiac arterial disease or constriction by the arcuate ligament of the diaphragm. When arterial flow seems inadequate in the absence of any clear anastomotic problem or anatomic injury to the artery, the common hepatic artery can be dissected proximally to the splenic artery. In some cases splenic artery ligation will increase inflow to the liver. We have also observed occasional respiratory variation in hepatic arterial inflow caused by occlusion of the celiac artery by the arcuate ligament of the diaphragm. In such cases, inflow can be restored by further proximal dissection and division of the diaphragmatic muscular fibers surrounding the origin of the celiac trunk off the aorta. When all these measures fail to achieve adequate arterial pulsation, the artery should be immediately revised using an aortic conduit for inflow.

Biliary anastomosis

The bile duct anastomosis is performed last. While there have been many variations in bile duct reconstruction that have been described, the two most commonly performed reconstructions are simple end-to-end choledochocholedochostomy and biliary–enteric drainage into a Roux-en-Y (defunctionalized) limb of intestine. End-to-end reconstruction is preferable because it avoids the need for an enteric anastomosis. In either case, cholecystectomy is performed first and the donor bile duct is prepared for anastomosis, usually above the cystic duct junction. End-to-end anastamosis is performed using fine monofilament absorbable suture. Size mismatches may be corrected by ducto-plasty with a running suture, or by spatulation of the smaller duct. In the past, a choledochal drainage tube (T-tube) was always left in the bile duct, with one limb of the tube stenting the anastomosis. The tube allowed collection of bile during the postoperative period, which facilitated clinical management of dysfunctional livers and allowed cholangiography. However, T-tubes are associated with complications in up to one-third of patients, most commonly bile peritonitis associated with tube removal several months after transplantation. This often requires hospitalization, endoscopic placement of biliary stents, and in some cases, operation. As part of a general trend toward greater operative simplicity, most centers have abandoned the routine use of T-tubes.

Hepatojejunostomy is preferred when primary end-to-end anastamosis is not possible, as in sclerosing cholangitis or when the recipient bile duct is too small to allow effective biliary drainage (**Fig. 38.12**). Hepatojejunostomy is also performed in almost all pediatric patients who may already have an existing Roux-en-Y limb from a Kasai procedure for biliary atresia. The original Roux limb can be revised for use in the hepatoenteric anastomosis. When a new Roux-en-Y must be constructed, the proximal jejunum is divided 20–30 cm distal to the ligament of Treitz with a stapler. The distal intestine is then used to construct a 40 cm defunctionalized limb. Bowel continuity is restored with a jejunojejunostomy. The jejunojejunostomy suture line is occasionally the source of gastrointestinal bleeding several days after transplantation, although these events are usually self limited. The Roux can be brought up to the donor liver through either an antecolic or retrocolic approach. The biliary–enteric anastomosis is performed with a single inter-rupted layer of absorbable suture to reapproximate mucosa to mucosa. If desired, a small stent can be left across the anastomosis, usually an infant feeding tube. Small stents almost invariably fall out if not secured with an absorbable suture. One end of the stent can also be brought out to the skin through a second enterotomy, allowing access for postoperative imaging. Before closure a final hemostatic survey is performed (**Fig. 38.13**). When the liver graft is functioning well, hemostasis is generally accomplished without much difficulty, but in cases of poor initial graft function the surgical surfaces and suture lines can bleed profusely from fibrinolysis, coagulopathy and hypothermia. Coagulopathy is treated with fresh frozen plasma, cryoprecipitate and platelets. Epsilon aminocaproic acid can be used to treat

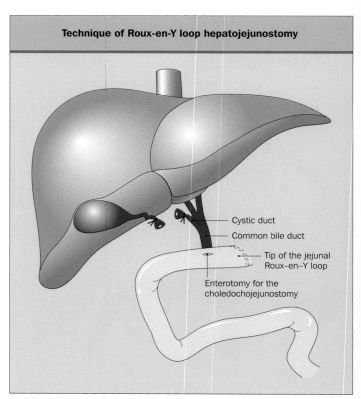

Technique of Roux-en-Y loop hepatojejunostomy

Cystic duct
Common bile duct
Tip of the jejunal Roux–en–Y loop
Enterotomy for the choledochojejunostomy

Figure 38.12 Technique of Roux-en-Y hepatojejunostomy.

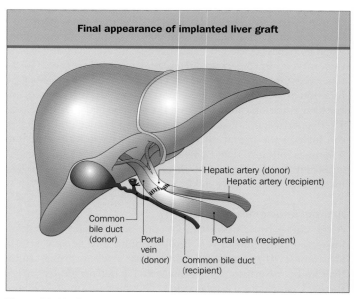

Final appearance of implanted liver graft

Hepatic artery (donor)
Hepatic artery (recipient)
Common bile duct (donor)
Portal vein (donor)
Portal vein (recipient)
Common bile duct (recipient)

Figure 38.13 Final appearance of implanted liver graft.

fibrinolysis. When hemostasis has been accomplished, closed suction drains are left in the peritoneum (**Fig. 38.14**). We generally use one or two drains, which are useful in evacuating postoperative serosanguinous fluid and facilitating early diag-nosis of a bile leak, but they are not reliable indicators of intra-peritoneal hemorrhage as their small size usually results in early occlusion by a clot.

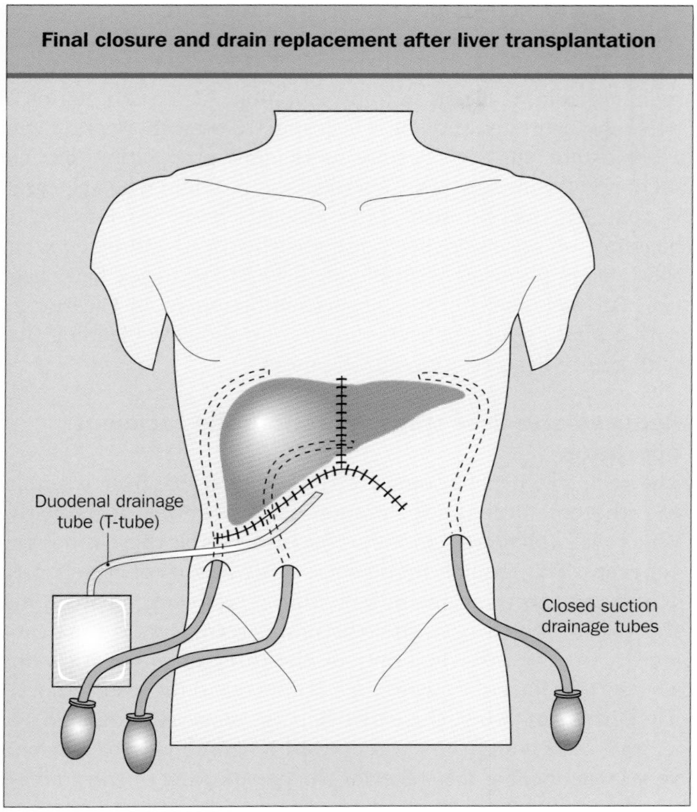

Final closure and drain replacement after liver transplantation

Duodenal drainage tube (T-tube)

Closed suction drainage tubes

Figure 38.14 Final closure and drain placement after liver transplantation.

SPECIAL OPERATIVE CONSIDERATIONS: PEDIATRIC AND REDUCED-SIZE LIVER TRANSPLANTATION

Standard cadaveric transplantation in children is quite similar to the adult transplant, utilizing smaller instruments and sutures. Bypass is not used in children, and hepatojejunostomy is the preferred method of biliary reconstruction in all except larger teenage children. Experienced anesthesiology is of paramount importance in successful pediatric transplantation. Because of the difficulty of establishing large volume access in infants, central venous and arterial lines may sometimes require open surgical placement before beginning the transplant operation.

Adult-sized children should be managed intraoperatively in the same way as adult transplant recipients, including availability of larger volume access and rapid transfusion devices. In this decade, techniques of reduced-size liver transplantation have become routine in the transplantation of children. The incentive for development of these techniques was the shortage of small donors, which leads to a waiting list mortality for children approaching 50%. Initially, when the adult waiting list was small in the 1980s, livers from adult donors could be readily diverted to children. A small liver was fashioned ex vivo on the back table, usually from the left lateral segment, while the remainder was discarded. Shortly thereafter, the technique was extended to create two grafts from a single liver, the 'split liver' procedure. The appeal of splitting livers was the possibility of doubling the organ supply, but initial experiences with split livers were fraught

with technical complications, thereby limiting application of this technique. More recently, there has been a renewed interest in split livers with the introduction of several innovations that have improved the results, most importantly the development of techniques to perform the dissection in vivo (in situ), borrowing directly from the experience with living donor liver transplantation.

We introduced living donors in children in the 1980s, with rapidly improving results throughout the 1990s. Living donation has now become routine in pediatrics, although with improvements in split liver transplantation more options are available to pediatric transplant surgeons than in the past. Widespread application of split liver transplantation as a replacement for living donor transplantation has been limited, however, by a lack of sharing between centers. Currently, in areas with multiple transplant centers there is little incentive on the part of non-pediatric centers to share their full size organs for splitting. Equitable resolution of this issue must be achieved before splitting can achieve its full potential, which could largely eliminate the need to perform living donor transplants in children. For the present time, however, we continue to rely on living donor transplantation to achieve optimal results for our pediatric patients.

More recently, increasing concern over liver transplant waiting time-related morbidity has fostered increased interest in the further development of living donation for adults, which requires a greater hepatic resection from the donor than living donation in pediatrics. Ethical issues over indications for adult living donation, patient selection, techniques and outcomes dominate debate in liver transplantation forums, although the overall role of this modality in improving outcomes remains controversial.

Technique of graft size reduction

Standard donor hepatectomy is performed in the cadaveric donor. The graft reduction (or splitting) is performed ex vivo (**Fig. 38.15**), or more recently, in situ, in which the liver is divided in the heart-beating cadaver donor to minimize ischemic time for the split liver. There are potential advantages to both ex vivo and in situ splitting, and the transplant surgeon should be prepared and comfortable with either approach. The size of liver required will determine the plane of the dissection. For a very small infant (with a donor to recipient size disparity of 10 to 1), the left lateral segment (Couinaud segments II and III) is used; whereas, if the disparity is less, the entire left lobe can be used. If the right lobe is to be discarded, the common structures of the porta hepatis are kept with the graft. When the liver is to be split into two grafts, the recipient team receiving the primary offer has the option of keeping the full length of portal structures with their graft. In practice, however, it is more optimal for the team receiving the extended right lobe (the larger portion of the liver) to receive the full length of the porta hepatis structures and vena cava, with the team receiving the left lateral segment receiving only the left portal vein, left bile duct, and left hepatic artery (same as in a live donor graft). In ex vivo splitting, the hilar structures and parenchymal division is performed on the back table, with the liver kept cold using ice slush. When the split is performed in vivo, usually in ideal hemodynamically stable donors, the hilar dissection and parenchymal division is performed like a living donor. The parenchymal division can be terminated at any point if the donor

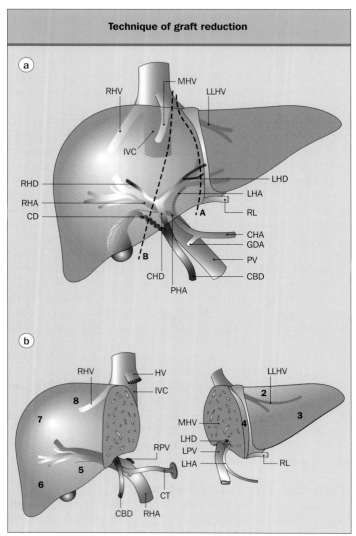

Technique of graft reduction

(a)

(b)

Figure 38.15 Technique of graft reduction. (a) There are two planes of potential parenchymal transection, for either a segment II/III graft (plane A) or for a full lobar split (plane B). (b) Dissected lobes. HV, hepatic vein; RHV, right hepatic vein; MHV, middle hepatic vein; LLHV, left lobe hepatic vein; IVC, inferior vena cava; CBD, common bile duct; CHD, common hepatic duct; CD, cystic duct; RHD, right hepatic duct; LHD, left hepatic duct; CHA, common hepatic artery; GDA, gastroduodenal artery; PHA, proper hepatic artery; LHA, left hepatic artery; RHA, right hepatic artery; GDA, gastroduodenal artery; CT, celiac trunk; PV, portal vein; RPV, right portal vein; LPV, left portal vein; RL, round ligament.

develops hemodynamic instability, and the liver can then be flushed and taken out whole, with the remainder of the transection continued ex vivo. In both techniques, the liver tissue is divided with clips or fine sutures being used to control the small vascular structures. As noted above, the hilar dissection is similar whether a left lateral or full left lobe graft is required. If the full left lobe is to be used, the liver is divided in the plane of the gallbladder fossa (Fig. 38.15a – plane B), and the parenchyma is transected to the right of the middle hepatic vein. If the lateral segment is used, the liver is divided just to the right of the round ligament (Fig. 38.15a – plane A). Superiorly, the dissection of the hepatic veins varies depending on whether the vena cava of the recipient is to be replaced by the donor vena cava. For lateral segment grafts, it is best to remove the vena

cava and the caudate lobe and position the graft directly on the recipient vena cava. If the whole left lobe is used, it is more convenient to preserve the entire vena cava and replace it in the recipient as in whole organ transplantation. At the completion of parenchymal transection, it is necessary to treat the section with a hemostatic surface. Despite meticulous preparation, the cut section will generally pose a hemostatic problem when the graft is split ex vivo. In situ splits are less prone to cut-section bleeding, because the vessels are identified and addressed while the liver is perfused with blood. Several strategies have been utilized, including fibrin glue, or reinforcement of the surface with a mesh, which permits direct control of the bleeding sites with suture ligatures through the mesh.

Reduced-size liver transplantation: the recipient operation

The recipient hepatectomy for the reduced size liver is similar to orthotopic liver transplantation with exception of the native vena cava, which must therefore be preserved if there is no graft vena cava. This requires meticulous suture ligation of each hepatic vein branch to the caudate lobe during recipient hepatectomy, the goal of which is to free the entire retrohepatic vena cava, leaving the liver attached only by the three main hepatic veins. The portal vein and cava are then clamped and the liver removed. The orifices of two of the native hepatic veins are combined into a single orifice and the caval opened longitudinally to fashion a very large opening that receives the hepatic vein of the graft for a wide unobstructed anastomosis. The portal vein is anastomosed end-to-end but requires careful positioning since the course of the vessel is altered by the shape of the partial graft. The artery is then reconstructed according to the local situation. If the recipient hepatic artery is of adequate caliber, it is used for the anastomosis, using the microscope if needed. Otherwise, an interposition graft can be taken to the aorta. Reconstruction of the bile duct requires a Roux-en-Y anastomosis since the orientation of the partial graft is generally distorted to the right.

Implantation of the left lobe of a split liver graft is comparable to the technique described above. The right lobe graft usually contains the vena cava and is implanted in a fashion that is nearly identical to a standard adult liver transplant. If common structures were allocated to the left lobe, reconstruction of the artery or bile duct may be more complex and require either an interposition graft or a microvascular anastomosis. Reconstruction of the bile duct may require creation of one or more anastomoses to segmental bile ducts. Although some authors favor use of small stents for these anastomoses, we perform a direct mucosa-to-mucosa anastomosis under high magnification without intubation. Two or, occasionally, three small ducts may be anastomosed. Whenever possible, small ducts are incorporated into a single anastomosis, but if they are too far apart separate anastomoses are constructed.

Abdominal closure

The use of reduced grafts often creates a scenario in which the graft is either too large or too small for the recipient. Both these situations can create lethal complications that must be detected and prevented at the time of abdominal closure. If the graft is too small, it can rotate on the axis of its vessels and acutely obstruct the circulation. Hepatic venous outflow is particularly prone to this complication. The graft's position must be assured

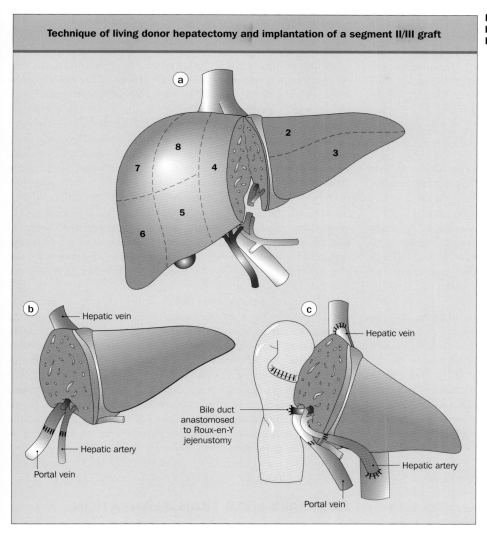

Technique of living donor hepatectomy and implantation of a segment II/III graft

Hepatic vein
Hepatic artery
Portal vein

Bile duct anastomosed to Roux-en-Y jejenustomy

Hepatic vein
Hepatic artery
Portal vein

Figure 38.16 Technique of living donor hepatectomy and implantation of a segment II/III graft.

by appropriate planning of the vascular anastomoses, and by positioning the intestines to occupy any empty space in the right upper quadrant into which the liver can rotate. Mechanical fixation of the liver is usually not helpful. If the liver is too large, closure under tension can result in a compression syndrome, leading to liver ischemia and renal and pulmonary compromise. This is managed by temporary prosthetic closure of the abdomen. The prosthetic material is subsequently removed at about 7–10 days after the transplant, a time when abdominal wall edema and ascites have abated in most patients thereby facilitating wound closure.

Living related donor transplantation
Living donor hepatectomy
Living donor hepatectomy has become common in pediatrics, since the initial description of the procedure in 1989. The graft is usually segments II and III of Couinaud, comprising 15–20% of the donor's hepatic volume, generally between 200 and 250 g of liver tissue. This is ideal for infants, but as the recipient becomes larger, outcomes are compromised by the small size of the graft. In the past 5 years, donation of the full right lobe has been performed with growing frequency for use in adult recipients.

Segmentectomy of segments II and III for a pediatric recipient can be readily performed through a midline incision (**Fig. 38.16a**). The porta hepatis is dissected to expose the origin of the left hepatic artery. The left portal vein is then encircled, and the posterior branches to the caudate lobe are divided. The left bile duct is approached anteriorly and encircled. The left duct should be divided with a minimum of dissection to preserve the blood supply of the duct wall. Superiorly, the confluence of the left and middle hepatic veins is exposed; this is the terminal point of the dissection. The parenchyma is then divided just to the right of the falciform ligament with meticulous division of the biliary and vascular branches to segment IV. If a larger graft is to be obtained, the parenchyma can be divided in the principal fissure just to the right of the middle hepatic vein. The full left lobe graft weighs between 350 and 500 g in adults and is sufficient for a small adult or an older child. After the parenchyma is divided the graft is attached only by its vessels, which are then divided, and the liver is rapidly flushed with heparinized preservation solution.

Right lobe donor hepatectomy
A graft of sufficient volume for an adult recipient can be obtained by right hepatectomy. Preoperatively, donor evaluation

is generally performed independently of the recipient evaluation, with a view towards optimizing risk by careful screening of anatomic, psychosocial and general medical conditions in potential donors. Donors undergo screening angiography and cholangiography (magnetic resonance imaging is used for this purpose at our center), and occasionally liver biopsy. While the donor evaluation and patient care pathways are not yet standardized, guidelines have been developed by the American Committee on Transplantation (ACOT) and by the New York State Department of Health.

Donor right hepatectomy requires an incision similar to that used for the transplant recipient. The portal dissection requires cholecystectomy and identification of the right hepatic artery near its origin. The right border of the common hepatic duct is exposed until the right bile duct is encountered. A single common trunk of the right bile duct is absent in the majority of cases. More commonly, the duct of segments V and VIII is encountered first, and then more superiorly and posteriorly, the duct to segments VI and VII. After the ducts are transected, the right portal vein is encircled at its origin. The liver is completely mobilized, and then the small hepatic vein branches to the caudate lobe are encircled and divided to free completely the right lobe from its attachments to the vena cava. The right hepatic vein is freed and encircled. After completion of the dissection the parenchyma is divided in the plane just to the right of the middle hepatic vein. Parenchymal division in a fully vascularized liver can be both tricky and tedious. The central venous pressure is kept low, with crystalloid infusion kept to a minimum during the division. Surgeons have adopted their own unique methods of parenchymal division in live donors to minimize blood loss but avoid unnecessarily long operations. A qualified assistant, preferably an attending surgeon or senior fellow, is advantageous during the parenchymal division. Our preference, which has worked well in over 100 live donor hepatectomies, is the use of the cavitron ultrasonic dissector together with electrocautery and metal clips. Operative sonography is used during parenchymal division to localize the vessels and guide the dissection. Most surgeons performing donor right hepatectomy perform the division to the right of the middle hepatic vein, preserving the middle vein in the donor. This may lead to relative engorgement of the medial segments of the graft, which in some cases may even require venous reconstruction of the outflow to these segments. Occasionally circumstances may require incorporation of the middle vein into the graft, for example when there is a relatively small right graft with a generous left lobe in the donor. The donor surgeon, in close communication with the recipient surgeon, should be prepared to address such contingencies at the time of operation. After completion of the parenchymal transection, the vessels are clamped and divided, and the graft flushed with heparinized preservation fluid.

Implantation of the lobe grafts

The left lobe graft is implanted as described above for reduced size liver transplantation. (Fig. 38.16b and c).

The right lobe graft is used if the donor is the same size, or smaller than the recipient. During implantation, the central venous pressure is maintained in a low normal range to avoid engorgement of the hemigraft after reperfusion. Reduced sized grafts are especially prone to engorgement injury due to limitations

in outflow in segments of the graft. The right hepatic vein of the graft is anastomosed end-to-side to the recipient hepatic vein orifice/vena cava. The orifice is fashioned into a large longitudinal opening that lessens the risk of torsional outflow obstruction, a common cause of graft failure in the early experience with live donor grafts. The portal vein is anastomosed end-to-end with reperfusion of the liver. A microvascular technique is used to anastomose the artery, but if needed the recipient's saphenous vein can be used to create an arterial conduit for a more convenient anastomosis to a larger vessel. The biliary anastomosis is most difficult in the adult recipient, particularly if the recipient had large volume losses and resuscitation leading to bowel edema. It is extremely difficult to create a fine anastomosis between the tiny segmental ducts and massively edematous jejunum. Multiple duct anastomoses are common, and the surgeon should be prepared to utilize all of the potential conduits for biliary drainage that are available, depending on the number and location of the bile ducts. When two ducts are present, both can usually be incorporated into a single or dual biliary enteric anastomosis. When more than two ducts are present, one of the ducts can sometimes be ligated. When three major ducts are present, we have sometimes utilized both primary duct-to-duct anastomosis in conjunction with biliary enteric anastomoses to obtain complete biliary drainage. Technical complications related to biliary anastomoses and the cut surface are common in live donor transplantation. A protocol for diagnosis and management should be in place before starting a live donor program, including assurances of the skills and availability of the diagnostic and interventional radiologists who are invaluable as partners in managing these difficult postoperative problems. Fortunately, these transplants can be done electively, with careful planning to minimize these technical difficulties (**Fig. 38.17**).

AUXILIARY LIVER TRANSPLANTATION

Replacement of part of the liver or the addition of a heterotopically placed partial liver graft has been used in cases of

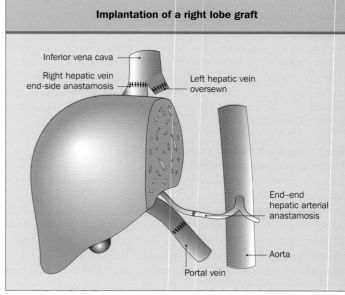

Figure 38.17 Implantation of a right lobe graft.

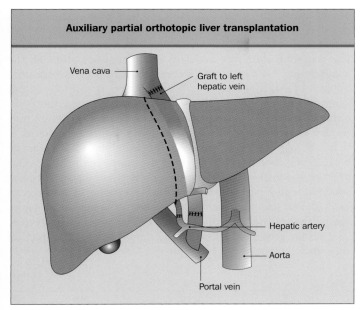

Figure 38.18 Auxiliary partial orthotopic liver transplantation. A left lobe graft has been implanted in the bed (orthotopically) of the resected native left lobe.

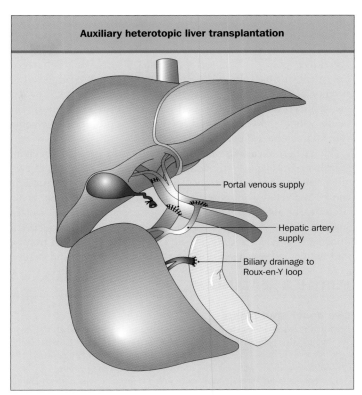

Figure 38.19 Auxiliary heterotopic liver transplantation.

fulminant hepatic failure or metabolic liver diseases. Auxiliary liver transplantation has also been proposed for living related liver transplantation in which a small left lobe graft is implanted next to the residual functioning native liver.

For fulminant hepatic failure, the addition of the functional liver mass is used to support the recipient hepatic function until hepatic regeneration of the native liver, if possible, or the graft occurs. In those individuals in which the native graft recovers adequately, immunosuppression can be discontinued and the auxiliary graft is allowed to atrophy via rejection. For the treatment of metabolic diseases, the addition of a functional liver mass producing specific proteins (e.g. factor VIII in hemophilia) or clearing metabolites or essential minerals (e.g. bilirubin in glucuronyltransferase deficiency or urea in urea cycle defects) can sustain an almost normal phenotype.

Auxiliary liver transplantation involves a group of diverse techniques that are too complex to be covered in this section. Early experiences established the need for portal blood and adequate hepatic venous outflow for successful grafting. This is most readily accomplished by placing the liver graft in an orthotopic position, in which a specific lobe is replaced by an anatomically similar graft (**Fig. 38.18**). Most commonly, the left lobe of the diseased liver is replaced with a left lobe graft from a cadaveric or living donor, requiring partial hepatectomy in the recipient as the first step. The hepatic vein is reconstructed in an end-to-end fashion, as are the portal vein and hepatic artery. The bile duct generally requires hepatojejunostomy. An older technique involves placement of the graft in the hepatic fossa inferior to the native liver with attachment of the portal and hepatic veins onto the side of the recipient vessels (**Fig. 38.19**). The principal technical challenge involves managing the competition for portal blood between the two livers. The recipient liver tends to be favored for portal perfusion and successful grafting depends upon modifying portal perfusion to favor the

graft, leading to relative hypertrophy of the graft. Optimal techniques for auxiliary liver transplantation remain under development as the eventual role of this technique remains uncertain.

IMMEDIATE POST-OPERATIVE MANAGEMENT OF LIVE DONOR RECIPIENTS – SPECIAL CONSIDERATIONS

The growing use of LDLT impacts postoperative care in several ways. In the immediate postoperative period, the reduced-size graft is especially prone to engorgement compared to whole grafts. The central venous pressure should be aggressively managed within a tight range of 5–10, sometimes with pharmacologic support of the blood pressure and the use of venodilators. Although most adults are in relatively good general condition prior to LDLT, the graft function may be poor initially because of the relatively small functional size of the donor liver in adult living donors. This can lead in some cases to a syndrome of cholestasis and persistent graft dysfunction which has been termed 'small for size syndrome'. Management of these patients must be meticulous to allow the livers to regenerate without the development of additional complications which can further injure the graft. Overall, however, the postoperative course of patients receiving LDLT has been smooth with a short intensive care unit and total length of stay and superb outcomes in experienced centers.

Vascular patency must be assessed postoperatively as well as during the transplant operation. The use of Doppler imaging is usually adequate for demonstrating hepatic artery and portal venous flow, however when there is doubt either magnetic resonance vascular imaging or direct angiography must be performed. In recent years, as the incidence of hepatic artery thrombosis has decreased, we have nonetheless continued an aggressive policy of sonographic surveillance of the artery. Emergent angiography with arterial stenting has replaced open surgery in our practice, since precise thrombolytic therapy can be administered, intimal flaps distant from the anastamosis can be identified and treated, and occult inflow problems like celiac stenoses can be addressed.

Biliary complications are more frequent in patients receiving split liver grafts and live donor grafts though they still occasionally complicate standard transplants. Both leaks and obstructions can be managed using interventional radiologic methods. Leaks occur early after surgery and are not always detected by the surgical drains. Aggressive use of sonography and cross-sectional imaging is needed to detect fluid collections. Bile leaks may be end fistulas. These need effective external drainage and control of sepsis, supplemented by diagnostic cholangiography and possible stenting to reduce leakage. Most biliary leaks will resolve with effective drainage, though open surgery is occasionally required as in the cases of complete disruption of the anastomosis. The anastomotic stenosis should always be suspected as part of the differential of graft dysfunction. Localized stenoses can be managed successfully with minimally invasive methods, either endoscopic or percutaneous. More complex stenoses may require a combination of interventional and open techniques.

In summary, surgical issues clearly impact hepatology practice both in selection and aftercare of the transplant patient. Our practice has evolved to full integration between hepatology and surgery for all aspects of the program. The course of the surgery, from donor selection and procurement to technical obstacles during the transplant, will determine the postoperative course. The outline presented herein attempts to describe, in a practical way, the conduct of the procedures.

FURTHER READING

Live donor transplants

Brown RS, Russo MW, Lai M, et al. A survey of liver transplantation from living adult donors in the United States. N Engl J Med 2003; 348:818–825. *A survey of transplant centers in the USA revealed that adult-to-adult liver transplantation from a living donor is being increasingly performed, but mainly in a few large-volume centers. Though mortality among donors is low, complications in the donor are relatively common and were more frequent in centers performing fewer operations.*

Raia S, Nery JR, Meis S. Liver transplantation from live donors. Lancet 1989; ii:497.

Singer PA, Siegler M, Whitington PF, et al. Ethics of liver transplantation with living donors. N Engl J Med 1989; 321:620–622.

Split/reduced-size liver transplant

Bismuth H, Azoulay D, Samuel D, et al. Auxiliary partial orthotopic liver transplantation for fulminant hepatitis: the Paul Brousse experience. Ann Surg 1996; 224:712–724.

Busuttil RW, Goss JA. Split liver transplantation. Ann Surg 1999; 229:13–21. *A review of the experience of ex vivo and in situ split liver transplantation. These techniques expand the pool of donor organs available and have been successful. The in situ splitting technique results in graft survival as good as that of whole organs.*

Emond JC, Whitington PF, Thistlethwaite JR, et al. Reduced size orthotopic liver transplantation: use in the management of children with chronic liver disease. Hepatology 1989; 10:867–872.

van Hoek B, de Boer J, Boudjema K, et al. Auxiliary versus orthotopic liver transplantation for acute liver failure, EURALT Study Group, European Auxiliary Liver Transplant Registry. J Hepatol 1999; 30:699–705.

Transplant general

Kalayoglu M, Sollinger HW, Stratta RJ, et al. Extended preservation of the liver for clinical transplantation. Lancet 1988; 1:617–619.

Millis JM, Melinek J, Csete M, et al. Randomized controlled trial to evaluate flush and reperfusion techniques in liver transplantation. Transplantation 1997; 63:397–403.

Randall HB, Wachs ME, Somberg KA, et al. The use of the T tube after orthotopic liver transplantation. Transplantation 1996; 61:258–261.

Shaked A, Busuttil RW. Liver transplantation in patients with portal vein thrombosis and central portacaval shunts. Ann Surg 1991; 214:696–702. *Portal vein thrombosis and portocaval shunts are not a contraindication to successful liver transplantation, although careful patient selection is needed.*

Shaw BW Jr, Martin DJ, Marquez JM, et al. Venous bypass in clinical liver transplantation. Ann Surg 1984; 200:524–534.

Soin AS, Friend PJ, Rasmussen A, et al. Donor arterial variations in liver transplantation: management and outcome of 527 consecutive grafts. Br J Surg 1996; 83:637–641.

Starzl TE, Marchioro TL, Von Kaulla KN, et al. Homotransplantation of the liver in humans. Surg Gynecol Obstet 1963; 117:659–676.

Starzl TE, Klintmalm GBG, Porter KA, et al. Liver transplantation with the use of cyclosporin A and prednisone. N Engl J Med 1981; 305:266–269.

Starzl TE, Miller C, Broznick B, et al. An improved technique for multiple organ harvesting. Surg Gynecol Obstet 1987; 165:343–348.

Todo S, Nery J, Yanaga K, et al. Extended preservation of human liver grafts with UW solution. JAMA 1989; 261:711–714. *This paper describes the major impact of the University of Wisconsin solution on graft preservation and subsequent successful grafting. This development was a major advance.*

Transplantation in children

Bismuth H, Houssin D. Reduced size orthotopic liver graft in hepatic transplantation in children. Surgery 1984; 95:367–370.

Broelsch CE, Whitington PF, Emond JC, et al. Liver transplantation in children from living related donors. Surgical techniques and results. Ann Surg 1991; 214:428–437. *A detailed description of hepatic segmented graft transplants in 20 young children. The early results show a 75% success rate in this difficult group of patients.*

the proteosome itself by alteration of subunit composition thus generating an 'immunoproteosome'.

MHC class II peptide generation and binding to MHC class II molecules is more complex than described for the peptide/MHC class I pathway (**Fig. 39.5**). As mentioned earlier, MHC class II molecules are α/β heterodimers. These are synthesized and form a nonameric complex with another molecule known as the invariant chain. This complex is targeted to the endocytic pathway within the transGolgi network via sorting signals that are present within the cytoplasmic tail of the invariant chain. It is here that the interaction with antigenic peptide takes place. Antigenic peptides become associated with MHC class II molecules and are usually generated by the endocytic pathway following the ingestion of extracellular antigen. The endocytic pathway where this interaction takes place has been defined as having multivesicular structures. Antigen is degraded by lysosomal type proteases into small peptides of varying lengths. At the same time, the MHC class II invariant chain complex is degraded by other proteases (including cathepsin) into single α/β structures with a small individual peptide of the invariant chain (clip) remaining associated in the MHC class II peptide binding groove. This clip peptide is then exchanged for antigenic peptides by a process catalyzed by human leukocyte antigen-DM (HLA-DM) molecules. The peptide requirements for binding to the MHC class II groove are not as stringent as that for class I ligands. The peptides are usually longer, ranging between 14 and 18 amino acids in length (even up to 28 amino acids). These peptides extrude from the binding groove at both the amino- and carboxyl-terminal ends. The peptides are anchored in the MHC class II groove by various anchor residues, the most important one being at the beginning of the groove where the amino acid at this position is often hydrophobic in nature (but may be charged, once again depending on the MHC class II allele with which it is actually associating). Once the α/β heterodimer and peptide complex is stabilized, this is then transported and appears on the cell surface where the antigenic determinants in the groove are recognized by the α/β T-cell receptor on CD4+ cells.

EARLY EVENTS IN ACTIVATION OF T CELLS BY ANTIGEN (G0–G1 TRANSITION)

Activation via the T-cell receptor

The recognition of antigen/MHC complex by the TCR occurs at what is known as the 'immunological synapse'. This consists of the central T-cell receptor, adhesion molecules, costimulation molecules, an intracellular signaling complex and cytoskeletal components. The engagement of this synapse activates complex signaling pathways that lead to the induction of lymphocyte activation, division and clonal proliferation. The T-cell receptor is associated at the cell surface with a group of molecules known as the CD3 complex (**Fig. 39.6**).

This complex consists of $\varepsilon/\gamma/\delta$ heterodimers and an important ζ/ζ homodimer. In particular, the ζ/ζ homodimer has a long cytoplasmic tail, part of which is a repetitive 16 amino acid motif known as the immunoreceptor tyrosine-base activation motif (ITAM). Following antigen binding to the receptor and oligomerization of the receptor and the CD3 complex, phosphorylation of the ITAM takes place by tyrosine kinase molecules associated with CD4 (lck) or the T-cell receptor itself (fym) (**Fig. 39.7**).

Phosphorylation of the ITAM leads to the generation of a specific binding site for other protein tyrosine kinase (PTK) molecules, in particular ZAP-70 and Syk. These molecules become activated, generating further multiple tyrosine phosphorylation sites that serve as binding sites for other proteins that regulate two major pathways of cellular activation, finally leading to transcription of IL-2 and other cytokine genes. One of the key mediators in one of the pathways is phospholipase Cg (PLCg). Following triggering of the T-cell receptor complex PLCg is recruited to the cell membrane, is phosphorylated and results in the hydrolysis of inositol phospholipids, generating inositol polyphosphates (IP-3) and diglycerols (DG) from the cell membrane. IP-3 stimulates the mobilization of calcium from intracellular stores. The increase in intracellular cytoplasmic calcium leads to the activation of the calmodulin-dependent serine phosphatase calcineurin. This is a

Figure 39.5 Schematic diagram of the generation of major histocompatibility complex (MHC) class II/peptide complexes.

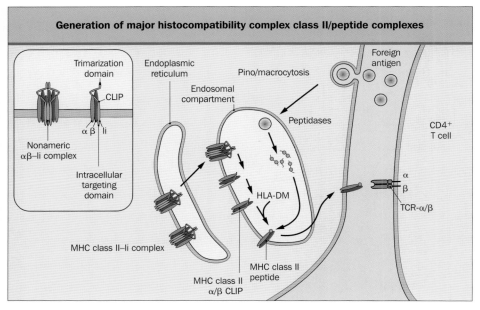

Generation of major histocompatibility complex class II/peptide complexes

Trimarization domain
CLIP
Nonameric $\alpha\beta$–li complex
α β li
Intracellular targeting domain
Endoplasmic reticulum
Endosomal compartment
Pino/macrocytosis
Foreign antigen
Peptidases
HLA-DM
CD4+ T cell
α
β
TCR-α/β
MHC class II–li complex
MHC class II peptide
MHC class II α/β CLIP

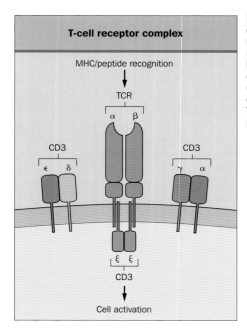

Figure 39.6 Schematic diagram of T-cell receptor complex that recognizes major histocompatibility complex (MHC)/peptide complexes resulting in T-cell activation and proliferation.

the mitogen-activated protein kinase (MAPK) cascade at the site of the JNK (JUN N-terminal kinase) molecule. The other product of phospholipid breakdown, DG, is important in the activation of another transcription factor nuclear factor-κB (NF-κB).

The second main pathway following the initial events at the TCR is activation of the MAPK cascade. This cascade is characterized by the successive phosphorylation of various cytoplasmic kinases which may act on themselves and finally lead to cytokine gene transcription. Mitogen-activated protein kinases phosphorylate at proline x-threonine/serine-proline sequences where x is often a leucine residue. They require dual phosphorylation at both serine/threonine and a tyrosine residue for activation. Activation through this cascade results in activation of c-JUN, c-FOS and NF-κB transcription factors, as well as optimally activating the NFAT transcription factor. Early activation of the MAPK cascade occurs via the RAS pathway and RAS-mediated recruitment of Raf-1 to plasma membrane. Raf-1 is one of the MAPKK (MAPK kinase) molecules that form part of the MAPK cascade itself. It is important to note that activation via both of these cascades (i.e. the PLCg/calcineurin pathway and the MAPK pathway) is needed for optimal T-cell activation.

Costimulatory pathways

Optimal activation via the T-cell receptor requires recruitment of other cell surface molecules as part of the immunogical synapse signaling complex. These include the CD8 and CD4 molecules themselves which interact with MHC class I and class II proteins respectively on the cell surface of the APC, the CD58/CD2 interaction, and the CD54/intercellular adhesion molecule (ICAM) interaction (**Fig. 39.8**).

However, the most important adhesion molecule is CD28, which interacts with the B7 (CD80/CD86) molecules on the APC. These molecules are both members of the immunoglobulin

crucial molecule in T-cell activation, and is a target for immunosuppressive drugs such as cyclosporine and tacrolimus. Activation of calcineurin has two main effects. It leads to the activation of the cytoplasmic form of nuclear factor for activated T cells (NFAT$_c$), resulting in its transfer to the nucleus where it combines with NFAT$_n$ to form an active nuclear transcription activator which binds to various gene promoters, including the promoter for the IL-2 gene. This transcription factor acts together with other transcription factors of the AP-1 family such as FOS and JUN. Calcineurin also plays a major role in the phosphorylation status of other pathways, in particular

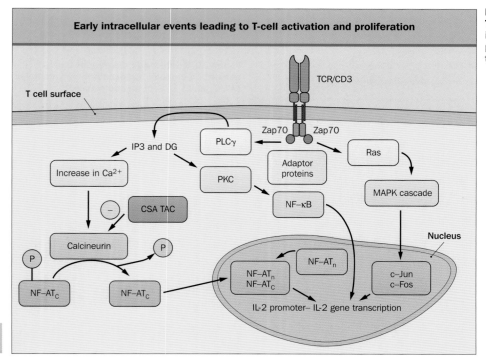

Figure 39.7 Early intracellular events leading to T-cell activation and proliferation. Sites of drug interactions outlined in the text are labeled. PKC, protein kinase C. CSA, cyclosporin; TAC, tacrolimus.

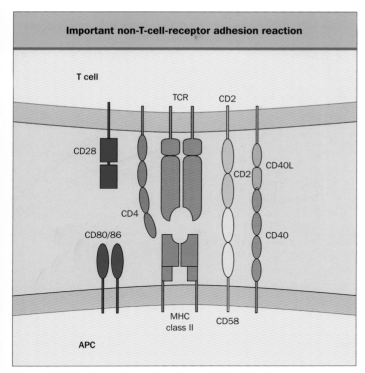

Important non-T-cell-receptor adhesion reaction

T cell

TCR CD2

CD28

CD40L

CD2

CD4

CD80/86

CD40

MHC
class II CD58

APC

Figure 39.8 Costimulatory molecules and their ligands.

superfamily. CD28 is a two-domain structure, while CD80/CD86 has a single immunoglobulin domain. Following T-cell receptor interaction, CD28 is rapidly expressed at increased levels on the cell surface, and ligation of CD28 with CD80/CD86 results in activation of the protein tyrosine kinase complex, including the MAPK cascade. It is at this point that the calcineurin pathway via the T-cell receptor and the activation pathway via CD28 meet. This process leads to the optimal activation of various gene transcription factors, which rapidly upregulate IL-2 itself, the IL-2 receptor, and the CD40 ligand. The pathway of CD28 signaling also leads to the upregulation of a molecule known as cytotoxic T-lymphocyte antigen (CTLA) 4. This molecule has approximately a 10- to 100-fold higher avidity for CD28 than for CD80/CD86. It has been recently recognized that CTLA4 may have an important negative influence on T-cell activation.

Another adhesion costimulatory pathway for T-cell activation is the CD40/CD40 ligand (CD40L/CD154) interaction. CD40/CD154 is a member of the TNF cytokine family, while CD40 is a member of the TNFR family. CD154 is expressed on T cells following activation via the TCR, while CD40 is widely expressed on cell types including antigen-presenting dendritic cells. This interaction is thought to be important in upregulating CD80/86 on APCs and in enhancing APC function itself. The CD40/CD154 interaction seems to be critical in T-cell-dependent macrophage activation.

Recently novel costimulatory molecules have been identified that make the above description somewhat simplified. These new molecules are part of the B7 or TNF family of molecules on APCs and part of the CD28 or TNFR family of T cells (Fig. 39.9). They include ICOS, PD-1, CD134 and CD27 on T cells with respective ligands on APCs. These interactions deliver both positive and negative signals in the context of T-cell receptor

stimulation. It is likely that the integration of these various costimulation signals may deliver different outcomes depending on the exact in situ environment.

LATER EVENTS IN ACTIVATION OF T CELLS BY ANTIGEN (G1–S PHASE TRANSITION)

The early activation steps and production and secretion of IL-2 lead to the induction of the IL-2 receptor and subsequent signaling through the IL-2 receptor. This signaling pathway and signaling through other cytokine receptors occurs via a different set of cytoplasmic molecules known as the Janus kinase (JAK) proteins and signal transducers and activation of transcription (STAT) molecules. This results in progression of lymphocyte activation in the cell cycle from the G1 to S phase. These latter events are important as the STAT/targets of rapamycin (TOR) molecules are important targets of the rapamycin group of immunosuppressant drugs.

HOW DO ACTIVATED CELLS ENTER TISSUES?

Following activation of T cells and the subsequent induction of other non-specific inflammatory cells, these cells circulate and enter tissues and, in the case of organ allografts, cause tissue damage and allograft rejection. The way in which these cells actually enter tissues has now been well defined. The process consists of three steps involving leukocyte-endothelial cell interactions. These steps are known as:

- the initial tethering and rolling step;
- step of adhesion of the leukocyte to the endothelium; and
- the extravasation of the leukocyte through the endothelium into the tissues (**Fig. 39.10**).

The initial rolling and tethering step is initiated by a group of molecules known as selectins. These are expressed on leukocytes themselves (L-selectin) and endothelial structures (E-selectin and P-selectin). Selectins are 'long' molecules that extend well out from the endothelial surface and have plant C-type lectin domains, which are positioned on the end of repetitive consensus repeat domains, these being homologous to the complement binding proteins. It is the presentation of this C-type lectin domain away from the cell surface that allows interaction with selectin ligands. The selectin ligands are a class of complex oligosaccharides known as lactosaminoglycans, and these contain the core tetrasaccharide structure sialyl Lewis-X (SLEX). Binding of selectins to their ligands is calcium dependent, and the initial tethering and rolling steps are relatively loose and reversible. Selectins are upregulated quite rapidly by various cytokines/chemokines which also lead to the induction of a high affinity group of molecules known as integrins, in particular lymphocyte function-associated antigen (LFA)-1, very late antigen (VLA)-4 and $\alpha 4\beta 7$ on the leukocyte cell surface. Integrins mediate the second step of leukocyte-endothelial interaction. The integrins bind to endothelial adhesion molecules such as the ICAMs (ICAM-1/ICAM-20), vascular adhesion molecule (VCAM-1) and mucosal addressing cell adhesion molecule (MAdCAM)-1. The interactions between integrins and the integrin receptors mediate firm adhesion of leukocytes to the vascular endothelium. Another molecule, vascular adhesion protein (VAP)-1, may play an important role in leukocyte–

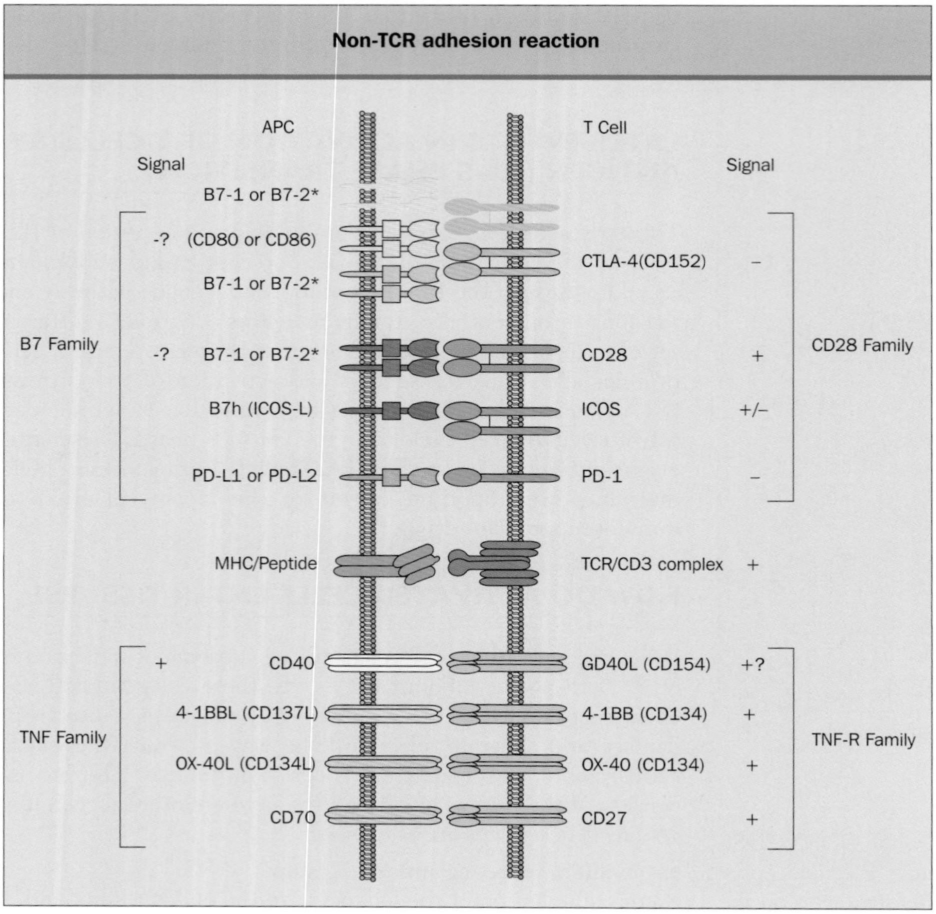

Non-TCR adhesion reaction

APC T Cell

Signal Signal

B7-1 or B7-2*

-? (CD80 or CD86) CTLA-4(CD152) –

B7-1 or B7-2*

B7 Family -? B7-1 or B7-2* CD28 + CD28 Family

B7h (ICOS-L) ICOS +/–

PD-L1 or PD-L2 PD-1 –

MHC/Peptide TCR/CD3 complex +

+ CD40 GD40L (CD154) +?

4-1BBL (CD137L) 4-1BB (CD134) +

TNF Family OX-40L (CD134L) OX-40 (CD134) + TNF-R Family

CD70 CD27 +

Figure 39.9 Important non-TCR adhesion reaction between the T-cell and the antigen-presenting cell (APC).

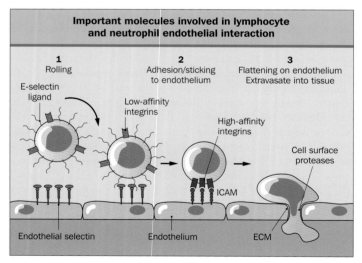

Important molecules involved in lymphocyte and neutrophil endothelial interaction

1	2	3
Rolling	Adhesion/sticking to endothelium	Flattening on endothelium Extravasate into tissue

E-selectin ligand

Low-affinity integrins

High-affinity integrins

Cell surface proteases

ICAM

Endothelial selectin   Endothelium   ECM

Figure 39.10 Important molecules involved in lymphocyte and neutrophil endothelial interaction resulting in cellular chemotaxis into inflamed tissues. ECM, extracellular matrix; ICAM, intercellular adhesion molecule; PCAM, platelet-cell adhesion molecule.

endothelial interactions within the liver. The second step of firm adhesion to the endothelium leads to leukocyte flattening, and the development of cell surface pseudopodia which insinuate themselves between endothelial junctions, and result in leukocyte extravasation into tissues. This last step involves the platelet endothelial cell adhesion molecule (PECAM)-1 and leukocyte cell surface proteinases, which are involved in the breakdown of endothelial cell junctions and extracellular matrix degradation. The above processes of extravasation and chemotaxis are driven particularly by the α and β chemokines.

MECHANISMS OF TISSUE INJURY

Once the activated cell enters tissues further activation of antigen-specific and non-specific effector mechanisms may take place resulting in tissue damage. One of the important cell interactions involved in tissue damage involves the cytotoxic T cell. CTLs are predominantly of the CD8+ phenotype, which interact with antigen in association with class I MHC expressed on tissue cells. Cell surface MHC class I is rapidly upregulated by any inflammatory response, particularly by mediators such as TNF and IFN-γ. This increased expression is important in clearance of viral antigen from tissues but also potentiates tissue damage in allograft rejection.

Cytotoxic T cells express important cell surface molecules such as Fas ligand, CD40 and cell-surface TNF. These molecules interact through their respective ligands such as Fas, CD154 and the TNFR and may induce cells to undergo programmed cell death or apoptosis. Activation of these pathways may also result in intracellular oxidative stress and cell necrosis. The pathways of apoptosis are similar in many cells, and have been described in great detail over the past 1–2 years. They are not discussed in detail here. Cellular apoptosis is triggered via a 'death domain' amino acid motif on the cytoplasmic tail of TNFRs (e.g. Fas), which are members of a larger family sharing these motifs. Cytotoxic T cells also produce various enzymes such as granzymes and perforin, which attack target cells and cause cell injury and death through apoptotic and necrotic pathways. Cells triggered in non-specific effector responses include NK cells, which were initially described in vitro and whose role in vivo has been difficult to define. They recognize and kill targets that do not express MHC class I molecules, and therefore their role in allograft rejection is probably minimal. They in fact carry receptors for MHC class I molecules, so that their activation is inhibited once the interaction between that receptor and MHC class I takes place.

Activated T cells, particularly of the CD4+ phenotype, produce significant amounts of IFN-γ and other molecules that turn on and activate macrophages. These cells are primarily involved in the DTH reaction, and they produce numerous cytokines such as TNF-α, IL-1, IL-6, IL-10 and TGF-β. All these molecules are important in cell injury via various mechanisms. The specific molecular pathways that are important in allograft rejection itself are discussed on the previous page.

Antibody production within non-lymphoid organs is probably minimal, but serum-derived antibody produced in lymph nodes and spleen may enter organs, activate complement and cause cellular injury. Such events are important in hyperacute allograft rejection and xenoallograft-associated rejection. The cellular target of serum antibody is likely to be the endothelial cell.

Th1 VERSUS Th2 CYTOKINE RESPONSE

One of the paradigms that is important in tissue injury, inflammation and regulation of the immune response, including outcomes from allograft rejection, has been the Th1/Th2 paradigm. This refers to the existence in some experimental systems of polarized cytokine responses following T-cell activation. The Th1 cytokine response involves the production of predominantly INF-γ, IL-2, and TNF-β (lymphotoxin), and results in macrophage activation and DTH reactions. In contrast, the Th2 response involves the production of IL-4, IL-5, IL-10 and IL-13, is associated with strong antibody responses including IgE production, and results in cross-inhibition of the Th1 response, predominantly via IL-4 and IL-10. Although the paradigm was initially worked out on isolated CD4+ T-cell clones in vitro, it has been observed in vivo following various immunization schedules and during experimental and clinical infectious states. For example, human tuberculoid leprosy is associated with a strong Th1 response at the site of the lesion, while lepromatous leprosy is associated with Th2-type responses. In experimental leishmaniasis, the BALB/c mouse is associated with systemic infection and progressive disease and a Th2-type response, while in the CH3B6 mouse leishmania is controlled and associated with a DTH Th1-type response. It is unclear how these responses are diverted at the early stages of T-cell activation. It is thought that IL-12 production and IFN-α production from perhaps macrophages and NK cells are important in the induction of the Th1 response. In contrast, IL-4, either produced from macrophages, T cells themselves, or mast cells, is crucial in directing the response towards a Th2 phenotype. In some experimental

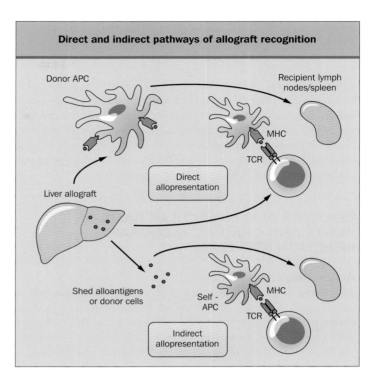

Figure 39.11 Direct and indirect pathways of allograft recognition.

situations, the Th1 response has been associated with allograft rejection, while the Th2 response has been associated with allograft tolerance.

ALLOANTIGEN RECOGNITION

The description of the immune response is formulated on the recognition of foreign antigen, consisting of foreign protein or infectious organisms, by the immune system. However, the response against an organ allograft is complicated by the presence of allo-MHC as well as self-MHC cell surface molecules. This has led to the concept that T-cell stimulation following allograft transplantation can occur by direct and indirect pathways (Fig. 39.11).

The direct T-cell response is defined as the stimulation of T cells by the allogeneic MHC antigen on allogeneic APCs. This response does not require intracellular processing and presentation of peptides in order to stimulate the T-cell response. Quite extraordinarily, when this response is measured in vitro, the frequency of precursor T cells for a direct alloimmune response is about 100-fold greater than that for a response to individual peptides derived from environmental antigens. The direct pathway is likely to involve two kinds of APCs. Initially, in tissues such as the liver, true APCs such as dendritic cells or macrophages are likely to be the main source of antigen presentation. Secondly, endothelial cells of the graft themselves which have been induced to express increased amounts of MHC, particularly class II and adhesion molecules, may also stimulate an allo-response. In contrast to direct T-cell activation, allostimulation may take place by normal physiological antigen processing. This is called indirect antigen presentation. In this situation, peptides derived from alloantigen combine with self- (recipient-) MHC molecules and are presented to the immune system as foreign antigen. Indirect T-cell activation is likely to depend more on the APCs in the recipient's draining lymph nodes and spleens, being primed either by soluble antigen or cellular antigen itself, following degradation into allopeptides.

Although it is thought that the direct pathway is crucial in allograft recognition, there is evidence that indirect antigen presentation actually does occur, as it is possible to immunize with allo-MHC peptides and induce recognition responses and even accelerate experimental rejection. The process may not be as efficient as the direct pathway and may play an important role in the processes of chronic allograft rejection.

CELLULAR AND MOLECULAR BASIS OF ACUTE AND CHRONIC ALLOGRAFT REJECTION (GENERAL)

Acute allograft rejection

The initial target of the acute allograft rejection response in vascularized allografts is the microvasculature. The microvasculature has high constitutive expression of MHC molecules and other adhesion molecules. Furthermore, the microvasculature has a very narrow lumen. This combination predisposes to leukocyte–endothelial cell interactions. The predominant cells that mediate acute rejection are T cells, particularly the T-helper CD4+ subset. The molecular mechanisms particularly involve a DTH reaction, with macrophage activation and production of cytokines such as IL-2, INF-γ, TNF-α and lymphotoxin. The T-helper subset also triggers alloreactive CTL production. Alloreactive CTLs have been isolated from allografts during rejection, and there is evidence of increased messenger RNA and protein for granzyme and perforin, major components of the CTL effector pathway. These CTLs are predominantly CD8+ and have been shown to be important, not so much in determining whether rejection occurs, but in the speed of the rejection process. As well as the recruitment of macrophages, there is evidence for the recruitment of other components of the non-specific immune system. In particular the presence of eosinophils and eosinophil protein products (eosinophilic cationic protein) and IL-5 have been correlated with acute rejection. Recently much interest has been shown in studying 'final common pathways' in tissue damage during acute rejection, particularly the role of nitric oxide and oxidative stress.

The role of antibody in causing tissue damage during acute allograft rejection has recently received more attention particularly in a subset of renal allograft recipients. This subset is identified by the deposition of the classical complement pathway component C4d. This form of rejection may be more severe and resistant to therapy than pure cellular rejection.

Chronic allograft rejection

Chronic allograft rejection usually results from uncontrolled acute rejection episodes, but it does have some distinct pathogenic mechanisms not seen in acute rejection. The microvasculature, an initial target during acute rejection, is totally obliterated in the chronic rejection process. In conjunction with obliteration of the microvasculature, there is the development of a process known as 'transplant vasculopathy' that affects medium-sized arteries. This vasculopathy is a result of antigen-specific and antigen non-specific damage to arterial endothelium. The initiating stimulus is a cell-mediated immune response directed against allo-MHC molecules. This results in the accumulation of CD4+- and CD8+-activated T cells within the vessel wall and the consequent activation of macrophages. The release of chemotactic factors such as membrane cofactor protein (MCP)-1, MIP-1α, and MIP-1β seems to be crucial in the resulting macrophage activation and proliferation. The release of platelet-derived growth factor from macrophages, adherent platelets and damaged endothelium is a major stimulator for smooth muscle proliferation. Transforming growth factor-β production by macrophages leads to the transition of smooth muscle cells to the myofibroblasts which secrete significant extracellular matrix protein resulting in vessel (subintimal) fibrosis. Similar processes also take place in the interstitium of various organs resulting in organ fibrosis.

DRUGS THAT INHIBIT THE IMMUNE SYSTEM: PHARMACOLOGY AND MECHANISMS OF ACTION

Corticosteroids

Corticosteroids are chemically modified derivatives of natural adrenal hormones and are used in various forms, such as prednisolone, hydrocortisone and methylprednisolone. They have similar efficacy apart from hydrocortisone, which acts at 1:5 strength compared with prednisolone and methylprednisolone. Corticosteroids have numerous mechanisms of action in inhibiting the immune system. At very high doses they cause lympholysis/apoptosis and margination of lymphocytes resulting in significant lymphopenia. They also inhibit macrophage/dendritic cell antigen-presenting function via inhibition of transcription of cytokines such as IL-1 and TNF-α, and by inhibiting arachidonic acid metabolism. Corticosteroids inhibit the first enzyme of the arachidonic acid metabolic pathway: phospholipase A2. This leads to blockage of the cyclo-oxygenase and 5-lipo-oxygenase pathways with the resulting inhibition of thromboxane and prostacyclin production. Corticosteroids also inhibit interferon-dependent adhesion molecule expression including MHC class II. Furthermore, there is some evidence that corticosteroids stimulate TGF-β production, a known inhibitory cytokine resulting in a more Th2-type cytokine profile (anti-inflammatory) rather than Th1 cytokine production.

Azathioprine

Azathioprine is an imidazole derivative of 6-mercaptopurine, and is well-absorbed and converted to 6-mercaptopurine and to 6-thio-ionosine monophosphate in the liver. Xanthine oxidase is required for azathioprine metabolism with conversion to 6-thiouric acid, followed by excretion in the urine. These chemicals are alkaloid DNA precursors and azathioprine leads to reduced bioavailability of purine molecules by inhibition of inosine monophosphate and the de novo purine pathway. Azathioprine also blocks phosphoribozyl pyrophosphate (PRPP), thus blocking purine synthesis via the salvage pathway. The overall affect of azathioprine is to inhibit lymphocyte proliferation at the G1–S phase transition (i.e. following signaling via the T-cell receptor/adhesion molecule cascade).

Cyclosporin

Cyclosporin was isolated from the fungus *Trichoderma polysporum*. It is a cyclic endecapeptide. It is currently available as a microemulsion (Neoral). Before this microemulsion form was available, absorption of cyclosporin (Sandimmune) showed large individual variation with an average oral bioavailability of only 30%, but varying between 5 and 90%. Cyclosporin (Sandimmune) is highly lipid-soluble, and dependent on bile salt availability in the gastrointestinal lumen. The microemulsion form (Neoral) has an improved overall bioavailability, with less individual variation and less dependence on bile salts for absorption. The 'area under the curve' profile increased by 1.5–3 fold with conversion to the microemulsified preparation of cyclosporin. Cyclosporin is highly metabolized in the gastrointestinal tract and the liver by the cytochrome P450 complex, mainly cytochrome P450 3A4. This results in numerous metabolites that are excreted in the bile. Less than 1% of cyclosporin is excreted unchanged. There is evidence of enterohepatic circulation.

Cyclosporin exerts its immunosuppressive actions by binding to a cytoplasmic protein called cyclophilin, the prototype member of the immunophilin family. Cyclophilin is a highly basic, abundant protein present in many tissues. It is an 18 kDa cis-transpeptidyl-propyl isomerase ('rotamase') which plays a role in protein folding. However, this action is not related to the drug's immunosuppressive property. Cyclosporin forms a complex with cyclophilin and this complex binds with high affinity to calcineurin (a cytoplasmic calcium-dependent phosphatase) resulting in inhibition of its phosphatase function. The phosphatase function of calcineurin is crucial in the activation of the $NFAT_c$ transcription factor resulting in its translocation into the nucleus to act as a transcription factor for the IL-2 molecule. This step is effectively blocked by the cyclosporin cyclophilin/calcineurin complex. Cyclosporin has two domains: one involved in the drug interaction with cyclophilin itself; and the effector domain that is a composite of the cyclosporin and the cyclophilin itself, which interacts with calcineurin. The interaction between cyclophilin and cyclosporin is highly dependent on the hydrophobic side chain of the 6-methyl leucine in cyclosporin. Also, it has been shown that tryptophan at position 121 in cyclophilin itself is required for calcineurin inhibition. The overall effect of cyclosporin is to block the early cytokine transcription gene and G0–G1 transition following T-cell activation.

Tacrolimus

Tacrolimus is a cyclic macrolide antibiotic similar to erythromycin. It was derived from the soil-based micro-organism *Streptomyces tsukubaensis*. It is well absorbed from the gastrointestinal tract, not influenced greatly by the presence or absence of bile in the gastrointestinal lumen, and like cyclosporin is extensively metabolized by the cytochrome P450 system and excreted in bile. The mechanism of immunosuppressive function is very similar to that of cyclosporin. It also binds to a cytoplasmic immunophilin. This immunophilin, known as FK-binding protein (FKBP), is a 12 kDa protein consisting of many isoforms, the most important of which is FKBP-12. In mice a recent isoform FKBP-51 has been shown to be mainly restricted to T cells. Its importance is currently under study. Like cyclosporin, the FK/FKBP complex then binds to calcineurin

resulting in inhibition of its phosphatase activity, inhibition of translocation of $NFAT_c$ to the nucleus, and inhibition of early transcription of genes such as IL-2. FK/FKBP and cyclosporin/cyclophilin bind at two overlapping but distinct sites within a region on calcineurin. Therefore, they do compete with each other for immunosuppressive function and thus are unable to be used simultaneously. There are three-dimensional crystal structures of the tacrolimus/immunophilin complex available, indicating a similar formation of an immunophilin-binding domain and an effector domain, as in the cyclosporin/immunophilin complex.

Rapamycin

Rapamycin is also a cyclic macrolide. It is also derived from a soil-based micro-organism, *Streptomyces hygroscopicus*. It is well-absorbed and metabolized by the cytochrome P450 system. Rapamycin, like cyclosporin and tacrolimus, mediates its action by binding to an immunophilin. In fact it binds to the FKBP immunophilin, particularly FKBP-12. However, it has no effect on the phosphatase activity of calcineurin. In contrast to tacrolimus, rapamycin does not undergo a dramatic conformational change when it binds to FKBP-12. Instead of binding to calcineurin, the complex of rapamycin/FKBP targets two cytoplasmic proteins associated with G1–S phase cell cycle progression. These molecules are known as targets of rapamycin TOR-1 and TOR-2. These 200 kDa proteins are highly expressed in human tissues, particularly in the testis and skeletal muscle. The two proteins have 67% identity but their exact function has not been totally defined. They seem to be cytoplasmic kinases involved in activation cascades that eventually turn on cytokine genes. The rapamycin/FKBP complex has been shown to bind to a 90 amino acid region adjacent to a lipid kinase domain within TOR-1/TOR-2. A crucial serine motif in this complex seems important in blocking TOR-1/TOR-2 function. Apart from the affect on TOR-1/TOR-2, there is evidence that rapamycin may also inhibit the promoter activity of proliferating cell nuclear antigen which is important in cell cycle progression within many cells. Apart from its effect on lymphocytes in blocking immune function, rapamycin also inhibits the proliferation of other cell types and, in terms of allograft rejection, inhibition of smooth muscle proliferation may be important in its effects on chronic rejection. Thus, rapamycin blocks the second set of phosphorylation events following the binding of IL-2 to the IL-2 receptor and the release of other cytokines, thereby acting later in the phase of lymphocyte activation than cyclosporin and tacrolimus.

Mycophenolate mofetil

Mycophenolic acid (MPA) was originally isolated from the fungal genus *Penicillium* and has been modified by a synthetic morpholinoethyl side chain ester resulting in the production of mycophenolate mofetil (MMF). This modification significantly improved oral bioavailability of MPA. Mycophenolate is converted back to MPA and undergoes conjugation in the liver. The drug is well-absorbed and primarily (87%) eliminated in the urine. Its half-life is approximately 12 h. MPA is a noncompetitive inhibitor of inosine monophosphate dehydrogenase (IMPDH), the key enzyme that converts inosine monophosphate (IMP) to adenosine monophosphate (AMP), thus effectively blocking the rate-limiting enzyme step in the de novo purine synthetic pathway. The drug seems more selective for lymphocytes because the IMPDH isoform-2 is five to six times more sensitive to MPA than the IMPDH isoform-1 enzyme. The IMPDH isoform-2 is predominantly expressed in lymphocytes and monocytes and this, in conjunction with the fact that lymphocytes tend not to use the salvage pathway for purine metabolism, results in the relative selective action of MMF on lymphocyte activation. The depletion of guanosine purine-type precursors also results in the inhibition of transfer of fructose and mannose to the cell surface of various glycoproteins. This seems particularly to affect adhesion molecules. Thus a further action of mycophenolate may be to inhibit lymphocyte binding to endothelium and extravasation into inflamed tissues. MMF not only has an affect on T- and B-cell proliferation, but also inhibits smooth muscle cell proliferation and thus has potential in the treatment of chronic rejection.

Antibodies (ALG, OKT3, IL-2 receptor)

Antibodies directed against antigens on human leukocytes are used as immunosuppressive therapy. Antithymocyte globulins (ATGs) or antilymphocyte globulins (ALGs) are raised in horses, goats or dogs and have been extensively used in human renal transplantation. Currently they have largely been replaced by the mouse monoclonal antibody OKT3 directed against the e-chain of the human CD3 complex and is thus specific for human T cells. OKT3 is given as a bolus intravenous injection and leads to the disappearance of all T cells in the peripheral blood within 30–60 min. This effect is due to a combination of cell apoptosis/lysis, cell marginalization, opsonization, and antigenic modulation of CD3/TCR from the cell surface. After 2–3 days of therapy, a small number of antigenically modulated cells appear in the peripheral blood, but these cells are non-functional. Other monoclonal antibodies (mAbs) against other T-cell antigens have been used experimentally, but have not met with significant clinical use.

The synthesis of 'humanized' mAb directed against the IL-2 receptor α-chain has resulted in high affinity reagents with powerful immunosuppressive properties. These are currently under study and preliminary evidence suggests that they result in a significant decrease in acute rejection episodes in renal transplant recipients. These agents are being mainly used in induction regimens and with a half-life of approximately 20 days can be administered monthly.

Future clinical therapies

A particularly interesting new drug is the molecule known as FTY 720. This compound acts on sphingosine-1-phosphate receptors leading to sequestration of lymphocytes to secondary lymphoid tissues and away from inflammatory organ responses such as allografts. It has been shown to be effective in experimental models of allograft rejection and in phase III trials in human non-liver transplantation. Side-effects are not prominent although some negative ionotrophic effects on the heart have been observed. A further new drug is on the horizon known as CP-690,550. This is a new JAK-3 inhibitor and it has been used to prolong renal allograft survival in non-human primates.

There is also considerable interest in the development of new mAbs against other adhesion molecules such as the CD28/

CD80 pathway and against molecules involved in lymphocyte endothelium interactions such as selectins. The humanized anti-CD52 mAb CAMPATH-1 is currently under study in both non-liver and liver transplantation. This mAb has profound lymphodepletion properties.

USE OF IMMUNOSUPPRESSIVE DRUGS TO PREVENT ACUTE REJECTION IN LIVER TRANSPLANATION

Currently the most common prophylactic therapeutic combination that has been used is based around initial triple immunosuppressive therapy with corticosteroids, azathioprine/mycophenolate, and tacrolimus/cyclosporin. High dose induction corticosteroid regimens usually consist of 500 mg at the time of transplant, reducing to 20–30 mg within 7–10 days. Lower dose regimens consist of just 1 mg/kg in tapering fashion. Some units withdraw corticosteroids at 3 months without any significant increase in acute rejection. Withdrawal of corticosteroids at varying time points post-transplant has received more support in recent times and is associated with improvement in side-effect profiles and little increase in frequency of allograft rejection. Corticosteroid-free protocols are being developed.

The calcineurin inhibitors, tacrolimus and cyclosporin, remain the pivotal drugs in the maintenance immunosuppression regimens. Tacrolimus usually starts at a dose of 0.1 mg/kg/day, while cyclosporin is given at a dose of 10 mg/kg day. Absorption of tacrolimus and cyclosporin in the first 24–48 h is variable, but this does not seem to decrease their effectiveness. Tacrolimus is given in two divided doses and the dose is titrated to maintain 12-h trough levels in the 8–12 ng/mL range initially and in the 4–8 ng/mL range after 3–6 months. Drug doses are also adjusted according to side-effects and allograft rejection status. Cyclosporin is also given twice daily and doses are adjusted according to either 12-h trough (C0) or 2-h post-intake (C2) levels. The latter has recently been advocated to minimize allograft rejection and side-effects. Target C2 levels in the early post-transplant phase are approximately 1600–1800 ng/mL, whilst later are in the 800–1000 ng/mL range. Trough drug levels are usually maintained in the 100–300 ng/mL level or lower in long-term patients. Two controlled trials have compared tacrolimus to cyclosporin therapy. One study compared tacrolimus to cyclosporin with C0 monitoring and showed better outcomes for tacrolimus therapy. The other compared tacrolimus to cyclosporin with C2 monitoring and showed no difference in the frequency of allograft rejection, but more diabetes and diarrhea was seen in the tacrolimus arm.

Although azathioprine is still used on a background of corticosteroid and tacrolimus/cyclosporin therapy, many units, particularly in the USA, have replaced it with MMF. The dose recommended in liver transplantation is 2 g/day. A multicenter international trial directly comparing mycophenolate and azathioprine in liver transplantation (in conjunction with corticosteroids and cyclosporin using C0 monitoring) showed no difference in patient or allograft survival but did find a 10% reduction in frequency of acute allograft ejection.

Rapamycin has been evaluated as a part of induction immunosuppression in liver transplant patients. In a randomized controlled trial, patients receiving rapamycin had worse patient and allograft survival, increased wound breakdown, increased infections and more vascular thromboses. Thus it is currently not recommended as part of primary induction immunosuppression in liver transplantation. It is however under study at lower doses than used in the initial trial.

The use of mAbs as part of immunosuppression induction protocols has not been common in liver transplantation. The addition of prophylactic OKT3 or ALG therapy, so-called 'quadruple therapy', did not lead to a significant decrease in rejection rates or alteration in outcomes. More recently the use of IL-2 receptor mAbs has been assessed. In a randomized controlled trial IL-2 receptor mAb induction was associated with a decrease in acute rejection in non-hepatitis C virus (HCV) infected patients but no difference in patient or allograft survival was seen.

USE OF IMMUNOSUPPRESSIVE DRUGS TO TREAT ACUTE REJECTION

Moderate to severe acute allograft rejection is usually treated with a 3-day pulse of corticosteroid therapy, at 1 g/day then tapering back to base line levels (**Fig. 39.12**).

Depending on the baseline regimen, calcineurin inhibitor doses may be increased and azathioprine may be replaced by MMF. Increasingly mild episodes of acute rejection are simply treated by increasing the doses of the maintenance immunosuppressive drugs. This is particularly the case in patients on tacrolimus therapy. In some instances, a patient on cyclosporin is converted to tacrolimus without a corticosteroid pulse. Patients who do not respond to pulsed corticosteroid therapy may undergo repeat therapy or receive OKT3 as a rescue strategy.

DRUGS THAT INHIBIT THE IMMUNE SYSTEM: SIDE-EFFECTS AND DRUG INTERACTIONS

General side-effects of immunosuppressive agents

All immunosuppressive drugs predispose the recipient to infection and the development of neoplastic disease, and it is important to remember the close correlation between suppression of the immune system to facilitate transplantation and these side-effects. The infections predisposed to by immunosuppressive drugs include the activation of the herpes viruses [cytomegalovirus (CMV), herpes simplex virus (HSV) and herpes zoster] and other opportunistic infections. There is also a predisposition to fungal and bacterial infections. General immunosuppression leads to the development of lymphoproliferative diseases and the development of epithelial tumors. Lymphoproliferative disease occurring relatively early post-transplant in the setting of immuno-suppression is often associated with Epstein-Barr virus (EBV). Apart from these general side-effects, each individual immuno-suppressive drug has particular side-effects that are exacerbated or decreased by certain drug interactions (**Table 39.2**).

Corticosteroids

The side-effects of corticosteroids are numerous and are to a significant degree dose-dependent. The most common effects involve the musculoskeletal problems of osteoporosis, osteo-necrosis and myopathy. Associated with these are the endocrine

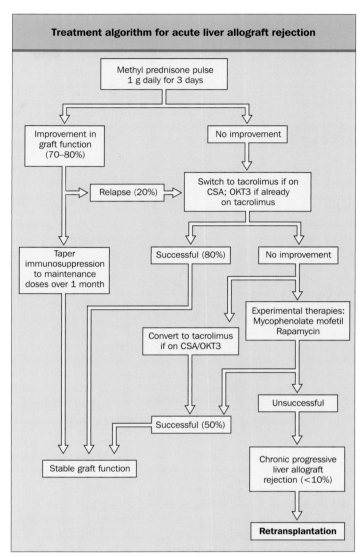

Figure 39.12 Treatment algorithm for acute liver allograft rejection.

effects of glucose intolerance with the development of overt diabetes, hypokalemia, and fluid retention and associated hyper-tension. There are effects on the neuropsychiatric system, such as psychosis, insomnia and depression, which are usually associ-ated with higher doses. Cataracts commonly occur with pro-longed use. The common gastrointestinal effects include dyspepsia and the predisposition to peptic ulceration. The skin bruises easily, atrophies and develops striae and acne. Corticosteroids are not contraindicated in pregnancy.

Azathioprine

The main side-effect of azathioprine is bone marrow depression, particularly leukopenia and thrombocytopenia. Other side-effects include mild alopecia, gastrointestinal upset and retinopathy. It should be also recognized that azathioprine may cause pancreatitis, cholestatic hepatitis and vascular abnormalities within the liver with the development of nodular regenerative hyperplasia and veno-occlusive disease. Its toxicity is increased by interaction with allopurinol, a xanthine oxidase inhibitor. Xanthine oxidase is involved in the metabolism of azathioprine

Summary of major side effects and drug interactions of immunosuppressive therapies		
Drug	Side effects	Drug interaction
Corticosteroids	Glucose intolerance, delirium, hypertension, osteoporosis, cataracts	N/A
Azathioprine	Thrombocytopenia, neutropenia 'allergic' reaction, pancreatitis	Allopurinol
Calcineurin inhibitors (cyclosporin or tacrolimus)	Hypertension, renal dysfunction, headaches, hair growth, central nervous system problems, hyperkalemia	Increased levels: diltiazem doxycycline erythromycin itraconazole omeprazole protease inhibitors (HAART)
		Decreased levels: rifampin phenytoin carbamazapine
Mycophenolate mofetil	Diarrhea, dyspepsia, neutropenia, thrombocytopenia, headache, skin rash	Not known
Rapamycin	Hyperlipidemia	Not known
OKT3/ALG	'Cytokine release' syndrome: aseptic meningitis bronchospasm fever, chills, rigors myalgias hypotension	Nil significant

Table 39.2 Summary of major side effects and drug interaction of main immunosuppressive therapies.

and these drugs should not be used in combination. Azathioprine may also cause an allergic reaction in <1% of individuals resulting in high fevers, arthralgia and myalgia. Re-introduction of azathioprine in these circumstances reproduces the syndrome. Azathioprine is not contraindicated in pregnancy.

Cyclosporin

Cyclosporin has quite a narrow therapeutic window. Its most common side-effects include hypertension (over 30% of cases) and nephrotoxicity. There is an almost universal decrease of 30% in the glomerular filtration rate, and a minority of patients gets more severe renal dysfunction. The nephrotoxicity is associated with structural changes within the kidney, particularly the development of interstitial fibrosis. Cyclosporin also has a tendency to cause hyperkalemia. Its other toxicities include effects on the central and peripheral nervous systems and it commonly causes tremor, headache, seizures (early complication) and may cause peripheral neuropathy. It has been associated with leukoencephalopathy, which mainly involves the occipital cortical pathways and may result in coma and the development of cortical blindness. Hirsutism and gingival hyperplasia commonly occur and can be distressing in females and children. It may also cause breast adenofibromatosis. Respiratory side-effects include sinusitis and sinus congestion.

The side-effects of cyclosporin are largely dose related, and toxicity can be enhanced by drug interactions that result in higher cyclosporin levels, including:

- calcium channel blockers, particularly diltiazem and verapamil;
- antibiotics such as doxycycline, clarithromycin and erythromycin;
- itraconazole and ketoconazole; and
- protease inhibitors.

Apart from these direct drug interactions on levels, neurotoxicity seems to be increased with the interaction with the antibiotic imipenem, and nephrotoxicity is increased with the use of aminoglycosides, non-steroidal anti-inflammatory drugs (NSAIDs), amphotericin, and intravenous bactrim. Angiotensin-converting enzyme inhibitors, used for the treatment of cyclosporin-associated hypertension, increase the hyperkalemic effect of cyclosporin.

Decreased cyclosporin levels can also result from drug interactions and this may predispose to allograft dysfunction. Cytochrome P450 enzyme inducers, such as the anticonvulsants (phenytoin, barbiturates), the antituberculous drugs [isoniazid (INAH) and rifampin (rifampicin)], octreotide and bactrim are particularly important in this regard. Cyclosporin is not contraindicated in pregnancy.

Tacrolimus

The side-effects of tacrolimus are very similar to those of cyclosporin, apart from a few significant differences. The renal nephrotoxicity is almost identical, although the neurotoxicity seems to be worse. Tacrolimus causes more diarrhea than cyclosporin. There seems to be less hypertension, but there is increased glucose intolerance with tacrolimus. There is certainly less gingival hyperplasia and hirsutism as compared with cyclosporin. Tacrolimus is thought to be associated with a 'lower cardiovascular risk' lipid profile than cyclosporin. The drug interactions with tacrolimus are very similar to those of cyclosporin. Concerns about the teratogenicity of tacrolimus are easing and it is now licensed for use during pregnancy in a number of countries.

Mycophenolate mofetil

The main side-effect is on the gastrointestinal tract, resulting particularly in diarrhea. There may be associated nausea and vomiting. Headache seems to be a common problem. Bone marrow suppression with anemia, leukopenia and thrombocytopenia is less common than with azathioprine, but does occur. MMF is contraindicated in pregnancy.

Rapamycin

The main side-effect of rapamycin is the development of hypertriglyceridemia, which may be quite profound. It also has effects on the gastrointestinal tract with nausea, vomiting and diarrhea. Rapamycin is also associated with a fibrosing pulmonary disease, despite its inhibitory effect on fibroblast proliferation that is clinically associated with impaired wound healing. It is contraindicated in pregnancy.

OKT3

The main effect of this drug is the development of the cytokine release syndrome, resulting in high fevers, arthralgia and myalgia. This syndrome can be quite severe and may be associated with aseptic meningitis, coma, adult respiratory distress syndrome and systemic hypotension. Cardiac arrest has been described with the use of OKT3. It is particularly important that the patient is not fluid overloaded at the time of administration. Side-effects are modified by the use of 1 g of methylprednisolone during the first injection and the regular use of antihistamines and acetaminophen (paracetamol) with each subsequent injection. The cytokine release syndrome is most severe during the first one or two injections. OKT3 causes profound immunosuppression. There is clinical reactivation of herpes viruses (HSV, CMV) in over 70% of cases. Total doses of >75 mg predispose to lymphoproliferative diseases.

IMMUNOSUPPRESSIVE STRATEGIES TO DECREASE CALCINEURIN INDUCED NEPHROTOXICITY

Probably the most common serious side-effect of immunosuppressive drugs is the nephrotoxicity associated with cyclosporin and tacrolimus therapy. The frequency of this problem increases with time post-transplant. There are now several studies that have shown that calcineurin inhibitors can be withdrawn in liver transplant patients and replaced with MMF resulting in improvement in renal function in some but not all patients. In this situation, MMF is usually used in combination with a low dose of corticosteroids in order to minimize the risk of rejection. Similar but less extensive data are available for sirolimus. However, access to this drug is more restricted.

LIVER ALLOGRAFT REJECTION

Hyperacute liver allograft rejection

This is an uncommon event in liver transplantation with only a small number of cases reported in the literature. It may come on within the first 1–2 days after transplantation, but usually does not appear until the second week (**Table 39.3**).

It is characterized by a rapid deterioration of graft function, often with the clinical picture of acute liver failure. There is usually a high fever, right upper quadrant pain, rapidly deteriorating liver function tests with asparate aminotransferase (AST) and alanine aminotransferase (ALT) at levels of >1000 IU/L. The international normalized ratio (INR) becomes rapidly prolonged and there is profound thrombocytopenia and acid/base disturbance.

Hyperacute rejection is an antibody and complement mediated attack on the vascular endothelium. The antibodies that result in the hyperacute rejection syndrome are either preformed HLA

Patterns of liver allograft rejection				
Type of rejection	Clinical	Biochemical changes	Biopsy features	Molecular/cellular pathways
Hyperacute	Within 10 days of transplant, acute liver failure	AST > 1000 μ/L AST > 1000 μ/L INR prolonged hypoglycemia	Hemorrhagic necrosis	Antibody and complement
Acute	Any time, commonest days 7–9 post-transplant, nonspecific symptoms (if any)	Any pattern	Mixed portal infiltrate, endotheliitis, bile duct damage	DTH, T cells, cytokines
Chronic	Any time after the first month post-transplant, jaundice and cholestasis	AP, γ-GT markedly elevated, hyper-bilirubinemia	Loss of inter-lobular bile ducts, portal tract fibrosis, a decrease in cellular filtrate	T cells, macrophages, growth factors, stellate cells

Table 39.3 Patterns of liver allograft rejection.

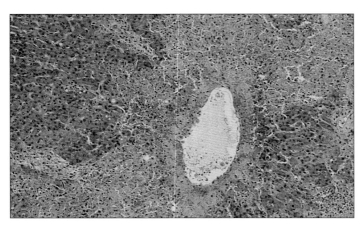

Figure 39.13 Liver biopsy features of hyperacute liver allograft rejection showing widespread hemorrhagic necrosis. (Hematoxylin and eosin)

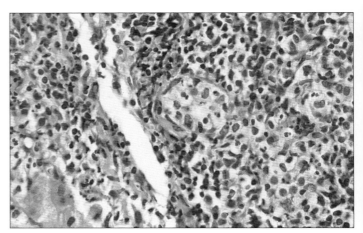

Figure 39.14 Liver biopsy features of acute liver allograft rejection with portal tract infiltrate and bile duct damage with invading inflammatory cells.

antibodies against the donor MHC antigens, or against blood group antigens. The characteristic pathologic finding is that of massive hemorrhagic necrosis associated with complement, fibrin and immunoglobulin deposition in arteries, veins and sinusoids (**Fig. 39.13**).

There may be segmental infarction of the graft, together with necrosis of the biliary tract. The management is very difficult. Plasmapheresis, cyclophosphamide and OKT3 therapies have been attempted with little success. The only really effective management is that of urgent re-transplantation.

Acute liver allograft rejection

Acute liver allograft rejection occurs in about 20–40% of patients. It occurs at a mean of 7–9 days after transplant, and is often clinically silent. Occasionally there may be right upper quadrant discomfort and fever. Biochemically there is derangement of the serum bilirubin, alkaline phosphatase (AP), γ-glutamyltranspeptidase (γ-GT), AST and ALT levels. However, these do not conform to a characteristic pattern, and cannot be used to definitively distinguish acute rejection from other causes of liver graft dysfunction. The coagulation status and platelet count is usually not disturbed.

The diagnosis of acute liver allograft rejection is made on liver biopsy and has been defined by an international panel as 'inflammation of the allograft, elicited by a genetic disparity between the donor and recipient, primarily affecting interlobular bile ducts and vascular endothelia, including portal veins and hepatic venules and occasionally the hepatic artery and its branches'. Hence, there are three predominant features:

- portal inflammation;
- bile duct damage; and
- endotheliitis.

At least two of these three features are required for a histopathologic diagnosis of acute rejection. First, a 'mixed' portal tract infiltrate consisting of lymphocytes, neutrophils, monocytes and eosinophils is present (**Fig. 39.14**). The percentage of eosinophils is usually determined by the corticosteroid dose at the time of the acute rejection. If the corticosteroid dose has been high and acute rejection occurs, then the eosinophils are not often seen.

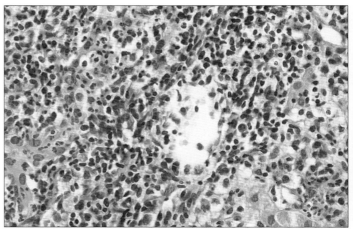

Figure 39.15 Liver biopsy features of acute liver allograft rejection showing endotheliitis.

The second feature is that of vascular endotheliitis, particularly of the portal tract venules, but sometimes including central veins (**Fig. 39.15**). This is characterized by activated lymphocytes and monocytes adhering to the vascular endothelium, invading underneath and sometimes lifting off the endothelial structures.

The third feature is inflammation of the interlobular bile ducts with infiltration of the epithelium with lymphocytes and monocytes (see Fig. 39.13). In more advanced cases, there is flattening of the epithelium and an increasing eosinophilic component to the cytoplasm and loss of nuclei from individual cells. Immunohistochemical studies have shown that the lymphocytic infiltrate within portal tracts is of both the CD4+ and CD8+ subsets, while infiltration of the biliary epithelium is predominantly by CD8+ cells. The molecular pathogenesis of acute liver allograft rejection is associated with increased intrahepatic expression of IL-2, INF-γ, and IL-5 (particularly if eosinophils are present). Studies have also indicated that there

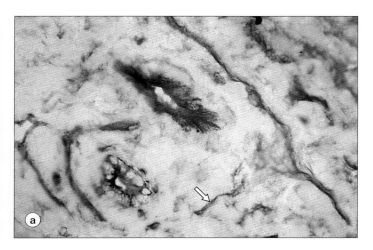

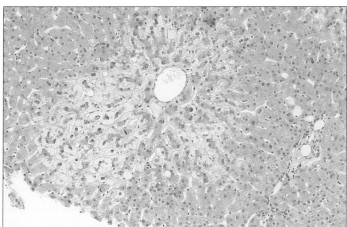

Figure 39.17 Centrizonal ballooning during acute liver allograft rejection suggesting vascular involvement and severe rejection.

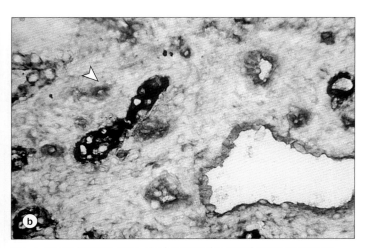

Figure 39.16 Identification of microvascular portal tract structures (brown staining). (a) In normal liver and (b) their reduction during acute liver allograft rejection.

Grading of acute liver allograft rejection	
Global assessment	*Criteria*
No rejection	No infiltrate present or the inflammation is related to other causes of dysfunction (viral hepatitis, biliary obstruction, etc).
Indeterminate for rejection	Rejection-type portal inflammatory infiltrate that fails to meet the criteria for the diagnosis of rejection because of lack of direct bile duct damage, or involvement of an insufficient percentage of portal triads.
Mild rejection	Evidence of a mixed portal infiltrate (usually lymphocytic with blasts and often with eosinophils and neutrophils) in at least one-third of the triads, that is generally mild and confined within the portal spaces. Clearly defined bile duct damage is present and subendothelial inflammation of portal or central vein branches is often seen.
Moderate rejection	As above for mild, with the rejection infiltrate expanding most or all of the triads.
Severe rejection	As above for moderate, with spillover of the infiltrate into the periportal areas and moderate to severe perivenular inflammation that extends into the hepatic parenchyma and is associated with hepatocyte necrosis.

Table 39.4 Diagnosis of acute graft rejection – Banff International Consensus Schema. This table shows the grading of acute liver allograft rejection.

is loss of portal tract microvascular structures during acute rejection (**Fig. 39.16**).

Although the three key pathologic changes described above are the basis of diagnosis, other changes may occur. In lobular areas there may be cell necrosis/apoptosis and a lobular portal tract infiltrate consisting mainly of CD8+ cells. The presence of centrizonal ballooning and particularly fallout of hepatocytes in zone 3 of the hepatic lobule suggests that the rejection is severe and may have a vascular component (**Fig. 39.17**).

Very rarely there may be arteritis of small arterioles in portal tracts.

Grading systems for acute liver allograft rejection have been provided by a number of groups. More recently a grading system has been developed by an international panel to classify and grade liver allograft rejection (**Table 39.4**).

This system essentially grades the level of acute rejection as indeterminate, mild, moderate or severe dependent on the degree of portal tract infiltrate. As part of this, a rejection activity index (RAI) can be derived by scoring each of the three main features (i.e. portal tract infiltrate, bile duct damage and endotheliitis) on a score of 0–3 (**Table 39.5**).

Acute allograft rejection and HCV infection

HCV infection in the liver allograft makes the diagnosis of acute allograft rejection somewhat more difficult. Features of mild/moderate acute rejection can be seen in HCV infection alone. These include the portal tract inflammation, some bile duct damage and interface hepatitis. A predominate allograft rejection

The acute liver allograft rejection activity index		
Category	Criteria	Score
Portal inflammation	Mostly lymphocytic inflammation involving, but not noticeably expanding, a minority of the triads.	1
	Expansion of most or all of the triads, by a mixed infiltrate containing lymphocytes with occasional blasts, neutrophils and eosinophils.	2
	Marked expansion of most or all of the triads by a mixed infiltrate containing numerous blasts and eosinophils with inflammatory spillover into the periportal parenchyma.	3
Bile duct inflammation damage	A minority of the ducts are cuffed and infiltrated by inflammatory cells and show only mild reactive changes such as increased nuclear cytoplasmic ratio of the epithelial cells.	1
	Most or all of the ducts infiltrated by inflammatory cells. More than an occasional duct shows degenerative changes such as nuclear pleomorphism, disordered polarity and cytoplasmic vacuolization of the epithelium.	2
	As above for 2, with most or all of the ducts showing degenerative changes or focal luminal disruption.	3
Venous endothelial inflammation	Subendothelial lymphocytic infiltration involving some, but not a majority of the portal and/or hepatic venules.	1
	Subendothelial infiltration involving most or all of the portal and/or hepatic venules.	2
	As above for 2, with moderate or severe perivenular inflammation that extends into the perivenular parenchyma and is associated with perivenular hepatocyte necrosis.	3
Total score	(Sum of components) =	9 (max)

Table 39.5 Diagnosis of acute graft rejection – Banff International Consensus Schema. This table shows the rejection activity index (RAI). Criteria that can be used to score liver allograft biopsies with acute rejection, as defined by the Banff International Consensus scheme.

Risk factors for chronic rejection
Persistently low CSA levels
Gender (M/F) allograft mismatch
CMV mismatch
Multiple episodes of acute rejection
Severe acute rejection
Late acute rejection
HCV infection and possibly interferon therapy
Positive lymphocytotoxic crossmatch with donor

Table 39.6 Risk factors for chronic rejection.

response is favored by a mixed portal tract infiltrate of neutrophils and eosinophils together with more severe bile duct injury or centrizonal cell loss.

Chronic liver allograft rejection

Chronic liver allograft rejection occurs at a low frequency in human liver transplantation. Currently, experience in most centers indicates a frequency of less than 3–5%. Several factors have been shown to predispose to chronic liver allograft rejection (**Table 39.6**). These include low cyclosporin levels, multiple episodes of acute rejection, late episodes of acute rejection, CMV infection, positive lymphotoxic antibody cross-matching,

HCV infection and gender mismatching between donor and recipient.

Clinically, chronic rejection is associated with progressive cholestasis, a rise in the serum bilirubin with clinical jaundice, an enlarged liver, increasing alkaline phosphatase and γ-GT with only moderate elevations in AST and ALT levels. The INR and the platelet count are usually normal. The diagnosis is based on liver histology and is characterized by two predominant lesions. First is the loss of interlobular bile ducts, the so-called 'vanishing bile duct syndrome'. This is associated with loss of microvasculature and arteriolar structures within the portal tract and a decreasing rather than increasing inflammatory infiltrate. The portal tracts often become small and fibrotic (**Fig. 39.18**).

The second major change occurs in the hepatic lobule with progressive ballooning in zone 3 of the hepatic lobule and cellular fallout with hepatocyte necrosis (**Fig. 39.19**).

There is marked upregulation of MHC and adhesion molecules on hepatocytes and remaining bile ducts. CD8+ T cells can still be found attacking bile duct remnants and in lobular zone 3 areas (**Fig. 39.20**).

Although often not seen on needle biopsy specimens, there is a marked transplant vasculopathy in medium-sized arteries in liver explants or at autopsy (**Fig. 39.21**). This consists of thickening of the arterial intimae, destruction of the internal elastic lamina, and the presence of macrophages (arterial foam cells), smooth muscle cells (myofibroblasts), and thickening and fibrosis of the intimae. There is also continuing infiltrate in these lesions of CD4+, and CD8+ cells, as well as macrophages (**Figs 39.22** and **39.23**).

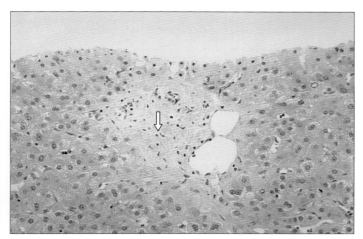

Figure 39.18 Liver biopsy features of chronic allograft rejection. Hematoxylin and eosin stained section of portal tract (arrow) showing lack of inflammatory infiltrate and portal tract fibrosis, severe bile duct damage, and loss of portal tract arterioles.

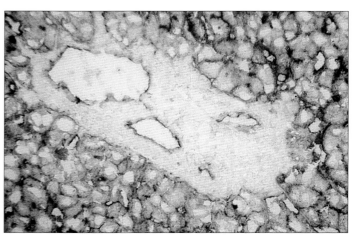

Figure 39.21 Liver biopsy features of chronic allograft rejection. Total loss of microvascular structures in chronic rejection.

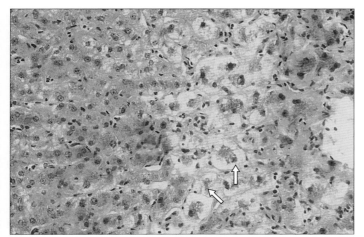

Figure 39.19 Liver biopsy features of chronic allograft rejection. Hematoxylin and eosin stained section of liver lobule showing ballooning of hepatocytes in zone 3 of hepatic lobule (arrows).

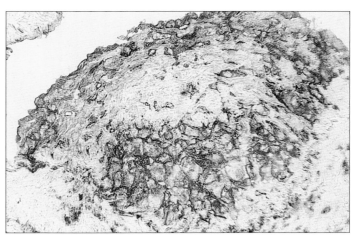

Figure 39.22 Liver biopsy features of chronic allograft rejection. Macrophage infiltrate in allograft atherosclerosis. Reproduced from Wiesner et al (91) by permission of Wiley-Liss, Inc.

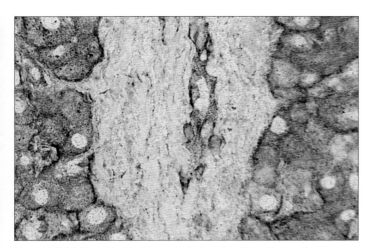

Figure 39.20 Liver biopsy features of chronic allograft rejection. Remnant of damaged bile duct (blue) being attacked by CD8+ T cells (pink). Reproduced from Wiesner et al (91) by permission of Wiley-Liss, Inc.

These lesions show increased expression of adhesion molecules on the endothelium. The process is not dissimilar to classic atherosclerosis, although the lesions tend to be concentric, affect medium-sized vessels, and have intact endothelium (**Figs 39.24** and **39.25**).

Once fully established, chronic rejection invariably progresses to graft failure. However, it is clear that there are intermediate cases where reversibility may occur. It is thought that tacrolimus therapy may be effective at early stages of chronic rejection, particularly when the serum bilirubin is <200 μmol/L. MMF may also be useful in this situation, although this has not yet been proven. Both these drugs inhibit smooth muscle, as well as T- and B-cell proliferation. Smooth muscle proliferation is an important feature of the chronic liver allograft response particularly at the level of the medium-sized arteries giving the transplant vasculopathy. Eventually rapamycin may also prove useful in chronic rejection.

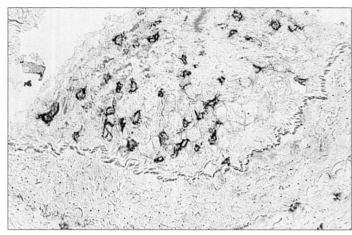

Figure 39.23 CD3+ T cells in allograft atherosclerosis. Reproduced from Wiesner et al (91) by permission of Wiley-Liss, Inc.

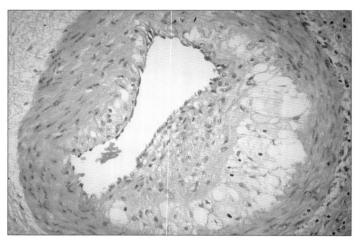

Figure 39.24 Liver biopsy features of chronic allograft rejection. Evidence of 'allograft atherosclerosis'.

Current approach to xenotransplantation	
Modification type	*Example*
Recipient	Depletion of anti-Galα1–3Gal antibodies
Donor	Knockout of α1,3-galactosyltransferase gene
	Creation of human CD55 (decay accelerating factor) transgenics
	Creation of human CD59 (membrane inhibitor of reactive lysis) transgenics
	Creation of combined human CD55/CD59 double transgenics

Table 39.7 Current approach to xenotransplantation.

XENOTRANSPLANTATION

The possibility of xenotransplantation (i.e. the transplantation of organs from one species to another) (**Table 39.7**) has been an ongoing area of research for several decades. The major problem with organ xenotransplantation has been hyperacute rejection characterized by interstitial hemorrhage and widespread vascular thrombosis leading to necrosis and destruction of the organ within minutes or hours after revascularization. This process is mainly mediated by the binding of xenoreactive antibodies to recipient endothelium, leading to the activation of the complement system. Natural inhibitors of the complement system are species specific and are unable to dampen down this process.

Recent studies have identified that 85% of xenoreactive antibodies (>90% of the IgM subclass) in human serum recognize a single structure: Galα1-3Gal. The synthesis of this sugar on various glycoproteins is catalyzed by α1,3-galactosyltransferase. Approaches to overcome hyperacute xenograft rejection have involved the depletion from recipient serum of these antibodies by various columns, and this has been shown to prevent hyper-

acute rejection of some xenografts. The other approach has been to produce 'knock-out' organ donors. In mice, xenografted organs in which the α1,3-galactosyltransferase gene has been ablated survive significantly longer than do 'normal' xenografts. A third approach has been the generation of transgenic xenograft donors which express a galactosyltransferase that catalyzes the addition of an extra sugar other than α-galactose onto the terminus of various oligosaccharide chains. Currently all of these processes remain at the experimental level, and have not been applied to the human situation.

Complement activation is a critical event during hyperacute xenograft rejection. This is regulated by complementary regulatory proteins such as decay-accelerating factor (CD55) and membrane inhibitor of reactive lysis (CD59). These control proteins are species specific. For example, pig CD55 and CD59 are unable to break down human complement. Thus, when human complement is activated on pig endothelium, the process is ongoing. Approaches to overcome this have included the production of transgenic animals that express human CD55 and CD59. Such experiments have recently shown that significant delays in hyperacute rejection after xenotransplantation can be obtained.

Apart from the problem of hyperacute rejection there are other layers of acute vascular rejection that are mediated by a significant cellular component, as well as an antibody/complement component. There is increasing interest in the possible role of NK cells in acute vascular xenograft rejection. Other hurdles to be overcome include further cellular responses resulting in T-cell-mediated xenograft rejection. Finally, concerns about infectious agents and the transfer of endogenous retroviral infections from other species into the human need to be overcome before xenotransplantation becomes a clinical reality.

LIVER ALLOGRAFT TOLERANCE

There are four main general mechanisms of tolerance:

- anergy, where the antigen is ignored by the immune system,
- regulation away from an active immune response towards a non-active immune response involving the induction of what are now known as T regulatory (Treg) cells,
- deletion of APCs, and
- activation-associated tolerance which may or may not be related to the deletional processes.

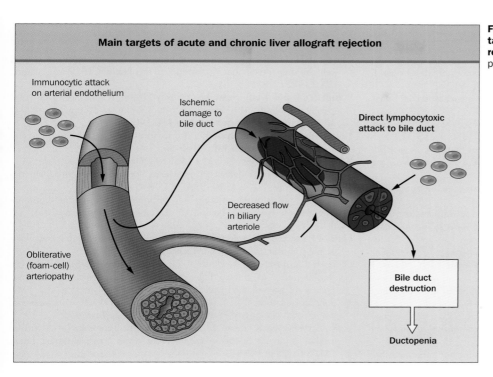

Main targets of acute and chronic liver allograft rejection

Immunocytic attack
on arterial endothelium

Ischemic
damage to
bile duct

Direct lymphocytoxic
attack to bile duct

Decreased flow
in biliary
arteriole

Obliterative
(foam-cell)
arteriopathy

Bile duct
destruction

Ductopenia

Figure 39.25 Schematic summary of the main targets of acute and chronic liver allograft rejection. Reproduced from Wiesner et al (91) by permission of Wiley-Liss, Inc.

It has been recognized in human clinical studies that a select group of patients can be weaned off immunosuppression without loss of their liver allograft, thus implying that a subset of humans in fact have become tolerant. The mechanisms of liver transplant tolerance have, however, been best studied in models of spontaneous tolerance, which have been identified between inbred rat strains, inbred mouse strains and some outbred pig strains. One of the important observations in clarifying the mechanisms of spontaneous liver allograft tolerance was the recognition that there was a migration of a significant number of donor leukocytes from the transplanted liver to the recipient lymph nodes and spleen. This led to the concept of the establishment of microchimerism and 'minigraft versus host disease' as a suppressor mechanism of the recipient immune response. While this process may definitely occur, it seems to evolve over a long period of time, while acceptance of livers in the experimental spontaneous tolerance systems occurs very rapidly within the first few days.

Recently, the mechanism of this early tolerance process has been defined to a significant extent. It seems that the early rapid migration of donor leukocytes from the liver allograft to recipient lymphoid tissues results in 'hyperactivation of recipient lymphocytes' (**Fig. 39.26**). This has been shown by the demonstration of increased messenger RNA production for IL-2 and IFN-γ by these cells. In subsequent events, it has been shown that within the liver allograft itself there is increased apoptosis of infiltrating lymphocytes in tolerant animals compared with animals undergoing rejection. These two observations imply that spontaneous liver allograft tolerance is an activation-associated event, resulting in apoptosis and probable deletion of alloreactive cells. The above concept has important implications

for approaches designed to increase the chances of liver allograft tolerance in the clinical setting. It would imply that donor leukocytes are crucial in establishing the process and that early heavy immunosuppression at the time of transplantation or in the 24–48 h afterwards may inhibit the tolerance process, rather than enhance it. Such concepts need to be tested in the clinical setting.

The above description applies to the induction of liver transplant tolerance. In long-term patients the presence of Treg cells may be important in the maintenance of tolerance. The study of these cells and their relationship to possible immunosuppressive drug withdrawal requires further investigation.

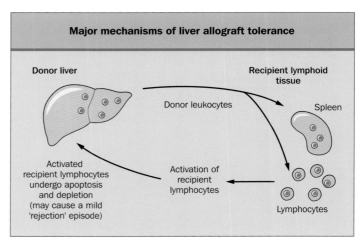

Major mechanisms of liver allograft tolerance

Donor liver

Recipient lymphoid
tissue

Donor leukocytes

Spleen

Activated
recipient lymphocytes
undergo apoptosis
and depletion
(may cause a mild
'rejection' episode)

Activation of
recipient
lymphocytes

Lymphocytes

Figure 39.26 Major mechanism of liver allograft tolerance.

FURTHER READING

Immunology

Antoniou AN, Powis SJ, Elliott T. Assembly and export of MHC class 1 peptide ligands. Curr Opin Immunol 2003; 15:75–81.

Auchincloss H, Sultan H. Antigen processing and presentation in transplantation. Curr Opin Immunol 1996; 8:681–687.

Brady LM, Watson SR. Lymphocyte migration into tissue: the paradigm derived from CD4 subsets. Curr Opin Immunol 1996; 8:312–320.

Bryant P and Ploegh H. Class 11 MHC peptide loading by the professionals. Curr Opin Immunol 2004:16:96–102. *Discussion of new data regarding MHC Class 11 antigen presentation.*

Hancock WW. Chemokine receptor-dependent alloresponses. Immunological Reviews 2003; 196:37–35.

Janssen E, Zhang W. Adaptor proteins in lymphocyte activation. Curr Opin Immunol 2003; 15:269–276. *Review of recent data of intracellular pathways following T cell activation.*

Koopman J-O, Hämmerling GJ, Momburg F. Generation, intracellular transport and loading of peptides associated with MHC Class I molecules. Curr Opin Immunol 1997; 9:80–88.

Pieters J. MHC Class II restricted antigen presentation. Curr Opin Immunol 1997; 9:89–95.

Rock Kenneth L. The ins and outs of cross-presentation. Nature Immunology 2003; 4:10. *Discussion of new data regarding cross antigen presentation mechanisms.*

Rossiter H, Alan R, Kupper TS. Selectins, T-cell rolling and inflammation. Mol Med Today 1997; 3:214–222.

Rothstein DM, Sayegh MH T cell costimulatory pathways in allograft rejection and tolerance. Immunol Rev 2003; 196;85–108.

Rumagnani S. The TH1/TH2 paradigm. Immunol Today 1997; 18:263–266.

Samelson L. Signal transduction mediated by the T-cell antigen receptor: Role of adapter proteins. Ann Rev Immunol 2002; 20:371–394.

Strom TB, Roy-Chaudhury P, et al. The TH1/TH2 paradigm and the allograft response. Curr Opin Immunol 1996; 8:688–693.

Su B, Karin M. Mitogen activated protein kinase cascades and regulation of gene expression. Curr Opin Immunol 1996; 8:402–411.

Takeda K, Kaisho T and Akira S. Toll-like receptors. Annu Rev Immmunol 2003; 21:335–376.

Trautmann A, Valitutti S. The diversity of the immunological synapses. Curr Opin Immunol 2003; 15;249–254.

Immunosuppressive therapy

Abraham RT, Wiedernecht GJ. Immunopharmacology of rapamycin. Ann Rev Immunol 1996; 14:483–510.

Brazelton T, Morris RE. Molecular mechanisms of action of new xenobiotic immunosuppressive drugs: tacrolimus (FK506), sirolimus (rapamycin), mycophenolate mofetil and leflunomide. Curr Opin Immunol 1996; 8:710–720.

Brinkmann V, Lynch KR. FTY720: targeting G-protein-coupled receptors for sphingosine 1-phosphate in transplantation and autoimmunity. 2002; 14:569–575.

Christians U, Jacbosen W, Benet L and Lampen A. Mechanisms of clinical relevant drug interactions associated with tacrolimus. Clin Pharmacokinet. 2002; 41;817–851.

European FK 506 Multicentre Liver Study Group. Randomised trial comparing tacrolimus (FK 506) and cyclosporine in prevention of liver allograft rejection. Lancet 1994; 344:423–428.

Holt DW, Johnstone A. Cyclosporin microemulsion. A guide to usage and monitoring. Biodrugs 1997; 7:175–197.

Kahan BD. Cyclosporine. N Engl J Med 1989;321:1725–1738.

Kirchner GI, Meier-Weidenbach I and Manns MP. Clinical pharmacokinetics of everolimus. 2004; 43:83–95.

Levy G. C_2 Monitoring strategy for optimising cyclosporine immunosuppression from the Neoral ®[1] formulation. BioDrugs 2001; 15:279–290.

Liu J. FK506 and cyclosporine molecular probes for studying intracellular signal transduction. Immunol Today 1993; 14:290–295.

O'Grady JG, Burroughs A, Hardy P, Elbourne D, Truesdale A and the UK and Republic of Ireland Liver Transplant Study Group. Tacrolimus versus microemulsified cyclosporin in liver transplantation: the TMC randomized control trial. Lancet 2002; 360:1119–1129. *Comparison of tacrolimus and cyclosporine therapy in liver transplantation.*

Scott L, McKeage K, Keam SJ and Plosker GL. Tacrolimus – A further update of it use in the management of organ transplantation. Drugs 2003; 63(12):1247–1297.

Sykes M. JAKing up immunosuppression. Nat Med 2003; 9:1458–1459. *Summary of new immunosuppressive drug.*

US Multicentre FK 506 Liver Study Group. A comparison of tacrolimus (FK506) and cyclosporine for immunosuppression in liver transplantation. N Engl J Med 1994; 331:1110–1115.

Rejection

McCaughan GW, Bishop GA. Atherosclerosis of the liver allograft. J Hepatol 1997; 27:592–598.

Rocha P N, Plumb TJ, Crowley SD, Coffman TM. Effector mechanisms in transplant rejection. Immunological Reviews 2003; 196:51–64.

Wiesner RH, Ludwig J, vanHaek B, Krom RAF. Current concepts in cell-mediated hepatic allograft rejection leading to ductopenia and liver failure. Hepatology 1991; 14:721–729.

Tolerance

Bishop GA, Sun JH, Sheil AGR, McCaughan GW. High dose/activation associated tolerance: a mechanism for allograft tolerance. Transplantation 1997; 64:1377–1383.

Lechler R, Bluestone J. Transplant tolerance – putting the pieces together. Curr Opin Immunol 1997; 9:631–633.

Walsh PT, Strom TB and Turka LA. Routes to transplant tolerance versus rejection: The role of cytokines. Immunity 2004; 20:121–131.

CHAPTER
40

Early Management

Federico G. Villamil and Andrés E. Ruf

INTRODUCTION

Orthotopic liver transplantation (OLT) is the most effective therapy for adults and children with decompensated cirrhosis, acute hepatic failure or primary liver cancer. Following this complex but formidable operation, the majority of patients are able to return to a productive life and resume pretransplant activities. However, the price of the new life offered by OLT is the morbidity and mortality associated with graft dysfunction, the adverse effects of immunosuppression or recurrence of the original disease in the allograft. Virtually all livers are injured after OLT and most patients develop at least one significant postoperative complication.

INTENSIVE CARE UNIT MANAGEMENT

Upon arrival at the intensive care unit (ICU) most patients are unconscious and intubated. Multiple interventions are usually required during the first 24 h to achieve hemodynamic, respiratory, metabolic and renal stability. However, patients with no surgical complications and adequate graft function recuperate rapidly allowing the progressive removal of intravascular lines and early extubation. Cirrhosis is associated with a hyperdynamic circulation characterized by a high cardiac output and decreased peripheral vascular resistance. Management of these pre-existing circulatory disturbances during surgery requires generous volume replacement and administration of vasoactive drugs to maintain hemodynamic stability. Volume replacement with crystalloid or colloid solutions and use of vasoactive drugs should be balanced to maintain a systolic blood pressure above 100 mmHg and a central venous pressure below 10 cm H$_2$O to avoid graft congestion.

Hypothermia is the rule early after OLT. It is due to the combined effects of prolonged surgery, the need for multiple transfusions and grafting of an organ preserved in cold solutions. Rapid correction of hypothermia is indicated to prevent its deleterious effects on tissue perfusion, and cardiac, renal and platelet functions.

Almost all patients develop oliguria or some degree of renal dysfunction during the first 48–72 h, especially those with hepatorenal syndrome before OLT. Hypotension during the operation and the toxic effects of antimicrobials and immunosuppressive agents are the most frequent causes of renal abnormalities in the first postoperative week. Management of early renal impairment requires generous volume replacement with colloids or crystalloids to maintain a diuresis >0.5 mL/kg/h and avoidance of nephrotoxic drugs. For example, less nephrotoxic immunosuppression is recommended for patients with persistent oliguria. Diuretics and/or dopamine are indicated in patients with persistent oliguria and normal filling pressures after volume replacement. Fortunately, renal dysfunction improves in the majority of patients within a few days.

Hyperglycemia is the most common metabolic abnormality encountered in OLT recipients and is usually related to the administration of high doses of corticosteroids or other diabetogenic drugs such as tacrolimus. Blood glucose should be frequently monitored and maintained below 200 mg/dL with regular insulin.

Patients who receive a large number of transfusions during surgery may develop citrate overload resulting in hypocalcemia. Correction of hypocalcemia is indicated to prevent complications such as myocardial dysfunction. Similarly, both citrate and the renal tubular effects of cyclosporin may cause significant hypomagnesemia which is a risk factor for seizures and other neurologic complications.

Close attention should be paid to the output and characteristics of fluids from the nasogastric, abdominal and biliary drains. The nasogastric tube allows early detection of gastrointestinal bleeding and enteral administration of drugs including immunosuppressive agents, which at present rarely require intravenous administration. The presence of blood or bile in the abdominal drains is often the first clue to the diagnosis of bleeding or bile leaks. Measurement of bilirubin levels and hematocrit in abdominal fluid samples is useful to confirm these diagnoses. Ascites occurs in almost all patients following OLT, but is greatest in those with poor graft function. It is important to adjust volume replacement to the output of ascitic fluid, minimizing the risk of hypovolemia and renal dysfunction. The quantity and quality of bile drainage through the T-tube in patients with duct-to-duct anastomosis is useful to assess graft function and to detect complications such as hemobilia.

Most patients are extubated within 48 h of surgery. Pleural effusions, especially on the right side, and atelectasis are common during the first week. For this reason, intense and frequent respiratory physiotherapy is part of the standard postoperative care.

The length of ICU stay is generally determined by the duration of mechanical ventilation and the need for vasopressors. On average, most patients are transferred out of ICU 2 or 3 days after OLT. The length of hospital stay ranges from 7 days to several weeks or even months depending on the severity of postoperative complications. However, most patients are discharged home during the second or third postoperative week.

ASSESSMENT OF EARLY GRAFT FUNCTION

The earliest parameters of successful engraftment are production of golden brown bile after the liver is reperfused, and

643

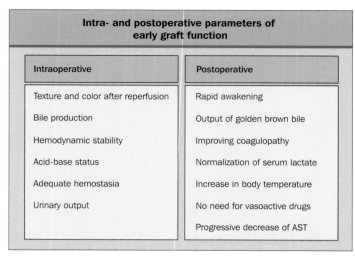

Figure 40.1 Intraoperative and postoperative parameters of early graft function. AST, aspartate aminotransferase.

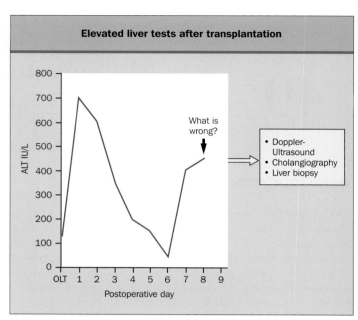

Figure 40.2 Elevated liver tests after the initial decline following liver transplantation. Requirement of specific studies to establish the diagnosis of graft dysfunction.

improvement in coagulopathy allowing satisfactory hemostasis (**Fig. 40.1**). Awakening of the patient shortly after arrival in the ICU reflects the rapid clearance of the anesthetic agents by a functioning liver. Serum lactate and international normalized ratio (INR) are the most valuable biochemical parameters to assess early graft function. Ideally, peak INR should be less than 2.0. However, the progressive improvement in coagulopathy rather than the absolute value is what indicates adequate function of the new liver. Serum lactate levels usually normalize within 12 h of OLT in patients with good allograft function (Fig. 40.1). Serum aminotransferases, aspartate aminotransferase (AST) and alanine aminotransferase (ALT) are indirect markers of the severity of preservation injury. In OLT recipients with good early function, AST peaks at less than 2000 IU/L and decreases rapidly over the subsequent days. Hyperbilirubinemia is not always indicative of graft dysfunction during the first days, but rather may reflect resorption of hematomas or blood in the abdomen or accelerated breakdown of transfused erythrocytes. Serum alkaline phosphatase (Alk Phos) and gamma-glutamyltransferase (GGT) usually remain within the normal range during the first days and are of little value in the differential diagnosis of early graft dysfunction.

MONITORING AND DIAGNOSTIC WORK-UP OF EARLY GRAFT DYSFUNCTION

A variety of insults can damage the allograft following early successful engraftment. The differential diagnosis of graft dysfunction is frequently challenging, even for experienced physicians, and relies on the combination of clinical parameters, serum biochemical tests, non-invasive and invasive radiologic procedures, and liver biopsy.

Clinical parameters

Clinical parameters are more important with respect to alerting the physician, rather than being a valuable tool for the diagnosis of a specific type of allograft dysfunction. As an example, fever, malaise, increasing jaundice and failure to thrive may be present in patients with rejection, infection with opportunistic organisms

or biliary complications. In addition, a large proportion of recipients with significant graft dysfunction remain completely asymptomatic.

Serum biochemical tests

After a successful transplant, serum bilirubin and liver enzymes decrease progressively over the following days and reach the normal range within 2–3 weeks. A rise in serum bilirubin, AST, ALT, Alk Phos or GGT after the initial postoperative decline is usually indicative of allograft injury. However, neither the degree of biochemical abnormalities nor the pattern of enzyme elevation is specific for any given cause of graft dysfunction. In addition, poor correlation exists between the degree of biochemical abnormalities and the severity of histologic findings. Significantly elevated liver tests are often found in patients with mild histologic disease and vice versa. Like clinical parameters, biochemical tests only alert one to allograft dysfunction while additional studies are needed to identify the specific cause of graft dysfunction (**Fig. 40.2**).

Non-invasive radiologic procedures

Ultrasonography (US) with Doppler examination is the most commonly utilized non-invasive imaging study following OLT due to its accuracy, low cost and availability at the bedside. Doppler-US allows assessment of the hepatic parenchyma, abdominal cavity, biliary tree and patency of the hepatic vasculature. US has good sensitivity for the detection of abdominal fluid collections, which are commonly present during the first weeks post-OLT. However, it is not very useful in differentiating loculated ascites from other types of fluids such as blood, bile or pus. The demonstration of bile duct dilatation on US is almost diagnostic of biliary obstruction. However, the US examination is normal in as many as 50% of patients with abnormal cholangiograms.

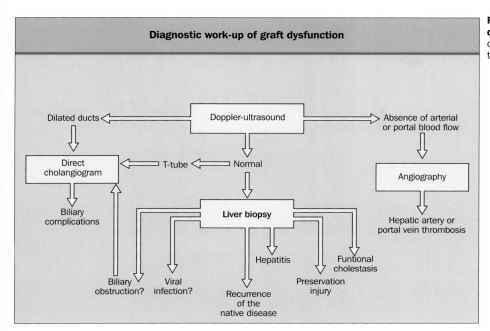

Figure 40.3 Diagnostic work-up of graft dysfunction. Simplified algorithm for the differential diagnosis of graft dysfunction in liver transplant recipients.

A bedside study is indicated during the first day in the ICU to detect as early as possible vascular problems that may require prompt surgical revision. Subsequently, it is performed whenever graft dysfunction is discovered. The accuracy of Doppler-US to detect vascular thrombosis or stenosis after OLT is around 90%. A confirmatory angiogram is required only when arterial or portal blood flow is not demonstrated by Doppler-US. Even a normal study is clinically relevant because it strongly suggests a non-vascular cause of graft dysfunction.

Direct cholangiography is the gold standard for the diagnosis of biliary complications. T-tubes, in patients with duct-to-duct anastomosis, and transjejunal catheters, in those with a Roux-en-Y choledochojejunostomy, provide easy access for visualization of the biliary system. However, a large proportion of duct-to-duct biliary anastomoses are currently performed without a T-tube. In these cases, magnetic resonance (MR) cholangiography may be used to diagnose biliary complications.

Invasive radiologic procedures

Diagnostic percutaneous transhepatic or endoscopic retrograde cholangiography may be indicated in OLT recipients without indwelling biliary catheters, if a non-invasive MR cholangiogram fails to provide an accurate diagnosis. The most appropriate technique is selected according to the type of biliary anastomosis and the suspected location of the complication. The percutaneous route is preferred in patients with a Roux-en-Y choledochojejunostomy or biliary lesions located at or above the confluence of the right and left ducts. The endoscopic route is indicated for more distal disease, i.e. at the anastomosis or below. If needed, percutaneous or endoscopic therapy can be performed at the time of the diagnostic procedure.

Liver biopsy

Liver biopsy is the single most valuable procedure for determining the cause of graft dysfunction and is indicated whenever graft dysfunction is suspected. Biopsies are processed using a rapid technique with a turnaround time of only 4–6 h. Most are performed percutaneously. The transjugular technique is reserved for patients with a contraindication to percutaneous biopsy such as severe coagulopathy or tense ascites. Alternatively, a small window in the abdominal wound provides good exposure of the graft surface for biopsy and the possibility of performing direct hemostasis. Most causes of graft dysfunction can be determined with hematoxylin and eosin stained specimens. Immunohistochemical studies may be useful to confirm specific causes of allograft injury such as viral infections.

Histopathologic interpretation in OLT recipients is more difficult than in non-transplant patients because more than one process may affect the allograft simultaneously. Examples of this are the frequent coexistence of rejection with preservation injury, biliary complications, cytomegalovirus (CMV) infection, or recurrent viral hepatitis. Therefore, a combined effort is required from both the pathologist and transplant physician, not only to determine the correct cause of graft dysfunction, but to establish the clinical relevance of histologic findings in order to select the best treatment strategy. Not infrequently, the biopsy findings do not fulfill diagnostic criteria for any specific cause of graft dysfunction. When doubt exists, it is generally preferable to adopt a conservative approach to therapy. A simplified algorithm for the differential diagnosis of graft dysfunction after OLT is shown in **Figure 40.3**.

CLASSIFICATION OF EARLY GRAFT DYSFUNCTION

The simplest and most practical classification of graft dysfunction is based on time of onset following OLT (**Fig. 40.4**). While specific complications tend to occur at different time intervals, significant overlap exists. As a general rule, preservation injury, vascular and biliary complications, acute cellular rejection, and most bacterial, fungal and viral infections are encountered within the first 3 postoperative months. In contrast, ductopenic rejection, biliary strictures, recurrent disease and de novo malignancies tend to occur later.

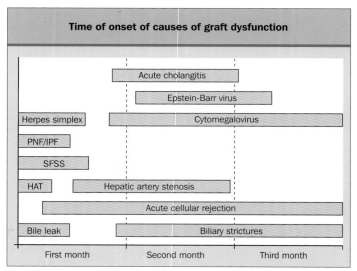

Time of onset of causes of graft dysfunction

Acute cholangitis

Epstein-Barr virus

Herpes simplex

Cytomegalovirus

PNF/IPF

SFSS

HAT

Hepatic artery stenosis

Acute cellular rejection

Bile leak

Biliary strictures

First month   Second month   Third month

Figure 40.4 Time of onset of causes of graft dysfunction during the first 3 months following liver transplantation. PNF, primary non-function; IPF, initial poor function; SFSS, small-for-size syndrome; HAT, hepatic artery thrombosis.

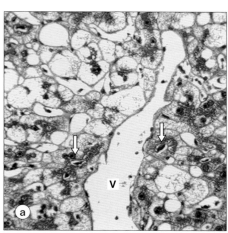

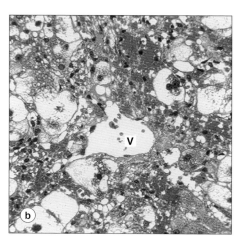

Figure 40.5 Preservation injury. Perivenular (V) area with (a) ballooning of hepatocytes and canalicular cholestasis (arrows) and (b) congestion and hemorrhagic necrosis.

PRESERVATION INJURY AND PRIMARY GRAFT DYSFUNCTION

The term preservation injury is used to describe the organ damage that results from the effects of cold and warm ischemia followed by reperfusion. Pre-existing donor diseases, including alcoholic steatosis, non-alcoholic steatosis or drug-induced hepatotoxicity can render the liver more susceptible to the effects of ischemia. Episodes of hypotension or hypoxia occurring after the declaration of brain death or during surgical removal of the donor organ may also result in graft injury. Cold preservation of the graft and rewarming during the interval from cold storage to resumption of hepatic circulation are the major events leading to ischemic injury. To minimize the risk of severe preservation injury, cold and warm ischemia times should be kept as short as possible. A good example of this is living-donor liver transplantation (LDLT), where cold ischemia time is minimal and primary non-function (PNF) is rare. The spectrum of preservation injury is quite variable and ranges from mild and rapidly reversible clinical and histologic abnormalities to PNF, a life-threatening complication leading to death or emergency retransplantation.

Initial poor function/primary non-function

Severe preservation injury leading to graft failure is called primary graft dysfunction, a syndrome with two similar although distinct variants: initial poor function (IPF) and PNF. In most reported series, IPF was defined as AST greater than 2000 IU/mL, and prothrombin time greater than 20 s during the first week after OLT. Despite borderline function, grafts with IPF are able to support life, although retransplantation may become necessary later. PNF is defined as death or need for emergency retransplantation within 2 weeks of surgery in patients with IPF and is usually associated with clinical features of severe acute liver failure such as persistence of encephalopathy or slowed awakening, absence of bile flow or production of 'white' bile, hypoglycemia,

lactic acidosis, hyperkalemia and renal dysfunction. Although PNF may be diagnosed immediately following OLT, it can also occur after several days following a period of adequate initial function. The reported incidences of IPF and PNF are 15% and 5–10% respectively. A major challenge for the transplant physician is to differentiate, as early as possible, reversible from irreversible primary graft dysfunction. In this dramatic scenario, a timely decision is required to establish the need for emergency retransplantation. PNF is the principal indication for regrafting during the first 2 weeks after OLT.

Histologic findings
Centrilobular hepatocyte ballooning and hemorrhagic necrosis are the main histologic features of preservation injury (**Fig. 40.5**) Submassive or massive coagulative necrosis is found in the explanted livers of patients with PNF. Portal tracts are usually unremarkable. Ductular proliferation and cholangiolitis, mimicking biliary obstruction, are frequently observed in patients who survive IPF without re-OLT. These findings are considered to be a non-specific portal reaction to the severity of parenchymal necrosis.

Risk factors for IPF
A number of donor and recipient risk factors for IPF have been identified. Donor and perioperative factors include donor age greater than 50 years, moderate or severe steatosis, cold preservation times greater than 12 h and warm ischemia times

greater than 1 h. Retransplantation and more advanced pretransplantation disease are the only recipient factors that have been found to be associated with poor outcome. Combining risk factors such as transplanting of old, steatotic grafts into medically unstable recipients should be avoided to minimize the risk of IPF. Despite the availability of better preservation solutions and the continuous search for more accurate risk identification, PNF remains unpredictable in most cases.

Other causes of early graft failure include hepatic artery thrombosis (HAT), portal vein thrombosis (PVT) and antibody-mediated rejection. The profound alteration of the liver microcirculation after cold storage and reperfusion may render the allograft more vulnerable to vascular thrombosis and biliary complications.

Adult-to-adult LDLT is today a universally accepted treatment modality. The volume of the reduced graft per se has a significant impact on outcome. Adult recipients of small reduced livers may develop early graft dysfunction, the so-called 'small-for-size syndrome', characterized by prolonged cholestasis, persistent ascites, coagulopathy and histologic features of ischemic injury, and may require retransplantation. Persistent portal hypertension and the relatively increased portal blood flow, due to the small volume of the right lobe graft, are the main factors involved in the pathogenesis of small-for-size syndrome.

FUNCTIONAL CHOLESTASIS

The term 'functional cholestasis' is used to describe progressive jaundice during the first weeks following OLT in the absence of biliary obstruction, rejection or viral hepatitis. Patients with this complication develop a gradual increase in serum bilirubin associated with normal or mildly elevated hepatocellular and canalicular enzymes. Histologic examination reveals prominent cellular and canalicular cholestasis without significant portal or lobular inflammation. Functional cholestasis is a benign and reversible condition of unknown cause for which there is no specific therapy.

TECHNICAL COMPLICATIONS AFTER LIVER TRANSPLANTATION

OLT is a highly complex operation and technical complications still occur in 10–30% of patients. The most frequent complications affect the biliary tree and to a much lesser degree the vasculature.

Postoperative hemorrhage

Severe coagulopathy and thrombocytopenia are prevalent in patients with end-stage cirrhosis and constitute the major risk factors for early postoperative hemorrhage. These patients often develop diffuse bleeding after reperfusion requiring prolonged and meticulous surgical hemostasis. The risk of hemorrhage further increases when graft function is poor due to coagulopathy. Postoperative bleeding may also result from technical problems during the harvesting procedure or the recipient's hepatectomy and grafting. Donor sources of bleeding include lacerations of the right lobe of the liver, the gallbladder bed, cystic artery or undetected small hepatic veins draining into the inferior vena cava (IVC). Injury to the adrenal gland during total hepatectomy and imperfect vascular anastomoses are the most common

surgical causes of bleeding during the recipient's operation. Finally, acute hemoperitoneum may result from the spontaneous rupture of splenic artery aneurysms or mycotic aneurysms located at the site of the hepatic arterial anastomosis. Clinical manifestations of abdominal hemorrhage after OLT range from an asymptomatic decrease in hematocrit to hypovolemic shock with hypotension and tachycardia. Patients with sustained and severe hypotension are at increased risk of ischemic damage to the allograft and renal failure, which adds significant morbidity. The presence of frank blood in the percutaneous drains or enlarging abdominal hematomas on imaging studies are sufficient to establish the diagnosis in most cases.

Hepatic artery thrombosis

The reported incidence of HAT ranges from 2.5 to 10% in adults and from 10 to 20% in children. Risk factors for HAT include recipient age, atypical recipient and donor hepatic artery anatomy, technical factors, underlying medical conditions and poor early graft function. Pediatric recipients are at higher risk of developing vascular complications due to the small diameter of the arterial vessels. Donor and recipient aberrant arteries require careful reconstruction to prevent HAT early after OLT. The need for vascular extension grafts is the main technical risk factor that may result in inadequate arterial blood supply to the transplanted liver. Hypercoagulable syndromes frequently found in patients with Budd-Chiari or pre-existing PVT predispose to HAT, especially if other anatomic or technical factors are present. Finally, graft edema associated with IPF and requirement of high doses of vasopressors may increase vascular resistance resulting in reduced arterial inflow. The impact of HAT on the allograft depends on the ability of the parenchyma and biliary system to survive on portal flow alone. OLT recipients with sufficient portal blood flow or rearterialization from collaterals can tolerate HAT without significant parenchymal changes. In contrast, bile ducts depend primarily on arterial flow from branches of the gastroduodenal and retroportal arteries that are divided in the transplant operation. The clinical presentation of HAT is variable. Early thrombosis in grafts that are unable to survive on portal blood flow alone results in infarction of the liver parenchyma and acute liver failure. In less dramatic cases, HAT produces necrosis of the extra- or intrahepatic biliary tree presenting as anastomotic bile leaks or intrahepatic bilomas, respectively. Patients who tolerate early HAT with no major sequelae have a more insidious clinical presentation with late development of multiple intrahepatic biliary strictures. Of note, HAT may be discovered incidentally in children, and to a lesser degree in adults, who remain asymptomatic with normal graft function and no biliary complications. Doppler-US accurately identifies HAT in around 90% of cases. Angiography is indicated to confirm the diagnosis and also in patients in whom HAT is strongly suspected on clinical grounds despite a normal Doppler study.

When HAT is detected very early after OLT, acute thrombectomy with or without reconstruction of the anastomosis may save the allograft. However, the majority of patients will require retransplantation some time later. Emergency regrafting is a life-saving procedure for patients with massive necrosis of the graft. In contrast, elective retransplantation is indicated only after the resolution of septic complications in patients with HAT presenting with hepatic abscesses or diffuse biliary strictures.

Hepatic artery stenosis

Hepatic artery stenosis is less frequent than HAT and usually occurs at the anastomotic site or within extension grafts utilized for the arterial reconstruction. Detection of high velocity flows across the anastomosis on Doppler-US is usually the first clue for the diagnosis. The clinical presentation of hepatic artery stenosis is similar to that of HAT but much less dramatic. The decreased arterial inflow affects the biliary tree more than the hepatic parenchyma. Although angioplasty is effective in some cases, surgical reconstruction of the anastomosis is the preferred therapy.

Portal vein thrombosis and stenosis

Inadequate portal vein perfusion is most detrimental in the early postoperative period and may lead to severe allograft dysfunction. The incidence of PVT following OLT is low and ranges from 0.3 to 2.2%. Prior splenectomy or large portosystemic shunts, pre-existing PVT or hypoplasia, hypercoagulable states, and size mismatch between donor and recipient portal veins are the principal risk factors for this complication. Early and complete PVT can be a catastrophic event with rapid onset of liver failure, shock and massive ascites. In this scenario, absent portal vein flow on Doppler examination is usually diagnostic although angiographic confirmation may be desired before surgery. Incomplete thrombosis or portal vein stenosis is associated with gradual development of portal hypertension. Splenomegaly and esophageal varices are the most frequent clinical findings. Development of hepatopetal venous collaterals may result in cavernous transformation of the portal vein. Stenosis of the portal vein is suspected whenever a Doppler examination shows turbulent flow, especially at the level of the anastomosis. Therapy should be tailored to each individual case. Among patients with early and complete PVT, emergency thrombectomy may salvage the graft, although many patients may still require retransplantation. Percutaneous angioplasty with balloon dilatation, transjugular intrahepatic portosystemic shunt (TIPS) and surgical reconstruction have been shown to be effective therapies for patients with partial PVT or stenosis.

Inferior vena cava thrombosis or stenosis

Stenosis or thrombosis of the infra- or suprahepatic IVC anastomoses occurs in only 1–2% of OLT recipients. The standard technique of liver grafting includes the removal of the intrahepatic IVC with the explant. In these cases, the superior end-to-end anastomosis is more susceptible to stenosis or thrombosis. Venous outflow problems are more frequent when the native IVC is preserved utilizing the so-called 'piggy-back' technique. Risk factors for venocaval obstruction or stenosis include use of large allografts for small recipients and OLT for Budd-Chiari syndrome. Clinical presentation is variable according to the location and degree of outflow obstruction. Most patients with stenosis or obstruction of the suprahepatic IVC anastomosis develop graft congestion with hepatomegaly, ascites and peripheral edema that may result in renal dysfunction. Complete obstruction is associated with severe graft failure and hemodynamic instability. In contrast, patients with stenosis or obstruction of the infrahepatic IVC anastomosis present with peripheral edema but no hepatomegaly, ascites or liver failure. Doppler-US is the most valuable screening procedure to identify decreased or absent blood flow as a result of IVC stenosis or thrombosis. However, contrast venography may be required to establish a precise anatomic diagnosis. Although surgical reconstruction of an obstructed suprahepatic IVC anastomosis is feasible, urgent retransplantation may be required. Balloon dilatation with or without insertion of expansile stents has been found to be an effective therapy both for supra- and infrahepatic venocaval stenoses and to correct venous outflow problems resulting from the use of the 'piggy-back' technique. Surgical reconstruction or retransplantation is indicated when the angiographic techniques fail. The key for success in patients transplanted for Budd-Chiari syndrome is immediate anticoagulation with heparin followed by conversion to warfarin a few days later.

Biliary complications

The biliary tract has been called the 'Achilles heel' of OLT. Biliary complications occur in 10–20% of patients transplanted with deceased donors. However, the incidence is significantly higher, up to 50%, in recipients of reduced-size grafts, especially in adult-to-adult LDLT. Major risk factors for biliary complications are bile duct ischemia resulting from HAT, ductopenic rejection, prolonged cold ischemia times, and use of organs from ABO incompatible donors. In general, bile leaks are more frequently observed after choledochojejunostomy and strictures after duct-to-duct anastomosis. The clinical spectrum of biliary tract complications ranges from an asymptomatic elevation of cholestatic enzymes to severe peritonitis and sepsis.

Bile leaks

Bile leaks in the early postoperative period are due to ischemic dehiscence of the anastomosis. In deceased-donor OLT, bile leaks may also occur from the insertion site of the T-tube, a cystic duct remnant or from an inadvertently transected aberrant bile duct. In recipients of LDLT the cut surface of the reduced graft is a frequent site of bile leakage. Bile leaks occurring several weeks post-OLT are most commonly related to T-tube removal. Bile leaks usually present as abdominal pain, jaundice, fever and leukocytosis. Detection of bile in the suction drains or abdominal fluid collections dictates the need for cholangiography to define the severity and location of the bile leak. Unclamping of the T-tube combined with percutaneous drainage of abdominal bilomas and antibiotic therapy is effective in most cases. When this strategy fails, or in patients without a T-tube, endoscopic or percutaneous biliary stenting may be necessary. Most severe anastomotic leaks require surgical revision, often with conversion of a duct-to-duct to a Roux-en-Y anastomosis.

Biliary strictures

Strictures are the most common cause of biliary obstruction following OLT. Aside from the surgical anastomosis itself, strictures may be located anywhere in the biliary tree from the intrahepatic ducts to the sphincter of Oddi. The reported incidence of biliary tract stenoses ranges from 3 to 20% in recipients of deceased donors. However, it is higher, 30–50%, following adult-to-adult LDLT, especially when more than one drains the right lobe graft. Most anastomotic strictures present within a few weeks of surgery, resulting from technical problems or ischemia, and are more common in patients with a duct-to-duct biliary reconstruction. Non-anastomotic strictures are strongly associated with prolonged cold ischemia or hepatic artery ischemia, and most commonly occur at the hilum. In most cases, these present after 2 months post-OLT. Sludge or stones may form as a result of bile duct strictures. In severe cases, large intrabiliary casts are found at the time of re-operation. OLT recipients with biliary obstruction can present in a variety of ways.

When biliary obstruction is incomplete, an asymptomatic rise in liver enzymes with a predominant cholestatic pattern is often the only abnormality. Jaundice, abdominal pain and signs of cholangitis usually indicate severe impairment of bile flow. US may show bile duct dilatation, particularly in patients with long-standing or complete biliary obstruction. However, a normal study does not exclude biliary complications. Most patients will eventually require MR cholangiopancreatography (MRCP) or direct cholangiography to assess the type, severity, number and location of the biliary strictures. Histologic abnormalities such as portal edema, ductular proliferation and centrilobular cholestasis may indirectly suggest the presence of biliary complications, although these findings lack specificity.

Re-establishment of biliary drainage is the therapeutic goal and should be urgently achieved when sepsis and secondary organ dysfunction are present. Percutaneous or endoscopic procedures are indicated both for diagnosis and therapy including removal of sludge, stones and biliary casts, balloon dilatation and stenting. Endoscopic papillotomy is the treatment of choice for patients with bile duct obstruction due to stenosis of the papilla of Vater. In most centers, surgical procedures are reserved for endoscopic or radiologic treatment failures. Diffuse ischemic-type strictures involving both the intra- and extrahepatic bile duct systems usually require multiple interventional procedures, and aggressive treatment of infection. Chronic administration of ursodeoxycholic acid may be of benefit. Although this strategy may provide several months or years of a good quality of life, some patients will develop biliary cirrhosis requiring retransplantation.

ALLOGRAFT REJECTION

Classically, allograft rejection has been classified as hyperacute, acute or chronic according to the time of onset following OLT. However, acute cellular rejection may occur at any time post-OLT, and chronic ductopenic rejection has been recognized within a few weeks following OLT.

Antibody-mediated rejection
Antibody-mediated or humoral rejection is extremely uncommon in OLT recipients. Binding of preformed antibodies to donor antigens expressed on the vascular endothelium results in diffuse small vessel thrombosis, widespread hemorrhagic necrosis, and rapid graft failure requiring emergency regrafting. OLT performed across the ABO blood group barrier is the major risk factor. Immunohistochemical demonstration of immunoglobulins and complement deposited along the sinusoids, veins and arteries, helps to differentiate antibody-mediated rejection from PNF or other causes of early graft failure.

Acute cellular rejection
Acute cellular rejection (ACR) is a frequent finding in OLT recipients. However, as the immunosuppressive agents and regimens have become more potent, the incidence of ACR has decreased over the last decade from 50–70% to only 20–30%, or even less. The vast majority of ACR episodes occur between

5 days and 8 weeks after surgery. Patients with ACR may be asymptomatic or present with a variety of symptoms and signs such as unexplained fever, malaise, increasing ascites or graft tenderness, associated with elevated serum bilirubin or liver enzymes.

Liver biopsy is the gold standard for the diagnosis of rejection. The histologic hallmarks of cellular rejection are portal inflammation, bile duct damage and endotheliitis (**Fig. 40.6**). Portal inflammatory infiltrates usually contain large activated or blastic lymphocytes, small lymphocytes, macrophages, neutrophils, plasma cells and a regular number of eosinophils (Fig. 40.6a). The mixed nature of the portal infiltrate is helpful in distinguishing rejection from recurrent or acquired viral hepatitis. Disruption of the limiting plate and bridging necrosis indicate severe cellular rejection. Non-suppurative cholangitis, also called rejection cholangitis or lymphocytic cholangitis, is characterized by infiltration of the epithelium of small interlobular bile ducts with lymphocytes or other inflammatory cells, producing degenerative changes or nuclear pyknosis (Fig. 40.6b). In severe cases, necrosis of epithelial cells results in bile duct loss. Endotheliitis is defined as the attachment of inflammatory cells to the endothelial surface of portal or terminal hepatic veins. Perivenular hepatocyte necrosis associated with central endotheliitis is regarded as a histologic feature of severe cellular rejection (Fig. 40.6c and d) Although no correlation exists between the exuberance of portal inflammation and response to therapy or outcome, severe bile duct damage or loss and centrilobular necrosis may announce the occurrence of irreversible rejection requiring re-OLT. Recent studies have shown that cellular rejection may not have a detrimental impact on overall patient survival. Moreover, mild ACR was significantly associated with increased patient survival suggesting that some level of alloreactivity may contribute to later immunologic hyporesponsiveness. These findings raise the question of whether complete elimination of all ACR should be a desirable goal in patients undergoing OLT.

Chronic ductopenic rejection
Early chronic ductopenic rejection (CDR), occurring weeks after OLT, usually follows episodes of severe or refractory cellular rejection. In this setting, duct loss is found in portal tracts with prominent inflammation. CDR diagnosed several months or years after OLT, one cause of vanishing bile duct syndrome, has a more indolent presentation with an asymptomatic increase in cholestatic enzymes, with or without increased serum bilirubin. Late CDR is characterized by duct loss in the absence of significant portal inflammation and is commonly associated with foam-cell arteriopathy. CDR has become increasingly uncommon occurring in only 1–2% of recipients.

INFECTIOUS COMPLICATIONS

Despite remarkable progress in liver transplantation, infection continues to be a significant cause of morbidity and mortality. The incidence of infectious complications in OLT recipients is up to 70% higher than that observed after kidney or heart transplantation. The majority of patients experience at least one episode of infection, particularly during the initial hospitalization when immunosuppression is maximal and surgical complications prevail. Sepsis is the leading cause of death the first 3 months

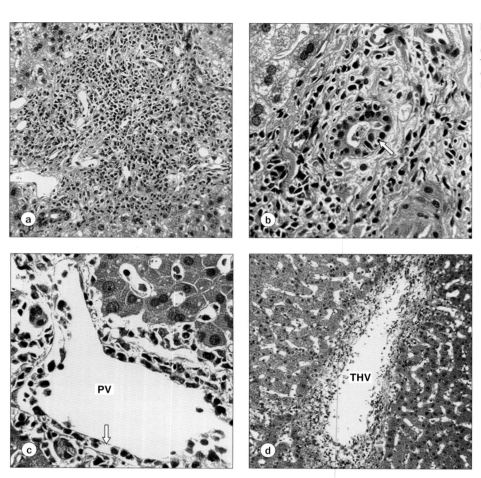

Figure 40.6 Cellular rejection. (a) Mixed portal inflammation. (b) Non-suppurative cholangitis (arrow). (c) Portal vein (PV) phlebitis with lifting of the endothelium (arrow). (d) Severe endotheliitis of terminal hepatic venule (THV) with perivenular necrosis.

after OLT. The transplant operation per se is a risk factor for infection because it is performed in a potentially contaminated environment within the abdominal cavity. The poor pre-operative medical and nutritional conditions of recipients and the intensity of immunosuppression are additional risk factors for the development of infection. Steroid boluses and use of antilymphocyte preparations significantly increase the risk of infection. Specific infectious complications tend to appear at different times after OLT, although overlap is frequent. As a general rule, bacterial and fungal infectious are more prevalent early after OLT and commonly involve extrahepatic organs, whereas viral infections occur later and frequently compromise the allograft. Infection-related mortality has decreased from 50% in the 1980s before the advent of selective immuno-suppression, to around 10% at the present time. This remarkable improvement was largely due to a therapeutic shift from management of established infection to prophylaxis.

Bacterial infections

Bacteria are the most common cause of infection in OLT recipients. The majority of episodes occurs within 2 months and originates mostly in the abdomen, especially among patients with surgical complications. Major risk factors for bacterial infection are prolonged surgery, high intraoperative transfusion requirements and the need for reoperations including retrans-plantation, CMV infection, renal impairment and the intensity of immunosuppression. The most common sites of infection are the biliary tree, abdominal cavity, intravascular catheters, lungs, surgical wounds and the urinary tract. Most early bacterial infections are due to Gram-positive organisms such as *Staphylococcus* spp. and *Streptococcus* spp. and aerobic Gram-negative bacilli such as *Enterobacteriaceae* and *Pseudomonas*. The spectrum of commonly isolated bacteria following OLT varies among patients treated preoperatively with oral non-absorbable antimicrobials such as the combination of norfloxacin and nistatin or selective bowel decontamination preparations. These regimens eliminate most aerobic Gram-negative bacilli and *Candida* species while preserving the anaerobic gut flora.

Ascending cholangitis is the most frequent bacterial infection affecting the allograft. Bile leaks or biliary obstruction may result in the formation of hepatic abscesses. In addition, infected liver tissue secondary to HAT frequently become seeded with bacteria leading to hepatic gangrene. Since sterile intrahepatic or abdominal collections are frequently found after OLT, aspiration under US or computed tomography guidance and culture are required to confirm the presence of infection. Nosocomial pneumonia is another common bacterial infection after OLT, particularly when there is need for prolonged mechanical ventilation. When examination of the sputum is not diagnostic, invasive procedures such as bronchoalveolar lavage or thoraco-centesis are often required to differentiate pneumonia from atelectasis and sterile pleural effusions which are common findings early after surgery. Infections with *Legionella* and *Nocardia* species are not uncommon after OLT and should be considered in patients with pulmonary infiltrates of unclear origin. Bacteremia in immunosuppressed transplant recipients is a serious infectious complication and is associated with increased mortality. Most commonly, it arises from abdominal collections or intravascular lines and to a lesser degree from wound, lung and urinary tract infections. Biliary or vascular complications and deep wound infection should always be considered whenever OLT recipients develop unexplained fever or bacteremia of unclear source. Infection with *Listeria monocytogenes* usually present as meningitis or encephalitis within 2 months of OLT. When suspected, a lumbar puncture should be performed without delay to prevent a fatal outcome. Fortunately, routine administration of trimethroprim-sulfamethoxazole to prevent *Pneumocystis carinii* is also effective against listerial and other bacterial infections.

Despite a paucity of randomized controlled trials demonstrating benefit from perioperative antibacterial prophylaxis, most centers administer intravenous antibiotics for the first 48–72 h after OLT. The antibiotics chosen are directed against organisms commonly found in the gastrointestinal flora and *Staphylococcus* such as cefoxitin, ceftizoxime, ampicillin-sulbactam, or cefotaxime plus ampicillin. The major concern about the use of antibiotic prophylaxis is selection of resistant organisms. When bacterial infection is suspected early after OLT, and before results of culture become available, empiric antimicrobial regimens are frequently used to cover the most likely pathogens according to the presumed site of infection. The susceptibility patterns of the microorganisms that prevail in each transplant center should also be considered for empiric therapy. However, once the offending organisms are identified, the antibiotics should be changed to those which have the narrowest spectrum coverage. Renal insufficiency is a frequent finding early after OLT due to the combined effects of underlying renal dysfunction, hypovolemia and nephrotoxic effects of calcineurin inhibitors. Therefore, empiric use of aminoglycosides and vancomycin should be avoided to prevent further nephrotoxicity. The most frequently used antibiotics to treat bacterial infections in OLT recipients are third or fourth generation cephalosporins, β-lactam/β-lactamase inhibitor combinations and quinolones.

Fungal infections

Fungal infections after OLT are less frequent than bacterial and viral infections but are associated with higher mortality. Major risk factors for fungal infection are similar to those described for bacterial infection and include advanced age, history of diabetes, emergency OLT, a prolonged transplant operation, transfusion of large amounts of blood products, repeated abdominal surgery, retransplantation, HAT, renal failure, CMV infection, intensity of immunosuppression and preoperative therapy with antibiotics or corticosteroids. OLT recipients are prone to develop opportunistic infections with fungi such as *Candida*, *Aspergillus* and *Cryptococcus* that rarely cause invasive disease in immunocompetent hosts. A high index of suspicion is required because the clinical presentation of fungal infections is frequently nonspecific and may also be obscured by other infectious or noninfectious complications. *Candida albicans* is the most prevalent fungi encountered following OLT. Although non-invasive mucocutaneous disease is the commonest presentation, candidal infections may produce many other complications such as pneumonia, abdominal abscesses, urinary tract infection, endo-

carditis and meningitis. Bloodstream invasion from these sites, or more frequently through intravascular catheters, results in disseminated disease in around half of the patients. Invasive infection with *Aspergillus fumigatus* characteristically involves the central nervous system and associated with this the mortality approaches 100%. Dissemination occurs through hematogenous spread and may compromise almost any organ. *Aspergillus* infection should be suspected in OLT recipients with persistent fever despite antibiotic therapy and in those with progressive pulmonary infiltrates of unclear origin.

Diagnosis relies on the identification of pathogenic fungi by staining and/or culture of blood or other specimens obtained through invasive procedures such as bronchoalveolar lavage or lung biopsy. Amphotericin B is currently the drug of choice to treat invasive fungal infections, however this may be changing. The benefits of amphotericin therapy are limited by its significant bone marrow and renal toxicities. This is particularly relevant in OLT recipients because renal dysfunction and cytopenias are common adverse effects of calcineurin inhibitors and antimetabolites. Liposomal formulations of amphotericin are less nephrotoxic and allow the administration of larger amounts of the active drug. However, because of the elevated cost, liposomal amphotericin is not routinely utilized in most countries as a first-line agent, unless significant nephrotoxicity is present. Prophylactic low-dose amphotericin is utilized in many centers to reduce the incidence and severity of fungal infections among high-risk patients. Azole antifungal agents such as fluconazole and itraconazole have been increasingly utilized to treat fungal infections in OLT recipients. Fluconazole is well absorbed and has good penetration in the central nervous system. It is effective both for *Candida* and *Cryptococcus* species but much less so for *Aspergillus*. The antifungal spectrum of itraconazole covers not only *Candida* species but also *Aspergillus*. The major drawback of this drug is its erratic absorption that often results in unpredictable plasma levels. Both fluconazole and itraconazole inhibit the hepatic metabolism of calcineurin inhibitors which may result in increased blood concentrations and overimmunosuppression. Two newer antifungals appear promising. Voriconzole is a new azole that has good activity against *Candida*, *Aspergillus* and *Cryptococcus neoformans*. Caspofungin is a good novel antifungal with good activity against *Candida* and *Aspergillus*. Most importantly they appear to have relatively little toxicity as compared to other antifungals.

Viral infections

Infection with opportunistic viruses such as cytomegalovirus (CMV), Epstein-Barr virus (EBV), herpes simplex virus (HSV), varicella-zoster virus (VZV) and adenovirus may produce graft dysfunction at variable time intervals following OLT (Fig. 40.4). Pediatric recipients without exposure to childhood illnesses before OLT have the highest risk of primary infection with opportunistic viruses. In contrast, reactivation of endogenous latent viral infections is more prevalent among adult recipients. Primary infection is usually more severe than reactivation. Diagnosis of viral infections in transplant recipients mostly relies on assays to detect viremia or antigenemia. Histologic examination of liver specimens with routine stains, immunohistochemistry, or in situ hybridization techniques may be helpful in some cases. However, serologic tests are unreliable because they lack sensitivity and specificity in immunosuppressed transplant recipients.

Cytomegalovirus infection

CMV is the single most common viral pathogen encountered in OLT recipients. When no antiviral prophylaxis is given, the incidence of CMV infection is 50–60% and CMV disease occurs in 20–30%. Without specific therapy, CMV disease is associated with high mortality. Main sources of infection are grafts from CMV-positive donors, transfusion of leukocyte-containing blood products and endogenous reactivation of latent infection. Risk factors for infection and disease include transplantation of a CMV-seropositive donor into a CMV-seronegative recipient, OLT for fulminant hepatic failure, intense baseline immunosuppression, use of antilymphocyte preparation and retransplantation. Most CMV infections occur between 4 and 12 weeks after surgery. Patients may develop primary infection, secondary infection (reactivation) and superinfection (reinfection). Primary infection occurs when CMV-seronegative recipients receive an organ or blood products from a seropositive donor. Reactivation is observed in seropositive recipients under the effects of immunosuppression. Superinfection is defined as reactivation of latent donor CMV infection after being grafted into a CMV-seropositive recipient. Clinical presentation of CMV infection is variable and ranges from asymptomatic viral shedding to lethal systemic disease with multiorgan involvement. Low-grade fever, malaise, arthralgias, myalgias, leukopenia with atypical lymphocytes, thrombocytopenia and elevated liver tests are the most common findings. Severe CMV disease is a tissue invasive disease involving the gastrointestinal tract, liver, retina or central nervous system. CMV has the ability to depress the host's immune response exerting an additive effect to that of immunosuppressive drugs. This overimmunosuppression induced by CMV increases the risk of superinfection with opportunistic bacterial or fungal pathogens.

Serologic tests are useful to assess donor and recipient past exposure to CMV. However, immunoglobulin M (IgM) and immunoglobulin G (IgG) antibodies lack sensitivity for the diagnosis of CMV infection after OLT. A number of sensitive and rapid diagnostic assays are now available to detect the presence of replicating CMV in serum samples or body fluids. The shell vial leukocyte culture technique utilizes a labeled monoclonal antibody that binds to an early viral antigen and has a turnaround time of only 24–48 h. CMV antigenemia is more sensitive than the shell vial culture and has the advantage of being more rapid, with results available in around 5 h, semiquantitative and of not requiring cell culture methodologies. Antigenemia assay is based on the reaction of a monoclonal antibody with a structural CMV antigen (pp65) located in the nuclei of polymorphonuclear leukocytes. Levels of antigenemia correlate with the severity of infection and decrease following effective therapy. Polymerase chain reaction (PCR) is the most sensitive diagnostic technique allowing the detection of even minimal concentrations of CMV DNA. The major drawback of qualitative PCR is the lack of specificity to differentiate CMV infection from CMV disease. Quantitative PCR is at present the diagnostic method of choice, especially to monitor the response to therapy. The demonstration of CMV viremia or antigenemia should strongly suggest active infection and the need for antiviral treatment. The modern diagnostic methodologies allow the detection of replicating virus several days before the onset of clinical disease and thus the initiation of pre-emptive therapy. Histologic diagnosis of CMV hepatitis mostly relies on the

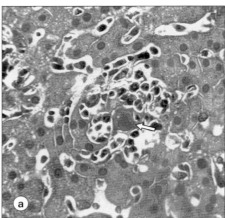

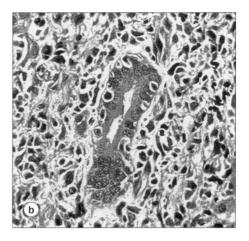

Figure 40.7 Coexistence of cytomegalovirus (CMV) hepatitis and allograft rejection. (a) Microabscess surrounding a necrotic hepatocyte with a CMV inclusion body (arrow). (b) Portal inflammation and rejection cholangitis.

presence of characteristic inclusion bodies in hepatocytes or mesenchymal cells, surrounded by clusters of neutrophils (microabscesses) or microgranulomas (**Fig. 40.7**a). Immunostaining of biopsy specimens with monoclonal antibodies that bind early CMV antigens or in situ hybridization with specific DNA probes are useful to confirm the diagnosis, especially when cytomegalic inclusion bodies are not present.

The advent of effective antiviral agents over the last decade has significantly decreased the CMV disease burden in OLT recipients. Ganciclovir and its analogs, foscarnet and cidofovir have excellent activity against CMV and other herpesviruses. CMV disease requires 2–3 weeks of intravenous ganciclovir, although the optimal length of therapy is still a matter of debate. The use of alternative drugs such as foscarnet and cidofovir should be restricted only to patients who develop viral resistance or fail to respond to ganciclovir. Both agents are nephrotoxic and therefore should be used with caution in OLT recipients. Intravenous or oral ganciclovir, intravenous immunoglobulin, CMV hyperimmune globulin and more recently oral valganciclovir have been successfully utilized for universal or selective prophylaxis of CMV infection. Use of valganciclovir, a valine ester prodrug of ganciclovir, appears to be practical and effective because it has a bioavailability up to 10-fold higher than that of oral ganciclovir. In most centers, ganciclovir prophylaxis is indicated in CMV-negative recipients grafted with CMV-positive donors or following administration of supplemental immunosuppression to treat cellular rejection. Another commonly used strategy is pre-emptive therapy in which ganciclovir is initiated at the time of the virologic diagnosis of CMV infection but before the onset of disease. Cellular rejection and CMV hepatitis often coexist (Fig. 40.7b). As the virus itself decreases the immune response, reduction of the level of immunosuppression is safe, and when combined with ganciclovir therapy, results in resolution of both rejection and CMV hepatitis in most cases.

Epstein-Barr virus infection

EBV produces a spectrum of abnormalities in OLT recipients ranging from asymptomatic infection to diffuse lymphomatous infiltration of multiple organs. Primary infection may be acquired from the allograft, transfusion of leukocyte-containing blood products and, less likely, from the community. Small children are at particular risk of developing primary EBV infection because around 50% lack previous exposure and are seronegative at the time of OLT. EBV infection is usually diagnosed from 2 to 6 months following OLT, but the risk of developing EBV-related post-transplant lymphoproliferative disease (PTLD) continues beyond that. Primary EBV infection often results in a mononucleosis-like syndrome with fever, malaise, circulating atypical lymphocytes and mild and reversible hepatitis. Diagnosis of EBV infection includes IgM and IgG antibodies to several viral antigens and molecular virologic tests to detect and quantitate viremia. EBV-related hepatitis is histologically characterized by polymorphous portal and sinusoidal inflammation, but with minimal hepatocellular necrosis. Endotheliitis of portal and central veins may be present, mimicking cellular rejection. The disproportion between the intensity of the portal infiltrate and mild or absent bile duct damage favors the diagnosis of EBV hepatitis over rejection. Demonstration of EBV antigens or genes in liver tissue by immunohistochemistry or in situ hybridization is useful to confirm the diagnosis in difficult cases. Uncomplicated EBV infection is self-limited and reversible unless supplemental immunosuppression is administered. EBV produces life-long latent infection, has unique tropism for B cells, and the ability to induce lymphocyte transformation and proliferation under the effects of immunosuppressive therapy. Around 2% of adults and up to 25% of EBV-seronegative children experience PTLD between 2 months and 2 years following OLT.

Herpes simplex virus infections

Primary HSV infection occurs via the allograft itself or from person-to-person contact. As 75% of adults are HSV-seropositive before OLT, the vast majority of infections result from re-activation of latent virus. The most common clinical presentation is the appearance of oral mucocutaneous or anogenital lesions within 4 weeks of OLT. Bacterial superinfections of orolabial lesions and esophageal involvement are frequent findings among heavily immunosuppressed patients. HSV pneumonia and central nervous system involvement are rare in OLT recipients. Serologic diagnosis of HSV infection is based on the detection of specific IgM antibodies or a fourfold rise in the serum concentration of IgG antibodies. However, direct immunofluorescence performed on swabs taken from mucocutaneous lesions is a rapid and sensitive methodology to confirm the diagnosis. Severe reactivation of virulent strains of HSV produces a rapidly progressive and fatal hepatitis early after OLT, with or without associated mucocutaneous lesions. Histologically, HSV hepatitis is characterized by circumscribed areas of coagulative necrosis with a non-zonal distribution and Cowdry-type nuclear inclusions in viable hepatocytes located at the periphery of necrotic areas. The presence of HSV antigens in infected hepatocytes can be confirmed by immunohistochemistry. Oral aciclovir is an effective therapy for most patients with mucocutaneous infections. Intravenous administration of aciclovir or ganciclovir is reserved for patients with disseminated disease. The routine use of prophylactic aciclovir or ganciclovir has resulted in a dramatic decrease in the incidence and severity of HSV infection after OLT over the last decade.

Human herpesvirus-6 and -7

Human herpesviruses (HHV) -6 and -7 are novel members of the β-herpesvirus family, agents known to maintain latency in the human host after primary infection. OLT recipients with HHV-6 infection may develop fever, encephalitis or other neurologic disorders, hepatitis, skin rash, pneumonitis and myelosuppression. In contrast, the clinical significance of HHV-7 infection following OLT remains unclear. The frequent association of HHV-6 and -7 infections with allograft rejection, CMV infection and other opportunistic infections suggest that these novel agents have immunomodulatory effects and trigger viral interactions. Diagnosis of HHV-6 and -7 infections mostly rely on antigenemia assays utilizing monoclonal antibodies that bind specific viral antigens in mononuclear cells. Molecular virologic assays are available for HHV-6 (HHV-6 DNA) but not for HHV-7. Viral antigens can also be detected in tissue with immunohistochemical methods.

Other viral infections

The large majority of adult patients, but not children, have antibodies to VZV before OLT. Reactivation in VZV-seropositive adults usually results in herpes zoster characterized by the appearance of painful vesicular lesions with a dermatomal distribution. In contrast, primary VZV infection occurs mostly in pediatric recipients and may cause severe illness with hemorrhagic skin lesions, pneumonia, hepatitis, encephalitis and pancreatitis leading to multiorgan failure and death. Direct immunofluorescence of swabs taken from cutaneous lesions, viral culture and Tzanc preparations are useful to certify the diagnosis. Intravenous aciclovir is the treatment of choice for VZV infections. Success of antiviral therapy largely relies on the early recognition of the disease. Varicella-zoster immunoglobulin is indicated in seronegative recipients whenever exposure to the virus is documented or strongly suspected. Vaccination pretransplant may also be effective.

Adenovirus infection is mostly restricted to pediatric recipients who usually present with fever associated with hepatitis or pneumonia within 1 month of OLT. The severity of hepatitis ranges from mild and self-limited disease to fulminant hepatic failure requiring urgent re-OLT. Liver biopsy shows areas of parenchymal necrosis with no particular zonal distribution, collections of inflammatory cells with a granulomatoid appearance, and nuclear inclusions in the periphery of necrotic areas. Immunostaining of specific viral antigens in liver specimens is required to confirm the diagnosis.

Papillomavirus infection in OLT recipients frequently causes extensive warty growths that may undergo malignant transformation or cervical lesions that may lead to squamous cell cancer.

Infection with human polyoma JC virus in immunosuppressed hosts produces multifocal leukoencephalopathy, a progressive demyelinating disease of the central nervous system.

Finally, many viruses that cause benign illness in the general population may have a serious impact in OLT recipients. Good examples of this are infections with the respiratory syncytial or influenza viruses.

FURTHER READING

Rejection

Demetris AJ, Batts KP, Dhillon AP and International Panel. Banff schema for grading liver allograft rejection: an international consensus document. Hepatology 1997; 25:658–663.

Hassoun Z, Shah V, Lohse CM, et al. Centrilobular necrosis after orthotopic liver transplantation association with acute cellular rejection and impact on outcome. Liver Transpl 2004; 10:480–487.

Ludwig J, Lefkowitch JH. Histopathology of the liver following transplantation. In: Maddrey WC, Schiff ER, Sorrell MF, eds. Transplantation of the liver. 3rd edn. Philadelphia: Lippincott Williams & Wilkins; 2001:229–250.

Wiesner RH, Demetris AJ, Belle SH, et al. Acute hepatic allograft rejection: incidence, risk factors, and impact on outcome. Hepatology 1998; 28:638–645. *Analysis of a large database describing incidence, timing, clinical risk factors and outcome of cellular rejection according to histologic severity.*

Biliary complications

Boraschi P, Braccini G, Gigoni R, et al. Detection of biliary complications after orthotopic liver transplantation with MR cholangiography. Magn Reson Imaging 2001; 19:1097–1105.

Moser MAJ, Wall WJ. Management of biliary problems after liver transplantation. Liver Transpl 2001; 7(suppl 1):46–52. *A detailed review of the diagnosis and management of biliary complications after OLT.*

Metabolic complications

Merritt WT. Metabolism and liver transplantation: review of perioperative issues. Liver Transpl 2000; 6(suppl 1):76–84.

Infection

Fung JJ. Fungal infection in liver transplantation. Transpl Infect Dis 2002; 4(suppl 3):18–23. *This report emphasizes that despite the reduced incidence observed in recent years and the availability of improved therapies, morbidity and mortality associated with fungal infections continues to be high.*

Holmes RD, Sokol RJ. Epstein-Barr virus and post-transplant lymphoproliferative disease. Pediatr Transplant 2002; 6:456–464. *A review of EBV-related PTLD in immunosuppressed children undergoing solid-organ transplantation.*

Ljungman P, Griffiths P, Paya C. Definitions of cytomegalovirus infection and disease in transplant recipients. Clin Infect Dis 2002; 34:1094–1097. *An update of the definitions of CMV infection and disease and of the indirect effects caused by this viral infection in OLT recipients.*

Razonable RR, Paya CV. The impact of human herpesvirus-6 and -7 infection on the outcome of liver transplantation. Liver Transpl 2002; 8:651–658.

Sampathkumar P, Paya CV. Management of cytomegalovirus infection after liver transplantation. Liver Transpl 2000; 6:144–156.

Wade JJ, Rolando N, Hayllar K, et al. Bacterial and fungal infections after liver transplantation: An analysis of 284 patients. Hepatology 1995; 21:1328–1336.

Miscellaneous complications

Crossin JD, Muradali D, Wilson SR. US of liver transplants: normal and abnormal. Radiographics 2003; 23:1093–1114.

Kiuchi T, Tanaka K, Ito T, et al. Small-for-size graft in living donor liver transplantation: How far should we go? Liver Transpl 2003; 9(suppl 1):29–35.

Ohkohchi N. Mechanisms of preservation and ischemic/reperfusion injury in liver transplantation. Transplant Proc 2002; 34:2670–2673.

Stange BJ, Glanemann M, Nuessler NC, et al. Hepatic artery thrombosis after adult liver transplantation. Liver Transpl 2003; 9:612–620.

Strasberg SM, Howard TK, Molmenti EP, et al. Selecting the donor liver: factors for poor function after orthotopic liver transplantation. Hepatology 1994; 20:829–838.

CHAPTER
41

Long-Term Management

James Neuberger

LONG-TERM MANAGEMENT

With the success of liver transplantation over the last two decades, the role of long-term care of the liver allograft recipient is becoming an area of increasing importance. Although the quality of life following liver transplantation is usually excellent, it can never be considered normal and regular monitoring is a requirement to maximize the recipient's opportunity to live as fulfilling a life as possible. Immunosuppressive regimens require surveillance and adjustment to maintain good graft function whilst minimizing the adverse effects. It should be remembered that the hepatic metabolic functions and profile will reflect the donor rather than the recipient, so that diverse metabolic conditions such as Gilbert syndrome, peanut allergy, protein C deficiency and alcohol-flush syndrome may be acquired following the transplant. In addition, some infectious and malignant complications may be derived from the donor.

Graft function must be carefully tracked and abnormalities investigated so appropriate intervention can be directed at limiting damage to the graft. The care of these patients requires close collaboration and cooperation between the recipient, the transplant unit, the local clinician and the primary healthcare provider. In the transplant recipients who die more than 5 years after transplantation, complications of immunosuppression (over-immunosuppression such as infection, renal failure, de novo malignancy and underimmunosuppression such as chronic rejection) account for just over half of all deaths, vascular disease (cardiovascular and cerebrovascular disease) account for about one-quarter, and recurrent disease or technical factors (biliary or vascular complications) account for the rest.

MAINTAINING GOOD GRAFT FUNCTION

The frequency of monitoring must balance the need for early detection and correction of abnormalities against the ambition to maximize the patient's quality of life. Most liver transplant programs monitor patients every 3 months during the second and third postoperative years and at a lower frequency thereafter. A template for follow-up is suggested in **Table 41.1**.

INVESTIGATION OF ABNORMAL LIVER FUNCTION

The finding of abnormal liver tests should prompt further investigation to identify the cause and extent of the graft dysfunction (**Table 41.2**). The cause of the liver dysfunction may be suspected from the clinical and biochemical features, but imaging and/or histologic evaluation are usually required to establish the precise diagnosis.

Suggested template for assessment of liver allograft recipients more than 1 year post-transplant	
Recipients should be assessed every 3–4 months or as clinically indicated	
Clinical	General health Hepatic problems
Examination	Weight Body mass index (BMI) Blood pressure Evidence of liver dysfunction Skin lesions
Investigations	Blood counts Renal function tests Liver tests Auto-antibodies* Immunoglobulins* Urine: creatinine clearance; urine albumin/creatinine ratio* Serum lipids*
Where appropriate	Viral hepatitis markers Bone densitometry[†] Liver ultrasound[†] Liver biopsy[†] Ophthalmologic examination[†]
*Annually. [†]As clinically indicated. [‡]For those on corticosteroids.	

Table 41.1 Suggested template for assessment of liver allograft recipients more than 1 year post-transplant.

ALLOGRAFT REJECTION

Acute rejection usually occurs within the first weeks after transplantation but it may also occur at any time after transplantation. However, in the majority of cases a precipitating event can be identified. These include:

- reduction in the dose of the immunosuppressive drugs as part of the process of defining the minimal immunosuppressive requirements in individual patients or in response to adverse effects of immunosuppression;
- poor patient compliance;
- inability to take medication e.g. vomiting; and
- changes in concomitant medication leading to accelerated metabolism of the calcineurin inhibitors (tacrolimus, cyclosporin) e.g. phenytoin or changes in the components of highly active retroviral treatment (HAART) therapy.

Some causes of graft dysfunction developing after 1 year post-transplant	
Immune mediated	Acute cellular rejection Ductopenic rejection De novo autoimmune hepatitis
Recurrent disease	Viral · Hepatitis B viral infection · Hepatitis C virus infection Autoimmune diseases · Primary biliary cirrhosis · Primary sclerosing cholangitis · Autoimmune hepatitis Cancer Alcohol associated liver disease Non-alcoholic fatty liver disease
Structural	Hepatic artery thrombosis Biliary strictures · Anastomotic · Non-anastomotic Cholangitis Portal venous thrombosis Hepatic venous thrombosis
Infections	
Drug toxicity	

Table 41.2 Some causes of graft dysfunction developing after 1 year post-transplant.

It has also been suggested that intercurrent viral infections may trigger rejection episodes in patients on stable and previously effective immunosuppression regimens. The biochemical and histologic features of rejection are very similar to that seen in the early post-transplant period (Ch. 40). The treatment of the rejection is also similar to that for early rejection although the response to therapy may be slower and less satisfactory and some cases progress inexorably to chronic rejection. In those patients with histologically mild rejection, merely increasing the dose of calcineurin inhibitor may be sufficient; for histologically moderate or severe rejection, the usual treatment is with a short course of high-dose corticosteroids. More than one episode of rejection or multiple episodes of rejection should prompt reassessment of the immunosuppressive regimen.

Chronic ductopenic rejection

Chronic ductopenic rejection usually develops during the first postoperative year but may occur at any time. In contrast to acute, cellular rejection, the time course of ductopenic rejection is slower. Risk factors for the development of chronic rejection include:

- prior retransplantation for chronic rejection;
- primary biliary cirrhosis (PBC) or primary sclerosing cholangitis (PSC) as original liver disease;
- recurrent episodes of acute cellular rejection;
- late (>3 months) acute rejection; and
- inadequate immunosuppression.

The clinical features include:

- progressive jaundice;

- symptoms associated with cholestasis (such as pruritus) in the later stages;
- cholestatic liver tests, initially the serum alkaline phosphatase and γ-glutamyltransferase levels rise followed by the serum bilirubin; and
- impaired synthetic function in advanced disease with reduction in the serum albumin level.

Abnormal coagulation tests may be due to vitamin K deficiency or impaired synthetic function.

Liver histology typically shows features of a 'vanishing bile duct syndrome', with progressive reduction in the intensity of the associated inflammatory infiltrate. Occasionally, a vascular pattern of damage is captured in the biopsy with occlusion of the arterial lumen by foamy macrophages. Chronic rejection may be reversible and is more likely to respond to treatment when more than 50% of portal tracts retain bile ducts.

Treatment is not always effective at reversing graft dysfunction. Increasing immunosuppression, by switching from cyclosporin to tacrolimus (where appropriate) or the institution of either mycophenolate or rapamycin/sirolimus may be of benefit if the damage is not too great. For those with end-stage disease, as shown by serum bilirubin in excess of 150 μmol/L or 20 mg/dL, liver replacement is the only effective therapeutic option.

HEPATIC ARTERY THROMBOSIS

The late or delayed presentation of hepatic artery thrombosis (HAT) differs from the early presentation in that ischemic hepatitis and graft infarction do not typically occur. Some cases are clinically silent and are detected on routine scanning. The usual presentations are with ischemic cholangiopathy, liver abscess or sepsis. The initial investigation should include ultrasound and Doppler examination of the artery. Occasionally, pulsation of the artery proximal to the thrombosis may give rise to the mistaken belief that the artery is patent. The diagnosis should be confirmed either by conventional angiography or computed tomography (CT)/magnetic resonance (MR) angiography (**Fig. 41.1**).

Treatment of the blockage by stenting, dilatation or use of thrombolysis is usually ineffective. Most cases of late HAT progress with the development of multiple intra- and extra-hepatic abscesses and biliary strictures. The only effective treatment is by liver transplantation. It is important that regrafting is not postponed while attempts are made to treat with systemic antibiotics, local drainage or biliary stenting since these approaches are rarely effective and procrastination results in the patient being in a worse clinical state when transplantation is eventually undertaken.

PORTAL VEIN THROMBOSIS

Portal vein thrombosis or stenosis is rare and is usually detected on routine examination at ultrasound. Occasionally it presents with complications of portal hypertension such as variceal hemorrhage or hypersplenism. The stenosis or thrombosis should be confirmed by vascular imaging (direct or with CT or MR). A stenosis can sometimes be dilated through an angiographic approach. Definitive treatment (with the construction of a shunt) is not always necessary, and varices treated either pharmacologically with β blockade (with propranolol or carvedilol), or endoscopic band ligation or sclerotherapy.

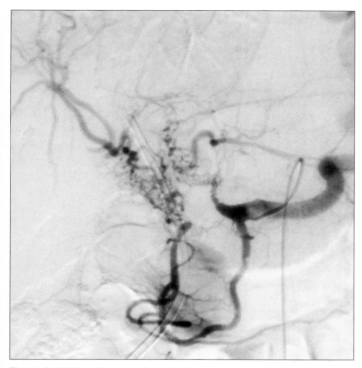

Figure 41.1 Hepatic artery thrombosis.

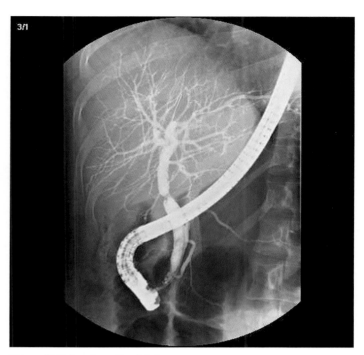

Figure 41.2 Anastomotic stricture.

BILIARY PROBLEMS

The biliary tract remains the Achilles heel of liver transplantation and is the source of most technical complications. The biliary tree is susceptible to ischemic damage because most of its blood supply is derived from a plexus of small collateral arteries that originate in the duodenum, with the remainder being supplied from the right hepatic artery. The use of cut-down and reduced sized livers, and livers derived from non-heart beating donors is more likely to be associated with late biliary strictures.

Anastomotic strictures
Anastomotic strictures (**Fig. 41.2**) usually present in the first few months after transplantation but may present later. The clinical history is of obstructive jaundice with pruritus, pale stools and dark urine. Sometimes there is associated cholangitis. Liver function tests typically show an obstructive pattern but it is important to appreciate that this may be subtle or even absent. Ultrasound may demonstrate dilated intrahepatic bile ducts, but the absence of duct dilatation does not reliably exclude a signifi-cant biliary obstruction in the liver transplant recipient. The diagnosis is confirmed by imaging the biliary tree, using magnetic resonance cholangiopancreatography (MRCP), endoscopic retro-grade cholangiopancreatography (ERCP) or percutaneous trans-hepatic cholangiography (PTC) (usually in patients with a Roux loop and a choledochojejunostomy).

The treatment of anastomotic strictures involves either endo-scopic dilatataion and stenting (which may be repeated) or formal biliary reconstruction with the fashioning of a Roux choledochojejunostomy. When the stricture arises at the Roux anastomosis, the optimal treatment is with percutaneous intra-hepatic dilatation. Sometimes, it is necessary to place a stent

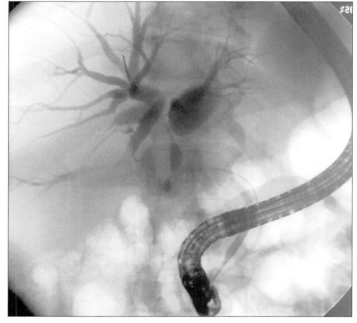

Figure 41.3 Non-anastomotic strictures.

across this anastomosis but this is best avoided as the long-term consequences are unknown.

Non-anastomotic strictures
The main causes of non-anastomotic strictures (**Fig. 41.3**) are:
- ischemic cholangitis;
- biliary sepsis;
- recurrent PSC.

Non-anastomotic strictures are usually multiple but solitary strictures can develop at the hilum. The treatment of single non-anastomotic strictures is similar to that of anastomotic strictures. However, mechanical intervention is usually futile in cases with multiple strictures and the initial management is usually directed at symptoms. Ursodeoxycholic acid (UDCA), at a dose of 10–15 mg/kg/day is usually given to help mitigate the effects of the retention of potentially toxic hydrophobic bile acids, although there is no strong evidence for a mitigating effect on the progression of liver damage. Most cases do progress leading to retransplantation because of uncontrolled symptoms or the consequences of secondary biliary cirrhosis.

RECURRENT DISEASES

Liver transplantation is curative in many indications (**Table 41.3**), but some diseases will recur in the graft. While this may not necessarily affect graft function and survival, it is important to recognize and, where appropriate, consider altering immunosuppression and offer specific treatment.

Metabolic diseases treated by liver transplantation	
Cured	α_1-Antitrypsin deficiency Antithrombin III deficiency Protein S deficiency Protein C deficiency Wilson disease Hemophilia type A and B Tyrosinosis Byler disease Galactosemia Crigler-Najjar syndrome
Recurrent/persistent	Amyloid Congenital protoporphyria Cystic fibrosis Gaucher disease* Hemochromatosis Niemann-Pick disease* Sea blue histiocyte disease*
*Commonly contraindications for liver transplantation.	

Table 41.3 Metabolic diseases treated by liver transplantation.

Viral infections

Recurrent hepatitis viral infection is covered in greater detail in Chapter 42, but de novo infection may also occur (**Table 41.4**). Many programs routinely offer immunization with hepatitis A and B virus prior to transplantation.

Hepatitis A virus

Hepatitis A viral infection may rarely affect the graft but the clinical picture is one of a mild, transient hepatitis occurring shortly after transplantation and is of little significance. De novo hepatitis A infection in the graft runs a similar pattern to that seen in the person with a native liver.

Hepatitis B virus

The management of hepatitis B virus (HBV) infected patients before and after transplantation is covered elsewhere. Infection of the graft with HBV may occur:

- when viral replication has not been suppressed prior to transplantation;
- when a non-immune, not infected recipient is transplanted with a graft from a donor who is anti-HBc-positive (hepatitis B core) in the absence of prophylaxis; and
- when HBV prophylaxis is inadequate or ineffective e.g. insufficient duration of treatment, non-compliance, viral mutation resulting in drug resistance.

In general, those who are at risk of developing HBV infection of the graft should be offered treatment with hyperimmune B immunoglobulin (HBIg) and lamivudine. The optimal dose and duration of HBIg treatment is unknown. Lamivudine should be given at 100 mg/day. Occasionally, viral mutations will occur so that the virus is not longer controlled by lamivudine. Therefore, those grafted for HBV-associated liver disease should be monitored with routine liver tests every 3 months together with assessment of serum HBV markers, including HBV DNA. Increases in serum HBV DNA levels suggest the development of viral mutations (such as the YMDD mutation). In this situation, adefovir 10 mg/day can be added to the regimen. Occasionally, HBV is resistant to adefovir but is sensitive to lamivudine.

Those who are given a graft from a donor who is anti-HBc positive should also receive long-term lamivudine and be screened for the development of HBV infection of the graft.

Hepatitis C virus

Recurrent infection of the graft by hepatitis C virus (HCV) is almost invariable. The patterns of damage associated with HCV

Recurrent viral hepatitis disease			
	Hepatitis A virus	*Hepatitis B virus (HBV)*	*Hepatitis C virus*
Frequency	Uncertain	Dependent on level of HBV DNA pre-orthotopic liver transplantation	Almost invariable
Outcome	Little significance	Little, if replication treated	Graft disease
Treatment	None needed	Lamivudine Adefovir	Interferon and ribavirin
Effect of immunosuppression	None	None	Worse with high dose steroids

Table 41.4 Recurrent viral hepatitis disease.

Recurrent autoimmune liver disease			
	Primary biliary cirrhosis	*Primary sclerosing cholangitis*	*Autoimmune hepatitis*
Incidence at 10 years	50%	40%	Uncertain
Effect on graft survival*	+/−	++	++
Treatment	UDCA	UDCA	Steroids
Diagnosis	Liver histology	MRCP/PTC	Serology and liver histology
Risk factors	Unknown	?Intact colon	Unknown
*+/− little effect, ++ significant effect; MRCP, magnetic resonance cholangiography and pancreatography; PTC, percutaneous transhepatic cholangiography; UDCA, ursodeoxycholic acid.			

Table 41.5 Recurrent autoimmune liver disease.

recurrence varies from a mild inflammation to severe fibrosis and cirrhosis. As with HBV, a form of cholestatic hepatitis may develop. The role of treatment with peginterferon and ribavirin is effective in a small minority as the treatment is usually poorly tolerated. The risk factors associated with HCV recurrence and its effects are discussed in detail in Chapter 42.

Autoimmune diseases
Autoimmune diseases may recur after liver transplantation (**Table 41.5**). Recognition is important because this may have an impact on the graft survival so recipients need to be advised. Furthermore, recognition is important with respect to understanding the pathophysiology of disease, managing the patient with allograft dysfunction and possible modification of the treatment.

Primary biliary cirrhosis
Following liver transplantation for PBC, the antimitochondrial and antinuclear antibodies show a transient fall but within 1 year reach or exceed titers measured before transplantation. Conditions associated with PBC, such as thyroid disease or sclerodactyly, may also develop for the first time after liver transplantation.

The diagnosis of recurrent PBC is made on the basis of

- cholestatic liver tests in the absence of biliary obstruction,
- granulomatous destruction of the middle-sized intrahepatic bile ducts on liver histology (**Fig. 41.4**).

It is now established that PBC may develop in the graft, affecting up to 60% by 10 years. The diagnosis is made on histologic examination of the liver. Risk factors have not been established but recent evidence suggests that recurrence is more rapid and more severe in those maintained on tacrolimus compared to those on cyclosporin-based immunosuppression. There is no effective treatment but most centers use UDCA (10–15 mg/kg/day). The effect of disease recurrence in the graft appears to be of little clinical significance within the first 10 years, although cirrhosis requiring retransplantation may develop in less than 3% at this time.

Autoimmune hepatitis and de novo autoimmune hepatitis
The reported incidence and risk factors for recurrence of autoimmune hepatitis (AIH) is conflicting. This is due partly to

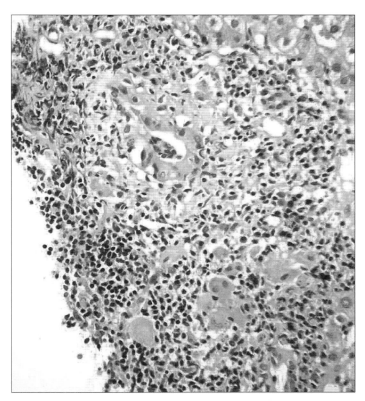

Figure 41.4 Liver biopsy showing recurrent primary biliary cirrhosis.

varying criteria for defining recurrent disease. Criteria for recurrent AIH include:

- hepatitic liver tests;
- elevated serum immunoglobulins;
- autoantibodies in significant titers;
- liver histology showing interface hepatitis (**Fig. 41.5**); and
- exclusion of other causes of graft dysfunction.

The likelihood of recurrent AIH is probably less than 30%. There is no consensus about risk factors or the response to corticosteroids. Many studies suggest that the majority of cases respond satisfactorily to increased doses of corticosteroids. However, there are other reports of progression to graft failure

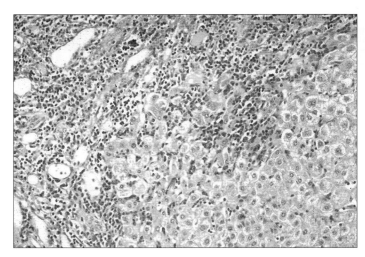

Figure 41.5 Liver biopsy showing recurrent autoimmune hepatitis.

despite additional immunosuppression. Because of the risk of recurrent disease, most centers advocate the continued use of a small dose of corticosteroids (such as prednisolone 5–10 mg/day) for at least 1 year and often longer term.

De novo autoimmune hepatitis

There have been several reports of a clinical and histologic appearance of AIH developing in patients transplanted for conditions other than AIH. This is more likely to occur in children but is seen in adults. Whether this represents a true 'autoimmune disease' or is a response to graft antigens (and therefore should be considered as a form of rejection) is unclear. The term 'graft dysfunction mimicking autoimmune hepatitis', while more cumbersome, is more accurate. Treatment is with increased immunosuppression and, where appropriate, introduction of corticosteroids, but this is not always effective in preventing progression of liver damage. Some patients develop graft cirrhosis and require regrafting.

Primary sclerosing cholangitis

The diagnosis of recurrent PSC in the graft may be difficult to substantiate as there are many causes for non-anastomotic strictures in the graft but the following criteria should be used:

- multiple non-anastomotic strictures;
- no severe reperfusion injury;
- no evidence of biliary tree ischemia;
- ABO identical graft; and
- no biliary obstruction.

Recurrent PSC presents with signs and symptoms of cholestasis. Liver ultrasound is usually normal but multiple intrahepatic strictures may be shown by PTC or MRCP (**Fig. 41.6**). ERCP is usually not technically possible since most, if not all, liver allografts recipients will have a Roux loop. Sometimes, the histologic features of PSC may be seen in the allograft (ductopenia, pericentral fibrosis).

Treatment is symptomatic. UDCA is usually offered but there is no evidence yet that this will affect the rate or severity of progression. Recurrent PSC is seen in about 40% by 10 years. Risk factors are unknown although it has been suggested that

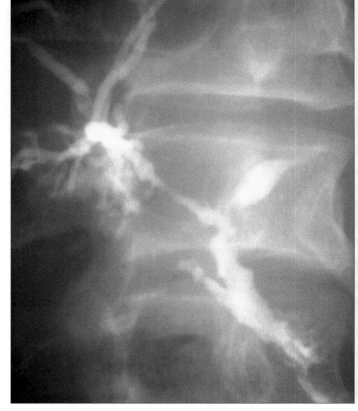

Figure 41.6 Recurrent primary sclerosing cholangitis.

those with a colectomy done before or during transplantation may be protected from recurrent disease.

Metabolic diseases

Transplantation will cure those metabolic diseases where the defect arises within the liver (such as protein C deficiency or Wilson disease) (Table 41.3). Where the defect arises mainly, or solely, outside the liver, transplantation will not be curative and the recipient must be screened, and where appropriate, treated.

Hemochromatosis

It is believed that the main defect in hemochromatosis lies in the gastrointestinal tract so that the liver graft may be at risk of accumulation of iron. It is recommended that the recipient be screened with serial estimation of iron, iron bonding capacity and ferritin.

Non-alcohol fatty liver disease

Non-alcohol fatty liver disease (NAFLD) may recur, or develop de novo in the allograft. The recipient should be advised to maintain ideal body weight and control diabetes (see below). Risk factors are as for fatty liver in the native liver, such as alcohol, obesity, diabetes and small bowel bypass surgery.

Malignancy

Refining the indications for transplantation for those with hepatic malignancy has meant that persisting disease (usually termed recurrent) is less likely. Rarely, malignancy in the donor may be transmitted to the recipient.

Hepatocellular carcinoma

Recurrent hepatocellular carcinoma (HCC) is usually apparent within the first 2 years but can present up to 10 years after transplantation. The tumor may arise in the graft, abdomen, chest or bones. The diagnosis may also be made on the basis of reappearance of raised α-fetoprotein levels in serum. Few centers routinely screen recipients for evidence of recurrence as there is currently no effective therapy available, except for the occasional case with isolated resectable lesions e.g. in the adrenal bed. The choice of immunosuppression may affect the rate of recurrence. While there is limited data in humans apart from retrospective analysis, it has been suggested that cyclosporin may be associated with more rapid tumor cell division, while, conversely, rapamycin may retard progression by inhibiting tumor angioneogenesis.

Cholangiocarcinoma

Few patients with cholangiocarcinoma are candidates for transplantation because of the high rates of recurrence as the tumor spreads early through the lymphatic system and nerves. The use of chemotherapy and brachytherapy may allow a selected group of patients to undergo transplantation but the risk of recurrence persists for at least 3–5 years after transplantation. There is no current effective treatment for recurrent cholangiocarcinoma.

Budd-Chiari syndrome

There are many factors that may underlie thrombosis of the hepatic veins. About 30–50% are associated with a myeloproliferative disorder and in these patients the risk of further thrombosis remains after transplantation. In other cases, the cause of the prothrombotic tendency is known and is considered to be corrected by liver transplantation (such as protein C deficiency), but nevertheless recipients are currently also routinely considered for long-term anticoagulation. Anticoagulation is commenced immediately after liver transplantation unless contraindicated by catastrophic bleeding. The diagnosis of recurrent hepatic venous outflow obstruction will present with right upper abdominal pain and the onset of ascites. The diagnosis is confirmed by demonstrating thrombosis of the hepatic veins. Stenting or local thrombolysis can be effective but regrafting may be required.

A Budd-Chiari-like syndrome can develop in patients transplanted for other indications in whom the cava is preserved and the hepatic veins are anastomosed using the 'piggy-back' technique. This presents with ascites, usually in the weeks immediately after liver transplantation. This phenomenon may be triggered by a separate cause of graft dysfunction if it causes swelling of the liver and distortion of the angles of drainage of the hepatic veins.

Sarcoidosis

Sarcoidosis may recur with florid granulomatous infiltration in the graft but it usually responds rapidly to increased corticosteroid therapy.

Alcoholic liver disease

The proportion of patients grafted for alcoholic liver disease who return to alcohol consumption varies greatly in reported series, in part because of the definition of recidivism. Less than 20% return to a pattern of drinking that is potentially harmful (more than 200 g/week) and fewer than 5% develop problems with graft damage or non-compliance, as a consequence of alcohol consumption.

All persons grafted for alcoholic liver disease should be counseled to avoid alcohol altogether since it is not possible to identify those who are able to return to a safe pattern of drinking. When relapse does occur, the patient should be counseled and offered help to abstain. Screening with markers such as carbohydrate-deficient transferrin or γ-glutamyltransferase levels, is not routinely done.

CONSEQUENCES OF IMMUNOSUPPRESSION

Lifelong immunosuppression is required for most liver allograft recipients. A small proportion of patients can stop immunosuppression with continued good graft function. A small number of transplant programs are currently attempting withdrawal of immunosuppression but this should not be attempted outside these experimental protocols and only after full and informed consent has been obtained from the patient. There are no accurate markers for the prospective identification of clinical tolerance. The advent of newer immunosuppressive regimens (such as those using Campath-1H) may be more effective in inducing tolerance and so permit either less intense immunosuppression or total withdrawal.

Consideration for withdrawal of immunosuppression should be confined to patients who:

- are 3 or more years post transplant;
- have stable and normal liver function; and
- have normal liver biopsies.

Those grafted for autoimmune diseases, such as PBC, PSC or AIH, are less likely to be withdrawn successfully. Immunosuppression should be withdrawn slowly and, any change in liver tests must indicate an increase in immunosuppression.

Immunosuppression is associated with toxicity and, as with any medication, the benefits must be balanced against the side-effects of treatment. Side-effects are either class related (such as increased risk of infection and malignancy) or drug-specific (for example, corticosteroid-associated osteoporosis). The introduction into clinical practice of newer immunosuppressive drugs allows the clinician to tailor the drugs used to the patient. Increasingly, immunosuppressive regimens are being changed over time. Immunosuppression, including choice of drug regimens and specific side-effects, are discussed in detail in Chapter 39.

GENERAL HEALTH ISSUES

Liver allograft recipients should be encouraged to return to a normal life but will need to be aware of the possible increased risks associated with a transplant and the consequences.

Medical problems
Cardiovascular risks

Most, but not all, studies have suggested that liver allograft recipients have a two- to threefold increased risk of cardiovascular morbidity and mortality. The reasons for this increased risk are multifactorial and include:

- weight gain and obesity post-transplantation;
- hypertension;

- hyperlipidemia;
- diabetes mellitus; and
- renal impairment.

Some of these risk factors may be affected by the immuno-suppression regimen. It is therefore important that regular assessment is made of these risk factors and recipients are counseled and treated appropriately.

Hypertension

The majority of liver allograft recipients are not hypertensive prior to transplantation, partly because of the vasodilatation that is characteristic of advanced cirrhosis. Significant hypertension develops in up to 70% of patients post-transplant. The etiology is multifactorial and is likely to be a consequence, in part, of the effects of the drugs, especially the calcineurin inhibitors and corticosteroids, and renal impairment. Important features of hypertension occurring in the liver allograft recipient include the loss of the nocturnal fall in blood pressure seen in non-grafted persons, and increased systemic vascular resistance.

Blood pressure is usually assessed at each clinic visit but it is well established that these readings correlate poorly with the patients' mean blood pressure readings. A high reading at a clinic should be followed by a series of readings in the community to get a better evaluation of the problem. Twenty-four hour blood pressure profiles are the best way of evaluating patients. Confirmed hypertension should be actively treated. The ideal target blood pressure is not clear in this situation but it seems reasonable to aim for a maximum systolic blood pressure of 140 mmHg and diastolic of 80 mmHg, and with more stringent control in patients with diabetes mellitus and renal impairment.

Drug therapy is usually required and most agents can be used in association with the typical immunosuppressive regimens. However, diuretics tend not to be very effective in this situation. First line therapy is often with a calcium channel blocker, despite a high incidence of dependent edema. Angiotensin-converting enzyme (ACE) inhibitors may be less effective in patients with a high systemic vascular resistance, but their action on the effect of the calcineurin inhibitors on renal blood flow can result in effective blood pressure control. For those who develop troublesome side-effects from ACE inhibitors, angiotensin II receptor antagonists can be used with good effect.

The threshold for treatment should be lowered in those with associated renal disease or proteinuria. In these patients, caution must be exercised with ACE inhibitors because of the potential for precipitating renal failure (**Table 41.6**). ACE inhibitors are the treatment of choice in patients with type I diabetes. Outside the context of liver transplantation, thiazides, β blockers, ACE inhibitors and the dihydropyridine class of calcium channel antagonists have been shown to be of benefit in slowing the progression of renal damage in patients with type 2 diabetes. However, this benefit has not been confirmed in a similar population of liver graft recipients. Caution must be observed with the use of antihypertensive drugs because of potential side-effects and drug interactions (see Table 41.6).

Hyperlipidemia

Hyperlipidemia is common after liver transplantation, as with other organ transplantations. The major risk factors include immunosuppressive drugs (especially sirolimus and cortico-steroids), coexisting renal damage, diabetes and obesity.

Treatment should be as for those without liver transplantation:

- general measures like avoidance of smoking and excessive alcohol consumption, increase in physical activity;
- pharmacologic treatments, e.g. the use of statins, should be considered in those with significant hyperlipidemia.

'Statins' should be used with caution in the liver allograft recipient because of possible drug interactions. There is an increased risk of rhabdomyolysis when combining a 'statin'

Drug treatment for hypertension in the liver allograft recipient	
β blockers	
Mode of action:	Reduce cardiac output Block peripheral adrenoreceptors Some depress plasma renin
Contraindications:	Asthma Uncontrolled heart failure
Side-effects:	Bronchospasm Bradycardia Peripheral vasoconstriction Fatigue Sleep disturbance
Interactions with immunosuppression:	None major Carvedilol may increase calcineurin inhibitor level
Angiotensin-converting enzyme inhibitors	
Mode of action:	Inhibits conversion of angiotensin I to angiotensin II
Contraindications:	Angioedema Reno-vascular disease
Side-effects:	Profound hypotension Renal impairment Persistent cough Gastrointestinal upset Blood dyscrasia Rarely hepatotoxicity
Interactions with immunosuppression:	Increased risk of hyperkalemia
Calcium channel blockers	
Mode of action:	Interfere with inward displacement of calcium ions through the slow channels of cell membranes
Contra-indications:	Pregnancy Unstable angina Severe left heart failure
Side-effects:	Flushing Headaches Gum hypertrophy
Interactions with immunosuppression:	Some may increase calcineurin inhibitor levels

Table 41.6 Drug treatment for hypertension in the liver allograft recipient.
Note: the list of drugs, side-effects and contraindications is not comprehensive

[3-hydroxy-3-methylglutaryl coenzyme A (HMGCoA) reductase inhibitors) with cyclosporin, nicotinic acid and a fibrate (especially gemfibrozil) so these combinations should be used only after full counseling and the introduction of suitable patient monitoring. Fenofibrate in combination with cyclosporin may increase the risk of renal toxicity.

Gout

Hyperuricemia is seen commonly after transplantation but actual gout is rare. The causes of hyperuricemia include renal impairment and the action of the calcineurin inhibitors on renal urate handling. Treatment of the acute attack of gout is a challenge since the non-steroidal anti-inflammatory drugs (NSAIDs) may precipitate renal failure in those taking calcineurin inhibitors, so colchicine is preferable. Colchicine may cause diarrhea, so drug doses need to be closely monitored. Preventative treatment is required when there are frequent, recurrent attacks, the presence of gouty tophi or signs of gouty arthritis. Treatment with allopurinol is contraindicated in those also taking azathioprine because of the high risk of neutropenia. Probenecid (note interaction with captopril) and sulfinpyrazone may be used.

Diabetes mellitus

New onset diabetes mellitus develops in about 15% of liver allograft recipients. The risk factors include the use of calcineurin inhibitors (especially tacrolimus), corticosteroids and concomitant HCV infection. Treatment is as for the diabetic with a native liver. Oral hypoglycemic agents of all classes are safe and effective although many patients will require insulin treatment.

Renal disease

There are many causes for renal impairment in the allograft recipient, and these include:

- calcineurin inhibitor toxicity;
- diabetic renal disease;
- hypertension;
- immunoglobulin A (IgA) nephropathy;
- HCV-associated glomerulonephritis;
- other pre-existing renal disease; and
- drug toxicity.

Calcineurin inhibitor toxicity remains the single greatest cause of renal failure in the liver allograft recipient. A retrospective analysis from the USA analyzed the probability of renal failure in just under 70 000 non-renal allograft recipients and found that during a median follow-up of 36 months, 16% developed end-stage renal disease (defined as a glomerular filtration rate of less than 29 mL/min/1.73 m^2 of body surface area). The risk factors for renal failure are shown in **Table 41.7**. Just under one-third of these patients required renal support or renal transplantation. The onset of renal failure was associated with a 4.5-fold increased risk of death. Several studies have shown that the risk of late renal failure is determined within the first postoperative year and levels and doses of calcineurin inhibitor are strong predictors of later renal failure. There does not appear to be a significant difference between cyclosporin and tacrolimus with respect to the incidence or severity of calcineurin inhibitor associated nephrotoxicity.

The probability of renal impairment and renal failure increases with time, so renal function should be regularly monitored. Simple measurement of serum creatinine and urea may be misleading and formal measurement of creatinine clearance is often impractical. The use of calculated measures of creatinine clearance (such as the Cockcroft-Gault formula) is less accurate but easier to perform. The mechanism of calcineurin inhibitor nephrotoxicity is not well understood but probably relates, at least in part, to renal ischemia. Kidney histology is not specific but shows interstitial fibrosis, tubular atrophy and vascular sclerosis.

The strategy for the prevention of renal failure is based on a combination of factors, including:

- avoidance of precipitating factors – avoid high levels of calcineurin inhibitor, especially during the first year, avoid concomitant use of drugs such as NSAIDs;
- treatment of exacerbating risk factors – aggressive treatment of hypertension and diabetes;
- early cessation of calcineurin inhibitors; and
- reduction of calcineurin inhibitor in combination with other agents, such as mycophenolate or rapamycin/sirolimus.

The level of creatinine clearance at which calcineurin inhibitor should be reduced or discontinued is not clear. Many programs are considering modification of calcineurin inhibitor regimens with creatinine clearance thresholds of 60–70 mL/min. Depending on the clinical situation, calcineurin inhibitor is either reduced or withdrawn. Many patients retain excellent graft function despite 'suboptimal' immunosuppression, probably reflecting tolerance or near-tolerance of the graft. These patients may get a satisfactory improvement in renal function with a reduction in cyclosporin levels <50 ng/mL or tacrolimus <3 ng/mL. In other patients, a similar outcome is achieved with additional immunosuppression from mycophenolate or sirolimus. When complete withdrawal of calcineurin inhibitors is contemplated, recipients are started on a combination of prednisolone (7.5–10 mg/day) and mycophenolate or sirolimus. Once the patients are stabilized on the new medications, the calcineurin inhibitor is gradually withdrawn completely. Renal function improves or stabilizes in about 70% of patients with these alterations to the immunosuppressive regimens.

Although some recipients can be maintained on monotherapy with mycophenolate, there is a risk of developing acute and chronic rejection and this approach is not recommended. The addition of a low dose of corticosteroids appears to reduce the risk of graft-threatening rejection.

Risk factors for the development of renal failure in non-renal allograft recipients	
Post-operative renal failure	2.13
Diabetes mellitus	1.42
Increasing age (per 10-year increment)	1.36
Hepatitis C virus infection	1.15
Hypertension	1.18
Female gender	0.744
Reproduced from Ojo et al (03) by permission of New Engl J Med.	

Table 41.7 Risk factors for the development of renal failure in non-renal allograft recipients.

Bone disease

Osteopenia is seen fairly commonly after liver transplantation and identified risk factors include pre-existing osteopenia, prolonged bed-rest, poor diet and use of corticosteroids. Management is aimed at prevention, early detection and intervention. Prevention should start during the management of chronic liver disease and continue after transplantation with early mobilization, curtailment of long-term use of corticosteroids, encouragement of active weight-bearing exercise, a diet adequate in calcium and vitamin D, avoidance of smoking and excess alcohol. There is no consensus as yet for the use of routine DEXA (dual energy X-ray absorptiometry) screening of the liver allograft recipient to screen for osteopenia. There should be a low threshold for the use of DEXA screening in those who are female and post-menopausal, with a family history of osteopenia or a history of non-traumatic fracture. Interventional studies are few but there is now some preliminary evidence that risedronate is effective in reversing the osteoporosis in liver transplant recipients. Spontaneous improvement in bone density has also been observed at 12–18 months after liver transplantation in patients with pre-existing chronic cholestatic disease.

Bowel disease

Patients with PSC and other cholestatic diseases have an increased risk of colitis. Following transplantation, the natural history of the colitis may change. In about one-third, the colitis will improve, in about one-third the colitis will remain unaltered and in the remainder, the colitis will deteriorate, requiring either increased treatment or even colectomy. In the liver allograft recipient with good liver function, colectomy is a safe procedure and is indicated in those with severe, recurrent flare-ups, severe dysplasia or malignancy. As indicated above, there is an increased risk of colon cancer in these patients. These cancers are often in the ascending colon.

Although there is no common consensus, it has been suggested that all patients with active colitis receive long-term treatment with UDCA as this has been shown in the non-transplant setting to be associated with a reduction in the rate of formation of colonic polyps and of colonic cancers. We also recommend annual colonoscopy, with multiple biopsies of the entire colon.

Neurologic problems

Most neurologic problems present in the first few weeks after transplantation but may be problematic in the long-term survivor. Neurologic problems may be seen as:

- cognitive problems;
- mood disorders e.g. anxiety or depression;
- tremor;
- headaches and migraine;
- dementia; and
- seizures.

In the liver allograft recipient, headaches are not uncommon and may be associated with calcineurin inhibitor use. There is also a risk of migraine, especially in those with a history prior to transplantation. Treatment is as for migraine in the non-transplant recipient e.g. with analgesia, propranolol, or proprietary drug combinations marketed for the treatment of migraine. In severe cases, it may be necessary to switch from calcineurin inhibitors to alternative immunosuppressive agents.

Some neurologic problems may be associated with co-morbid conditions, such as a peripheral neuropathy associated with alcohol excess or diabetes, cerebrovascular disease which may be related to age and exacerbated by drug treatment, and rarely progressive multifocal leukoencephalopathy. When neurologic changes develop, drug effects should be considered and treatment amended. Investigation, including magnetic resonance imaging (MRI) examination, is not often helpful except for when it demonstrates structural problems such as abscess, large or small infarcts or metastatic deposits.

GENERAL HEALTH AND LIFESTYLE ISSUES

Quality of life post-transplant

Although the quality of life following liver transplantation is usually very good, it cannot be considered normal. The physical and psychologic sequelae are discussed below.

Weight gain and obesity

Weight gain occurs in up to 70%. There are many factors responsible for the weight gain, including the use of corticosteroids, the loss of anorexia associated with liver failure, liberation from dietary restrictions and better absorption and utilization of foods. There is also evidence of a reduction in the basal metabolic rate after liver transplantation. Weight gain is greatest in the first post-transplant year and in those who were overweight prior to the onset of liver disease. The obesity may cause fatty liver disease in the allograft and may even lead to cirrhosis. Liver allograft recipients should be counseled about sensible eating habits and lifestyle activity. Weight should be monitored and dietary advice given early.

Skin and dental problems

Many liver allograft recipients have poor dentition as a consequence of their previous liver disease. Dental work may carry a risk of bacteremia. There is no consensus about the need for antibiotic prophylaxis in the liver allograft recipient. If antibiotic therapy is indicated, then care must be taken to ensure there is no interaction with the immunosuppression.

Gum hypertrophy is sometimes seen and may be associated with the use of cyclosporin and with nifedipine. Treatment is of the hypertrophy itself and consideration should be given to switching from cyclosporin to another regimen.

Hirsutism is seen in some of those on cyclosporin treatment and may be distressing to women. Sometimes the hirsutism will resolve after 6 months. If not, treatment is either with topical treatments or by switching to an alternative treatment regimen. Hair loss may occur either as a result of the trauma of the surgery or from the use of immunosuppressive treatment, especially azathioprine.

As discussed above, skin cancers are seen in those on immunosuppression. Any suspicious skin lesion should be biopsied and treatment given accordingly. Basal cell carcinoma is the commonest skin malignancy but squamous cell carcinoma, melanoma and Kaposi sarcoma all occur with higher frequency than in the general population.

Sexual health and reproduction

The number of liver allograft recipients who become pregnant is still relatively low but clear trends are emerging. There is a return to normal menstrual pattern with the return of good liver

CHAPTER 42

Recurrent Viral Hepatitis in Liver Transplant Recipients

Scott W. Biggins and Norah A. Terrault

INTRODUCTION

The majority of liver transplants performed worldwide are for complications of chronic viral hepatitis. Medical and surgical advances over the last two decades have made long-term survival after liver transplant a reality. However, recurrent disease due to viruses accounts for a significant proportion of the cost, morbidity and mortality post-transplantation, and the prevention and treatment of recurrent viral hepatitis is one of the most critical areas for improvement in liver transplant outcomes.

Hepatotropic viruses resulting in recurrent infection following liver transplantation are listed in **Table 42.1**. In terms of magnitude, hepatitis B virus (HBV), hepatitis C virus (HCV) and cytomegalovirus (CMV) account for the vast majority of infections and are the main contributors to post-transplant morbidity and graft loss. Less frequently, herpes simplex virus (HSV), herpes

zoster virus (HZV), Epstein-Barr virus (EBV), can recur. In this latter group, EBV infection is most serious, resulting in post-transplant lymphoproliferative disease (PTLD). Uncommon causes of recurrent viral infection manifesting as hepatitis include adenovirus, human herpesvirus-6 (HHV-6) and HHV-7.

In the USA, chronic HBV infection accounts for 8% of liver transplants performed. Initial results were poor, with 5-year survival rates of 50% in the early 1990s. The advent of effective prophylactic therapies to prevent recurrent HBV infection led to significant improvements in outcome and current survival rates at 5 years are 80% or greater. The importance of preventing recurrent infection to ensure prolonged graft survival is highlighted by the HBV experience. HCV is the most common indication for liver transplantation in the USA and Europe accounting for up to 50% of transplants in some programs. Unlike HBV, there are presently no effective prophylactic

Recurrent hepatotropic viruses in liver transplant recipients			
Virus	Prevalence %[a] US LT 2003	% Recurrent disease	References
HBV	2.6 5–10	2.7–10 (with combination HBIg/antiviral prophylaxis)[c]	UNOS[b] Roche[c]
HCV	26.4	100	UNOS[b]
HDV	NA, <0.1[b]	80 (if HBV recurrence)[d]	Samuel[d]
CMV	7.9[b] (IgG+) 27[a] 60[a]	4.8[d] (all) with Rx 18[d] (all) without Rx 14.8[d] (D+R-) with Rx 44[d] (D+R-) without Rx 0.7[e] (D+R+) with Rx 5.2[e] (D+R-) with Rx	Burak[a] Gane[f] Seehofer[e]
EBV	54[b] (IgG+), 4.2[b] (DNA+) 58 (DNA+)	NA (adults) 69 (peds)	Barkholt[g] Krieger[h]
HSV	35[i]	1 (liver), 53 (oral)[i]	Singh[i]
VZV	7[i]	3 (1 year)[i], 14 (5 years)[j]	Singh[i] Herrero[j]
Adenovirus	5.8[k]	3.6[k]	McGrath[k]
HHV-6, -7	14–82[l]	1–6.7[l]	Razonable[l]

HBIg, hepatitis B immunoglobulin; HBV, hepatitis B virus; HCV, hepatitis C virus; HDV, hepatitis D virus; CMV, cytomegalovirus; EBV, Epstein-Barr virus; HSV, herpes simplex virus; VZV, varicella-zoster virus; HHV-6, -7, human herpes virus-6 and -7; LT, liver transplantation; Rx, prophylactic treatment; D/R, donor CMV antibody and recipient CMV antibody status
[a]Burak et al (02); [b]Based on OPTN data as of January 1, 2004; [c]Roche & Samuel (04); [d]Samuel et al (97); [e]Seehofer et al (02); [f]Gane et al (97); [g]Barkholt et al (96); [h]Krieger et al (00); [i]Singh et al (88); [j]Herrero et al (04); [k]McGrath et al (98); [l]Razonable & Paya (02).

Table 42.1 Recurrent hepatotropic viruses in liver transplant recipients.

Therapeutic strategies used in the management of recurrent viral infections		
Timing/Type	*Definition*	*Examples*
Pretransplant	Initiated before transplantation and continued for variable periods post-transplantation with the goal to prevent recurrent infection	ADV or LAM for HBV decompensated cirrhosis LADR protocol of interferon α2b plus ribavirin for HCV cirrhosis
Prophylactic	Initiated at the time of transplantation and continued for variable periods post-transplantation with the goal of preventing recurrent infection	HBIg begun in anhepatic phase of transplant for HBV; Ganciclovir for CMV negative recipient of CMV positive donor liver
Pre-emptive	Initiated early in the post transplant period, typically within the first 4 weeks following transplantation, and before biochemical and histological disease is manifest	PEG-IFN and RBV after transplant for HCV with normal ALT without biopsy
Recurrent disease	Initiated after biochemical and histological evidence of recurrent disease	PEG-IFN and RBV for HCV with elevated ALT and stage ≥2 fibrosis on biopsy ADV for HBV recurrence with elevated ALT and progressive histology Ganciclovir for CMV hepatitis after transplant
ADV, adefovir; CMV, cytomegalovirus; HBIg, hepatitis B immunoglobulin; HBV, hepatitis B virus; HCV, hepatitis C virus; IFN, interferon; LADR, low accelerating dose regimen; LAM, lamivudine; PEG-IFN, pegylated IFN; RBV, ribavirin.		

Table 42.2 Therapeutic strategies used in the management of recurrent viral infections.

therapies to prevent graft reinfection. Recurrent infection is universal in those with viremia pretransplantation, and progressive histologic disease leading to cirrhosis occurs in up to 30% within 5–10 years of transplantation.

Therapeutic approaches for the management of viral hepatitis in the setting of transplantation generally fall in one of several categories (**Table 42.2**). Pretransplant therapies include those focused on achieving viral eradication prior to transplantation and are most applicable to HBV and HCV. Prophylactic therapies are given from the time of transplantation for defined risk periods or indefinitely. Prophylactic approaches have been used successfully to prevent recurrent HBV and CMV infections. Pre-emptive therapies are used when recurrent viral infection has occurred but before liver disease is manifest. This strategy has been used in the management of HCV-infected patients. Finally, for those with established recurrent infection and evidence of graft or other organ injury, antiviral therapies have been used to eradicate infection and control disease progression.

HEPATITIS B VIRUS

Successful treatment advances in the last decade have significantly improved outcomes of liver transplantation for HBV. The early experience of liver transplantation for HBV was vexed by recurrent HBV infection in the majority of patients with often aggressive disease leading to high rates of graft loss. Hepatitis B immunoglobulin (HBIg) given perioperatively and for prolonged periods post-transplantation, markedly reduced HBV recurrence with 5-year survival rates increasing from 50 to 75%. Nucleoside/nucleotide agents including lamivudine, tenofovir and adefovir dipivoxil, given pre- or post-transplantation have further contributed to improvements in graft and patient survival (**Fig. 42.1**). Current graft survival rates for patients with HBV are comparable or superior to other indications for transplantation.

Diagnosis and pathology of recurrent HBV

Recurrence of HBV is defined typically by the reappearance of HBsAg in the serum and is associated with variable levels of HBV DNA in serum and liver. The reappearance of these serologic and virologic markers is accompanied by clinical evidence of hepatitis with elevation of serum aminotransferase levels and acute or chronic hepatitis on liver biopsy (**Fig. 42.2a**). Immunohistochemical staining for hepatitis B surface (HBs) antigen (HBsAg) and hepatitis B core (HBc) antigen (HBcAg) are positive in those with histologic evidence of recurrent HBV and active replication (**Fig. 42.2b**). In most patients the histologic features are the same as those found in non-transplant patients. Early changes are those of acute hepatitis with a predominance of lobular necroinflammation evolving to portal-based disease with variable degrees of hepatocyte necrosis, mononuclear inflammation and fibrosis. The remarkable features of post-transplant HBV infection are the more rapid rate of fibrosis progression, with evolution to cirrhosis occurring in as short a period as 2 years. In approximately 5% of transplanted patients with recurrent HBV, a variant form of hepatitis, called fibrosing cholestatic hepatitis or FCH, develops. FCH is a hyperaggressive form of HBV infection unique to the transplant setting. The variant is associated with very high levels of HBV DNA in serum and high expression of HBsAg and HBcAg in hepatocytes, together with cholestasis, ballooned hepatocytes and a paucity of inflammatory cells (**Fig. 42.2c**). These findings suggest a direct cytopathic injury to hepatocytes by HBV.

Natural history of recurrent HBV after liver transplantation

Without prophylactic therapy, HBV recurrence occurs in 80–100% which, without treatment, leads to cirrhosis and graft loss within 5 years in 50% of patients. Predictors of a more favorable outcome after transplant are hepatitis D virus co-infection, fulminant hepatic failure, absence of HBeAg and low levels of HBV DNA

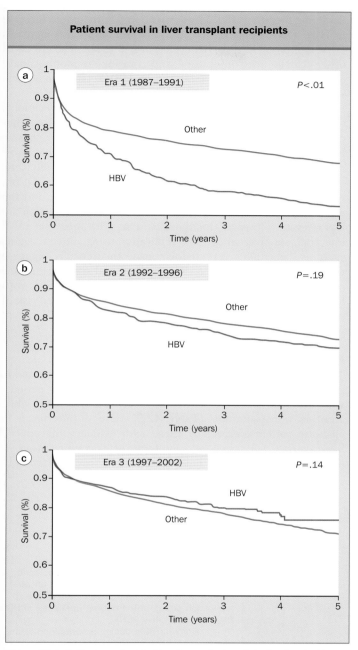

Figure 42.1 Patient survival in liver transplant recipients. Survival in transplant recipients with HBV versus other diagnoses. A progressive improvement in survival is seen in patients transplanted for chronic HBV in the past 15+ years. While patient survival was significantly lower in HBV patients versus other diagnoses in era 1, these differences are not apparent in subsequent cohorts. The improvement in survival coincides with improvements in therapies to prevent and treat HBV infection. (a) Era 1 (1987–1991), (b) era 2 (1992–1996), and (c) era 3 (1997–2002). Reproduced from Kim et al (04) by permission of Wiley-Liss, Inc.

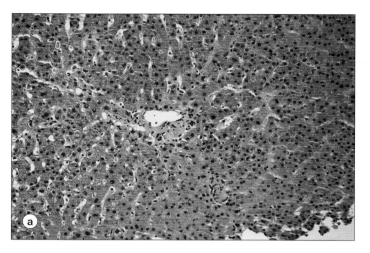

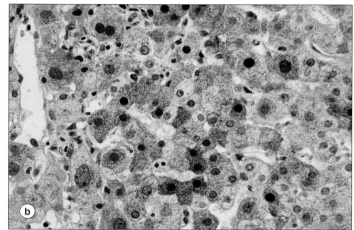

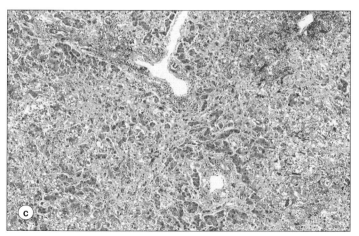

Figure 42.2 Histologic features of recurrent HBV infection after liver transplantation. (a) Recurrent HBV, chronic hepatitis; (b) Immunohistochemical stains for HBcAg and HBsAg in acute recurrent HBV; (c) recurrent HBV, fibrosing cholestatic variant. (Courtesy of Dr Linda Ferrell, University of California San Francisco.)

before transplantation (**Fig. 42.3**). For those who develop FCH, the mortality rate is essentially 100% in the absence of antiviral 'rescue therapy'. With current therapies to prevent and treat recurrent HBV infection, survival rates are currently 85% overall. The treatment approaches utilized prior to and following liver transplantation to prevent and treat HBV infection are detailed in **Figure 42.4** and discussed below.

The natural history of HBV after transplantation is accelerated, presumably in large part, due to the effects of immunosuppressive therapy. In the absence of prophylaxis therapies to prevent HBV recurrence, HBV DNA levels increase after transplantation. There is a corticosteroid responsive element on the hepatitis B core protein which upregulates HBV replication. Lymphocyte-

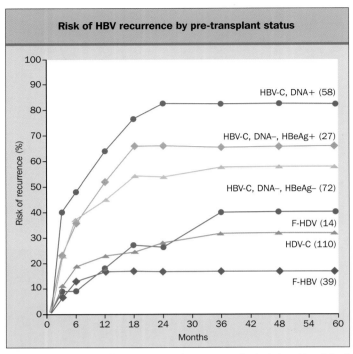

Figure 42.3 Risk of HBV recurrence by pretransplant status. The risk of HBV recurrence, defined by presence of HBsAg in serum, is highest among those with indices of active viral replication pretransplantation (HBeAg-positive and HBV DNA-positive by hybridization assay) and lowest in patients with low levels of HBV DNA pretransplantation, including those with fulminant hepatitis and hepatitis D co-infection. Reproduced from Samuel et al (93) by permission of the Massachusetts Medical Society. F-HDV, fulminant HDV; HDV-C, HDV cirrhosis; F-HBV, fulminant HBV; HBV-C, HBV cirrhosis.

depleting therapy (OKT-3) was associated with a rapid increase in HBV DNA levels in one study. Azathioprine also increases HBV replication in vitro, but cyclosporin does not. The effects of other calcineurin inhibitors and inosine monophosphate dehydrogenase (IMPDH) inhibitors on HBV replication are less well characterized.

Acute rejection is less common in liver transplant recipients with chronic HBV compared to those transplanted for other causes of cirrhosis. The immunosuppressive effects of chronic HBV infection are cited as the probable reason for this lower rate of rejection. With the widespread use of prophylactic therapies to prevent HBV recurrent post-transplantation, recurrent HBV infection is now an uncommon event, and the effects of chronic HBV infection on risk of acute rejection are less relevant. However, for those patients with recurrent HBV infection, suppression of HBV replication using antiviral agents such as lamivudine or adefovir may theoretically increase the risk for acute rejection. Recovery of viral-specific immune responses has been documented in patients treated with lamivudine therapy. While a consideration, an enhanced risk of rejection in liver transplant recipients with recurrent HBV disease on treatment with antivirals has not been reported.

Pretransplant management of HBV

The antiviral drugs lamivudine and adefovir are well tolerated in patients with decompensated liver disease allowing patients with advanced disease to be treated safely and effectively while awaiting transplantation (**Table 42.3**). Use of interferon in cirrhotic patients, especially those with evidence of reduced liver synthetic function or symptoms of decompensation, is limited by cytopenias, a heightened risk of bacterial compli-

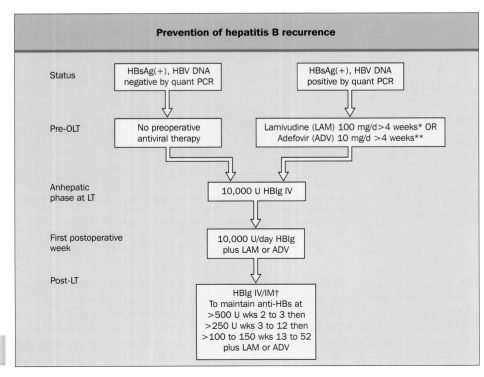

Figure 42.4 Prevention of hepatitis B recurrence. Most transplant programs use a combination of HBIg and nucleoside/nucleotide analogs as prophylaxis. The duration of antiviral therapy pretransplantation is dictated by the replication status of the patient (presence of HBV DNA by quantitative PCR).
†Post-transplant HBIg dosing is variable in terms of dose and duration. The doses presented here represent a more conservative approach of indefinite combination therapy. However, lower doses of HBIg and discontinuation of HBIg with or without vaccination, plus continued nucleoside/nucleotide analog therapy have been used with some success.
*Patients with lamivudine resistance require treatment with adefovir.
**Patients with adefovir resistance require treatment with lamivudine.

Treatment options in patients with decompensated cirrhosis awaiting liver transplantation			
	Lamivudine	*Adefovir*	*Entecavir*
Current status	FDA-approved for HBV	FDA-approved for HBV	FDA-approved for HBV
Dose (q.d.)	100 mg	10 mg	0.5 mg 1.0 mg lamivudine-resistant
Route of administration	oral	oral	oral
Duration of treatment	12 months + (HBeAg+) 12 months ++ (HBeAg–)	12 months + (HBeAg+) 12 months ++ (HBeAg–)	12 months + (HBeAg+) 12 months ++ (HBeAg–)
HBeAg seroconversion	16% at 1 year 27% at 2 years 40% at 3 years	12% at 1 year	21% at 1 year
HBsAg loss	0% at 1 year	0% at 1 year	0% at 1 year
Histological improvement	55% at 1 year	53–64% at 1 year	55–72% at 1 year
Side-effects	Elevated amylase, CK but pancreatitis rare	Renal toxicity with higher doses	Rare
Frequency of contraindications	± Dose adjustment for renal insufficiency	± Dose adjustment for renal insufficiency	± Dose adjustment for renal insufficiency
Risk of drug resistance	20% at 1 year 70% at 5 years	~2–3% at 2 years	0% at 1 year if wild-type HBV 7% at 1 year lamivudine-resistant
Cost[†]	Moderate ($7 per day)	High (~$18 per day)	High (~$20 per day)

CK, creatinine; FDA, federal drug administration; HBeAg, hepatitis B e antigen; HBsAg, hepatitis B surface antigen; HBV, hepatitis B virus.
[†]Average wholesale price.

Table 42.3 Treatment options in patients with decompensated cirrhosis awaiting liver transplantation.

cations, and the potential to precipitate worsening of liver function. Tenofovir fumarate has been used in patients with HIV and HBV infection, and appears to be a safe and effective anti-HBV agent. Lamivudine, adefovir and tenofovir require dose-adjustment in patients with renal dysfunction. Adefovir has been associated with elevated creatinine levels in 3% of treated patients and these changes are usually reversible. Renal dysfunction, manifested by Fanconi syndrome and elevation in creatinine, has also been described with tenofovir.

By achieving suppression of HBV replication pretransplantation, the risk of recurrent HBV infection post-transplantation is reduced. In addition, important and significant biochemical and clinical improvements can be achieved, leading to a delay in the need for liver transplantation in some patients. Since clinical and biochemical improvements tend to lag behind virologic response, patients with severely decompensated liver disease may die before the clinical benefits of antiviral treatment can be realized. In a multicenter study of 154 North American patients with decompensated chronic hepatitis B treated with lamivudine for a median of 16 months, 78% of deaths occurred within the first 6 months of treatment and were due to complications of liver failure. In contrast, those treated patients surviving at least 6 months had an actuarial 3-year survival of 88%.

Lamivudine was the first nucleoside analog to be used in the treatment of decompensated cirrhotics and there is abundant evidence attesting to its benefits in this population. In a study of 23 patients with severely decompensated HBV cirrhosis, defined as a Child-Pugh-Turcotte (CPT) score of 10, treated with lamivudine, the median change in CPT scores was –3.0 versus +1.0 in an untreated historical control group ($P = 0.016$). Liver transplantation was performed in 34.8% of treated patients versus 73.9% of controls ($P = 0.04$) and the time to death or transplantation was significantly longer in treated patients than in controls ($P < 0.001$). Adefovir offers similar clinical benefits. In a large multicenter trial, 128 patients with decompensated cirrhosis and lamivudine resistant HBV treated with adefovir, 81% became aviremic by quantitative polymerase chain reaction (PCR) and 90% had improved CPT scores. Tenofovir is another nucleoside analog like adefovir, with activity against both wild-type and lamivudine-resistant HBV. Since tenofovir has not been approved for treatment of chronic HBV, information on efficacy and long-term safety in liver transplant recipients is largely lacking. Entecavir has activity against wild-type, lamivudine-resistant and adefovir-resistant HBV. Since this drug was only recently approved, data on efficacy in liver transplant patients is not yet available.

Hepatitis 'flares' during lamivudine and adefovir treatment occur in about 10% of treated patients after 1 year of therapy and are also frequent with treatment discontinuation. Consequently in cirrhotic patients, especially those with evidence of reduced hepatic reserve or frank decompensation, prolonged treatment is used. Prolonged therapy, however, is associated with an increased frequency of resistance and the consequences of drug resistance in cirrhotic patients can be significant. The risk of drug resistance is around 20% after 1 year with lamivudine and 2% after 2 years with adefovir. The emergence of drug resistant HBV has been linked with an increased frequency of hepatitis flares, worsening of histology, and clinical deterioration in patients with cirrhosis, including liver decompensation and liver-related death. The emergence of drug-resistant HBV pre-transplantation also increases the risk of recurrent HBV after transplantation. Thus, careful monitoring of HBV DNA levels is warranted in cirrhotic patients and changes in antiviral therapy should be considered when HBV DNA levels increase by $1.0 \log_{10}$ or more and before clinical decompensation occurs. Considering the risks associated with the development of drug resistance with prolonged therapy, combination nucleoside/nucleotide analogs would appear to be a good strategy. Studies to date, however, have not determined the optimal drug combinations nor have the benefits of combination therapy been established.

Post-transplant treatment strategies
Prophylactic HBIg therapy
While HBIg monotherapy is largely of historical interest since the current practice is to use HBIg in combination with one or more antivirals, the factors influencing treatment efficacy and failure with HBIg monotherapy are relevant to today's prophylactic strategies. Before the use of HBIg, many transplant programs considered 'active' HBV infection a relative or absolute contra-indication to liver transplantation. HBIg was the first therapy shown to prevent HBV recurrence in the transplant setting. While short-term HBIg given for 6 months or less was not effective prophylaxis, subsequent studies using longer duration, higher dose HBIg demonstrated a significant decrease in HBV recurrence and a parallel improvement in survival. In the largest study of 334 transplant recipients with HBV, patients treated with HBIg at least 6 months post-transplant had a recurrence rate of 36% compared to 75% in patients not receiving HBIg.

Pretransplant replication status was and remains an important determinant of the success of prophylactic therapy. Active HBV replication, defined by presence of HBeAg and/or serum HBV DNA levels $>10^5$ copies/mL, predicts a higher risk of treatment failure with HBIg than 'inactive' chronic HBV disease. Most protocols administer high dose HBIg (typically 10 000 IU) intraoperatively during the anhepatic phase and for the first postoperative week. Dosing after this immediate postoperative period is more variable; some protocols titrating HBIg to maintain specific anti-HBs titers while others providing a fixed monthly dose of HBIg. Pharmacokinetic studies demonstrate that 'effective prophylaxis' requires HBIg doses titrated to achieve anti-HBs titers of 500 IU/L during the first week, of 250 IU/L during weeks 2–12, and of 100 IU/L thereafter. Thus both prolonged treatment periods and high anti-HBs titers, especially in the first 12 weeks post-transplantation are important in achieving high treatment efficacy. A recent pharmacokinetic study of patients receiving pretransplant lamivudine followed by combination lamivudine and HBIg therapy post-transplantation reaffirms that importance of pretransplant replication status in determining HBIg requirements. Recipients with low levels of HBV DNA ($<10^5$ copies/mL) pretransplantation had lower HBIg requirements than those with higher levels of HBV DNA. Interestingly, the HBIg requirements of native non-replicators (i.e. low levels of HBV DNA prior to receipt of antiviral therapy) were lower than patients with low HBV DNA levels due to

lamivudine suppression, who in turn, had lower HBIg requirements than patients with high levels of HBV DNA (despite lamivudine therapy) at the time of liver transplantation. These data suggest that the pretreatment replication status and pre-transplant success of antiviral therapy are both factors influencing HBIg requirements and the risk of HBV recurrence post-transplantation.

Prophylaxis using HBIg monotherapy failed to prevent recurrent HBV in 20% of patients on average, with very low rates (5% or less) in those with low level HBV replication pre-transplantation but up to 50% in those with active replication pretransplantation. Early failures were due to inadequate suppression of HBV replication due to high pretransplant HBV DNA levels, inadequate dosing of HBIg, or both. Treatment failures occurring later (after at least 6 months of HBIg) were due to the development of HBV surface escape mutants. Escape mutations were located in the immunodominant epitope of the surface protein, the 'a' determinant, most commonly at amino acid positions 134, 144 and 145 (**Fig. 42.5**) and associated with reduced binding of anti-HBs in vitro. Given the reduced binding affinity, continuing HBIg after the emergence of escape mutants is ineffective and alternative therapies are needed to prevent progressive HBV disease. HBIg escape mutants are sensitive to lamivudine and adefovir.

Studies have evaluated whether transplant recipients on HBIg monotherapy who are HBsAg-negative and HBV DNA-negative can be transitioned from HBIg to lamivudine monotherapy. In a study of 16 HBsAg-negative, HBV DNA-negative transplant recipients who switched from HBIg to lamivudine 2 years after transplantation, none developed recurrent HBV with average follow-up of 51 months. Another study reported less success with this strategy with 4 of 12 patients developing recurrent HBV viremia after 34 months of follow-up. The failure or success of this strategy may be related to the pretransplant replication status of the patient. Patients who have active replication pre-transplantation are at higher risk for treatment failure with either HBIg monotherapy and with lamivudine monotherapy. In those patients on long-term HBIg prophylactic therapy who are HBsAg-negative and without clinical evidence of HBV recurrence, HBV DNA has be identified in serum, lymphocytes or liver in nearly half of the patients 10 years post-transplantation, but at low levels only detectable by PCR methods. This suggests the risk of recurrent HBV persists for years, even in the presence of effective prophylactic therapy. Such data suggest long-term and possibly indefinite treatment may be required in these transplant recipients. Whether those patients lacking HBV DNA in all compartments can be safely discontinued from anti-HBV therapy is unknown.

Lamivudine monotherapy prophylaxis
In the search for prophylactic therapies which were safe and well-tolerated in transplant recipients, easy to administer and of lower cost, lamivudine monotherapy was initially examined as an alternative to HBIg monotherapy. The largest study was of 77 HBV-infected patients awaiting transplantation, given lamivudine 100 mg daily pretransplantation and continued up to 2 years after transplantation. HBV recurrence rates were similar to historical controls treated with HBIg monotherapy after 2 years (**Fig. 42.6**). As seen with HBIg monotherapy, pretransplant replication status strongly influenced the success of

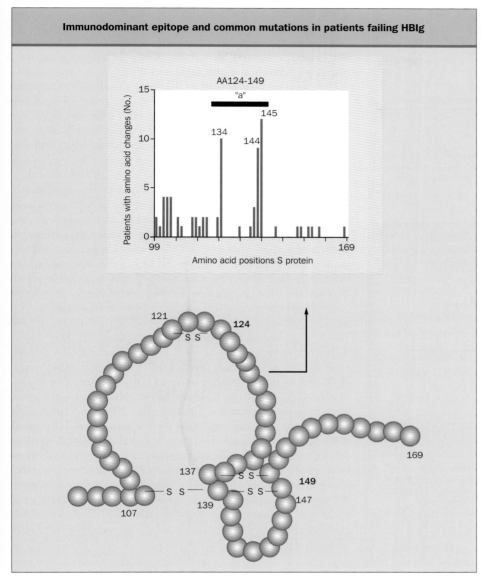

Immunodominant epitope and common mutations in patients failing HBIg

Figure 42.5 Immunodominant epitope and common mutations in patients failing HBIg. The region of the surface protein involved in binding of HBs antibody is described as a cysteine-rich web and single amino acid changes in the immunodominant "a" determinant (amino acids 124–149) result in reduced binding of anti-HBs in vitro. The most common escape mutations reported in patients failing HBIg monotherapy are at amino acid positions 134, 144 and 145 of the surface protein.

lamivudine monotherapy. At 2 years post-transplantation, none of the patients who were HBeAg and HBV DNA-negative pre-lamivudine therapy had recurrent HBV infection compared to 61% of patients who were HBeAg and HBV DNA-positive before starting treatment. A limitation of lamivudine monotherapy is the development of drug resistance during prolonged therapy. In transplant recipients receiving prophylactic lamivudine mono-therapy, resistance developed in 20–40% after 1 year.

Combination prophylaxis with HBIg and lamivudine or other antivirals

In the majority of transplant programs, combination immuno-prophylaxis, with HBIg and an antiviral agent such as lamivudine or adefovir, is the current standard of care for patients with HBV undergoing liver transplantation. The combination of HBIg and lamivudine is more efficacious then either agent alone and high efficacy is reported for both HBeAg-positive and HBeAg-negative (presumed precore mutation) chronic HBV. With follow-up periods of 13–30 months post-transplantation, HBV recurrence

rates in patients receiving prophylactic treatment with lamivudine plus HBIg range from 0–10%.

High dose HBIg protocols can cost up to $100 000 in the first year post-transplantation and $10 000–$50 000 in subsequent years depending upon the doses given. Several different HBIg preparations are available (**Table 42.4**). The significant cost of long-term HBIg therapy has spurred investigation of alternative protocols using lower doses of HBIg in combination with anti-viral agents, short-term HBIg with long-term antivirals and alternative immunoprophylaxis agents (see below). In general, protocols that give HBIg to maintain anti-HBs trough titers at a specified level (usually 100 IU/mL) are more cost-effective than regimes giving a fixed monthly dose of HBIg, and intramuscular administration of HBIg is less costly than intravenous adminis-tration. Intramuscular administration of HBIg has a 40–45% reduction in the delivery of anti-HBs to the intravascular space, but titer levels >100 IU/L can be achieved and maintained. Protocols using lower doses of HBIg in combination with lamivudine have similar efficacy rates as protocols using higher

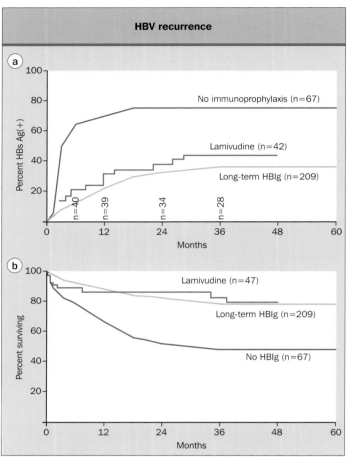

Figure 42.6 HBV recurrence. Patients treated with lamivudine monotherapy pre and post-transplantation were compared to historical data from patients treated with HBIg monotherapy post-transplantation (for <6 months and >6 months). (a) Rate of HBV recurrence post-transplantation, (b) Actuarial rate of patient survival. Reproduced from Perrillo et al (2001) by permission of Wiley-Liss, Inc.

doses of HBIg, suggesting that the use of HBIg in conjunction with a nucleoside/nucleotide analog may allow lower doses of HBIg to be administered. Alternative forms of HBs antibody are also being evaluated in clinical trials including hepatitis B immune plasma and monoclonal anti-HBs.

Combination therapy using HBIg plus a nucleoside/nucleotide analog for an indefinite duration may not be required in all liver transplant recipients with pretransplant HBV infection. In patients with naturally occurring low level HBV replication (i.e. inactive chronic HBV infection) awaiting transplantation, treatment with HBIg monotherapy, lamivudine monotherapy or combination therapy are similarly successful. Whether the small risk of treatment failure with monotherapy warrants long-term combination therapy in this population is unknown. In contrast, patients with active HBV replication pretransplantation have high rates of treatment failure with HBIg and lamivudine monotherapies and combination therapy provides superior benefits. Recent studies has evaluated whether HBIg can be stopped after a defined period of combination therapy and lamivudine monotherapy be used to provide ongoing prophylaxis. In a study comparing long-term HBIg and lamivudine versus short-term (1 month) HBIg and long-term lamivudine, all patients were HBsAg-negative at 18 months post-transplant and there was no difference in recurrence of HBV DNA by group (3/14 on long-term combination therapy versus 1/15 in short-term HBIg group). HBV vaccination as an alternative to HBIg has been also studied (**Table 42.5**). In HBsAg-negative, HBV DNA-negative transplant recipients on combination therapy with HBIg and lamivudine, the success of inducing and maintaining anti-HBs levels >10 IU/L with vaccination was variable (18–64%), possibly related to the vaccination preparation or dosing schedule. However, among the vaccine responders, HBIg was discontinued with no evidence of recurrent HBV with follow-up periods up to 40 months. Lamivudine was continued as prophylaxis in all vaccine responders. Longer-term studies are needed to define the subsets of patients who may be suitable for HBIg discontinuation.

Licensed hepatitis B immunoglobulin (HBIg) preparations				
Product	*Protein IgG%*	*Anti-HBs (IU/L)*	*Manufacturer/Reference*	*Country*
HBIg (before 1999)	16.5	200	NABI	USA
NABI-HB	5	300	NABI-Rockville	USA
Hyperhep/Bayhep	16.5	200	Cutter/Miles/Bayer	USA
Hep-B-Gammagee	16.5	>100	Merck, Sharp and Dome	USA
Hepatect	5	50	Biotest Pharma	Europe
Hepatitis B IG	5	50	BioProduct Lab	UK
Uman-B IG	–	200/50	Farma Biagini	Italy/Europe
Hebagam IM	–	100	Natal Bioproducts Institute	South Africa
Hepuman	–	200	Berna	Europe

anti-HBs, antibody to hepatitis B surface antigen; IgG, immunoglobulin G.
Modified from Terrault & Vyas (03) by permission of Elsevier.

Table 42.4 Licensed hepatitis B immunoglobulin (HBIg) preparations.

HBV vaccination as alternative to HBIg							
			% Response at Specific Anti-HBs Cut-off				*Duration Follow-up after HBIg Stopped*
Reference	*N*	*Vaccine Strategy*	*>10 IU*	*>100 IU*	*>500 IU*	*Recurrence N*	
Barcena, 1999	5	3 doses, 0, 1, and 2 mos + 3 add'n doses if needed	80	23	NA	0/4	5–8 mos
Angelico, 2002	17	Double doses, 3 courses	18	12	6	NA	40 mos
Sanchez-Fueyo, 2002	22	3 doses, routine schedule	63	23.5	9.1	0/14 (2 had fall in anti-HB titer to <10 IU/L)	14 mos
Bienzie, 2003	20	Adjuvant + vaccine ×3 and prn*	80	NA	NA	0/16	13.5 mos
Albeniz-Arbizu, 2003	12	3 doses, 0, 1 and 2 mos	75	17	NA	1/12	19 mos

*Additional doses given if initial anti-HBs titer <10 IU/L
Abbreviations: anti-HBs = anti-hepatitis B surface antibody titer, HBIg = hepatitis B immunoglobulin
Roche B, Samuel D. Liver Transplantation 2004.

Table 42.5 HBV vaccination as alternative to HBIg.

The development of lamivudine-resistant HBV prior to transplantation presents additional challenges in the post-transplant period. Variable success has been reported using high-dose HBIg monotherapy to prevent reinfection in these patients. With the availability of antiviral agents with efficacy against lamivudine-resistant HBV, the preferred strategy is adefovir, entecavir or tenofovir in combination with HBIg. An additional concern is the potential for cross-resistance in patients receiving HBIg and nucleoside/nucleotide analogs in combination or sequentially. Due to the overlapping reading frames of HBV, mutations in the polymerase potentially can cause changes in the surface gene and vice versa. Thus, the selection of resistance mutations in the polymerase with pretransplant treatment with lamivudine or adefovir may be associated with mutations in the surface gene, which may limit the efficacy of subsequent HBIg treatment, at least theoretically.

The ideal time to begin antiviral therapy pretransplantation is determined primarily by liver disease severity and the replication status of the patient. For those with inactive HBV disease (normal serum aminotransferase levels and low levels of HBV DNA, typically $\leq 10^4$ copies/mL), antiviral therapy can be started at or near the time of transplantation. For those with active HBV disease (HBeAg-positive or HBV DNA $>10^4$ copies/mL or abnormal liver enzymes), the duration of nucleoside/nucleotide therapy should be sufficient to achieve viral suppression, achieve the desired clinical benefits and yet minimize emergence of drug resistance. To achieve reductions in HBV DNA levels to of $\leq 10^4$ copies/mL usually requires a period of 3–6 months of lamivudine or adefovir treatment depending upon baseline HBV DNA levels, and clinical improvements in patients with decompensated disease requires at least 6 months of treatment. Since the timing of transplantation is usually not known, prolonged treatment with antiviral agents is common in patients awaiting transplantation and drug resistance may develop in this population. Antiviral agents that have a low rate of viral resistance may be better suited for patients with decompensated liver disease requiring prolonged periods of pretransplant therapy.

Management of recipients of anti-HBc-positive allografts

Due to the discrepancy between the static number of donor organs and increasing number of patients awaiting liver transplantation, use of anti-HBc-positive allografts to expand the donor pool is a common practice. Most anti-HBc-positive, HBsAg-negative allografts have normal or near normal liver enzymes and histology, but there is a risk of de novo HBV infection in recipients. HBV-naïve and anti-HBs-negative recipients are at highest risk of de novo HBV with receipt of an anti-HBc-positive organ with a reported incidence of 33–78%. The lowest risk is seen in anti-HBs-positive recipients. Prophylactic therapies reduce the risk of de novo infection in patients receiving anti-HBc-positive grafts. Prophylaxis must take into account the pretransplant serologic status of the recipient (**Table 42.6**). For recipients with pre-existing chronic HBV infection, a combination of HBIg and a nucleoside/nucleotide analog is used as prophylaxis. Lamivudine alone with or without HBIg has been used to prevent de novo HBV in HBsAg-negative recipients of anti-HBc-positive allografts. Pretransplant vaccination, even when anti-HBs titers are successfully induced and maintained, does not prevent de novo HBV post-transplant in all patients. Therefore, prophylaxis is generally undertaken even if pretransplant HBV vaccination was successful. For patients with pre-existing immunity against HBV infection (anti-HBc-positive with or without anti-HBs), the risk of de novo infection is so low some experts suggest that an alternative to long-term prophylaxis may be close serologic and virologic monitoring and initiation of nucleoside analog therapy at the first signs of infection. Larger-scale studies to determine the optimal treatment algorithms in these patients with different levels of risk are needed.

Treatment of recurrent HBV in transplant recipients

Graft survival is less in those who develop recurrent HBV than those who remain HBsAg-negative post-transplantation. In patients with recurrent HBV infection, the goals of therapy are to suppress viral replication, stabilize graft function and prevent histologic progression. Challenges associated with the treatment of recurrent HBV infection in transplant patients include the presence of immunosuppression, which may affect treatment efficacy, the frequent presence of drug-resistant HBV, and the rapid development of recurrent cirrhosis in the absence of effective antiviral therapy. Emergence of resistance with single drug therapy occurs with prolonged treatment, albeit at a different rate with each drug (**Fig. 42.7**). Sequential use of anti-HBV therapies can lead to an accumulation of polymerase and surface gene mutations and an increasingly drug-resistant form of HBV infection. Knowledge of the preceding drug exposure history is critical in making treatment decisions. In general, the treatment options for drug-experienced patients with recurrent HBV are more limited than those with wild-type HBV infection (recurrent or de novo). Despite the theoretical advantages of combination nucleoside/nucleotide analog therapy, the optimal combination of available antivirals that will achieve the desired benefits of high efficacy and low toxicity has not been established.

Lamivudine and adefovir are the mainstays of therapy for those with recurrent disease (**Table 42.7**). Experience with entecavir is limited, but the safety and efficacy data in non-transplant patients suggest this drug will be useful in treatment of recurrent HBV disease. Famciclovir, ganciclovir (intravenous) and interferon were used for the management of patients with recurrent disease prior to the availability of lamivudine, but the antiviral effects of these agents were modest and less consistently achievable than with lamivudine and adefovir. Thus famciclovir, ganciclovir and interferon should be considered second-line agents for use in patients failing first-line therapies with lamivudine, entecavir and/or adefovir. Tenofovir was used to treat lamivudine-resistant HBV infection prior to the availability of adefovir and entecavir; although experience is limited, tenofovir appears to be another treatment option for patients with lamivudine-resistant recurrent HBV infection. Given the limited data on long-term safety and efficacy of tenofovir in transplanted patients, tenofovir should be considered second-line therapy. Future agents may include the new nucleoside/nucleotide analogs currently under study such as clevudine, emtricitabine and telbivudine.

Lamivudine is effective in liver transplant recipients with recurrent HBV due to wild-type HBV, those who have failed HBIg therapy and those with adefovir-resistant HBV. Additionally, lamivudine has been shown to have efficacy in FCH. In the largest clinical study in North America of 52 liver transplant recipients with recurrent HBV (including 50% who had failed HBIg prophylaxis), lamivudine 100 mg daily for a median of 49 weeks resulted in normalization of liver enzymes in 72%, decline in HBV DNA levels in 60%, HBeAg loss in 50% and HBsAg loss in 6%. However, 27% had a virologic breakthrough and 36% of these patients experienced clinical deterioration with the development of drug resistance. Other studies show similar results; while the majority of patients respond initially, emergence of lamivudine resistance limits long-term efficacy and monitoring for virologic breakthrough is essential. There is cross-resistance between lamivudine and

Management of recipients of anti-HBc positive allografts		
Recipient status	Risk of de novo HBV in absence of prophylaxis	Prophylaxis regimes reported to be effective
HBsAg+	Unknown	HBIg plus antiviral (same as HBsAg+ patient not receiving anti-HBc + organ)
HBsAg–, anti-HBc–, anti-HBs–	33–78%	Lamivudine (or other antiviral) monotherapy HBIg (short or long term) plus antivirals
HBsAg–, anti-HBc+, anti-HBs+	0–13%	Lamivudine (or other antiviral) monotherapy No prophylaxis – treat if de novo HBV
anti-HBc, anti-hepatitis B core antibody; anti-HBs, anti-hepatitis B surface antibody; HBeAg, hepatitis B e antigen; HBIg, hepatitis B immunoglobulin; HBsAg, hepatitis B surface antigen; HBV DNA, hepatitis B virus DNA.		

Table 42.6 Management of recipients of anti-HBc positive allografts.

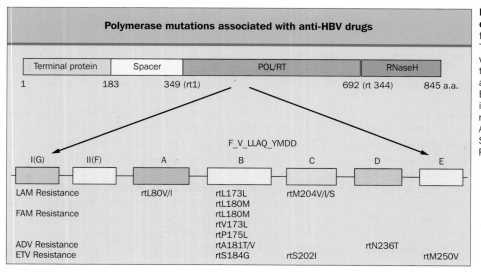

Figure 42.7 Mutations associated with anti-HBV drugs. Genotype-independent numbering scheme for the HBV polymerase/RT domain is shown. The primary location for mutations associated with LAM-resistance in domains B and C; similar to those for FAM. The signature mutation associated with ADV-resistance is in domain D. Entecavir resistance mutations have only been identified in patients with preexisting lamivudine-resistance mutations. LAM: lamivudine, ADV: adefovir, FAM: famciclovir. (Courtesy of S. Locarnini, Victoria Infectious Diseases Reference Laboratory, Melbourne, Australia.)

Treatment options for patients with recurrent HBV			
Patient population	First-line agents	Second-line agents	Comments
No prior therapy	Lamivudine, adefovir, entecavir	Tenofovir i.v., ganciclovir, interferon	Risk of resistance with prolonged therapy higher with lamivudine than adefovir or entecavir. Adefovir and entecavir are more costly than lamivudine.
HBIg treatment failure	Lamivudine, adefovir, entecavir	Tenofovir i.v., ganciclovir, interferon	Lamivudine and adefovir are effective against surface gene mutants.
Lamivudine resistance	Adefovir, entecavir	Tenofovir i.v., ganciclovir, interferon	Case report of patients treated with sequential HBIg and lamivudine resistance who had increased viral replication in the presence of lamivudine.
Famciclovir resistance	Adefovir, entecavir	Lamivudine, tenofovir i.v., ganciclovir, interferon	Lamivudine is effective in short-term, but lamivudine resistance emerges more rapidly if prior famciclovir exposure.
Adefovir resistance	Lamivudine, entecavir	Tenofovir, interferon	Only lamivudine has been demonstrated to be effective. IFN likely to be option; efficacy of other antiviral unknown.

Table 42.7 Treatment options for patients with recurrent HBV.

famciclovir and prior treatment with famciclovir increases the risk of lamivudine resistance.

Adefovir is effective against wild-type and lamivudine-resistant HBV. In 196 liver transplant recipients with recurrent and lamivudine-resistant HBV disease, treatment with adefovir 10 mg daily for 52 weeks led to undetectable HBV DNA (<200 copies/mL) levels in 35%, normalization of liver enzymes in 46%, and improvement in CPT score in over 90%. Adefovir was well tolerated but renal toxicity was a concern. A total of 13% of treated patients had a 0.5 mg/dL increase in serum creatinine during treatment but all patients had other potential risk factors for abnormal creatinine levels including concurrent use of calcineurin inhibitors. Dose adjustments in patients with reduced creatinine clearance and close monitoring of renal function are recommended during adefovir therapy. Adefovir resistance is seen in 2 and 4% of patients after 2 and 3 years of treatment. Adefovir-resistant HBV is sensitive to lamivudine and entecavir.

Entecavir is now available and is active against both HBeAg-positive and HBeAg-negative hepatitis B, including lamivudine-refractory disease. Little is known about its effectiveness and safety in the transplant setting.

Retransplantation for recurrent HBV

Retransplantation for graft failure due to recurrent HBV was associated with dismal outcomes in the pre-HBIg and pre-nucleoside era, with mortality rates of 68–95%. The contemporary experience is significantly better. Using prophylactic regimes of HBIg with and without antiviral agents, low rates of recurrent HBV disease in the second graft and prolonged survival are achievable. For patients who are HBV DNA-positive and requiring retransplantation, high dose HBIg with anti-HBs target titers >500 IU/L appear more successful than lower dose HBIg using target titers of 100 IU/L. The addition of pretransplant nucleoside/nucleotide analogs to reduce HBV DNA levels pre-transplantation enhances the efficacy of prophylaxis further and prevents recurrent HBV in the majority of these patients. The optimal dose of HBIg therapy and choice of antiviral agent(s) must be individualized and based upon the patient's prior drug exposures and likelihood of harboring specific surface and polymerase mutations.

HEPATITIS C VIRUS

More than 20 000 patients worldwide have undergone liver transplantation for HCV cirrhosis, and in North America, HCV accounts for 25–50% of the liver transplants performed. Unfortunately, recurrent HCV is essentially universal in patients who are viremic pretransplantation and is associated with a more rapid progression to cirrhosis in the transplanted liver. The risk of death and allograft failure are increased in HCV-positive transplant recipients [hazard ratio (HR) 1.23 and HR 1.30] compared HCV-negative recipients (**Fig. 42.8**). Further limiting graft outcomes in transplant patients are a poor response to and limited tolerability of interferon and ribavirin therapy. High baseline viral load and a predominance of genotype 1 infection reduce even further the likelihood of achieving viral clearance. However, in selected patients, viral eradication or slowing of disease progression appears to be achievable. For the remaining patients with progressive histologic disease and non-response to treatment, retransplantation is the only current option. Unfortunately, retransplantation for recurrent HCV is associated with 5-year survival rate of 50%, making this a controversial indication for retransplantation.

Natural history of recurrent HCV after transplantation

Liver transplant recipients with HCV have increased viral replication, increased risk of fibrosis and an accelerated time to cirrhosis compared to patients not on immunosuppressive therapy (**Table 42.8**). Viral kinetic studies of the early events following transplantation have shown that HCV RNA levels drop abruptly during the anhepatic phase and again during the 8–24 h after reperfusion. By 24–72 h there is an increase of

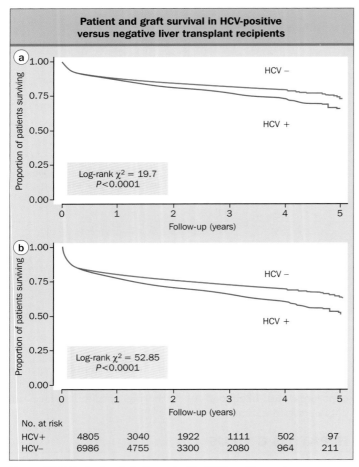

Figure 42.8 Patient and graft survival in HCV-positive and HCV-negative liver transplant recipients. (a) Kaplan-Meier estimates of patient survival according to HCV infection status. (b) Kaplan-Meier estimates of allograft survival according to HCV infection status. Reproduced from Forman et al (02) by permission of Elsevier.

Natural history of hepatitis C post-transplantation

	Post-transplantation	Non-immunosuppressed persons with chronic HCV
Fibrosis progression (units fibrosis/year)	0.3/year (0.004–2.19/year)	0.2/year (0.09–0.8/year)
Median time to cirrhosis	8–12 years	20–30 years
Decompensation rate after cirrhosis	50% at 1 year	4% per year
Survival after decompensation	41% at 1 year	50% at 5 years

The natural history of HCV disease post-transplantation is truncated compared to that of non-immunosuppressed persons with chronic HCV (i.e. disease progression prior to transplantation). Modified from Berenguer (03).

Table 42.8 Natural history of hepatitis C post-transplantation.

patients with chronic HCV infection (**Fig. 42.9b**). Approximately 20% of patients develop chronic hepatitis without acute hepatitis; this presentation appears to have a more favorable outcome in terms of disease progression. The majority, 70%, develops acute hepatitis and evolves to chronic hepatitis. In 10% or less of transplant recipients, a severe and rapidly progressive form of hepatitis, termed cholestatic hepatitis, develops.

Cholestatic hepatitis is characterized by serum bilirubin >6 mg/dL, high serum HCV RNA levels ($>10^6$ copies/mL), and a characteristic histologic pattern of perivenular ballooning hepatocytes, confluent necrosis, bile duct proliferation and cholestasis, but with minimal inflammation (**Fig. 42.9c**). This form of recurrent disease has been historically associated with a poor prognosis, with mortality rates as high as 50% at 1 year and 18% at 3 years. However, stabilization of liver disease and prolonged survival has been achieved in some patients with use of antiviral therapy.

Immunosuppression, acute rejection and HCV

Excessive immunosuppression and rapid changes in immuno-suppression are thought to be key factors influencing the severity of recurrent HCV disease. Steroid-free immunosuppressive regimens have shown some benefits in HCV infected recipients. When steroids are used, the rate of withdrawal rather than the absolute dose of steroids appears to be of importance. In contrast to HCV-negative recipients, who have reduced mortality if they experience an episode of acute cellular rejection, HCV infected recipients have a threefold increase in mortality after an episode of rejection. Rapid changes in immunosuppression, such as occurs with boluses of corticosteroids and lymphocyte-depleting agents like OKT-3 in treatment of acute rejection, are associated with increased risk of severe HCV disease and decreased time to HCV recurrence.

In terms of specific immunosuppressive agents, none has been identified as being harmful to HCV disease progression per se. Retrospective analyses of patients receiving tacrolimus versus

serum HCV RNA to detectable levels, with levels increasing over postoperative weeks 2–4 and peaking between weeks 4 and 16 before stabilizing. At 1-year post-transplantation, viral levels are typically 1.0 $\log_{10}$ higher than pretransplant levels. While the correlation between post-transplant HCV viral titer and histologic severity of recurrent disease is poor, some studies have found an association between pretransplant viral load and risk of cirrhosis and/or graft loss post-transplantation.

Recurrent infection defined by the presence of detectable HCV RNA in serum and liver occurs universally and early in patients who are viremic pretransplantation. Clinical and histologic presentations among infected transplant recipients are more variable. Acute recurrent HCV disease, when manifest, usually occurs within 3 to 6 months after transplantation and is characterized by elevated serum aminotransferase levels and histologic findings of lobular hepatitis, focal hepatocellular necrosis, and acidophilic bodies (**Fig. 42.9a**). Chronic recurrent HCV disease occurs with or without a preceding acute hepatitis phase. The histologic changes of chronic HCV disease include mixed portal and periportal inflammation with or without peri-portal fibrosis, similar to the histologic picture of non-transplant

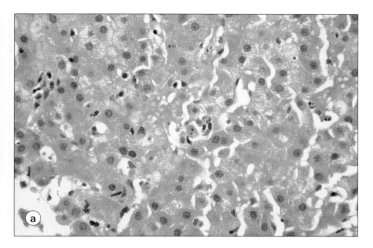

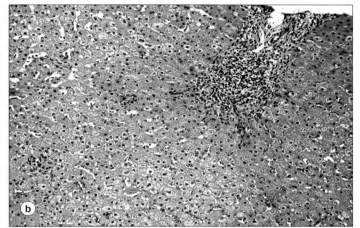

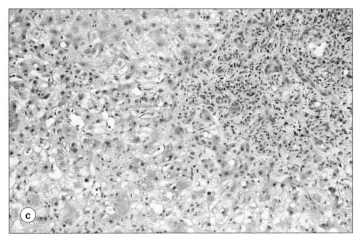

Figure 42.9 Histologic features of HCV infection in liver transplant recipients. (a) Acute hepatitis, (b) chronic hepatitis, (c) cholestatic variant. (Courtesy of Dr Linda Ferrell, University of California San Francisco.)

Factors associated with increased severity of HCV recurrence	
Consistently linked with disease severity	*Conflicting studies on relationship to disease severity*
High pre-LT HCV viral load Necroinflammation at initial biopsy Acute rejection Later year of transplantation CMV infection	HCV Genotype I Older donor age Peak AST level HLA incompatibility
Non-white race	Live donor liver transplant
	Prolonged warm ischemia time
OKT-3 use	–
AST, aspartate aminotransferase; CMV, cytomegalovirus; HCV, hepatitis C virus; HLA, human lymphocyte antigen; LT, liver transplantation; MMF, mycophenolate mofetil; OKT-3; anti-CD3 monoclonal antibody.	

Table 42.9 Factors associated with increased severity of HCV recurrence.

cyclosporin-based immunosuppression show no difference in disease severity between groups. Mycophenolate mofetil use was implicated in early multivariate analyses predicting disease severity, but two large prospective studies found no difference in HCV recurrence or outcomes in those transplant recipients who did and did not receive mycophenolate mofetil. The limited data on induction therapy using lymphocyte-depleting therapy indicate no adverse effects on disease progression. Sirolimus has not been studied sufficiently to draw conclusions.

The histologic features of early recurrent HCV and acute cellular rejection overlap and make the diagnosis of acute cellular rejection in the setting of recurrent HCV disease difficult. In a retrospective study of 285 liver transplant recipients, HCV was associated with an increased risk of early (<6 months after transplant) acute cellular rejection compared to other transplant indications (HR 1.7). In this same study, 49% of transplant recipients with HCV had at least one episode of early acute cellular rejection. In light of this difficulty and due to the reported association between treatment of acute rejection and increased risk of HCV disease progression, some experts have recommended that only acute rejection of moderate or severe degree should be treated. Corticosteroid boluses and leukocyte depleting agents should be used judiciously. Additionally, expert panels recommend against rapid withdrawal of immuno-suppression. An exception to these guidelines may be cholestatic hepatitis in which rapid reduction in the level of immuno-suppression has been considered the cornerstone to therapy.

Factors associated with recurrent HCV

Several recipient, donor and viral factors have been associated with increased severity of HCV recurrence and reduced graft survival and patient survival (**Table 42.9**). The factors most firmly associated with high risk of progression to cirrhosis and graft loss due to HCV include: liver biopsy histology at 1 year, acute cellular rejection, use of OKT-3 for rejection, presence of CMV viremia and non-white race. Whether recipients of live donor allografts are at risk of earlier and more severe HCV recurrence than deceased donor recipients is controversial. A concerning trend is the decreasing graft and patients survival rates over time for patients with HCV; this contrasts sharply with the increasing survival rates seen for non-HCV indications during the same time period. Two changes in clinical practice have been implicated as the cause for this trend in patients with HCV: the use of newer and more potent immunosuppressive agents, and the increasing use of older donors, particularly those over 50 years of age.

Anti-HCV-positive donors

HCV antibody-positive donors are increasingly being used for patients whose urgency for an allograft precludes waiting for an antibody-negative donor allograft. Since spontaneous clearance of HCV virus can occur in up to 45% of those exposed to HCV, a sizeable portion of otherwise healthy potential donors who are HCV antibody-positive may not have an active HCV infection. Additionally, 80% of persons with chronic HCV infection and persistently normal liver enzymes have mild or minimal histologic disease. Since only antibody results are available at the time of transplantation, all anti-HCV-positive organs must be considered a source of HCV RNA and a risk for HCV disease post-transplantation. In general, anti-HCV organs should be restricted to HCV RNA-positive patients with a high need awaiting liver transplantation. Use of anti-HCV-positive organs in HCV un-infected persons is not recommended currently, as the organ presents a risk for de novo HCV infection and no effective prophylactic therapy is available. Similarly, since spontaneous or treatment-induced clearance for HCV RNA does not protect against future HCV infection, anti-HCV-positive, HCV RNA-negative patients awaiting transplantation should not receive organs from anti-HCV-positive donors.

Virologic analyses of the organs of anti-HCV-positive recipients of anti-HCV-positive organs indicate that the majority are in-fectious and that the recipient viral strain typically predominates post-transplantation. However, the possible negative consequences of giving a recipient infected with a favorable HCV genotype for treatment (e.g. HCV genotype 2 or 3) a donor organ which may be infected with a less variable genotype, must be fully dis-cussed with potential recipients. To date, the outcome data available indicate that patient and graft survival are at least as good and perhaps better for anti-HCV-positive recipients receiving an allograft from an anti-HCV-positive donor compared to those receiving an anti-HCV-negative donor (**Fig. 42.10**). Thus, the use of allografts that are anti-HCV-positive represents a reasonable expansion of the donor pool in selected anti-HCV-positive patients who are well informed and HCV RNA-positive.

Pretransplant antiviral therapy

Recurrent HCV after liver transplantation requires the presence of HCV RNA pretransplantation and limited studies suggest the severity of HCV disease after transplantation is related to pretransplant levels of HCV RNA. The impact of a treatment-induced reduction in viral load pretransplantation on the risk of HCV recurrence is unknown, but if a sustained virologic response is achieved pretransplantation, HCV recurrence is rare post-transplantation.

In advanced liver disease, treatment with interferon and ribavirin is associated with reduced tolerability, frequent dose reductions and possible precipitation of clinical decompensation. However, with the selection of appropriate candidates and using a low accelerating dosage regimen (LADR) of interferon plus

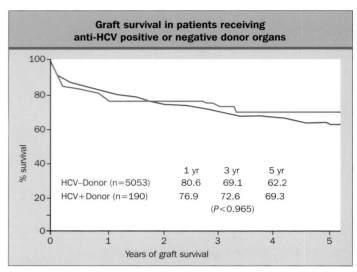

Figure 42.10 Graft survival. Graft survival in patients receiving anti-HCV-positive and anti-HCV-negative donor organs. Number of grafts analyzed each year is indicated. There was no difference in survival between groups. Reproduced from Velidedeoglu et al (02) by permission of Lippincott, Williams and Wilkins.

ribavirin, sustained responses can be achieved. In a study of 102 patients awaiting liver transplant with mean CPT score of 7.1 +/– 2.0, 40 patients achieved an end-of-treatment response, 21 achieved a sustained viral response, and only 16 of 102 could not tolerate treatment. The sustained virologic response (SVR) rates were genotype-dependent, 11% and 50% for genotypes 1 and non-1, respectively. None of the 10 patients who were HCV RNA-negative pretransplantation had recurrent HCV after trans-plantation but all 22 patients who were HCV RNA-positive had recurrence. In this study, interferon α2b was started at half dose with ribavirin 200 mg daily, and if tolerated, the doses were increased incrementally every 2 weeks (interferon first, then ribavirin) until target doses were achieved. Adverse events in this study were common with thrombocytopenia (<45 000/mL) and leukopenia (neutrophil count <1000/mL) the most frequent. In contrast to these results, another study of patients with more severe liver disease (mean CPT score 11.9 +/– 1.2) using inter-feron α2b 1 MU thrice weekly with ribavirin, 1 MU daily alone or 3 MU thrice weekly alone reported greater intolerance to treatment regimens and a high rate of serious adverse events. Whether growth factors such as granulocyte-macrophage colony stimulating factor (GM-CSF) and erythropoietin can increase the tolerability of interferon and ribavirin in this population is unknown. While additional studies to define the optimal treat-ment strategy are needed, the available data suggest patients with mildly decompensated liver disease may be appropriate candidates for pretransplant antiviral therapy, whereas the risk of complications may outweigh benefits in those with more advanced stages of decompensation.

Post-transplant management of HCV infection

Treatment approaches can be divided into three general categories (prophylactic, pre-emptive and treatment of established disease) based upon the timing of the intervention (**Table 42.2**). Prophyl-actic therapy is started at the time of transplantation and continued for variable periods post-transplantation. As with any form of 'post-exposure' prophylaxis, the goal of prophylaxis is to prevent infection. Pre-emptive treatment of recurrent HCV refers to initiating antiviral therapy early in the post-transplant period, typically within the first 4 weeks following transplantation, and before biochemical and histologic disease is manifest. Treatment of recurrent HCV disease refers to initiating antiviral therapy for biochemical and histologically evidence of recurrent disease.

Dose reductions are more common in transplant patients receiving antiviral therapy for recurrent HCV than in non-transplant populations. Dose reductions, in turn, likely contribute to the lower response rates seen in this population. Cytopenias are frequent due to concurrent use of immunosuppressive agents and alterations in renal function related to calcineurin inhibitor therapy or other post-transplant factors affecting ribavirin clearance. Indeed, the optimal dose of ribavirin in transplant patients has not been determined. Growth factors may be an important method of managing cytopenias and improving quality of life during antiviral treatment.

As interferon has immunomodulatory effects, specifically upregulation of human leukocyte antigen (HLA) expression on bile duct epithelia, there has been persistent concern regarding the risk of rejection related to use of interferon in liver transplant recipients. Additionally, this risk of acute rejection may be greater if interferon is used pre-emptively rather than later post-transplantation, since the risk of acute rejection is highest in the first 3 months after transplantation. In uncontrolled retrospective studies, rates of acute cellular rejection reported in patients on antiviral therapy range from 11 to 34%. In controlled studies, the frequency of acute rejection has not been significantly different in interferon-treated patients compared to untreated controls.

Prophylactic therapy

There are no established prophylactic therapies for HCV. In the transplant setting, HCV antibody therapy is being evaluated as a potential means of preventing HCV infection post-transplantation. Preclinical and retrospective cohort data support this approach. In a retrospective observational study of transplant recipients with HBV and HCV receiving HBIg, the prevalence of recurrent HCV disease after transplantation was lower in those who received HBIg prior to screening for HCV compared to those who received HBIg after screening for HCV began. These results suggested that the HCV antibodies in HBIg prior to HCV screening reduced the risk of recurrent disease. In a study of two chimpanzees treated with high dose hepatitis C immune globulin (HCIG) immediately before and continued after HCV inoculation, both were initially viremic but subsequently had undetectable HCV RNA and had no evidence of biochemical hepatitis.

At least three HCV antibody preparations are being studied in prospective clinical trials. A preliminary report of the Canadian HCV immune globulin study (Cangene Corp, Canada) found no benefit with HCV RNA detectable in all treated patients post-transplantation and no appreciable difference in level of viremia or histologic disease in patients receiving HCIG prophylaxis versus controls. Other studies using different antibody products and alternative dosing schedules are underway, but at the present time, prophylactic therapy has no established role in the management of patients with HCV undergoing liver transplantation.

Pre-emptive antiviral therapy

The lower HCV viral loads present in the early post-transplant period and the absence of significant histologic disease may favorably affect the success of antiviral therapy in the transplant setting. This rationale underlies the pre-emptive therapy strategy. Studies have shown that pre-emptive antiviral therapy can lead to eradication of HCV infection, but tolerability of therapy can be limiting. Unlike non-transplant and acutely infected patients, liver transplant recipients are typically on multiple immunosuppressants, prophylactic antimicrobial agents, have variable renal function, and are recovering from a major operative procedure in the setting of advanced liver disease. In a study of 110 patients transplanted for HCV, only 60% were found to be candidates for interferon and ribavirin therapy at 8 weeks post-transplantation by traditional criteria. Patients with a high pre-transplant model of end-stage liver disease (MELD) and CPT scores were less suitable for this therapeutic approach.

Clinical trials using pre-emptive interferon monotherapy, though generally positive, demonstrated a modest benefit, primarily in delaying time to histologic recurrence. Sustained virologic responses were infrequent, occurring in 0–22%. More recent studies using interferon and ribavirin suggest combination therapy is more efficacious. An uncontrolled study from Italy of 36 patients (83% genotype 1b) treated with combination standard interferon α2b 3 MU thrice weekly and ribavirin 10 mg/kg/day initiated within 3 weeks after transplant and continued for 52 weeks, reported sustained virologic responses in 33%, all of whom had normal serum aminotransferase levels and histology after completion of therapy. Viral clearance was more frequent in patients with non-1 HCV genotypes (100%) compared to those with genotype 1b (20%).

In contrast to the Italian experience, a US study of pre-emptive standard or pegylated (PEG)-interferon α2b, 3 MU thrice weekly or 1.5 μg/kg/week, or interferon/peginterferon α2b plus ribavirin, 600 mg daily increasing to 1.0–1.2 g daily, for a total of 48 weeks, reported sustained virologic responses in only 9.1%, with most responders in the combination therapy group. Dose reductions and discontinuations were required in 85% and 37% of patients, respectively. The inability to achieve full-dose therapy may explain the low rate of sustained virologic response. The differences in applicability and tolerability of pre-emptive therapy in the Italian and US studies may reflect the clinical status of the patients in the early post-transplant period. The subgroups of patients for which pre-emptive therapy is best suited is unknown, and whether pre-emptive treatment is better than delaying treatment until recurrent disease is established also requires study.

Treatment of established HCV disease

Study protocols for the treatment of established recurrent HCV disease have generally initiated treatment between 6 and 24 months after transplantation. Theoretical advantages of initiating treatment when recurrent disease is clinically or histologically apparent rather than as pre-emptive treatment include lower doses of immunosuppression (may enhance response to antiviral therapy), improved clinical status to better tolerate treatment, lower risk of acute rejection, and cost savings since only those with progressive disease are treated. Potential disadvantages of the 'wait and treat recurrent disease' approach include higher viral load and more fibrosis which may reduce likelihood of response.

Treatment of established disease with interferon or ribavirin monotherapy has been disappointing. The combination interferon and ribavirin resulted in sustained virologic responses in approximately 20% of treated patients. Histologic improvements were reported in both responders and non-responders.

Most of the studies evaluating combination therapy for established recurrent HCV disease were uncontrolled and of small sample size, and with variable interferon and ribavirin doses and treatment duration. Doses of interferon α were typically 3 MU trice weekly (range 1.5–5 MU) with ribavirin typically 600–1000 mg daily (range 400–1200 mg daily). Duration of therapy typically was 1 year. End of therapy biochemical and virologic responses ranged from 25% to 100% and 9% to 64%, respectively. There was a wide range of reported sustained virologic responses (assessed at 6 months after completion of therapy), 5–56%. Generally, adverse events during combination treatment were common with withdrawal of treatment required in up to 50% of patients; anemia, leukopenia and thrombocytopenia were the most common causes.

Peginterferon has not been compared directly to standard interferon in combination therapy for established recurrent HCV disease and published data using peginterferons are limited. The reported rates of sustained viral response with peginterferon and ribavirin were at least as good as standard interferon and ribavirin, ranging from 26% to 37.5%. Despite titrated regimens using low initial doses of peginterferon and ribavirin, dose reductions and discontinuations were frequent.

The optimal duration of treatment for recurrent HCV disease is unknown. In an immunosuppressed population of liver transplant recipients, longer treatment periods may be necessary to enhance sustained virologic responses. Prolonged low dose 'maintenance' interferon is being evaluated for histologic and clinical benefits in patients who fail to clear HCV after combination interferon and ribavirin therapy in several clinical trials (HALT-C, EPIC and CO-PILOT). There are no data regarding whether this strategy is effective in the transplant setting.

The cost-effectiveness of antiviral therapy for recurrent HCV disease was examined in one study. Using a Markov-based decision analytic model to simulate costs and health outcomes, treatment of recurrent HCV with antiviral therapy (interferon and ribavirin) was cost effective. Treatment of 100 men, aged 55 years, with recurrent HCV would prevent 29 cases of cirrhosis, seven deaths, and had an incremental cost effectiveness ratio of $29 100 per year of life saved.

Retransplantation for recurrent HCV

In the USA, 8–9% of all transplants performed are retransplants, with recurrent HCV accounting for approximately 40%. Compared to primary transplantation, retransplantation for all indications is associated with longer hospital stays, 40% greater costs and a 10–20% reduction in survival. Outcomes of retransplantation for recurrent HCV disease are at best similar to other indications yet most studies report inferior results. In a large study of over 10 000 patients in the UNOS database, anti-HCV-positive retransplant recipients had reduced survival compared to anti-HCV-negative retransplant recipients, with 5-year survival rates of 61% and 54%, respectively. Studies specifically evaluating retransplantation for recurrent HCV disease (not just

HCV-positive status) are smaller and from single centers but show similar or worse outcomes. Predictors of poor outcome following retransplantation included recipient age over 50 years, serum creatinine greater than 2.0 mg/dL, and serum bilirubin greater than 10 mg/dL. In general, outcomes are predicted to be best if retransplantation occurs before the onset of liver decompensation or significant renal dysfunction. Additionally, those with a longer period of time from first to second transplant appear to have a better outcome. Overall, however, retransplantation for recurrent HCV disease remains controversial. Currently, most transplant programs use a selective approach, choosing HCV infected patients with favorable clinical characteristics for retransplantation.

CYTOMEGALOVIRUS

CMV is an important pathogen in liver transplant recipients, contributing directly to morbidity and mortality. Infection usually develops within the first 3 months after transplantation. Without antiviral prophylaxis, the overall incidence of CMV infection is 50–60%, and of CMV disease is 20–30%. The clinical impact of CMV in transplant recipients relates to the direct effects of the infectious disease syndromes, and the indirect effects of viral-associated immune modulation leading to an increased risk of superinfection with other opportunistic pathogens, chronic allograft rejection, and possibly EBV-associated lymphoproliferative disease.

Diagnosis of CMV in liver transplant recipients

The diagnosis of CMV infection can be established by serologic and virologic techniques. Serology is most useful in assessing past exposure to CMV in both the donor and recipient. Serial testing with documentation of either seroconversion or rising immunoglobulin G (IgG) titers is an indirect measure of active viral infection, but these are not routinely tested after transplantation. The cornerstone for CMV diagnosis is the demonstration of the virus in the blood, respiratory specimens, urine or tissue. The gold standard for CMV diagnosis has been the growth of the virus in cultures with demonstration of cytopathic effect. Typical histologic features in tissue biopsies include the presence of 'cytomegalic' cells with intranuclear inclusions and associated acute, focal inflammation. However, more rapid methods are available (**Table 42.10**). The sensitive CMV antigen test, which detects a structural protein of CMV, pp65, is usually the diagnostic test of choice. Alternatively, detection of virus in blood or tissues using PCR can identify presence of infection but has lower specificity in identifying patients with CMV disease. However, since viremia precedes the clinical symptoms by 2–5 days, the PCR detection of viremia may be useful in situations in which pre-emptive therapy is desirable. Additionally, the presence of CMV antigens in tissues using monoclonal antibody staining or in situ hybridization supports the diagnosis of CMV organ involvement.

Natural history and clinical presentation

Three patterns of viral transmission are observed. Primary CMV infection develops in a CMV-seronegative individual who receives blood products and/or an organ from a seropositive donor or acquires de novo infection from a community source. Secondary CMV infection or reactivation occurs when latent CMV re-

Crippin JS, McCashland T, Terrault N, et al. A pilot study of the tolerability and efficacy of antiviral therapy in hepatitis C virus-infected patients awaiting liver transplantation. Liver Transpl 2002; 8:350–355.

Everson G. Treatment of patients with hepatitis C virus on the waiting list. Liver Transpl 2003; 9:S90–94.

Forman LM, Lewis JD, Berlin JA, et al. The association between hepatitis C infection and survival after orthotopic liver transplantation. Gastroenterology 2002; 122:889–896.

Garcia-Retortillo M, Forns X, Feliu A, et al. Hepatitis C virus kinetics during and immediately after liver transplantation. Hepatology 2002; 35:680–687.

Manzarbeitia C, Tepermann L, Chalasani. N, et al. 40 kDa peginterferon as prophylaxis against HCV recurrence after liver transplantation: Preliminary results of a randomized, multicenter trial. Hepatology 2001; 34:406A.

McCaughan G, Zekry A. Impact of immunosuppression on immunopathogenesis of liver damage in hepatitis C virus-infected recipients following liver transplantation. Liver Transpl 2003; 9:S21–27.

McTaggart R, Terrault N, Vardanian A, et al. Hepatitis C etiology of liver disease is strongly associated with early acute rejection following liver transplantation. Liver Transpl 2004; 10:975–985.

Rosen HR, Madden JP, Martin P. A model to predict survival following liver retransplantation. Hepatology 1999; 29:365–370.

Saab S, Ly D, Han S, et al. Is it cost-effective to treat recurrent hepatitis C infection in orthotopic liver transplantation patients? Liver Transpl 2002; 8(5):449–457.

Samuel D, Bizollon T, Feray C, et al. Interferon- α2b plus ribavirin in patients with chronic hepatitis C after liver transplantation: a randomized study. Gastroenterology 2003; 124:642–650. *The first randomized controlled study of interferon and ribavirin in liver transplant recipients with recurrent HCV infection. Tolerability of full-dose therapy was limited with discontinuation of treatment in 43% and the sustained response rates with 48 weeks treatment was only 21%.*

Terrault N. Prophylactic and preemptive therapies for hepatitis C virus-infected patients undergoing liver transplantation. Liver Transpl 2003; 9:S95–100.

Vargas HE, Laskus T, Wang LF, et al. Outcome of liver transplantation in hepatitis C virus-infected patients who received hepatitis C virus-infected grafts. Gastroenterology 1999; 117:149–153.

Velidedeoglu E, Desai NM, Campos L, et al. The outcome of liver grafts procured from hepatitis C-positive donors. Transplantation 2002; 73(4):582–587.

Other viral agents and general transplantation issues

Barkholt LM, Dahl H, Enbom M, et al. Epstein-Barr virus DNA in serum after liver transplantation – surveillance of viral activity during treatment with different immunosuppressive agents. Transpl Int 1996; 9(5):439–445.

Basgoz N, Preiksatis J. Post-transplant lymphoproliferative disorder. J Infect Dis North Am 1995; 9:901–923.

Burak KW, Kremers WK, Batts KP et al. Impact of cytomegalovirus infection, year of transplantation, and donor age on outcomes after liver transplantation for hepatitis C. Liver Transpl 2002; 8(4):362–369.

Clark D. Human herpesvirus 6 and human herpesvirus 7: emerging pathogens in transplant patients. Int J Hematol 2002; 76:246–252.

Couchoud C. Cytomegalovirus prophylaxis with antiviral agents for solid organ transplantation. Cochrane Database Syst Rev 2000; 2:CD001320.

Evans P. An association between cytomegalovirus infection and chronic rejection after liver transplantation. Transplantation 2000; 69:30–35.

Falagas M, Snydman D, Ruthazer R, et al. Effect of cytomegalovirus infection status on first-year mortality rates among orthotopic liver transplant recipients. The Boston Center for Liver Transplantation (CMVIG) Study Group. Ann Intern Med 1997; 126:275–279.

Freeman R. Valganciclovir: oral prevention and treatment of cytomegalovirus immunocompromised host. Expert Opin Pharmacother 2004; 5:2007–2016.

Gane E, Saliba F, Valdecasas GJ, et al. Randomised trial of efficacy and safety of oral ganciclovir in the prevention of cytomegalovirus disease in liver-transplant recipients. The Oral Ganciclovir International Transplantation Study Group [corrected]. Lancet 1997; 350(9093):1729–1733.

Griffiths P, Ait-Khaled M, Bearcroft C, et al. Human herpes viruses 6 and 7 as potential pathogens after liver transplant: prospective comparison with the effect of cytomegalovirus. J Med Virol 1999; 59:496–501.

Herrero J, Quiroga J, Sangro B, et al. Herpes zoster after liver transplantation: incidence, risk factors, and complications. Liver Transpl 2004; 10:1140–1143.

Krieger NR, Martinez OM, Krams SM, et al. Significance of detecting Epstein-Barr-specific sequences in the peripheral blood of asymptomatic pediatric liver transplant recipients. Liver Transpl 2000; 6(1):62–66.

McGrath D, Falagas M, Freeman R, et al. Adenovirus infection in adult orthotopic liver transplant recipients: incidence and clinical significance. J Infect Dis 1998; 177:459–462.

Pereyra F, Rubin R. Prevention and treatment of cytomegalovirus infection in solid organ transplant recipients. Curr Opin Infect Dis 2004; 17:357–361. *Comprehensive review of the natural history of CMV infection in transplant recipients, risk factors for disease, monitoring strategies and treatment options.*

Razonable R, Paya C. The impact of human herpesvirus-6 and -7 infection on the outcome of liver transplantation. Liver Transpl 2002; 8:651–658.

Razonable R, Paya C. Herpesvirus infections in transplant recipients: current challenges in the clinical management of cytomegalovirus and Epstein-Barr virus infections. Herpes 2003; 10:60–65.

Samuel D, Feray C, Bismuth H. Hepatitis viruses and liver transplantation. J Gastroenterol Hepatol 1997; 12(9–10):S335–341.

Seehofer D, Rayes N, Tullius S, et al. CMV hepatitis after liver transplantation: incidence, clinical course, and long-term follow-up. Liver Transpl 2002; 8:1138–1146.

Singh N, Dummer JS, Kusne S, et al. Infections with cytomegalovirus and other herpesviruses in 121 liver transplant recipients: transmission by donated organ and the effect of OKT3 antibodies. J Infect Dis 1988; 158(1):124–131.

Index

abdominal compartment
    (compression) syndrome,
    607–8, 617
abdominal discomfort, 61–2
abdominal examination, 68–9
abdominal pain, 61
    biliary colic, 437
    in cholecystitis, 440
    in fatty liver disease, 334
    in hepatocellular carcinoma,
        456
    in porphyria, 371
abdominal trauma, 578
abdominal wall, prominent veins,
    68–9
abetalipoproteinemia, 330–1
ABO incompatible liver grafts, in
    acute liver failure, 529
abscesses, liver, 256–9
    amebic, 258–9
    in ascariasis, 260
    in echinococcosis, 256–8
    in listeriosis, 250, 251
    in melioidosis, 251
    post-liver transplant, 650
    pyogenic, 577–8
    tuberculous, 255
absorption, in cirrhosis, 178
acamprosate, 319
acanthocytosis, 201
acetaldehyde, 312, 313, 314
acetaminophen (paracetamol)
    biotransformation, 508–9
    dose
        in hepatitis A, 207
        in NAFLD, 188, 339
    hepatotoxicity, 55, 508–9
        in alcoholics, 313, 519
        in childhood, 409
        clinical features, 520, 521
        pathogenesis, 500, 508–9
        risk factors, 499, 508
    induced acute liver failure,
        519
        clinical features, 520, 521
        liver transplantation, 528,
            532
        management, 527–8
        prognostic indicators, 526
    overdose, 508
        indications for referral, 525
        jaundice, 89
        management, 527–8

acetate, 312, 313
acetazolamide, 50
acetic acid injection,
    percutaneous ablation, 133
acetoacetate, 329
acetone, 329
acetyl-coenzyme A (acetyl-CoA),
    29, 329
acetylation rate, isoniazid, 508
aciclovir, 653, 666, 687
acid–base disturbances, in acute
    liver failure, 521
acid lipase, 387
    deficiency, 387
acinus, hepatic, 6, 7, 45–6
    complex, 6
    simple, 6, 7
    zone 1 see periportal region
    zone 2 see mid-zonal area
    zone 3 see perivenular region
    zones, 6, 7, 12, 45–6
ackee fruit, unripe, 330, 333
acrodermatitis, 183
    Gianotti papular, 216
actin, 9–10, 24–5, 44–5
activated partial thromboplastin
    time (APTT), 199
acute fatty liver of pregnancy
    (AFLP), 490–1
    acute liver failure, 519
    clinical features, 490–1
    diagnosis, 494
    jaundice, 90
    liver biopsy, 102, 491
    pathogenesis, 330, 333, 490
    prognosis, 495
    treatment, 495
acute hepatitis
    acute liver failure, 518
    histology, 104, 105
    in listeriosis, 250
    in pediatric patients, 406, 416
    in pregnancy, 492
    in Wilson disease, 354–5
    see also specific types
acute intermittent porphyria
    (AIP), 370, 371
acute liver allograft rejection see
    under rejection, liver
    allograft
acute liver failure, 517–36
    in childhood, 413, 416–17
    causes, 416–17, 520

clinical features, 417
liver transplantation, 417,
    418, 419
    management, 417
clinical features, 72, 520–2
definitions, 517
diagnosis, 522–3, 524, 525
drug-induced, 497, 519
in Epstein–Barr virus infection,
    253
etiology, 72, 518–20
hepatic encephalopathy, 169,
    173, 520
in hepatitis B, 215, 216,
    518–19
    and hepatitis D co-infection,
        231, 518
in hepatitis C, 239, 519
in hepatitis E in pregnancy,
    210, 211, 212, 519
of indeterminate etiology see
    seronegative hepatitis
in infancy, 413–16
King's College criteria, 525–6,
    529
liver transplantation, 527,
    528–32
    auxiliary, 530–1, 619
    bridging measures, 527, 528
    in childhood, 417, 418, 419
    grafts and graft allocation,
        528–9
    indications, 586
    numbers of operations, 585,
        587
    operative techniques, 530–2
    patient selection, 529–30
    results, 532
in lymphoma, 520, 523, 546
management, 527–36
nutritional management,
    185–7, 536
pathogenesis, 518–20
in pregnancy, 495, 519–20
prognosis, 523–7
in Wilson disease, 354–5, 365,
    520, 523
acute sickle hepatic crisis
    (ASHC), 541
acyl coenzyme A (acyl-CoA), 329
acyl coenzyme A (acyl-CoA):
    cholesterol acyltransferase,
    53

adefovir dipivoxil
    HBV resistance, 674
    in hepatitis B, 224, 225–7
        lamivudine combination, 229
        lamivudine-resistant HBV,
            225, 226
        post-transplant recurrence,
            226–7, 594–5, 678, 679
        pretransplant prophylaxis,
            672–4, 677
adenocarcinomas, metastatic, 469
adenomas
    bile duct, 115, 426–7
    liver cell see hepatocellular
        adenomas
adenovirus infections,
    post-transplant, 653, 669,
    688
adherens (intermediate)
    junctions, 22, 44
adrenal nest tumors, 433
Adriamycin see doxorubicin
aflatoxins, 455–6, 513–14
AFP see α-fetoprotein
African iron overload, 341, 373
age, liver transplant recipients,
    532, 591
AIDS see HIV infection/AIDS
AIH see autoimmune hepatitis
AIRE gene mutations, 270
Alagille syndrome, 65, 403–4
    liver transplantation, 403–4,
        603
alanine aminotransferase (ALT),
    serum, 74
    in alcoholic liver disease, 75,
        315
    causes of raised, 75–7
    evaluation of isolated mild
        elevation, 73, 74, 77
    interpretation of raised, 74–5
    in jaundice, 94
albumin
    ascitic fluid, 155
    bilirubin binding, 50
    fatty acid transport, 328
    infusion
        in hepatorenal syndrome, 163
        in spontaneous bacterial
            peritonitis, 162, 165,
            166
        with therapeutic
            paracentesis, 157

albumin *(Continued)*
  serum, 79
    in jaundice, 94
    liver transplant candidates,
      418
    in pregnancy, 487
    reduced *see*
      hypoalbuminemia
  synthesis, 56
  thyroid hormone binding, 538
alcohol (ethanol), 311–13
  abstinence, 319–20, 323
    liver transplant recipients,
      324, 597
  content of beverages, 311
  enzyme induction, 498
  metabolism, 312–13
  nutritional effects, 178, 185
  percutaneous injection, 133
    in hepatocellular carcinoma,
      465–6
  in porphyrias, 370, 377, 378
  toxic effects on mitochondria,
    313–14, 333
alcohol abuse *see* alcoholism
alcohol consumption, 311–12
  assessment, 315
  cirrhosis risk and, 311–12
  hepatitis C and, 317
  hepatocellular carcinoma and,
    317
  liver allograft recipients, 665
  per capita, 311, 312
alcohol dehydrogenase, 312–13
alcoholic cirrhosis (and fibrosis),
  311
  alcohol consumption and, 312
  cardiomyopathy, 194–5
  clinical features and diagnosis,
    316–17
  liver transplantation, 324,
    596–7
    numbers of operations, 587
    timing, 589–90
  pathology, 319
  pathophysiology, 314–15
  treatment, 323–4
  vs hepatic encephalopathy, 174
alcoholic fatty liver (steatosis),
  311
  clinical features and diagnosis,
    315
  pathology, 318
  pathophysiology, 313, 332–3
  treatment, 319–20
alcoholic foamy degeneration,
  315, 318
alcoholic hepatitis, 311
  clinical features, 91, 315
  diagnosis, 315–16
  hepatorenal syndrome
    prevention, 162, 322
  liver transplantation, 597
  Maddrey Discriminant
    Function (DF), 320

nutritional management, 185,
  320, 321, 322
pathology, 318–19
pathophysiology, 313–14
treatment, 320–3
alcoholic liver disease, 311–25
  alcohol use and risk, 311–12
  clinical features and diagnosis,
    69–70, 315–17
  hematologic changes, 201
  hepatitis C and, 317
  hepatocellular carcinoma, 317
  histopathology, 114, 318–19
  iron abnormalities, 348
  jaundice, 89, 90, 315
  liver transplantation, 324,
    596–7
  malnutrition, 177–8, 315
  natural history, 319
  osteoporosis, 196
  pathophysiology, 313–15
  post-transplant recurrence, 661
  serum aminotransferases, 75,
    315, 316
  treatment, 319–24
alcoholism (alcohol abuse/
  dependence)
  acetaminophen toxicity, 313,
    519
  assessment, 315
  CAGE questions, 315
  hepatitis B, 217
  management, 319, 320
  natural history, 319–20
aldehyde dehydrogenase, 312–13
aldolase B, 387–8, 410
aldosterone, raised, in ascites,
  153, 156
alendronate, 197
alkaline phosphatase (ALP),
  serum, 77–9
  in alcoholic liver disease, 315
  causes of low, 78
  causes of raised, 73, 78
  in cystic fibrosis, 384, 412
  evaluation of isolated mild
    elevation, 78
  in jaundice, 93–4
  in neonatal liver disease, 398,
    401, 403
  normal/abnormal ranges, 74
  in pregnancy, 487
  in primary sclerosing
    cholangitis, 292
  in steatosis and NASH, 335
alkaline phosphatase–total
    bilirubin ratio, in fulminant
    Wilson disease, 355, 357
alkaloids, hepatotoxic, 512
alkaptonuria, 386
alkylating agents, 512
alloantigen recognition, 629–30
allograft rejection, liver *see*
  rejection, liver allograft
allograft tolerance, liver, 640–1

ALP *see* alkaline phosphatase
Alpers disease, 333, 416
α-fetoprotein (AFP)
  in childhood liver tumors, 412,
    468
  in chronic hepatitis B, 216
  fetal production, 1
  in hepatocellular carcinoma,
    459–60, 571
  in hereditary tyrosinemia type
    1, 385
α tocopherol *see* vitamin E
α$_1$-antitrypsin (A$_1$AT), 378
  genotypes, 378–9
  immunostaining, 103
  serum, 379, 381
α$_1$-antitrypsin deficiency, 378–81
  clinical features, 379
  diagnosis, 379–81, 402
  differential diagnosis, 263
  epidemiology, 378–9
  laboratory diagnosis, 77
  liver histology, 112, 379, 380,
    381, 402
  liver transplantation, 381, 421,
    601
  neonatal hepatitis, 401, 402
  pathophysiology, 378–9, 380
  in pediatric patients, 405
  treatment, 381, 402
ALT *see* alanine aminotransferase
Amanita phalloides poisoning,
  513, 520, 528
amatoxins, 49, 513
amebiasis, 258–9
American Association for the
    Study of Liver Diseases
    (AASLD), Wilson disease
    guideline, 361
amiloride, 50
  in ascites, 156, 157
amineptine, 333
amino acids
  aromatic/branched-chain ratio,
    172, 175
  in bile, 47
  branched-chain (BCAA)
    enriched formulations, 183,
      188
    in hepatic encephalopathy,
      175, 185, 187
  fatty acid synthesis from,
    329
  metabolism
    in cirrhosis, 178–9
    zonation, 58
  non-essential, 185
5-aminolevulinic acid (ALA),
  369, 385
5-aminolevulinic acid (ALA)
    dehydratase
  deficiency (ADDP) (severe),
    370–1
  inhibition, tyrosinemia type 1,
    370, 385, 386

δ aminolevulinic acid (ALA)
    synthase, 369
aminopyrine breath test, 80
aminotransferases, serum, 73,
    74–7
  in alcoholic liver disease, 75,
    315, 316
  in fatty liver disease, 74, 75,
    76, 334–5
  in hepatitis A, 207, 208
  in hepatitis B, 216
  in hepatitis E, 211
  interpretation, 74–5
  isolated mild elevation, 73, 74
  in jaundice, 94
  liver graft function and, 644
  in neonatal liver disease, 398,
    401
  in pregnancy, 487
  in primary biliary cirrhosis, 280
  in primary sclerosing
    cholangitis, 292
  in thyroid disease, 538
amiodarone
  hepatotoxicity, 334, 510, 511,
    516
  in NAFLD, 188
amitriptyline, 506
ammonia
  hepatic encephalopathy
    pathogenesis, 170–2, 173,
      520
  metabolism, 56, 170
    in liver disease, 171
    zonation, 58
  neurotoxic effects, 171–2
  serum
    elevated levels *see*
      hyperammonemia
    measurement, 174
ammonium tetrathiomolybdate,
    in Wilson disease, 361, 362
amoxicillin-clavulanic acid, 166,
    507
amphotericin, 249, 250, 651
ampicillin, 507
ampulla of Vater, 12, 14
amyl alcohol test, 375
amylo-1,4→1,6 transglucosidase
    deficiency, 389, 390
amylo-1,6-glucosidase deficiency,
    389, 390, 410
amyloidosis, 541–2
  familial, with polyneuropathy
    (FAP), 541, 603
  jaundice, 91
  liver biopsy, 104
  sinusoidal infiltration, 484
anabolic steroids
  in alcoholic hepatitis, 321,
    322
  hepatocellular adenoma and,
    424
  hepatotoxicity, 91, 504–5
analgesics, hepatotoxic, 508–10

anatomy, liver, 3–14
Elias three-dimensional model, 5, 6
functional organization, 5–6, 7, 17, 18
gross, 3–6
intrahepatic organization, 5, 6
microscopic, and ultrastructure, 6–14
segmental *see* segments, liver
surgical resection and, 567
vessels and functional anatomy, 3–5
ANCA *see* anti-neutrophil cytoplasmic antibodies
Andersen disease (glycogen storage disease II), 389, 390, 410
anemia
in acute liver failure, 522
causing jaundice, 86
in childhood liver tumors, 412
iron overload, 341, 342
in liver disease, 200–1
in non-cirrhotic portal fibrosis, 552
see also hemolytic anemia
anesthetic agents, hepatotoxic, 512–13
anesthetist, in liver transplant surgery, 605, 609
angiography, 132
in Budd-Chiari syndrome, 481
in focal nodular hyperplasia, 431
hemangiomas, 428
hepatocellular adenomas, 425
hepatocellular carcinoma, 462
infantile hemangioendothelioma, 429
in non-cirrhotic portal hypertension, 553, 555, 561, 563
angiomyolipoma, histopathology, 115
angioplasty
in Budd-Chiari syndrome, 481–2
portal vein, 478
angiosarcoma, 467–8
differential diagnosis, 429
histopathology, 116, 117
angiotensin-converting enzyme (ACE) inhibitors, 510, 662
anorexia, 61, 178
anthropomorphic measures, 181
anti-anginal agents, hepatotoxic, 511
anti-gp210 antibodies, 278, 281
anti-liver-kidney microsomal antibodies *see* liver–kidney microsomal (LKM) antibodies
anti-M2 antibodies, in primary biliary cirrhosis, 277–8, 281

anti-neutrophil cytoplasmic antibodies (ANCA)
in autoimmune hepatitis, 268–9
cytoplasmic (cANCA), 268
perinuclear (pANCA)
in autoimmune hepatitis, 268–9, 293
in primary sclerosing cholangitis, 291, 293
anti-smooth muscle antibodies (anti-SMA)
in autoimmune hepatitis, 266, 267
in primary sclerosing cholangitis, 293
anti-soluble liver antigen/liver pancreas (SLA/LP) antibodies, 267–8, 271
anti-Sp100 antibodies, 278, 281
anti-tumor necrosis factor (TNF) therapy, alcoholic hepatitis, 321, 322
antiarrhythmic agents, hepatotoxic, 510–11
antibiotics
in acute cholangitis, 441
in acute liver failure, 534–5
in alcoholic liver disease, 320
in brucellosis, 252
in hepatic encephalopathy, 175
hepatotoxic, 506–8
in leptospirosis, 254
in listeriosis, 251
in melioidosis, 251
post-liver transplant prophylaxis, 532, 651
in primary sclerosing cholangitis, 298
in spontaneous bacterial peritonitis, 166–7
in syphilis, 255
antibodies
in allograft rejection, 630, 649
autoreactive *see* autoantibodies
immunosuppressive monoclonal (mAbs), 632, 633
xenoreactive, 640
anticentromere antibodies, 278, 282, 540
anticoagulation
in acute liver failure, 535
in Budd-Chiari syndrome, 481
in portal vein thrombosis, 478, 563–5
anticonvulsant (antiepileptic) drugs
acetaminophen toxicity and, 519
in acute liver failure, 534
hepatotoxicity, 505–6
P450 induction, 498
antidepressants, 506
antifibrinolytic agents, 200

antifibrotic therapy
in primary sclerosing cholangitis, 306
see also colchicine
antifungal agents
in acute liver failure, 535
hepatotoxicity, 507–8
in liver transplant recipients, 532, 651
antigen-presenting cells (APCs), 621
in alloantigen recognition, 629–30
T cell interaction, 626–7, 628
antigen recognition, T cell, 624–5
antihelminthic agents, 260
antihistamines, for pruritus, 99
antihyperlipidemic agents, hepatotoxic, 511
antihypertensive agents
hepatotoxic, 510
in liver allograft recipients, 662
antilymphocyte globulins (ALGs), 632, 633
antimalarial agents, in porphyria cutanea tarda, 377
antimetabolites, hepatotoxic, 511–12
antimitochondrial antibodies (AMA)
in primary biliary cirrhosis, 277–8, 280, 281
in primary sclerosing cholangitis, 293
antinuclear antibodies (ANA), 278
in autoimmune hepatitis, 265–6
in primary biliary cirrhosis, 278, 281
in primary sclerosing cholangitis, 293
antioxidants
in alcoholic hepatitis, 321, 322–3
in NASH, 339
in neonatal hemochromatosis, 414
in Wilson disease, 363
antiphospholipid antibodies, 540
nodular regenerative hyperplasia and, 565
antiphospholipid syndrome (APS), 540
portal vein thrombosis/ Budd-Chiari syndrome, 476, 481
sinusoidal dilatation, 483
antipurines, hepatotoxicity, 511–12
antipyrimidines, hepatotoxic, 512
antithrombin III, 56, 198
deficiency, 476–7, 478, 559
therapy in acute liver failure, 535

antithymocyte globulins (ATGs), 632
antithyroid therapy
in alcoholic liver disease, 321, 322, 324
hepatotoxicity, 538, 539
antituberculous agents, hepatotoxic, 508
antiviral agents
in cytomegalovirus disease, 252, 652–3
in hepatitis B, 224–8, 593–5, 672–9
in hepatitis C, 244–6, 682–4
hepatotoxic, 512
see also specific agents
Apaf-1, 38
apical sodium-dependent bile acid transporter (ASBT), 52
aplastic anemia, in acute liver failure, 522
apoceruloplasmin, 353, 357
apolipoprotein B-48 (apoB-48), 330–1, 332
apolipoprotein B-100 (apoB-100), 330, 332
gene mutations, 330–1, 339
partial loss of function, 76, 331
polymorphisms, 332
synthesis, 330
apolipoprotein E (apoE), 332
polymorphisms, 332
apoptosis
hepatic stellate cells, 40
hepatocyte, 37–9
in alcoholic liver disease, 314, 318
in liver allograft tolerance, 641
liver regeneration and, 39
signaling pathways, 37–8
T cell-mediated, 628–9
apoptosome, 38
aprotinin, 200, 608
arginine vasopressin (AVP), 159–60
arsenic, 513, 550
arterial vasodilation theory
ascites, 153–4
hepatorenal syndrome, 161–2
arteriography, hepatic, 132
arterioportal fistula, solitary, 475
arteriovenous fistulae, in hereditary hemorrhagic telangiectasia, 475–6
arthrogryposis, cholestasis, renal tubular dysfunction (ARC), 404
arthropathies/arthralgias, in primary biliary cirrhosis, 282
ascariasis, 260
ascites, 153–8
in alcoholic cirrhosis, 316
antimicrobial activity of fluid, 164
classification, 154

ascites (Continued)
  clinical features, 61–2, 69, 154–5
  in congestive heart failure, 543–4
  definition, 153
  diagnostic approach, 155–6
  diuretic-intractable, 158
  diuretic-resistant, 158
  in extrahepatic portal vein obstruction, 560
  fluid evaluation, 155
  hepatorenal syndrome risk factors, 163
  in hypothyroidism, 539
  nutritional assessment and, 181–2
  pathogenesis, 153–4
  post-liver transplantation, 643
  in primary sclerosing cholangitis, 300
  prognosis, 158, 159
  refractory, 154, 157–8
  spontaneous bacterial peritonitis, 153, 164–7
  treatment, 156–8
ascorbic acid (vitamin C), 183
asialoglycoprotein (ASGP) receptors (ASGPR), 33
  autoantibodies, 268
L-asparaginase, 512
aspartate aminotransferase (AST), serum, 74
  in alcoholic liver disease, 75, 315
  causes of elevated, 75–6
  evaluation of isolated mild elevation, 73, 74, 77
  interpretation of raised, 74–5
  in jaundice, 94
aspartate aminotransferase: alanine aminotransferase (AST:ALT) ratio, 75, 94
  in alcoholic liver disease, 75, 315, 316
  in NASH, 334–5
Aspergillus infections, 651
aspirin
  in hepatopulmonary syndrome, 193
  hepatotoxicity, 333, 409, 509
  in liver transplant surgery, 608–9
associated systemic conditions, 191–203
Association for the Study of Liver Disease (AASLD), hepatitis B guidance, 229, 230
AST see aspartate aminotransferase
asterixis, 70, 174
astrocytes
  Alzheimer type II, 170
  ammonia-induced damage, 171

changes in hepatic encephalopathy, 170
atelectasis, post-liver transplant, 643
atherosclerosis-like lesions, in chronic allograft rejection, 639
atox1, 353
ATP7B (Wilson disease protein), 351, 352–3
auscultation, abdominal, 69
autoantibodies
  in autoimmune hepatitis, 265–9, 293
    post-transplant, 274
  in drug-induced liver disease, 263, 267, 268, 501
  in primary biliary cirrhosis, 266, 277–8
    post-transplant, 274
  in primary sclerosing cholangitis, 291, 293
  in viral hepatitis, 271
autoimmune cholangitis (AIC)
  liver biopsy, 107–8, 109
  vs autoimmune hepatitis, 271
  see also overlap syndromes
autoimmune disorders
  autoimmune hepatitis-associated, 270
  non-cirrhotic portal fibrosis and, 551
  post-transplant recurrence, 659–60
  primary sclerosing cholangitis-associated, 300–2
  see also autoantibodies; specific disorders
autoimmune hemolytic anemia, giant cell hepatitis with, 421
autoimmune hepatitis (AIH), 263–75
  acute liver failure, 520
  autoantibodies, 265–9, 293
  in childhood, 271, 405, 407–8, 416–17
  cirrhosis, 271, 597
  clinical features, 270
  definition, 265
  diagnosis, 264, 265, 407–8
  differential diagnosis, 92, 263, 281–2
  epidemiology, 265
  etiology, 207, 269–70
  extrahepatic associations, 270, 539
  liver graft dysfunction mimicking, 660
  liver histology, 105, 106, 265
  liver transplantation, 274, 597
  natural history and prognosis, 271–2
  overlap syndromes, 271
  pathogenesis, 265

post-transplant
    de novo development, 421, 660
    recurrence, 421, 659–60
  pregnancy in, 492
  primary sclerosing cholangitis and, 301–2
  relapse, 273
  remission, 273
  stabilization, 273
  subclassification, 270–1
  systemic lupus erythematosus and, 539
  treatment, 272–4, 408
    failure, 273
  type 1, 265, 270–1, 407
  type 2, 265, 271, 407
  type 3, 265, 271
autoimmune polyendocrine syndrome (APECED), 270
  autoantibodies, 267, 268, 270
autonomic dysfunction, in extrahepatic portal vein obstruction, 561
autumn fever, 253
auxiliary liver transplantation, 605
  in acute liver failure, 530–1, 619
  heterotopic technique, 619
  operative technique, 618–19
  orthotopic technique, 530, 619
  in pediatric patients, 419
avascular necrosis, in primary sclerosing cholangitis, 297–8
azathioprine, 630
  in autoimmune hepatitis, 272–3, 408
  drug interactions, 633–4
  hepatotoxicity, 482, 511–12
  mechanism of action, 630
  in pregnancy, 492
  in primary biliary cirrhosis, 285
  in primary sclerosing cholangitis, 306
  side-effects, 273, 633–4
azygous vein, 138

B cells, 621
B7 (CD80/CD86), 626–7, 628
Bacillus cereus emetic toxin, 333
bacteremia, post-liver transplant, 651
bacteria
  intestinal
    hepatic encephalopathy pathogenesis, 170, 172
    translocation into systemic circulation, 164
  in primary biliary cirrhosis etiology, 278
  in primary sclerosing cholangitis etiology, 289–90
bacterial infections
  in acute liver failure, 522, 534–5

jaundice, 91
  non-cirrhotic portal fibrosis and, 550
  post-liver transplant, 650–1
  susceptibility in liver disease, 64–5, 201
  systemic, with hepatic manifestations, 250–2
  see also sepsis; spontaneous bacterial peritonitis
balloon cells see hepatocytes, ballooning
balloon tamponade, bleeding varices, 144, 147
band ligation, variceal see endoscopic variceal band ligation
Bantus, South African, 373
barbiturates
  in cerebral edema, 533
  see also phenobarbital
bare area, 3, 4
Bartonella infections, 255, 483
basal ganglia, in hepatic encephalopathy, 172–3
basement membrane
  formation in cirrhosis, 44
  lack of, 33, 39, 43–4
BCS see Budd-Chiari syndrome
Behçet disease, 476
Bengal splenomegaly, 549
benign liver tumors, 423–34
  of childhood, 413
  epithelial, 424–7
  histologic classification, 423
  histopathology, 114–15
  investigation and management, 423
  non-epithelial, 427–30
  radiology, 129, 423–4
  surgical management, 573–4
  tumor-like lesions, 430–4
β blockers
  hepatotoxicity, 511
  in liver allograft recipients, 662
  portal hypotensive effects, 142
  prevention of variceal rebleeding, 148–9
  primary prevention of variceal bleeding, 145, 146, 150
β-carotene, in protoporphyria, 378
β_2-microglobulin (β_2m), 623
  in antigen recognition, 624
  HFE protein interaction, 342, 343
betaine, in NAFLD, 188, 339
bevacizumab, 470
beverages, alcoholic, 311
bicarbonate (HCO_3^-)
  secretion into bile, 51, 52
  transport, 49–50
bile
  cholesterol supersaturation, 436

bile *(Continued)*
  composition, 46–7
  enterohepatic circulation, 52, 54
  formation, 12, 46–52, 53
    bile acid transport, 48–9
    bilirubin metabolism and transport, 50–1
    ductular events, 51, 52
    electrolyte and solute transport, 46–50
    fetus, 1
    gallbladder function, 51–2
    newly transplanted liver, 643–4
    zonation, 57
  gallbladder function, 51–2
  gallstone formation, 436
  intrahepatic transport, 44
bile acid(s), 47
  canalicular secretion, 49
  conjugated, 47
  enterohepatic circulation, 52, 54
  metabolism, 47, 48
  primary, 47, 48
  in primary sclerosing cholangitis etiology, 290
  secondary, 47, 48, 52
  serum, in primary biliary cirrhosis, 280
  synthesis, 52
    inherited disorders, 401, 404
  therapy of gallstones, 438
  transport, 48–9
  see also ursodeoxycholic acid
bile acid-dependent bile flow (BADBF), 48–9
bile acid diarrhea, idiopathic, 52
bile acid-independent bile flow (BAIBF), 48, 49–50
bile canaliculi, 12, 14
  bile acid secretion, 49
  bile plugs, 107, 108
  development, 1
  hepatocyte relations, 7, 22, 44
  microscopic anatomy, 7, 8, 9
  structural organization, 5, 6, 17
bile duct(s)
  adenomas, 115, 426–7
  anastomoses
    in liver transplantation, 614, 616, 618
    stenotic complications, 620, 657
  cystadenomas, 426
  development, 1, 3
  epithelial cells, 12, 13
    in cysts of polycystic disease, 444
    secretory activity, 51, 52
  extrahepatic
    anatomy, 12, 14
    arterial supply, 14
    development, 1, 17

extrinsic compression, 92
  primary sclerosing cholangitis, 293, 294
  fibrous stenoses *see* biliary strictures
  interlobular, 12, 13, 14, 44
    in allograft rejection, 636, 638, 639
    paucity *see* ductopenia
  intrahepatic
    anatomy, 5, 6, 87
    Caroli disease, 449–50
    destruction in PBC, 278–9, 280, 281
    development, 1, 17
    drug-induced destruction, 504
    hypoplasia, 402–4
    microscopy, 12, 13
    primary sclerosing cholangitis, 293, 294
  ischemic injury, 473–4
  microhamartomas, 426–7, 447
  obstruction *see* biliary obstruction
  paucity *see* ductopenia
  portal biliopathy, 561, 563, 564
  septal, 12, 13
  spontaneous perforation, 400
  stones *see* choledocholithiasis
bile ductules, 12, 14
  disorders causing jaundice, 91
  secretory activity, 51, 52
bile infarcts, 107, 108, 474
bile leaks
  live donor graft recipients, 620
  pediatric liver transplantation, 420
  post-liver transplantation, 648
bile plugs
  canalicular, 107, 108
  zone 1 canals of Hering, 107
bile salt export pump (bsep), 49, 404
bile salts *see* bile acid(s)
biliary atresia, 398–9
  clinical features, 398
  diagnosis, 398, 399
  liver transplantation, 399, 417, 603
  management, 398–9
biliary cirrhosis
  in cystic fibrosis, 382, 384
  primary *see* primary biliary cirrhosis
  in sarcoidosis, 542
  secondary, liver transplantation, 593
biliary colic, 437
biliary disease, 435–42
  in cystic fibrosis, 382–3
  extrahepatic, in neonates, 398–400

in extrahepatic portal vein obstruction, 561, 562, 563, 564
  imaging, 130–1
  jaundice, 92
  post-liver transplantation, 648–9, 657–8
  in pregnancy, 494
biliary dyskinesis, postcholecystectomy, 438–9
biliary hypoplasia, intrahepatic, 402–4
biliary obstruction
  biliary reconstruction surgery, 580
  differential diagnosis, 92, 93
  in extrahepatic portal vein obstruction, 563
  imaging, 95–7, 131
  in inspissated bile syndrome, 400
  jaundice, 88, 92
  liver biopsy, 97–8
  in lymphoma, 545
  management, 98
  post-liver transplantation, 648–9, 657
  in primary sclerosing cholangitis, 298
  see also cholestasis/cholestatic liver disease, extrahepatic
biliary reconstruction surgery, 580–1, 582
  in living donor liver transplantation, 618
  in orthotopic liver transplantation, 614
  in primary sclerosing cholangitis, 307
  in reduced-size liver transplantation, 616
biliary sludge, 440
  in pregnancy, 491–2
biliary strictures (fibrous stenoses)
  after hepatic artery occlusion, 474
  biliary reconstruction surgery, 580–1
  in cystic fibrosis, 383
  post-liver transplantation, 420, 648–9, 657–8
  in primary sclerosing cholangitis, 293, 298
biliary system
  development, 1, 3
  intrahepatic, anatomy, 87
bilirubin
  conjugation, 51, 84
  excretion, 84, 86
  formation, 83, 84, 85
    disorders causing increased, 86–7
  metabolism, 50, 83–6
    inherited disorders, 51, 84–6, 87–8, 89

serum, 79, 83
    after liver transplantation, 644
    in alcoholic liver disease, 315, 316
    in jaundice, 62, 65
    liver transplant candidates, 418
    in primary biliary cirrhosis, 280, 283–4
    prognostic value, 79, 83
    see also hyperbilirubinemia
  transport, 50–1, 84
  unconjugated, measurement, 95
bilirubin diglucuronide transferase deficiency, 397
bilirubin-UDP-glucuronosyl-transferase (UDP-GT; bilirubin UGT-1), 51, 84
  deficiency, 84–6
  gene, 86
biliverdin, 83, 85
biliverdin reductase, 83, 85
bilomas, 474, 647
bioartificial liver (BAL), 528
bioelectrical impedence analysis (BIA), 181–2
biotin, 183
biotransformation, 53–5, 498
  zonation, 57, 58
bisphosphonates, 197, 297
bleeding *see* hemorrhage/bleeding
bleeding time, prolonged, 199, 201
bleomycin, 512
blood pressure
  in liver allograft recipients, 662
  in liver disease, 68
  see also hypertension
blood transfusion
  iron overload, 341
  massive, 87, 643
  viral hepatitis transmission, 206, 214, 237
body cell mass (BCM), assessment, 182
body mass index (BMI), 177
  liver transplant outcome and, 181
  see also obesity
bone disease
  in chronic liver disease, 195–8
  in Gaucher disease, 393–4, 395
  in liver allograft recipients, 664
  see also hepatic osteodystrophy
bone marrow transplantation (BMT), 120–1, 482–3
bone mineral density (BMD), 196
bosentan, 194
Bouveret syndrome, 437

bowel disease, in liver allograft recipients, 664
brachiocephalic vein, 138
brain
copper accumulation, in Wilson disease, 351
damage, in acute liver failure, 521, 523
edema *see* cerebral edema
imaging, in Wilson disease, 356
pathology, hepatic encephalopathy, 170
brain natriuretic peptide (BNP), 195
brainstem herniation, in acute liver failure, 521
breast cancer, in primary biliary cirrhosis, 283
bromocriptine, in hepatic encephalopathy, 175
brucellosis, 251–2, 255
bruising, easy, 65–6
bruits, hepatic arterial, 69, 315
Budd-Chiari syndrome (BCS), 479–82
acute liver failure, 520
caudate lobe hypertrophy, 5, 482
clinical features, 480
course and prognosis, 481
diagnosis, 480–1
etiology, 476, 479–80
hepatocellular carcinoma, 456, 481
imaging, 130, 480–1
jaundice, 89–90
liver histology, 109, 110, 480
liver transplantation, 600, 661
management, 481–2
pathogenesis, 479–80
pregnancy and, 492
secondary, 479
steroid-related, 505
budenoside, in autoimmune hepatitis, 273
Burkholderia pseudomallei, 251
Bush Tea, 514
busulfan, hepatotoxicity, 512
Byler disease *see* progressive familial intrahepatic cholestasis (PFIC), type 1

C-reactive protein, 515
cadherins, 44
caffeine breath test, 80
CAGE questions, 315
calcineurin, 625–6, 627
cyclosporin/tacrolimus actions, 631
inhibitors *see* cyclosporin; tacrolimus
calcitonin therapy, 197, 297
calcium
intracellular, 625–6

metabolism, abnormalities, 196–7
supplements, 197–8
calcium channel blockers, 194
in alcoholic hepatitis, 323
hepatotoxicity, 510–11
in liver allograft recipients, 662
caloric test, Gilbert syndrome, 87
CAMPATH-1, 632
canaliculi *see* bile canaliculi
canals of Hering (periportal cholangioles), 12, 14, 44
electron microscopy, 14
light microscopy, 13
three-dimensional organization, 5, 6
cancer *see* malignant disease
Candida albicans, 249, 651
Candida glabrata, 249
Candida tropicalis, 249
candidiasis
hepatosplenic (HSC), 249
in liver transplant recipients, 651
capsule of Glisson, 3
caput medusae, 69
carbamazepine, hepatotoxicity, 505, 506
carbamoylphosphate synthetase, 56
carbimazole, hepatotoxicity, 538, 539
carbohydrates
dietary requirements, in cirrhosis, 183, 184
hepatocyte cell coat, 22
metabolism, 55
in cirrhosis, 178–9
zonation, 56, 57
non-absorbable, in hepatic encephalopathy, 175
plasma membrane, 18, 20
carbon tetrachloride, 90, 513
carbonic anhydrase (CAH), 50, 51, 52
carcinoembryonic antigen (CEA), 460, 469
carcinoid syndrome, 470, 471
carcinoid tumors, metastatic, 470–1
pharmacological control, 471
prognosis, 470
surgical resection, 573
'cardiac cirrhosis,' 543–4
cardiac dysfunction
in acute liver failure, 522
in Alagille syndrome, 403
in cirrhosis, 194–5
in Wilson disease, 355
cardiomyopathy, 68
alcoholic, 195
cirrhotic, 194–5
cardiorespiratory dysfunction, 62, 191–5
liver transplantation, 609

see also pulmonary dysfunction
cardiovascular drugs, hepatotoxic, 510–11
cardiovascular examination, 68
cardiovascular risks, liver allograft recipients, 661–3
carnitine, 56, 329
shuttle, 329
carnitine palmitoyl transferase I (CPTI), 329, 330
deficiency, 330, 333
carnitine palmitoyl transferase II (CPTII), 329, 333
Caroli disease, 448, 449–50
liver transplantation, 600
Carrel patch, donor hepatic artery, 607, 613
caspases, 37, 38
caspofungin, 651
catenins, 44
caudate lobe, 3, 4
Couinaud functional segment, 5
hypertrophy, in Budd-Chiari syndrome, 5, 482
venous drainage, 4, 5
caveolae, 26–7, 28
cavernous hemangiomas *see* hemangiomas
CD3 complex, 625, 626
CD4, 626
CD4+ T cells, 621
in allograft rejection, 630, 636
antigen recognition, 624, 625
mechanisms of tissue injury, 629
in primary biliary cirrhosis, 277, 278
CD8, 626
CD8+ T cells, 621
in allograft rejection, 630, 636, 638, 639, 640
antigen recognition, 624–5
mechanisms of tissue injury, 628–9
see also cytotoxic T lymphocytes
CD28, 626–7, 628
CD40/CD40 ligand, 627
CD55, 640
CD59, 640
CD80/CD86 (B7), 626–7, 628
celiac disease
hepatic manifestations, 546
in primary biliary cirrhosis, 178, 282–3
cell cycle, 35–7
cell division, 30, 35
cell junctions, hepatocyte, 22, 44–5
cells
fetal liver, 17
non-parenchymal, 39–41
parenchymal *see* hepatocytes

relative numbers of different types, 17, 18
cellular biology, 17–41
central pontine myelinolysis, 170
central venules, lobular, 5, 7
centrilobular zone, 6, 7
drug-induced necrosis, 502–3
see also perivenular region
cephalosporins, in spontaneous bacterial peritonitis, 166
cerebral edema
in acute liver failure, 173, 521, 530
in childhood acute liver failure, 417
management, 533–4
cerebral perfusion pressure
in acute liver failure, 521, 533
during liver transplantation, 530
cerebrohepatorenal syndrome *see* Zellweger syndrome
ceruloplasmin
physiologic role, 353
serum, 356, 357, 358
charcoal
hemoperfusion, in acute liver failure, 527, 528
oral, in protoporphyria, 378
Charcot triad, 441
chelation therapy
in Wilson disease, 361–2
see also penicillamine
chemoembolization, hepatic artery *see* transcatheter arterial chemoembolization
chemokines, 623
chemotherapy
hepatoblastoma, 468
hepatocellular carcinoma, 466–7
intra-arterial, metastatic tumors, 470, 471
metastatic tumors, 470, 471
sinusoidal obstruction syndrome, 482
chenodeoxycholic acid, 47, 48
in cholelithiasis, 438
cherry red spots, esophageal varices, 141
chickenwire fibrosis, 113, 114, 318–19, 338
Child-Pugh grading of disease severity, 71
hepatocellular carcinoma therapy and, 461, 464
in primary sclerosing cholangitis, 305
Chinese herbal remedies, 514
chlorambucil, 512
chloride (Cl⁻) transport, 50, 51
chloroquine, in porphyria cutanea tarda, 377
chlorpromazine, 506

cholangiectasis, in primary
    sclerosing cholangitis, 293
cholangiocarcinoma (CCA)
    in choledochal cysts, 448
    histopathology, 116, 117
    liver transplantation, 299–300,
        592, 599
        recurrence after, 661
    in primary sclerosing
        cholangitis, 292, 293,
        298–300
cholangiocytes, 12, 44
    destruction, in PBC, 278–9
cholangiography
    post-liver transplantation, 645
    in primary sclerosing
        cholangitis, 289, 292, 293
    see also endoscopic retrograde
        cholangiopancreatography;
        magnetic resonance
        cholangiography;
        percutaneous transhepatic
        cholangiography
cholangiohepatocellular
    carcinoma, combined, 116
cholangitis
    acute, 441–2
        in biliary atresia, 398–9
        in primary sclerosing
            cholangitis, 298
    fibrous, 294
    fibrous obliterative, 294
    non-suppurative destructive,
        280, 281
    post-liver transplant, 650
    recurrent pyogenic
        after hepatic artery
            occlusion, 474
        in Caroli disease, 449
        in choledocholithiasis, 92
        in congenital hepatic
            fibrosis, 447–8
    sclerosing see sclerosing
        cholangitis
cholecystectomy
    in cholecystitis, 440–1
    in gallstone pancreatitis, 442
    indications, 438
    laparoscopic, 438, 439
    in liver transplant operation,
        614
    open, 438
    postcholecystectomy
        syndrome, 438–9
    prophylactic, asymptomatic
        gallstones, 437
    symptomatic gallstones, 438
cholecystitis
    acalculous, 440
    acute, 439–41
        diagnosis, 440
        imaging, 131, 132
        management, 440–1
    calculous, 440
    in neonates, 400

choledochal cysts, 399–400,
    448–9
choledochocholedochostomy
    alternative to, 608
    end-to-end technique, 614
choledochoduodenostomy, 580–1
choledochojejunostomy,
    Roux-en-Y, 608
choledocholithiasis
    acute cholangitis, 441
    in Caroli disease, 449
    diagnosis, 441
    endoscopic sphincterotomy,
        438
    in extrahepatic portal vein
        obstruction, 563
    gallstone pancreatitis, 442
    imaging, 130–1, 132
    jaundice, 92
    management, 441–2
    in primary sclerosing
        cholangitis, 298
choledochus see common bile
    duct
cholelithiasis see gallstones
cholestasis/cholestatic liver
    disease, 90–2
    in Alagille syndrome, 403
    benign postoperative, 91–2
    benign recurrent, 91
    bland, pure or canalicular, 503,
        504
    clinical features, 90
    differential diagnosis, 92, 93,
        295
    drug-induced, 282, 502, 503–4
    ductal, 504
    ductopenic, 504
    ductular or cholangiolar, 504
    extrahepatic (acute), 90, 92
        liver biopsy, 107, 108
        see also biliary obstruction
    functional, post-liver
        transplantation, 647
    hepatocanalicular, 503
    intrahepatic (chronic), 90–1,
        107
        atypical presentations, 91
        complications, 296–8
        disorders of bile ductules, 91
        infiltrative diseases, 90–1
        liver biopsy, 107–8, 109
        with minimal histologic
            abnormalities, 91
        of pregnancy see intrahepatic
            cholestasis of pregnancy
        progressive familial see
            progressive familial
            intrahepatic cholestasis
        in sarcoidosis, 542
        sickle cell (SCIC), 541
    laboratory tests, 77–9
    liver biopsy, 107–8
    liver transplantation, 585, 587,
        591–3

in lymphoma, 545
    management, 98, 99
        in neonates, 403
    osteoporosis, 196
    primary sclerosing cholangitis,
        292, 296–8
    steroid-related, 504
    subclinical, in pregnancy, 487
cholestatic hepatitis
    drug-induced, 507, 510, 512
    fibrosing see fibrosing
        cholestatic hepatitis
    in recurrent hepatitis C, 680,
        681
cholesterol
    in bile, 47
    bile acid synthesis from, 47,
        48, 52
    esterification defect, 331
    esters, 53
    gallstones, 92, 435, 436
        pregnancy and, 491–2
    membrane, 18–20, 21
    metabolism, 52–3
    serum
        in Alagille syndrome, 403
        in primary biliary cirrhosis,
            280
        in steatosis/NASH, 335
        see also
            hypercholesterolemia
    supersaturation of bile, 436
    synthesis, zonation, 57
cholesterol ester hydrolase, 53
cholesterol ester storage disease
    (CESD), 333, 387
cholestyramine, for pruritus, 99,
    489
cholic acid, 47, 48
choline deficiency, 331, 339
choluria, in hepatitis A, 207
chondrocalcinosis, in Wilson
    disease, 356
chromatin, 30
chromium, 183
chronic hepatitis
    autoimmune hepatitis, 265,
        270
    in children, 405
    cryptogenic, 271
    differential diagnosis, 263
    drug-induced, 502, 503
    hepatitis B, 216
    histology, 104–6
    Wilson disease, 355
chronic liver allograft rejection
    see under rejection, liver
    allograft
chronic liver disease
    causes, 72
    clinical features, 61–70, 72
    drug-induced, 502, 504
    end-stage, liver
        transplantation, 585, 586
    grading, 71

hepatic encephalopathy, 169,
    173–4
    pregnancy in pre-existing,
        492–3, 495
    in sickle cell disease, 541
    survival, 71
    see also cirrhosis
chronic lobular hepatitis (CLH),
    221
chronic obstructive pulmonary
    disease, 378, 379
chylomicrons, 329, 332
    remnants, 330, 332
cidofovir, 652, 686
cimetidine, 536
ciprofloxacin, 166–7, 507
circulatory function
    in acute liver failure, 521–2,
        535
    evaluation in cirrhosis/ascites,
        156
    in liver disease, 62, 68
cirrhosis
    alcohol consumption and,
        311–12
    alcoholic see alcoholic cirrhosis
    ascites, 153–8, 159
    in autoimmune hepatitis, 271,
        597
    basement membrane
        formation, 44
    biliary see biliary cirrhosis
    'cardiac,' 543–4
    cardiac dysfunction, 194–5
    cryptogenic, 339, 405
    in cystic fibrosis, 382, 384
    dilutional hyponatremia, 153,
        159–60
    drug-induced, 504
    esophageal varices, 140
    gastric varices, 141–2
    HBV-related, 216, 221, 222
        adefovir dipivoxil therapy,
            226–7
        lamivudine therapy, 225
        management guidelines, 230
    HCV-related, 240, 246–7
    HDV-related, 231
    hepatic encephalopathy, 173–4
    hepatocellular carcinoma and,
        453, 457, 461–2
    hepatorenal syndrome, 153,
        161–4
    in hereditary
        hemochromatosis, 346,
        347
    imaging, 126, 127
    liver palpation, 69
    liver resection in, 461–2,
        569–70
    liver transplantation, 417–18,
        585, 587
    malnutrition, 177–90
    in NASH, 339
    nutritional assessment, 181–2

cirrhosis (Continued)
  nutritional management, 185, 323–4
  nutritional requirements, 183–4
  portal hypertension, 140
  pregnancy in, 492–3
  in primary sclerosing cholangitis, 295, 300
  in protoporphyria, 378
  sodium retention, 153
  spontaneous bacterial peritonitis, 153, 164–7
  vs non-cirrhotic portal fibrosis, 553, 557
  see also chronic liver disease
cis-Golgi network (CGN), 25, 26
cisplatin, chemoembolization, 464
citrate overload, post-liver transplantation, 643
citric acid cycle, 29
classification, severity of liver disease, 70–1
clathrin, 26, 28
clay-pipe-stem fibrosis, 259
clevudine, in chronic hepatitis B, 228
clofibrate, 511
Clonorchis, 260–1
clotting factors see coagulation factors
clubbing, finger, 67–8, 195, 196
CMV see cytomegalovirus
coagulation disorders, 198–200
  in acute liver failure, 522, 535–6
  clinical features, 62, 65–6
  in extrahepatic portal vein obstruction, 561
  laboratory evaluation, 199
  liver transplant surgery, 608–9
  in non-cirrhotic portal hypertension, 552–3, 555
  treatment, 200
coagulation factors
  changes in liver disease, 198
  serum levels, 79–80
  synthesis, 56
  see also specific factors
coated pits, 26, 28
coated vesicles, 26, 27, 28
cocaine, 506
coccidiomycosis, 255
colchicine, 24
  in alcoholic liver disease, 323
  in liver allograft recipients, 663
  in primary biliary cirrhosis, 285, 287
  in primary sclerosing cholangitis, 306
colectomy, in chronic hepatic encephalopathy, 176
colestyramine, in protoporphyria, 378

colitis
  in liver allograft recipients, 664
  see also ulcerative colitis
collagen vascular disorders, 539–41
collagens, 10–11, 32, 33
collateral circulation
  in Budd-Chiari syndrome, 480, 481
  in extrahepatic portal vein obstruction, 477, 559
  in hepatic artery occlusion, 473
  in splenic vein thrombosis, 479
  see also portosystemic communications
colorectal cancer
  in liver allograft recipients, 664
  metastases, 469
    radiofrequency ablation, 571
    surgical resection, 470, 572–3
  primary sclerosing cholangitis and, 301
coma, hepatic, 70
common bile duct, 12, 14
  anastomosis, liver transplant operation, 614
  stones see choledocholithiasis
common hepatic duct, 12, 14
complement activation, 629, 640
computed tomography (CT), 124
  arterial portography (CTAP), 127, 132
  arteriography (CTA), 132
  benign liver tumors, 424
  in focal nodular hyperplasia, 431
  hemangiomas, 427, 428
  hepatic cysts, 434
  hepatic metastases, 468–9
  hepatocellular adenomas, 425
  hepatocellular carcinoma, 457–8, 459, 462, 571
  infantile hemangioendothelioma, 429
  in jaundice, 95, 96, 97
  lipiodol, 132
  mesenchymal hamartoma, 432, 433
  multiphasic imaging, 124
  multislice, 124
  in non-cirrhotic portal hypertension, 553, 556
  spiral or helical, 124
  in steatosis/NASH, 336, 337
congenital hepatic fibrosis, 447–8, 565
congestive heart failure, 543–4
congestive hepatopathy, 543–4
congo red, 103
conjugation
  bilirubin, 51, 84
  drugs and toxins, 54–5, 498
  zonation, 58
conjunctival pallor, 65

connective tissue, 10–11, 32–3
connexins, 22, 44
connexon, 22, 23
constipation, 62
continuous ambulatory peritoneal dialysis (CAPD), in diabetes, 537
contraception
  hepatocellular adenomas and, 424, 456
  in liver allograft recipients, 665
  see also oral contraceptive steroids
contrast agents
  iodinated, 124
  magnetic resonance, 125
  ultrasonic, 123
copper
  24 h urinary excretion, 356, 357, 363
  accumulation, in Wilson disease, 351
  dietary intake, 352
  functions, 352
  hepatic content, 356, 357–8
  hepatic metabolism, 352–3
  intracytoplasmic, 107, 108
  in primary sclerosing cholangitis etiology, 290
  radioactive (^{64}Cu), test, 359
  serum, 356, 357
  supplements, 183
  toxic effects, 351
copper transporter 1 (Ctr1), 352–3
coproporphyria, hereditary, 370, 371–2
coproporphyrinogen oxidase, 371, 372
cords see liver cell plates
Cori disease (glycogen storage disease III), 389, 390, 410
coronary artery bypass grafting (CABG), 195
coronary artery disease (CAD), 195
coronary ligament, 3, 4
corticosteroids, 630
  in acute liver allograft rejection, 633
  in acute liver failure, 527
  in alcoholic hepatitis, 321–2
  in autoimmune hepatitis, 272–3, 274, 408
  in liver transplantation, 632, 633
  mechanism of action, 630
  osteoporosis and, 196, 197–8
  in primary biliary cirrhosis, 285, 287
  in primary sclerosing cholangitis, 305–6
  in recurrent post-transplant hepatitis C, 680
  side-effects, 273, 633, 634

costimulatory pathways, T cell activation, 626–7, 628
Couinaud liver segments see segments, liver
covalent binding, hepatotoxins, 500
CP-690,550, 632
creatinine
  clearance, 663
  height index, 181
  serum, 162, 316
CREST syndrome, 66, 278, 282, 540
Crigler–Najjar syndrome, 87–8
  type I, 51, 86, 87–8, 89, 397
    auxiliary liver transplantation, 419
    liver transplantation, 421, 601
  type II, 51, 86, 87–8, 89, 397
Crohn colitis, primary sclerosing cholangitis and, 300
Cruveilhier-Baumgarten syndrome, 69
cryoablation, 133
  hepatocellular carcinoma, 466
cryoglobulinemia, in chronic hepatitis C, 240–1
cryoglobulins, serum, 240, 241
cryoprecipitate, 200
Cryptococcus infections, 651
cryptogenic cirrhosis, 339, 405
cryptogenic hepatitis, 271
cryptosporidiosis, 295
crystal violet, 103
CT see computed tomography
CTLA-4 see cytotoxic T-lymphocyte antigen 4
cyanosis, 68
cyclic adenosine monophosphate (cAMP), 51, 328–9
cyclic guanosine monophosphate (GMP), 33
cyclin-dependent kinases (cdks), 36, 37
cyclins, 36, 37
cyclophilin, 631
cyclophosphamide
  in autoimmune hepatitis, 274
  hepatotoxicity, 482, 512
cyclosporin, 631
  adverse effects, 420, 421, 634
  in autoimmune hepatitis, 273–4, 408
  drug interactions, 634
  hepatotoxicity, 512
  in liver transplantation, 632, 633
  mode of action, 626, 631
  nephrotoxicity, 634, 635, 663
  in primary biliary cirrhosis, 285
  in primary sclerosing cholangitis, 306
cystadenocarcinoma, hepatic, 576–7

cystadenomas
  bile duct, 426
  hepatic, 576–7
cystic duct, 12, 14
cystic fibrosis (CF), 382–5
  biliary tract and gallbladder, 382–3
  clinical features, 382–3
  diagnosis, 383–4
  epidemiology, 382
  liver disease, 411–12
    clinical features, 412
    diagnosis, 383–4, 405, 412
    management, 384–5, 405, 412
    in neonates, 405
    pathophysiology, 382, 412
  liver transplantation, 385, 412, 600
  pathophysiology, 382, 383
  treatment, 384–5
cystic fibrosis transmembrane conductance regulator (CFTR), 382, 383
  gene mutations, 382
  hepatic function, 51, 52
cystic liver diseases, 442–50
cysts
  in Budd-Chiari syndrome, 479–80
  choledochal, 399–400, 448–9
  hydatid see hydatid cysts
  intrahepatic biliary, in Caroli disease, 450
  neoplastic, 576–7
  in polycystic liver disease, 447, 575–6
    aspiration and sclerosis, 446
    clinical features, 444–5
    fenestration, 446, 447, 576
    medical therapy, 445–6
    natural history, 442–3
    pathogenesis, 444
    resection, 446, 576
  simple hepatic, 433–4, 447, 575
    aspiration, 447, 575
    unroofing, 575
cytochalasin B, 10
cytochrome c, 38
cytochrome P450 enzymes, 498
  drug metabolism, 54–5, 498
  induction, 55, 498, 499
  intracellular localization, 9
cytochrome P4501A2 (CYP1A2), 499
  autoantibodies, 267, 268
cytochrome P4502A6 (CYP2A6), autoantibodies, 267, 268
cytochrome P4502C (CYP2C), 499
cytochrome P4502C9 (CYP2C9), autoantibodies, 267, 268, 501

cytochrome P4502D6 (CYP2D6), 269, 499
  autoantibodies, 266–7
  deficiency, 498
cytochrome P4502E1 (CYP2E1), 498, 499
  acetaminophen metabolism, 508
  metabolism of alcohol, 313
cytochrome P4503A4 (CYP3A4), 498, 499
cytokeratins, 103
  bile duct, 1, 24
  hepatocyte, 10, 24
cytokine release syndrome, 635
cytokines
  in alcoholic liver disease, 313–14
  in anti-allograft responses, 621–3
  in drug-induced liver injury, 500
  role in tissue injury, 629
  Th1/Th1 response, 629
cytokinesis, 35
cytomegalovirus (CMV), 252
  childhood acute hepatitis, 416
  diagnosis, 263
  granulomatous hepatitis, 255
  immunostaining, 103
  liver donor–recipient mismatch, 685
  in liver transplant recipients, 652–3, 669, 684–6
    clinical manifestations, 652, 685–6
    diagnosis, 652, 684, 685
    histopathology, 118, 652
    pediatric patients, 420
    primary infection, 652, 684
    prophylaxis, 686
    secondary infection (reactivation), 652, 684–5
    superinfection, 652, 685
    treatment, 686
  neonatal hepatitis, 401
  post-transplant lymphoproliferative disorder and, 687
  primary sclerosing cholangitis and, 290
cytoskeleton, hepatocyte, 9–10, 22–5
cytotoxic T-lymphocyte antigen 4 (CTLA-4), 627
  polymorphisms, 270, 314
cytotoxic T lymphocytes (CTL), 621
  in allograft rejection, 630
  in hepatitis B, 215
  mechanisms of tissue injury, 628–9
  see also CD8+ T cells

death receptor pathway, 37–8
debrisoquin metabolizer phenotypes, 498
δ agent see hepatitis D virus
demyelination, in hepatic encephalopathy, 170
dental problems, 418, 664
deoxycholic acid, 47, 48, 52
dermatan sulfate, 392
desmosomes, 22, 44
development
  hepatic cells, 17
  liver, 1
developmental assessment, 418
dexamethasone, in intrahepatic cholestasis of pregnancy, 489
diabetes mellitus (DM), 537
  complications of biliary disease, 438, 439
  hepatic steatosis/ steatohepatitis, 327, 537
  hepatogenous, 202
  in liver allograft recipients, 663
  liver histology, 113, 537
  management, 338–9
  non-insulin-dependent (NIDDM) (type 2), 202, 537
  serum aminotransferases, 76
diglycerols (DG), 625, 626
diacytosis, 21, 24, 26
diagnosis, liver disease, 70–1
dialysis
  in acute liver failure, 535
  in diabetes, 537
  in polycystic liver disease, 445
  see also hemodialysis
diarrhea, 62
  idiopathic bile acid, 52
diastolic dysfunction, in cirrhotic cardiomyopathy, 195
diazepam, in acute liver failure, 534
diclofenac hepatotoxicity, 501, 509–10
diet
  in hepatic encephalopathy, 175, 184–5
  protein restricted, 175, 185
  sodium restricted, 156–7, 185
  weight loss, 188, 189
  see also nutritional management
dietary supplements, 188
dihydralazine-induced hepatitis, 267, 268
dimethyl iminodiacetic acid (HIDA) scintigraphy, 440
4,6-dioxoheptanoic acid, 385, 386
diphenhydramine, 99
disaccharides, non-absorbable, in hepatic encephalopathy, 175

Discriminant Function (DF), alcoholic hepatitis, 320
Disse, space of see space of Disse
disseminated intravascular coagulation (DIC), 198, 199
  in acute liver failure, 522
  management, 200
distal splenorenal shunts (DSRS), 144, 150
diuretics
  in ascites, 156–7, 158
  complications in cirrhosis, 157
  hepatotoxic, 510
divalent metal transporter 1 (DMT1), 344
DNA, 30
  damage, cell cycle checkpoints, 36
  synthesis, regenerating liver, 37
donor livers
  ABO incompatible, 529
  allocation, 528–9, 585–90
  preservation injury, 646–7
  rejection see rejection, liver allograft
  size matching, 607–8
  see also liver allografts
donors, liver
  anti-HCV positive, 682
  deceased, hepatectomy, 606–7, 608
  extended criteria (ECD), 606
  living related, 617–18
    see also living related donor liver transplantation
  reduction hepatectomy, 419, 615–16
  selection, 606
  shortages, 585
dopamine, in acute liver failure, 535
doxorubicin, 464, 466–7, 512
doxycycline, 252, 254
drains, surgical, after liver transplantation, 614, 615, 643
drepanocytosis, 484
drug(s)
  to avoid in porphyrias, 377
  history, 63
  prescribing, liver allograft recipients, 666
drug-induced liver disease, 497–516
  acute liver failure, 497, 519
  acute liver injury, 502
  autoantibodies, 263, 267, 268, 501
  in childhood, 409, 416
  cholestasis, 282, 502, 503–4
  chronic liver injury, 502, 504
  clinical features, 514
  diagnosis, 514–16
  by drug class, 504–14
  epidemiology, 497

drug-induced liver disease
(Continued)
hepatitis, 502, 503
jaundice, 89, 91
liver biopsy, 108–9, 502–4, 516
management, 516
NASH, 328
necrosis, 502–3
pathogenesis, 499–501
patterns, 501–4
phospholipidosis, 333–4, 502,
503
risk factors, 498–9
sinusoidal obstruction
syndrome, 482
steatosis, 330, 333, 503
drug metabolism, 53–5, 497–8
phase I, 55, 498
phase II, 55, 498
phenotypes, 498
zonation, 57, 58
see also xenobiotic metabolism
drug metabolizing enzymes,
54–5, 498
induction, 55, 498, 499
see also cytochrome P450
dual-energy X-ray
absorptiometry (DEXA),
182, 197, 664
Dubin–Johnson syndrome, 51,
86, 88, 89
ductal plate, hepatic, 1, 3
ductopenia (vanishing bile duct
syndrome; bile duct paucity)
in chronic allograft rejection,
118, 638, 639, 649
differential diagnosis, 295
drug-induced, 504
idiopathic adulthood see
idiopathic adulthood
ductopenia
pediatric liver transplantation,
603
in primary biliary cirrhosis,
280, 281
in primary sclerosing
cholangitis, 294, 301, 302
ductus venosus, 1, 2
duodenal crypt cell programming
hypothesis, hereditary
hemochromatosis, 344
duodenal papilla, 12, 14
Dupuytren's contracture, 67
dynamin, 45
dynein, 24, 45
dysfibrinogenemia, 199
dysgeusia, 178
dysplastic hepatocellular nodule,
115, 459
dyspnea, 62, 68, 191
in ascites, 154
in hepatopulmonary syndrome,
192
in portopulmonary
hypertension, 193

E2F, 36
EBV see Epstein–Barr virus
ecchymoses, 62
echinococcosis, 256–8
see also hydatid cysts
Echinococcus granulosus, 257
Echinococcus multilocularis, 257
echinocytes, 201
echocardiography
in cirrhotic cardiomyopathy,
195
contrast (CE), in
hepatopulmonary
syndrome, 192
eclampsia, 489
acute liver failure, 519–20
diagnosis of liver disease, 494
ecstasy, 506, 519
edema, 62
in cirrhosis, 153, 154
nutritional assessment and,
181–2
pitting, 66
treatment, 156–7
see also ascites
EHPVO see extrahepatic portal
vein obstruction
elderly patients
autoimmune hepatitis, 271–2
drug-induced hepatotoxicity,
499
electroencephalogram (EEG), in
hepatic encephalopathy, 174
electrolytes
in acute liver failure, 521
bile, 47
diuretic-induced disturbances,
157
transport, in bile formation,
49–50
electron transport chain, 29–30
enzyme deficiencies, 414
Elias three-dimensional model, 5,
6
embolization, catheter
arterioportal fistulas, 475
in hereditary hemorrhagic
telangiectasia, 476
infantile
hemangioendothelioma,
430
liver cell adenomas, 426
metastatic carcinoid tumors,
471
see also transcatheter arterial
chemoembolization
empyema, spontaneous bacterial,
164
emtricitabine, in chronic
hepatitis B, 227
endocrine disorders, 537–9
in hepatocellular carcinoma,
456
in liver disease, 63, 69–70
neonatal hepatitis, 401, 402

endocrine signaling, 33
endocytosis, 26–7
receptor-mediated (RME), 26,
649, 650
endometriosis, hepatic, 433
endoplasmic reticulum (ER),
7–9, 25
compartments, 25
membrane protein synthesis,
21
nuclear envelope and, 30, 31
rough (RER), 7, 8, 9, 19, 25
smooth (SER), 7–9, 19, 25, 45
endoscopic injection
sclerotherapy (EIS), 143
in acute variceal hemorrhage,
147
effects on gastric varices, 142
in non-cirrhotic portal
hypertension, 555–6, 562
prevention of variceal
rebleeding, 149
primary prevention of variceal
bleeding, 145–6
endoscopic retrograde
cholangiopancreatography
(ERCP)
in acute cholangitis, 441–2
in Caroli disease, 450
in choledocholithiasis, 441–2
in cholelithiasis, 438
in jaundice, 95–6, 97
in primary sclerosing
cholangitis, 292, 293
endoscopic sphincterotomy,
438–9
endoscopic therapy
in acute variceal hemorrhage,
147
in portal hypertension, 143–4
prevention of variceal
rebleeding, 149
primary prevention of variceal
bleeding, 145–6
in primary sclerosing
cholangitis, 298
endoscopic ultrasonography
(EUS), 96–7
endoscopic variceal band ligation
(EVL), 143–4
in acute hemorrhage, 147
in non-cirrhotic portal
hypertension, 555–6, 562
prevention of rebleeding, 149
primary prevention of
bleeding, 146, 150
endosomes, 19, 21, 26
endothelial cells
alloantigen recognition, 629–30
in chronic allograft rejection,
630
leukocyte interaction, 627–8
sinusoidal, 39
development, 17
fenestrae, 39, 43–4

microanatomy, 8, 9, 10,
43–4
molecular barrier, 43–4
relative numbers/volume, 18
endotheliitis, in acute allograft
rejection, 636
endothelin receptor antagonists,
194
endotoxin, 313, 550
energy
expenditure, in cirrhosis,
179–80, 184
requirements, in cirrhosis,
183–4
stores, 330
substrates, in cirrhosis, 183
enflurane, 513
Entamoeba dispar, 258
Entamoeba histolytica, 258–9
entecavir
in chronic hepatitis B, 227, 673
in recurrent hepatitis B, 679
enteral nutrition, 185, 187
acute liver failure, 536
alcoholic cirrhosis, 323–4
alcoholic hepatitis, 320, 322
post-transplant, 187
specialized formulations, 188
enterohepatic circulation, 52, 54
enzyme-linked receptors, 33
enzyme replacement therapy, in
Gaucher disease, 394
eosinophils, in allograft rejection,
630, 636
ephedrine, 188
epidermal growth factor (EGF)
receptors, 33, 34
epinephrine, in acute liver
failure, 535
epithelioid
hemangioendothelioma see
hemangioendothelioma,
epithelioid
epoprostenol, 194
Epstein–Barr virus (EBV), 252–3
diagnosis, 253, 263
granulomatous hepatitis, 255
post-liver transplant infections,
420, 653, 666, 669, 687
post-transplant
lymphoproliferative
disorder and see
post-transplant
lymphoproliferative
disorder
ERCP see endoscopic retrograde
cholangiopancreatography
Erlenmeyer flask deformity, 394,
395
erythema
diffuse, esophageal varices,
141
palmar, 67, 487
erythritol, 48
erythrocytes see red blood cells

erythrocytosis, in hepatocellular carcinoma, 456
erythrohemophagocytosis, 522
erythromycin, 507
erythropoiesis, ineffective, 341
erythropoietic protoporphyria *see* protoporphyria
erythropoietin, 200
Escherichia coli, in primary biliary cirrhosis etiology, 278
esophageal transection surgery, 144
esophageal varices, 140–1
    band ligation, 143–4
    bleeding
        cessation, 141
        prediction of risk, 140–1
        recurrence risks, 141
        see also variceal bleeding
    grading, 139
    in pregnancy, 487
    pressure measurement, 140–1
    'red signs,' 141
    sclerotherapy *see* endoscopic injection sclerotherapy
esophageal veins
    extrinsic plexus, 138
    intrinsic, 138
estrogen
    hepatotoxicity, 504–5
    induced jaundice, 91
    induced NASH, 328
    intrahepatic cholestasis of pregnancy and, 488
    in polycystic liver disease, 443, 445–6
    therapy, 188, 197, 297
etanercept, in alcoholic hepatitis, 321, 322
ethanol *see* alcohol
ethinyl estradiol, 50
ethnic variations *see* racial variations
etidronate, 197
examination, physical, 63–70
exercise, physical, 77, 338
exocytosis, 26–7
extended criteria donors (ECD), 606
extracellular matrix (ECM), 10–11, 32–3
    cell interactions, 32
    components, 32–3
    functions, 32
    stellate cells, 40
extracellular space, liver, 17, 18
extracorporeal liver assist device (ELAD), 528
extracorporeal liver support systems, 528
extracorporeal shock-wave lithotripsy, 438
extrahepatic portal vein obstruction (EHPVO), 476–8, 549, 557–65

clinical features, 477, 555, 559–61
definition, 557
diagnosis, 477–8, 561–2
differential diagnosis, 557
etiology and pathogenesis, 476–7, 551, 558–9
hemodynamics, 555, 561
management, 478, 562–5
pathology, 559
pathophysiology, 559
eye
    in Alagille syndrome, 403
    signs of liver disease, 65

F-actin, 24
facial signs
    Alagille syndrome, 65, 403
    liver disease, 65
factor II gene mutation, 476
factor V, 198, 199
    in acute liver failure, 525–6
    Leiden, 476, 480, 551, 559
factor VII, 198, 199
factor VIIa, recombinant, 200, 536, 608
factor VIII, 198
falciform ligament, 3, 4
false neurotransmitter hypothesis, hepatic encephalopathy, 172
famciclovir, 678, 679
familial amyloidosis with polyneuropathy (FAP), 541, 603
family history, 63
Fas-associated protein with death domain (FADD), 38, 314
Fas/Fas ligand-mediated apoptosis, 37–8, 314
Fasciola hepatica, 260–1
fat
    dietary requirements, in cirrhosis, 183, 184
    focal deposition, 335, 337, 433
    stores in liver, 329
    see also fatty acids; lipids
fat-storing cells *see* hepatic stellate cells
fatigue, 61
    in primary biliary cirrhosis, 283
    in primary sclerosing cholangitis, 296
fatty acid-binding protein (FABP), 58, 84, 331
fatty acids
    β-oxidation, 329–30
    in acute fatty liver of pregnancy, 490
    defects, 330, 333
    delivery to liver from periphery, 328–9
    essential, deficiency, 331
    fate in liver, 329–31
    free, 328–9, 332

in hepatic encephalopathy pathogenesis, 172
metabolism, 55–6, 328–32
    in alcoholic fatty liver, 313, 332–3
    zonation, 58
peroxisomal oxidation, 55–6, 330
synthesis in liver, 329
fatty liver, 327–40
    alcoholic *see* alcoholic fatty liver
    in cystic fibrosis, 382
    focal, 335, 337, 433
    focal sparing, 337
    imaging, 335–7
    liver biopsy, 113–14
    of pregnancy *see* acute fatty liver of pregnancy
    serum aminotransferases, 74, 75–6, 334–5
    see also non-alcoholic fatty liver disease; non-alcoholic steatohepatitis; steatosis, hepatic
fenofibrate, 663
ferric reductase, Dcytb, 344
ferritin, serum, 201
    in hemochromatosis, 345, 346, 347, 348
ferrochetalase, 371, 373–4
    gene abnormalities, 373–4
    genetic polymorphisms, 374
ferroportin 1, 341, 344
fetal liver, 1, 2, 17
fetor hepaticus, 63, 65, 174
fever (pyrexia), 64–5
    in alcoholic hepatitis, 315, 316
    spontaneous bacterial peritonitis, 165
    of unknown origin (PUO), 456, 577
fibrin degradation products, 199
fibrinogen, 199
fibrinolysis, 198, 199
fibroblasts, 10, 40
fibrocystic liver diseases, 442–50
fibrocystin, 443, 444, 447
fibrolamellar carcinoma *see* hepatocellular carcinoma (HCC), fibrolamellar
fibronectin, 11, 33
fibrosing cholestatic hepatitis (FCH), 120
    antiviral therapy, 678
    in recurrent hepatitis B, 120, 215, 593, 670, 671
fibrosis, hepatic
    alcoholic *see* alcoholic cirrhosis (and fibrosis)
    bridging, 239, 319
    centrilobular, 319
    chickenwire, 113, 114, 318–19, 338
    in chronic hepatitis, 105
    clay-pipe-stem, 259

congenital, 447–8, 565
in cystic fibrosis, 382, 384
HBV-related, 221
HCV-related, 237, 239, 240
    effect of antiviral therapy, 242–3
in hereditary hemochromatosis, 346
non-cirrhotic portal *see* non-cirrhotic portal fibrosis
pericellular, 318–19
periportal, 319
perisinusoidal, 483
in primary biliary cirrhosis, 279
sinusoidal, 484
in steatohepatitis, 113–14, 338
stellate cell activation, 40
FIC1 (PFIC1) gene, 91, 404
Fitz-Hugh-Curtis syndrome, 69
FK-binding protein (FKBP), 631
flavin adenine dinucleotide (FADH$_2$), 29
floxuridine, 512
flucloxacillin, 507
fluconazole, 249, 651
fluid management
    in dilutional hyponatremia, 160
    post-liver transplantation, 643
fluid retention, 62, 64
    in children, 419
    nutritional assessment and, 181–2
    solute-free, in cirrhosis, 159–60
    see also ascites; edema
flukes, liver, 260–1
flumazenil, in hepatic encephalopathy, 533
[18]F-fluorodeoxyglucose (FDG), 132
5-fluorodeoxyuridine (FUDR), intra-arterial, 464, 471
fluoroquinolones, hepatotoxicity, 507
5-fluorouracil (5-FU)
    hepatotoxicity, 512
    intra-arterial, 464, 470
    metastatic tumors, 470
foamy degeneration, 333
    alcoholic, 315, 318
    see also microvesicular steatosis
focal nodular hyperplasia (FNH), 430–2
    Budd-Chiari syndrome, 479–80
    clinical features, 431–2
    hepatocellular adenoma and, 424
    management, 431–2, 574
    pathology, 115, 430
    radiology, 129, 130
folate deficiency, 183, 184, 201
folic acid supplements, 183
folinic acid (FA), 470

formiminotransferase cyclodeaminase (FTCD), 268
Fort Bragg fever, 253
foscarnet, 652, 686
fractures, pathological, 196, 297
free radicals, in alcoholic hepatitis, 313
fresh frozen plasma (FFP), 200, 535–6
friction rubs, 69
fructose
  intolerance (fructosemia), hereditary (HFI), 387–8
    neonates, 401
    older children, 405, 410–11
  metabolism, 55, 388
fructose-1-phosphate aldolase B, 387–8, 410
FTY 720, 632
fucose receptor, 33
fulminant hepatic failure see acute liver failure
fumaryl acetoacetate (FAA), 385
fumaryl acetoacetate (FAA) hydrolase (fumarylacetoacetase), 385, 414
functions, liver, 43–59
  bile formation, 46–52
  hepatocyte heterogeneity, 56–8
  metabolism, 52–6
  morphologic aspects, 43–6
fungal infections, 65, 249–50
  in acute liver failure, 522, 534–5
  post-liver transplant, 420, 532, 651
fungicides, 513
furosemide, in ascites, 156, 157, 158

G-protein-linked receptors, 33
GABAergic neurotransmission hypothesis, hepatic encephalopathy, 172, 520
galactokinase deficiency, 391
galactose
  elimination capacity (GEC), 80
  metabolism, 55, 391
galactose-1-phosphate uridyl transferase (GALT) deficiency, 391, 413
¹⁴C-galactose breath test, 80
galactosemia, 391
  acute liver failure, 413–14
  neonatal hepatitis, 401
gallbladder
  anatomical relations, 3, 4
  calcified (porcelain), 442
  cancer, 300, 442
  in cystic fibrosis, 382–3
  development, 17
  function, 51–2

motility, gallstone formation and, 436–7
mucus secretion, 52
polyps, 442
sludge see biliary sludge
varices, 561
gallbladder disease, 435–42
  epidemiology and risk factors, 435, 436
  indications for cholecystectomy, 438
gallstones (cholelithiasis), 435–9
  asymptomatic, 437
  black pigment, 92, 435
  brown pigment, 92, 435–6
  cholecystitis and, 439–40
  cholesterol see cholesterol, gallstones
  clinical features, 437
  complications, 437, 438
  in cystic fibrosis, 383
  endoscopic sphincterotomy, 438
  epidemiology and risk factors, 435
  in hypothyroidism, 539
  imaging, 130–1, 132
  in neonates, 400
  obstructive jaundice, 92
  pancreatitis, 442
  pathogenesis, 435–7
  in pregnancy, 491–2, 494
  in primary biliary cirrhosis, 283
  in primary sclerosing cholangitis, 298
  in protoporphyria, 374, 378
  in sickle cell disease, 541
  treatment, 438–9
  see also choledocholithiasis
γ-glutamyltransferase (GGT), serum, 79
  in alcohol abuse, 315
  normal/abnormal ranges, 74
  in steatosis/NASH, 335
ganciclovir
  in cytomegalovirus infection, 252, 652–3, 686
  in herpes simplex infections, 653
  in post-transplant lymphoproliferative disorder, 687
  in recurrent hepatitis B, 678
gangliosides, 20
gangrene, post-liver transplant, 650
gap junctions, 22, 23, 44
garlic, in hepatopulmonary syndrome, 193
gastric antral vascular ectasia (GAVE), 139, 142
gastric varices, 139
  after splenic vein thrombosis, 479

bleeding
  prediction of risk, 142
  treatment of active, 147, 148
isolated (IGV), 139
  bleeding risks, 142
  type 1 (IGV1), 139
  type 2 (IGV2), 139
natural history, 141–2
in non-cirrhotic portal fibrosis, 556
gastric vein, left, 137, 138
gastroesophageal junction devascularization surgery, 144
veins, 138–9
gastroesophageal varices (GEV; GOV), 139, 140–2
  anatomy and classification, 138–40
  bleeding risks, 142
  type 1 (GOV1), 139
  type 2 (GOV2), 139
  see also esophageal varices; gastric varices; varices
gastrointestinal hemorrhage, 61, 137–51
  after TIPS, 149
  in extrahepatic portal vein obstruction, 477, 478, 560
  in hepatocellular carcinoma, 456
  in non-cirrhotic portal hypertension, 552, 555–6
  in primary biliary cirrhosis, 283
  in splenic vein thrombosis, 479
  spontaneous bacterial peritonitis and, 164, 166–7
  upper (UGI), non-variceal causes, 146
  see also variceal bleeding
gastrointestinal symptoms, 61–2
gastropathy, portal hypertensive (PHG), 139, 142
gastrostomy feeding tubes, 187
Gaucher cells, 393, 394
Gaucher disease, 393–4, 411
  clinical features, 393–4, 395
gender differences
  autoimmune hepatitis, 265, 407
  drug-induced hepatotoxicity, 499
  fulminant Wilson disease, 355
  gallbladder disease, 435, 436
  hereditary hemochromatosis, 345
  NASH risk, 328
  primary biliary cirrhosis, 277
gene therapy, 381, 385, 387
genetic factors
  in alcoholic liver disease, 314
  in autoimmune hepatitis, 269–70
  in primary biliary cirrhosis, 277

in primary sclerosing cholangitis, 290–1
  see also HLA haplotypes
germander, 514
giant cell arteritis, 540–1
Gilbert syndrome, 87, 89
  drug-induced hepatotoxicity, 499, 508
  pathogenesis, 51, 86
gingival hyperplasia, 420, 634, 664
Glisson, capsule of, 3
globus pallidus, in hepatic encephalopathy, 172
glomerulonephritis, 216, 241
glucagon
  challenge test, 388
  therapy, 321, 323, 527
β glucocerebrosidase, 393, 394
glucocerebroside accumulation, 393, 394
glucosamine, 188
glucose
  in acute porphyria, 376
  fatty acid synthesis from, 329
  infusion, in fulminant hepatic failure, 187
  metabolism, 55
    in cirrhosis, 178–9
    zonation, 56, 57
  requirements, 187
glucose-6-phosphatase, 388, 410
  deficiency, 388–9, 410
  transport defects, 388, 389, 410
glucuronidation, 55, 58
glutamic oxaloacetic transaminase, serum (SGOT) see aspartate aminotransferase
glutamic pyruvic transaminase, serum (SGPT) see alanine aminotransferase
glutamine
  brain, in hepatic encephalopathy, 170
  neurotoxic effects, 171, 173
  synthesis, 56, 170
  zonation, 57, 58
glutamine synthetase, 56, 170
glutathione (GSH)
  in acetaminophen metabolism, 508–9
  in alcoholic liver disease, 313–14
  in bile, 47
  in bile formation, 49, 50, 51
  conjugation of drugs, 54–5
  in drug-induced hepatotoxicity, 500
glutathione S-transferase, 51, 55
gluten intolerance, in primary biliary cirrhosis, 282–3
glycerophospholipids, membrane, 18, 20
glycine, 47

glycocalyx (cell coat),
   hepatocyte, 21–2
glycogen
   within hepatocytes, 8, 10
   nuclei, 338
   synthesis and breakdown, 55
   zonation, 56, 57
glycogen storage diseases (GSD),
   388–90, 409–10
   type I, 388–90, 410
   types II–IX, 389, 390, 410
glycolipids, membrane, 20
glycolysis, 55
glycosaminoglycans, 32–3
glypressin (terlipressin), 143,
   147, 163
Golgi complex, 7, 25, 45
   compartments, 25
   endocytotic/exocytic
      pathways, 26
   microscopy, 8, 9
gout, in liver allograft recipients,
   663
grading, severity of liver disease,
   70–1
graft versus host disease
   (GVHD), 91, 120, 121
grafts, liver see liver allografts
granulomas, 106
   in sarcoidosis, 542
granulomatous hepatitis
   drug-induced, 503
   histopathology, 106
   infectious causes, 255–6
   in schistosomiasis, 255, 259
granulomatous liver diseases
   cholestasis, 91
   histopathology, 106, 107
   infectious causes, 255–6
griseofulvin, hepatotoxicity, 507–8
ground substance, 32
growth
   in extrahepatic portal vein
      obstruction, 560, 561
   in liver transplant recipients,
      421
gynecomastia, 63, 70
   diuretic-induced, in cirrhosis,
      157

hair, signs of malnutrition, 183
halothane hepatitis, 512–13
   autoantibodies, 267, 268, 501
hamartoma, mesenchymal, 432,
   433
HAMP gene mutations, 341
hand signs, liver disease, 67–8
Hansen disease, 256
haplotype analysis, in Wilson
   disease, 359–61, 362
HAV see hepatitis A virus
Havrix®, 209
HBV see hepatitis B virus
HCC see hepatocellular
   carcinoma

HCV see hepatitis C virus
HDV see hepatitis D virus
headache, in liver allograft
   recipients, 664
healthcare workers, viral
   hepatitis risk, 215, 237
heart disease, ischemic, 195
heart failure
   in cirrhotic cardiomyopathy,
      195
   congestive, 543–4
HELLP syndrome, 484, 489–90
   acute liver failure, 519
   prognosis, 495
   treatment, 495
hemangioendothelioma
   epithelioid, 468, 505
      liver histology, 117
      liver transplantation, 599
   infantile, 413, 428–30
      management, 429–30
      pathology, 429
      radiology, 429
hemangiomas (cavernous), 427–8
   in childhood, 413
   clinical presentation, 428
   in fatty liver, 335
   management, 428, 573, 574
   pathology, 427
   radiology, 129, 424, 427–8
   vs hepatocellular carcinoma,
      459
hematemesis, 61
   in extrahepatic portal vein
      obstruction, 560
   see also gastrointestinal
      hemorrhage
hematobilia, 456
hematocystic spots, esophageal
   varices, 141
hematologic disorders, 62, 200–1
   in acute liver failure, 522
hematoma, subcapsular
   in pregnancy, 490, 495
   traumatic, 578
hematopoietic cells, fetal liver, 17
heme
   biosynthetic defects in
      porphyrias, 369–70, 371
   biosynthetic pathway, 371
   containing proteins, 83
   intravenous therapy, 376–7
   metabolism, 83, 85, 372
heme arginate, 376–7
heme oxygenase, 83, 85
hemochromatosis, hereditary
   (HH), 341–9
   clinical features, 344–5
   diagnosis, 77, 345–6
   differential diagnosis, 263
   HFE-related, 341, 342–4
      genetics, 342–3
      pathophysiology, 343–4
   stages of recognition, 342
   imaging, 126–7

jaundice, 90
   juvenile, 341, 342
   liver histology, 102, 111–12,
      345–6, 347
   liver transplantation, 601, 660
   neonatal, 414, 520
   non-HFE-related, 341, 342
   screening, 348
   treatment, 346–7
hemodialysis
   in hepatorenal syndrome, 164
   liver function tests and, 75, 76
hemodynamic changes
   in acute liver failure, 521–2,
      535
   in extrahepatic portal vein
      obstruction, 561
   in liver disease, 68
   in liver transplantation, 643
   in non-cirrhotic portal fibrosis,
      551–2, 554, 555
hemoglobin
   in alcoholic liver disease, 315,
      316
   degradation, 83
hemoglobinuria, paroxysmal
   nocturnal, 476, 480, 481
hemojuvelin, 341
hemolysis
   in liver disease, 201
   ribavirin-induced, 246
hemolytic anemia
   autoimmune, giant cell
      hepatitis with, 421
   jaundice, 86
   in Wilson disease, 90, 355,
      356–61, 365
hemoperitoneum
   post-liver transplantation, 647
   tumor rupture, 425, 456
hemophagocytic
   lymphohistiocytosis, familial,
      416
hemophagocytosis, 118
hemopoiesis, fetal liver, 1
hemorrhage/bleeding
   after liver biopsy, 101
   disorders, 62, 65–6
   gastrointestinal see
      gastrointestinal
      hemorrhage
   intraoperative, liver resections,
      569
   liver cell adenoma, 424–5, 426
   in liver trauma, 578–80, 581
   portal hypertensive
      gastropathy, 142
   post-liver transplantation, 647
   variceal see variceal bleeding
   see also coagulation disorders
hemostasis
   during liver resections, 570
   during liver transplantation,
      614
hemostatic disorders, 198–200

heparan sulfate, 11, 33, 392
heparin, 535, 608–9
hepatectomy
   deceased donor, 606–7, 608
   definitions, 567
   extended right, 462
   liver graft recipient
      orthotopic procedure,
         610–11
      reduced size liver, 616
   living donor, 617
      right lobe, 617–18
      segmentectomy of segments
         II/III, 617
   partial (PH)
      liver regeneration, 37
      techniques, 567–9
   reduction, pediatric
      transplantation, 419,
         615–16
   total, in acute liver failure,
      530–2
   see also resection, liver;
      surgery, hepatic
hepatic adenomas see
   hepatocellular adenomas
hepatic arterioles, 5, 12, 13, 14
hepatic artery, 3, 4
   anastomoses
      in living donor
         transplantation, 618
      in orthotopic liver
         transplantation, 613–14
      in reduced-size liver
         transplantation, 616
   anatomical variations, 608
   aneurysms, 474–5
      false, 474, 475
   chemoembolization see
      transcatheter arterial
      chemoembolization
   diseases, 473–6
   functional distribution of
      blood supply, 3–5
   intrahepatic anatomy, 5, 6
   ligation
      donor hepatectomy, 607
      infantile
         hemangioendothelioma,
         430
      recipient hepatectomy, 611
   occlusion, 473–4
   post-transplant surveillance,
      619–20
   stenosis, post-liver
      transplantation, 648
hepatic artery thrombosis (HAT)
   diagnosis, 474
   imaging, 130, 657
   post-liver transplant, 474, 620,
      647
      late/delayed presentation,
         656
      pediatric patients, 420, 647
      prevention, 613

hepatic diverticulum, 1, 17
hepatic ductal plate,
    development, 1, 3
hepatic ducts, 12, 14
hepatic encephalopathy, 63,
    169–76
  in acute liver failure, 169, 173,
    517, 520
    diagnosis, 522
    management, 533–4
    prognosis and, 523
  in alcoholic liver disease, 315,
    316
  in childhood, 417
  chronic intractable, 175–6
  classification, 169–70
  clinical features, 70, 173–4
  clinical grading, 70
  definition, 169
  diuretic-induced, in cirrhosis,
    158
  history taking in, 61
  minimal, 174
  neuropathology, 170
  nutritional management, 175,
    184–5, 187
  pathogenesis, 170–3
  persistent, 174
  precipitant-induced, 173–4
  precipitating factors, 70, 173
    control measures, 174–5
  in primary sclerosing
    cholangitis, 300
  stages, 173
  TIPS-related, 174, 175
  treatment, 174–6
hepatic iron concentration
    (HIC), 346
hepatic iron index (HII), 346
hepatic osteodystrophy
    (metabolic bone disease),
    195–8
  incidence and prevalence, 196
  management, 197–8, 297
  post-transplant, 196, 197–8,
    297
  in primary biliary cirrhosis,
    196, 283, 288
  in primary sclerosing
    cholangitis, 296–7
hepatic phosphorylase deficiency,
    389, 390, 410
hepatic stellate cells (HSCs) (Ito
    cells), 10, 39–40, 43
  activated, 40
    in alcoholic liver disease,
      314–15, 318
  microscopy, 9, 11
  quiescent, 40
  relative numbers/volume, 18
hepatic surgery see surgery,
    hepatic
hepatic veins, 4, 5
  causes of outflow obstruction,
    110

intrahepatic branches, 5, 6
  membranous obstruction of
    ostium, 480
  in reduced-size liver
    transplantation, 616
  thrombosis, 480
hepatic venous outlet
    obstruction, 109, 110,
    479–82
  see also Budd-Chiari syndrome
hepatic venous pressure
  free (FHVP), 139–40
  wedged see wedged hepatic
    venous pressure
hepatic venous pressure gradient
    (HVPG), 137, 139–40
  in non-cirrhotic portal
    hypertension, 479, 549
hepatic venous system,
    development, 1, 2
hepatic venules, terminal, 5, 6
hepaticojejunostomy see
    Roux-en-Y
    hepaticojejunostomy
hepatitis
  cryptogenic, 271
  drug-induced, 502, 503
  histology, 104–6
  interface, 104, 105
  non-A, non-B, 235
  non-A-E see seronegative
    hepatitis
  nutritional requirements,
    183–4
  see also specific types
hepatitis A, 205–9
  acute liver failure, 518
  in childhood, 416
  clinical features, 207
  diagnosis, 77, 207, 263
  epidemiology, 205–6
  in liver transplant recipients,
    658
  neonatal jaundice, 402
  pathogenesis, 206
  prevention, 208–9
  treatment and prognosis, 207–8
  vaccine, 208–9
    in NAFLD, 339
  vertical transmission, 493
hepatitis A and B combined
    vaccine (Twinrix®), 209
hepatitis A virus (HAV), 205
  genome, 205
  IgG antibody (IgG anti-HAV),
    207, 208
  IgM antibody (IgM anti-HAV),
    207, 208
  replication cycle, 206
  transmission, 205–6
hepatitis B, 213–30
  acute, 216
    in children, 216
    HDV co-infection, 231, 232
    serodiagnosis, 217, 218, 219

acute liver failure, 215, 216,
    518
  chronic, 216
    acute liver failure-like
      syndromes, 518–19
    in children, 217, 406–7
    HBeAg-negative see under
      hepatitis B e antigen
    HBeAg-positive see under
      hepatitis B e antigen
    HBV mutants, 216
    HDV superinfection, 231,
      232
    hepatocellular carcinoma,
      215, 216, 221, 454, 455
    in immunocompromised
      patients, 217
    liver histology, 105, 106, 221
    management see hepatitis B,
      management (below)
    natural history, 221
    prognosis, 221, 222
    serodiagnosis, 217, 218,
      219–20
  clinical features, 216–17
  diagnosis, 77, 217–21, 263
  epidemiology, 213–15
  extrahepatic manifestations,
    216
  hepatitis C co-infection, 217,
    246, 455
  hepatitis D co-infection, 230,
    231, 518, 595
  high-risk groups, 214–15
  HIV co-infection, 217, 225,
    227
  liver histology, 220–1
  liver transplantation, 229,
    593–5
    antiviral therapy, 225,
      226–7, 594–5
    de novo infection after, 677,
      678
    reinfection after see
      post-transplant
      recurrence (below)
    survival after, 594, 671
  management, 221–9
    combination therapies,
      228–9
    future treatment strategies,
      229
    guidelines, 229, 230
    interferon therapy, 223–4
    nucleoside/nucleotide
      analogs, 224–8
    objectives, 221–3
  neonatal jaundice, 402
  pathogenesis, 215–16
  polyarteritis nodosa, 216, 540
  post-transplant recurrence,
    593–5, 658, 669, 670–9
    diagnosis, 670
    drug treatment, 225, 226–7,
      658, 677–9

in hepatitis D co-infection,
    595, 596
  histopathology, 119–20,
    670, 671
  natural history, 670–2
  post-transplant prophylaxis,
    593–5, 672–7
  pretransplant prophylaxis,
    594, 672–4
  recipients of anti-HBc-
    positive allografts, 677,
    678
  retransplantation for, 679
  prevalence, 213–14, 215
  vaccination, 230
    adverse reactions, 230
    in childhood, 230, 407, 493
    hepatitis D prevention, 233
    hepatocellular carcinoma
      prevention, 454
    indications, 230
    in liver allograft recipients,
      676, 677
    neonates, 230, 493
    serologic markers, 217
  vaccines, 230
hepatitis B core antigen
    (HBcAg), 213
  expression, 215
  IgG antibody (IgG anti-HBc),
    218
  IgM antibody (IgM anti-Hbc),
    217–18, 518
  immunostaining, 103
  liver histology, 105, 106
  -positive liver allografts, 677,
    678
  in serodiagnosis, 217–18
hepatitis B e antigen (HBeAg),
    213
  antibody (anti-HBe), 217,
    218–19
  expression, 215, 216
  -negative chronic hepatitis B,
    218–19, 220, 221
    adefovir dipivoxil therapy,
      226
    combination therapy, 228–9
    interferon therapy, 223,
      224
    lamivudine therapy, 225
    new nucleoside analogs,
      227
  -positive chronic hepatitis B,
    218, 220, 221
    adefovir dipivoxil therapy,
      226
    combination therapy, 228,
      229
    interferon therapy, 223, 224
    lamivudine therapy, 224–5
    new nucleoside analogs,
      227–8
  seroconversion, 218, 221
  in serodiagnosis, 217, 218–19

hepatitis B immunoglobulin (HBIg)
costs, 675
post-exposure prophylaxis, 230
post-transplant prophylaxis, 593–4, 595, 674, 675–7
preparations, 676
hepatitis B surface antigen (HBsAg)
antibodies (anti-HBs), 217, 232
expression, 215
in hepatitis D, 232
immunostaining, 103
post-transplant reappearance, 593, 670
in serodiagnosis, 217
hepatitis B virus (HBV), 213
direct cytopathic effects, 215
DNA, 213
integration into host genome, 216, 454
post-transplant recurrence, 593, 670, 671–2
pretransplant status, 593, 672, 674
serum assays, 217, 218, 219–20
drug resistance, 225, 226, 673–4, 677, 678
genome, 213
genotypes, 220
immune-mediated liver injury, 215
inactive carriers
serologic markers, 217, 219, 220
transition to, 221
mutants, 216, 218–19, 221
HBIg treatment failure, 674, 675
lamivudine-resistant, 225, 226
in liver allograft recipients, 678
vaccine-escape, 230
replication cycle, 213, 214
transmission, 214–15
vertical transmission, 213–14, 406, 493
hepatitis B X protein (HBX), 213
hepatitis C, 235–48
acute, 239
liver biopsy, 105
recurrent post-transplant, 680, 681
treatment, 246
acute liver failure, 239, 519
alcohol and, 317
chronic, 235
autoantibodies, 267, 268, 271
in childhood, 407
clinical features, 239–40

complications, 240–1
extrahepatic manifestations, 240–1
hepatocellular carcinoma, 454–5
HFE gene mutations, 348
liver histopathology, 105, 239
porphyria cutanea tarda and, 65, 241, 373, 377
pregnancy in, 492
prognosis, 240
recurrent post-transplant, 680, 681
scoring systems, 239, 240
serum aminotransferases, 75–6, 77
treatment see below
clinical features, 239–40
diagnosis, 77, 238–9, 263
epidemiology, 237–8
future outlook, 247
in hemodialysis patients, 75
hepatitis B co-infection, 217, 246, 455
HIV co-infection, 237, 246
liver transplantation, 595–6, 679, 680
natural history, 240
neonatal jaundice, 402
post-transplant recurrence, 658–9, 669–70, 679–84
anti-HCV-positive donors, 682
factors influencing severity, 681–2
histopathology, 119–20, 680, 681
immunosuppression, acute rejection and, 680–1
natural history, 679–81
post-transplant management, 246–7, 682–4
pre-emptive antiviral therapy, 683
pretransplant antiviral therapy, 682
prophylactic therapy, 683
retransplantation, 684
treatment of established, 246–7, 683–4
vs acute rejection, 637–8, 681
prevention, 247
schistosomiasis co-infection, 259
treatment, 241–7
antiviral agents, 243–6
co-infected patients, 246
combination therapy, 245
decompensated cirrhosis, 246–7
effect on hepatic fibrosis, 242–3

goals, 241
non-responders, 246
patient selection, 243
patterns of response, 241–2
post-transplant disease, 246–7, 682–4
predictability of response, 243
relapse, 246
side-effects, 245–6
sustained virologic response (SVR), 241, 242
vaccine, 247
hepatitis C immune globulin (HCIG), in liver transplant recipients, 683
hepatitis C virus (HCV)
antibodies (anti-HCV), 238–9
autoimmune hepatitis and, 269
discovery, 235
genome, 235, 236
genotypes, 235, 236
pathogenetic mechanisms, 237
positive liver donors, 682
RNA
post-transplant recurrence, 595–6, 679–80
serum assays, 239
transmission, 237
vertical transmission, 237, 407, 493
virology, 235–7
hepatitis D, 230–3
acute liver failure, 518
autoantibodies, 267, 268, 271
clinical features, 231
diagnosis, 77, 231–2, 263
epidemiology, 230–1
liver transplantation, 233, 595, 596
natural history, 231
post-transplant recurrence, 669
prevention, 233
treatment, 233
hepatitis D antigen (HDAg), 230, 231
serum assay, 232
tissue markers, 232
hepatitis D virus (HDV), 230
antibodies, 231, 232
latent infection, 231
RNA, 232
superinfection, 231, 232
hepatitis E, 209–12
acute liver failure, 519
clinical features, 211
diagnosis, 77, 211, 263
epidemiology, 210
pathogenesis, 210–11
in pregnancy, 210, 211, 212, 492
prevention, 212
treatment and prognosis, 211–12
vaccine, 212

hepatitis E virus (HEV), 209–10
genome, 209
genotypes, 209–10
IgG antibody (IgG anti-HEV), 211
IgM antibody (IgM anti-HEV), 211
replication cycle, 210–11
hepatitis G virus (HGV), 77, 688
hepatoblastoma, 412–13, 467, 468
hepatocellular adenomas (HA), 424–6
in childhood, 413
clinical features, 425–6
in glycogen storage disease I, 388, 390
management, 426, 573–4
pathology, 114–15, 424
pregnancy and, 493
radiology, 129, 424–5
steroid-related, 504–5
hepatocellular carcinoma (HCC), 453–67
in alcoholic liver disease, 317
α_1-antitrypsin deficiency and, 379
in autoimmune hepatitis, 272
Budd-Chiari syndrome and, 456, 481
chemoembolization, 128, 133
in childhood, 412–13
clinical presentations, 456–7
diagnosis, 457–60, 571
epidemiology and pathogenesis, 453–6
fibrolamellar (FLHCC)
clinical features, 456–7
histopathology, 116, 117
liver transplantation, 599
pediatric patients, 412, 413
surgical management, 572
HBV-related, 215, 216, 221, 454, 455
HCV-related, 454–5
HDV-related, 231
in hereditary tyrosinemia type 1, 385
histopathology, 116, 460
imaging, 124, 127–9, 457–9
intra-arterial therapy, 464–5
liver transplantation, 462–3, 598–9
operative technique, 609
recurrence after, 598, 599, 661
management, 461–7
inoperable disease, 463–7
surgical approaches, 461–3, 571–2
Milan criteria, 598
natural history and prognosis, 460–1
non-cirrhotic, 457

hepatocellular carcinoma (HCC)
  (Continued)
  percutaneous alcohol injection,
    133, 465–6
  in porphyrias, 370
  in primary biliary cirrhosis, 283
  in primary sclerosing
    cholangitis, 300
  radiotherapy, 466
  sclerosing variant, 457
  screening, 467
  staging, 460–1, 571–2
  steroid-related, 504–5
  thermal and laser ablation,
    133, 466
  tumor rupture, 456
hepatocellular injury
  acute, 89–90
  chronic, 90
  drug/toxin-induced, 500–1, 502
hepatocellular plates see liver cell
  plates
hepatocerebral degeneration,
  acquired (AHCD), 70, 170,
  202–3
  clinical features, 174
  liver transplantation, 176, 203
hepatocystin, 444
hepatocyte specific antigen
  (hepatocyte paraffin-1,
  HepPar-1), 9, 460
hepatocytes, 6–10, 17–39
  apoptosis, 37–9
    in alcoholic hepatitis, 314,
    318
  ballooning
    in alcoholic hepatitis, 318,
    319
    in allograft rejection, 638,
    639
    in preservation injury, 646
  bile canalicular (apical)
    membrane, 7, 21, 22, 44
    bile acid secretion, 49
    bilirubin secretion, 51
    lipid secretion, 53
  bile formation, 46–52
  in biopsy specimens, 12
  cell coat (glycocalyx), 21–2
  cell cycle regulation, 35–7
  cell surface, 21–2
  cytoplasmic organelles, 7–9,
    22–30, 45
  cytoskeleton, 9–10, 22–5
  development, 1, 17
  extracellular matrix
    interactions, 32
  fat accumulation see steatosis,
    hepatic
  fatty acid metabolism, 55–6,
    328–32
  ground-glass inclusions, 105,
    106
  heterogeneity (zonation), 56–8
    metabolic pathways, 56–8

physiologic significance, 58
  regulation, 58
intercellular (lateral) domain,
  7, 21, 22
intercellular junctions, 22, 23,
  44–5
intracellular compartment
  volumes, 19
metabolic functions, 52–6
microscopy and ultrastructure,
  6–10
nuclear envelope, 30–1
nuclear pore complex, 31
nucleocytoplasmic transport,
  31
nucleus, 7, 12, 19, 30–1
  function, 30
  morphology, 30
plasma membrane, 17–21, 44
  biogenesis and turnover, 21
  domains, 21
  lipids, 18–21
  potential difference, 46, 49
  proteins, 21
  receptors, 33–4
plates see liver cell plates
polarity, 17, 22
regeneration, 37–9
relative numbers/volume, 17,
  18
signal transduction, 33–5
sinusoidal (basolateral)
    membrane, 7, 8, 21, 22,
    44
  bile acid transport, 48–9
  bilirubin uptake, 51, 83–4
  transport proteins, 46
structural organization, 17, 18
transplantation, 419
volume of viable, in acute liver
  failure, 526
zones 1, 2 and 3, 46
hepatoduodenal ligament, 3
hepatogenous diabetes, 202
hepatolenticular degeneration,
  acquired, 170, 202–3
hepatoma see hepatocellular
  carcinoma
hepatomegaly, 69
  causes, 69
  in cystic fibrosis, 382
  in fatty liver disease, 334
  in glycogen storage disease I,
    388, 390
  in hepatocellular carcinoma,
    456
hepatoportal sclerosis
  historical perspective, 549–50
  liver histology, 110, 111
  see also non-cirrhotic portal
    fibrosis
hepatopulmonary syndrome
  (HPS), 68, 191–3
  diagnostic criteria, 192
  natural history, 192–3

in primary biliary cirrhosis,
    283
  treatment, 193
hepatorenal syndrome (HRS),
    153, 161–4
  in alcoholic liver disease, 316
  clinical features and diagnosis,
    162
  definition, 161
  pathophysiology, 161–2
  prevention, 162, 322
  prognosis, 164
  treatment, 163–4
  type 1, 162
  type 2, 162
hepatorrhaphy, mesh, in liver
  trauma, 579, 580
hepatosplenic candidiasis (HSC),
  249
hepatosplenomegaly
  in Gaucher disease, 393
  in mucopolysaccharidoses, 392
hepatotoxicity, 497–516
  see also drug-induced liver
    disease
hepatotoxins
  classification, 499, 500
  type A, 499–500
  type B (idiosyncratic), 500,
    501
hepcidin, 341
  gene mutations, 341, 344
  hypothesis, hereditary
    hemochromatosis, 344
hephaestin, 344
Her disease (glycogen storage
  disease VI), 389, 390, 410
herbal medicines, 514
herbicides, 513
hereditary hemochromatosis see
  hemochromatosis,
  hereditary
hereditary hemorrhagic
  telangiectasia (HHT), 66,
  475–6
hereditary tyrosinemia see
  tyrosinemia, hereditary
hernias, abdominal, in ascites,
  154, 156
herpes simplex virus (HSV)
  in autoimmune hepatitis
    etiology, 269
  hepatitis
    acute liver failure, 519
    in childhood, 416
    diagnosis, 263
    in neonates, 401, 402
    post liver transplant, 118,
      120, 653
    in pregnancy, 492, 494
  immunostaining, 103
  post-transplant infections,
    653, 666, 669, 687
herpes zoster (shingles), 666,
  687

HFE gene, 341, 342–4
  C282Y heterozygotes, 341,
    344, 348
  C282Y homozygotes, 342–3,
    344–5
  compound (C282Y/H63D)
    heterozygotes, 342, 343
  mutation analysis, 345, 346,
    348
  mutations, 341, 342–3
    in porphyria cutanea tarda,
      348, 373
    in other liver diseases, 348
HFE protein, 342, 343–4
HH see hemochromatosis,
  hereditary
hirsutism, 420, 634, 664
Hispanic Americans, gallbladder
  disease, 435, 436
histiocytoma (inflammatory
  pseudotumor), 433
histochemical stains, 102, 103
histoplasmosis, 250, 255
history, clinical, 61–3
HIV infection/AIDS
  AIDS-related sclerosing
    cholangitis, 295
  cholangiopathy, 92, 106
  cytomegalovirus infection,
    252
  drug-induced hepatotoxicity,
    499, 507
  hepatitis A vaccination, 209
  hepatitis B co-infection, 217,
    225, 227
  hepatitis C co-infection, 237,
    246
  liver biopsy, 107
  Mycobacterium avium
    intracellulare, 255, 256
  neonatal jaundice, 402
  peliosis hepatis, 483
  syphilis co-infection, 255
HJV gene mutations, 341
HLA haplotypes
  in autoimmune hepatitis, 266,
    269, 274
  in cystic fibrosis liver disease,
    411
  in drug-induced
    hepatotoxicity, 501
  in primary biliary cirrhosis,
    277
  in primary sclerosing
    cholangitis, 290–1
HMG-CoA reductase inhibitors
  (statins)
  hepatotoxicity, 511
  in liver allograft recipients,
    662–3
  in NAFLD management, 188,
    339
Hodgkin disease, 118, 545
Hoesch test, 375
homosexual men, 206, 214

hormone replacement therapy (HRT)
in hepatic osteodystrophy, 197, 198
in polycystic liver disease, 443, 445–6
HSV *see* herpes simplex virus
HUG-Br1 gene defects, 86
human herpesvirus-6 (HHV-6), 653, 669, 687–8
human herpesvirus-7 (HHV-7), 653, 669, 687–8
human herpesvirus-8 (HHV-8), 666
human immunodeficiency virus infection *see* HIV infection/AIDS
human papillomavirus infection, post-transplant, 653, 666
Hunter syndrome (type II MPS), 392, 393
Hurler syndrome (type 1H MPS), 392, 393
hydatid cysts (hydatid disease), 257–8, 576
Budd-Chiari syndrome, 479
surgical management, 576
hydralazine, 510
hydrothorax, hepatic, 154–5, 164
3-hydroxy-3-methylglutaryl (HMG)-coenzyme A (CoA) reductase, 53, 58
inhibitors *see* HMG-CoA reductase inhibitors
D-3-hydroxybutyrate, 329
5-hydroxyindoleacetic acid (5-HIAA), 470–1
7-α-hydroxylase, 47
hydroxylethyl free radicals, 313
hydroxyquine, in porphyria cutanea tarda, 377
hydroxyzine, 99
hyperacute liver allograft rejection *see under* rejection, liver allograft
hyperacute liver failure, 517
intracranial hypertension, 520–1
liver transplantation, 529
pathology, 524
referral criteria, 526
hyperacute xenograft rejection, 640
hyperammonemia, 56
pathogenesis, 171–2
treatment, 175
hyperbilirubinemia, 79
conjugated, 51, 88, 95
in neonatal liver disease, 398, 401, 403
in jaundice, 83
non-hepatic causes, 73
in primary biliary cirrhosis, 280, 283–4
indicating need for transplant, 288, 591

unconjugated, 88, 95
in neonates, 397
hypercalciuria, in Wilson disease, 355
hypercholesterolemia, 65, 339
hyperdynamic circulation, 68, 521–2
hyperemesis gravidarum, 488, 494, 495
hypergammaglobulinemia
in alcoholic liver disease, 314
in primary sclerosing cholangitis, 291, 292–3
hyperglycemia, post-liver transplantation, 643
hyperinsulinemia, 202
hyperkalemia
diuretic-induced, in cirrhosis, 157, 158
in liver transplant operation, 612
hyperlipidemia
in glycogen storage disease I, 388
in liver allograft recipients, 421, 662–3
NASH risk, 327–8
hyperoxaluria, primary, 601–2
hyperpigmentation, 65, 280
hypersensitivity reactions
delayed-type (DTH), 629, 630
drug-induced liver injury, 501
hypersplenism
in extrahepatic portal vein obstruction, 560, 562, 563
in liver disease, 200, 201
hypertension, 68
in liver allograft recipients, 420, 662
in pre-eclampsia, 489
hyperthyroidism, 538
hypertrophic pulmonary osteopathy, 68, 195, 196
hyperuricemia, in liver allograft recipients, 663
hyperventilation, in cerebral edema, 533
hypoalbuminemia, non-hepatic causes, 73, 79
hypobetalipoproteinemia, 76, 331
hypocalcemia, post-liver transplantation, 643
hypoglycemia
in acute liver failure, 187, 521
in cirrhosis, 187
in glycogen storage diseases, 388, 410
in hepatocellular carcinoma, 456
in neonatal liver disease, 401, 402
hypoglycin (methylenecyclo-propylalanine), 330, 333

hypogonadism, 70
hypokalemia, diuretic-induced, in cirrhosis, 157, 158
hyponatremia
in acute intermittent porphyria, 371
in acute liver failure, 521
dilutional, in cirrhosis, 153, 159–60
diuretic-induced, in cirrhosis, 157, 158
hypophosphatemia, in acute liver failure, 521
hypopituitarism, neonatal hepatitis, 401, 402
hypotension
in acute liver failure, 535
in chronic liver disease, 68
hypothermia, post-liver transplant, 643
hypothyroidism
liver abnormalities, 538–9
neonatal, 401, 402
hypoxemia, in hepatopulmonary syndrome, 191, 192

ibuprofen, 509, 510
icterus, 65
see also jaundice
idiopathic adulthood ductopenia (IAD)
differential diagnosis, 282, 295
liver biopsy, 107–8, 109
L-iduronidase deficiency, 392
ileal lipid-binding protein, 52
ileal pouch-anal anastomosis (IPAA), 307
pouchitis, 301, 307
ileostomy, peristomal variceal bleeding, 300
ill health, general, 61
imaging, 123–35
benign liver tumors, 129, 423–4
biliary abnormalities, 130–1
cystic fibrosis, 384
diffuse liver diseases, 125–7
drug-induced liver disease, 516
hepatic steatosis/NASH, 335–7
hepatocellular carcinoma, 124, 127–9, 457–9
in jaundice, 95–7
masses, 127–9
modalities, 123–5, 132–3
non-cirrhotic portal hypertension, 553, 556
post-liver transplantation, 644–5
primary sclerosing cholangitis, 293
vascular abnormalities, 129–30
Wilson disease, 356
see also specific modalities
iminodiacetic acid scintigraphy, 97, 131

immune serum globulin (ISG), hepatitis A prevention, 208
immune system, 621–3
immunizations, pre-liver transplant, 419
immunocompromised patients
cytomegalovirus infection, 252
hepatitis B, 217
histoplasmosis, 250
liver allograft recipients, 661
Mycobacterium avium intracellulare, 255
immunoglobulin, intravenous
CMV prophylaxis in transplant recipients, 686
hepatitis A prevention, 208
immunoglobulin A (IgA), 12, 33
immunoglobulin light chains, 484, 541
immunoglobulin M (IgM)
in primary biliary cirrhosis, 280, 281
in primary sclerosing cholangitis, 293
immunoglobulin (Ig) superfamily, 621
immunohistochemical stains, 102, 103
immunologic abnormalities
in extrahepatic portal vein obstruction, 561
in non-cirrhotic portal fibrosis, 550–1
in primary biliary cirrhosis, 277–9
in primary sclerosing cholangitis, 291
immunologic idiosyncrasy, in drug-induced hepatotoxicity, 501, 502
immunologic mechanisms
in alcoholic hepatitis, 314
in childhood acute liver failure, 416–17
in drug-induced hepatotoxicity, 501
immunological synapse, 625
immunology, transplant, 621–42
immunomodulatory drugs, hepatotoxic, 511–12
immunophilins, 631
immunoreceptor tyrosine-base activation motif (ITAM), 625
immunosuppressive drugs, 630–5
adverse effects, 420, 421, 633–5, 661
in autoimmune hepatitis, 272–4, 408
drug interactions, 633–5
in liver allograft recipients, 632–5
long-term management, 661
non-compliance, 421, 666

immunosuppressive drugs
(Continued)
to prevent acute rejection,
632–3
to treat acute rejection, 633
pharmacology and mechanisms
of action, 630–2
in primary biliary cirrhosis,
285–6
in primary sclerosing
cholangitis, 305–6
in recurrent post-transplant
hepatitis C, 680–1
importins, 31
inborn errors of metabolism,
369–94
childhood, 405, 409–12
drug-induced hepatotoxicity,
499
liver histology, 102, 110–13
liver transplantation, 418
outcome, 421
neonatal jaundice, 397, 401,
402–5
see also metabolic liver
diseases; specific disorders
indinavir, 86
indocyanine green (ICG),
hepatic clearance, 80
infants
acute liver failure, 413–16
newborn see neonates
infarction, hepatic
in Budd-Chiari syndrome, 480
in hepatic artery occlusion,
473–4
in hyperacute allograft
rejection, 636
in pregnancy, 490
infections, 249–61
in acute liver failure, 522,
534–5
in alcoholic liver disease, 316,
320
granulomatous hepatitis, 255–6
hepatic encephalopathy and,
172
immunosuppressed patients,
633
intrauterine, neonatal
hepatitis, 401–2
in liver allograft recipients,
649–54, 666
pediatric patients, 420
prophylaxis, 532, 651
liver histopathology, 102
parasitic, 259–61
susceptibility in liver disease,
64–5, 201
systemic, with hepatic
manifestations, 249–55
see also abscesses, liver; viral
hepatitis; specific
infections
infectious mononucleosis, 253

inferior mesenteric vein, 137
inferior thyroid vein, 138
inferior vena cava (IVC)
anastomoses, in liver
transplant surgery, 612
ligation, liver transplant
operation, 607, 611
membranous obstruction, 480
in reduced-size liver
transplantation, 616
stenosis, post-liver
transplantation, 648
thrombosis, 480, 648
infertility, 63
inflammation
in acute allograft rejection,
636
in alcoholic hepatitis, 318
in drug-induced liver injury,
500
in hepatitis, 104, 105
in NASH, 113, 334, 338
in primary biliary cirrhosis, 280
inflammatory bowel disease,
primary sclerosing
cholangitis and, 289, 300–1
inflammatory pseudotumor, 433
infliximab, in alcoholic hepatitis,
321, 322
influenza virus, 654
injection drug users see
intravenous drug users
inositol polyphosphates (IP-3),
625
insecticides, 513
inspissated bile syndrome, 400
insulin
fatty acid metabolism and,
328, 330
in NASH pathogenesis, 335–6
resistance, 184, 202
in childhood, 409
clinical features, 334
fatty acid metabolism and,
328, 332
measurement, 335
therapy
in acute liver failure, 527
in alcoholic hepatitis, 321,
323
insulin-like growth factor, 179
insulin receptors, 33, 34
integrins, 32, 33, 627–8
intensive care unit (ICU),
post-transplant care, 643
intercellular adhesion molecule-1
(ICAM-1), 10, 291
interferon α
in acute hepatitis C, 246
in acute liver failure, 527
adverse effects, 224, 245–6,
539
in chronic hepatitis B, 220,
222, 223–4
in childhood, 406

lamivudine combinations,
228–9
long-term outcome, 223
predictors of non-response,
223
pretransplant patients, 672–3
in chronic hepatitis C, 243–4
in children, 407
effect of antiviral therapy,
242–3
pretransplant therapy, 682
ribavirin combination, 243,
245
special patient groups,
246–7
in chronic hepatitis D, 233
in HBV/HCV co-infection,
246
pegylated see pegylated
interferons
in recurrent hepatitis B, 678
in recurrent hepatitis C, 683,
684
interferon-α (IFN-α), 623, 629
interferon-β, 623
interferon-γ (IFN-γ), 622, 623
in antigen recognition, 624–5
in Th1 response, 629
interleukin-1 (IL-1), 313, 622
interleukin-1β, 91
interleukin-2 (IL-2), 622
in T-cell activation, 625, 626,
627
in Th1 response, 629
interleukin-2 (IL-2) receptor,
622, 627
α-chain monoclonal antibody
(mAb), 632, 633
interleukin-4 (IL-4), 622, 629
interleukin-5 (IL-5), 622, 630
interleukin-6 (IL-6), 622
in alcoholic hepatitis, 313, 322
interleukin-8 (IL-8), 622
in alcoholic hepatitis, 313,
314, 322
interleukin-10 (IL-10), 622
promoter polymorphisms, 314
in Th2 response, 629
interleukin-12 (IL-12), 215, 622,
629
interleukin-13 (IL-13), 622–3
interleukin-15 (IL-15), 623
interleukin-18 (IL-18), 623
intermediate-density lipoprotein
(IDL), 330, 332
intermediate filaments, 10, 23,
24
intermittent inflow occlusion, for
liver resections, 569
international normalized ratio
(INR), 199
in acute liver failure, 525, 526
liver graft function and, 644
liver transplant candidates,
418

interventional radiology, 133–4
intracranial pressure
monitoring, 530, 534
raised
in acute liver failure, 173,
520–1
management, 533–4
intrahepatic cholestasis of
pregnancy (ICP), 487, 488–9
diagnosis, 494
prognosis, 495
treatment, 495
intrauterine growth retardation,
400, 401
intrauterine infections, neonatal
hepatitis, 401–2
intravenous drug users
hepatitis A, 205–6
hepatitis B, 214
hepatitis C, 237, 247
signs, 65–6
iodine-131 (^{131}I), intra-arterial
administration, 466
ion-channel-linked receptors, 33
iproniazid, 506
irenotecan, 470
iron
absorption, in hereditary
hemochromatosis, 343
binding capacity, total, 201
concentration, hepatic (HIC),
346
deficiency (anemia)
increased bilirubin, 86
in liver disease, 183, 201
in protoporphyria, 374,
377–8
deposits, in hemochromatosis,
111, 346, 347
index, hepatic (HII), 346
in liver disease, 348
metabolism, role of HFE
protein, 343
serum, 201
supplements, 188
iron overload
African, 341
imaging, 126–7
inherited see
hemochromatosis,
hereditary
neonatal, 342
parenteral, 341, 342
in porphyria cutanea tarda,
348, 370, 373, 377
secondary, 341–2
liver histology, 111–12, 346
in sickle cell disease, 541
syndromes, 341–2
ischemia, hepatic
in Budd-Chiari syndrome, 480
donor livers, 646
hepatic artery occlusion,
473–4
jaundice, 89–90

ischemia, hepatic *(Continued)*
liver biopsy, 109–10, 111
in pre-eclampsia/eclampsia, 489
ischemic heart disease, 195
ischemic hepatitis
acute liver failure, 520
in congestive heart failure, 544
islet cell tumors of pancreas, metastatic, surgical resection, 573
isoniazid, 508
isosorbide dinitrate (ISDN), 143
isosorbide mononitrate (ISMN), 143, 145, 146
Ito cells *see* hepatic stellate cells
itraconazole, 651

Jag 1 gene mutations, 403
Jarisch-Herxheimer reaction, 255
jaundice, 62, 65, 83–99
in acute liver failure, 520
in alcoholic liver disease, 315
causes, 86–92
in choledochal cyst, 400, 448
clinical features, 92–3
in congestive heart failure, 543
in cystic fibrosis, 382–3
diagnosis and evaluation, 93–8
decision analysis, 95
imaging studies, 95–7
liver biopsy, 97–8
screening laboratory tests, 93–5
serologic testing, 97
differential diagnosis, 88
in extrahepatic portal vein obstruction, 560
in hepatitis A, 207
in hepatitis B, 216
in hepatocellular carcinoma, 456
in hypothyroidism, 539
in intrahepatic cholestasis of pregnancy, 488
in leptospirosis, 254
in liver disease, 88–92
in lymphoma, 545
management, 98, 99
neonatal *see* neonatal jaundice
obstructive, 88, 92
in choledocholithiasis, 442
liver biopsy, 97–8
see also biliary obstruction
pathophysiology, 83–6
physiologic, of newborn, 86
postoperative, 91–2
in pregnancy, 91, 487
in primary biliary cirrhosis, 91, 279
in syphilis, 254
JC virus, post-transplant infection, 654, 666
jejunojejunostomy, in liver transplantation, 614
jejunostomy feeding tubes, 187

karyopherins, 31
Kasabach-Merritt syndrome, 573
Kasai portoenterostomy, 398–9, 603
Katayama fever, 259
Kayser–Fleischer rings, 65, 354, 356
keratan sulfate, accumulation, 392
ketoconazole, hepatotoxicity, 507
ketone bodies, 329
Kiernan lobules *see* lobules, liver
kinesin, 24, 45
King's College criteria, acute liver failure, 525–6, 529
Kupffer cells, 39
in alcoholic hepatitis, 313
development, 17
microscopy, 8, 9, 10
pigmented, 104, 105
relative numbers/volume, 18
kwashiorkor, 177, 330

labetalol, 511
laboratory tests, 73–81
lactate, serum
in acetaminophen overdose, 526
in acute liver failure, 521
liver graft function and, 644
lactate dehydrogenase, ascitic fluid, 166
lactitol, in hepatic encephalopathy, 175
lactulose, in hepatic encephalopathy, 175, 178
lamellar bodies, 333
laminin, 11, 33
lamins, 24, 266, 278
lamivudine
HBV resistance, 225, 226, 674
in hepatitis B, 224–5
adefovir combination, 229
in childhood, 406
peginterferon combination, 228–9
post-transplant prophylaxis, 674–7
post-transplant therapy, 225, 678–9
in pretransplant management, 594, 672–4
laparoscopic surgery
cholecystectomy, 438, 439
polycystic liver disease, 446, 447
laparoscopy, presurgical, 567
laser thermal ablation, hepatocellular carcinoma, 466
lecithin, 47, 53
left lateral segment liver grafts, donor organ reduction, 615–16

left lobe
anatomic, 3, 4
Couinaud functional segments, 5
grafts
donor organ reduction, 615–16
implantation technique, 616, 618
physiologic, 3, 4
venous drainage, 5
lepromatous hepatitis, 256
leprosy, 256
Leptospira interrogans, 253
leptospirosis, 253–4
anicteric, 254
icteric, 254
lethargy, 61
see also fatigue
leucine aminopeptidase, 77–8, 487
leukemia, 249, 481
leukocyte function-associated antigen-1 (LFA-1), 10, 291, 627
leukocytes (white blood cells)
ascitic fluid, 155
donor, in liver allograft tolerance, 641
endothelial cell interaction, 627–8
see also lymphocytes; macrophages; neutrophils; polymorphonuclear (PMN) leukocytes
leukonychia, 67
LFA-1 *see* leukocyte function-associated antigen-1
libido, reduced, 63
lichen planus, 65, 241
lifestyle modification, in NAFLD, 338
ligamentum teres (round ligament)
anatomy, 3, 4
development, 1, 2
ligamentum venosum, 1, 2
ligandins, 51, 84
limbs, examination, 66
limiting plate, 5, 6
Linton-Nachlas tube, 144
lipids
biliary secretion, 53, 54
membrane, 17, 18–20
bilayers, 17, 19
phases, 20
raft model, 20–1
peroxidation, 334, 351, 500
see also fat; fatty acids
lipiodol, 132, 464, 466
lipodystrophies, 327–8
lipolysis, adipocyte, 328
lipomatous tumors, 430
lipopolysaccharide (LPS), 313, 550

lipoprotein lipase (LPL), 332
lipoproteins
metabolism, 52–3, 332
modification of circulating, 332
release of fatty acids, 332
Listeria monocytogenes, 250, 651
listeriosis, 250–1
lithocholic acid, 47, 48, 52
lithotripsy, extracorporeal shock-wave, 438
liver
anatomy *see* anatomy, liver
architecture, 17, 18
cellular biology, 17–41
development, 1
functions, 43–59
volume *see* volume, liver
liver allografts
anti-HBc-positive, 677, 678
anti-HCV-positive, 682
assessment of early function, 643–4
dysfunction mimicking autoimmune hepatitis, 660
early dysfunction, 644–7
classification, 645, 646
live donor graft recipients, 619
monitoring and diagnostic work-up, 644–5
risk factors, 646–7
initial poor function (IPF), 646–7
late dysfunction, 655, 656
long-term monitoring of function, 655
preservation injury, 646–7
primary dysfunction, preservation injury and, 646–7
primary non-function (PNF), 646, 647
rejection *see* rejection, liver allograft
tolerance, 640–1
see also donor livers
liver biopsy, 101–21
in AIDS, 106
in bone marrow transplantation, 120–1
in cholestatic liver disease, 107–8
complications, 101–2
contraindications, 101
in drug-induced liver disease, 108–9, 502–4, 516
in fatty liver diseases, 113–14, 337–8
in hepatitis, 104–6
indications, 76, 101
interpretation, 12, 102–4
in liver transplantation, 118–20

liver biopsy *(Continued)*
  allograft rejection, 636–7,
    638–9, 649, 650
  early graft dysfunction, 645,
    646
  routine, 667
  in metabolic liver disease,
    110–13
  percutaneous (PLB)
    technique, 101
    ultrasound guidance, 101–2
  space-occupying lesions,
    114–18
  stains, 102, 103
  tissue processing, 102
  transjugular (TJB), 101
  vascular lesions, 109–10
liver cell adenomas *see*
  hepatocellular adenomas
liver cell cancer, primary
  (PLCC) *see* hepatocellular
  carcinoma
liver cell plates, 5, 46
  development, 1
  hepatocyte heterogeneity
    along, 56–8
  microanatomy, 43–4
  microscopy, 6, 7, 12
liver cytosol type 1 (LC-1)
  antibodies, 268
liver function tests (LFTs), 73–80
  cholestatic liver injury, 77–9
  hepatic synthetic function,
    79–80
  hepatobiliary injury, 74–7
  in jaundice, 93–5
  non-hepatic causes of
    abnormal, 73
  in pregnancy, 487, 488
liver–kidney microsomal (LKM)
  antibodies, 266–7, 271
  type 1 (LKM-1), 266–7, 268
  type 2 (LKM-2), 267, 268,
    501
  type 3 (LKM-3), 267, 268
liver-kidney transplantation, 447,
  601–2
liver microsomal (LM) antibodies,
  268
liver pancreas (LP) antibodies,
  267–8, 271
liver segments of Couinaud *see*
  segments, liver
liver transplant operation, 605–20
  auxiliary grafts, 618–19
  deceased donor hepatectomy,
    606–7
  history, 605
  operating room organization,
    605–6
  orthotopic, 607–14
    anhepatic phase, 611–12
    arterial anastomoses,
      613–14
    biliary anastomosis, 614

donor liver selection, 607
factors increasing difficulty,
  608–9
final closure and drain
  placement, 614, 615
general approaches, 609
hepatectomy phase, 610–11
piggyback technique, 609,
  612, 661
reperfusion phase, 612–13
technical complications,
  647–9
three phases, 609–13
in pediatric patients, 615–17
postoperative care of live
  donor recipients, 619–20
reduced-size grafts, 615–18
  abdominal closure, 616–17
  early postoperative care,
    619–20
  implantation of lobe grafts,
    618
  living related donor
    hepatectomy, 617–18
  recipient operation, 616
  technique of size reduction,
    615–16
liver transplantation
  in acetaminophen overdose,
    526
  in acute liver failure *see under*
    acute liver failure
  in Alagille syndrome, 403–4,
    603
  in alcoholic liver disease, 324,
    596–7
  allograft rejection *see*
    rejection, liver allograft
  in α₁-antitrypsin deficiency,
    381, 421, 601
  in autoimmune hepatitis, 274,
    597
  auxiliary *see* auxiliary liver
    transplantation
  in biliary atresia, 399, 417,
    603
  in cirrhosis with ascites, 156
  contraindications, 590–1
  coronary artery disease (CAD)
    and, 195
  in cystic fibrosis, 385, 412,
    600
  cytomegalovirus infection
    after, 252
  early complications
    allograft rejection, 647–9
    detection, 643
    functional cholestasis, 647
    graft dysfunction *see under*
      liver allografts
    infections, 649–54
    live donor graft recipients,
      620, 647
    pediatric patients, 420
    technical, 647–9

early management, 643–54
  assessment of graft function,
    643–4
  intensive care unit, 643
in hepatic encephalopathy, 176
in hepatitis B *see under*
  hepatitis B
in hepatitis C, 595–6, 679, 680
in hepatitis D, 233, 595, 596
in hepatocellular carcinoma *see*
  under hepatocellular
  carcinoma
in hepatocerebral
  degeneration, 176, 203
in hepatogenous diabetes, 202
in hepatopulmonary syndrome,
  191, 193
in hepatorenal syndrome, 163
in hereditary tyrosinemia type
  1, 386, 421, 601
immunology, 621–42
immunosuppressive therapy
  see immunosuppressive
  drugs, in liver allograft
  recipients
indications and patient
  selection, 585–604
late complications, 655–67
  allograft rejection, 655–6
  biliary problems, 657–8
  bone disease, 196, 197–8,
    297, 664
  disease recurrence *see below*
  general health and lifestyle
    issues, 664–7
  hepatic artery thrombosis,
    656
  immunosuppression, 661
  medical problems, 661–4
  in pediatric patients, 420
  portal vein thrombosis, 656
latent HDV infection, 231
liver biopsy *see under* liver
  biopsy
living related donor *see* living
  related donor liver
  transplantation
long-term management,
  655–68
in malignant disease, 418,
  597–600
MELD score *see* MELD score
in non-alcoholic fatty liver
  disease, 339, 660
numbers of operations, 585,
  586
nutritional management, 187,
  419
nutritional requirements,
  183–4
obesity and, 178, 181
orthotopic (OLT), 607–14
pathology, 118–20
pediatric *see* pediatric liver
  transplantation

in polycystic liver disease,
  446–7
for portal hypertension/
  variceal bleeding, 144–5,
  150, 151
in portopulmonary
  hypertension, 193, 194,
  609
pregnancy after, 493, 664–5
in primary biliary cirrhosis *see*
  under primary biliary
  cirrhosis
in primary sclerosing
  cholangitis *see under*
  primary sclerosing
  cholangitis
protein energy malnutrition
  and, 178, 181
in protoporphyria, 378
recurrent disease after,
  658–61
  hepatocellular carcinoma,
    598, 599, 661
  pediatric patients, 421
  viral hepatitis, 658–9,
    669–89
  see also under specific
    diseases
reduced-size, 419, 615–18
retransplantation, 603–4
  recurrent hepatitis B, 679
  recurrent hepatitis C, 684
split-liver *see* split-liver
  transplantation
surgical technique *see* liver
  transplant operation
timing, 585–90
in Wilson disease, 363, 421,
  600–1
xenografts, 640
see also liver allografts
living related donor liver
  transplantation (LDLT)
  in acute liver failure, 528
  adults, 615, 617–18
    early complications, 619, 647
  donor segmentectomy of
    segments II/III, 617
  early postoperative care of
    recipients, 619–20
  pediatric patients, 419, 615,
    617–18
  right lobe donor hepatectomy,
    617–18
LKM antibodies *see* liver–kidney
  microsomal (LKM)
  antibodies
lobar hyperplasia, compensatory,
  433
lobectomy, 462, 463, 567
  see also resection, liver
lobes, liver
  anatomy, 3, 4
  physiologic division, 3, 4
  see also specific lobes

lobular hepatitis, in obesity, 327
lobules, liver (Kiernan), 5–6, 7, 18
long chain hydroxyacyl-CoA dehydrogenase (LCHAD), 330, 333
  deficiency, 490
loop diuretics, in ascites, 156
low-density lipoprotein (LDL), 330, 332
low-density lipoprotein (LDL) receptors, 33, 34, 332
lung perfusion scanning, radionuclide, 192
lupus erythematosus, systemic (SLE), 539–40
luteinizing hormone-releasing hormone (LHRH) analogs, in acute porphyria, 377
lymph, hepatic, 11
lymphangioma, hepatic, 430
lymphatics, 11–12
lymphocytes
  endothelial cell interaction, 627–8
  large granular, 41
  liver-associated, 10
  see also T cells
lymphohistiocytosis, familial hemophagocytic, 416
lymphoma, 544–6
  acute liver failure, 520, 523, 546
  hepatic radiation injury, 546
  hepatitis C-related, 455
  histopathology, 118
  in liver allograft recipients, 665–6
  liver involvement, 545
  primary hepatic, 468, 545
lymphoproliferative disorder
  post-transplant see post-transplant lymphoproliferative disorder
  X-linked (XLP), 253
lysosomal acid lipase see acid lipase
lysosomal acid maltase deficiency, 389, 390
lysosomes, 25–6
  endocytotic pathway, 26
  hepatocyte, 9, 19
  membrane protein degradation, 21
  phospholipid accumulation, 333–4

macroaggregate albumin particles, technetium-labeled (^{99m}TcMAA), 192
macrocytosis, 201
macrophage inflammatory protein 1 (MIP-1), 313

macrophages
  in allograft rejection, 630, 638, 639
  in drug-induced liver injury, 500
  mechanisms of tissue injury, 629
  role of cytokines, 622, 623
  in Th1/Th2 response, 629
macrovesicular steatosis, 113
  causes, 328, 332
  drug-induced, 503
  in NASH, 338
macula adherens see desmosomes
Maddrey Discriminant Function (DF), alcoholic hepatitis, 320
magnetic resonance angiography (MRA), 125
  in non-cirrhotic portal hypertension, 553, 557
magnetic resonance cholangiography (MRC), 125
  gallstones, 131, 132
  jaundice, 96
magnetic resonance cholangiopancreatography (MRCP)
  choledochal cysts, 448
  choledocholithiasis, 441
magnetic resonance imaging (MRI), 124–5
  benign liver tumors, 424
  focal nodular hyperplasia, 431
  hemangiomas, 428
  hepatic cysts, 434
  hepatocellular adenomas, 425
  hepatocellular carcinoma, 459, 571
  infantile hemangioendothelioma, 429
  steatosis/NASH, 337
  Wilson disease, 356, 359
magnetic resonance spectroscopy (MRS), 126
magnetic resonance venography (MRV), 125
major histocompatibility complex (MHC), 623–4
  in alloantigen recognition, 629–30
  in allograft rejection, 630
  class I molecules, 623–4
    in antigen recognition, 624–5
  class II molecules, 624
    in antigen recognition, 625
  gene complex, 623–4
  see also HLA haplotypes
malabsorption
  in biliary atresia, 399
  as cause of malnutrition, 178
  in cystic fibrosis, 411–12
  management, 98
  in primary sclerosing cholangitis, 296
malaise, general, 61

maleyl acetoacetate, 385
malignant disease
  acute liver failure, 520, 522–3
  biliary reconstruction/bypass, 580, 581
  Budd-Chiari syndrome, 479
  contraindicating liver transplant, 418, 590, 609
  infiltration of sinusoids, 484
  jaundice, 92
  in liver allograft recipients, 665–6
  non-tumor liver lesions in extrahepatic, 118
  screening, in liver allograft recipients, 666
malignant liver tumors, 453–74
  of childhood, 412–13, 468
  histopathology, 116–18
  interventional radiology, 133–4
  liver transplantation, 418, 597–600
    numbers of operations, 585, 587
    recurrence after, 660–1
  primary, 453–68
  radiology, 127–9
  secondary see metastases, hepatic
  surgical management, 571–3
Mallory bodies, 10, 24
  in alcoholic liver disease, 114, 314, 319
  in chronic cholestasis, 108
  in NASH, 113, 338
  in Wilson disease, 112
malnutrition, 177–90
  in alcoholic liver disease, 177–8, 315
  clinical features, 64, 182–3
  definition, 177
  drug-induced hepatotoxicity and, 499
  nutritional assessment, 181–2
  pathophysiology, 178–80
  prevalence, 177–8
  prognosis, 180–1
  protein energy see protein energy malnutrition
  see also obesity
Malta fever, 251
manganese
  in hepatic encephalopathy pathogenesis, 172–3
  supplements, 183
mannitol, 48, 533
mannose 6-phosphate (M6P) receptors, 26, 33
mannose receptors, 33
marasmus, 177
Maroteaux-Lamy syndrome, 392
masses
  histopathology, 114–18
  imaging, 127–9
  see also tumors, liver

mastocytosis, 484
maternal–infant transmission see vertical transmission
Mayo risk score, primary biliary cirrhosis, 284, 588–9
MDR3 (ABCB4; mouse mdr2) gene
  function, 53, 54
  mutations, 282, 404, 488
mean corpuscular volume (MCV), 201, 315
mean pulmonary artery pressure (MPAP), 193
medical history, past, 63
Mediterranean fever, 251
medium chain acyl-CoA dehydrogenase (MCHAD), defects, 330
medium chain triglycerides, 183, 412
mefenamic acid, 509
megaloblastic anemia, 86
megamitochondria, in alcoholic liver disease, 318, 319
MELD score, 71, 79
  calculation equation, 588
  efficacy of liver transplantation and, 588, 589
  in hepatocellular carcinoma, 598
  liver transplant timing and, 585–8
  pediatric liver transplantation, 603
  TIPS and, 144
melena, 62
melioidosis, 251
membranes, cell, 17–21
  bilayer structure, 17, 19
  fluidity, 20
  lipids and proteins, 17–20
  phases, 20
  see also hepatocytes, plasma membrane
membranous glomerulonephritis, HBV-related, 216
mercaptans, in hepatic encephalopathy, 172
6-mercaptopurine, 482, 511–12, 630
mesenchymal hamartoma, 432, 433
mesh hepatorrhaphy, in liver trauma, 579, 580
messenger RNA (mRNA), 30, 31
metabolic acidosis
  in acetaminophen overdose, 526
  in acute liver failure, 521
metabolic bone disease see hepatic osteodystrophy
metabolic disorders
  in acute liver failure, 521
  post-liver transplantation, 643

metabolic idiosyncrasy, in drug-induced hepatotoxicity, 501, 502
metabolic liver diseases, 369–96
  auxiliary liver transplantation, 419
  childhood, 409–12, 416–17
  liver histology, 110–13
  liver transplantation, 418, 600–2
  outcome, 421
  recurrence after, 658, 660
  see also inborn errors of metabolism
metabolic rate, in cirrhosis, 180
metabolism, hepatic, 52–6
  ammonia, 56
  carbohydrate, 55
  cholesterol and lipoproteins, 52–3
  drug see drug metabolism
  fatty acid, 55–6
  important pathways, 54
  protein synthesis, 56
  zonation, 56–8
metallothionein, 352, 353, 363
metastases, hepatic, 453, 468–71
  clinical features, 468
  diagnosis, 468–9
  histology, 469
  imaging, 127, 128
  liver transplantation, 599–600
  management, 133, 470
  natural history and prognosis, 469–70
  neuroendocrine tumors see neuroendocrine tumors, metastatic
  surgical resection, 470, 572–3
metformin, 188, 202
methimazole, hepatotoxicity, 538, 539
methionine, acetaminophen metabolism and, 509
methionine adenosyltransferase (MAT), 323
methotrexate
  hepatotoxicity, 484, 511
  in primary biliary cirrhosis, 285–6, 287
  in primary sclerosing cholangitis, 306
methyldopa
  in carcinoid syndrome, 471
  toxicity, 501, 510
methylene blue, in hepatopulmonary syndrome, 193
methylene tetrahydrofolate reductase (MTHFR), C677T gene mutation, 476, 559
methylenecyclopropylalanine (hypoglycin), 330, 333
methylenedioxymethamphetamine (ecstasy), 506, 519

metoprolol, 511
metronidazole, 175, 259
Mexican Americans, gallbladder disease, 435
MHC see major histocompatibility complex
micelles, bile salt, 47
microagglutination test (MAT), 254
microfilaments, 9–10, 24–5
microhamartomas, bile duct, 426–7, 447
microsatellite markers, Wilson disease, 361
microscopic liver anatomy, 6–14
microsomal autoantibodies, 266–7, 268
microsomal epoxide hydrolase (mEH), 49
microsomal triglyceride transfer protein (MTTP), 330, 331
microtubules, 10, 23, 24, 45
microvesicular steatosis, 332
  acute fatty liver of pregnancy, 490, 491
  alcoholic, 315, 318
  causes, 333
  drug-induced, 330, 333, 503
  histopathology, 102, 114
  pathogenesis, 329, 330, 332
microvilli, hepatocyte, 7, 21, 22, 44
mid-zonal area (acinar zone 2), 6, 7, 12, 46
  drug-induced necrosis, 503
midodrine, in hepatorenal syndrome, 163
Milan criteria, hepatocellular carcinoma, 598
milk thistle see silymarin
Minnesota tube, 144
minocycline, hepatotoxicity, 501, 507
Mirizzi syndrome, 92, 440–1
mistletoe, 514
mitochondria
  alcohol toxicity, 313–14, 333
  apoptotic pathway, 38–9
  DNA, 29
    depletion syndromes, 414
  energy metabolism, 29–30
  disorders, 414
  fatty acid oxidation, 55–6, 329–30
  hepatocyte, 19, 27–30
  functions, 27, 29–30
  microscopy, 8, 9, 29
  structure, 29
  in Wilson disease, 351, 358
mitogen-activated protein kinases (MAPK), 626, 627
mitogens, hepatic, in alcoholic hepatitis, 321, 323
mitosis, 35, 37

Model for End-stage Liver Disease score see MELD score
molecular mimicry, 269, 501
monoamine oxidase inhibitors (MAOIs), 506
monoclonal antibodies (mAbs), immunosuppressive, 632, 633
monocyte chemoattractant protein 1 (MCP-1), 313
mononucleosis
  infectious, 253
  sporadic fatal, 253
Monospot test, 253
Morquio syndrome (type IV MPS), 392, 393
movement disorder, in Wilson disease, 355
MRI see magnetic resonance imaging
MTHFR gene, C677T mutation, 476, 559
mucins, gallbladder, 436
mucopolysaccharidoses (MPS), 391–3
mud fever, 253
Muehrcke lines, 67
multidrug resistance-associated protein 2 (mrp2/MRP2), 49, 51, 86
  gene mutations, 86, 88
multidrug resistance-associated protein 3 (mrp3), 49
multifocal leukoencephalopathy, progressive, 654, 666
muralium (simplex), 5, 17
murine mammary tumor virus, 278–9
Murphy sign, 131, 440
muscle
  ammonia detoxification, 171
  wasting, 61, 64, 179, 180
mushroom (Amanita) poisoning, 513, 520, 528
c-Myc, 37
Mycobacterium avium intracellulare (MAI), 255–6
Mycobacterium leprae, 256
Mycobacterium tuberculosis (MTB), 255
mycophenolate mofetil (MMF), 631–2
  in autoimmune hepatitis, 274, 408
  in liver transplantation, 632, 633, 639
  mechanism of action, 631–2
  side-effects, 634, 635
myeloablative therapy, sinusoidal obstruction syndrome, 482–3
myelofibrosis, 481
myeloma, multiple, 484, 541
myelopathy, hepatic, 70, 202–3

myeloproliferative disorders
  Budd-Chiari syndrome, 476, 480, 481
  extrahepatic portal vein obstruction, 559
  portal vein thrombosis, 476–7, 478
myofibroblasts, 10, 40
  in alcoholic liver disease, 314–15
  in allograft rejection, 630
myopathy, proximal, 66
myosin microfilaments, hepatocyte, 9–10
myostatin, 179, 180
myxedema ascites, 539

N-acetyl-p-benzoquinoneimine (NAPQI), 313, 508–9
N-acetylcysteine
  in acetaminophen-induced liver failure, 527–8
  acetaminophen metabolism and, 509
  in acute liver failure, 533–4, 535
  in alcoholic hepatitis, 322–3
  in neonatal hemochromatosis, 414
N-acetylglucosamine (GlcNAc) receptors, 33
Na+-taurocholate cotransporting polypeptide (NTCP), 49
NAD, 312–13
NADH
  alcohol-induced production, 312–13
  mitochondrial production, 29, 329
NADH/NAD ratio, in alcoholism, 313
nadolol, 142, 145, 146
NAFLD see non-alcoholic fatty liver disease
nail signs, liver disease, 67–8
naloxone, in alcoholism, 319
naltrexone, for pruritus, 98, 99
naproxen, 509
NASH see non-alcoholic steatohepatitis
native Americans, gallbladder disease, 435
natural killer (NK) cells, 621, 629
nausea and vomiting, 61
  as cause of malnutrition, 178
  in hepatitis A, 207
  in pregnancy, 494
NCPF see non-cirrhotic portal fibrosis
necrosis
  in acute hepatitis, 104
  in alcoholic hepatitis, 314, 318, 319
  in Budd-Chiari syndrome, 480

necrosis (Continued)
  in chronic hepatitis B, 221
  in drug-induced hepatotoxicity, 109, 502–3
  in hepatic ischemia, 109, 111
  in hyperacute rejection, 636
  ischemic bile duct, 474
  in preservation injury, 646
  sclerosing hyaline (SHN), 114
neomycin, 175, 178
neonatal hepatitis syndrome, 400–2
  endocrine disorders, 401, 402
  inborn errors of metabolism, 401, 402
  intrauterine infections, 401–2
neonatal jaundice, 397–405
  breast-fed babies, 397
  inherited disorders, 397, 401, 402–5
  investigation, 399
  physiologic, 86, 397
  unconjugated hyperbilirubinemia, 397
neonates, 397–405
  extrahepatic biliary disease, 398–400
  HBV vaccination, 230, 493
  hemochromatosis, 414, 520
  intrahepatic biliary hypoplasia, 402–4
  iron overload, 342
  management of liver disease, 403
  umbilical sepsis, 558, 559
  see also vertical transmission
nephrocalcinosis, in Wilson disease, 355
nephrotoxicity, cyclosporin/tacrolimus, 634, 635, 663
nerve supply, hepatic, 12
neuroendocrine tumors, metastatic, 470–1
  intraoperative management, 609
  liver transplantation, 599–600
  pharmacological control, 471
  surgical resection, 573
neurologic complications, 63
  acute liver failure, 521, 533–4
  cyclosporin, 634
  Gaucher disease, 394
  hepatic encephalopathy, 174
  liver allograft recipients, 664
  porphyrias, 371
  Wilson disease see Wilson disease, neurologic
  see also hepatic encephalopathy
neurologic examination, 70
neuronal degeneration of childhood, progressive (Alpers disease), 333, 416
neutropenia, 201, 249

neutrophils
  in alcoholic hepatitis, 314
  in drug-induced hepatotoxicity, 500
  dysfunction, in liver disease, 201
  endothelial cell interaction, 627–8
  in NASH, 338
  see also polymorphonuclear leukocytes
niacinamide, 183
nicotinamide adenine dinucleotide see NAD
Niemann-Pick disease, 333
  type A, 401
  type C, 401, 405
nifedipine, hepatotoxicity, 511
nimesulide, 510
nitisinone (NTBC), in hereditary tyrosinemia type 1, 386, 415–16
nitric oxide (NO), 142, 194
2(2-nitro-trifluoromethylbenzoyl)-1,3-cyclohexenedione see nitisinone
nitrofurantoin hepatotoxicity, 501, 507
nitrogen, requirements in cirrhosis, 183
nitroglycerin (NTG), in acute variceal hemorrhage, 147
nitrosovasodilators (nitrates), 142–3
  in acute variceal hemorrhage, 147
  prevention of variceal rebleeding, 148–9
  primary prevention of variceal bleeding, 145, 146
nocturia, 62
nodular regenerative hyperplasia (NRH), 432, 565
  antiphospholipid antibodies and, 540
  in Budd-Chiari syndrome, 480
  pathology, 110, 111, 432, 558
  radiology, 432
  sinusoidal dilatation and, 483
nodular transformation, partial, 565
nodules
  dysplastic hepatocellular, 115, 459
  regenerating
    in acute liver failure, 522, 524, 530
    in alcoholic cirrhosis, 319
    in Budd-Chiari syndrome, 480, 481
    in nodular regenerative hyperplasia, 432, 565
    in partial nodular transformation, 565
    in Wilson disease, 359

non-A, non-B hepatitis, 235
non-A-E hepatitis see seronegative hepatitis
non-alcoholic fatty liver disease (NAFLD), 327–40
  clinical features, 334
  in diabetes, 327, 537
  diagnosis, 337–8
  epidemiology, 327–8
  imaging, 335–7
  jaundice, 90
  laboratory tests, 334–5
  liver transplantation, 660
  nutritional supplements and medications, 188
  obesity and, 178, 181, 327
  pathophysiology, 328–34
  serum aminotransferases, 74, 75, 76, 334–5
  treatment and prognosis, 338–9
  weight loss, 187, 188
non-alcoholic steatohepatitis (NASH), 327–40
  in childhood, 409
  clinical features, 334
  diagnosis, 337–8
  epidemiology/risk factors, 327–8
  HFE gene mutations, 348
  imaging, 335–7
  laboratory tests, 334–5
  liver biopsy, 113–14, 337–8
  pathogenesis, 334
  serum aminotransferases, 74, 76, 333–5
  treatment and prognosis, 338–9
non-cirrhotic portal fibrosis (NCPF) (obliterative portal venopathy), 478–9, 549, 550–7
  clinical features, 479, 552
  diagnosis, 479
  differential diagnosis, 553, 557
  epidemiology, 550
  etiology, 504, 550–1
  hemodynamics, 551–2, 554, 555
  histology, 110, 479, 551, 552, 553
  historical perspective, 549–50
  hypothesis for pathogenesis, 551
  imaging, 553
  laboratory features, 552–3
  management, 555–7
  pathology, 551, 552
  prognosis, 479
  sinusoidal fibrosis, 484
  vs idiopathic portal hypertension, 550
non-cirrhotic portal hypertension (NCPH), 5, 549–66
non-compliance, liver allograft recipients, 421, 667

non-Hodgkin lymphoma (NHL), 545
non-steroidal anti-inflammatory drugs (NSAIDs)
  acute liver failure, 519
  hepatotoxicity, 497, 509–10
  induced microvesicular steatosis, 333
norepinephrine (noradrenaline), 163, 535
norethandrolone, 10
norfloxacin, 166–7
Normosang, 376–7
North Italian Endoscopic Consortium (NIEC) index, variceal bleeding risk, 141
NTBC see nitisinone
nuclear envelope, 30–1
nuclear factor -κB (NF-κB), 626
nuclear factor for activated T cells (NFAT), 625–6, 631
nuclear medicine see scintigraphy
nuclear pore complex (NPC), 31
nucleocytoplasmic transport, 31
nucleolus, 30
nucleosides/nucleotide analogs
  in chronic hepatitis B, 224–8
  hepatitis B, 222–3
  hepatotoxic, 333, 512
5' nucleotidase, 77–8, 79
nutrients
  inadequate intake, 178
  malabsorption see malabsorption
  requirements, 183–4
nutritional assessment, 181–2
nutritional management, 177, 183–9
  acute liver failure, 185–7
  in acute liver failure, 536
  alcoholic cirrhosis, 323–4
  alcoholic hepatitis, 185, 320, 321, 322
  cystic fibrosis, 384, 412
  galactosemia, 391, 414
  glycogen storage diseases, 389, 410
  goals, 185, 186
  hepatic encephalopathy, 175, 184–5, 187
  hereditary tyrosinemia type 1, 415
  liver transplantation, 187, 419
  neonatal liver disease, 403
  nutrient requirements, 183–4
  principles and practice, 187–8
  route of nutrient administration, 187–8
  specific alterations in liver disease, 184–5
  specific patient populations, 185–7
  weight loss, 187
  see also malnutrition

obesity, 185
  benign hepatic steatosis, 327
  childhood, 409
  definition, 177
  drug-induced hepatotoxicity
    and, 499
  in liver allograft recipients,
    187, 664
  liver transplantation and, 178,
    181
  NASH associated, 178, 181
  NASH risk, 327
  prevalence, 178
  serum aminotransferases, 76
  weight loss, 187, 188, 189
obstetric cholestasis *see*
    intrahepatic cholestasis of
    pregnancy
occludin, 44, 45
OCT1, 54, 55
octanoic acid, 172
octopamine, 172
octreotide
  in acute variceal hemorrhage,
    147, 150
  in carcinoid syndrome, 471
  in hepatorenal syndrome, 163
  in portal hypertension, 143
  scintigraphy, 471
ofloxacin, 166, 507
Oil red O stain, 103
OKT3 monoclonal antibody,
    632, 633
  side-effects, 634, 635
oliguria, 62
  in hepatorenal syndrome, 162
  post-liver transplantation, 420,
    643
operating rooms, liver transplant,
    605–6
opiates, endogenous, in pruritus,
    98, 296
Opisthorchis, 260–1
opportunistic infections
  HIV infection/AIDS, 106
  immunosuppressed patients,
    633
  post-transplant, 118, 119, 120,
    651–4
oral contraceptive steroids
    (OCS)
  in acute porphyria, 377
  hepatocellular adenomas and,
    424
  hepatotoxicity, 504–5
  jaundice, 91
  sinusoidal dilatation and, 483
oral mucosa, signs of
    malnutrition, 183
orcein, 103
organic acidemias, liver
    transplantation, 421
organic anion transporting
    polypeptide 1 (oatp1), 49,
    51

organic anion transporting
    polypeptide 2 (OATP2),
    83–4
organic anion transporting
    polypeptide 3 (oatp3), 52
organic cations, hepatic uptake,
    54, 55
ornithine-aspartate, in hepatic
    encephalopathy, 175
ornithine transcarbamylase
    deficiency, 333
orthodeoxyia, 68
osteoarthritis, in Wilson disease,
    356
osteocalcin, 196
osteodystrophy, hepatic *see*
    hepatic osteodystrophy
osteomalacia, 195, 196–7
osteopenia, 196
  in liver allograft recipients,
    664
  management, 197–8
  in primary biliary cirrhosis,
    196, 283, 288
  in primary sclerosing
    cholangitis, 296–7
osteoporosis, 195–6
  in hepatoblastoma, 412
  incidence and prevalence, 196
  in liver allograft recipients,
    196, 664
  management, 197–8, 297
  in primary biliary cirrhosis,
    196, 283, 288
  in primary sclerosing
    cholangitis, 296–7
overlap syndromes, 271, 282,
    286
  see also autoimmune
    cholangitis
oxaliplatin, 470
oxandralone, in alcoholic
    hepatitis, 322
oxidative stress
  in alcoholic liver disease,
    313–14
  in drug-induced
    hepatotoxicity, 500
oxygen
  administration, in
    hepatopulmonary
    syndrome, 191, 192
  debt, in acute liver failure, 535
  tension, arterial (PaO_2), in
    hepatopulmonary
    syndrome, 191, 192, 193

P-glycoprotein (MDR1), 55
p33ING1, 37
p53 protein, 36, 37
p107, 36
PACK syndrome, 540
packing, perihepatic, in liver
    trauma, 579
palmar erythema, 67, 487

palpation, abdominal, 69
pancreas
  abnormalities, in primary
    biliary cirrhosis, 283
  carcinoma of head, 92
  in cystic fibrosis, 383, 384
pancreatitis, 92, 442
Panhematin, 376
pantothenic acid, 183, 339
paper money skin, 65, 66
papillomavirus infection,
    post-transplant, 653, 666
paracentesis
  diagnostic, 155, 165
  therapeutic, 157–8
paracetamol *see* acetaminophen
parachlorophenylalanine, 471
paracrine signaling, 33
paraneoplastic syndromes,
    hepatocellular carcinoma,
    456
paraquat, 513
parasitic infections, 259–61
parasympathetic nerves, 12
parenchymal cells, hepatic *see*
    hepatocytes
parenteral iron overload, 341, 342
parenteral nutrition
  in acute liver failure, 536
  in liver disease, 187–8
  total (TPN)
    induced cholestasis, 91
    induced hepatic steatosis,
      339
parotid enlargement, 63, 65
paroxysmal nocturnal
    hemoglobinuria, 476, 480,
    481
partial nodular transformation,
    565
PBC *see* primary biliary cirrhosis
pediatric end-stage liver disease
    (PELD) score, 603
pediatric liver transplantation,
    417–21, 602–3, 605
  in acute liver failure, 417, 418,
    419
  contraindications, 418
  early complications, 420
  evaluation, 418
  indications, 417–18, 602–3
  late complications, 420–1
  living donor, 419, 615, 617–18
  operative techniques, 419,
    615–18
    abdominal closure, 616–17
    graft size reduction, 615–16
    implantation of lobe grafts,
      618
    living donor hepatectomy,
      617–18
    reduced-size liver recipient
      operation, 616
  postoperative management,
    419–20

preparation for, 419
quality of life after, 421
survival, 421
pediatric patients, 397–422
  acute liver failure *see* acute
    liver failure, in childhood
  acute viral hepatitis, 406, 416
  α_1-antitrypsin deficiency, 379,
    401, 402
  autoimmune hepatitis, 271,
    405, 407–8, 416–17, 421
  chronic hepatitis, 406–9
  clinical features of liver
    disease, 406
  drug-induced liver disease, 409
  extrahepatic portal vein
    obstruction, 557, 558–9,
    559–60
  hepatic tumors, 412–13
  hepatitis A, 207, 416
  hepatitis A vaccination, 208,
    209
  hepatitis B, 213–14, 215,
    216–17, 406–7
  hepatitis B vaccination, 230,
    407, 493
  hepatitis C, 407
  liver disease in older, 405–13
  malignant liver tumors,
    412–13, 468
  metabolic liver disease,
    409–12
  valproic acid toxicity, 416,
    506
  Wilson disease, 353, 405, 411
  see also neonates
pegylated interferons
    (peginterferons)
  in hepatitis B, 223–4, 228–9
  in hepatitis C, 243–4, 245,
    246, 247
  in hepatitis D, 233
  in recurrent hepatitis C, 683,
    684
PELD score, 603
peliosis hepatis, 483
  bacillary, 483
  hepatocellular adenoma and,
    424
  steroid-related, 505
pellagra, 183
penicillamine (D-penicillamine)
  adverse effects, 362
  in alcoholic hepatitis, 323
  in pregnancy, 364, 492
  in primary biliary cirrhosis, 285
  in primary sclerosing
    cholangitis, 290, 305
  in Wilson disease, 361–2, 365,
    411
pentoxifylline (PTX), 162, 321,
    322
percussion, abdominal, 69
percutaneous ablation methods,
    133–4

percutaneous transhepatic
  cholangiography (PTC)
  in Caroli disease, 450
  in jaundice, 96
  in primary sclerosing
    cholangitis, 292
perhexiline maleate, 334, 511
peribiliary gland hamartoma, 115
peribiliary glands, 12, 13
peribiliary plexus, 473–4
pericarditis, constrictive, 544,
  545
perilobular zone, 6
perinatal transmission see vertical
  transmission
periportal cholangioles see canals
  of Hering
periportal region (acinar zone 1),
  6, 7, 45–6
  changes in cholestasis, 107,
    108
  light microscopy, 12, 46
  metabolic specialization, 56–8
  sinusoidal blood composition,
    57
perisinusoidal cells see hepatic
  stellate cells
perisinusoidal fibrosis, 483
peritoneal dialysis, continuous
  ambulatory (CAPD), 537
peritoneal lavage, diagnostic, 578
peritoneum, 3
peritonitis
  secondary, 166
  spontaneous bacterial see
    spontaneous bacterial
    peritonitis
perivenular region (acinar zone 3),
  7, 46
  changes in cholestasis, 107,
    108
  drug-induced necrosis, 502–3
  light microscopy, 12, 46
  metabolic specialization, 56–8
  sinusoidal blood composition,
    57
peroxisomes, 9, 19, 30
  fatty acid oxidation, 55–6, 330
  in Wilson disease, 358
pesticides, 513
petechiae, 62
PFIC see progressive familial
  intrahepatic cholestasis
PFIC1 (FIC1) gene, 91, 404
phagocytosis, 26, 27
phenobarbital
  in cerebral edema, 533
  in Crigler–Najjar syndrome II,
    51, 88, 397
  in intrahepatic cholestasis of
    pregnancy, 489
  for pruritus, 98
phenols, in hepatic
  encephalopathy, 172
phenylbutazone, 509

phenylethanolamine, in hepatic
  encephalopathy, 172
phenylketonuria, 386
phenytoin, 505, 534
phlebothrombosis, intrahepatic
  portal veins, 559
phlebotomy therapy
  in hereditary
    hemochromatosis, 346–7,
    348
  in other liver diseases, 348
  in porphyria cutanea tarda, 377
phosphate/pyrophosphate
  translocase T-2, 388, 389
phosphatidylcholine (PC), biliary
  secretion, 53, 54
phosphatidylcholine transfer
  protein (PC-TP), 53, 54
phosphatidylserine (PS), 20
phospholipase Cγ (PLCγ), 625
phospholipidoses, 333–4
  drug-induced, 333–4, 502,
    503
phospholipids
  biliary secretion, 53, 54
  as cause of steatosis, 333–4
  leaflets, 18
  membrane, 18, 19, 20
phosphorus, yellow, 513
phosphorylase kinase deficiency,
  389, 390, 410
photosensitivity, in porphyria,
  372, 373, 374, 378
phototherapy, 98, 397
physical examination, 63–70
PIAF chemotherapy regimen, 467
pica, 550
piggyback technique, donor liver
  implantation, 609, 612, 661
pigment gallstones, 435–6
pinocytosis, 26, 27
pit cells, 10, 40–1
pitressin, in portal hypertension,
  143
PKD-1 gene mutations, 442,
  443, 444
PKD-2 gene mutations, 442,
  443–4
PKD-3 gene, putative, 442
PKHD 1 gene mutations, 443,
  447
PLADO chemotherapy regimen,
  467
plasma cell granuloma
  (inflammatory
    pseudotumor), 433
plasmalemmal vesicles
  (caveolae), 26–7, 28
platelet(s)
  counts, 198, 199
  in acute liver failure, 536
  in alcoholic liver disease,
    315, 316
  dysfunction, 198–9, 201
  in acute liver failure, 522

in non-cirrhotic portal
  hypertension, 552–3,
  555
transfusions, 200
platelet derived growth factor,
  314, 630
plates, liver cell see liver cell plates
plectin, 23, 24
pleural effusions, 62, 68
  in cirrhosis, 154–5
  post-liver transplant, 643
Pneumocystis carinii, 651
pneumonia, 64, 650–1
polyarteritis nodosa (PAN), in
  hepatitis B, 216, 540
polycystic kidney disease (PKD)
  autosomal dominant
    (AD-PKD), 442–3, 444
  autosomal recessive (AR-PKD),
    443, 447
  congenital hepatic fibrosis and,
    447, 565
polycystic liver disease, 433,
  442–7, 575–6
  classification, 442
  clinical features, 444–5
  complications, 445, 446
  genetics, 443–4
  isolated autosomal dominant
    (PCLD), 443–4, 444
  molecular diagnostics, 444, 445
  natural history, 442–3
  treatment, 445–7
polycystic ovary syndrome, 388,
  390
polycystin-1 (PC-1), 443, 444
polycystin-2 (PC-2), 443, 444
polycythemia vera, 86
polyenoyl phosphatidylcholine
  (PPC), in alcoholic liver
  disease, 323
polymerase chain reaction (PCR)
  cytomegalovirus DNA assay,
    652
  HBV DNA assays, 219
  Wilson disease test, 359, 360
polymorphonuclear (PMN)
  leukocytes, 621
  in alcoholic hepatitis, 318
  ascitic fluid, 155, 165, 166
  see also neutrophils
polymyalgia rheumatica, 540–1
polyoma JC virus, post-
  transplant infection, 654,
  666
Pompe disease, 389, 390
porphobilinogen (PBG), 369–70
  urinary, 375
porphobilinogen (PBG)
  deaminase, 371
porphyria(s), 369–78
  acute hepatic, 369, 370
  clinical features, 370–2
  prevention of attacks, 377
  treatment, 376–7

chronic hepatic, 372–3
  treatment, 376, 377–8
clinical features, 370–5
diagnosis, 375–6
epidemiology, 369
erythropoietic, 369, 373–5
hepatic, 369, 370
  clinical features, 370–3
  liver biopsy, 113
  pathophysiology, 369–70, 371
  treatment, 376–8
see also specific types
porphyria cutanea tarda (PCT),
  370, 372–3
  in chronic hepatitis C, 65,
    241, 373, 377
  HFE C282Y mutations, 348,
    373
  iron overload, 348, 370, 373,
    377
  liver biopsy, 102, 113, 373,
    374
  pathophysiology, 370
  prevention, 378
  treatment, 377–8
  type I, 372
  type II, 372
  type III, 373
porphyrins
  blood, 370
  plasma fluorescence, 376
  stool, 370, 376
  urinary, 370, 375
porta hepatis, 3, 4
portacaval fistula, spontaneous,
  476
portacaval shunts, 144, 148
  hepatic encephalopathy
    complicating, 174, 175
portal biliopathy, in extrahepatic
  portal vein obstruction, 561,
  563, 564
portal cavernoma (cavernous
  transformation), 477, 559
  imaging, 131, 477, 562, 563
  management, 478
portal cholangiopathy, 553, 564
portal fibrosis, non-cirrhotic see
  non-cirrhotic portal fibrosis
portal hypertension, 137–51
  ascites, 153
  classification, 137–8
  clinical features, 68–9, 140–2
  in congenital hepatic fibrosis,
    448
  in cystic fibrosis, 382, 385, 412
  drug-induced, 504
  idiopathic (IPH), 549–50
    epidemiology, 550
    etiology, 550–1
    hemodynamics, 551–2, 555
    management, 556–7
    pathology, 551, 552
    vs non-cirrhotic portal
      fibrosis, 550

portal hypertension (Continued)
see also non-cirrhotic portal fibrosis
interventional radiology, 133
natural history, 140–2
in nodular regenerative hyperplasia, 432
non-cirrhotic, 5, 549–66
pathophysiology, 137–40
pharmacological therapy, 142–3
in portal vein thrombosis, 477, 478
postsinusoidal, 137, 138
presinusoidal, 137–8
in primary biliary cirrhosis, 283
in primary sclerosing cholangitis, 300
in sarcoidosis, 542–3
sinusoidal, 137, 138
therapeutic opportunities, 145–50
therapeutic strategies, 142–5
see also variceal bleeding
portal hypertensive gastropathy (PHG), 139, 142
portal-systemic encephalopathy, 170, 476
portal tracts, 5, 6
fibrous tissue, 12, 13
light microscopy, 12, 13
liver lobule concept, 6, 7
lymphatic plexus, 11
portal vein
anastomoses
in living donor transplantation, 618
in orthotopic liver transplantation, 612
in reduced-size liver transplantation, 616
anatomy, 3, 4, 137
functional, 3–5
intrahepatic, 5, 6
aneurysm, 476
bacteremia
occult, 550
in primary sclerosing cholangitis, 289–90
cavernous transformation see portal cavernoma
'congenital absence,' 476
congenital defects, 558–9
development, 1, 2
disease, 476–9
embolization (PVE), in hepatocellular carcinoma, 572
extrahepatic obstruction see extrahepatic portal vein obstruction
hepatocellular carcinoma involving, 599
intrahepatic obstruction, 478–9

ligation
donor hepatectomy, 607
recipient hepatectomy, 611
percutaneous remobilization, 462
post-transplant surveillance, 619–20
pressure, 139–40
stenosis, liver graft recipients, 648
portal vein thrombosis (PVT), 476–8, 557
acute, 477
chronic, 477, 478
differential diagnosis, 553
in hepatocellular carcinoma, 464
imaging, 477, 558
during liver transplant surgery, 609, 611
non-cirrhotic portal fibrosis and, 551
post-liver transplantation, 648, 656
see also extrahepatic portal vein obstruction
portal venopathy, obstructive see non-cirrhotic portal fibrosis
portal venules, 5, 14
inlet, 5, 6, 13
light microscopy, 12, 13
portoportal shunts, 479
portopulmonary hypertension, 191, 193–4
diagnostic criteria, 192, 193
liver transplantation, 193, 194, 609
treatment, 193–4
portosystemic communications, 138–9
portosystemic shunts
after splenic vein thrombosis, 479
hepatic myelopathy, 203
isolated
spontaneous/congenital, 169–70, 174
spontaneous portacaval fistula, 476
surgical
in acute variceal bleeding, 148
in α1-antitrypsin deficiency, 381
in Budd-Chiari syndrome, 482
hepatic encephalopathy complicating, 174
in non-cirrhotic portal hypertension, 556–7, 562–3
in portal hypertension, 144
prevention of variceal rebleeding, 149–50
positron emission tomography (PET), 132–3

post embolization syndrome, 464
post-transplant
lymphoproliferative disorder (PTLD), 633, 653, 665–6
in children, 420
EBV-associated, 253, 653, 665, 666, 687
pathology, 118, 120
postcholecystectomy syndrome, 438–9
postoperative care
live donor graft recipients, 619–20
liver resection, 569–70
liver transplantation, 643
postoperative patients
benign cholestasis, 91–2
jaundice, 91–2
pouchitis, in primary sclerosing cholangitis, 301, 307
praziquantel, 259, 261
pre-eclampsia, 484, 489–90
acute liver failure, 519–20
diagnosis of liver disease, 494
in liver transplant recipients, 493
prognosis, 495
treatment, 495
prealbumin, 79, 538
variant, 541, 602
prednis(ol)one
in alcoholic hepatitis, 321–2
in autoimmune hepatitis, 272–3, 408
in primary biliary cirrhosis, 285
pregnancy
acute fatty liver see acute fatty liver of pregnancy
acute liver failure, 495, 519–20
in autoimmune hepatitis, 492
hepatitis E, 210, 211, 212, 492
intrahepatic cholestasis see intrahepatic cholestasis of pregnancy
jaundice, 91, 487
in liver allograft recipients, 493, 664–5
liver diseases, 487–96
classification, 487
coincidental, 487, 492–3
differential diagnosis, 493–5
epidemiology, 487
occurring more commonly, 487, 491–2
pathophysiology and clinical features, 488–93
prognosis, 495–6
unique, 487, 488–91
normal changes, 487–8
in pre-existing liver disease, 492–3
in primary biliary cirrhosis, 283
in Wilson disease, 363–4, 492

preservation injury, liver grafts, 646–7
preservation solution, liver transplant surgery, 605, 607, 612
primary biliary cirrhosis (PBC), 277–88
associated disorders, 282–3, 539
autoantibodies, 266, 277–8
clinical features, 279–80
complications, 283
diagnosis, 280–1
differential diagnosis, 263, 271, 281–2, 295
epidemiology, 277
histopathology, 107–8, 109, 280, 281
jaundice, 91, 279
laboratory tests, 280
liver transplantation, 287–8
autoantibody persistence after, 274
indications, 588–9, 591
outcome, 288, 591
recurrence after, 659
malnutrition, 178
Mayo risk score, 284, 588–9
mechanism of progression, 279
osteodystrophy, 196, 288
pathogenesis/immunologic abnormalities, 277–9
prognosis, 283–4, 588–9
scleroderma and, 282, 540
Sjögren syndrome and, 282, 540
treatment, 284–7
UDCA-resistant, 286–7
primary sclerosing cholangitis (PSC), 196, 289–309
associated diseases, 300–2, 539
clinical features, 291–2
complications, 295–300
cryptogenic, 405
diagnosis, 292–5
differential diagnosis, 263, 271, 282, 295
epidemiology, 289
jaundice, 92
liver histology, 107–8, 109, 292, 294–5
liver transplantation, 307
bone disease after, 297–8
cholangiocarcinoma and, 299–300, 592
indications, 589–90, 591–3
outcome, 307, 308, 592
recurrence after, 659, 660
malnutrition, 178
management, 305–7
medical therapy, 305–7
natural history, 302, 303
osteoporosis, 196
pathophysiology, 289–91

primary sclerosing cholangitis
(PSC) *(Continued)*
prognosis, 302–5, 589
small duct variant, 293
surgical therapy, 307
Pringle maneuver
for liver resections, 569
in liver trauma, 579, 581
PRKCSH gene mutations, 442,
443, 444
procoagulant factors, in non-
cirrhotic portal fibrosis, 551
proctocolectomy
peristomal varices, 300
pouchitis after, 301
in primary sclerosing
cholangitis, 307
progenitor cells, 12, 37
prognosis, assessing, 70–1
programmed cell death, 37–9
liver regeneration and, 39
signaling pathways, 37–8
see also apoptosis
progressive familial intrahepatic
cholestasis (PFIC), 404
type 1 (Byler disease), 404
liver transplantation, 421,
603
type 2, 49, 404
type 3, 282, 404
progressive multifocal
leukoencephalopathy, 654,
666
progressive neuronal
degeneration of childhood
(Alpers disease), 333, 416
propranolol
portal hypotensive effects, 142
prevention of variceal
rebleeding, 148–9
primary prevention of variceal
bleeding, 145
propylthiouracil (PTU)
in alcoholic liver disease, 321,
322, 323
hepatotoxicity, 538, 539
prostaglandin I₂ (prostacyclin), in
acute liver failure, 533–4,
535
proteasome, 26S, 625
protein(s)
ascitic fluid, 155, 164, 166
bile, 47
dietary
in hepatic encephalopathy,
175, 185
requirements in cirrhosis,
179, 183
restriction, 185
extracellular matrix, 32, 33
import into nucleus, 31
membrane, 17, 19, 20, 21
biogenesis and turnover, 21
integral (intrinsic), 21
peripheral (extrinsic), 21

metabolism, in cirrhosis, 178–9
plasma, synthesis, 56
synthesis, 30, 56
transmembrane, 19, 21
protein C, 56, 198
deficiency, 476–7, 478, 480,
551, 559
protein energy malnutrition
(PEM)
assessment, 181–2
clinical features, 182–3
definition, 177
hepatic steatosis, 330
liver transplantation and, 178,
181
pathophysiology, 178–80
prevalence, 177–8
prognosis, 180, 181
protein kinases, 33–4
protein S, 56, 198
deficiency, 476–7, 551, 559
protein tyrosine kinases (PTK),
625
proteoglycans, 11, 32–3, 33
prothrombin gene, G20210A
mutation, 559
prothrombin time (PT), 79–80,
199
in acute liver failure, 522, 525,
526
in alcoholic liver disease, 315,
316
in hepatitis A, 207
in hepatitis B, 216
international differences, 525
in jaundice, 94
prolonged, 56, 79
management, 200
non-hepatic causes, 73
prothrombotic disorders *see*
thrombogenic disorders
protoporphyria (PP)
(erythropoietic
protoporphyria), 370, 373–5
clinical features, 374–5
diagnosis, 376
genetics, 373–4
liver transplantation, 601
prevention, 378
treatment, 377–8
protoporphyrin, 374–5
erythrocyte, 375–6
protoporphyrinogen oxidase,
371, 372
pruritus, 62, 65
in hepatitis C, 240
in intrahepatic cholestasis of
pregnancy, 488
management, 98, 99
in neonates, 403
in pregnancy, 489
in primary biliary cirrhosis,
279, 280, 283
in primary sclerosing
cholangitis, 296

PSC *see* primary sclerosing
cholangitis
pseudo-Cushing's syndrome, 65,
70
pseudolipoma, 433
pseudolymphoma, 433
pseudotumor, inflammatory, 433
psychiatric disorders
interferon-induced, 224, 245
in Wilson disease, 355
psychoactive drugs, hepatotoxic,
506
psychologic assessment, children,
418
psychologic preparation,
pediatric liver
transplantation, 419
psychosocial development, post-
liver transplant, 421
pulmonary angiography, in
hepatopulmonary syndrome,
192
pulmonary dysfunction
in acute liver failure, 522
in α₁-antitrypsin deficiency,
378, 379
causes in liver disease, 191
in cystic fibrosis, 382
physical signs, 68
post-liver transplant, 643,
650–1
in primary biliary cirrhosis,
283
see also hepatopulmonary
syndrome;
portopulmonary
hypertension
pulmonary hypertension, 68
in portopulmonary
hypertension, 193
primary, 193, 194
pulmonary osteopathy,
hypertrophic, 68, 195, 196
purpura, 65–6
pylephlebitis, acute, 477
pyrexia *see* fever
pyridoxine
deficiency, 184
supplements, 183, 362
pyridoxine-5-phosphate, 75, 184
pyrimethamine-sulfadoxine, 507
pyrrolizidine, 482, 512, 514
pyruvate dehydrogenase complex
E2 subunit (PDC-E2),
277–8, 281, 501

Q fever, 255
quadrate lobe, 3, 4
quality of life, liver graft
recipients, 421, 664–5
quantitative insulin sensitivity
check index (QUICKI), 335
quinidine, 510
quinolone antibiotics, 166–7,
507

racial variations
gallbladder disease, 435, 436
hepatocellular carcinoma, 453
radiation-induced liver damage,
482, 546
radiocopper test, in Wilson
disease, 359
radiofrequency ablation (RFA)
hepatocellular carcinoma, 466
percutaneous, 133, 570–1
surgical, 570–1
radioisotopes, intra-arterial
therapy, 466, 467
radiology, 123–35
interventional, 133–4
see also imaging
radionuclide imaging *see*
scintigraphy
radiotherapy, hepatocellular
carcinoma, 466
Raf-1, 626
raft model, membrane lipids,
20–1
rapamycin, 631
in liver transplantation, 632–3
mode of action, 627, 631
side-effects, 634, 635
RAS, 626
Raynaud phenomenon, 282, 540
Raynold pentad, 441
receptor-mediated endocytosis
(RME), 26, 649, 650
receptors, cell surface, 33–4
red blood cells
ascitic fluid, 155
morphological and membrane
changes, 201
protoporphyrin detection,
375–6
radiolabeled, 123–4
red signs, esophageal varices, 141
red wale marks, esophageal
varices, 141
redox state, in alcoholic fatty
liver, 313
reduced-size liver
transplantation, 419, 615–18
abdominal closure, 616–17
graft size reduction technique,
615–16
postoperative care of
recipients, 619–20
recipient operation, 616
regeneration, liver, 37–9
in acute liver failure, 522, 524,
530
auxiliary liver transplantation
and, 530, 531
see also nodules, regenerating
rejection, liver allograft, 635–9,
649, 655–6
acute (cellular), 635, 636–8,
641, 649
activity index, 637, 638
in chronic hepatitis B, 672

rejection, liver allograft
    (Continued)
    drug treatment, 632–3
    grading, 637
    histopathology, 118, 119,
        636–7, 649, 650
    immunology, 630
    interferon therapy and, 683
    late presentation, 655–6
    in pediatric patients, 420
    precipitating factors, 655–6
    prophylactic drug therapy,
        632–3
    vs HCV recurrence, 637–8,
        681
    chronic (ductopenic), 635,
        638–9, 641, 656
    early presentation, 649
    histopathology, 118, 119,
        638–9
    immunology, 630
    in pediatric patients, 420
    risk factors, 638, 656
    hyperacute (antibody-
        mediated), 635–6, 649
    histopathology, 118, 119,
        636
    in pediatric patients, 420
    immunology, 621–30
renal failure/impairment
    in acute liver failure, 521, 532,
        535
    in chronic hepatitis B, 673
    in cirrhosis, 156
    diuretic-induced, in cirrhosis,
        157, 158
    in hepatorenal syndrome, 162
    in liver allograft recipients,
        421, 643, 663
    liver transplant surgery in, 608
    in polycystic kidney disease,
        445
    in spontaneous bacterial
        peritonitis, 165, 166
    see also hepatorenal syndrome
renal function
    abnormalities in cirrhosis, 153
    evaluation in cirrhosis/ascites,
        155–6
    post-liver transplant recovery,
        532
renal replacement therapy
    in acute liver failure, 535
    see also dialysis; hemodialysis
renal transplantation see liver-
    kidney transplantation
renal tubular acidosis, in primary
    biliary cirrhosis, 283
renal vasoconstriction, in
    hepatorenal syndrome,
        161–2
renin–angiotensin–aldosterone
    system, in arterial
    vasodilation theory, 153, 161
reovirus type 3, 290

reperfusion injury, transplanted
    liver, 612–13
reperfusion syndrome, 612
reproductive health, liver
    allograft recipients, 664–5
resection, liver
    anatomy and terminology,
        463, 567, 568
    benign tumors, 573–4
    in cirrhosis, 461–2, 569–70
    in cystic disease, 574–7
    in hepatocellular carcinoma,
        461, 462, 572
    metastatic tumors, 470, 572–3
    non-anatomic, 462
    in polycystic liver disease, 446,
        576
    postoperative care, 569–70
    surgical techniques, 567–9
    in trauma, 579–80
    see also hepatectomy; surgery,
        hepatic
respiratory disorders see
    pulmonary dysfunction
respiratory examination, 68
respiratory exchange ratio
    (quotient), in cirrhosis, 180
respiratory syncytial virus, 654
resuscitation
    in acute variceal hemorrhage,
        146, 147
    in hepatic surgery, 567
retention mechanism, nuclear
    uptake, 31
reticulin collapse, 104, 105
reticulocytosis, 201
reticuloendothelial system
    (RES), spontaneous
    bacterial peritonitis and, 164
retinoblastoma protein (pRb),
        36–7
retinoids, 39–40, 514
retinol, 39–40
retinol-binding protein (RBP), 39
Reye syndrome, 333, 409, 509
    jaundice, 90
    liver biopsy, 102
rheumatic diseases, 539–41
rheumatoid arthritis (RA), 540
    juvenile, 417
rheumatoid factor, 241
rhodanine, 103
ribavirin
    in chronic hepatitis C, 244–5,
        247
    in children, 407
    combination therapy, 243,
        245
    pretransplant therapy, 682
    special patient groups,
        246–7
    in recurrent hepatitis C, 683,
        684
    side-effects, 245–6
riboflavin, supplements, 183

ribosomal RNA (rRNA), 30
ribosomes, 25, 29
Riedel's lobe, 69
rifampin (rifampicin), 51, 83
    in brucellosis, 252
    hepatotoxicity, 508
    in mycobacterial infections,
        255, 256
    P450 induction, 498
    for pruritus, 98, 99
rifaximin, in hepatic
    encephalopathy, 175
right lobe
    anatomic, 3, 4
    Couinaud functional segments,
        5
    grafts
        donor organ reduction,
            615–16
        implantation technique,
            616, 618
        living donor hepatectomy,
            617–18
    physiologic, 3, 4
    venous drainage, 5
right ventricular systolic
    pressure, in portopulmonary
    hypertension, 193
risedronate, 197
RNA, 30
v-ros receptor, 34
Rotor syndrome, 88, 89
round ligament see ligamentum
    teres
Roux-en-Y
    choledochojejunostomy, 608
Roux-en-Y hepaticojejunostomy,
        580–1
    in choledochal cyst, 400, 449
    in liver transplantation, 614
    operative technique, 581, 582
rubella, neonatal hepatitis, 401
rubs, friction, 69
rupture
    hepatic, in pregnancy, 490, 495
    hepatic tumor, 425, 456

S-adenosylmethionine (SAMe),
        188, 323, 489
salicylate hepatotoxicity, 509,
        540
Salmonella minnesota, 278
salt restriction, 156–7, 185
Sanfilippo syndrome (type III
    MPS), 392, 393
sarcoidosis, 542–3
    differential diagnosis, 282
    jaundice, 91
    post-transplant recurrence,
        661
sarcomas, 117, 467–8
satellitosis, in alcoholic hepatitis,
        318
SBP see spontaneous bacterial
    peritonitis

ribosomal RNA (rRNA), 30
Scheie syndrome (type IS MPS),
        392, 393
Scheuer scoring system, chronic
    hepatitis, 240
schistosomiasis, 259–60
    granulomatous hepatitis, 255,
        259
    portal vein obstruction, 478
scintigraphy (radionuclide
    imaging), 123–4
    benign liver tumors, 424
    in biliary atresia, 398, 399
    in cholecystitis, 440
    in focal nodular hyperplasia,
        431, 574
    hemangiomas, 428
    hepatobiliary, 97, 131
    lung perfusion scanning, 192
    in non-cirrhotic portal
        hypertension, 553
    in steatosis/NASH, 337
sclerae, yellow, 65
scleroderma, 282, 540
    see also CREST syndrome
sclerosing cholangitis
    AIDS-related, 295
    in childhood, 408–9
    in cystic fibrosis, 383
    primary see primary sclerosing
        cholangitis
sclerosing hyaline necrosis
    (SHN), 114
sclerotherapy, variceal see
    endoscopic injection
    sclerotherapy
screening
    cancer, in liver allograft
        recipients, 666
    hepatocellular carcinoma, 467
    hereditary hemochromatosis,
        348
    Wilson disease, 360, 361, 362
SEC63 gene mutations, 442, 444
secretin, 51, 444
segments, liver, 3–5, 567, 568
    II/III grafts, 615
    resections, 463, 567
seizures, in acute liver failure,
        534
selectins, 627, 628
selenium, hepatotoxicity, 513
Sengstaken-Blakemore tube, 144
sepsis
    in acute liver failure, 522,
        534–5
    jaundice, 91
    in liver disease, 64–5
    neonatal, 397
    post-liver transplantation, 420,
        649–50
    prophylaxis, 532
septa, interlobular, 5–6, 7
septicemia, 64
septo-optic dysplasia, 401, 402
septum transversum, 1

serologic testing
 cytomegalovirus, 652
 Epstein–Barr virus, 253
 hepatitis A, 207
 hepatitis B, 217–20
 hepatitis C, 238–9
 hepatitis D, 231–2
 hepatitis E, 211
 in jaundice, 97
 syphilis, 254
seronegative (non-A-E) hepatitis,
  518
 acute liver failure, 519
 in childhood, 416
serum sickness-like syndrome,
  hepatitis B, 216
7-day fever, 253
sexual dysfunction, 63, 665
sexual health, liver allograft
  recipients, 664–5
sexual transmission, viral
  hepatitis, 214, 237
shingles (herpes zoster), 666, 687
shunt surgery see portosystemic
  shunts, surgical
shuttle vesicles, 25
sialadenitis, HCV-related, 241
sick euthyroid state, 539
sickle cell disease, 541
sickle cell intrahepatic cholestasis
  (SCIC), 541
sickle hepatic crisis, acute
  (ASHC), 541
sideroblastic anemia, 86
sieve plates, 10, 39
signal-mediated vectorial
  transport, 31
signal transducers and activators
  of transcription (STATs),
  627
signal transduction, 33–5
signs, liver disease, 64–70
 in normal pregnancy, 487
sildenafil, 194
silymarin (milk thistle), 188,
  324, 528
single photon emission computed
  tomography (SPECT), 123,
  124
sinus venosus, 1, 2
sinusoidal obstruction syndrome
  (SOS) (veno-occlusive
  disease), 479, 482–3
 in bone marrow transplant
  recipients, 120–1, 482
 histology, 109, 110, 482
 jaundice, 90
sinusoidal plexus, primitive
  hepatic, 1, 2
sinusoids, hepatic, 5, 6
 capillarization, 318
 cells, 8, 10, 39–41
 development, 1, 17
 dilatation, 483–4
 disorders, 482–4

fibrosis, 484
 hepatocyte relations, 7, 8, 22,
  44
 infiltration, 484
 microscopic anatomy, 10, 43
 vascular relations, 5, 6
 zonation of blood composition,
  57
sirolimus, adverse effects in
  children, 421
Sjögren syndrome, 282, 540
skeletal abnormalities, in Alagille
  syndrome, 403
skin
 cancer, in liver allograft
  recipients, 664
 hyperpigmentation, 65, 280
 paper money, 65, 66
 problems, liver allograft
  recipients, 664
 side-effects of penicillamine,
  362
 yellow discoloration, 65, 83
skin manifestations
 alcoholic liver disease, 315, 316
 liver disease, 65–6
 malnutrition, 183
 porphyria, 370, 372, 373, 374
  management, 377, 378
SLC40A1 gene mutations, 341
sleep–wake patterns, in cirrhosis,
  173
slow acetylators, 507, 508
sludge, biliary see biliary sludge
small for size syndrome, 619, 647
small intestine
 bile acid absorption/transport,
  52
 chylomicron synthesis, 332
snacks, night-time, in cirrhosis,
  180, 324
SNARE protein, 404
social history, 63
sodium (Na$^+$)
 in bile, 47
 dietary restriction, 156–7, 185
 retention, in ascites, 153–4
 serum
  in alcoholic liver disease,
   315–16
  see also hyponatremia
 transport, 49–50, 51
 urine, 162, 316, 317
sodium benzoate, in hepatic
  encephalopathy, 175
sodium fluoride, 297
soluble liver antigen (SLA)
  antibodies, 267–8, 271
somatostatin (and analogs)
 in acute variceal hemorrhage,
  147, 150
 in carcinoid syndrome, 471
 in polycystic liver disease, 445
 in portal hypertension, 143
 see also octreotide

South African porphyria see
  variegate porphyria
space-occupying lesions see masses
space of Disse, 7, 8, 10
 cells interacting with, 39
 extracellular matrix, 11
spastic paraparesis, 170, 174, 203
spgp gene, 49
sphincter of Oddi dysfunction,
  438–9
sphingolipids, membrane, 18, 20
sphingomyelin, 20, 21
spider nevi, 63, 65, 66
 in pregnancy, 487
spirochete infections, 253–5
spironolactone, in ascites, 156–7,
  158
splanchnic circulation, in
  cirrhosis, 153, 154, 161
spleen, palpation, 69
splenectomy
 in extrahepatic portal vein
  obstruction, 562, 563
 in splenic vein thrombosis, 479
splenic vein, 137
 thrombosis, 479
splenomegaly, 69
 Bengal, 549
 in extrahepatic portal vein
  obstruction, 560, 562
 in non-cirrhotic portal
  hypertension, 552
 tropical, 549, 553
 see also hepatosplenomegaly
split-liver transplantation, 419,
  605, 615–16
 operative technique, 615–16
spontaneous bacterial empyema,
  164
spontaneous bacterial peritonitis
  (SBP), 153, 164–7
 clinical features and diagnosis,
  165–6
 culture negative, 165
 definition, 164
 pathophysiology, 164, 165
 prevention, 166–7
 in primary sclerosing
  cholangitis, 300
 prognosis, 166
 treatment, 162, 166
spur cell anemia, 201
St John's wort, 188
stains, histochemical and
  immunohistochemical, 102,
  103
starvation, accelerated, in
  cirrhosis, 184
statins see HMG-CoA reductase
  inhibitors
STATs, 627
steatohepatitis (SH), 113–14
 see also alcoholic liver disease;
  non-alcoholic
  steatohepatitis

steatorrhea, 62
 as cause of malnutrition, 178
 management, 98
 in primary sclerosing
  cholangitis, 296
steatosis, hepatic, 327
 alcoholic see alcoholic fatty
  liver
 causes, 537
 clinical features, 334
 in diabetes, 327, 537
 drug-induced, 330, 333, 503
 epidemiology, 327
 imaging, 125–6, 335–7
 inflammation and, 334
 laboratory tests, 334–5
 macrovesicular see
  macrovesicular steatosis
 microvesicular see
  microvesicular steatosis
 pathophysiology, 328–34
 risk factors, 327–8
stellate cells see hepatic stellate
  cells
stem cells, in liver regeneration,
  37
stents, biliary–enteric
  anastomosis, 614
steroids
 hepatotoxic effects, 504–5
 see also anabolic steroids;
  corticosteroids; estrogen;
  oral contraceptive steroids
sterol carrier protein 2, 53
streptozocin, 471
striae, 66
subacute liver failure, 517
 auxiliary liver transplantation,
  531
 intracranial hypertension,
  520–1
 liver histology, 522, 524
 referral criteria, 526
subconjunctival hemorrhage, 62,
  65
subjective global assessment, in
  protein energy malnutrition,
  182
succinylacetone (SA), 385, 386,
  415
sucralfate, 536
Sugiura procedure, 144
sulfation, 55, 58
sulfonamides, hepatotoxicity,
  507
sulfotransferases, 55
sulfoxidation, abnormal, in PBC,
  279
sulfur colloid, technetium-99m
  (^{99m}Tc)-labeled, 123, 337
 in focal nodular hyperplasia,
  431, 574
sulindac, 509, 510
sump syndrome, 581
superior mesenteric vein, 137

superoxide anions, 313
surgery, 567–83
  biliary reconstruction see biliary reconstruction surgery
  emergency, in acute variceal bleeding, 147–8
  hepatic, 567–80
    anatomical aspects, 567, 568
    history, 567
    intraoperative monitoring and resuscitation, 567
    in liver trauma, 578–80
    metastatic tumors, 572–3
    postoperative care, 569–70
    pyogenic abscess, 577–8
    radiofrequency ablation, 570–1
    techniques, 567–9
    see also hepatectomy; resection, liver
  in portal hypertension, 144
  prevention of variceal rebleeding, 149–50
  in primary sclerosing cholangitis, 307
  prior, liver transplantation after, 608, 610–11
  shunts see portosystemic shunts, surgical
  see also specific procedures
sustained virologic response (SVR), hepatitis C therapy, 241, 242
swineherd disease, 253
sympathetic nervous system
  in arterial vasodilation theory, 153, 161
  liver innervation, 12
symptoms, liver disease, 61–3
synaptic signaling, 33
syphilis, 254–5
  congenital, 401, 402
systemic disorders
  associated with liver disease, 191–203
  in liver allograft recipients, 661–4
  liver involvement, 537–47
systemic lupus erythematosus (SLE), 539–40

T-cell receptors (TCR), 621, 624
  α/β, antigen recognition, 624–5
  complex, 625, 626
  costimulatory pathways, 626–7, 628
  signaling pathways, 625–6
T cells, 621
  activated, entry to tissues, 627–8
  alloantigen recognition, 629–30
  in allograft rejection, 630

antigen-mediated activation
  early events (G0-G1 transition), 625–7, 628
  later events (G1-S transition), 627
antigen recognition, 624–5
mechanisms of tissue injury, 628–9
in primary biliary cirrhosis, 277, 278
in primary sclerosing cholangitis, 291
role of cytokines, 622
Th1/Th1 cytokine response, 629
T-tubes
  cholangiography, 645
  in liver transplantation, 614, 643
TACE see transcatheter arterial chemoembolization
tacrine, 514
tacrolimus, 631
  adverse effects, 634–5
    in children, 420, 421
  in autoimmune hepatitis, 274
  drug interactions, 635
  hepatotoxicity, 512
  in liver transplantation, 420, 632, 633, 639
  mode of action, 626, 631
  nephrotoxicity, 635, 663
  in primary sclerosing cholangitis, 306
tamoxifen, 157, 188, 328
TAP-1/TAP-2, 624
target cells, 201
targets of rapamycin (TOR-1/TOR-2), 631
tattoos, 66
taurine, in cystic fibrosis, 385, 411
telangiectasia, 65
  hereditary hemorrhagic, 66, 475–6
telbivudine, in chronic hepatitis B, 227–8
tenofovir, in hepatitis B, 673, 678, 679
terlipressin see glypressin
testicular atrophy, 63, 70
tetracycline toxicity, 333, 506–7
tetrahydroaminoacridine, 514
tetrathiomolybdate, in Wilson disease, 361, 362
Th1/Th1 cytokine response, 629
thermal ablation, hepatocellular carcinoma, 466
thiamine
  deficiency, 184
  supplements, 183, 184, 320
thiazide diuretics, 510
thiazolidinediones, 188
thioflavin-T, 103
6-thioguanine, 482, 512

thiopentone, in cerebral edema, 533
thorotrast, 467–8
threonine deficiency, 330, 331
thrombocytopenia, 198–9, 201
  in extrahepatic portal vein obstruction, 563
  management, 200
thrombocytosis, in childhood liver tumors, 412
thromboelastography (TEG), 199
thromboendarterectomy, portal vein, 611
thrombogenic (prothrombotic) disorders
  Budd-Chiari syndrome, 476, 480
  extrahepatic portal vein obstruction, 476–7, 478, 559
  liver transplant surgery, 608–9
thrombolysis
  in Budd-Chiari syndrome, 482
  in portal vein thrombosis, 478
thrombopoietin, 198
thyroid disease, 537–9
  autoimmune
    interferon-induced, 246, 539
    liver disease-associated, 539
  in chronic liver disease, 539
  liver abnormalities, 537–9
  in primary biliary cirrhosis, 282
thyroid hormones
  changes in liver disease, 539
  hepatic function, 538
  metabolism, 537–8
thyroid transcription factor 1 (TTF1), 460
thyrotoxicosis, 538
thyroxine (T$_4$), 538, 539
thyroxine-binding globulin (TBG), 537–8, 539
ticrynafen-induced hepatitis, 267, 268
tienilic acid, 501
tight junctions, 22, 44, 45
TIPS see transjugular intrahepatic portosystemic shunting
tissue plasminogen activator (tPA), 199
tissues
  entry of activated cells, 627–8
  mechanisms of injury, 628–9
TNF receptor-associated death domain protein (TRADD), 314
tocopherol see vitamin E
tolerance, liver allograft, 640–1
Toll receptors, 621, 622
TOR-1/TOR-2, 631
total vascular exclusion (TVE)
  for liver resections, 569
  in liver trauma, 580
toxic shock syndrome, 333

toxin-induced liver disease, 497–516
  childhood acute liver failure, 416
  jaundice, 89, 90, 91
  non-cirrhotic portal fibrosis and, 550
  specific toxins, 513
  steatosis, 330, 333
  see also drug-induced liver disease
toxins
  metabolism, 497–8
  primary sclerosing cholangitis and, 289–90
toxoplasmosis, neonatal hepatitis, 401, 402
trace metals
  non-cirrhotic portal fibrosis and, 550
  supplements, 183
tranexamic acid, 200
trans-Golgi network (TGN), 25, 26
aminotransferases see aminotransferases
transcatheter arterial chemoembolization (TACE), 133
  hepatocellular carcinoma, 464–5, 572
  metastatic carcinoid tumors, 471
transcobalamin-1, in fibrolamellar hepatocellular carcinoma, 412
transfer RNA (tRNA), 30, 31
transferrin
  carbohydrate deficient, 315
  saturation, in hemochromatosis, 345, 346, 347, 348
  serum, in hemochromatosis, 346
transferrin receptors, 33, 34
  type 1 (TfR1), 343, 344
  type 2 (TfR2) gene mutations, 341
transforming growth factor-β (TGF-β), 34–5, 37, 623
  in alcoholic hepatitis, 313
  in allograft rejection, 630
transforming growth factor-β (TGF-β) receptors, 34–5
transfusion see blood transfusion
transhepatic cholangiography see percutaneous transhepatic cholangiography
transition vesicles, 25
transjugular intrahepatic portosystemic shunting (TIPS), 133, 144
  in acute variceal bleeding, 147–8
  in α$_1$-antitrypsin deficiency, 381

transjugular intrahepatic
portosystemic shunting
(TIPS) *(Continued)*
in ascites, 157–8
in Budd-Chiari syndrome, 482
in children, 419
in cirrhotic cardiomyopathy,
195
complications, 144, 149
in cystic fibrosis, 385
"endogenous," 169
hepatic encephalopathy
complicating, 174, 175
in hepatopulmonary syndrome,
193
in hepatorenal syndrome, 164
liver transplantation after, 150,
609, 611
prevention of variceal
rebleeding, 149
in primary sclerosing
cholangitis, 300
stents, 144
transplant vasculopathy, 630,
638, 639
transport proteins, hepatocyte,
46, 49
transporters associated with
antigen processing (TAPs),
624
transthyretin, variant, 541, 602
trauma
liver, 578–80, 581
major, jaundice, 87
travelers
hepatitis A, 206
hepatitis A vaccination, 208,
209
tremor, flapping *see* asterixis
triacylglycerols (TAG)
(triglycerides), 328, 330
in alcoholic steatosis, 313,
332–3
cycling, 329
delivery from periphery, 328
fate of plasma, 332
medium chain, 183, 412
plasma, in steatosis/NASH,
335
secretion by liver, 330
sources of plasma, 331–2
synthesis in liver, 329, 330
triamterene, in ascites, 156
triangular ligaments, 3
tricyclic antidepressants, 506
trientine
in pregnancy, 364
in Wilson disease, 361, 362,
365, 411
triglycerides *see* triacylglycerols
triiodothyronine (T₃), 538, 539
trimethoprim-sulfamethoxazole,
507
trisegmentectomy, 462, 463
triskelion, 26, 28

tropical splenomegaly syndrome
(TSS), 549, 553
tryptophan, 172
tuberculoma, 255
tuberculosis, 91, 255, 508
tuberous sclerosis, 430
tubulins, 24
tuftsin, 201
tumor-like lesions, liver, 430–4
tumor necrosis factor-α
(TNF-α), 91, 623
in alcoholic hepatitis, 313,
314, 322
hepatotoxicity, 500
promoter polymorphisms, in
autoimmune hepatitis,
269–70
therapy targeting, in alcoholic
hepatitis, 321, 322
tumor necrosis factor-β (TNF-β),
629
tumor necrosis factor (TNF)
family, 627, 628
tumors, liver
benign *see* benign liver tumors
of childhood, 412–13
drug-induced, 504
imaging, 127–9
liver biopsy, 114–18
malignant *see* malignant liver
tumors
Twinrix®, 209
tyrosine, metabolism, 385, 386
tyrosinemia, hereditary (HT),
385, 386
type 1 (HT1), 385–7, 405
acute liver failure, 414–16
gene therapy, 381, 387
liver transplantation, 386,
421, 601
neonatal hepatitis, 401
pathophysiology, 385, 386
porphyric crises and, 370
treatment, 386–7, 415–16

UDCA *see* ursodeoxycholic acid
UGA suppressor serine
tRNA–protein complex, 268
ulcerative colitis, chronic
(CUC), primary sclerosing
cholangitis and, 289, 290,
300–1, 307
ultrasonic dissector, 569, 570
ultrasonography (US), 123
benign liver tumors, 424
in cholecystitis, 440
endoscopic (EUS), 96–7
focal nodular hyperplasia, 431
gallstones, 437
hemangiomas, 427
hepatic metastases, 469
hepatocellular adenomas, 425
hepatocellular carcinoma, 457,
458
hydatid cysts, 257

infantile
hemangioendothelioma,
429
in jaundice, 95, 96, 97
liver biopsy guidance, 101–2
in non-cirrhotic portal
hypertension, 553, 556
in polycystic liver disease, 444
post-liver transplantation,
644–5
solitary hepatic cysts, 447
in steatosis/NASH, 336
ultrastructure, liver, 6–14, 17, 18
umbilical hernia, 64
umbilical sepsis, neonatal, 558,
559
umbilical veins, 1, 2
catheterization, 558, 559
fissure, 3
umbilicus, everted, 62, 69
undulant fever, 251
United Network for Organ
Sharing (UNOS), 305, 528,
599
University of Wisconsin
preservation solution, 605
urea, synthesis, 56, 57, 58
uridine diphosphate (UDP)-
glucuronyl transferases, 55
family 1 (UGT1A),
autoantibodies, 267, 268
see also bilirubin-UDP-
glucuronosyl-transferase
uridine diphosphoglucose
4-epimerase deficiency, 391
urinary tract infections, 64
urine, osmolality, 162, 316
urine talc test, 375
urobilinogens, 86
uroporphyrinogen decarboxylase
(Uro-D), 371, 372, 373
ursodeoxycholic acid (UDCA;
ursodiol), 47, 48, 50
in autoimmune hepatitis, 274
in cholelithiasis, 438
in cystic fibrosis, 384–5, 405,
412
in NAFLD, 188, 339
in post-transplant biliary
strictures, 658
in primary biliary cirrhosis,
277, 285, 286–7
in primary sclerosing
cholangitis, 306–7
for pruritus, 98, 99, 489
in sclerosing cholangitis of
childhood, 409
ursodiol *see* ursodeoxycholic acid

V₂ receptor antagonists, in
dilutional hyponatremia, 160
vaccinations
liver allograft recipients, 666,
667
pre-liver transplant, 419

valacyclovir, 687
valerian, 514
valganciclovir, in cytomegalovirus
infection, 252, 652–3, 686
valproic acid (valproate) toxicity,
330, 333, 506
in childhood, 416, 506
jaundice, 90
liver histology, 522
valtorcitabine, 228
vanishing bile duct syndrome *see*
ductopenia
variceal bleeding, 137
active, treatment, 146–8, 150
gastric varices, 148
general principles, 146, 147
pharmacological measures,
147
TIPS and emergency
surgery, 147–8
balloon tamponade, 144, 147
in congenital hepatic fibrosis,
448, 565
in extrahepatic portal vein
obstruction, 478, 559–60,
562–3
in non-cirrhotic portal fibrosis,
552, 555–6
pediatric, management, 419
peristomal, in primary
sclerosing cholangitis, 300
predictive factors, 140–2, 145
in pregnancy, 492–3
primary prevention, 145–6, 150
endoscopic therapy, 145–6
pharmacological agents, 145,
146
recurrence risks, 141, 146, 148
recurrent, treatment and
prevention, 148–51
endoscopic therapy, 149
liver transplantation, 150,
151
pharmacological agents,
148–9
surgery, 149–50
TIPS, 149
spontaneous cessation, 141,
146
surgical approaches, 144
therapeutic strategies, 142–5
varicella zoster virus (VZV), 263
pediatric acute liver failure,
416
post-transplant infections,
653, 666, 669, 687
varices
anatomy, 138–9
band ligation *see* endoscopic
variceal band ligation
classification, 139–40
ectopic, 139
esophageal *see* esophageal
varices
gastric *see* gastric varices

varices (Continued)
likelihood of rupture, 140
in non-cirrhotic portal fibrosis, 553
pediatric, management, 419
peristomal, in primary sclerosing cholangitis, 300
pressures, in non-cirrhotic portal hypertension, 551, 555
resistance to flow, 140
sclerotherapy see endoscopic injection sclerotherapy
transmural pressure gradient, 140
wall tension, 140
see also gastroesophageal varices
variegate porphyria (VP), 370, 372, 376
vascular adhesion protein (VAP)-1, 627–8
vascular diseases, 473–85
imaging, 129–30
liver biopsy, 109–10
vasculitis
hepatitis B-associated, 216
leukocytoclastic, 66
systemic, 540–1
vasculopathy, transplant, 630, 638, 639
vasoconstrictor drugs, in hepatorenal syndrome, 163
vasopressin, 143, 147
vasopressor agents, in acute liver failure, 535
veins, dilated abdominal, 68–9
venesection therapy see phlebotomy therapy
veno-occlusive disease see sinusoidal obstruction syndrome
venography, hepatic
in Budd-Chiari syndrome, 481
in non-cirrhotic portal hypertension, 553
venous hums, 69
venovenous bypass
for liver transplantation, 605, 609, 610, 611
in liver trauma, 580
ventilation, mechanical, after liver transplantation, 643
verapamil
in alcoholic hepatitis, 323
hepatotoxicity, 510–11
vertical transmission, 493
hepatitis B, 213–14, 406, 493
hepatitis C, 237, 407, 493
very-low-density lipoprotein (VLDL), 53
in alcoholic fatty liver, 313, 332–3
defects in synthesis, 330–1
modification of circulating, 332

release of fatty acids, 332
remnants, 330, 332
synthesis and secretion, 330–1
triacylglycerol, 330, 331–2
vesicles, 45
coated, 26, 27, 28
plasmalemmal (caveolae), 26–7, 28
secretory, 26
shuttle, 25
transition, 25
Vierhoff Van Gieson stain, 103
vimentin, 24
vinyl chloride (VC), 467, 513
viral hepatitis, 252–3
acute liver failure, 518–19
autoantibodies, 271
in childhood, 406–7, 416
cholestasis, 91
differential diagnosis, 92, 93, 263, 265
jaundice, 89
laboratory diagnosis, 77
liver transplantation, 585, 587, 593–6
timing, 590
malnutrition in chronic, 178
post-transplant recurrence, 658–9, 669–89
histopathology, 119–20
therapeutic strategies, 670
in pregnancy, 487, 492, 494
trends in incidence, 237, 238
see also specific types
viral infections
in liver transplant recipients, 651–4
vertical transmission see vertical transmission
see also viral hepatitis; specific infections
virus-associated autoimmunity, 271
viruses
in autoimmune hepatitis etiology, 269
in primary biliary cirrhosis etiology, 278–9
in primary sclerosing cholangitis etiology, 290
vitamin A
chronic intoxication, 484
in cystic fibrosis, 384
deficiency, 183, 184
storage, 10, 39
supplements, 183, 184, 188
vitamin B complex, deficiencies, 183, 184
vitamin B$_6$ see pyridoxine
vitamin B$_{12}$
deficiency, 184, 201
supplements, 183
vitamin C (ascorbic acid), 183

vitamin D
metabolism, abnormalities, 196–7
supplements, 183, 184, 197–8
vitamin deficiencies, 182, 183, 184
in primary biliary cirrhosis, 283
in primary sclerosing cholangitis, 296
vitamin E (α tocopherol)
deficiency, 184
in NASH, 339
supplements, 183, 184, 188
in Wilson disease, 363
vitamin K, 56, 198
deficiency, 198
in intrahepatic cholestasis of pregnancy, 488, 489
in jaundice, 94
replacement, 200
vitamin supplements, 183, 184, 188
in alcoholic liver disease, 320
in cystic fibrosis, 384, 412
in neonatal liver disease, 403
vitelline veins, 1, 2
vitiligo, 65
VLDL see very-low-density lipoprotein
volume, liver
assessment, in acute liver failure, 526–7
future (post-resection), 462
vomiting see nausea and vomiting
von Gierke disease (glycogen storage disease I), 388–90, 410
von Meyenburg complexes (VMCs), 426–7, 447
voriconzole, 651

water load test, 155–6
water retention see fluid retention
Watson–Schwartz test, 375
weakness, 61
wedged hepatic venous pressure (WHVP), 137, 139–40
in extrahepatic portal vein obstruction, 561
in non-cirrhotic portal fibrosis, 551, 554
weight gain, in liver allograft recipients, 664
weight loss
diets, 188, 189
in liver disease, 61, 182
in NAFLD, 338
in obesity, 187
in type 2 diabetes, 339
Weil disease, 253, 254
West Nile virus, 666
white blood cell (WBC) count,
in alcoholic liver disease, 315, 316–17, 320

white blood cells see leukocytes
Wilson disease, 351–67
acute liver failure, 354–5, 365, 520, 523
in childhood, 353, 405, 411
clinical presentations, 353–6
definition, 351
diagnosis, 356–61
diagnostic scoring system, 359
differential diagnosis, 263
epidemiology, 351
family screening, 360, 361, 362
gene, 351–2
mutation analysis, 359
mutations, 352
hemolytic anemia, 90, 355, 356–61, 365
hepatic
diagnosis, 356–61
pathogenesis, 351, 353
presentations, 353, 354–5
prognosis, 364–5
response to therapy, 361–2, 363
jaundice, 90
Kayser–Fleischer rings, 65, 354, 356
laboratory tests, 77, 356, 357–8
liver biopsy, 102, 112, 113, 358, 360
liver transplantation, 363, 421, 600–1
neurologic, 351, 353–4, 355
diagnosis, 356
pathogenesis, 351
prognosis, 365–6
response to therapy, 361–2, 363
pathogenesis, 351–3
phenotype–genotype correlations, 352
pregnancy in, 363–4, 492
prognosis, 364–6
protein see ATP7B
treatment, 361–3
Wolman disease, 333, 387, 401

X-linked lymphoproliferative disorder (XLP), 253
xanthelasmata, 65, 280
xanthomas, 65, 66, 93
xanthomatous transformation, hepatocytes, 107, 108
xenobiotic metabolism, 497–8
abnormal, in PBC, 279
zonation, 57, 58
see also drug metabolism
xenon-133 (^{133}Xe) scanning, 337
xenotransplantation, 640
xiao-chai-hu-tang, 514

Y9 bile acid binders, 49
yellow phosphorus, 513

yttrium-90 (^{90}Y), intra-arterial
administration, 466, 467

Zellweger syndrome, 401, 404–5
zidovudine (AZT), 512

Zieve syndrome, 201
zinc
  deficiency, 183
  in hepatic encephalopathy,
    175

  in pregnancy, 364
  supplements, 183
  in Wilson disease, 361, 363
ZO1, 44, 45
ZO2, 44, 45

zonula adherens *see* adherens
  junctions
zonulae occludens *see* tight
  junctions